Rome III

The Functional
Gastrointestinal
Disorders

Senior Editor

DOUGLAS A. DROSSMAN, MD

Professor of Medicine and Psychiatry
Co-Director, UNC Center for Functional GI and Motility Disorders
Division of Gastroenterology and Hepatology
University of North Carolina at Chapel Hill, NC, USA

Editors

ENRICO CORAZZIARI, MD
Professor of Gastroenterology
Dipartimento di Scienze Cliniche
Universita degli Studi "La Sapienza," Rome, Italy

MICHEL DELVAUX, MD, PhD
Department of Internal Medicine and Digestive Pathology
CHU de Nancy
Vandoeuvre-les-Nancy, France

ROBIN C. SPILLER, MD
Professor of Gastroenterology
Nottingham University Hospital
Wolfson Digestive Diseases Centre
Nottingham, UK

NICHOLAS J. TALLEY, MD, PhD, FRACP, FRCP
Professor of Medicine
Mayo Clinic College of Medicine
Consultant, Division of Gastroenterology and Hepatology,
    Mayo Clinic, Rochester, MN
Director, Motility Interest Group, Mayo Clinic, Rochester
Visiting Professor of Medicine, University of Sydney,
    Nepean Hospital, Sydney, Australia

W. GRANT THOMPSON, MD, FRCPC
Emeritus Professor of Medicine
Division of Gastroenterology
University of Ottawa, Ottawa, Canada

WILLIAM E. WHITEHEAD, PhD
Professor of Medicine
Division of Gastroenterology and Hepatology
Co-Director, UNC Center for Functional GI and Motility Disorders
University of North Carolina at Chapel Hill, NC, USA

Rome III

The Functional Gastrointestinal Disorders

THIRD EDITION

Degnon Associates, Inc.
McLean, Virginia

Managing Editor, Carlar J. Blackman
Copy Editor, Patrice Ferriola
Graphic Design, Jerry Schoendorf
Design and Composition by BW&A Books, Inc., Durham, NC
Printed by Allen Press, Inc., Lawrence, KS

ISBN 0-9656837-6-1 cloth library edition
ISBN 0-9656837-5-3 paper board edition
Library of Congress Control Number: 2006928484

Printed in the United States of America

Third Edition
First Printing

This book is dedicated to our families who have supported us through this process, our staff for their contributions in our effort, Professor Aldo Torsoli whose vision has made Rome III a reality, and our fellows and trainees who will carry on the work.

Contents

Members of the Rome III Committees

Rome III Committees

Fundamentals of Neurogastro-enterology: Basic Science

Jackie (Jack) D. Wood, Msc, PhD, *Chair*
Professor of Physiology and Cell Biology
  and Internal Medicine
The Ohio State University
College of Medicine
Columbus, OH, USA

David Grundy, PhD, *Co-Chair*
Professor of Biomedical Science
University of Sheffield
Sheffield, UK

Elie D. Al-Chaer, MS, PhD, JD
Associate Professor
Departments of Pediatrics, Neurobiology,
  and Developmental Sciences
Director, Center for Pain Research
College of Medicine
University of Arkansas for Medical
  Sciences
Little Rock, AR, USA

Qasim Aziz, PhD, FRCP
Professor of Gastroenterology
University of Manchester
GI Sciences
Hope Hospital
Salford, Manchester, UK

Stephen M. Collins, MD
Professor of Medicine
Head of Gastroenterology
McMaster University Medical Center
Hamilton, Ontario, CANADA

Meiyun Ke, MD
Professor of Medicine
Department of Gastroenterology
Peking Union Medical College Hospital
Chinese Academy of Medical Science
Chief of Gastrointestinal Motility Group
Chinese Gastroenterology Association
Chinese Association of Medicine
Beijing, CHINA

Yvette Taché, PhD
Professor of Medicine
Division of Digestive Diseases
David Geffen School of Medicine at UCLA
Director, CURE: Digestive Diseases
  Research Center—Animal Core
Co-Director, Center for Neurovisceral
  Sciences & Women's Health
University of California at Los Angeles,
  CA, USA
VA Greater Los Angeles Healthcare
  System, Los Angeles, CA USA

Fundamentals of Neurogastroenterology: Physiology/Motility/Sensation

John E. Kellow, MD, FRACP, *Chair*
Associate Professor of Medicine
University of Sydney
Royal North Shore Hospital
Sydney, AUSTRALIA

Fernando Azpiroz, MD, PhD, *Co-Chair*
Chief, Section GI Research
University Hospital Vall d'Hebron
Barcelona, SPAIN

Michel Delvaux, MD, PhD
Department of Internal Medicine and
  Digestive Pathology
CHU de Nancy
Vandoeuvre-les-Nancy, FRANCE

Gerald F. Gebhart, PhD
Professor and Head, Dept. of
    Pharmacology
Carver College of Medicine
University of Iowa
Iowa City, IA, USA

Howard M. Mertz, MD
Clinical Associate Professor
Department of Medicine
Vanderbilt University
St. Thomas Hospital
Nashville, TN, USA

**Eamonn M. M. Quigley, MD, FRCP,
    FACP, FACG, FRCPI**
Professor of Medicine and Human
    Physiology
Head of the Medical School
Principal Investigator
Alimentary Pharmabiotic Centre
National University of Ireland, Cork
Cork, IRELAND

André J.P.M. Smout, MD, PhD
University Hospital
Utrecht, GA, THE NETHERLANDS

**Pharmacological and Pharmacokinetic
Aspects of Functional GI Disorders**

Michael Camilleri, MD, *Chair*
Atherton and Winifred Bean Professor
Professor of Medicine and Physiology
Mayo Clinic College of Medicine
Director, Clinical Enteric Neuroscience
    Translational and Epidemiological
    Research
Mayo Clinic
Rochester, MN USA

Lionel Bueno, Dr. Ing, PhD, Dr.es Sc.,
    Co-Chair
Head of Research
Unité de Neurogastroentérologie
Institut National de la Recherche
    Agronomique
Toulouse, FRANCE

Fabrizio De Ponti, MD, PhD
Professor of Pharmacology
Department of Pharmacology
University of Bologna
Bologna, ITALY

Jean Fioramonti, PhD
Institut National de la Recherche
    Agronomique
NeuroGastroenterology and Nutrition
    Unit
Toulouse, FRANCE

R. Bruce Lydiard PhD, MD
Director, Southeast Health Consultants,
    LLC
Charleston, SC, USA
Clinical Professor of Neuropsychiatry and
    Behavioral Science
Medical University of South Carolina
Columbia, SC, USA

Jan Tack, MD, PhD
Professor of Medicine
Department of Gastroenterology
University Hospitals Leuven
Chair, Department of Pathophysiology
University of Leuven
Leuven, BELGIUM

**Gender, Age, Society, Culture and the
Patient's Perspective in the Functional
Gastrointestinal Disorders**

Brenda B. Toner, PhD, *Chair*
Professor and Head
Women's Mental Health Program
Director, Fellowship Program
Department of Psychiatry
University of Toronto
Head, Women's Mental Health and
    Addiction Research Section
Centre for Addiction and Mental Health
Toronto, CANADA

Lin Chang, MD, *Co-Chair*
Associate Professor of Medicine
Co-Director, Center for Neurovisceral
  Sciences and Women's Health
Division of Digestive Diseases
David Geffen School of Medicine at UCLA
Los Angeles, CA, USA

Shin Fukudo, MD, PhD
Professor
Tohoku University Graduate School of
  Medicine
Behavioral Medicine
Sendai, JAPAN

Elspeth A. Guthrie, MD
Professor of Psychological Medicine
University of Manchester
Manchester, UK

G. Richard Locke, III, MD
Professor of Medicine
Mayo Clinic College of Medicine
Consultant, Division of Gastroenterology
  and Hepatology
Director, Esophageal Interest Group
Director, GIH Outcomes Research Unit
Rochester, MN, USA

Nancy Norton, BS
President and Founder
International Foundation for Functional
  Gastrointestinal Disorders
Milwaukee, WI, USA

Ami D. Sperber, MD, MSPH
Associate Professor of Medicine
Department of Gastroenterology
Soroka Medical Center
Faculty of Health Sciences
Ben-Gurion University of the Negev
Beer-Sheva, ISRAEL

Psychosocial Aspects of Functional
Gastrointestinal Disorders

Francis C. Creed, MD, *Chair*
Professor of Psychological Medicine
University of Manchester
University Department of Psychiatry
Manchester Royal Infirmary
Manchester, UK

Rona L. Levy, MSW, PhD, MPH,
  Co-Chair
Professor of Social Work, Psychology and
  Medicine
Director, Behavioral Medicine Research
  Group
University of Washington
Seattle, WA, USA

Laurence A. Bradley, PhD
Professor of Medicine
University of Alabama at Birmingham
Division of Clinical Rheumatology &
  Immunology
Birmingham, AL, USA

Carlos Francisconi, MD
Associate Professor of Medicine
Department of Internal Medicine,
  Universidade Federal do Rio Grande do
  Sul Gastroenterology Division Hospital
  de Clínicas de Porto Alegre Rio
Grande do Sul, BRAZIL

Bruce D. Naliboff, PhD
Professor, Department of Psychiatry and
  Biobehavioral Sciences
Co-Director, Center for Neurovisceral
  Sciences and Women's Health
David Geffen School of Medicine at UCLA
VA Great Los Angeles, Healthcare System
Los Angeles, CA, USA

Kevin W. Olden, MD
Professor of Medicine & Psychiatry
Division of GI
University of South Alabama
Mobile, AL, USA

Functional Esophageal Disorders

Jean Paul Galmiche, MD, *Chair*
Professor of Gastroenterology and
  Hepatology
Research Dean
Director of "Institut des Maladies
  de l'Appareil Digestif"
Nantes University
Nantes, FRANCE

Ray E. Clouse, MD, *Co-Chair*
Professor of Medicine and Psychiatry
Division of Gastroenterology
Washington University
St. Louis, MO, USA

András Bálint, MD, PhD
Assistant Professor of Surgery
Deputy-Director, 3rd Department of
  Surgery
Semmelweis University Medical School
Budapest, HUNGARY

Ian J. Cook, MD, FRACP
Professor of Medicine
University of New South Wales
Director, Dept of Gastroenterology
St. George Hospital
Sydney, AUSTRALIA

Peter J. Kahrilas, MD
Gilbert H Marquardt Professor of
  Medicine
Chief Division of Gastroenterology
Northwestern University's Feinberg School
  of Medicine
Chicago, IL, USA

William G. Paterson, MD
Professor of Medicine, Biology and
  Physiology, Queen's University
Division of Gastroenterology and Queen's
  University Research Chair
Kingston, Ontario, CANADA

André J.P.M. Smout
University Hospital
Utrecht, GA, THE NETHERLANDS

Functional Gastroduodenal Disorders

Jan Tack, MD, PhD, *Chair*
Professor of Medicine, Department of
  Gastroenterology
University Hospitals Leuven
Chair, Department of Pathophysiology
University of Leuven
Leuven, BELGIUM

**Nicholas J. Talley, MD, PhD, FRACP,
  FRCP,** *Co-Chair*
Professor of Medicine
Mayo Clinic College of Medicine
Consultant, Division of Gastroenterology
  and Hepatology, Mayo Clinic, Rochester,
  MN, USA
Director, Motility Interest Group, Mayo
  Clinic, Rochester, MN, USA
Visiting Professor of Medicine, University
  of Sydney, Nepean Hospital, Sydney,
  AUSTRALIA

Michael Camilleri, MD
Atherton and Winifred Bean Professor
Professor of Medicine and Physiology
Mayo Clinic College of Medicine
Director, Clinical Enteric Neuroscience
  Translational Epidemiological Research
Mayo Clinic
Rochester, MN, USA

Gerald Holtmann, MD
Professor of Medicine
Royal Adelaide Hospital
Department of Gastroenterology
Hepatology and General Medicine
Adelaide, AUSTRALIA

Pin-Jin Hu, MD
Professor of Medicine
Director, Department of Gastroenterology
The First Affiliated Hospital
Sun Yat-Sen University
Guangzhou, CHINA

Juan-R. Malagelada, MD, PhD
Hospital General Vall d'Hebron
Digestive Diseases
Barcelona, SPAIN

Vincenzo Stanghellini, MD
Professor of Medicine
Department of Internal Medicine and
 Gastroenterology
Policlinico S.Orsola-Malpighi
University of Bologna, ITALY

Functional Bowel Disorders

George F. Longstreth, MD, *Chair*
Chief of Gastroenterology, Kaiser
 Permanente San Diego
Clinical Professor of Medicine
University of California San Diego School
 of Medicine
San Diego, CA, USA

W. Grant Thompson, MD, FRCPC,
 Co-Chair
Emeritus Professor of Medicine
Division of Gastroenterology
University of Ottawa
Ottawa, CANADA

William D. Chey, MD, FACG, FACP
Associate Professor of Internal Medicine
Director—GI Physiology Laboratory
University of Michigan Health System
Ann Arbor, MI, USA

Lesley A. Houghton, PhD
Neurogastroenterology Unit
Academic Division of Medicine and
 Surgery
University of Manchester
Wythenshawe Hospital
Manchester, UK

Fermín Mearin, MD, PhD
Director of the Gastroenterology Service
Institute of Functional and Motor
 Digestive Disorders
Centro Médico Teknon
Barcelona, SPAIN

Robin C. Spiller, MD
Professor of Gastroenterology
Wolfson Digestive Diseases Centre
University of Nottingham
Nottingham, UK

Functional Abdominal Pain Syndrome

Ray E. Clouse, MD, *Chair*
Professor of Medicine and Psychiatry
Division of Gastroenterology
Washington University
St. Louis, MO, USA

Emeran A. Mayer MD, *Co-Chair*
Director, Center for Neurovisceral
 Sciences & Women's Health
University of California, Los Angeles
Los Angeles, California, USA

Qasim Aziz, PhD, FRCP
Professor of Gastroenterology
University of Manchester
GI Sciences
Hope Hospital
Salford, Manchester, UK

Douglas A. Drossman, MD
Professor of Medicine and Psychiatry
Co-Director, UNC Center for Functional
 GI and Motility Disorders
Division of Gastroenterology and
 Hepatology
University of North Carolina at Chapel
 Hill, NC, USA

Dan L. Dumitrascu, MD
Associate Professor
University of Medicine and Pharmacy
 Iuliu Hatieganu
Third Medical Department
Cluj, ROMANIA

Hubert Mönnikes, MD, PhD
Professor of Medicine
Charité—Medical Center and School of
  Medicine Campus Virchow
Department of Medicine
Division of Hepatology, Gastroenterology,
  and Endocrinology
Freie Universität and Humboldt-
  Universität
Berlin, GERMANY

Bruce D. Naliboff, PhD
Professor, Department of Psychiatry and
  Biobehavioral Sciences
Co-Director, Center for Neurovisceral
  Sciences and Women's Health
David Geffen School of Medicine at UCLA
VA Great Los Angeles, Healthcare System
Los Angeles, California, USA

Functional Gallbladder and Sphincter
of Oddi Disorders

Jose Behar, MD, *Chair*
Rhode Island Hospital
Brown University School of Medicine
Chair, Division of Gastroenterology
Providence, RI, USA

Enrico Corazziari, MD, *Co-Chair*
Professor of Gastroenterology
Head, Gastroenterologia A
Dipartimento di Scienze Cliniche
Universita degli Studi "La Sapienza"
Rome, ITALY

Moises Guelrud, MD
Tufts-New England Medical Center
Tufts University School of Medicine
Boston, MA, USA

Walter J. Hogan, MD
Professor of Medicine & Radiology
Medical College of Wisconsin
Milwaukee, Wisconsin USA

Stuart Sherman, MD
Professor of Medicine and Radiology
Clinical Director, Division of
  Gastroenterology and Hepatology
Director, ERCP Service
Indiana University School of Medicine
Indianapolis, IN, USA

James Toouli, MBBS, FRACS, PhD
Professor of Surgery
Flinders University Adelaide
Department of Surgery
Flinders Medical Center
Bedford Park, AUSTRALIA

Functional Anorectal Disorders

Arnold Wald, MD, *Chair*
Professor of Medicine
University of Wisconsin Medical School
Section of Gastroenterology and
  Hepatology
Madison, WI, USA

Adil E. Bharucha, MBBS, MD, *Co-Chair*
Associate Professor of Medicine
Mayo Clinic College of Medicine
Consultant, Division of Gastroenterology
  and Hepatology
Mayo Clinic
Rochester, MN, USA

Paul Enck, PhD
Director of Research
University Hospitals Tuebingen
Department of Internal Medicine VI
Tuebingen, GERMANY

Satish S. C. Rao, MD, PhD, FRCP (LON)
Professor of Medicine
University of Iowa Hospitals and Clinics
Center for Digestive Diseases
Iowa City, Iowa, USA

Childhood Functional Gastrointestinal Disorders: Neonate/Toddler

Peter J. Milla, MD, *Chair*
Professor of Paediatric Gastroenterology
  and Nutrition
Institute of Child Health
University College London
London, UK

Paul E. Hyman, MD, *Co-Chair*
Professor of Pediatrics
Chief, Pediatric Gastroenterology
University of Kansas
Kansas City, Kansas, USA

Marc A. Benninga, MD, PhD
Director, Pediatric Gastrointestinal
  Motility Lab
Emma Kinderziekenhuis AMC
Amsterdam, THE NETHERLANDS

Geoffrey Davidson, MBBS, MD, FRACP
Director, Centre for Paediatric and
  Adolescent Gastroenterology
Women's and Children's Hospital
North Adelaide, AUSTRALIA

David R. Fleisher, MD
Associate Professor of Child Health
Pediatric Gastroenterology
University of Missouri Health Care
Columbia, MO, USA

Jan Taminiau, MD
Emma Kinderziekenhuis AMC
Department of Pediatrics
Amsterdam, THE NETHERLANDS

Childhood Functional Gastrointestinal Disorders: Child/Adolescent

Carlo Di Lorenzo, MD, *Chair*
Professor of Pediatrics
The Ohio State University
Chief, Division of Pediatric
  Gastroenterology
Children's Hospital of Columbus
Columbus, OH, USA

Andrée Rasquin, MD, *Co-Chair*
Professor of Pediatrics
Division of Gastroenterology, Hepatology
  and Nutrition
University of Montreal
Montreal, Quebec, CANADA

David Forbes, MBBS
Associate Professor
School of Paediatrics & Child Health
University of Western Australia
Princess Margaret Hospital for Children
Perth, AUSTRALIA

Ernesto Guiraldes, MD
Profesor Titular
Departmento de Pediatria
Escuela de Medicina
Pontificia Universidad Catolica de Chile
Santiago, CHILE

Jeffrey S. Hyams, MD
Head, Division of Digestive Diseases and
  Nutrition
Connecticut Children's Medical Center
Professor of Pediatrics
University of Connecticut School of
  Medicine
Hartford, CT, USA

Annamaria Staiano, MD
Professor of Pediatrics
Dipartimento di Pediatria
Universita' Federico II
Napoli, ITALY

Lynn S. Walker, PhD
Professor of Pediatrics
Director, Division of Adolescent Medicine
  and Behavioral Science
Vanderbilt University Children's Hospital
Nashville, TN, USA

Design of Treatment Trials for
Functional Gastrointestinal Disorders

E. Jan Irvine, MD, FRCP(C), MSc, *Chair*
Professor of Medicine, University of
  Toronto
Head, Division of Gastroenterology,
  St. Michael's Hospital
Toronto, Ontario, CANADA

William E. Whitehead, PhD, *Co-Chair*
Professor of Medicine
Division of Gastroenterology and
  Hepatology
Co-Director, UNC Center for Functional
  GI and Motility Disorders
University of North Carolina at Chapel
  Hill, NC, USA

William D. Chey, MD, FACG, FACP
Associate Professor of Internal Medicine
Director—GI Physiology Laboratory
University of Michigan Health System
Ann Arbor, MI, USA

Kei Matsueda, MD, PhD
Director, NHO Saigata National Hospital
NCNP, Division of GI
Ohgata-ku Johetsu-city, Niigata, JAPAN
Ichikawa-city Chiba, JAPAN

Michael Shaw, MD
Associate Clinical Professor of Medicine
University of Minnesota
Park Nicollet Clinic
Minneapolis, MN, USA

**Nicholas J. Talley, MD, PhD, FRACP,
  FRCP**
Professor of Medicine
Mayo Clinic College of Medicine
Consultant, Division of Gastroenterology
  and Hepatology, Mayo Clinic, Rochester,
  MN, USA
Director, Motility Interest Group, Mayo
  Clinic, Rochester, MN, USA
Visiting Professor of Medicine, University
  of Sydney, Nepean Hospital, Sydney,
  AUSTRALIA

**Sander J. O. Veldhuyzen van Zanten, MD,
  PhD**
Associate Professor
Dalhousie University Medicine
Queen Elizabeth II Health Sciences Center
Halifax, Nova Scotia, CANADA

Foreword I

"The Road to Rome" ends this third edition of *The Functional Gastrointestinal Disorders*, as it did the second edition. It is appropriate for me to begin with this ending since it is actually the beginning—the start of a journey that spans two decades. To all those who made this journey over the past 20 years, up or down the Road to Rome depending whether their interests lie above or below Treitz's ligament, congratulations. To paraphrase an old Chinese proverb "the journey is its own reward." The published labor of these travelers is surely personally rewarding. But their travelogue is also our reward—all of us stakeholders in *The Functional Gastrointestinal Disorders*—scientists, clinicians, the pharmaceutical industry, and most important our patients and their families. Fueled by modern technology and applied science of neurogastroenterology, molecular biology, genetics, functional imaging, psychology, and pharmacology, the current journey to Rome defines new mechanisms by which the gut and the enteric nervous system interact and communicate within the local and distant internal environment. It also provides direction how to reinstate a sense of balance when the interaction and communication become disrupted and lead to symptoms. This third edition travelogue explores new childhood, gender, cultural, and patient centered vistas. It revisits more familiar functional landscapes such as definition, testing, clinical outcome, and management recommendations through the eyes of stringent study design, validated assessment methods, and evidenced based medicine. At the end of the road what specific rewards can the stakeholders claim?

For scientists whose path is forged by basic and translational research of the brain-gut axis, a veritable highway of investigation has been opened to keep them speeding ahead for years to come. A mechanistic understanding of visceral hypersensitivity and pain, the ability to integrate functional imaging with neurophysiology and neuropharmacology, identifying the implications of transmitter and receptor genetic polymorphisms, and comprehending signal processing within the enteric and central nervous systems are among the destinations to which scientists are headed.

The account of this expedition provides clinicians with simpler (duration of symptoms), more realistic (functional dyspepsia, IBS subtyping and gallbladder and sphincter of Oddi), and practical (pediatric categories and functional abdominal pain syndrome) classification of functional disorders. In addition, the novel insights offered into the pathogenesis, psychosocial impact, and pharmacologic and non-pharmacologic management are important vehicles for those of us who regularly journey side by side with patients who suffer from functional gastrointestinal disorders.

Since "one size does not fit all," the pharmaceutical industry travels a challenging and often uncharted route. A beacon to guide their journey lies in the exciting prospect that pharmacogenetics might predict treatment response, the various novel therapeutic approaches (e.g., serotonin, tachykinins, opioiods, cannabinoids, anti-inflammatories, and antibiotics) and the practical design for clinical trials outlined in this book.

Patients and their families are the biggest beneficiaries of this excursion. They after all are not tourists but live their lives on this road that is ". . . characterized by long-term courses, unpredictable symptom episodes, and disabling effects that are often accompanied by minimally effective treatments, social stigma, and isolation." It is a perpetually ". . . demanding road for families as well as patients. . . ." Empathy, education, encouragement, and expectation line the Road to Rome and augment the therapeutic pavement, smooth the potholes, and straighten the curves making for an easier, more palatable journey.

Sri Sathya Baba, an Indian spiritual leader, wrote, "Small minds select narrow roads; expand your mental vision and take to the broad road of helpfulness, compassion, and service." Thank you, Doug, Enrico, Michel, Robin, Nick, Grant, Bill, and everyone else who took the broad road on this Rome III journey. We the stakeholders appreciate your efforts, insights, recommendations, and directions for the future. We wish you continued gratifying and rewarding travel when you begin a fourth trip along the *Via Appia*. For *The Functional Gastrointestinal Disorders*, all roads must continue to lead to Rome.

David A Peura, MD
President, American Gastroenterological Association
Professor of Medicine, University of Virginia Health
Science Center, Charlottesville, Virginia

Foreword II

I am deeply honored to have been asked to write a foreword for the third version of this unique contribution to our specialty focused on the functional gastrointestinal disorders (FGIDs). Dr. D. Drossman, his team of co-editors, and the 87 internationally recognized specialized clinicians and investigators are to be commended for a truly superb achievement in advancing the field of the FGIDs, an area in gastroenterology of immense importance that remains insufficiently valued.

The Rome process started over 15 years ago and rapidly became the vehicle driving research and patient care of the FGIDs. The Rome process superseded by far any other attempt to enhance the recognition and categorization of FGIDs as real clinical entities, and to disseminate new and evolving pathogenetic, clinical, and therapeutic knowledge. The Rome process has matured through three generations with increasing evidence-based quality. The classification system remains based on the assumption and premise that for each disorder there are identifiable symptom clusters that emerge across clinical and population groups. From the beginning, the academic environment was receptive of the need for a mechanism to classify the FGIDs, both for research and clinical care.

The mission of Rome III has not changed and reflects a further expansion of its activities with a global dimension to improve knowledge of the science and practice relating to the FGIDs. Indeed, the mission remains pure and simple by fostering innovation and ensuring that the practice of gastroenterology is scientifically based and provides care and value to patients. It was therefore logical to expect that there would be a need to revise the diagnostic criteria as well as information on patho-physiology and treatment since new scientific data about functional disorders continue to accumulate. Rome III remains faithful to the basic principle of the process encapsulated in the premise that diagnosis, differential diagnosis, and therapy of functional GI disorders might and should be facilitated by a precise symptom-based categorization of patient groups.

What is truly unique about the Rome process, particularly for Rome III, is the amount of effort that went into its creation and the amount of forethought that has gone into deciding how to implement the plan, set objectives and goals, measure outcomes, and provide the backbone structure that guarantees current and future successful achievements. Twenty-eight adult and seventeen pediatric FGIDs are covered in extenso. The adult FGIDs are categorized in esophageal, gas-troduodenal, bowel, functional abdominal pain, biliary, and anorectal domains. Functional dyspepsia and irritable bowel syndrome (IBS) are obviously dominant entities, with substantial overlap with other related functional disorders. The pe-diatric domains relate functional disorders in neonates and toddlers and the child and adolescent populations. The changes from Rome II to Rome III largely reflect updates in the literature. An important change is the simplification of the time frame during which symptoms should be present. Functional dyspepsia is de-emphasized as an entity for research due to the heterogeneity of the symptom complex. Instead, postprandial distress syndrome and epigastric pain syndrome are proposed. Diarrhea-, constipation-, and mixed-IBS subtypes are largely based on stool consistency. Also noteworthy of mentioning is the fact that Rome III abounds with novelties such as the ongoing work to capture the whole book and related scientific data into a CD slide-set module for self-learning and for lectur-ing on the subject.

To me, it is overwhelmingly clear that the overall impact of the Rome pro-cess is tremendous. The Rome criteria are now adopted as the gold standard (e.g., for epidemiological studies) for the FGIDs. New questionnaires are being devel-oped framing the questions to be consistent with the Rome criteria. Uniformity is mandatory for studies of ethnic and geographical differences, for information on health care utilization, therapeutic and alimentary-dietary approaches, etc. But there is more concerning the worldwide impact of the Rome process. A major spin-off is the undeniable increased awareness, understanding, and appreciation of the importance of the FGIDs. The educational impact is impressive as clini-cians increasingly use the various criteria for proper diagnosis and, ultimately, proper therapy and improved patient care. Moreover, authorities almost without exception request patient selection according to the Rome criteria for pharma-ceutical investigations. The ultimate reason to explain the perhaps unforeseen success of the Rome process was, and is, the fact that there was indeed an unmet need to bring order to the complexity of FGIDs and the necessity to have stan-dard guidelines for patient selection, investigation, and therapy, particularly with a multinational dimension. If you want to convince yourself of Rome's impact, just compare the old GI textbooks with the current ones. With the Rome criteria now generally adopted as the gold standard in epidemiological studies of FGIDs, more data should be forthcoming relating to ethnic and geographical differences in the frequency of IBS, chronic constipation, diarrhea etc.

Is this the end? By no means. As insights into functional aberrations deepen, as more sophisticated technology becomes available for more accurate analysis, so will, in parallel, our concepts evolve, together with the need for adaptation, amendment, and updating of our concepts. This will again translate into further advanced guidelines for diagnosis, staging, and grading. Challenges remain, particularly in the need for deeper understanding of the complexities of the mind-gut relationship and the translation of neurochemical disturbances into clinical symptomatology.

I am confident that Rome III will be highly successful: The Rome team deserves our deepest congratulations for yet another jewel in the crown. Their ability to select worldwide top researchers and clinicians who are active in the respective fields and well versed in the stringent rules of evidence-based medicine is truly remarkable. The end product is another classic. The World Gastroenterology Organization recognizes the enormous value and impact of the Rome process and expresses its wishes for a megasuccess for the benefit of our specialty and the patients troubled with functional disorders.

Guido NJ Tytgat, MD, PhD
Professor Emeritus
Past President of the World
Gastroenterology Organization

Man should strive to have his intestines relaxed all the days of his life.
—Moses Maimonides, 1135–1204 A.D.

A good set of bowels is worth more to a man than any quantity of brains.
  —Josh Billings (Henry Wheeler Shaw), 1818–1885 A.D.

For centuries, physicians and historians have recognized that it is common for maladies to afflict the intestinal tract, producing symptoms of pain, nausea, vomiting, diarrhea, constipation, difficult passage of food or feces, or any combination. When persons experience these symptoms as severe enough, or that they impact on daily life, they define the symptoms as an illness and may seek medical care. In modern times, the physician caring for these patients seeks to identify metabolic, infectious, neoplastic and other structural abnormalities. If they are not found, the patient is (often by exclusion) considered to have a functional gastrointestinal (GI) disorder. This book is dedicated to helping the clinician and investigator to: (1) make a positive diagnosis of these disorders, (2) understand their pathophysiology, and (3) make effective treatment decisions.

It is with great pleasure that we introduce the first edition of the *Functional Gastrointestinal Disorders.* This book, the culmination of over 7 years' effort by 30 internationally recognized investigators in the field, provides the first categorization of the

25 functional GI disorders from esophagus to anorectum. Also included is the most comprehensive discussion available of the epidemiology, physiology, psychosocial features, and clinical evaluation and treatment recommendations for these disorders.

Perhaps the most unique component of this book is the inclusion of the symptom-based ("Rome") diagnostic criteria for the functional GI disorders. The efforts of seven multinational Working Team Committees have, through careful review of the literature and consensus, developed a standard for diagnosis that can be used in research and clinical care. In effect, the methods leading to these criteria (see Chapter 1) duplicate the processes that eventuated in the successful development of diagnostic classifications in psychiatry (DSM-III) and rheumatology (ARA Criteria). For easy retrieval of information, these criteria are listed not only in the chapters for each organ system, but are also compiled into a single section (Appendix A). We are hopeful that their inclusion in this book will encourage the use of standardized diagnostic methods for epidemiological surveys and clinical trials. We also expect that their use by physicians in practice will reduce the need for costly and unnecessary diagnostic studies occasionally done to "rule out organic disease."

Some additional features of this book are worth noting. First, it is well recognized that most studies in this field are methodologically flawed because of difficulties relating to patient selection, efficacy and outcome assessment, and statistical analysis. So, for investigators interested in clinical trials, we include a chapter that not only reviews the limitations of previous studies, but also makes recommendations for the optimal design of future protocols (Chapter 7). Second, we recognize the need for epidemiologists, health policy planners and clinicians to refer to population-based frequency data for these disorders. In Chapter 8, we include tabular data and summary information from a recently published U.S. national study using our recommended "Rome" criteria. This chapter includes information on the prevalence of all these disorders with breakdown by gender, age and other sociodemographic factors, as well as health care use and disability statistics. Finally, since these criteria were originally developed for physician assessment, they are not easily adapted to surveys or self-report questionnaires. Therefore, the authors have produced a matched set of question items (Appendix B) as used in the national survey for clinical investigators to use in their research.

We expect that as new scientific data about these disorders accumulate, there will be a need to revise the diagnostic criteria as well as information on pathophysiology and treatment. Therefore, we have set up a process for future committee meetings that will permit ongoing review and modification of our current recommendations. These changes and enhancements will be included in future editions of this book.

The editors would like to thank Professor Aldo Torsoli for his foresight and support of the Working Team process, the many committee members and reviewers who helped in the creation of these documents, Ms. Sandy Hall for her assistance in the preparation of the manuscript, and Ms. Lynne Herndon whose professional commitment and tireless efforts made the publication of this book a reality.

Douglas A Drossman, MD and
the Working Team Committees
1994

Preface to the
Second Edition

It is with great enjoyment and anticipation that we offer this second edition of *The Functional Gastrointestinal Disorders.* This book is the culmination and most visible product of the Rome II project, a 3-year effort organized by a dedicated Coordinating Committee, and implemented with the assistance of over 60 international investigators, a tireless administrative staff, and the support and interest of many pharmaceutical sponsors and regulatory agencies.

This edition improves upon the first edition, published in 1994, in several ways: (1) All previous chapters (esophageal, gastroduodenal, bowel, biliary and anorectal disorders, design of treatment trials) have been completely updated and expanded to accommodate the rapid growth in the field of functional GI disorders; (2) Several new committees have been formed to contribute chapters on the physiological, (motility/sensation) basic science (brain-gut), and psychosocial aspects of these disorders, as well as on a new classification system for the pediatric functional GI disorders; (3) We have added a historical piece ("The Road to Rome") that catalogues the evolution in thinking and process of the Rome I and II projects; (4) We include a summary and recommendations from the recent Clinical Outcomes Conference, held at the World Congress of Gastroenterology (Vienna) in 1998. This conference began the process of collaboration among the Rome committee members, pharmaceutical companies, international expert advisors and regulatory agencies; (5) Finally, we provide a new questionnaire and coding scheme for the ROME II criteria that can be used both for epidemiological and clinical studies.

Possibly the most important component of the book is the inclusion of symptom-based diagnostic criteria for clinical investigation and practice. Since publication of the original criteria 5 years ago, there has been enthusiastic support, and also well-founded criticism. The criticism relates to concerns that the criteria are not physiologically based, that they were determined by consensus ("Delphi" approach) rather than through validation studies, and that they are likely to change over time. With regard to the first concern, to date, no physiologic criteria have emerged to diagnose these disorders. In addition, these symptom-based criteria have stood the test of time. They have proven their value in clinical trials and hopefully have reduced patient care costs by curtailing the tendency to order unneeded diagnostic studies to "rule out organic disease." Second, we recognize and accept the need for validation studies, and over the last few years several studies using factor analysis or clinical validation by experts have supported these criteria (primarily for IBS). In addition, we have set up a research fund, and have awarded several grants to encourage clinical investigators to test the validity of these new criteria. Whatever the results, the information obtained will be used either to support or lead to modification of the criteria. Finally, we have also set up a rigorous, yet conservative, process for changes to the previous criteria (See Chapter 1). All prior criticisms against the inclusion of specific items, and recommendations for new items were collected and communicated to the committees so they could be addressed and commented upon. In some cases, this led to changes in the criteria. In addition, the peer review process for the criteria and the chapters were expanded to include external and internal academic reviewers, and had to be evidence-based, and/or acceptable to all parties. The changes made in the criteria in most cases do not eliminate the use of the previous criteria, but enhance them, and they are more consistent with the new knowledge in our pathophysiological understanding of these disorders.

This book is part of a larger effort by the ROME II Committees to help advance the field of functional GI disorders, and to legitimize these conditions for our patients. I would like to outline some of the projects underway:

1. *Publication of criteria in Gut supplement.* The recent publication of the criteria, and an abridged version of these chapters in a supplemental issue of *Gut* is a way to communicate our findings and recommendations to a much larger audience. This book provides a more in-depth treatment of the topic.

2. *Formation of an International Resource Committee.* We have formed a committee of pharmaceutical sponsors and regulatory agencies, and have met biennially to address the shared interests and concerns relating to the design of treatment trials. One outcome of this group has been the Clinical

Outcomes Conference in Vienna, which set the stage for future dialog to develop consensus recommendations for study design.

3. *Research funds to support validation studies.* As noted, we have set up a peer review process to evaluate applications that test the utility and validity of the ROME II criteria for functional GI disorders. To date we have awarded five grants, and expect to continue this process.

4. *Establish an epidemiological database.* We have begun the process of administering international surveys in order to set up a database for future studies.

We are grateful for the support and encouragement from our sponsors and supporters, and believe that we can make a difference in increasing awareness and understanding for the field of functional GI disorders both to physicians and patients alike. In addition, we hope that the criteria and other information presented in this book will help physicians and other health care workers in their investigation and care of patients with these troubling disorders. Many thanks go to Ms. Carlar Blackman for her creative intelligence and enthusiasm in keeping the numerous projects and activities underway, to George Degnon for his skills in coordinating the meetings, and for his sound advice, and to Ms. LouAnn Brower for her assistance in the production of this book.

Douglas A Drossman, MD
and the Rome II Coordinating Committee
March 2000

You cannot reason with a hungry belly; it has no ears.
—Greek Proverb

*To be a social success, do not act pathetic, arrogant, or
bored. Do not discuss your unhappy childhood, your visit
to the dentist, the shortcomings of your cleaning woman,
the state of your bowels, or your spouse's bad habits.
You will be thought a paragon of good behavior.*
—Mason Cooley, 1927

*When I began practice ... I was relatively safe in assum-
ing that abdominal pain was appendicitis or green apples.
Today it is also highly probable that the patient is suffering
from the fact that his wife of 40 years wants to leave him
for the Peace Corps or Richard Burton.*
—Dr. Gunnar Gunderson, AMA President, 1962

Throughout recorded history, the bowels have had
meanings that go beyond their usual function. They
are shrouded in mystery, their dysfunction is linked
to emotion and shame, and proper functioning is required for general well-being. The functional gastrointestinal disorders (FGIDs) continue to have many
of these attributes simply because they defy an understanding within traditional pathologically based medicine, and in the past have been considered "2nd class."
Perhaps, what is not seen is not believed. Yet over the
last few decades, a great deal of scientific knowledge
coming from basic science research, neurophysiology,
and clinical and behavioral investigation have helped
us to understand the mechanisms behind the function

and dysfunction of the gastrointestinal system. The FGIDs are best understood as dysfunctions of highly integrated biobehavioral systems within the individual, and with this new understanding they are amenable to study and treatment.

Over the last 15 years, the Rome organization sought to legitimize and update our knowledge of the FGIDs by bringing together scientists and clinicians from around the world to classify and critically appraise the science of gastrointestinal function and dysfunction. This knowledge permits clinical scientists to make recommendations for diagnosis and treatment.

We are most pleased to offer you this third edition of *Rome III: The Functional Gastrointestinal Disorders*. Through the work of the editors, 14 committees, and our administrative staff, this volume provides the culmination of a 5-year process. This preface highlights some of the enhancements and updates of Rome III since the 2nd edition was published in 2000.

- *New chapters.* Given the development and release of new pharmaceutical agents, Rome III includes a chapter that addresses the pharmacological and pharmacokinetic aspects of medications for the FGIDs. The globalization of research has increased the need to understand the sociodemographic aspects of the FGIDs, and the interests and needs of our patients. These are addressed in a unique chapter on gender, age, society, culture and the patient's perspective that embraces a world view for these disorders. Recognizing that functional abdominal pain syndrome involves primarily dysregulation of the central nervous system, rather than intestinal function, we have removed this condition from the functional bowel disorders chapter, and recruited international experts involved in pain and behavioral research to produce a new document tailored specifically to this condition. Finally, since the developmental level of the child influences diagnosis and treatment, Rome III includes two pediatric chapters. One deals with the disorders unique to neonates and toddlers, another covers child/adolescent disorders. While it is unclear as to when a child medically becomes an adult, (most would accept from 15–18 years), the child/adolescent chapter offers a transition, since it possesses features similar to, but not the same as, the adult disorders. Thus, the reader will note that the diagnostic categories may differ across these chapters, and there may be differences in the criteria items, or the time frame of occurrence. For example, the time requirement for identification of FGIDs in neonates and toddlers is shorter than in adults, and functional dyspepsia in children and adolescents retains the Rome II classification. These will be adjusted when pediatric studies evaluate the new adult criteria in children.

- *New appendices.* Since the diagnosis of an FGID requires not only the Rome criteria, but also evidence to exclude other disease, we have compiled a list of alarm signs or "red flags" for clinical practice and research. These items were developed by the committees based on evidence in the literature and consensus of the experts. The alarm signs and symptoms are intended as guides to alert the clinician/investigator when additional testing may be indicated, so their endorsement does not necessarily exclude a diagnosis of a FGID. Also included is a brief set of items for clinicians to consider when deciding when to refer a patient to a mental health professional. The Rome III criteria are now presented alone and in a separate appendix that compares Rome II to Rome III. The proximity of the two sets of criteria may assist clinical or industry investigators to reconcile similarities and differences in clinical trials. Also, we are pleased to provide the new Rome III questionnaire for epidemiological and clinical research, which was developed by a committee chaired by W. Grant Thompson. Finally, a new chapter presents the results of a validation study for this questionnaire coordinated by William Whitehead and an international team of investigators. These new data permit better estimation of threshold determinations for the diagnostic criteria and represent an important new dimension of the Rome process.

— *Expanded new areas of research relevant to the field.* With the growth of new research areas over the last six years, we have expanded sections on brain imaging and CNS regulation of gut function (Chapters 2, 3, and 6), mucosal immunology and inflammation, including postinfectious FGID (Chapters 2, 3, and 9), pharmacokinetics (Chapter 4), and psychosocial and sociocultural aspects of the FGIDs (Chapters 5 and 6).

The Rome process aims to respond to new developments in the field. New information is carefully appraised, discussed, and communicated to the reader. However, changes in criteria or recommendations for treatment occur only if the available data compels the committees to do so. Thus, we have retained the key elements of Rome II, but improve upon them by providing new information based on evaluation of the evidence. The rationale for change is included in each chapter. As in the past, when the committee needs to make recommendations with insufficient evidence, the "Delphi" consensus method is used.

The Rome committees recommend that studies can still be conducted using Rome II criteria (i.e., "grandfathered") because most of the changes in Rome III, while supported, have yet to be validated. Nevertheless, a gradual shift to Rome III criteria is recommended. In some cases, with incomplete knowledge to make decisions, we may have made mistakes in Rome II, and Rome III seeks to correct or improve upon the past. Some of the changes and their rationale include:

— *A change in the time frame for diagnosis of the FGIDs.* Rome I required a time frame of 3 months to exclude acute or transient symptoms of gastrointestinal distress. Rome II introduced a frequency domain to the criteria, and lengthened the required time of onset ("At least 12 weeks, which need not be consecutive in the preceding 12 months of . . .”). Soon after publication, we learned that this concept is difficult to remember, is cumbersome in a questionnaire, and may be too restrictive. The Rome III time frame is easier to understand and is more amenable to research and clinical care. In Rome III, symptoms should originate 6 months earlier (½ the onset time of Rome II) and current activity should be met for 3 months (“Criteria present for the last 3 months and onset at least 6 months prior to diagnosis.”).

–   *A change in functional dyspepsia.* Functional dyspepsia has been one of the most difficult set of symptoms to understand and classify. No doubt this relates to the heterogeneous determinants of the symptom stem as previously defined. Rome I identified dyspepsia among all patients with upper abdominal pain or discomfort without definite structural or biochemical findings. It then subclassified this condition into ulcer-like dyspepsia based on a cluster of pain-related symptoms, or dysmotility-like dyspepsia based on a collection of symptoms related to early satiety, fullness, and bloating, among others. Rome II refined these criteria: “Persistent or recurrent dyspepsia (pain or discomfort centered in the upper abdomen) in the absence of organic disease and IBS symptoms” and attempted to subclassify based solely on the predominant symptom, i.e., pain defining ulcer-like, and discomfort defining dysmotility-like dyspepsia. It has since become clear that no single symptom is present in all patients with functional dyspepsia, and there is considerable variation and overlap of pain and discomfort among patients over time and across cultures. These observations reduce the utility of this classification scheme. Recent data based on factor analyses of general populations and patients, physiological studies, and clinical experience led to a new classification of a “dyspepsia symptom complex” for Rome III. Now “functional dyspepsia” is merely an “umbrella” term with limited utility for research (though it can still be used in clinical practice). This complex is now defined by two subsets that may overlap: (1) meal-induced dyspeptic symptoms (postprandial distress syndrome or PDS) and (2) epigastric pain (epigastric pain syndrome or EPS). Further studies will be needed to validate this change.

–   *More restrictive criteria for functional disorders of the gallbladder and sphincter of Oddi.* One of the more complex and controversial areas of the FGIDs relates to the diagnosis and treatment of patients with functional biliary tract disorders. In part this relates to the low prevalence of these disorders relative to other FGIDs and the iatrogenic risk associated with diagnosing these non-life threatening conditions with invasive studies like endoscopic retrograde cholangiopancreatography (ERCP) and sphincter of Oddi manometry, or treating them with unnecessary surgery or endoscopic sphincterotomy. Furthermore, the chapter is written primarily by and for the interventionalist who sees a highly selective patient population who are severely disabled from their recurrent pain episodes, and who already have undergone full diagnostic evaluation and treatment trials. For these highly experienced endoscopists and surgeons, the procedures may be warranted, though this too remains controversial. Thus there is a "gap" between the diagnosis and treatment approach of the practicing gastroenterologist or primary care physician, our primary audience, and the guidelines needed for the interventional endoscopist. The committee sought to address this issue and improve upon Rome II by making the Rome III criteria more restrictive. This change reduces the population susceptible to the invasive studies needed to confirm these diagnoses. Furthermore, the new criteria are considered as only the first step in the recommended diagnostic process. Once criteria are met, other diagnostic studies must be done (e.g., endoscopic ultrasound or MRI) to exclude other disorders. Following this, an adequate therapeutic trial of medications (e.g., nifedipine, antidepressants) is recommended. Only if this is unsuccessful is referral recommended specifically to centers dedicated to the study and treatment of these conditions. We hope that attention to these refinements will reduce the number of unneeded and potentially risky procedures, and identify a patient population more likely to benefit from an intervention.

— *Revision of IBS subtyping.* The Rome II subtype classification for IBS with constipation (IBS-C) and IBS with diarrhea (IBS-D) has proven difficult to use in clinical practice. In addition, it is unclear how to classify patients who may not meet criteria for these two subtypes, yet still have IBS. For these reasons, the bowel committee simplified the subtype classification by using the one criterion most closely tied to intestinal transit: stool consistency. Using this system, IBS-C is defined as hard or lumpy stools at least 25% of bowel movements with loose (mushy) or watery stools with fewer than 25% of bowel movements, and IBS-D is defined as loose (mushy) or watery stools at least 25% of bowel movements and hard or lumpy stool with fewer than 25% of bowel movements. Furthermore, patients who fulfill both of these criteria are considered to have mixed IBS (IBS-M) and those who meet neither are considered unspecified (IBS-U). Although further studies are needed to confirm the validity of this recommendation, it is logical. Meanwhile, the Rome II proposal for identifying subtypes remains a legitimate subject of continuing research. The bowel committee, supported by recent research, stresses the instability of the IBS subtypes and cautions against considering them static in a person's medical experience.

We are hopeful that this 3rd edition, like its predecessors, will be a valuable resource to students and other trainees, clinicians, investigators, and our patients.

Douglas A Drossman, MD
and the Rome III Editors,
August 2006

Acknowledgments

The Editorial Board is most grateful to the 87 authors representing 18 countries whose knowledge, experience, and hard work led to this final product. We thank our industry sponsors for helping bring the Rome III project to fruition. The sponsors are: Astellas, Astra Zeneca, Axcan, Forest, GlaxoSmithKline, Microbia, Novartis, Procter & Gamble, Solvay, Sucampo/Takeda, and Vela Pharmaceuticals. We also thank the Rome Foundation Staff and Rome III Book Administration for their tireless contributions: George Degnon of Degnon Associates, Executive Director of the Rome Foundation, for his vision and direction; Carlar Blackman, Administrative Director of the Rome Foundation and Managing Editor of Rome III, for her creativity and ability to keep our many activities going and move us ahead; Kathy Haynes of Degnon Associates for her efficiency and care in meeting and sponsorship organization; Chris Dalton for her assistance in the Rome III meeting; Patrice Ferriola of KZEPharm-Associates for copyediting; Julie Allred of BW&A Books, Inc. for design and publication advice; Diane Feldman for her careful proofreading and coordination of final revisions; Spencer Dorn, MD for his technical assistance; and Jerry Schoendorf for his graphic design. We also want to acknowledge the 60 external peer reviewers whose expertise helped us to improve on the manuscripts, and Erin Dubnansky and the *Gastroenterology* journal administrative staff for helping us process the document reviews. In addition, we acknowledge the following professionals and organizations for their support or assistance: The US Food and Drug Administration (FDA); the International Foundation for Functional Gastrointestinal Disorders (IFFGD); the Clinical Practice and Motility Nerve-Gut Interactions Sections of the American Gastroenterological Association (AGA); the World Congress of Gastroenterology in Montreal, 2005 (WCOG); and the Functional Brain-Gut Research Group (FBG).

Rome III

The Functional Gastrointestinal Disorders

Chapter 1

The Functional Gastrointestinal Disorders and the Rome III Process

Douglas A. Drossman

A Perspective on the Functional Gastrointestinal Disorders

Throughout recorded history and alongside structural diseases of the intestinal tract are maladies that have produced multiple symptoms of pain, nausea, vomiting, bloating, diarrhea, constipation, or difficult passage of food or feces [1]. While structural diseases can be identified by pathologists and at times cured by medical technology, the nonstructural symptoms that we describe as "functional" remain enigmatic and less amenable to explanation or effective treatment. Often considered "problems of living," there are physiological, intrapsychic, and sociocultural factors that amplify perception of these symptoms so they are experienced as severe, troublesome, or threatening, with subsequent impact on daily life activities. Those suffering from such symptoms attribute the symptoms to an illness and self-treat or seek medical care. Traditionally trained physicians then search for a disease (inflammatory, infectious, neoplastic and other structural abnormalities) in order to make a diagnosis and offer treatment specific to the diagnosis. In most cases [2], no structural etiology is found, the doctor concludes that the patient has a "functional" problem, and the patient is evaluated and treated accordingly.

This clinical approach results from a faulty conceptualization of functional gastrointestinal disorders (FGIDs) and to the inaccurate, demeaning, and potentially harmful implications that some physicians, patients, and the general public attribute to them [3]. Some clinicians feel ill at ease when making a diagnosis of an FGID since they are trained to seek pathology [4]. In a random sample survey of 704 members of the American Gastroenterological Association [5], the most common endorsement of a functional GI disorder was: ". . . no known structural (i.e., pathological or radiological) abnormalities, or infectious, or metabolic causes" (81%). Next came "a stress disorder" (57% practitioners and 34% academicians and trainees), and last was a "motility disorder" (43% practitioners and 26% academicians/trainees [6]. Although this study is almost 20 years old, the widespread belief that the FGIDs are disorders of exclusion and/or are caused by stress remains. More recently, 13 international investigators agreed that in their countries, physicians view the FGIDs as psychological disorders or merely the absence of organic disease, and often ascribe pejorative features to the patient [3]. Some physicians deny the very existence of the functional GI disorders [7], while others exhibit dismissive or negative attitudes toward patients [4, 8, 9]. Some physicians may pursue unneeded diagnostic studies to find something "real" [10], resulting in increased health care costs, and possibly inappropriate care [11]. These types of beliefs and behaviors can "delegitimize" the FGIDs and the patients who experience them.

What is missing in these attitudes and behaviors is a proper understanding of the true genesis of FGID symptoms, an acknowledgment of their impact on patients, and a rational basis for diagnosing and treating them. In the last few decades several important events have occurred that brought these common disorders into the forefront of clinical care, scientific investigation, and public awareness, and in the process have made them scientifically exciting and clinically legitimate.

The first event began 3 decades ago with a paradigm shift that moved away from conceptualizing illness and disease based on a 3-century old reductionistic model of disease, where the effort was to identify a single underlying biological etiology, to a more integrated, biopsychosocial model of illness and disease [12–14]. The former reductionistic disease-based model had its roots with Descartes' separation of mind and body and at the time was a concept that harmonized prevailing societal views of separation of church and state [1, 13]. What resulted was permission to dissect the human body (which was previously forbidden), so disease was defined by what was seen (i.e., pathology based on abnormal morphology). This approach led to centuries of valuable research producing effective treatments for many diseases. However, the concept of the mind (i.e., the central nervous system, CNS) as being amenable to scientific study or as playing a role in illness and disease was marginalized: the mind was considered the seat of the soul, and was not to be tampered with. I believe that this has had a profound effect on Western society where mental illness or even the effects of stress on physiological function became unavailable for study and even stigmatized. More recent scientific studies link the mind and body as part of a system where their dysregulation can produce illness (the person's experience of ill health) and disease. By embracing this integrated understanding, the biopsychosocial model allows for symptoms to be both physiologically multidetermined and modifiable by sociocultural and psychosocial influences.

Figure 1 illustrates the relationships between psychosocial and physiological factors and functional gastrointestinal symptoms and clinical outcome. Early in life, genetics (e.g., serotonin reuptake transporter (SERT) [15], IL-10 [16] and other genetic polymorphisms) in addition to environmental factors (e.g., family influences on illness expression [17, 18], or abuse [19, 20], major losses, or exposure to infections [21]) may affect one's psychosocial development (susceptibility to life stress, psychological state, coping skills, social support) and/or the development of gut dysfunction (i.e., abnormal motility, visceral hypersensitivity, inflammation, or altered bacterial flora). Furthermore, these brain-gut variables can reciprocally influence their expression. Therefore an FGID is the clinical product of the interaction of psychosocial factors and altered gut physiology via the brain-gut axis [22]. For example, an individual with a bacterial gastroenteritis or other bowel disorder who has no concurrent psychosocial difficulties and good coping skills may not develop the clinical syndrome (or be aware of it) or, if it does develop, may not perceive the need to seek medical care. Another individual with coexistent psychosocial comorbidities, high life stress, abuse history, or maladaptive coping, may develop a syndrome (e.g., postinfectious IBS or dys-

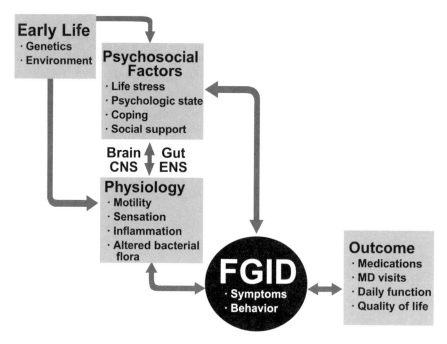

Figure 1. A biopsychosocial conceptualization of the pathogenesis and clinical expression of the functional GI disorders. It shows the relationships between psychosocial and physiological factors, functional gastrointestinal symptoms, and clinical outcome.

pepsia), go to the physician frequently, and have a generally poorer outcome [20, 23–26]. It is also noted that the clinical outcome will, in turn, affect the severity of the disorder (note double-sided arrow in Figure 1). Thus, a family that addresses the illness behavior adaptively and attends to the individual and his or her psychosocial concerns may reduce the impact of the illness experience and resultant behaviors. Conversely, a family that is overly solicitous to the person's illness [27] or a societal group that interprets certain symptoms with threat may amplify the symptoms and illness behaviors [28]. In the health care field, when the physician acknowledges the reality of the patient's complaints, provides empathy, and engages in an effective physician-patient interaction symptom severity and health care seeking are reduced [29]. Conversely, another physician who repeatedly performs unneeded diagnostic studies to rule out pathological disease, dismisses the patients concerns, or does not effectively collaborate in the patient's care is likely to promote a vicious cycle of symptom anxiety and health care seeking [11, 30].

The second change, over the last two decades, has been the remarkable growth in investigative methods that provide evidence for the FGIDs as disorders of brain-gut interactions: (1) motility assessment has improved [31–33]; (2) the barostat has become the standard for testing visceral hypersensitivity [34]; (3) imaging of the brain—positron emission tomography (PET), functional magnetic resonance imaging (fMRI)—provide a window into the central modulation of GI function and its linkages to emotional and cognitive areas [35]; (4) standardized psychological instruments permit the categorization and quantification of emotions, stress, and cognitions (see Chapter 6) to help us determine their influences on symptoms and health outcomes; and most recently (5) the molecular investigation of brain and gut peptides, mucosal immunology, inflammation, and alterations in the bacterial flora of the gut provide the translational basis for gastrointestinal symptom generation. (See Chapters 2 and 3.)

A third event over the last decade has been the development and release of new pharmacological agents to treat altered motility, visceral hypersensitivity, and their stress-mediated effects in patients with FGIDs. These include 5-HT agonists and antagonists and other gut receptor active agents for constipation and diarrhea [36–38], more centrally acting agents to treat stress-mediated effects of CNS modulation of the gut [39–41], and many others covering a vast array of putative mechanisms. For better or worse, increasing media attention to newer pharmaceutical agents has also heightened awareness of the FGIDs within the medical community and general public.

We have come a long way since the 1980s. The FGIDs are now recognized as clinical entities. Researchers and clinicians world wide are more involved with these disorders, and the Rome process has played an important role in categorizing and disseminating the new and evolving knowledge. These disorders are now a prominent part of undergraduate and postgraduate medical curricula, clinical training programs, and international symposia. The number of papers in peer-reviewed journals has skyrocketed, as has attention to these disorders through public media, including television and cinema. There are now future challenges to be faced, which include improved understanding of the relationships between mind and gut, and the translation of basic neurotransmitter function into clinical symptoms and their impact on the patient. The need remains to educate clinicians and the general public on this rapidly growing knowledge and, in the process, continue to legitimize these disorders to society. We are hopeful that the information provided in the Rome III book will continue the process that helps us to achieve these goals.

The Rome III Classification System for Functional Gastrointestinal Disorders

The 28 adult and 17 pediatric FGIDs are presented in Table 1. These are symptom-based diagnostic criteria that are not explained by other pathologically based disorders. However, in recent years histological findings have been identified that

Table I. Functional Gastrointestinal Disorders

A. Functional Esophageal Disorders

A1. Functional heartburn
A2. Functional chest pain of presumed esophageal origin
A3. Functional dysphagia
A4. Globus

B. Functional Gastroduodenal Disorders

B1. Functional dyspepsia
   B1a. Postprandial distress syndrome (PDS)
   B1b. Epigastric pain syndrome (EPS)
B2. Belching disorders
   B2a. Aerophagia
   B2b. Unspecified excessive belching
B3. Nausea and vomiting disorders
   B3a. Chronic idiopathic nausea (CIN)
   B3b. Functional vomiting
   B3c. Cyclic vomiting syndrome (CVS)
B4. Rumination syndrome in adults

C. Functional Bowel Disorders

C1. Irritable bowel syndrome (IBS)
C2. Functional bloating
C3. Functional constipation
C4. Functional diarrhea
C5. Unspecified functional bowel disorder

D. Functional Abdominal Pain Syndrome (FAPS)

E. Functional Gallbladder and Sphincter of Oddi (SO) Disorders

E1. Functional gallbladder disorder
E2. Functional biliary SO disorder
E3. Functional pancreatic SO disorder

F. Functional Anorectal Disorders

F1. Functional fecal incontinence
F2. Functional anorectal pain
   F2a. Chronic proctalgia
      F2a1. Levator ani syndrome
      F2a2. Unspecified functional anorectal pain
   F2b. Proctalgia fugax
F3. Functional defecation disorders
   F3a. Dyssynergic defecation
   F3b. Inadequate defecatory propulsion

G. Functional Disorders: Neonates and Toddlers

G1. Infant regurgitation
G2. Infant rumination syndrome
G3. Cyclic vomiting syndrome
G4. Infant colic
G5. Functional diarrhea
G6. Infant dyschezia
G7. Functional constipation

H. Functional Disorders: Children and Adolescents

H1. Vomiting and aerophagia
   H1a. Adolescent rumination syndrome
   H1b. Cyclic vomiting syndrome
   H1c. Aerophagia
H2. Abdominal pain-related FGIDs
   H2a. Functional dyspepsia
   H2b. Irritable bowel syndrome
   H2c. Abdominal migraine
   H2d. Childhood functional abdominal pain
      H2d1. Childhood functional abdominal pain syndrome
H3. Constipation and incontinence
   H3a. Functional constipation
   H3b. Nonretentive fecal incontinence

blur the distinction between "functional" and "organic" [3, 10, 42]. The FGIDs are better categorized by their motor and sensory physiology and CNS relationships that produce disorders of GI functioning; as such there can be clinical overlap of FGIDs with other disorders.

The FGIDs are classified into 6 major domains for adults: esophageal (category A), gastroduodenal (category B), bowel (category C), functional abdominal pain syndrome (category D), biliary (category E), and anorectal (category F). The pediatric system is classified first by age range (neonate/toddler: category G, and child/adolescent, category H), and then by symptom pattern or area of symptom location. Each category site contains several disorders, each having relatively specific clinical features. So, the functional bowel disorders (category C) include irritable bowel syndrome (IBS) (C1), functional bloating (C2), functional constipation (C3) and functional diarrhea (C4), which anatomically are attributed to the small bowel, colon, and rectum. Thus, while symptoms (e.g., diarrhea, constipation, bloating, pain) may overlap across these disorders, IBS (C1) is more specifically defined as pain associated with change in bowel habit, and this is distinct from functional diarrhea (C4), characterized by loose stools and no pain, or functional bloating (C2), where there is no change in bowel habit. Each condition also has different diagnostic and treatment approaches.

The symptoms of the FGIDs relate to combinations of several known physiological determinants: increased motor reactivity, enhanced visceral hypersensitivity, altered mucosal immune and inflammatory function (which includes changes in bacterial flora), and altered CNS-enteric nervous system (ENS) regulation (as influenced by psychosocial and sociocultural factors and exposures). For example, fecal incontinence (category F1) may primarily be a disorder of motor function, while functional abdominal pain syndrome (category D) is primarily understood as amplified central perception of normal visceral input. IBS (category C1) is more complex, and results from a combination of dysmotility, visceral hypersensitivity, mucosal immune dysregulation, alterations of bacterial flora, and CNS-ENS dysregulation. The contribution of these factors may differ across different individuals or within the same individual over time. Thus, the clinical value of separating the functional GI symptoms into discrete conditions as shown in Table 1 is that they can be reliably diagnosed and more specifically treated.

Scientific Observations on the Pathophysiology of Functional GI Disorders

Using Figure 1 as a template, what follows is a more detailed description of these associations.

— Genetic Predispositions

Genetic factors may predispose some individuals to develop FGIDs, while in others environmental factors contribute to the phenomic expression of these conditions, as well as patient attitudes and behaviors (including health care seeking) relating to it. Genetic factors may play a role in several pathways, including lower levels of IL-10—an anti-inflammatory cytokine—in some patients with IBS [16] that may effect gut mucosal neural sensitivity, SERT polymorphisms that can effect levels of 5-HT neurotransmitter or the response to 5-HT blocking agents[15] [43], G-protein polymorphisms that can affect both CNS and gut related actions [44], and α2 adrenoreceptor polymorphisms that affect motility[45]. An area for future study is the role of CNS-related genetic abnormalities as identified in other conditions, for example with regard to hypothalamic-pituitary-adrenal (HPA)-corticotropin-releasing hormone (CRH) reactivity or linkages between IBS and commonly observed comorbidities like post-traumatic stress disorder (PTSD), depression and anxiety disorders. For example, SERT polymorphisms have effects on mood disturbances[46] and thus may be a genetic link to disorders of brain-gut function like IBS.

— Early Family Environment

The aggregation of FGIDs in families [47] is not only genetic. What children learn from parents may contribute to the risk of developing an FGID [17]. In fact, children of adult IBS patients make more health care visits (and incur more health care costs) than the children of non-IBS parents [48, 49]. In addition, children with recurrent abdominal pain have higher levels of anxiety and depression than healthy children [50] and these psychosocial features predict later symptoms [51].

— Psychosocial Factors

While psychosocial factors do not define the FGIDs and are not required for diagnosis, they are modulators of the patient's experience and behavior, and ultimately, the clinical outcome. Research on the psychosocial aspects of patients with FGIDs yields three general observations (see Chapter 6): (1) *Psychological stress exacerbates gastrointestinal symptoms.* Psychological stress or one's emotional responses to stress can affect gastrointestinal function and produce symptoms in healthy subjects, but do so to a greater degree in patients with functional gastrointestinal disorders. This is evident by the high association of psychosocial comorbidities, life stress, and abuse among patients with FGIDs, which predict poorer outcomes; (2) *Psychosocial factors modify the experience of illness and illness behaviors such as health care seeking.* While patients with FGIDs show greater psychological disturbance than otherwise healthy subjects and patients with medical disease, the data are drawn from patients seen at referral centers. Among FGID sufferers who are non-health care seekers there are no differences in psychological disturbances from the general population. This explains why psychosocial trauma (e.g., sexual or physical abuse history) is more common in referral centers than in primary care, may lower pain threshold and symptom reporting, and is associated with a poorer clinical outcome. These factors can be reduced or "buffered" by adaptive coping skills and social support. Thus, it follows that the psychosocial response of family, society, and culture can also have a palliative effect on the illness experience; (3) *A functional GI disorder may have psychosocial consequences.* Any chronic illness has psychosocial consequences on one's general well-being, daily function status, one's sense of control over the symptoms, and the implications of the illness in terms of future functioning at work and at home. This is understood in terms of one's health-related quality of life (HRQOL).

— Abnormal Motility

It is well recognized that vomiting, diarrhea, acute abdominal pain, incontinence, and many other GI symptoms are generated by disturbed gastrointestinal motility. Furthermore, in healthy subjects, strong emotion or environmental stress can lead to increased motility in the esophagus, stomach, small intestine, and colon. The FGIDs are characterized by having an even greater motility response to stressors (psychological or physiological) when compared to normal subjects [32, 52–54]. These motor responses are only partially correlated with symptoms and are not sufficient to explain reports of chronic or recurrent abdominal pain.

— Visceral Hypersensitivity

The poor association of pain with GI motility with many of the functional GI disorders—e.g., functional chest pain of presumed esophageal origin (A2), epigastric pain syndrome (functional dyspepsia, B1b), irritable bowel syndrome (C1), functional abdominal pain syndrome (D)—is explained by more recent studies relating to abnormalities in visceral sensation [55, 56]. These patients have a lower pain threshold with balloon distension of the bowel (visceral hyperalgesia), or they have increased sensitivity even to normal intestinal function (e.g., allodynia), and there may be an increased area of somatic referral of visceral pain. Visceral hypersensitivity may be amplified in patients with FGIDs, a process called sensitization or stimulus hyperalgesia. Repetitive balloon inflations in the colon leads to a progressive though transient increase in pain intensity in healthy subjects [57], but this occurs to a greater degree and for a longer period in patients with FGIDs [58]. Hypersensitivity and sensitization may be amplified at all levels of the neuraxis. It may occur through altered receptor sensitivity at the gut mucosa and myenteric plexis, which may be enabled by mucosal inflammation [42], degranulation of mast cells close to enteric nerves [59], or increased serotonin activity [60, 61], possibly enhanced by alteration of the bacterial environment or infection [21, 62]. There may also be increased excitability via central sensitization [63], and possibly growth of the spinal cord dorsal horn neurons due to chronic or repetitive visceral stimulation, thus amplifying throughput to the CNS. Finally, as discussed below, there may be altered central down-regulation of visceral afferent transmission, thus reducing pain [35, 64].

— Inflammation

For almost 15 years, investigators have proposed that increased inflammation in the enteric mucosa or neural plexi may contribute to symptom development [65], and only a few years ago was it recognized that about one half of patients with IBS have increased activated mucosal inflammatory cells [42]. This observation is concurrent with clinical observations that about one third of patients with IBS or dyspepsia describe that their symptoms began after an acute enteric infection, and also, up to 25% of patients presenting with an acute enteric infection will go on to develop IBS-like or dyspeptic symptoms [66–68]; the mucosa of these individuals typically do have increased inflammatory cells and inflammatory cytokine expression [24, 69]. It is likely that mucosal inflammation may be at least in part a determinant of visceral hypersensitivity and sensitization as noted above.

— Bacterial Flora

Following from work showing a possible contribution of bacterial overgrowth in at least a subset of patients with IBS [70], there is growing interest in the role of altered bacterial flora contributing to the development of IBS. For example, in one study [71] improvement in IBS symptoms in response to *bifidobacter infantis* was associated with alteration of IL-10/IL-12 ratios, thus converting a more inflammatory cytokine environment seen in IBS to a more normal one as seen in healthy individuals. Future studies are needed to support this growing area of research in the FGIDs.

— Brain-Gut Interactions Via the CNS-ENS

Bidirectional "hardwiring" of brain-gut axis. The brain-gut axis allows bidirectional input and thus links emotional and cognitive centers of the brain with peripheral functioning of the GI tract and vice versa. So, extrinsic (vision, smell, etc.) or enteroceptive (emotion, thought) information have, by nature of their neural connections from higher centers, the capability to affect gastrointestinal sensation, motility, secretion, and inflammation. Conversely, viscerotopic effects (e.g., visceral afferent communications to the brain) reciprocally affect central pain perception, mood, and behavior. For example, spontaneously induced contractions of the colon in rats lead to activation of the locus coeruleus in the pons, an area closely connected to pain and emotional centers in the brain [72]. In turn, increased arousal or anxiety is associated with a decrease in the frequency of migrating motor complex (MMC) activity of the small bowel [73] and of heightened visceral hypersensitivity and autonomic reactivity among patients with IBS [74].

Stress and postinfectious FGID. A feature of the FGIDs is their increased motor and sensory reactivity to environmental stimuli and this also leads to greater gut physiological reactivity to stress [74] or its neurochemical mediators like CRH [39, 75–77]. A good model for brain-gut interactions relates to postinfectious IBS (PI-IBS). In two studies [61, 67] that compared patients who develop PI-IBS to those who recover from infection without developing IBS (recovered group) and to a nonsymptomatic control group, the distinguishing features relate to increased mucosal inflammation and higher levels of psychological distress occurring at the onset of the infection. In fact, there were no significant differences in visceral sensation thresholds or motility between the PI-IBS and the recovered group. This suggests that CNS amplification of peripheral signals occurring in the psychologically distressed PI-IBS group raised them to conscious awareness, thereby perpetuating the symptoms [78]. Furthermore, it is possible that the CNS contributed to the increased expression of peripheral inflammatory/cytokine activity via altered HPA axis reactivity to stress as is seen in IBS [79]. These data suggest that for postinfectious IBS to become clinically expressed, there must be evidence for brain-gut dysfunction with both visceral sensitization and high levels of psychological distress.

Brain imaging. Brain imaging provides a window to brain physiology in response to visceral stimulation [80, 81] of healthy subjects and patients with FGIDs. This can be done with PET, fMRI and related imaging modalities [35, 82, 83]. These studies may help us to understand the role of the CNS in modulating visceral pain and motility. In general, there is an association of anterior cingulate cortex (ACC) activation to rectal distension in IBS relative to controls [82]. Studies using both fMRI and PET show increases in activity of the ACC compared to controls [84–89]. Preliminary data also show that in IBS ACC activation to rectal distension correlates with anxiety [90], stressful life events, maladaptive coping

[91], and a history of abuse [92]. Furthermore, abuse history and IBS diagnosis appear to have synergistic effects causing even greater activation of the perigenual ACC [93]. The future may help us view the responses to CNS treatments like psychological [94] and antidepressant [95] therapies in IBS, thus predicting agents more amenable to such treatments.

Brain-gut peptides. A treatment approach consistent with the concept of brain-gut dysfunction is likely to involve the neuropeptides and receptors present in the ENS and CNS. Putative agents include primarily 5-HT and its congeners, the enkephalins and opioid agonists, substance P, calcitonin gene-related polypeptide (CGRP), and cholecystokinin (CCK), neurokinin (NK) receptor and CRH antagonists, among others. These neuropeptides have integrated activities on gastrointestinal function and human behavior depending upon their location. Ongoing Phase II and III pharmacological treatment trials using agents active at these receptor sites will hopefully address the diverse, but interconnected symptoms of pain, bowel dysfunction, and psychosocial distress so commonly associated with the FGIDs.

An Approach to the Care of Patients with Functional GI Disorders

This section provides general care guidelines for patients with FGIDs. Further information can be found elsewhere [96–100].

— The Therapeutic Relationship

The basis for implementing an effective physician-patient relationship is supported by growing evidence of improved patient satisfaction, adherence to treatment, symptom reduction, and other health outcomes [29, 100–102]. The following are guidelines for the establishment of a therapeutic relationship [103]:

1. Obtain the history through a nondirective, nonjudgmental, patient centered interview.
2. Conduct a careful examination and cost-efficient investigation.
3. Determine the patient is understanding of the illness and his or her concerns (*"What do you think is causing your symptoms?"*).
4. Then provide a thorough explanation of the disorder that takes into consideration the patient's beliefs.

5. Identify and respond realistically to the patient's expectations for improvement (*"How do you feel I can be helpful to you?"*).
6. When possible, provide a link between stressors and symptoms that are consistent with patient's beliefs (*"I understand you don't think stress is causing your pain, but the pain itself is so severe and disabling that it's causing you a great deal of distress"*).
7. Set consistent limits (*"I appreciate how bad the pain must be, but narcotic medication is not indicated"*).
8. Involve the patient in the treatment (*"Let me suggest some treatments for you to consider"*).
9. Make recommendations consistent with patient interests (*"Antidepressants can be used for depression, but they are also used to "turn down" the pain, and in doses lower than that used for depression"*).
10. Establish a long-term relationship with a primary care provider.

Because the FGIDs are chronic, it is important to determine the immediate reasons for the patient's visit: (*"What led you to see me at this time?"*) and to evaluate the patient's verbal and nonverbal communication. Possible causes include:

1. New exacerbating factors (dietary change, concurrent medical disorder, side effects of new medication),
2. Personal concern about a serious disease (recent family death),
3. Environmental stressors (e.g., major loss, abuse history),
4. Psychiatric comorbidity (depression, anxiety),
5. Impairment in daily function (recent inability to work or socialize), or
6. A "hidden agenda" such as narcotic or laxative abuse, or pending litigation or disability

Once the reasons for the visit are determined, treatment may be based on the severity and nature of the symptoms, the physiologic and psychosocial determinants of the patient's illness behavior, and the degree of functional impairment. Although illness severity exists on a continuum, it is arbitrarily separated into mild, moderate, and severe categories:

Mild Symptoms

Patients with mild or infrequent symptoms are usually seen in primary care practices and do not have major impairment in function or psychological disturbance. They may have concerns about the implications of their symptoms, but do not make frequent visits and usually maintain normal activity levels. Here, treatment is directed toward:

1. *Education.* Indicate that the FGIDs are very real and the bowels are overly responsive to a variety of stimuli such as food, hormonal changes, medication, and stress. Pain resulting from spasm or stretching of the gut, from a sensitive gut, or both, can be experienced anywhere in the abdomen and can be associated with changes in gastrointestinal function leading to symptoms (e.g., pain, nausea, vomiting, diarrhea). The physician should emphasize that both physiologic and psychological factors interact to produce symptoms.

2. *Reassurance.* The physician should elicit patient worries and concerns and provide appropriate reassurance. While this can be an effective therapeutic intervention, the patient will not accept it if it is communicated in a perfunctory manner and before necessary tests are completed.

3. *Diet and medication.* Offending dietary substances (e.g., lactose, caffeine, fatty foods, alcohol, etc.) and mediations that adversely cause symptoms should be identified and possibly eliminated. Sometimes a food diary is helpful.

Moderate Symptoms

A smaller proportion of patients, usually seen in primary or secondary care, report moderate symptoms and have intermittent disruptions in activity, for example, missing social functions, work, or school. They may identify a close relationship between symptoms and inciting events such as dietary indiscretion, travel, or distressing experiences. They may be more psychologically distressed than patients with mild symptoms. For this group, additional treatment options are recommended.

1. *Symptom monitoring.* The patient can keep a symptom diary for one to two weeks to record the time, severity, and presence of associated factors. This may help to identify inciting factors such as dietary indiscretions or specific stressors not previously considered. The physician can then review possible dietary, lifestyle, or behavioral influences with the patient. This encourages the patient's participation in treatment, and as symptoms improve, increases his or her sense of control over the illness.

2. *Pharmacotherapy directed at specific symptoms.* Medication can be considered for symptom episodes that are distressing or that impair daily function. The choice of medication will depend on the predominant symptoms and is outlined in later chapters of this book. In general, prescription medications should be considered as ancillary to dietary or lifestyle modifications for chronic symptoms, but can be used during periods of acute symptoms exacerbation.

3. *Psychological treatments.* Psychological treatments may be considered for motivated patients with moderate to severe GI symptoms and for patients with pain. It is more helpful if the patient can associate symptoms with stressors. These treatments, which include cognitive-behavioral therapy, relaxation, hypnosis, and combination treatments, help to reduce anxiety levels, encourage health promoting behaviors, and give the patient greater responsibility and control in the treatment and improve pain tolerance. See Chapter 6 for more details.

Severe Symptoms

Only a small proportion of patients with FGIDs have severe and refractory symptoms. These patients also have a high frequency of associated psychosocial difficulties including diagnoses of anxiety, depression or somatization, personality disturbance, and chronically impaired daily functioning. There may be a history of major loss or abuse, poor social networks or coping skills, and "catastrophizing" behaviors. These patients may see gastroenterology consultants frequently and hold unrealistic expectations to be "cured." They may deny a role for psychosocial factors in the illness and may be unresponsive to psychological treatment or to pharmacological agents directed at the gut.

1. *The physician's approach.* These patients need an ongoing relationship with a physician (gastroenterologist or primary care physician) who provides psychosocial support through repeated brief visits. In general the physician should (a) perform diagnostic and therapeutic measures based on objective findings rather than in response to patient demands, (b) set realistic treatment goals, such as improved quality of life rather than complete pain relief or cure, (c) shift the responsibility for treatment to the patient by giving therapeutic options, and (d) change the focus of care from treatment of disease to adjustment to chronic illness.
2. *Antidepressant treatment.* The tricyclic antidepressants (TCA) (e.g., desipramine, amitriptyline), and more recently the serotonin-noradrenergic reuptake inhibitors (SNRIs) (e.g., duloxetine) have a role in controlling pain via central analgesia as well as relief of associated depressive symptoms. The selective serotonin reuptake inhibitors (SSRIs) (e.g., citalopram, fluoxetine, paroxetine) may have an ancillary role as they are less effective for pain but can help reduce anxiety and associated depression. Antidepressants should be considered for patients with chronic pain and impaired daily functioning, coexistent symptoms of major or atypical depression, symptom anxiety or panic attacks. Even without depressive symptoms, these agents may help when the pain is dominant and consuming. A poor clinical response

may be due to insufficient dose or failure to adjust the dosage based on therapeutic response or side effects. Treatment should be instituted for at least 3 to 4 weeks. If effective, it can be continued for up to a year and then tapered.

3. *Pain treatment center referral.* Pain treatment centers provide a multi-disciplinary team approach toward rehabilitation of patients who have become seriously disabled.

The Rome Committees and Criteria Development

Beginning about 15–20 years ago, and with growing awareness of the FGIDs, the academic environment was receptive to a classification system that could be used for research and clinical care. At this time the Rome working teams began, and have since served as the nidus to modify and update information on these disorders for research and patient care. Beginning by necessity as a group that developed criteria by consensus (via the "Delphi Approach" [104, 105]), the process has matured through three generations, producing a series of publications (Rome I, II, and III), with an increased evidence-based approach to the recommendations. The Rome organization was incorporated in 1996 as the Working Teams for Diagnosis of Functional GI Disorders, became a 501(c)3 tax-exempt organization in 1997, and was renamed the Rome Foundation in 2003 to reflect the expansion of its activities globally. The Foundation continues its mission to improve knowledge of the science and practice relating to the functional GI disorders, and has received support from academic organizations, investigators and clinicians, pharmaceutical regulatory agencies, pharmaceutical companies, and federal research agencies. See Chapter 17 ("The Road to Rome") for a historical account of the Rome committee work.

This part of the chapter will review the rationale and limitations of a symptom-based diagnostic classification system, and discuss the process with which the Rome III criteria were developed.

— Rationale for Symptom-Based Diagnostic Criteria

The Rome III classification system is based on the premise that for each disorder there are symptom clusters that "breed true" across clinical and population groups. This presumption provides a framework for identification of patients for research that is modified as new scientific data emerges. The rationale for classifying the functional GI disorders into symptom-based subgroups has several bases [106].

Site-Specific Differences

Patients with functional GI disorders report a wide variety of symptoms affecting different regions of the gastrointestinal tract. These symptoms have in common disturbances in sensory and/or motor gastrointestinal function, or similarities in CNS processing of visceral and somatic signals. Despite overarching similarities in CNS functioning amenable to central treatments, many, if not most of the FGIDs have peripherally generated symptoms that require more specific treatments (e.g., for diarrhea or constipation). Furthermore, epidemiological studies using factor analysis and other methods provide the evidence for the existence of site-specific syndromes [107–109].

Symptoms Resulting from Multiple Influencing Factors

Unlike motility criteria that define motor dysfunction with varying or no symptoms (examples being gastroparesis, and pseudo-obstruction or "nutcracker esophagus"), symptom-based criteria may be influenced by abnormal motility, visceral hypersensitivity, or brain-gut dysfunction. Thus functional abdominal pain syndrome (D) relates to dysfunction of central pain regulation in the absence of motility disturbances of the gut. Each condition may have varying contributions from these pathophysiological determinants.

Epidemiologic Data

Epidemiological studies show similar frequencies for these conditions across various studies and populations in Western countries including the USA, Australia, England, and France [110, 111], but may be lower in Asian countries and among African-Americans [112, 113]. In addition, a factor analysis study using two community samples [114] identified an irritable bowel factor, and these symptoms were very similar to those developed from a clinical population of irritable bowel patients using discriminant function analysis ("Manning" criteria) [115]. When differences do exist, these may relate to the type of criteria used, which may over- or under-represent the population being tested [116].

Treatment Implications

A critical value to the use of symptom-based diagnostic criteria relates to the ability to define patient subsets amenable to treatment trials. Thus, centrally acting treatments can have overarching effects on pain in most all the FGIDs, while treatments for diarrhea or constipation can be targeted to appropriate subgroups using the specified criteria.

Need for Diagnostic Standards in Clinical Care and Research

Since there are no unique physiological features that can characterize all the disorders, and because it is symptoms that patients bring to physicians, the use of a symptom-based classification system is rational for clinical care and research. Symptom-based criteria are used in psychiatry (e.g., the Diagnostic and Statistical Manual of Mental Disorders IV, or DSM-IV) [117], and rheumatology [118], and are becoming increasingly accepted within gastroenterology. Symptom-based criteria can help guide the diagnostic and treatment approach, reduce the ordering of unneeded diagnostic studies, and standardize the selection of patients for clinical trials.

— Qualifications for the Use of Symptom-Based Criteria

There are several limitations and qualifications to the use of symptom-based criteria [106].

Other Diseases May Coexist that Need to be Excluded

The high frequency of the FGIDs assures their coexistence with other diseases. If 10–15% of the population has IBS, then at least as many with inflammatory bowel disease (IBD) will have IBS, and new evidence suggests that there is more than a chance association [119]. In fact, IBD may even predispose to IBS [120, 121]. Similarly, *H. Pylori* needs to be excluded and/or treated among patients with functional dyspepsia. So, for research purposes, it is necessary to exclude other diseases before a functional GI designation can be applied. However, physicians are well aware that in clinical situations one must consider the presence of two or more conditions and make judgments on the proper treatments for both. One example would be a patient with IBS-IBD having predominant pain and diarrhea not explained by the morphological findings.

Symptoms May Overlap with Other Functional GI Disorders

It is common for functional GI disorders to coexist, and the criteria permit the coexistence of more than one FGID. Examples would be esophageal chest pain (A2) or globus (A4), with IBS (C1) or fecal incontinence (F1). However, there are situations where a hierarchical classification of the FGIDs is required. For example, when criteria for both IBS (C1) *and* epigastric pain syndrome (B1b) are fulfilled, the diagnosis of IBS only is made when the epigastric pain is relieved by defecation. Similarly functional bloating (C2) exists only when IBS and the dyspeptic conditions are excluded, since bloating is common to both these other conditions, and a diagnosis of functional constipation (C3) is made only if IBS criteria are not met.

Symptoms Must Have Begun 6 Months Prior to Diagnosis and Be Active for 3 Months

This is a modification of the Rome II criteria and is less restrictive. Thus, onset of symptoms should begin at least 6 months before clinical presentation and the diagnostic criteria must be fulfilled for the last 3 months (rather than 1 year, as for Rome II).

Diagnostic Categories Do Not Include Psychosocial Criteria

Although psychosocial disturbances can affect the onset, course, severity, and outcome of the FGIDs, they are not required for diagnosis. Psychosocial disturbances are more common in patients seen in referral practices over primary care or in the community of nonconsulters.

Criteria Are Determined by Clinical Consensus and Existing Evidence

The proposed diagnostic criteria were originated by the consensus of experts in the field and have since been modified only if there is compelling evidence to do so. All changes in criteria relate to a rationale that is provided in the chapter. In some cases, recommendations for changes (e.g., dyspeptic criteria, subtypes of IBS) are not yet proven but are supported by compelling evidence. New criteria will be tested in future studies now underway, and this will form the basis for future modifications of the criteria.

— The Rome Committee Process

The process for developing these criteria is a rigorous one. The consensus process was initiated by Professor Aldo Torsoli for the International Congress of Gastroenterology in Rome (Roma '88). Dr. Torsoli charged the committees [104] to use a "Delphi" method [105] of decision-making, which fosters a team effort to produce consistency in opinion, or consensus, (although not necessarily total agreement) for difficult questions not easily addressed. The Rome II committees and more recently the Rome III board took on the responsibility to enhance these activities further using a rigorous 4-year, 13-step process:

1. The Editorial Board identified individuals who fulfilled pre-set criteria (academic research record, name recognition, ability to work in groups, and diversity issues related to discipline, geographic location, and gender) to chair and co-chair each of the 14 subcommittees. The chair and co-chair were charged to coordinate their committee to develop a manuscript for the *Gastroenterology* journal and a larger manuscript for the Rome III book.

2. The chair and co-chair, with consultation from the Board, recommended an international panel of up to six additional members fulfilling the same criteria noted above to join the subcommittee.

3. The chair and co-chair designated each committee member to produce an initial document covering their particular area of expertise. The members are charged to critically synthesize the literature regarding the physiological, psychological, and diagnostic and treatment aspects of a particular functional disorder or scientific content area.

4. The chair and co-chair then incorporated all documents into a manuscript that was sent back to the entire committee for review (Document A).

5. This process of modification and re-review by the committee was repeated 2 more times (Documents B and C) over a 2-year period; it is associated with critical appraisal and modification by all members of the information presented.

6. The committee met for two days in November-December, 2004 to revise the documents. This face-to-face meeting led to consensus on the diagnostic criteria and scientific content.

7. The information was summarized and presented to the full committee of chairs and co-chairs over one day for feedback and harmonization of content across committees.

8. The chair and co-chair then revised the documents again (Document D) and sent them to up to six outside international experts, in addition to scientists in the pharmaceutical industry, for their review and commentary. This process was handled in collaboration with the Rome Foundation and the *Gastroenterology* journal administrative staff.

9. Concurrently, the copy editor identified areas that required revisions relating to style and format and sent it to the chairs and co-chairs for modification.

10. The Editorial Board served as editors to facilitate and respond to the review process. Each board member was responsible for two committees.

11. The committee chairs responded to the editor's and reviewers' comments either by modifying the manuscripts as requested, or providing a written response that addressed the reviewers' concerns. In some cases the manuscripts were reviewed and modified 3 times before final acceptance.

12. The revised manuscripts and the commentaries by the reviewers and authors were then sent to the Editorial Board who met in September and again in December, 2005 to critically review these materials and submit any final comments back to the authors. In some cases, edits were made by the editors and were sent for approval to the chairs and co-chairs.

13. Finally, when the documents were completed, all members signed off their approval, before it was sent to the copyeditor for a final check on content and style prior to publication.

— Changes Made in Rome III

The changes from Rome II to Rome III reflect mainly updates in the literature and committee recommendations derived from these new data. In addition, a few modifications in the categories and criteria were made. The following summarizes the changes, and the reader is referred to the relevant chapter for details.

1. *Time frame change for FGIDs.* Symptoms are now recommended to originate 6 months prior to diagnosis and be currently active (i.e., meet criteria) for 3 months. This time frame is less restrictive when compared to Rome II (12 weeks of symptoms over 12 months) and is easier to understand and apply in research and clinical practice.

2. *Changes in classification categories:*
   a. *Rumination syndrome moved from functional esophageal (Category A) to functional gastroduodenal disorders (Category B).* This reflects the evidence that this disorder originates from disturbances in the stomach and abdomen.
   b. *Removal of functional abdominal pain syndrome (FAPS) from functional bowel disorders (Category C) into its own category (Category D).* This is based on growing evidence that FAPS relates more to CNS amplification of normal regulatory visceral signals rather than functional abnormalities *per se* within the GI tract.
   c. *Creation of two pediatric categories.* The Rome II category of Childhood Functional GI Disorders is now classified as Childhood Functional GI Disorders: Neonate/Toddler (Category G) and Childhood Functional GI Disorders: Child/Adolescent. This is due to the different clinical conditions that arise between these two categories relating to growth and development of the child.

3. *Criteria changes:*
   a. *Functional Dyspepsia.* For Rome III, functional dyspepsia is de-emphasized as an entity for research due to the heterogeneity of this symptom complex as defined. Instead, the committees recommend

two conditions that are subsumed under the functional dyspepsia "umbrella": (a) postprandial distress syndrome, and (b) Epigastric pain syndrome. These are similar to dysmotility-like and ulcer-like dyspepsia of Rome II. However, they are now defined by a complex of symptom features with physiological support rather than being based on the previous requirement of the predominant symptom of epigastric discomfort or pain respectively.

b. *More restrictive criteria for functional disorders of the gallbladder and sphincter of Oddi.* There are more defining features and exclusions required for symptom-based diagnosis of these conditions. In doing so, we have reduced the patient population who would then receive invasive studies like endoscopic retrograde cholangiopancreatography (ERCP) and manometry to confirm the diagnosis and be treated.

c. *Revision of IBS subtyping.* The committees are recommending that diarrhea, constipation and mixed subtypes be based on a simple classification related to stool consistency. However, the bowel subtyping used in Rome II for diarrhea-predominant IBS (IBS-D) and constipation-predominant IBS (IBS-C) is still acceptable.

We are hopeful that these changes will make the Rome III criteria more useful for research and clinical care. Future studies will be needed to confirm the validity of these changes.

Concluding Comments

It is with great anticipation that we introduce this 3rd edition: *Rome III, The Functional Gastrointestinal Disorders.* We hope that the information will help the reader gain a better understanding of these disorders, and help clinicians in the diagnosis and care of our patients. This book is the culmination of a 5-year effort of 87 internationally recognized investigators representing 18 countries. As we look back on the process, the information we have obtained is comprehensive, though certainly not complete. It is likely that the next 6 years will bring considerable advances in our understanding and treatment of these disorders, and when that occurs, we plan to revise the information as we move to Rome IV. As we look forward, we have taken on several new initiatives to continue our mission. This includes new working team committees that have been instituted to develop standardization of brain imaging assessment and to make recommendations relating to symptom severity for research and clinical care. We have also begun to capture this book and future scientific data into a CD slide set module for self-learning and lectures. Finally, we are looking to disseminate this knowledge through additional educational products on a global scale. The Rome process is a dynamic one and we look forward to future activities to help improve the science of the FGIDs and care of patients.

References

1. Drossman DA. Psychosocial and Psychophysiologic Mechanisms in GI Illness. In: Kirsner JB, ed. *The Growth of Gastroenterologic Knowledge in the 20th Century.* 1 ed. Lea & Febiger, Philadelphia, 1993, pp. 419–432.
2. Kroenke K, Mangelsdorff AD. Common symptoms in ambulatory care: incidence, evaluation, therapy, and outcome. Am J Med 1989; 86:262–266.
3. Drossman DA. Functional GI Disorders: What's in a Name? 1. Gastroenterology 2005; 128(7):1771–1772.
4. Drossman DA. Challenges in the physician-patient relationship: Feeling "drained." Gastroenterology 2001; 121(5):1037–1038.
5. Mitchell CM, Drossman DA. Survey of the AGA membership relating to patients with functional gastrointestinal disorders. Gastroenterology 1987; 92:1282–1284.
6. Russo MW, Gaynes BN, Drossman DA. A National Survey of Practice Patterns of Gastroenterologists with Comparison to the Past Two Decades. J Clin Gastroenterol 1999; 29(4):339–343.
7. Christensen J. Heraclides or the physician. Gastroenterology Int 1990; 3:45–48.
8. Dalton CB, Drossman DA, Hathaway MD, Bangdiwala SI. Perceptions of physicians and patients with organic and functional gastroenterological diagnoses. Clin Gastroenterol Hepatol 2004; 2(2):121–126.
9. Heitkemper M, Carter E, Ameen V, Olden K, Cheng L. Women with irritable bowel syndrome: differences in patients' and physicians' perceptions. Gastroenterology Nurs 2002; 25(5):192–200.
10. Drossman DA. The "organification" of functional gi disorders: Implications for research. Gastroenterology 2003; 124 :6–7.
11. Longstreth GF, Drossman DA. Severe Irritable Bowel And Functional Abdominal Pain Syndromes: Managing The Patient And Health Care Costs. Clin Gastroenterol Hepatol 2005; 3:397–400.
12. Engel GL. The need for a new medical model: A challenge for biomedicine. Science 1977; 196:129–136.
13. Drossman DA. Presidential Address: Gastrointestinal Illness and Biopsychosocial Model. Psychosom Med 1998; 60(3):258–267.
14. Engel GL. The clinical application of the Biopsychosocial model. Am J Psychiatry 1980; 137:535–544.
15. Yeo A, Boyd P, Lumsden S et al. Association between a functional polymorphism in the serotonin transporter gene and diarrhoea predominant irritable bowel syndrome in women. Gut 2004; 53(10):1452–1458.

16. Gonsalkorale WM, Perrey C, Pravica V, Whorwell PJ, Hutchinson IV. Interleukin 10 genotypes in irritable bowel syndrome: evidence for an inflammatory component? Gut 2003; 52(1):91–93.

17. Levy RL, Jones KR, Whitehead WE et al. Irritable bowel syndrome in twins: Heredity and social learning both contribute to etiology. Gastroenterology 2001; 121(4):799–804.

18. Hotopf M, Carr S, Mayou R, Wadsworth M, Wessely S. Why do children have chronic abdominal pain, and what happens to them when they grow up? Population based cohort study. BMJ 1998; 316(7139):1196–1200.

19. Leserman J, Li Z, Drossman DA, Hu JB. Selected symptoms associated with sexual and physical abuse history among female patients with gastrointestinal disorders: the impact on subsequent helath care visits. Psychol Med 1998; 28:417–425.

20. Drossman DA, Li Z, Leserman J, Toomey TC, Hu Y. Health status by gastrointestinal diagnosis and abuse history. Gastroenterology 1996; 110(4):999–1007.

21. Spiller RC. Post infectious irritable bowel syndrome. Gastroenterology 2003; 124(5): 1662–1671.

22. Jones MP, Dilley JB, Crowell MD, Drossman D. The mind-body connection in the GI disorders of function: Anatomic and physiologic relationships between the central nervous system and digestive tract. Neurogastroenterol Motil 2006;18:91–103.

23. Gwee KA, Leong YL, Graham C et al. The role of psychological and biological factors in postinfective gut dysfunction. Gut 1999; 44(3):400–406.

24. Dunlop SP, Jenkins D, Neal KR, Spiller RC. Relative importance of enterochromaffin cell hyperplasia, anxiety, and depression in postinfections IBS. Gastroenterolgy 2003; 125(6):1651–1659.

25. Drossman DA, Li Z, Leserman J et al. Effects of coping on health outcome among female patients with gastrointestinal disorders. Psychosom Med 2000; 62:309–317.

26. Drossman DA, Whitehead WE, Toner BB et al. What determines severity among patients with painful functional bowel disorders? Am J Gastroenterol 2000; 95(4): 974–980.

27. Levy RL, Whitehead WE, Walker LS et al. Increased somatic complaints and health-care utilization in children: effects of parent IBS status and parent response to gastrointestinal symptoms 2. Am J Gastroenterol 2004; 99(12):2442–2451.

28. Kleinman A, Eisenberg L, Good B. Culture, illness and care. Clinical lessons from anthropologic and cross-cultural research. Ann Intern Med 1978; 88:251.

29. Stewart M, Brown JB, Donner A et al. The impact of patient-centered care on outcomes. J Fam Pract 2000; 49(9):796–804.

30. Keefer L, Sanders K, Sykes MA et al. Towards a better understanding of anxiety in irritable bowel syndrome: A preliminary look at worry and intolerance of uncertainty. J Cognitive Psychother 2005; 19(2):163–172.

31. Azpiroz F, Enck P, Whitehead WE. Anorectal functional testing: Review of collective experience. Am J Gastroenterol 2002; 97(2):232–240.

32. Parkman HP, Hasler WL, Fisher RS. American Gastroenterological Association technical review on the diagnosis and treatment of gastroparesis. Gastroenterology 2004; 127(5):1592–1622.

33. Pandolfino JE, Kahrilas PJ. AGA technical review on the clinical use of esophageal manometry. Gastroenterology 2004; 128(1):209–224.

34. Whitehead WE, Delvaux M, Working Team. Standardization of procedures for test-

ing smooth muscle tone and sensory thresholds in the gastrointestinal tract. Dig Dis Sci 1994; 42(2):223–241.

35. Drossman DA. Brain Imaging and its Implications for Studying Centrally Targeted Treatments in IBS: A Primer for Gastroenterologists. Gut 2005; 54(5):569–573.

36. Evans BW, Clark WK, Moore DJ, Whorwell PJ. Tegaserod for the treatment of irritable bowel syndrome 1. Cochrane Database Syst Rev 2004;(1):CD003960.

37. Lembo A, Weber HC, Farraye FA. Alosetron in irritable bowel syndrome: strategies for its use in a common gastrointestinal disorder. Drugs 2003; 63(18):1895–1905.

38. Galligan JJ, Vanner S. Basic and clinical pharmacology of new motility promoting agents 1. Neurogastroenterol Motil 2005; 17(5):643–653.

39. Sagami Y, Shimada Y, Tayama J et al. Effect of a corticotropin releasing hormone receptor antagonist on colonic sensory and motor function in patients with irritable bowel syndrome. Gut 2004; 53(7):958–964.

40. Drossman DA, Toner BB, Whitehead WE et al. Cognitive-Behavioral Therapy vs. education and Desipramine vs. Placebo for Moderate to Severe Functional Bowel Disorders. Gastroenterology 2003; 125(1):19–31.

41. Creed F, Fernandes L, Guthrie E et al. The cost-effectiveness of psychotherapy and paroxetine for severe irritable bowel syndrome. Gastroenterology 2003; 124 (2):303–317.

42. Chadwick VS, Chen W, Shu D et al. Activation of the mucosal immune system in irritable bowel syndrome. Gastroenterology 2002; 122(7):1778–1783.

43. Camilleri M, Atanasova E, Carlson PJ et al. Serotonin-transporter polymorphism pharmacogenetics in diarrhea-predominant irritable bowel syndrome. Gastroenterology 2002; 123(2):425–432.

44. Holtmann G, Siffert W, Haag S et al. G-protein beta3 subunit 825 CC genotype is associated with unexplained (functional) dyspepsia. Gastroenterology 2004; 126(4):971–979.

45. Kim HJ, Camilleri M, Carlson PJ et al. Association of distinct alpha(2) adrenoceptor and serotonin transporter polymorphisms with constipation and somatic symptoms in functional gastrointestinal disorders. Gut 2004; 53(6):829–837.

46. Caspi A, Sugden K, Moffitt TE et al. Influence of life stress on depression: moderation by a polymorphism in the 5-HTT gene 57. Science 2003; 301(5631):386–389.

47. Locke GR, III, Zinsmeister A, Talley NJ, Fett SL, Melton J. Familial association in adults with functional gastrointestinal disorders. Mayo Clin Proc 2000; 75:907–912.

48. Levy RL, Whitehead WE, Von Korff MR, Saunders KW, Feld AD. Intergenerational transmission of gastrointestinal illness behavior. Am J Gastroenterol 2000; 95 (2):451–456.

49. Levy RL, Von Korff M, Whitehead WE et al. Costs of care for irritable bowel syndrome patients in a health maintenance organization. Am J Gastoenterol 2001; 96(11):3122–3129.

50. Walker LS, Garber J, Greene JW. Psychosocial correlates of recurrent childhood pain: a comparison of pediatric patients with recurrent abdominal pain, organic illness, and psychiatric disorders. J Abnorm Psychol 1993; 102(2):248–258.

51. Walker LS, Garber J, Smith CA, Van Slyke DA, Claar RL. The relation of daily stressors to somatic and emotional symptoms in children with and without recurrent abdominal pain. J Consult Clin Psychol 2001; 69(1):85–91.

52. Quigley EMM, Hasler WL, Parkman HP. AGA technical review on nausea and vomiting. Gastroenterology 2001; 120(1):263–286.

53. Locke GR, III, Pemberton JH, Phillips SF. AGA Technical Review on Constipation. Gastroenterology 2000; 119(6):1766–1778.

54. Drossman DA, Camilleri M, Mayer EA, Whitehead WE. AGA Technical Review on Irritable Bowel Syndrome. Gastroenterology 2002; 123(6):2108–2131.

55. Delgado-Aros S, Camilleri M. Visceral hypersensitivity 2. J Clin Gastroenterol 2005; 39(4 Suppl 3):S194–S203.

56. Mayer EA, Gebhart GF. Basic and clinical aspects of visceral hyperalgesia. Gastroenterology 1994; 107(1):271–293.

57. Ness TJ, Metcalf AM, Gebhart GF. A psychophysiological study in humans using phasic colonic distension as a noxious visceral stimulus. Pain 1990; 43:377–386.

58. Munakata J, Naliboff B, Harraf F et al. Repetitive sigmoid stimulation induces rectal hyperalgesia in patients with irritable bowel syndrome. Gastroenterology 1997; 112(1): 55–63.

59. Barbara G, Stanghellini V, DeGiorgio R et al. Activated mast cells in proximity to colonic nerves correlate with abdominal pain in irritable bowel syndrome. Gastroenterology 2004; 126(3):693–702.

60. Gershon MD. Nerves, reflexes, and the enteric nervous system: pathogenesis of the irritable bowel syndrome 2. J Clin Gastroenterol 2005; 39(4 Suppl 3):S184–S193.

61. Dunlop SP, Coleman NS, Blackshaw E et al. Abnormalities of 5-hydroxytryptamine metabolism in irritable bowel syndrome. Clin Gastroenterol Hepatol 2005; 3(4):349–357.

62. Dunlop SP, Jenkins D, Neal KR, Spiller RC. Relative importance of enterochromaffin cell hyperplasia, anxiety and depression in post-infectious IBS. Gastroenterology 2003; 125(6):1651–1659.

63. Stam R, Ekkelenkamp K, Frankhuijzen AC et al. Long-lasting changes in central nervous system responsivity to colonic distention after stress in rats. Gastroenterology 2002; 123(4):1216–1225.

64. Mayer EA. The neurobiology of stress and gastrointestinal disease. Gut 2000; 47(6): 861–869.

65. Collins SM. Is the irritable gut an inflamed gut? Scand J Gastroenterol 1992; 27 Suppl 192:102–105.

66. McKendrick W, Read NW. Irritable bowel syndrome—post salmonella infection. J Infection 1994; 29:1–4.

67. Gwee KA, Leong YL, Graham C et al. The role of psychological and biological factors in post- infective gut dysfunction. Gut 1999; 44:400–406.

68. Mearin F, Perez-Oliveras M, Perelló A et al. Dyspepsia after a Salmonella gastroenteritis outbreak: One-year follow-up cohort study. Gastroenterology 2005; 129(1):98–104.

69. Gwee KA, Collins SM, Read NW et al. Increased rectal mucosal expression of interleukin 1beta in recently acquired post-infectious irritable bowel syndrome. Gut 2003; 52(4):523–526.

70. Pimentel M, Chow EJ, Lin HC. Eradication of small intestinal bacterial overgrowth reduces symptoms of Irritable Bowel Syndrome. Am J Gastroenterol 2000; 95(12):3503–3506.

71. O'Mahony L, McCarthy J, Kelly P et al. Lactobacillus and Bifidobacterium in Irritable Bowel Syndrome: Symptom Responses and Relationship to Cytokine Profiles. Gastroenterology 2005; 128(3):541–551.

72. Svensson TH. Peripheral, autonomic regulation of locus coeruleus noradrenergic

neurons in brain: Putative implications for psychiatry and psychopharmacology. Psychopharmacology 1987; 92:1–7.

73. Valori RM, Kumar D, Wingate DL. Effects of different types of stress and or "prokinetic" drugs on the control of the fasting motor complex in humans. Gastroenterology 1986; 90:1890–1900.

74. Murray CD, Flynn J, Ratcliffe L et al. Effect of acute physical and psychological stress on gut autonomic innervation in irritable bowel syndrome 1. Gastroenterology 2004; 127(6):1695–1703.

75. Fukudo S, Nomura T, Hongo M. Impact of corticotropin-releasing hormone on gastrointestinal motility and adrenocorticotropic hormone in normal controls and patients with irritable bowel syndrome. Gut 1998; 42(6):845–849.

76. Tache Y. Corticotropin releasing factor receptor antagonists: potential future therapy in gastroenterology? Gut 2004; 53(7):919–921.

77. Tache Y, Martinez V, Million M, Maillot C. Role of corticotropin releasing factor subtype 1 in stress-related functional colonic alterations: Implications in irritable bowel syndrome. Eur J Surg 2002; 168(11(Supplement 587)):16–22.

78. Drossman DA. Mind over matter in the postinfective irritable bowel. Gut 1999; 44 (3):306–307.

79. Dinan TG, Quigley EMM, Ahmed S et al. Hypothalamic-pituitary-gut axis dysregulation in irritable bowel syndrome: Plasma cytokines as a potential biomarker? Gastroenterology 2006;130:304–311.

80. Yaguez L, Coen S, Gregory LJ et al. Brain response to visceral aversive conditioning: a functional magnetic resonance imaging study 1. Gastroenterology 2005; 128(7):1819–1829.

81. Kern MK, Shaker R. Cerebral cortical registration of subliminal visceral stimulation. Gastroenterology 2002; 122:290–298.

82. Hobson AR, Aziz Q. Brain imaging and functional gastrointestinal disorders: has it helped our understanding? Gut 2004; 53(8):1198–1206.

83. Hobson AR, Furlong PL, Worthen SF et al. Real-time imaging of human cortical activity evoked by painful esophageal stimulation. Gastroenterology 2005; 128:610–619.

84. Mertz H, Morgan V, Tanner G et al. Regional cerebral activation in irritable bowel syndrome and control subjects with painful and nonpainful rectal distention. Gastroenterology 2000; 118:842–848.

85. Naliboff BD, Derbyshire SWG, Munakata J et al. Cerebral activation in irritable bowel syndrome patients and control subjects during rectosigmoid stimulation. Psychosom Med 2001; 63(3):365–375.

86. Drossman DA, Ringel Y, Vogt B et al. Alterations of brain activity associated with resolution of emotional distress and pain in a case of severe IBS. Gastroenterology 2003; 124(3):754–761.

87. Chang L, Berman S, Mayer EA et al. Brain responses to visceral and somatic stimuli in patients with irritable bowel syndrome with and without fibromyalgia. Am J Gastroenterol 2003; 98(6):1354–1361.

88. Hobday DI, Aziz Q, Thacker N et al. A study of the cortical processing of ano-rectal sensation using functional MRI. Brain 2001; 124(Pt 2):361–368.

89. Verne GN, Himes NC, Robinson ME, Briggs RW, Gopinath KS, Weng L et al. Central representation of cutaneous and visceral pain in irritable bowel syndrome. Gastroenterology 120[5 (1)], A713. 2001.

90. Morgan V, Pickens D, Shyr Y. Anxiety is associated with increased anterior cingulate but not thalamic activation during rectal pain in IBS and controls. Gastroenterology 120[5 (1)]. 2001.

91. Ringel Y, Drossman DA, Leserman J, Lin W, Liu H, Vogt B et al. Association of anterior cingulate cortex (ACC) activation with psychosocial distress and pain reports. Gastroenterology 124[4], A-97. 2003.

92. Ringel Y, Drossman DA, Turkington TG et al. Regional Brain Activation in Response to Rectal Distention in Patients with Irritable Bowel Syndrome and the Effect of a History of Abuse. Dig Dis Sci 2003; 48(9):1774–1781.

93. Ringel Y, Drossman DA, Leserman J, Lin W, Liu H, Smith JK et al. IBS diagnosis and a history of abuse have synergistic effect on the perigenual cingulate activation in response to rectal distention. Gastroenterology 124[4], A-531. 2003.

94. Lackner JM, Coad ML, Mertz HR et al. Cognitive therapy for irritable bowel syndrome is associated with reduced limbic activity, GI symptoms, and anxiety. Behav Res Ther 2005; 43(7):943–957.

95. Morgan V, Pickens D, Gautam S, Kessler R, Mertz H. Amitriptyline reduces rectal pain-related activation of the anterior cingulate cortex in patients with irritable bowel syndrome. Gut 2005; 54(5):601–607.

96. Drossman DA. Diagnosing and treating patients with refractory functional gastrointestinal disorders. Ann Intern Med 1995; 123(9):688–697.

97. Drossman DA, Chang L. Psychosocial factors in the care of patients with GI disorders. In: Yamada T, ed. *Textbook of Gastroenterology*. Lippincott-Raven, Philadelphia, 2003, pp. 636–654.

98. Chang L, Drossman DA. Optimizing patient care: The psychosocial interview in the irritable bowel syndrome. Clin Persp Gastroenterol 2002; 5(6):336–341.

99. Drossman DA. The Physician-Patient Relationship. In: Corazziari E, ed. *Approach to the Patient with Chronic Gastrointestinal Disorders*. Messaggi, Milan, 1999, pp. 133–139.

100. Lipkin MJr, Putnam SM, Lazare A. The Medical Interview: Clinical Care, Education, and Research. 1 ed. Springer-Verlag, New York, 1995, pp. 1–643.

101. Roter DL, Hall JA, Merisca R et al. Effectiveness of interventions to improve patient compliance: a meta-analysis. Med Care 1998; 36(8):1138–1161.

102. Ilnyckyj A, Graff LA, Blanchard JF, Bernstein CN. Therapeutic value of a gastroenterology consultation in irritable bowel syndrome. AlimentPharmacol Ther 2003; 17(7):871–880.

103. Drossman DA, Thompson WG. The irritable bowel syndrome: Review and a graduated, multicomponent treatment approach. Ann Intern Med 1992; 116(12 (Pt 1)): 1009–1016.

104. Torsoli A, Corazziari E. The WTR's, the Delphic Oracle and the Roman Conclaves. Gastroenterol Int 1991; 4:44–45.

105. Milholland AV, Wheeler SG, Heieck JJ. Medical assessment by a delphi group opinion technic. New Engl J Med 1973; 298:1272–1275.

106. Drossman DA. Do the Rome Criteria Stand Up? In: Goebell H, Holtmann G, Talley NJ, eds. *Functional Dyspepsia and Irritable Bowel Syndrome: Concepts and Controversies (Falk Symposium 99)*. 1 ed. Kluwer Academic Publishers, Dordrecht, 1998, pp. 11–18.

107. Whitehead WE. Functional bowel disorders: Are they independent diagnoses? In:

Corazziari E, ed. *NeUroGastroenterology*. 1 ed. Walter de Gruyter, Berlin, 1996, pp. 65–74.

108. Whitehead WE, Bassotti GA, Palsson O et al. Factor analysis of bowel symptoms in U.S. and Italian populations. Dig Liver Dis 2003; 35(11):774–783.

109. Camilleri M, Dubois D, Coulie B et al. Prevalence and Socioeconomic Impact of Upper Gastrointestinal Disorders in the United States: Results of the US Upper Gastrointestinal Study 1. Clin Gastroenterol Hepatol 2005; 3(6):543–552.

110. Müller-Lissner SA, Bollani S, Brummer RJ et al. Epidemiological aspects of irritable bowel syndrome in Europe and North America. Digestion 2001; 64(3):200–204.

111. Saito YA, Schoenfeld P, Locke GR, III. The epidemiology of irritable bowel syndrome in North America: A systematic review. Am J Gastroenterol 2002; 97(8):1910–1915.

112. Wigington WC, Johnson WD, Minocha A. Epidemiology of irritable bowel syndrome among African Americans as compared with whites: A population-based study. Clin Gastroenterol Hepatol 2005; 3:647–653.

113. Gwee KA. Irritable bowel syndrome in developing countries—a disorder of civilization or colonization? 2. Neurogastroenterol Motil 2005; 17(3):317–324.

114. Whitehead WE, Crowell MD, Bosmajian L et al. Existence of irritable bowel syndrome supported by factor analysis of symptoms in two community samples. Gastroenterology 1990; 98:336–340.

115. Manning AP, Thompson WG, Heaton KW, Morris AF. Towards positive diagnosis of the irritable bowel. Br Med J 1978; 2:653–654.

116. Thompson WG, Irvine EJ, Pare P, Ferrazzi S, Rance L. Functional gastrointestinal disorders in Canada: First population-based survey using Rome II criteria with suggestions for improving the questionnaire. Dig Dis Sci 2002; 47(1):225–235.

117. American Psychiatric Association. Diagnostic and Statistical Manual of Mental Disorders—DSM-IV. 4 ed. American Psychiatric Association, Washington, D.C., 1994, pp. 1–886.

118. Schumaker HR, Klippel JH, Robinson DR. Primer on the Rheumatic Diseases. Atlanta, Georgia: Arthritis Foundation; 1988.

119. Bayless TM. Inflammatory bowel disease and irritable bowel syndrome. Med Clin North Am 1990; 49:21–28.

120. Isgar B, Harman M, Kaye MD, Whorwell PJ. Symptoms of irritable bowel syndrome in ulcerative colitis in remission. Gut 1983; 24:190–192.

121. Quigley EMM. Irritable bowel syndrome and inflammatory bowel disease: Interrelated diseases? Chinese Journal of Digestive Diseases 2005; 6:122–132.

Chapter 2

Fundamentals of Neurogastroenterology: Basic Science

Jackie D. Wood

and David Grundy, Co-Chairs

Elie D. Al-Chaer

Qasim Aziz

Stephen M. Collins

Meiyun Ke

Yvette Taché

Introduction

Current topics in neurogastroenterology, as related to functional gastrointestinal disorders (FGIDs), are the focus of this chapter. Neurogastroenterology continues to be an emerging area of scientific and clinical subspecialization that began in the early 1990s. It is a spin-off from neurologically oriented research in the basic medical sciences and advances in the understanding of FGIDs in clinical gastroenterology.

Neurogastroenterology encompasses the investigative sciences dealing with functions, malfunctions, and malformations in the brain and spinal cord and the sympathetic, parasympathetic, and enteric divisions of the autonomic innervation of the musculature, glands, and blood vasculature of the digestive tract. Somatomotor systems are included insofar as pharyngeal phases of swallowing and pelvic floor involvement in defecation and continence are of concern. Psychological and psychiatric relations to gastrointestinal (GI) disorders are significant components of neurogastroenterology, especially in relation to perception of GI-related discomfort and pain. Neurogastroenterology as the descriptor for a specialized sector of gastroenterology has evolved by combining research in the basic medical sciences with the study of the diagnosis and treatment of FGIDs in clinical medicine. Basic neurogastroenterological research integrates physiology, biochemistry, neurobiology, anatomy/histology, endocrinology, microbiology, immunology, and pharmacology into a unified subspecialty focused on the innervation of the digestive system. Clinical gastroenterology translates basic research to the diagnosis and treatment of FGIDs, examples of which are the irritable bowel syndrome (IBS), relations of FGIDs to inflammatory states, functional dyspepsia, and brain-gut relations in physical and emotional stress.

Visceral Pain and Sensation

— Peripheral Sensory Physiology

The GI tract has a rich sensory afferent innervation that mediates reflex control of GI functions including motility, secretion, blood flow, and modulation of immune responses. Both intrinsic (enteric) and extrinsic sensory endings detect mechanical, chemical, and thermal stimuli. In addition, sensory information reaching the CNS from the gut can give rise to both painful and nonpainful sensation and can influence feeding and illness behavior. Sensations from the GI tract tend to be vague and poorly localized; nevertheless, some individuals have heightened visceral sensitivity, which is a hallmark of FGIDs. Whether the hypersensitivity reflects transmission of aberrant sensory signals to the brain, normal signals that are interpreted inappropriately by the brain, or a combination of both is an unresolved question.

Sensory Neurons, AH-Type Neurons, and Intestinofugal Neurons

The enteric nervous system (ENS) contains all the elements necessary for assimilation of information and coordination of motor output. The sensory neurons that initiate enteric reflexes have not been identified unequivocally. A population of multipolar neurons that electrophysiologically are characterized by long-lasting after-hyperpolarization following generation of an action potential (hence the acronym AH neuron) may function as intrinsic primary afferent neurons (IPAN). However, these neurons behave very differently from spinal or vagal sensory afferents described below, which faithfully encode stimulus energy into the firing of action potentials and represent the sensory detector for intramural axon reflexes. (See: section on axon reflexes below.) Instead, variability in excitability of the AH neurons and their synaptic interconnections suggest that they may be multifunctional interneurons and play an important role in determining the output of, as well as the input to, enteric reflex circuits. Other enteric neurons project out from the bowel wall to the prevertebral sympathetic ganglia and are referred to as intestinofugal fibers. These mediate "local" sympathetic reflexes without being directly involved in visceral perception.

Extrinsic afferents from the GI tract consist of vagal and spinal afferents. Vagal afferents have cell bodies in nodose ganglia and projections into the brain stem. Cell bodies of spinal afferents are located in dorsal root ganglia and project to the dorsal horn of the spinal cord and the dorsal column nuclei. Spinal afferents are broadly subdivided into splanchnic and pelvic afferents that follow the path of sympathetic and parasympathetic efferents that project to the gut wall. Somatic afferents that innervate the striated musculature of the pelvic floor project to the sacral spinal cord via the pudendal nerve.

Vagal and spinal afferent fibers are predominantly unmyelinated C-fibers or thinly myelinated A-delta fibers that transmit different modalities of sensory information at low conduction velocity. Broadly speaking, vagal afferents transmit physiological information on the nature and composition of the luminal contents, on the presence or absence of motility, and on contractile tension in the musculature, while spinal afferents convey pathophysiological information related to potentially noxious mechanical or chemical stimuli arising through tissue injury, ischemia, or inflammation. However, there is some overlap in their sensitivity, particularly between vagal and pelvic afferents, and there is also some interplay between the different populations of extrinsic afferents. Nevertheless, patients with spinal cord injury experience little or no sensations of GI origin; whereas conscious perception of sensations is preserved after vagotomy (i.e., a common procedure for treatment of peptic ulcer disease in the 1950s and 60s).

Sensory Endings

Endings of vagal and spinal sensory neurons terminate within the musculature, mucosa, and ganglia of the ENS [1]. Spinal afferents terminate also in the serosa and mesenteric attachments and form a dense network around mesenteric blood vessels and their intramural tributaries. All sensory neurons have at least one generator region where changes in stimulus energy are converted into action potential codes for transmission of information to central processing networks. The frequency and patterning of action potential transmission from the generator region to the central nervous system (CNS) represent coded information that the CNS interprets as stimulus intensity and rate of change of stimulus intensity. The various kinds of sensory endings generate a steady flow of afferent traffic to the CNS that contains information on activity both within and outside the gut wall.

Vagal Afferents

Vagal afferent endings in the mucosa are in close association with the lamina propria adjunct to the mucosal epithelium where they directly monitor the chemical nature of luminal contents, either directly following passage of molecules across the epithelium or indirectly via input from enteroendocrine cells in the epithelium. Enteroendocrine cells, in these cases, respond to luminal content by releasing mediators that diffuse in paracrine fashion to stimulate receptors on the sensory endings.

Vagal afferent endings in the musculature are classified as intramuscular arrays and in the ENS as intraganglionic laminar endings (IGLEs). Intramuscular arrays are distributed within the muscle sheets running parallel to the long axes of the muscle fibers. They appear to make direct contact with the muscle fibers and also form appositions with intramuscular interstitial cells of Cajal, which might have a role in mechanosensory transduction. IGLEs are basket-like structures associated with myenteric ganglia in the ENS. The location of IGLEs between the circular and longitudinal muscle layers exposes them to the shearing forces generated during stretching of the intestinal and contraction of the musculature. IGLEs are low threshold mechanoreceptors. They are also present in the pelvic supply to the rectal musculature. Their location in regions in which graded sensations arise in response to stimulation (e.g., balloon distension) has led to the suggestion that these endings may transmit signals that are interpreted by the brain as nonpainful sensations of fullness. In view of a close association of IGLEs with the chemical microenvironment within myenteric ganglia, IGLEs are suggested to be a site of "cross talk" between the ENS and extrinsic afferents.

Spinal Afferents

Spinal afferents have multiple receptive fields extending over relatively wide areas of bowel. Those in the serosa and mesenteric attachments respond to distortion of the viscera during distension and contraction. Other endings detect changes in the submucosal chemical milieu following injury, ischemia, or infection and may play a role in generating algesic hypersensitivity.

Axon Reflexes

Intramural spinal afferent fibers give off collateral branches that innervate blood vessels and enteric ganglia. These contain and release neurotransmitters during local axon reflexes that influence GI blood flow, motility, and secretory reflexes. Spinal afferents on route to the spinal cord also give off collaterals that innervate neurons in prevertebral sympathetic ganglia. The same sensory information is thereby transmitted to information processing circuits in the spinal cord, ENS, and prevertebral ganglia. The main transmitters are calcitonin gene-related peptide (CGRP) and substance P (SP) and both peptides are implicated in the induction of neurogenic inflammation. A small proportion of vagal afferents express CGRP and SP. Nevertheless, there is little functional evidence for axon reflexes mediated by vagal afferents.

Adequate Stimuli

Gastrointestinal pain is described anecdotally as dull, aching, ill-defined and diffusely localized. Stimuli (e.g., cutting, crushing, and burning) that evoke cutaneous pain are not perceived when applied to the GI tract of conscious subjects. Whereas the adequate stimuli for cutaneous pain are damage or threat of damage, adequate stimuli for visceral discomfort and pain are hollow organ distension and traction on the mesentery. Ischemia and inflammation, which alter the extracellular milieu, stimulates and sensitizes the afferent nerve terminals.

Sensory transduction ultimately depends upon the modulation of ion channels and/or receptors in the membranes of the sensory nerve terminal. Cutaneous and visceral afferents share many of the same channels and receptors; however, their activation is processed differently when it reaches the CNS. GI afferents express transient receptor potential (TRP) proteins. One such protein, TRPV1 (also called VR1) has been well characterized as a heat- (42°C) and pH- (<6.8) sensitive ion channel that is also activated by capsaicin, which is the pungent component of "hot" peppers. TRPV1 is expressed by most GI afferents where protons (i.e., lowered pH) may be the most functionally relevant stimulus. Low pH, which might occur as a consequence of tissue injury, ischemia, or gastroesophageal reflux, potentiates the thermal sensitivity of TRPV1.

Excessive distension and powerful muscle contraction are adequate stimuli for GI mechanosensitive afferents that lead to abdominal pain. Mechanosensitivity can arise indirectly following the release of chemical mediators such as adenosine triphosphate (ATP) that in turn acts on purinergic receptors present on afferent nerve terminals. Alternatively, there may be direct activation via mechanosensitive ion channels in the afferent nerve terminals. Mechanical deformation of the nerve ending leads to the opening or closing of the ion channels, which depolarize the terminal to threshold for action potential firing and transmission of the sensory information to the CNS.

Stimulus-Response Functions

Vagal mechanoreceptors have low distension thresholds of activation as indicated by responses to increases in distending pressures of a few mmHg and maximal firing frequencies occurring within the physiological range of distension. Spinal mechanoreceptors are classified as low-threshold, high-threshold or silent receptors. Low-threshold mechanoreceptors respond to physiological levels of distension and will continue to encode higher levels of distension that cause pain in humans or pain behavior in animals. High-threshold mechanosensitive afferents respond to higher levels of distension that can be considered noxious. Silent nociceptors do not respond at all in the normal intestine, but become responsive to distension when the intestine is injured or inflamed. This kind of receptor behavior illustrates how mechanosensitivity is not fixed either in terms of the threshold for sensory activation or the relationship between stimulus and response. Injury and inflammation decrease the threshold and increase the magnitude of the response for a given stimulus; a phenomenon known as peripheral sensitization. This sensitization underlies the perception of an innocuous stimulus as painful and exaggerates the intensity of pain experienced during a painful stimulus (i.e., hypersensitivity).

Chemotransduction

Chemosensitivity also arises as part of a modality specific mechanism for detecting luminal content (e.g., pH, osmolarity, nutrients, bacterial toxins, etc.). Luminal nutrients, for example, cross the epithelium by various transport mechanisms to reach the afferent nerve terminals in the lamina propria. Prior to absorption, luminal nutrients cause the release of messenger molecules [e.g., cholecystokinin (CCK) and serotonin (5-HT)] from enteroendocrine cells in the mucosa and these molecules in turn act on afferent terminals that lie in close proximity in the lamina propria. Apical tufts of microvilli on enteroendocrine cells project into the intestinal lumen and monitor luminal contents. Release of different mediators into the lamina propria is selective for distinct subpopulations of vagal mucosal afferents. Members of each distinct subpopulation are "labeled lines" for a specific modality as they transmit information to the brain via vagal afferents.

Serotonin acts at 5-HT$_3$ receptors on vagal afferent fibers to signal the brain when threatening agents (e.g., noxious substances or toxins) appear in the lumen. The brain recognizes the threat and programs defensive responses that include nausea and vomiting. Whereas 5-HT action on vagal afferents is related to defense, release of CCK and its action on a subpopulation of vagal afferents plays a pivotal role in the control of food intake and gastric emptying. Several other mediators involved in food intake regulation (e.g., leptins, orexins, and ghrelin) appear to interact with CCK signaling at the level of vagal afferent terminals.

Promiscuous Chemosensitivity

Chemosensitivity is involved in the process leading to peripheral sensitization. Sensitizing mediators are released by a plethora of cell types including platelets, leukocytes, lymphocytes, macrophages, mast cells, glia, fibroblasts, blood vessels, muscle cells, and neurons [2]. Several mediators can be released from a single cell type to either act directly on the sensory nerve terminal or indirectly by stimulating release of agents from other cells in a series of cascades.

A battery of chemical mediators, including biogenic amines, purines, prostanoids, proteases, and cytokines, act in a promiscuous manner on a range of receptors expressed upon any one sensory ending. Three distinct processes are involved in the actions of these substances on visceral afferent nerves. Firstly, by direct activation of receptors coupled to the opening of ion channels present on nerve terminals, the terminals are depolarized and firing of impulses is initiated. Secondly, sensitization develops in the absence of direct stimulation and results in hyperexcitability to both chemical and mechanical modalities. Sensitization may involve postreceptor signal transduction that includes G-protein coupled alterations in second messenger systems, which in turn lead to phosphorylation of membrane receptors and ion channels that control excitability of the afferent endings. Thirdly, genetic changes alter the phenotype of mediators, channels, and receptors expressed by the afferent nerve. For example, a change in the ligand-binding characteristics or coupling efficiency of newly expressed receptors could alter the sensitivity of the afferent terminals. Neurotrophins such as nerve growth factor and glial-derived neurotropic factor influence different populations of visceral afferents and play an important role in adaptive responses to nerve injury and inflammation.

Promiscuous chemosensitivity accounts in part for the plasticity of visceral afferent sensitivity in pathological states. Increased sensitivity of spinal afferents to both mechanical and chemical stimulation might contribute to chronic pain.

Moreover, sensitization may lead to hyper- or dysreflexia because the same sensory neurons trigger reflexes that control and coordinate gut motility, secretion, and blood flow. Peripheral sensitization can occur rapidly and be short-lived because the changes taking place at the level of the sensory nerve terminal are dependent upon release of one or more algesic mediators. However, in the event of sustained tissue injury or inflammatory states, changes in gene expression can occur that prolong peripheral sensitization. Alterations in genes that determine the amount and pattern of neurotransmitters released from the sensory nerve terminals in the spinal cord and the brain result in altered CNS processing of sensory information. Peripheral sensitization integrated with central sensitization of this nature is undoubtedly a significant factor determining the sensations of abdominal pain and discomfort associated with FGIDs.

— The Spinal Cord

After entering the dorsal horn of the spinal cord, visceral afferents terminate in laminae I, II, V, and X [3]. Visceral afferents constitute 10% of all afferent inflow into the spinal cord, which is small considering the large surface area of most visceral organs. Sensory input from the visceral and somatic bodily regions converges at the same neurons in both the dorsal horn and supraspinal centers [3, 4, 5, 6]. Viscero-visceral convergence of sensory information also occurs at second-order spinal neurons. Examples include the convergence of pelvic visceral inputs from colon and rectum, bladder, uterine cervix, and vagina onto the same second-order neurons [3, 7]. Along with the low density of visceral nociceptors and the functional divergence of visceral input within the CNS, viscero-visceral convergence explains the poor localization of visceral pain. Visceral information carried by pelvic afferents converges onto spinal neurons in the lumbosacral segments of the cord and those carried by splanchnic afferents converge onto neurons in thoracolumbar segments [8].

Ascending Spinal Pathways

Ascending spinal pathways involved in the transmission of visceral nociceptive information include the spinothalamic, spinohypothalamic, spinosolitary, spinoreticular, and spinoparabrachial tracts (Figure 1). A pathway in the dorsal columns involving largely postsynaptic neurons is also involved in viscerosensory processing and visceral pain transmission [5, 6, 9–12]. The pain signals are then transmitted via the ipsilateral dorsal column nuclei (i.e., nucleus gracilis and nucleus cuneatus) to the contralateral ventroposterolateral nucleus of the thalamus [4, 5, 13, 14]. This pathway is now considered more important in visceral noci-

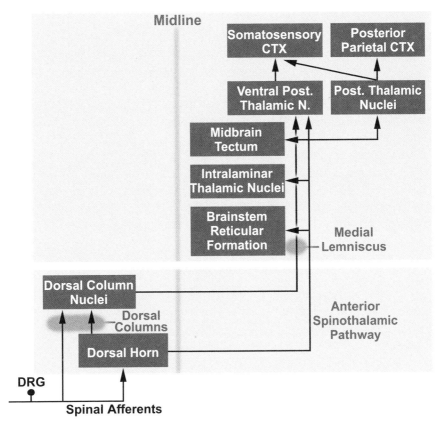

Figure 1. Multiple ascending spinal pathways transmit nociceptive information to processing centers in the brain. CTX = Cortex; N. = Nucleus; Post. = Posterior; DRG = Dorsal Root Ganglion.

ceptive transmission than the spinothalamic and spinoreticular tracts. Moreover, downwardly directed traffic in the dorsal columns may modulate the descending control of visceral nociceptive processing [15, 16].

A midline myelotomy that severs axons in the human posterior columns attenuates otherwise intractable visceral pain [11, 12]. Stimulation of the posterior columns in patients with severe IBS evokes an immediate increase in the intensity of their abdominal pain [17]. These observations in humans are consistent with experimental results in animals. Severing the axons of the dorsal columns in rats or monkeys reduces the neuronal responses to colorectal distension in the ventral posterolateral nucleus of the thalamus and of neurons in the dorsal column nuclei, particularly in the nucleus gracilis [4, 6].

Central Sensitization

Central sensitization is believed to be the neural mechanism underlying secondary hyperalgesia; a phenomenon which describes increased pain sensitivity in regions distant to the site of injury or inflammation. Sensitization occurring within the spinal cord is due to a decrease in neuronal firing threshold, enhanced neuronal responsiveness, and an expansion of spinal neuronal receptive fields [18]. These changes can persist beyond the period of injury or inflammation and be associated with altered bowel function [19]. Glutamate and substance P are the main neurotransmitters in the spinal processing of visceral pain. Alterations of N- methyl-d-aspartate (NMDA) and non-NMDA glutamate receptors and neurokinin receptors are implicated in central sensitization. Central sensitization might explain symptoms of visceral hypersensitivity found in patients with IBS.

Spinal Modulation

The brain contains regulatory circuits that function to modulate the perception of pain. Several modulatory systems within the CNS affect the conscious perception of sensory stimuli, including pain. At the level of the spinal cord, input from nonnociceptive and nociceptive afferent pathways can interact to modulate transmission of nociceptive information to higher brain centers.

Descending Spinal Modulatory Pathways

Spinal visceral nociceptive transmission is subject to descending modulatory influences from supraspinal structures (e.g., periaqueductal gray, nucleus raphe magnus, locus ceruleus, nuclei reticularis gigantocellularis, and the ventrobasal complex of the thalamus). Descending modulation can be inhibitory, facilitatory, or both, depending on the context of the visceral stimulus or the intensity of the descending signal. Serotonergic, noradrenergic and, to a lesser extent, dopaminergic projections are major components of descending modulatory pathways (Figure 2).

The descending influence from the ventromedial medulla is mediated mainly by pathways traveling in the dorsolateral spinal cord [20] and can be inhibitory or facilitatory based on stimulus intensity. In contrast, descending control from the thalamus is context-specific in that it may facilitate or inhibit spinal nociceptive processing depending upon the presence or absence of central sensitization.

Aside from descending inhibitory influences, spinal visceral input is subject to tonically active supraspinal facilitating modulation, which may be a mechanism that enhances conscious perception of visceral sensations in the absence of noxious stimulation. Exaggeration of descending facilitating signals from the brain

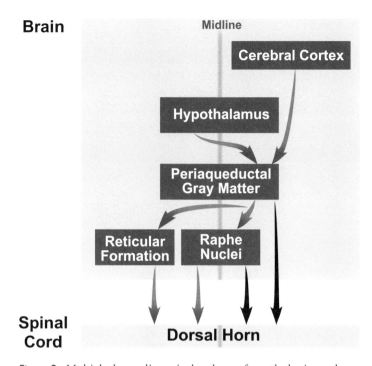

Figure 2. Multiple descending spinal pathways from the brain modulate the transmission of nociceptive signals after they enter the spinal cord.

might also partly explain the visceral hypersensitivity that is found in a subset of IBS patients.

The Representation of Sensation in the Brain

Conscious experience of sensation within the brain is a multifaceted process that involves a complex interaction between sensory-discriminative, affective, and cognitive dimensions. Afferent input passes via the brainstem nuclei and midbrain structures to the cerebral cortex where processing in sensory discriminative areas establish the intensity of sensation and its site of origin in the body. Further processing in limbic structures of the brain allows sensation to be judged in light of current physical and psychological status and memories of similar past experiences. Finally, an emotional response is generated and cognitive judgments are made about coping with the sensation.

Functional brain imaging techniques make it possible to study the complex interaction between a number of cortical and subcortical areas involved in sensory experience. Cortical evoked potentials (CEP) and magnetoencephalography

(MEG) provide temporal resolution in the millisecond time domain and permit study of brain activity in real time, but with limited spatial resolution. The spatial resolution of MEG is far superior to CEP because the magnetic fields, unlike the electrical fields, are not distorted by conduction through the skull. Brain imaging using functional magnetic resonance imaging (fMRI) and positron emission tomography (PET) provide excellent spatial resolution, but poor temporal resolution, which precludes their use for studying neurophysiological characteristics (e.g., conduction velocities) of sensory pathways. Both fMRI and PET rely on measurements of blood flow in cortical and subcortical areas where increased metabolic activity occurs in response to sensory experience. The PET requirement for isotopes makes repeated studies, particularly in clinical situations, less feasible than fMRI. For a review of the pros and cons of using different functional brain imaging techniques, see reference 21.

Studies show that CEPs can be evoked from different regions of the GI tract (e.g., esophagus and rectum) and that the characteristics of the responses from each organ are shaped by their innervation and function (Figure 3). Because earlier clinical studies of visceral sensation relied on subjective methods of grading the stimulus intensity and this had the potential for introducing bias in the interpretation of the responses, visceral sensation can now be studied objectively by examining the effect of increasing stimulus intensity on the amplitude and latency of the components of the CEP waveform. Results obtained in this manner show that as stimulation intensity and sensory perception increases, a corresponding reduction in the latency and increase in amplitude of the CEP occurs (Figure 4). This phenomenon is common across all evoked potential modalities and reflects the recruitment of an increasing number of afferent inputs. A significant value of CEP is the ability to correlate the reported sensation with an objective neurophysiological measure and this reduces the response bias commonly encountered in clinical evaluation of visceral pain.

Viscerocortical Pain Matrix

Application of fMRI and PET techniques has identified a network of brain areas that process some of the sensory information evoking sensations localized to the GI tract. Unlike somatic sensation, which has a strong homuncular representation in the primary somatosensory cortex, visceral sensation is primarily represented in the secondary somatosensory cortex. Representations in the primary somatosensory cortex are vague and diffuse, which might account for visceral sensation being poorly localized in comparison with somatic sensation. Nevertheless, visceral sensation is represented in paralimbic and limbic structures (e.g., anterior insular cortex, amygdala, anterior and posterior cingulate cortex), and prefrontal and orbitofrontal cortices. These are the areas that process the affective and cognitive components of visceral sensation (Figure 5). Systematic

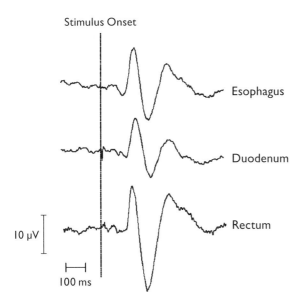

Figure 3. Cortical evoked potentials in response to stimulation of the esophagus, duodenum, or rectum. Despite similarity of waveforms, latencies for each of the potentials differ, with rectally-evoked responses having the shortest latency despite the longest distance separating the site of stimulation and positions of the cortical recording electrodes. Adapted from [218] with permission.

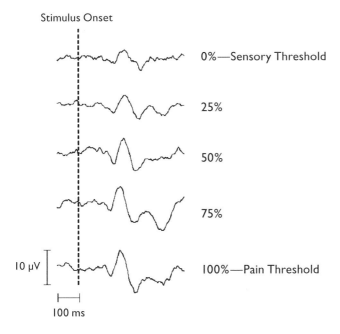

Figure 4. Effects of increasing stimulation intensity on the latency and amplitude of cortical evoked potential from the esophagus. The amplitude progressively increases with a reduction in latency as the stimulus intensity increases. Adapted from [218] with permission.

review of neuroimaging data for visceral sensation suggests that differences also exist in the cortical representation of the upper and lower GI tract, with the primary sensory motor cortex demonstrating more prominent upper gut representation and prefrontal and orbitofrontal cortices demonstrating greater lower gut representation.

Functional brain imaging techniques have also been used to compare the brain processing of visceral and somatic sensation. Direct comparison of brain processing of esophageal and anterior chest wall sensation found that processing for both modalities occurred in a common brain network consisting of secondary somatosensory and parietal cortices, thalamus, basal ganglia, and cerebellum [22]. However, differential processing of sensory information from the two modalities occurred within the insular, primary sensory, motor, anterior cingulate, and prefrontal cortices. This is consistent with knowledge that similarities exist for visceral and somatic pain experience and might also explain the individual's ability to distinguish between the two modalities and generate differential emotional, autonomic, and motor responses when each modality is individually stimulated.

Gender differences in cortical representation of rectal sensation occur among healthy volunteers. While activation in the sensory-motor and parieto-occipital areas is common in men and women, greater activation in the anterior cingulated / prefrontal cortices occurs in women. Moreover, the volume of cortical activity in females was greater than in men at all perception levels. The functional significance of these findings is unclear and will require further study. Nevertheless, the gender differences in the processing of sensory input are reminiscent of reports that perceptual responses are exaggerated in female patients with FGIDs.

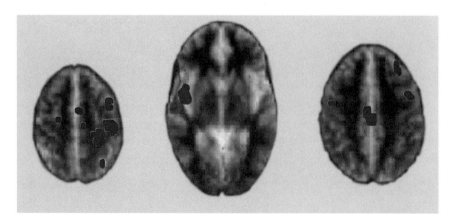

Figure 5. Functional MRI scans showing cortical activation to esophageal distension. (A) Primary and secondary sensory cortices. (B) Insular cortex. (C) Anterior cingulate and prefrontal cortex. The horizontal sections represent different levels of the brain and therefore differ in the size of the cross-section.

Prospective Brain Studies

Brain-imaging research has laid the foundation for future studies in FGID patients that might determine whether sensory dysfunction in these patients is due to disordered sensory detection and transmission in the periphery (e.g., tissue injury or inflammation), aberrant processing of sensory information in the brain, or a combination of peripheral and central factors. The challenge for the future will be to design appropriate studies to identify the dysfunctional sites.

Central Efferent Control of GI Function

— Vagal Innervation

The motor supply to the upper digestive tract is derived from two nuclei in the brainstem [23]. One, the nucleus ambiguus, contains the motor neurons that supply the striated muscle of the upper tract, including esophagus and upper-esophageal sphincter. Parasympathetic neurons supplying the smooth muscles of the upper gut originate in the dorsal motor nucleus of the vagus (DMN), which is a spindle-shaped nucleus extending rostrocaudally through the medulla oblongata on either side of the central canal as it emerges into the 4th ventricle. The DMN is organized anatomically into longitudinal columns of neurons that ultimately give rise to the vagal efferent fibers that supply the various abdominal organs. Vagal motor nerve fibers transmit efferent input to the ENS where they make synaptic contact with the excitatory and inhibitory motor neurons that innervate the musculature of the stomach. Most of the vagal efferents release acetylcholine (ACh) to stimulate nicotinic excitatory receptors on the postsynaptic neurons. Stimulation of vagal efferents evokes a mixture of contraction and relaxation as a consequence of activating parallel pathways to excitatory and inhibitory motor neurons. Contractile responses to vagal stimulation are largely cholinergic and are blocked by drugs that act at muscarinic receptors on the musculature. Vagally-evoked relaxation is mediated by release of nitric oxide, adenosine triphosphate (ATP), and vasoactive intestinal peptide from the inhibitory motor innervation of the musculature.

— Brainstem Reflexes

A diverse array of neurotransmitters is expressed in the synaptic neuropil surrounding the DMN neurons [23]. Brain regions with a prominent input to the DMN include the nucleus tractus solitarius (NTS), medullary raphe nuclei, the paraventricular nucleus of the hypothalamus and the central nucleus of the amygdala. These connections underlie emotional and behavioral influences on vagal outflow to the gut and, in particular, the effects of stress on GI function that involve central mediators, which include thyrotropin-releasing hormone (TRH), corticotropin-releasing factor (CRF) and CCK. (See the section on CRF and stress, later in this chapter.)

Vagal efferent activity is modulated by sensory input from both vagal (via the NTS) and spinal afferents and as such can be augmented or suppressed to initiate reflex responses. Because vagal pathways connect to both excitatory and inhibitory motor neurons in the ENS, these pathways are suggested to be reciprocally controlled such that contraction of the gastric musculature arises from activation of cholinergic pathways and simultaneous inhibition of inhibitory pathways. (See the section on neural control of the gastric reservoir, later in this chapter.) Accordingly, vagally-evoked relaxation of the musculature would involve simultaneous activation of inhibitory pathways and suppression of excitatory pathways. The reflex circuits in the brainstem may therefore be hardwired for reciprocal control with a complex interplay of inhibitory and excitatory synaptic mechanisms.

Gastrointestinal vagal afferents synapse with second order neurons in the NTS. The NTS is composed of various subnuclei of which the subnucleus gelatinosus and the medial and commissural nuclei are the principal targets for gastric afferents, although an afferent projection to the area postrema has also been reported [23]. The projection to the area postrema is associated with input from GI afferents that evoke emesis. Neurons in the NTS project to other nuclei within the brainstem (e.g., DMN) that are involved in the vago-vagal reflex control of gastric function. Additional sensory pathways ascend through the midbrain and reticular nuclei to innervate higher brain centers and, in particular, hypothalamic nuclei involved in mechanisms of satiety and regulation of food intake (Figure 1).

Enteric Nervous System

Fundamentals of Neurogastroenterology in *Rome II* provided a review of the neurophysiology of the ENS that was up-to-date at the time [24, 25]. Advances since *Rome II* appear in subsequent reviews [26–30] and are summarized in brief in this section. Attention to the ENS continues to have central importance for neurogastroenterology and FGIDs because the digestive tract does not work without the integrative functions of the ENS. Normal functioning of the neural networks of the ENS is necessary for effective motility, secretion and blood flow, and coordination of these functions into organized patterns of behavior at the level of the integrated organ system. As expected, malfunctions of integrative ENS control of the gut's effector systems are increasingly recognized as underlying factors in gastrointestinal disorders, especially in the functional gastrointestinal disorders, and therefore become a target for drug therapy [29, 31–34].

— Enteric Neural Signaling

Fundamental mechanisms for chemically mediated signaling in the ENS are the same as elsewhere in the nervous system and may occur in the form of neurocrine (i.e., synaptic transmission), endocrine, or paracrine signals. Transmitters at chemical synapses are released by Ca^{2+}-triggered exocytosis from stores localized in vesicles at axonal terminals or transaxonal varicosities. Release is triggered by the depolarizing action of action potentials when they arrive at the release site and open voltage-activated Ca^{2+} channels. Once released, enteric neurotransmitters bind to their specific postsynaptic receptors to evoke ionotropic or metabotropic synaptic events. When the receptors are directly coupled to the ionic channel, they are classified as "ionotropic." They are "metabotropic" receptors when their effects to open or close ionic channels are indirectly mediated by guanosine triphosphate (GTP)-binding proteins and the induction of cytoplasmic second messengers (e.g., cyclic adenosine monophosphate (AMP), inositol trisphosphate and diacylglycerol) [35].

The kinds of synaptic events in the ENS are basically the same as in the brain and spinal cord. Fast and slow excitatory postsynaptic potentials (EPSPs) and inhibitory postsynaptic potentials (IPSPs) are principal synaptic events in the ENS. An enteric neuron may express mechanisms for both slow and fast synaptic neurotransmission. Fast synaptic potentials have durations in the millisecond range; slow synaptic potentials last for several seconds, minutes or longer. Fast synaptic potential are usually EPSPs. The slow synaptic events may be either EPSPs or IPSPs.

— Fast Excitatory Postsynaptic Potentials (EPSPs)

Fast EPSPs were reported for the earliest intracellular studies of myenteric neurons, but were found only in S-neurons in the early work of Hirst et al. and Nishi and North [36, 37]. Fast EPSPs are rapidly activating depolarizing responses with durations of less than 50 milliseconds. Fast EPSPs were later reported to occur in AH- and S-type neurons in both myenteric and submucosal plexuses [27]. Fast EPSPs appear to be the sole mechanism of transmission between vagal efferents and enteric neurons [38]. Most of the fast EPSPs are mediated by ACh acting at nicotinic postsynaptic receptors. The actions of 5-HT at the 5-HT$_3$ serotonergic receptor subtype and purine nucleotides at P2X purinergic receptors behave much like fast EPSPs and it is possible that some fast EPSPs are purely serotonergic or purinergic or reflect a summation of purinergic and serotonergic input [39–44]. P2X receptors are potential therapeutic targets [45]. Antagonists at 5-HT$_3$ receptors have proved effective in treatment of diarrhea-predominant IBS [46].

Nicotinic Receptors

Different combinations of alpha and beta subunits assemble in different combinations to form nicotinic receptors in general. Functional receptors are formed by five subunits. Eight different alpha subunits (i.e., alpha$_{2-9}$) and nine beta subunits (i.e., beta$_{2-4}$) have been identified. The properties of a specific nicotinic receptor are determined by the kinds of subunits that form the pentameric receptor. The main mediator of nicotinic fast EPSP-like responses in enteric neurons is a receptor composed of apha$_3$ and beta$_4$ subunits [43].

Purinergic Receptors

P2X receptors are trimeric proteins formed by subunits with two transmembrane domains. There are at least seven subtypes of P2X receptors ranging from P2X$_1$ to P2X$_7$. Immunohistochemical studies using specific P2X receptor antibodies found at least three P2X receptor subunits in the ENS that were identified as P2X$_2$, P2X$_3$ and P2X$_7$ [47–50]. The P2X$_2$ receptor is expressed in neurons that express immunoreactivity for the chemical codes of inhibitory musculomotor neurons, noncholinergic secretomotor neurons and calbindin-immunoreactive neurons [49]. Loss of the purinergic component of fast EPSPs in P2X$_2$ knockout mice supports the suggestion that the P2X$_2$ receptor is a major player in purinergic fast transmission in enteric neurons [42]. P2X$_3$ subunits form heteromers with P2X$_2$ subunits in aborally projecting inhibitory musculomotor neurons. Calbindin-immunoreactive enteric neurons do not express P2X$_3$ receptor immunoreactivity [48, 50].

Serotonergic 5-HT$_3$ Receptors

Responses mediated by 5-HT$_3$ receptors are found on neurons in both plexuses throughout the gastrointestinal tract, including the stomach [51]. Neither purinergic nor serotonergic fast EPSPs occur in each and every class of neurons (i.e., based on chemical codes) in the guinea-pig colon and elsewhere [44].

Results obtained with patch clamp recording methods show that both the nicotinic and 5-HT$_3$ serotonergic receptors connect directly to nonselective cationic channels. Opening of these channels is responsible for the depolarizing event [52]. Rapid desensitization, within seconds in vitro, is a characteristic of both the nicotinic and 5-HT$_3$ operated channels, both of which are ionotropic. Purinergic "fast" depolarizing responses, like serotonergic 5-HT$_3$ receptor-mediated responses, reflect opening of ligand-gated nonselective cationic channels [53].

Fast Excitatory Postsynaptic Potentials Rundown

Amplitudes of nicotinic fast EPSPs in the intestine become progressively smaller when they are evoked repetitively by focal electrical stimulation applied to the surface of the ganglion or interganglionic fiber tract in vitro. Decrease in EPSP amplitude occurs at stimulus frequencies as low as 0.1 Hz, and the rate of decline is a direct function of stimulus frequency. Rundown of this nature does not occur at the synapses in the stomach or gallbladder [54–56]. The rundown phenomenon reflects presynaptic inhibition of ACh release by additional transmitter substances broadly released by the electrical stimulus or by negative feedback involving auto-inhibition of ACh release mediated by presynaptic inhibitory muscarinic receptors [57]. Rundown cannot be attributed to postsynaptic changes, because no decrease in the amplitude of the EPSPs occurs during repetitive applications of ACh from microejection pipettes.

Significance of Fast Excitatory Postsynaptic Potentials

The importance of fast EPSPs emerges from their function in the rapid transfer and transformation of neurally coded information between axons and neuronal cell bodies and axons and dendrites that form the enteric neural networks. Fast EPSPs may or may not depolarize the membrane to its threshold for discharge of an action potential. Summation of multiple inputs increases the probability of reaching firing threshold. Fast EPSPs do not reach threshold when the neuronal membranes are hyperpolarized during slow IPSPs. They are most likely to reach spike threshold when the membranes are depolarized during slow EPSPs or depolarizing action of modulators released in paracrine fashion from non-neuronal cells. This effect of slow EPSPs and of slow EPSP-like paracrine mediators is an example of neuromodulation whereby the input-output relationship of a neuron to one input (i.e., fast EPSPs) is modified by a second synaptic or other kind of modulatory input.

— Slow Excitatory Postsynaptic Potentials

Slow EPSP and slow EPSP-like excitation evoked by substances released in endocrine or paracrine fashion are major signaling events in the ENS microcircuitry, where many research advancements have been made. Slow EPSPs in enteric neurons with S-type electrophysiological behavior and uniaxonal morphology differ from neurons with AH-type electrophysiological behavior and multipolar Dogiel Type II morphology [35]. Slow EPSPs in AH-type enteric neurons are associated with slowly activating membrane depolarization, suppression of hyperpolarizing after-potentials, decreased membrane conductance, and elevated excitability. Postreceptor signal transduction in AH neurons involves stimulation of adenylate cyclase and elevation of intraneuronal cyclic AMP. Slow EPSPs in S-type uniaxonal neurons are also slowly activating, depolarizing potentials associated with elevated excitability; however, unlike AH-neurons, membrane conductance either increases or does not change during the EPSP. The postreceptor signal transduction cascade in these neurons involves stimulation of phospholipase C and elevation of intraneuronal Ca^{2+} [35]. Exposure to bradykinin, serine proteases, ATP, CRF or angiotensin II has been reported to mimic slow EPSPs in the ENS, and expanded insight into the signaling role of serotonin has occurred during the time since publication of *Rome II* in 1999 and 2000 [24, 25].

Serotonin

Serotonin is the predominant paracrine mediator expressed by mucosal enterochromaffin cells [58]. Many of the GI responses to 5-HT arise from activation of receptors on enteric neurons and sensory afferent neurons. Several distinct families of receptors mediate the excitatory actions of 5-HT. Metabotropic G protein-coupled receptors of the $5-HT_4$ and $5-HT_{1P}$ subtypes and ionotropic $5-HT_3$ receptors mediate the actions of 5-HT on enteric neurons and sensory afferents. A selective antagonist for the $5-HT_7$ receptor subtype suppresses stimulus-evoked slow EPSPs in the ENS and the slow EPSP-like action of exogenously applied 5-HT [59]. Slow EPSP-like actions of 5-HT were attributed to stimulation of $5-HT_{1P}$ receptors in the past [51, 60–63]. The $5-HT_{1P}$ receptor now appears to be a hetero-oligomeric combination of $5-HT_{1B}$ and dopamine D_2 receptors [64]. Elevated levels of 5-HT in the hepatic portal circulation in the postprandial state reflect stimulated release from mucosal enterochromaffin cells. The postprandial release of 5-HT is reported to be augmented in IBS patients and has been suggested to underlie the IBS symptoms of cramping abdominal pain, diarrhea, and fecal urgency in diarrhea-predominant patients [65]. This observation is reinforced by findings of elevated numbers of enterochromaffin (EC) cells in rectal mucosal biopsies from IBS patients [66].

Application of 5-HT evokes increased firing in extrinsic afferents via $5-HT_3$ receptors that can be blocked by selective antagonists (e.g., alosetron) [67, 68, 69]. Intramural terminals of both spinal and vagal afferents express $5-HT_3$ receptors. Reported efficacy of alosetron in the treatment of abdominal pain and discomfort in the diarrhea-predominant form of IBS in women suggests that these symptoms reflect disordered endogenous release of 5-HT [70]. Similarly, ligands acting at

5-HT_4 receptors might also modulate afferent sensitivity [71] and might contribute to the efficacy of such ligands in constipation-predominant IBS [72].

Serotonergic signaling in the mucosa and the ENS is terminated by a transmembrane 5-HT reuptake transporter called "SERT" (seratonin reuptake transporter) [73]. The mucosal epithelium and enteric neurons express SERT. Mucosal SERT expression is reported to be decreased in experimental inflammation, constipation-predominant IBS, diarrhea-predominant IBS, and ulcerative colitis [72]. Potentiation of the action of 5-HT due to decreased expression of SERT and persistence of 5-HT at its receptors might account for the discomfort and diarrhea in diarrhea-predominant IBS. Symptoms, which are reminiscent of the alternation of diarrhea and constipation in a subgroup of IBS patients, are found in transgenic mice that lack SERT [72].

Genetic polymorphisms in the DNA promotor region for SERT are associated with psychogenic disorders (e.g., depression, schizophrenia, and bipolar disorder) and may underlie expression of one or the other of the IBS phenotypes (constipation, diarrhea, or alternator) [74–76]. Genetic polymorphisms at the SERT promoter appear to influence the response of diarrhea-predominant IBS patients to treatment with a 5-HT_3 receptor antagonist [77].

Bradykinin

Bradykinin (BK) is an established inflammatory mediator derived from proteolytic action on plasma proteins as a result of tissue injury, anoxia, or inflammation. Application of BK evokes slow EPSP-like excitation in AH- and S-type neurons [78–80]. The selective B_2 BK receptor antagonist Hoe 140, but not the selective B_1 receptor antagonist des-arg^{10}-Hoe 140, suppresses responses to BK. Reverse transcriptase-polymerase chain reaction (RT-PCR) and Western blot analysis confirms the existence of B_2 receptor mRNA and protein in guinea-pig myenteric and submucosal plexuses and binding of fluo-HOE 140 (HOE741) reveals that the neurons are endowed with the B_2 receptors and not the B_1 receptor [78]. The mechanism of excitatory action of BK is somewhat unique in that it acts at the neuronal B_2 receptor to stimulate the neuron to synthesize and release prostaglandin E_2, which feeds back and acts at EP_1 receptors to evoke excitation in the same neuron [79]. Prostaglandin feedback accounts for an earlier finding that BK releases ACh from the myenteric plexus by a prostaglandin-mediated mechanism [81]. Exposure to bradykinin also suppresses the amplitude of both stimulus-evoked slow EPSPs and fast nicotinic EPSPs in the ENS.

Serine Proteases and Protease-Activated Receptors

Serine proteases can be released from enteric mast cells to mimic slow EPSPs by stimulating protease-activated receptors (PARs) on the neurons [82–

84]. Application of thrombin, trypsin, or mast cell tryptase evokes slow EPSP-like excitatory responses in AH- and S-type enteric neurons. Synthetic activating peptides for PAR-1, PAR-2 and PAR-4 receptors mimic these actions. The depolarizing responses evoked by a majority of PARs-sensitive uniaxonal enteric neurons express immunoreactivity (IR) for nitric oxide synthase [82]. IR for nitric oxide synthase (i.e., labeled antibodies raised against nitric oxide label the neurons) suggests that these neurons are descending inhibitory motor neurons to the intestinal circular muscle.

Adenosine Triphosphate

Secretomotor neurons with vasoactive intestinal peptide-IR in the submucosal plexus of guinea-pig intestine receive slow EPSP input that is mediated by synaptic release of ATP and its action at $P2Y_1$ receptors expressed by the neurons [85]. MRS2179, a selective $P2Y_1$ purinergic receptor antagonist, blocks both the slow EPSP and mimicry of the EPSP by exogenously-applied ATP. The submucosal secretomotor neurons receive their purinergic excitatory input from neighboring neurons in the same plexus, from neurons in the myenteric plexus, and from sympathetic postganglionic neurons. The ATP-mediated EPSPs occur coincident with fast nicotinic synaptic potentials evoked by projections from both myenteric neurons and other submucosal neurons and with noradrenergic inhibitory postsynaptic potentials (IPSPs) that are evoked by firing of sympathetic fibers that innervated the same neurons.

The $P2Y_1$ receptors on secretomotor neurons are metabotropic receptors that are linked to activation of phospholipase C, synthesis of inositol 1,4,5-trisphosphate, and mobilization of Ca^{2+} from intracellular stores. The purinergic neurons that synapse with and release ATP at postsynaptic $P2Y_1$ receptors on submucosal secretomotor neurons themselves express excitatory serotonergic $5\text{-}HT_3$ receptors that respond to exogenously applied 5-HT and might be stimulated by release of 5-HT from mucosal enterochromaffin cells [85]. Purinergic $P2Y_1$ signaling to secretomotor neurons is currently recognized as an important aspect of the functional regulation of intestinal mucosal secretion [86, 87].

Corticotropin Releasing Factor (CRF)

A later section on mechanisms underlying the impact of stress on intestinal motor, secretory, and immune functions presents evidence from animal models that stimulation of CRF receptors in the brain and ENS is a factor in stress-induced alteration of GI functions and the exacerbation of FGID symptoms in humans [88]. IR for CRF is expressed in both the myenteric and submucosal plexuses of all regions of the large and small intestine and the myenteric plexus of the stomach of the guinea pig [89, 90]. Most of the CRF-IR myenteric neurons have uniaxonal morphology; the remainder have Dogiel Type II multipolar morphology. CRF-IR cell bodies in the myenteric plexus of the ileum express IR for choline acetyltransferase, substance P and nitric oxide synthase. CRF-IR never colocalizes with IR for calbindin, calretinin, neuropeptide Y, serotonin or somatostatin in the myenteric plexus. CRF-IR cell bodies are more abundant in the submucosal plexus than in the myenteric plexus. All CRF-IR neurons in submucosal ganglia express vasoactive intestinal polypeptide (VIP)-IR and are likely to be secretomotor/vasodilator neurons.

Exposure to CRF evokes slowly activating, depolarizing responses associated with elevated excitability in both myenteric and submucosal neurons [89]. Histological analysis of biocytin-filled neurons finds that both uniaxonal neurons with S-type electrophysiological behavior and neurons with AH-type electrophysiological behavior and Dogiel II morphology respond to CRF. The CRF-evoked depolarizing responses are suppressed by the CRF_1/CRF_2 receptor antagonist astressin, and the selective CRF_1 receptor antagonist NBI 27914, and are unaffected by the selective CRF_2 receptor antagonist antisauvagine-30 [89]. RT-PCR reveals expression of mRNA transcripts for the CRF_1 receptor, but not the CRF_2 receptor in both myenteric and submucosal plexuses of guinea pigs. Immunoreactivity for the CRF_1 receptor is distributed widely in the myenteric plexus of the stomach and small and large intestine, and in the submucosal plexus of the small and large intestine. CRF_1 receptor-IR is co-expressed with calbindin, choline acetyltransferase, and substance P in myenteric plexus neurons. In the submucosal plexus, CRF_1 receptor-IR immunoreactivity is found in neurons that express calbindin, substance P, choline acetyltransferase, or neuropeptide Y. The evidence implicates the CRF_1 receptor as the mediator of the excitatory actions of CRF on neurons in the ENS.

CRF-IR neurons do not express IR for the CRF_1 receptor. CRF_1-IR is expressed in neuronal neighbors of those with CRF-IR, which suggests that secretomotor neurons expressing CRF-IR might provide synaptic input to CRF_1 receptors on neighboring cholinergic neurons. A general conclusion is that actions on enteric neurons might underlie the neural mechanisms by which stress-related release of CRF in the periphery alters intestinal propulsive motor function, mucosal secretion, and mucosal barrier function. (See the section on corticotropin-releasing factor and stress, later in this chapter.)

Angiotensin

Two enzymes catalyze the conversion of angiotensin I to angiotensin II (AT-II), which is the biologically active form in the intestine. One of the enzymes, angiotensin-converting enzyme (ACE), is expressed in a variety of tissues and organs, including the brush border of the small intestinal epithelium [91, 92]. Mast cell alpha kinases are a second set of converting enzymes. Alpha-chymase is the major non-ACE producer of AT-II in humans [93, 94]. Release of alpha-chymase accounts for the appearance of AT-II as one of the main products associated with degranulation of mast cells [94]. Significantly elevated levels of AT-II are found in mucosal biopsies from patients with Crohn's colitis, which suggests that elevated levels might be associated with inflammatory states, which include mast cell hyperplasia [95].

The predictable hypertensive action of systemically administered AT-II is well known. Systemic dosing with AT-II evokes vasoconstriction and reduced blood flow in the intestinal mesenteric vasculature in parallel with whole-body hypertension. Elevated vascular resistance and decreased flow in the inferior mesenteric vascular bed leads to ischemic colitis in pigs receiving pathophysiological doses of AT-II [96].

AT-II also alters intestinal absorption of Na^+ and H_2O. Low doses of AT-II (e.g., $0–60$ ngkg^{-1}min^{-1}) stimulate Na^+ and H_2O absorption [97, 98]. Stimulation of absorption is secondary to elevated release of norepinephrine (NE) from intramural sympathetic nerves in concert with suppression of neuronal reuptake of NE [99]. Intracerebroventricular administration of AT-II stimulates descending spinal pathways, which activate sympathetic outflow to the bowel [100].

Inhibitory actions of NE on enteric secretomotor neurons explain the action of AT-II to suppress mucosal secretion and induce an absorptive state. Secretomotor neurons are well recognized as excitatory motor neurons in the submucosal division of the ENS, which innervate the intestinal crypts of Lieberkühn [101]. Firing of secretomotor neurons releases ACh and/or VIP as neurotransmitters at their junctions in the crypts. Secretomotor axons also send collaterals to innervate submucosal arterioles [102–104]. Collateral innervation of the blood vessels links blood flow to secretion by releasing ACh and simultaneously at neuro-epithelial and neurovascular junctions. Once released, ACh acts at the blood vessels to dilate the vessels and increase blood flow in support of stimulated secretion.

Secretomotor neurons have receptors that receive excitatory and inhibitory synaptic input from neurons in the integrative circuitry of the ENS and from sympathetic postganglionic neurons. Activation of the excitatory receptors on secretomotor neurons stimulates the neurons to fire and release their transmitters at the junctions with the crypts and regional blood vessels. The overall result of secretomotor firing is stimulation of the secretion of H_2O, electrolytes, and mucus from the crypts. Elevated firing of secretomotor neurons converts the intestine in situ from an absorptive state to a secretory state with increased liquidity of the luminal contents.

Inhibitory inputs decrease the probability of secretomotor firing. The physiological effect of inhibiting secretomotor activity is suppression of mucosal secretion. Postganglionic neurons of the sympathetic nervous system are one of the important sources of inhibitory input to the secretomotor neurons [105, 106]. Submucosal somatostatinergic neurons are another source of inhibitory input [105]. Norepinephrine released from sympathetic axons acts at alpha$_{2a}$ noradrenergic receptors to inhibit the secretomotor neurons [106]. Inhibition of secretomotor firing reduces the release of excitatory neurotransmitters at the neuro-epithelial junctions. The end result is conversion to an absorptive state with reduced secretion of water and electrolytes. Suppression of secretion in this manner is postulated to be part of the mechanism by which low-dose AT-II stimulates absorption in association with augmented intramural sympathetic nervous activity.

Results of electrophysiological studies in secretomotor neurons suggest that AT-II enhances inhibitory sympathetic noradrenergic neurotransmission to secretomotor neurons and thereby suppresses mucosal secretion [107]. Exposure to AT-II depolarizes the membrane potential and elevates neuronal excitability in small numbers of myenteric neurons (~25%) and submucosal neurons (~32%). On the other hand, hyperpolarizing responses (i.e., inhibitory responses) are evoked by AT-II in nearly one half of the neurons in both plexuses. The hyperpolarizing responses are suppressed by alpha$_2$ noradrenergic receptor antagonists, which suggests that the hyperpolarizing responses reflect stimulation of NE release from sympathetic neurons. Exposure to AT-II enhances the amplitude and prolongs the duration of noradrenergic IPSPs in secretomotor neurons and suppresses the amplitude of both fast and slow EPSPs. The selective AT-II$_1$ receptor (AT$_1$R) antagonists ZD-7115 and losartan, but not a selective AT$_2$R antagonist (PD-123319), suppress the actions of AT-II. Western blot analysis and RT-PCR find expression of AT$_1$R protein and the mRNA transcript for the AT$_1$R in the ENS. No expression of AT$_2$R protein or mRNA can be found in the guinea-pig ENS [107]. AT$_1$R-IR is expressed by a majority of enteric neurons in the gastric antrum and small and large intestines.

The evidence suggests that formation of AT-II might have paracrine-like actions in the ENS, which would include alterations in neuronal excitability and facilitated release of NE from sympathetic postganglionic axons. The enhanced presence of NE is expected to suppress fast and slow excitatory neurotransmission in the enteric microcircuits and to suppress neurogenic mucosal secretion. Hard, dry stools and chronic constipation in some patients might reflect enhanced sympathetic nervous activity and elevated release of NE. In such cases, it might be predicted that treatment with an ACE inhibitor would relieve the constipation.

— Inflammation

Work to understand the actions of inflammatory/immune mediators in the ENS began with histamine in 1975 when exposure to it was found to excite neurons in the myenteric plexus of cat small intestine [108]. Since then, several putative mediators expected to be present in the inflamed bowel, or to be released in response to sensitizing antigens in atopic bowel, have been tested for their electrophysiological actions on neuronal excitability and neurotransmission in the ENS. These include histamine, 5-HT, adenosine, interleukin-1β (IL-1β), interleukin-6 (IL-6), leukotrienes, prostaglandins, nitric oxide, and mast cell proteases, actions of which have been reviewed in detail elsewhere [26]. Most act to mimic slow EPSPs in AH-type enteric neurons, an action that includes membrane depolarization, decreased membrane conductance, elevated excitability, and suppression of hyperpolarizing after-potentials. Moreover, most of the inflammatory/ immune mediators act to suppress fast nicotinic EPSPs and noradrenergic IPSPs. The inflammatory mediators also act to elevate excitability in submucosal secretomotor neurons. The elevation of excitability, which occurs coincident with suppression of noradrenergic IPSPs and removal of sympathetic braking action on secretomotor neurons, undoubtedly underlies the neurogenic secretory diarrhea associated with inflammatory states and responses to allergens.

Animal models for intestinal inflammation, parasitic infection (e.g., *Trichinella spiralis* or *Nippostrongylus brasiliensis*), and food allergy (e.g., milk protein or ovalbumin) have proved useful for translating to the pathological state of the whole bowel the observations that have been obtained with experimental application of inflammatory/immune mediators to single enteric neurons [26, 109–115]. Preparation of the inflammatory models involves rectal injection of agents (e.g., trinitrobenzene sulphonic acid (TNBS), acetic acid, turpentine, or mustard oil) that results in local mucosal inflammation or transmural inflammation depending on the agent used.

Neuronal excitability of single enteric neurons is enhanced during the inflammatory phase of infection with *Trichinella spiralis* as compared with uninfected animals [116, 117]. Decreased resting membrane potentials, increased membrane input resistance, decreased threshold for action potential discharge, and suppression of the amplitude and duration of hyperpolarizing after-potentials occur in AH-type neurons in preparations from infected guinea pigs. The state of augmented excitability in AH neurons, which is found with electrophysiological recording in single neurons, is reflected by increased cytochrome oxidase activity and expression of *c-fos*-IR in the neurons [117]. Excitability in S-type enteric neurons is also elevated in preparations from *T. sprialis*-infected animals as reflected by elevated levels of spontaneous action potential discharge [116].

Mast Cells

Mastocytosis occurs in *T. spiralis* infection and the excitatory effects of application of *T. spiralis* antigens to enteric neurons in preparations from infected guinea pigs in vitro reflect mast cell release of histamine and its excitatory action at histamine H_2 receptors on the neurons [26, 116]. The situation is the same in the small and large intestine of guinea pigs that are sensitized to a food antigen [118, 119]. Exposure to the antigen evokes mast cell release of histamine, which acts at histamine H_2 receptors to elevate neuronal excitability. The overlay of histamine on the neural networks also acts at presynaptic inhibitory histamine H_3 receptors on postganglionic sympathetic nerve terminals to suppress release of norepinephrine [118, 119]. Mast cells in the stomachs from the same animals do not become sensitized to the food antigen (i.e., milk protein) and histamine has no excitatory action on neurons in the gastric myenteric plexus [119].

Human Mast Cells

Mast cells from human intestines appear to behave in a manner similar to that of mast cells in animal models. Mast cells, enzymatically dispersed from human intestines and maintained in culture, can be stimulated to degranulate and simultaneously release multiple mediators by cross-linking of their IgE receptors with an antibody that binds the Fcε α-chain [120]. The culture media, with the released mast cell products, are then centrifuged and stored frozen to await study of effects when applied to enteric neurons. Application of supernatants containing mast cell secretory products to either guinea-pig or human ENS preparations in vitro evokes excitatory responses in single neurons that are reminiscent of the effects of mast cell degranulation in food allergy and animal models for parasitic infection [116–120]. Unlike the findings in animal models, the products of human mast cell degranulation appeared not to suppress fast nicotinic neurotransmission in the ENS preparations as determined by application of imaging technology with voltage-sensitive dyes [120].

Chemically Induced Inflammatory Models

A minor loss of enteric neurons occurs in the animal models with TNBS-induced colitis [109]. Elevated excitability of enteric neurons in this model is a constant finding when electrical and synaptic behavior are recorded with intracellular microelectrodes [109–113]. Hyperexcitability is especially prominent in AH-type neurons in the TNBS guinea-pig model. AH neurons, which generally fire only once or not at all in response to long-lasting depolarizing current pulses in their resting state in the normal intestine, fire repetitively in response to the same depolarizing pulses in the TNBS-inflamed intestine [113]. Elevated excitability in the AH neurons in the TNBS models is associated with shortening of the action potential duration and suppression of the characteristic hyperpolarizing after-spike potentials. Surprisingly, no statistically significant change in either the membrane potential or input resistance of the AH neurons was reported for the TNBS model [111, 113].

Some of the electrophysiological changes in AH neuronal behavior in the TNBS model are essentially the same as the behavior during slow synaptic excitation and the actions of putative paracrine inflammatory mediators (e.g., histamine, prostaglandins, platelet activating factor, etc.) [26]. A "cocktail" of inflammatory mediators is undoubtedly "flooding" the ENS microcircuitry in the TNBS model and can be postulated to account for the observed alterations in neuronal activity. Separate identification of each of the involved mediators remains as a project for the future. Nevertheless, Linden et al. [112] reported that activation of cyclooxygenase and associated prostaglandin production was one of the factors associated with the hyperexcitability in the AH neurons. Prostaglandins are known to evoke slow EPSP-like responses in AH neurons when applied exogenously to freshly dissected preparations in vitro and to mimic the electrophysiological changes found in TNBS colitis when stable analogs are applied over 2-day periods [78, 115, 121].

Whereas fast nicotinic neurotransmission is found to be suppressed by mast cell degranulation during exposure to sensitizing antigens, fast and slow EPSPs are reported to be significantly larger in the TNBS-inflamed colon of guinea pigs [111, 113]. Selective inflammatory mediators in TNBS inflammation might suppress the release of norepinephrine and remove its braking action from the excitatory synapses and thereby account for the enhanced EPSPs. Stimulus-evoked fast EPSPs in submucosal neurons lose some of their sensitivity to blockade by hexamethonium in S-type neurons in the inflamed intestine [111], which could reflect elevation of ACh at nicotinic receptors. Fast EPSPs in the submucosal plexus of the inflamed intestine develop sensitivity to suppression by purinergic P2X and 5-HT$_3$ receptor antagonists that is not readily evident in normal controls. Presynaptic facilitation of neurotransmitter release was proposed as the mechanism underlying augmentation of neurotransmission in the TNBS-inflamed mucosa [111].

Postinfectious IBS

Following an acute bout of infectious enteritis, a significant proportion of patients develop IBS-like symptoms [122–124]. Hypochondriasis and adverse life events are reported to double the risk for development of postinfective IBS [65, 122–124]. Nevertheless, the question of whether the association between acute infectious enteritis and IBS reflects low-level inflammation (e.g., microscopic enteritis) and chronic exposure of the neural and glial elements of the ENS to elevated levels of 5-HT, histamine, or other inflammatory mediators is suggested, but remains to be fully resolved.

— Enteric Glial Cells

Enteric glial cells (EGCs) were until recently a generally overlooked component of the ENS. They are now becoming a focus of increasing attention in neurogastroenterology, especially in terms of mucosal protection, inflammatory responses, and signaling [125].

EGCs express many of the properties of the astroglia in the CNS and represent one of the several criteria often evoked as justification for reference to the ENS as a "brain-in-the-gut." Contrary to past assumptions, accumulating evidence suggests that EGCs are more than passive scaffolding that supports the neurons in ENS ganglia. When positioned outside of the ganglia in the lamina propria, they are associated with submucosal blood vessels and the mucosal epithelium. EGCs form a dense latticework of cells in close apposition to the basal side of the intestinal mucosal epithelium. Current evidence and concepts now interpret the EGCs as being actively involved in the integrated functions of the whole organ [125]. They are believed to be necessary for the structural and functional integrity of the ENS, necessary for maintenance of the mucosal epithelial barrier, and to be participants in inflammatory/immune responses.

Protective Functions

Fulminant and fatal inflammation of the intestine, which is unrelated to bacterial overgrowth, occurs in transgenic mouse models after ablation of their EGCs [126]. The earliest pathological sign in the mice is a submucosal vasculitis followed by inflammatory disruption of the mucosa. These observations were among the first to implicate EGCs in regulation of permeability of the vascular endothelium and the mucosal epithelium. Recent findings suggest that EGCs are important factors in the maintenance of the integrity of epithelial tight junctions and their role in establishing mucosal barrier function [127, 128]. Perturbation of EGCs in animal models in vivo results in increases in paracellular permeability of the mucosal epithelium and changes in the expression of synthetic enzymes for neurotransmitters in enteric neurons (e.g., nitric oxide synthase and choline acetyltransferase). Inclusion of EGCs in cocultures with intestinal epithelial cells (i.e., Caco-2, HT29 or IEC-6 cells) increases electrical resistance as the epithelial cells become confluent in monolayers, which is indicative of sealing of "tight" epithelial cell junctions and tightening of the "epithelial barrier" to movement of larger molecules. EGCs also exert strong antiproliferative effects on the various epithelial cell lines in culture and this is dependent on secretion of transforming growth factor (TGF)-β1. The presence of EGCs after 2 days in coculture with the Caco-2 epithelial cell line significantly increases the surface area of the monolayers in the absence of Caco-2 cellular hypertrophy or mitosis.

The influence of EGCs on the formation of an epithelial barrier appears to provide protection against transepithelial invasion by pathogens. In in vitro coculture models, the presence of EGCs decreases crossing of the epithelial barrier by *Shigella flexneri* and also suppresses the inflammatory response to this organism [128].

Results obtained from studies in which EGCs are cocultured with enteric neurons suggest that the EGCs protect the neurons against neurodegeneration under inflammatory conditions (e.g., elevation of nitric oxide). Cytokine signals involving EGCs are central events underlying the inflammation. Selective activation of EGCs by proinflammatory cytokines reflects their role in intestinal inflammation [129, 130]. Exposure to proinflammatory cytokines activates *c-fos* expression in EGCs in vitro and *c-fos* expression is known to be up-regulated in intestinal inflammation induced by intramural injection of formalin in rat colons [131]. Exposure of EGCs in purified primary cultures to IL-1β stimulates the synthesis and release of IL-6. This action of IL-1β is at IL-1 receptors that are expressed by the EGCs [132]. At the level of the ENS, IL-1β and IL-6 act synergistically both to excite submucosal secretomotor neurons and to suppress the braking action of norepinephrine release from sympathetic postganglionic terminals in submucosal ganglia [132–134].

Signaling in Glial Networks

EGCs are linked one to another into networks by gap junctions that conduct ions and larger organic molecules [135]. Mechanical or chemical stimulation of a single glial cell in an EGC network in culture evokes a wave of Ca^{2+} release that travels from cell to cell throughout the network [136]. The propagation of the Ca^{2+} waves in the EGC networks appears as the same phenomenon in CNS astroglia in culture [137] and is reminiscent of the transmission of impulses in nerve fibers.

Like the networks of astroglia in the CNS, neurocrine, endocrine, or paracrine signaling to the ECG networks is suggested by the expression of receptors for a number of known signal molecules. ECG networks respond to ATP, UTP, 5-HT, histamine, and bradykinin [138]. Like ENS neurons, ECG networks also express the protease-activated receptors, PAR-1 and PAR-2, and can respond to mast cell proteases with propagating Ca^{2+} waves [82, 83, 139]. Application of endothelin to ECG networks likewise stimulates endothelin B receptors to evoke elevation of intracellular Ca^{2+}. The dynamics of Ca^{2+} homeostasis in this case involves release from intracellular stores followed by capacitative Ca^{2+} entry into the cells from the extracellular milieu [140].

Gastrointestinal Neuromotor Control

The musculature of the stomach and small and large intestine is unitary-type smooth muscle. Unitary-type smooth muscles contract spontaneously in the absence of neural or endocrine influence and contract in response to stretch. There are no structured neuromuscular junctions, and neurotransmitters diffuse over extended distances to influence relatively large numbers of muscle fibers. The muscle fibers in unitary-type smooth muscles are connected to their neighbors by gap junctions [141]. Gap junctions are permeable to ions and thereby transmit electrical current from muscle fiber to muscle fiber and account for the spread of slow waves and accompanying myogenic contractions from points of initiation (e.g., pacemaker regions) in three dimensions throughout the smooth muscle syncytium [142].

Networks of specialized pacemaker cells, called interstitial cells of Cajal (ICCs), are associated with the gastric and intestinal musculature [143, 144]. Pacemaker potentials, also called electrical slow waves, originate in the ICC networks and appear as rhythmic oscillations consisting of depolarization and repolarization phases. Gap junctions connect the ICC networks to the bulk musculature. During the depolarizing phase of each slow wave in the ICC network, electrical current flows across the gap junctions to depolarize the membrane potential of the muscle fibers to their threshold for action potential discharge, which in turn triggers contraction. ICCs also function as relays for transmission from enteric motor neurons to the GI musculature. Images obtained from histological studies show ICCs interposed between excitatory and inhibitory motor nerve axons and muscle fibers in both stomach and intestine [144, 145]. Mutant mice with malformed ICC networks have impaired neuromuscular transmission [146]. Abnormal ICCs have been reported to occur in achalasia of the lower esophageal sphincter and cardia, infantile hypertrophic pyloric stenosis, chronic intestinal pseudo-obstruction, Hirschsprung's disease, inflammatory bowel diseases, and slow-transit constipation [147].

— Neural Control of Gastric Motility

Functionally, the stomach is divided into a proximal reservoir and a distal antral pump. The reservoir incorporates the anatomically defined fundus and proximal corpus; the antral pump includes the caudal corpus, the antrum, and the pylorus. Differences in motility between the reservoir and antral pump reflect their different functions. The musculature of the reservoir is specialized for maintaining continuous contractile tone (tonic contraction) and relaxes to accommodate increases in volume during gastric filling. Phasic contractions generated by the musculature of the antrum pump, mix, grind, and propel the gastric contents toward the gastroduodenal junction.

Neural Control of the Antral Pump

Gastric action potentials that originate in a dominant pacemaker region located in the corpus distal to the midregion evoke the phasic contractions of the antral pump. The gastric action potential lasts for 5–10 s and has a rising depolarization phase, a plateau phase, and a falling repolarization phase. The amplitude of the plateau phase is neurally controlled to determine the strength of antral pump contractions [148]. The pacemaker continuously generates gastric action potentials; nevertheless, a propagating contraction occurs only when the plateau phase is above a threshold voltage, which in turn is dependent upon the balance of excitatory and inhibitory transmitters released by enteric motor neurons. From its site of origin, the action potential propagates rapidly around the gastric circumference and triggers a ring-like contraction. The action potential and associated ring-like contraction then travel more slowly to the gastroduodenal junction [149]. When the rising phase reaches the terminal antrum and spreads into the pylorus, contraction of the pyloric muscle closes the partition between the stomach and duodenum. The following contraction forces gastric contents into an antral compartment of ever-decreasing volume and progressively increasing pressure. This results in jet-like retropulsion through the orifice formed by the trailing contraction. Trituration and reduction in particle size occur as the material is forcibly retropulsed through the advancing orifice and back into the gastric reservoir to wait for the next propulsive cycle. Repetition at 3 cycles per min in humans reduces particle size to the 1–7 mm range that is necessary before a particle can be emptied into the duodenum. Dysrhythmia of electrical and contractile behavior in the antral pump is associated with nausea and vomiting, delayed gastric emptying, and gastroparesis.

Neural Control of the Gastric Reservoir

The gastric reservoir has two primary functions. One accommodates the arrival of a meal without a significant increase in intragastric pressure and intramural tension. Failure of accommodation underlies the uncomfortable sensations of early satiety, bloating, epigastric pain, and nausea. (See Chapter 7.) The second function is constant compression of the contents of the reservoir, which forces the contents into the antral pump.

The musculature of the gastric reservoir is innervated by enteric excitatory and inhibitory motor neurons [23]. Vagal efferent nerves and intramural enteric neural networks control the firing frequencies of the motor neurons. Increased activity of excitatory motor neurons coordinated with decreased activity of inhibitory motor neurons results in increased contractile tone in the reservoir, a decrease in its volume, and an increase in intraluminal pressure. Increased activity of inhibitory motor neurons in coordination with decreased activity of excitatory motor neurons results in decreased contractile tone in the reservoir, expansion of its volume, and a decrease in intraluminal pressure. Inhibitory motor neurons in the gastric reservoir express the $5\text{-}HT_1$ receptor, which when activated, stimulate neuronal firing and release of inhibitory neurotransmitters that relax the musculature of the reservoir [51]. Stimulation of the 5-HT$_1$ receptors on inhibitory motor neurons by sumatriptan has reported efficacy in treatment of dyspeptic symptoms of early postprandial fullness and satiety [150]. Animal studies also suggest that the 5-HT receptor on gastric inhibitory motor neurons might be the 5-HT$_1$ subtype [151].

Gastric Reservoir Relaxation

Neurally mediated decreases in tonic contracture of the musculature are responsible for relaxation in the gastric reservoir (i.e., increased volume). Three kinds of relaxation are recognized: (1) *Receptive relaxation* is initiated by the act of swallowing. It is a reflex triggered by stimulation of mechanoreceptors in the pharynx followed by transmission over afferents to the dorsal vagal complex (i.e., the nucleus tractus solitarius and dorsal motor nucleus of the vagus) and subsequent activation of efferent vagal fibers to inhibitory motor neurons in the gastric ENS. (2) *Adaptive relaxation* is triggered by distension of the gastric reservoir. It is a vago-vagal reflex triggered by stretch receptors in the gastric wall, transmission over vagal afferents to the dorsal vagal complex, and efferent vagal fibers to inhibitory motor neurons in the gastric ENS. (3) *Feedback relaxation* is evoked by the presence of nutrients in the small intestine and is mediated by both vagal and enteric reflexes triggered by paracrine signaling actions of CCK and/or 5-HT on vagal afferent terminals [152]. Adaptive relaxation is impaired in patients who have suffered iatrogenic injury to the vagus nerves during procedures such as laparoscopic fundoplication surgery. The loss of adaptive relaxation following vagal injury is associated with a lowered threshold for sensations of fullness and pain during gastric filling. Increased sensitivity to gastric distension in these cases may be explained by enhanced stimulation of the spinal mechanoreceptors that sense distension of the gastric wall. (See the section on visceral pain and sensation at the beginning of this chapter.) Descending influences from higher brain regions modulate vago-vagal transmission and account for emotional and behavioral influences on gastric function, for example during stress. These influences can extend throughout the GI tract.

— Neural Control of Small Intestinal Motility

Four fundamental patterns of small intestinal motility are the interdigestive migrating motor complex (MMC) pattern, the postprandial pattern of mixing movements, power propulsion, and neurally programmed musculomotor quiescence (sometimes called physiological ileus). The integrative microcircuitry of the ENS contains the programs for each of these patterns.

Migrating Motor Complex

The MMC is a specific pattern of motor activity in the stomach and small intestine during fasting in most mammalian species, including humans [153]. The MMC continues in the small intestine after a vagotomy or sympathectomy, but stops when it reaches a region of the intestine where the ENS has been interrupted [154]. Presumably, command signals to the enteric neural circuits are necessary for initiating the MMC. The relative contributions of neural and hormonal (e.g., the hormone motilin) mechanisms as command signals remain to be determined. Levels of the hormone motilin reach a peak in the plasma coincident with the onset of the MMC in the antrum [155].

Gallbladder contraction and delivery of bile into the duodenum are coordinated with the onset of the MMC in the antroduodenal region [156]. As bile enters the duodenum, the activity front of the MMC propels it to the terminal ileum, where it is reabsorbed into the hepatic portal circulation. This mechanism minimizes the accumulation of concentrated bile in the gallbladder and increases the movement of bile acids in the enterohepatic circulation during the interdigestive state.

The adaptive significance of the MMC appears also to be a mechanism for clearing indigestible debris from the intestinal lumen during the fasting state. Large indigestible particles are emptied from the stomach only during the interdigestive state.

Bacterial overgrowth in the small intestine is associated with absence of the MMC [157, 158]. This condition suggests that the MMC may play a "housekeeper" role in preventing the overgrowth of microorganisms that might occur in the small intestine if the contents were allowed to stagnate in the lumen. Small intestinal bacterial overgrowth was recently proposed as the underlying pathophysiology of IBS symptoms [159, 160].

Postprandial Pattern

A mixing pattern of motility (segmentation) replaces the MMC when the small intestine is in the digestive state following ingestion of a meal [161]. Volume and caloric content of the meal determines the duration of the postprandial motility pattern. Lipids, particularly medium-chain triglycerides, are most effective in suppressing the neural program for the MMC and calling up the program for the segmentation pattern of the digestive state [162]. During the postprandial pattern, peristaltic contractions, which propagate for only very short distances, account for the segmental appearance of the bowel on X-ray film. Signals transmitted from the brain stem by vagal efferent nerves to the ENS interrupt the MMC and initiate the neural mixing program during ingestion of a meal. Interruption of the MMC by a meal does not occur in extrinsically denervated segments of small intestine in dog models [163]. Blockade of vagal nerve conduction prevents the conversion from the interdigestive to the postprandial motility state in all regions of extrinsically innervated small intestine [164, 165].

Power Propulsion

The power propulsion motor pattern is relevant for understanding the symptoms of cramping abdominal pain, diarrhea, and fecal urgency in infectious enteritis, inflammatory bowel disease, radiation-induced enteritis, and functional GI disorders. It is peristaltic propulsion characterized by strong, long-lasting contractions of the circular muscle that propagate for extended distances along the small and large intestine. The circular muscle contractions during power propulsion are sometimes referred to as "giant migrating contractions" because they are considerably stronger than the phasic contractions during the MMC or mixing pattern [166]. Giant migrating contractions last 18 to 20 s and span several cycles of the electrical slow waves. They are a component of a highly efficient propulsive mechanism that rapidly strips the lumen clean as it travels rapidly over long lengths of bowel.

Power propulsion occurs in the retrograde direction during emesis in the small intestine and in the orthograde direction in response to noxious stimulation in both the small and the large intestine. Abdominal cramping pain sensations and sometimes diarrhea are associated with this motor pattern [167]. Application of irritants to the mucosa, the introduction of luminal parasites, enterotoxins from pathogenic bacteria, allergic reactions, and exposure to ionizing radiation each activates the powerful propulsive motor program. These characteristics suggest that power propulsion is a defensive adaptation for rapid clearance of noxious or threatening contents from the intestinal lumen. It also accomplishes mass movement of intraluminal contents in normal states, especially in the large intestine.

— Neural Control of Large Intestinal Motility

The large intestine is subdivided into functionally distinct regions that correspond approximately to the ascending colon, transverse colon, descending colon, rectosigmoid region, and internal anal sphincter. The transit of small radio opaque markers through the large intestine occurs in 36 to 48 h, on average with the remnants of several meals ingested over 3- to 4-day periods being intermixed and eliminated together in the stool.

Ascending Colon

Neuromuscular mechanisms analogous to adaptive relaxation in the gastric reservoir permit cecal filling without excessive increases in intraluminal pressure. After instillation of radio-labeled chyme into the cecum in humans, half of the instilled volume empties in <90 min. This suggests that the ascending colon is not the primary site for the large intestinal functions of storage, mixing, and removal of water from the feces. The motor patterns of the ascending colon consist of orthograde or retrograde peristaltic propulsion. The significance of backward propulsion in this region is uncertain; it may be a mechanism for temporary retention of the chyme in the ascending colon. Forward propulsion in the ascending colon might be controlled by feedback signals on the fullness of the transverse colon.

Transverse Colon

Radioscintigraphic markers are retained in the transverse colon for about 24 h, which suggests that this is the primary location for the removal of water and electrolytes from the feces [168]. The ENS programs a segmentation pattern of motility that accounts for the ultraslow forward movement of feces in the transverse colon. Ringlike contractions of the circular muscle divide the colon into pockets called haustra that repeat uniformly along the colon. Formation of each contracting and receiving haustral segment no doubt reflects operation of the fundamental peristaltic polysynaptic reflex circuit with the timing, spacing, and migration of the haustra programmed at higher levels of the hierarchy of enteric neural network control [169]. Haustrations are dynamic in that they form and reform at different sites. The most common pattern in the fasting individual is for the contracting segment to propel the contents in both directions into receiving segments. This mechanism mixes and compresses the semiliquid feces in the haustral pockets and probably facilitates the absorption of water with minimal net forward propulsion. Precisely how the ENS programs the dynamics of haustral behavior remains one of the intriguing aspects of enteric neurobiology.

Net forward propulsion occurs when sequential migration of the haustra occurs along a length of bowel. The contents of one haustral pocket are propelled into the next region, forming a second pocket, and from there to the next segment, where the same events occur. This pattern results in slow forward progression and may reflect a mechanism for compression of the stored feces.

Power propulsion is another of the programmed motor events in the transverse and descending colon. This motor pattern transiently replaces haustral programming and fits the general pattern of neurally coordinated peristaltic propulsion [166, 169]. Operation of the power propulsion program results in the mass movement of feces over long distances. Mass movements may be triggered by increased delivery of ileal chyme into the ascending colon following a meal. The increased incidence of mass movements and generalized increase in segmental movements following a meal is called the gastrocolic reflex. Irritant laxatives (e.g., castor oil or senna) act to initiate the motor program for a more robust form of power propulsion in the colon that can be accompanied by cramping lower abdominal pain. The presence of threatening agents in the colonic lumen, such as parasites, enterotoxins, and food antigens, also initiate this kind of power propulsion [26]. Haustration returns in the normal bowel after the passage of the power contraction and associated mass movement reaches the rectosigmoid region. In contrast, in the colon of patients with ulcerative colitis, power propulsion associated with cramping pain occurs at repetitive intervals and haustrations are absent [170].

Descending Colon and Rectosigmoid Regions

Propagation of power propulsion from the transverse colon to the descending colon is responsible for mass movements of feces into the sigmoid colon and rectum. The sigmoid colon and rectum are reservoirs with a capacity of up to 500 ml in humans. Distensibility in this region is an adaptation for temporarily accommodating the mass movements of feces from above. The rectum begins at the level of the third sacral vertebra and follows the curvature of the sacrum and coccyx for its entire length. It connects to the anal canal, which is surrounded by the internal and external anal sphincters (Figure 6.)

Innervation of the Anorectum and Pelvic Floor

Mechanoreceptors in the rectum detect distension and transmit the coded information to the neural networks of the ENS and spinal cord on a moment-to-moment basis. Sensory innervation of the anal canal and perianal skin differ from the rectum in that somatosensory nerves transmit multiple modalities of sensory information from these areas to interneuronal processing circuitry in sacral segments of the spinal cord and in the brain. (See the section on representation of sensation in the brain, earlier in this chapter.) Sensory receptors detect touch, pain, and temperature with high sensitivity in the anal canal and at the anal verge. Processing of information from these receptors in the spinal cord and higher brain centers allows the individual to discriminate consciously between the presence of gas, liquid, and solids in the anal canal.

Mechanoreceptors in the muscles of the pelvic floor detect changes in the orientation of the anorectum as feces are propelled into the region and transmit the information to the CNS for processing that leads to conscious awareness of a threat to continence and an urge to defecate. Signals to the brain from mechanoreceptors in the pelvic floor musculature provide the first conscious warning of the arrival of stool in the rectum. The sensory mechanisms associated with the pelvic floor musculature account for the ability of an individual to experience the movement of feces in the anal canal and maintain fecal continence after surgical resection of the rectosigmoid region (e.g., surgical correction for Hirschsprung's disease). Sensory mechanisms in the rectum differ from the anal canal and perianal skin in that de-

A Pelvic Floor Musculature

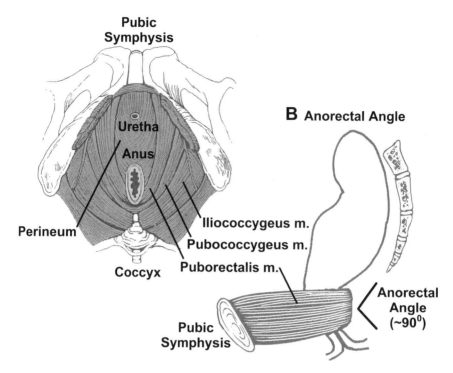

B Anorectal Angle

Figure 6. The musculature of the pelvic floor maintains fecal continence. (A) Pelvic floor muscle groups. The levator ani muscles form the floor of the pelvis and are divided into pubococcygeus and iliococcygeus muscles. Both muscles arise from anterior regions of the pelvis. The iliococcygeus inserts into the coccyx. Divisions of the pubococcygeus from either side join to form the puborectalis. The puborectalis forms a loop around the rectum that becomes important in the maintenance of the anorectal angle and fecal continence. (B) Tonic contraction of the puborectalis muscle in conditions of rest closes the distal rectum and works in conjunction with the anal sphincters in the maintenance of continence. Contractile tension in the puborectalis is relaxed during defecation. Contraction of the puborectalis muscle forms an anorectal angle of approximately 90°, which opens to a more obtuse angle of about 120° when muscle tension is relaxed during defecation.

tection of distension is the primary stimulus parameter. Ability of patients to experience generally satisfactory defecation and continence after colectomy and surgical construction of an ileo-anal pouch suggests that the presence of rectal sensory function is unnecessary for defecation or continence.

Overlapping sheets of skeletal muscle termed the *levator ani* form the pelvic floor. The levator ani muscles include the pubo, ilio, and ischiococcygeus. They work in concert with the puborectalis and the external anal sphincter as components of a functioning unit necessary for the maintenance of fecal continence and normal defecation. The pelvic floor musculature exhibits physiological and histological properties like those of the tonic somatic muscles that maintain upright bodily posture against the forces of gravity [171–173]. Weakening of the pelvic floor musculature (e.g., in advanced age) or traumatic damage to the musculature or its innervation (e.g., during childbirth) can underlie fecal incontinence and disordered defecation [174]. Like other skeletal muscles, weakening of the pelvic floor musculature can often be corrected through targeted isometric exercise [175].

The puborectalis sling and the upper margins of the internal and external sphincters form the anorectal ring, which marks the boundary of the anal canal and rectum. Surrounding the anal canal over a length of about 2 cm are the internal and external anal sphincters. The external anal sphincter is skeletal muscle attached to the coccyx posteriorly and the perineum anteriorly. When contracted, it compresses the anus into a slit, thereby closing the orifice. The internal anal sphincter is a modified extension of the circular muscle coat of the rectum. It is comprised of fatigue-resistant smooth muscle that, like other sphincteric muscles in the digestive tract, contracts tonically to sustain closure of the anal canal. Timed activation of the inhibitory innervation relaxes muscle tension and transiently opens the sphincter to permit forward passage of luminal contents. Sphincteric achalasia occurs when enteric inhibitory motor neurons to the sphincter are lost or fail to function (e.g., Hirschsprung's disease).

Rectoanal Reflex

Tonic contraction of the internal anal sphincter and the puborectalis muscle blocks the passage of feces into the anal canal and maintains continence with small volumes in the rectum. Rapid influx of feces and consequent distension of the rectum activates the rectoanal reflex, which relaxes the internal sphincter and simultaneously contracts the external sphincter. Like other enteric reflexes, the rectoanal reflex involves stimulation of distension receptors in the rectal wall and processing of the sensory information by neural networks in the ENS and spinal cord. Processing in the ENS leads to reflex excitation of inhibitory motor neurons to relax tension in the smooth muscle of the internal anal sphincter. Processing in the spinal cord leads to excitation of spinal motor neurons to contract the external anal sphincter. Conscious sensation of rectal fullness in the lower abdomen is experienced as the rectum fills and reflects CNS processing of information from the mechanoreceptors in the pelvic floor musculature. Sensory physiology of afferents from the pelvic floor differs significantly from splanchnic afferents [176, 177]. Pelvic mechanosensitive afferents respond to lower stimulus intensities, have larger response magnitudes, and adapt less completely to sustained stimulation. Pelvic floor afferents also differ from intestinal afferents by having a lack of sensitivity to application of inflammatory mediators. Most intestinal afferents are stimulated by application of bradykinin or ATP, while pelvic floor afferents are resistant to these agents as well as to stimulation by capsaicin.

Relaxation of the internal anal sphincter allows contact of the rectal contents with the sensory receptors in the lining of the anal canal. Sensory signals that reach the brain from the anal canal serve as an early warning of the possibility of a breakdown of maintenance of continence. Continence in this situation is maintained by involuntary reflex contraction of the external anal sphincter and puborectalis muscle and by conscious voluntary effort to contract the same muscles. The external sphincter closes the anal canal and the puborectalis sharpens the anorectal angle to form a mechanical barrier to onward movement of the feces.

Power propulsion in diarrheal states (e.g., diarrhea-predominant IBS or infectious enteritis) moves large volumes of liquid stool with high velocity into the rectum with potential for overwhelming the mechanisms of continence and the embarrassment of soiling [167, 178]. Sensory detection of rectal distension by rapid influx of large volumes of liquid stool, transmission to the spinal cord, and supraspinal processing of the information underlie the sensations of fecal urgency and fear of an accident in diarrheal states.

Spinal Motor Control

Individual pools of motor neurons in the sacral spinal cord innervate the levator ani, puborectalis, and external anal sphincter muscle groups. A pool of small motor neurons in the ventral horn of the sacral spinal cord at S2, named *Onuf's nucleus*, project their axons in the pudendal nerve. Branches of the pudendal nerve directly innervate the external anal sphincter in humans. Branches of sacral nerves 3 and 4 that do not project in the pudendal nerve innervate the puborectalis [171, 172]. Nerves projecting from one side of the sacrum innervate the puborectalis muscle only on the same side [179]. Due to their separate innervation, interference with pudendal nerve conduction does not alter voluntary contraction of the puborectalis, but abolishes voluntary and reflex contraction of the external anal sphincter.

The external anal sphincter, puborectalis, and levator ani are each innervated by distinct pools of spinal motor neurons, which suggests that each of these muscles is a functionally distinct entity that can be controlled independently by the integrative circuitry in the spinal cord. The external anal sphincter is stimulated to maintain tone by low-frequency spontaneous firing in its motor innervation that continues in awake and sleeping humans. Muscle spindles are present in the external anal sphincter and puborectalis muscle of animals and humans. However, their role in the generation of the tonic motor input to the muscle is not understood. The tonic motor input to the external sphincter is abolished experimentally by eliminating the sensory input to the cord following bilateral transection of the spinal dorsal roots. This underlies the unproven suggestion that gamma motor input to muscle spindles in the external anal sphincter might be part of the spinal reflex loop that maintains contractile tone in the sphincter. Supraspinal pathways in addition to spinal reflexes undoubtedly come into play in the neural control of the external anal sphincter as reflected by individual ability to voluntarily initiate sphincteric "squeeze."

Supraspinal Motor Control

Descending spinal pathways transmit the commands from the brain for voluntary contraction of the external anal sphincter and puborectalis muscle. Descending pathways provide monosynaptic excitatory synaptic input and polysynaptic inhibitory input to the spinal motor neurons in Onuf's nucleus that innervate the external sphincter. The ventromedial reticulospinal tract transmits the excitatory input and the ventrolateral reticulospinal tract carries the inhibitory signals to the motor neurons. Contraction of the external anal sphincter occurs in response to rectal distension in both normal and paraplegic subjects. Nevertheless, normal subjects have a significantly lower threshold for evoking the reflex than paraplegics. Enhancement of the reflex in normal subjects is postulated to reflect a descending excitatory influence from the brain [180]. In young children, voluntary control of the external sphincter is undeveloped, and rectal distension evokes relaxation in the sphincter. When the children advance to an age where they gain voluntary control of the sphincter, rectal distension evokes a brief contraction of the sphincter similar to what is found in adults. The changes in the distension reflex as the child matures are attributed to myelinization of the spinal pyramidal tracts [181].

Suprasegmental input to the reflex circuitry in the sacral spinal cord determines both the amplitude of sensory evoked spinal reflexes and the kind of reflex response that occurs. For example, voluntary straining evokes relaxation of the external anal sphincter and the puborectalis sling. On the other hand, increases in abdominal pressure during coughing or heavy lifting evoke an increase in the contractile activity of the two muscles [182].

Voluntary straining to defecate normally evokes relaxation of tension in the puborectalis sling. Paradoxical contraction of the puborectalis muscle during voluntary straining to defecate is sometimes identified as a causative factor in a subgroup of chronically constipated patients [183]. The association of paradoxical puborectalis contraction in patients with Parkinson's disease or multiple sclerosis led to the suggestion that the paradoxical behavior of the pelvic floor musculature reflects defective transmission in descending suprasegmental pathways [184, 185]. Successful use of biofeedback techniques to train patients to avoid the paradoxical behavior of the puborectalis and external anal sphincter in a subgroup of constipated patients is consistent with disordered descending control from the brain as an underlying cause [186].

Defecation

Defecation requires neural coordination of smooth muscles in the colon and rectosigmoid region and the skeletal muscles of the pelvic floor. Distension of the rectum by the mass influx of feces or gas evokes the urge to defecate or release flatus. CNS processing of mechanosensory information from distension receptors in the rectum is the mechanism underlying this sensation. Local processing of the mechanosensory information in neural networks of the ENS activates the reflex for relaxation of the internal anal sphincter. At this stage of rectal distension, voluntary and involuntary contraction of the external anal sphincter and the puborectalis muscle prevents leakage. The decision to defecate at this stage is voluntary. When the decision is made, commands from the brain to the sacral spinal cord "shut off" the excitatory input to the external sphincter and levator ani muscles. Additional skeletal motor commands contract the abdominal muscles and diaphragm to increase intra-abdominal pressure. Coordination of the skeletal muscle components of defecation results in a straightening of the anorectal angle, descent of the pelvic floor, and opening of the anal canal and anus.

Programmed behavior of the smooth muscle during defecation includes shortening of the longitudinal muscle layer in the sigmoid colon and rectum, followed by strong contraction of the circular muscle layer [187]. This behavior corresponds to the basic stereotyped pattern of peristaltic propulsion [28, 169]. It is the endpoint for intestinal peristalsis in that the circular muscle of the distal colon and rectum become the final propulsive segment, while the outside environment receives the forwardly propelled luminal contents.

A voluntary decision to resist the urge to defecate is eventually accompanied by relaxation of the circular muscle of the rectum. This form of adaptive relaxation accommodates the increased volume in the rectum. As wall tension relaxes, the stimulus for the rectal distension receptors is removed, and the urge to defecate subsides. Receptive relaxation of the rectum is accompanied by a return of contractile tension in the internal anal sphincter, relaxation of tone in the external sphincter, increased pull by the puborectalis muscle sling and sharpening of the anorectal angle. When this occurs, the feces remain in the rectum until the next mass movement further increases the rectal volume and stimulation of mechanoreceptors again signals the neural mechanisms for defecation.

Stress and Gastrointestinal Function

Brain-gut interactions are reflected by the perturbations of GI motor and mucosal function and visceral sensitivity that are associated with a variety of psychological stressors and mental states [188]. Stress in experimental animal models (e.g., acoustic stress, repeated handling, restraint, surgery, immune mediators) causes inhibition of gastric emptying and small intestinal transit [189, 190]. Similarly in humans, fear, anger, anxiety, painful stimuli, and physical stress are all associated with delayed gastric emptying and intestinal transit [190]. In contrast to these inhibitory effects on the upper gut, stress stimulates colonic motor function as reflected by decreased colonic transit time, increased contractile activity, and induction of defecation and diarrhea [191].

Stress also disrupts mucosal secretory and barrier functions [192]. Exposure to restraint or water avoidance stress stimulates colonic mucosal secretion as reflected by elevated secretion of electrolytes, mucus, and H_2O coincident with enhanced permeability and translocation of macromolecules across the intestinal epithelium by both transcellular and paracellular routes in the rat [192]. Stress-induced breakdown of the colonic mucosal barrier permits penetration of antigens and commensal microbes into the lamina propria where contact with the mucosal immune system occurs [193].

Exposure to fecal antigens initiates inflammatory responses that resemble ulcerative colitis in a primate stress model [194, 195]. Stress-evoked inflammatory responses in the colon might underlie the sustained alteration of colonic motility and increased visceral sensitivity to colorectal distention that appears after acute exposure to stress in animal models [196]. Experimentally induced inflammation of the colonic mucosa continues to potentiate diarrhea in response to restraint stress for several days after the histological features of inflammation and basal colonic transit have returned to normal.

The evidence suggests that genetic or environmental (e.g., early life experiences) factors or previous visceral inflammation influence the impact of acute stress on colonic function [190, 197, 198]. Rats that genetically express an enhanced endocrine response to stress are more susceptible to stress-induced inhibition of intestinal transit and stimulation of colonic motor activity than other strains [190, 197, 199]. Rat strains that are genetically prone to anxiety display enhanced visceral pain responses to colorectal distension [200]. In both rodents and primates, the stress of neonatal maternal deprivation results in long-term alterations of colonic epithelial barrier function, mucosal immunity, and enhanced colonic motor and visceral sensitivity to stress in adult life [196, 200, 201, 202].

Psychological stress exacerbates the symptoms of IBS, of which cramping abdominal pain associated with urgency and explosive watery diarrhea predominate [203]. The association with stress is further reflected by observations that psychotherapy and treatment with low-dose antidepressants (e.g., tricyclic antidepressants and selective serotonin reuptake inhibitors) are often effective [203–206]. The simultaneous impact of stress on colonic motor, secretory, and immune functions and the partial dependence on stimulation of CRF receptors in the brain and ENS of animal models support a hypothesis that CRF neural signaling is a contributory factor in the stress-related exacerbation of symptoms in patients with IBS.

— Corticotropin-Releasing Factor and Stress

Corticotropin-releasing factor (CRF) and three related peptides (urocortin 1, 2, and 3) bind to CRF_1 and CRF_2, which are distinct G protein-coupled receptors [207]. CRF interaction with the pituitary CRF_1 receptor is essential for the glucocorticoid rise induced by stress [208]. Activation of brain CRF_1 receptors mediates stress-induced colonic motor responses and visceral sensitization to colorectal distension [88, 188]. Intestinal CRF_1 receptors on enteric cholinergic neurons also contribute to colonic motor responses to stress [188]. The augmentation of colonic mucosal secretion and disruption of mucosal barrier function induced by stress are also mediated by intramural CRF receptors and related degranulation of enteric mast cells [188]. Immunoreactivity (IR) for CRF is expressed in nerve cell bodies and fibers in both the myenteric and submucosal plexuses in most regions of the GI tract [90]. CRF-IR nerve fibers in the intestine are all derived from enteric neurons; neither sympathetic postganglionic fibers nor sensory afferent fibers express CRF-IR. Only the CRF_1 receptor subtype is expressed by enteric neurons [89]. Activation of central CRF-CRF_1 signaling has emerged as a key factor for understanding stress-induced behavioral changes in animal models [209]. These include anxiousness, impairment in cognitive performance and locomotor activity, altered sleep patterns and addictive behaviors, all of which take place independently of the adrenal cortical endocrine response [210, 211].

Likewise, in humans, stress-associated dysfunction of the CRF-CRF_1 neuronal circuitry in the brain is implicated in the onset and persistence of affective disorders such as anxiety, major depression, and early stress [209]. Comorbidity of IBS with anxiety and depression might be explained in the context of hyperactivity of CRF-CRF_1 signaling pathways in the brain. Activation of specific hypothalamic (e.g., paraventricular nucleus) or pontine areas (e.g., locus ceruleus and Barrington's nucleus) by exogenously applied CRF, or by exposure to stress, results in behavior symptomatic of anxiety and/or depression coincident with colonic motor dysfunction [191, 24]. Administration of CRF_1 receptor antagonists alleviates these effects in rodents [188, 212]. Of interest in this respect are reports that activation of neurons in the locus ceruleus by colorectal distention in rats involves stimulation of the CRF_1 receptor [213]. Increased firing of neurons in the locus ceruleus, in response to exteroceptive or interoceptive stressful input, results in widespread activation of noradrenergic neurons, which project to forebrain sites associated with arousal and focused attention [214, 215]. Enhanced activity in these forebrain projections is postulated to underlie the stress-related alterations in perceptual threshold to colorectal distention and the hyperreactivity associated with stress in IBS patients [209]. The collective evidence from animal models suggests that blockade of CRF_1 receptor signaling in the brain has the beneficial effect of preventing stress-related gut dysfunction and visceral hypersensitivity [209].

Future Directions

Basic translational research in the immediate and extended future can be expected to maintain ongoing progress in each of the following areas:

1. Integration of CNS imaging technology and classical neurophysiological and neuropharmacological approaches for improved understanding of the neurobiology of the brain-gut axis.
2. Continued mechanistic focus on the basic science of visceral hypersensitivity and pain that includes the molecular basis for peripheral sensitization of sensory receptors by inflammatory mediators, selectivity of central pain-related transmission pathways and higher order central processing of nociceptive information from the viscera.
3. Expanded investigation of the neuroendocrine pathways, which connect the brain with the gut and are responsible for alteration of function during psychogenic stress.
4. Application of genomic chip technology in searches for genetic polymorphisms in receptors, enzymes, and steps in signal transduction cascades in elements of the ENS.
5. Focus on identification of drug targets on neural elements of the ENS and CNS and on nonneural cell types, such as mast cells and enterochromaffin cells, which release substances that alter the activity of neurons.

References

1. Berthoud HR, Kressel M, Raybould HE, Neuhuber WL. Vagal sensors in the rat duodenal mucosa: distribution and structure as revealed by in vivo DiI-tracing. Anat Embryol (Berl) 1995;191:203–12.

2. Kirkup AJ, Brunsden AM, Grundy D. Receptors and transmission in the brain-gut axis: potential for novel therapies. I. Receptors on visceral afferents. Am J Physiol 2001;280:G787–94.

3. Ness TJ, Gebhart GF. Visceral pain: a review of experimental studies. Pain 1990;41:167–234.

4. Al-Chaer ED, Lawand NB, Westlund KN, Willis WD. Pelvic visceral input into the nucleus gracilis is largely mediated by the postsynaptic dorsal column pathway. J Neurophysiol 1996;76:2675–90.

5. Al-Chaer ED, Lawand NB, Westlund KN, Willis WD. Visceral nociceptive input into the ventral posterolateral nucleus of the thalamus: a new function for the dorsal column pathway. J Neurophysiol 1996;76:2661–74.

6. Al-Chaer ED, Feng Y, Willis WD. A role for the dorsal column in nociceptive visceral input into the thalamus of primates. J Neurophysiol 1998;79:3143–50.

7. Berkley KJ, Hubscher CH, Wall PD. Neuronal responses to stimulation of the cervix, uterus, colon, and skin in the rat spinal cord. J Neurophysiol 1993;69:545–56.

8. Traub RJ. Evidence for thoracolumbar spinal cord processing of inflammatory, but not acute colonic pain. Neuroreport 2000;11:2113–6.

9. Willis WD, Al-Chaer ED, Quast MJ, Westlund KN. A visceral pain pathway in the dorsal column of the spinal cord. Proc Natl Acad Sci U S A 1999;96:7675–9.

10. Al-Chaer ED, Feng Y, Willis WD. Comparative study of viscerosomatic input onto postsynaptic dorsal column and spinothalamic tract neurons in the primate. J Neurophysiol 1999;82:1876–82.

11. Hirshberg RM, Al-Chaer ED, Lawand NB, Westlund KN, Willis WD. Is there a pathway in the posterior funiculus that signals visceral pain? Pain 1996;67:291–305.

12. Kim YS, Kwon SJ. High thoracic midline dorsal column myelotomy for severe visceral pain due to advanced stomach cancer. Neurosurgery 2000;46:85–90.

13. Al-Chaer ED, Westlund KN, Willis WD. Nucleus gracilis: an integrator for visceral and somatic information. J Neurophysiol 1997;78:521–7.

14. Ness TJ. Evidence for ascending visceral nociceptive information in the dorsal midline and lateral spinal cord. Pain 2000;87:83–8.

15. Broussard RF, Kawasaki M, Al-Chaer ED. The dorsal column of the spinal cord facilitates spinal neuronal sensitization associated with colorectal hypersensitivity in an animal model of the irritable bowel syndrome. Gastroenterology 2000;118 (Supp. 2):A1164.

16. Saab CY, Arai YCP, Al-Chaer ED. Modulation of visceral nociceptive processing in the lumbar spinal cord following thalamic stimulation or inactivation and after dorsal column lesion in rats with neonatal colon irritation. Brain Res 2004; 1008(2):186–92.

17. Malcolm A, Phillips SF, Kellow JE, Cousins MJ. Direct clinical evidence for spinal hyperalgesia in a patient with irritable bowel syndrome. Am J Gastroenterol 2001; 96:2427–31.

18. Al-Chaer ED, Westlund KN, Willis WD. Sensitization of postsynaptic dorsal column neuronal responses by colon inflammation. Neuroreport 1997;8:3267–73.

19. Ma H, Park Y, Al-Chaer ED. Functional outcomes of neonatal colon pain measured in adult rats. J Pain 2002; 3(2) Supp.1: page 27, #707.

20. Zhuo M, Gebhart GF. Facilitation and attenuation of a visceral nociceptive reflex from the rostroventral medulla in the rat. Gastroenterology 2002;122:1007–19.

21. Hobson AR, Aziz Q. Brain imaging and functional gastrointestinal disorders: has it helped our understanding? Gut 2004;53:1198–206

22. Strigo IA, Duncan GH, Boivin M, Bushnell MC. Differentiation of visceral and cutaneous pain in the human brain. J Neurophysiol 2003;89:3294–303.

23. Rogers RC, Hermann GE, Travagli RA. Brainstem control of gastric function In: Johnson LR, Barrett KE, Ghishan FK, Merchant JL, Said HM, Wood JD, eds. Physiology of the Gastrointesinal Tract 4th ed. San Diego, Elsevier, 2006 (In Press)

24. Wood JD, Alpers D.H., Andrews PLR. Fundamentals of neurogastroenterology: Basic Science. In: Drossman DA, Talley NJ, Thompson WG, Corazziari E, and Whitehead WE, eds. *The Functional Gastrointestinal Disorders: Diagnosis, Pathophysiology and Treatment*: A Multinational Consensus. McLean, Virginia: Degnon Associates, 2000:31–90.

25. Wood JD, Alpers DH, Andrews PLR. Fundamentals of neurogastroenterology. *Gut* 1999;45 (Suppl II):II6–II16.

26. Wood JD. Enteric neuroimmunophysiology and pathophysiology. Gastroenterology 2004;127:635–57.

27. Wood JD. Cellular neurophysiology of enteric neurons. In: Johnson LR, Barrett KE, Ghishan FK, Merchant JL, Said HM, Wood JD, eds. Physiology of the Gastrointestinal Tract 4th ed. San Diego, Elsevier, 2006:629–664.

28. Wood JD. Integrative functions of the enteric nervous system. In: Johnson LR, Barrett KE, Ghishan FK, Merchant JL, Said HM, Wood JD, eds. Physiology of the Gastrointesinal Tract 4th ed. San Diego, Elsevier, 2006.

29. Wood JD. Neuropathophysiology of the irritable bowel syndrome. J Clin Gasterology 2002;35:S11–S22.

30. Wood JD. Neurobiology of the enteric nervous system. In: Dyck PJ, Thomas PK, eds. Peripheral Neuropathey 4th ed. Philadelphia, W.B. Saunders, 2005, pp. 249–77.

31. Camilleri M. Pharmacogenomics and functional gastrointestinal disorders. Pharmacogenomics 2005;6:491–01.

32. Camilleri M, Talley NJ. Pathophysiology as a basis for understanding symptom complexes and therapeutic targets. Neurogastroenterol Motil 2004;16:135–42.

33. De Giorgio R, Camilleri M. Human enteric neuropathies: morphology and molecular pathology. Neurogastroenterol Motil 2004;16:515–31.

34. De Giorgio R, Guerrini S, Barbara G, Stanghellini V, De Ponti F, Corinaldesi R, Moses PL, Sharkey KA, Mawe GM. Inflammatory neuropathies of the enteric nervous system. Gastroenterology 2004;126:1872–83.

35. Wood JD, Kirchgessner A. Slow excitatory metabotropic signal transmission in the enteric nervous system. Neurogastroenterol Motil 2004;16 Suppl 1:71–80.

36. Holman ME, Hirst GDS, Spence I. Preliminary studies of the neurones of Auerbach's plexus using intracellular microelectrodes. Aust J Exp Biol Med Sci 1972;550:795–01.

37. Nishi S, North RA. Intracellular recording from the myenteric plexus of the guinea-pig ileum. J Physiol 1973;231:471–91.

38. Schemann M, Grundy D. Electrophysiological identification of vagally innervated enteric neurons in guinea pig stomach. Am J Physiol. 1992;263:G709–G18.
39. Galligan JJ, LePard KJ, Schneider DA, Zhou X. Multiple mechanisms of fast excitatory synaptic transmission in the enteric nervous system. J Auton Nerv Syst 2000; 81:97–03.
40. Hu HZ, Gao N, Lin Z, Gao C, Liu S, Ren J, Xia Y, Wood JD. P2X(7) receptors in the enteric nervous system of guinea-pig small intestine. J Comp Neurol 2001;440: 299–10.
41. Galligan JJ, Bertrand PP. ATP mediates fast synaptic potentials in enteric neurons. J Neurosci 1994;14:7563–71.
42. Ren J, Bian X, DeVries M, Schnegelsberg B, Cockayne DA, Ford AP, Galligan JJ. P2X2 subunits contribute to fast synaptic excitation in myenteric neurons of the mouse small intestine. J Physiol 2003;552:809–21.
43. Galligan JJ, North RA. Pharmacology and function of nicotinic acetylcholine and P2X receptors in the enteric nervous system. Neurogastroenterol Motil 2004;16 Suppl 1:64–70.
44. Nurgali K, Furness JB, Stebbing MJ. Analysis of purinergic and cholinergic fast synaptic transmission to identified myenteric neurons. Neuroscience 2003;116:335–47.
45. Galligan JJ. Enteric P2X receptors as potential targets for drug treatment of the irritable bowel syndrome. Br J Pharmacol 2004;141:1294–1302.
46. Camilleri M, Northcutt AR, Kong S, Dukes GE, McSorley D, Mangel AW. Efficacy and safety of alosetron in women with irritable bowel syndrome: a randomised, placebo-controlled trial. Lancet 2000;355:1035–40.
47. Xiang Z, Burnstock G. P2X2 and P2X3 purinoceptors in the rat enteric nervous system. Histochem Cell Biol 2004;121:169–79.
48. Poole DP, Castelucci P, Robbins HL, Chiocchetti R, Furness JB. The distribution of P2X3 purine receptor subunits in the guinea pig enteric nervous system. Auton Neurosci 2002;101:39–47.
49. Castelucci P, Robbins HL, Furness JB. P2X(2) purine receptor immunoreactivity of intraganglionic laminar endings in the mouse gastrointestinal tract. Cell Tissue Res 2003;312:167–74.
50. Van Nassauw L, Brouns I, Adriaensen D, Burnstock G, Timmermans JP. Neurochemical identification of enteric neurons expressing P2X(3) receptors in the guinea-pig ileum. Histochem Cell Biol 2002;118:193–203.
51. Tack JF, Janssens J, Vantrappen G, Wood JD. Actions of 5-hydroxytryptamine on myenteric neurons in guinea pig gastric antrum. Am J Physiol 1992;263:G838–G46.
52. Derkach V, Surprenant A, North RA. 5-HT3 receptors are membrane ion channels. Nature 1989;339:706–09.
53. Galligan JJ. Ligand-gated ion channels in the enteric nervous system. Neurogastroenterol Motil 2002;14:611–23.
54. Schemann M, Wood JD. Synaptic behaviour of myenteric neurones in the gastric corpus of the guinea-pig. J Physiol 1989;417:519–35.
55. Tack JF, Wood JD. Synaptic behaviour in the myenteric plexus of the guinea-pig gastric antrum. J Physiol 1992;445:389–06.
56. Mawe GM. Intracellular recording from neurones of the guinea-pig gall-bladder. J Physiol 1990;429:323–38.
57. North RA, Slack BE, Surprenant A. Muscarinic M1 and M2 receptors mediate depo-

larization and presynaptic inhibition in guinea-pig enteric nervous system. J Physiol 1985;368:435–52.

58. Erspamer V, Asero B. Identification of enteramine, the specific hormone of the enterochromaffin cell system, as 5-hydroxytryptamine. Nature 1952;169:800–01.

59. Monro RL, Bornstein JC, Bertrand PP. Slow excitatory post-synaptic potentials in myenteric AH neurons of the guinea-pig ileum are reduced by the 5-hydroxytrytamine(7) receptor antagonist SB 269970. Neuroscience 2005;134:975–86.

60. Mawe GM, Branchek TA, Gershon MD. Peripheral neural serotonin receptors: identification and characterization with specific antagonists and agonists. Proc Natl Acad Sci U S A 1986;83:9799–803.

61. Wood JD, Mayer CJ. Serotonergic activation of tonic-type enteric neurons in guinea pig small bowel. J Neurophysiol 1979;42:582–93.

62. Nemeth PR, Ort CA, Zafirov DH, Wood JD. Interactions between serotonin and cisapride on myenteric neurons. Eur J Pharmacol 1985;108:77–83.

63. Wade PR, Wood JD. Actions of serotonin and substance P on myenteric neurons of guinea-pig distal colon. Eur J Pharmacol 1988;148:1–8.

64. Liu M, Gershon MD. Homo- and heterooligomerization involving 5-HT$_{1B}$ receptors in mouse enteric neurons creates novel receptor activities that contribute to the serotonergic regulation of intestinal motility. Neurogastroenterol Mot 2005;17: 614A.

65. Spiller RC. Postinfectious irritable bowel syndrome. Gastroenterology 2003;124:1662–71.

66. Spiller RC, Jenkins D, Thornley JP, Hebden JM, Wright T, Skinner M, Neal KR. Increased rectal mucosal enteroendocrine cells, T lymphocytes, and increased gut permeability following acute Campylobacter enteritis and in post-dysenteric irritable bowel syndrome. Gut 2000;47:804–11.

67. Beyak, MJ, Bulmer DCE, Jiang W, Keating CD, Rong W, Grundy D. Extrinsic sensory afferent nerves innervating the gastrointestinal tract. In: Johnson LR, Barrett KE, Ghishan FK, Merchant JL, Said HM, Wood JD, eds. Physiology of the Gastrointesinal Tract 4th ed. San Diego, Elsevier, 2006 (In Press)

68. Kirkup AJ, Brunsden AM and Grundy D. Receptors and transmission in the brain-gut axis: potential for novel therapies I. Receptors on visceral afferents. Am J Physiol 2001; 280:G787–G794.

69. Kozlowski CM, Green A, Grundy D, Boissonade FM, Bountra C. The 5-HT(3) receptor antagonist alosetron inhibits the colorectal distention induced depressor response and spinal c-fos expression in the anaesthetised rat. Gut 2000;46:474–80.

70. Camilleri M, Northcutt AR, Kong S, Dukes GE, McSorley D, Mangel AW. Efficacy and safety of alosetron in women with irritable bowel syndrome: a randomised, placebo-controlled trial. Lancet 2000;355:1035–40.

71. Schikowski A, Thewissen M, Mathis C, Ross HG, Enck P. Serotonin type-4 receptors modulate the sensitivity of intramural mechanoreceptive afferents of the cat rectum. Neurogastroenterol Motil 2002;14:221–27.

72. Novick J, Miner P, Krause R, Glebas K, Bliesath H, Ligozio G, Ruegg P, Lefkowitz M. A randomized, double-blind, placebo-controlled trial of tegaserod in female patients suffering from irritable bowel syndrome with constipation. Aliment Pharmacol Ther 2002;16:1877–88.

73. Chen JJ, Li Z, Pan H, Murphy DL, Tamir H, Koepsell H, Gershon MD. Maintenance of serotonin in the intestinal mucosa and ganglia of mice that lack the high-affinity

serotonin transporter: Abnormal intestinal motility and the expression of cation transporters. J Neurosci 2001;21:6348–61.

74. Pata C, Erdal ME, Derici E, Yazar A, Kanik A, Ulu O. Serotonin transporter gene polymorphism in irritable bowel syndrome. Am J Gastroenterol 2002;97:1780–84.

75. Wang BM, Wang YM, Zhang WM, Zhang QY, Liu WT, Jiang K, Zhang J. [Serotonin transporter gene polymorphism in irritable bowel syndrome]. Zhonghua Nei Ke Za Zhi 2004;43:439–41.

76. Yeo A, Boyd P, Lumsden S, Saunders T, Handley A, Stubbins M, Knaggs A, Asquith S, Taylor I, Bahari B, Crocker N, Rallan R, Varsani S, Montgomery D, Alpers DH, Dukes GE, Purvis I, Hicks GA. Association between a functional polymorphism in the serotonin transporter gene and diarrhoea predominant irritable bowel syndrome in women. Gut 2004;53:1452–58.

77. Camilleri M, Atanasova E, Carlson PJ, Ahmad U, Kim HJ, Viramontes BE, McKinzie S, Urrutia R. Serotonin-transporter polymorphism pharmacogenetics in diarrhea-predominant irritable bowel syndrome. Gastroenterology 2002;123:425–32.

78. Hu HZ, Liu S, Gao N, Xia Y, Mostafa R, Ren J, Zafirov DH, Wood JD. Actions of bradykinin on electrical and synaptic behavior of neurones in the myenteric plexus of guinea-pig small intestine. Br J Pharmacol 2003;138:1221–32.

79. Hu HZ, Gao N, Liu S, Ren J, Xia Y, Wood JD. Metabotropic signal transduction for bradykinin in submucosal neurons of guinea pig small intestine. J Pharmacol Exp Ther 2004;309:310–19.

80. Hu HZ, Gao N, Liu S, Ren J, Wang X, Xia Y, Wood JD. Action of bradykinin in the submucosal plexus of guinea pig small intestine. J Pharmacol Exp Ther 2004;309: 320–27.

81. Yau WM, Dorsett JA, Youther ML. Bradykinin releases acetylcholine from myenteric plexus by a prostaglandin-mediated mechanism. Peptides 1986;7:289–92.

82. Gao C, Liu S, Hu HZ, Gao N, Kim GY, Xia Y, Wood JD. Serine proteases excite my-enteric neurons through protease-activated receptors in guinea pig small intestine. Gastroenterology 2002;123:1554–64.

83. Reed DE, Barajas-Lopez C, Cottrell G, Velazquez-Rocha S, Dery O, Grady EF, Bun-nett NW, Vanner SJ. Mast cell tryptase and proteinase-activated receptor 2 induce hyperexcitability of guinea-pig submucosal neurons. J Physiol 2003;547:531–42.

84. Linden DR, Manning BP, Bunnett NW, Mawe GM. Agonists of proteinase-activated receptor 2 excite guinea pig ileal myenteric neurons. Eur J Pharmacol 2001;431:311–14.

85. Hu HZ, Gao N, Zhu MX, Liu S, Ren J, Gao C, Xia Y, Wood JD. Slow excitatory syn-aptic transmission mediated by P2Y1 receptors in the guinea-pig enteric nervous system. J Physiol 2003;550:493–04.

86. Christofi FL, Wunderlich J, Yu JG, Wang YZ, Xue J, Guzman J, Javed N, Cooke H. Mechanically evoked reflex electrogenic chloride secretion in rat distal colon is trig-gered by endogenous nucleotides acting at P2Y1, P2Y2, and P2Y4 receptors. J Comp Neurol 2004;469:16–36.

87. Cooke HJ, Xue J, Yu JG, Wunderlich J, Wang YZ, Guzman J, Javed N, Christofi FL. Mechanical stimulation releases nucleotides that activate P2Y1 receptors to trigger neural reflex chloride secretion in guinea pig distal colon. J Comp Neurol 2004;469:1–15.

88. Tache Y, Martinez V, Million M, Wang L. Stress and the gastrointestinal tract III. Stress-related alterations of gut motor function: role of brain corticotropin-releas-ing factor receptors. Am J Physiol 2001;280:G173–77.

89. Liu S, Gao X, Gao N, Wang X, Fang X, Hu HZ, Wang GD, Xia Y, Wood JD. Expression of type 1 corticotropin-releasing factor receptor in the guinea pig enteric nervous system. J Comp Neurol 2005;481:284–98.

90. Liu S, Gao N, Hu H-Z, Wang X-Y, Fang X, Gao X, Xia Y, Wood JD. Distribution and chemical coding of corticotropin releasing factor-immunoreactive neurons in the guinea-pig enteric nervous system. J Comp Neurol 2005; (In Press)

91. Stevens BR, Fernandez A, Kneer C, Cerda JJ, Phillips MI, Woodward ER. Human intestinal brush border angiotensin-converting enzyme activity and its inhibition by antihypertensive Ramipril. Gastroenterology 1988;94:942–47.

92. Yoshioka M, Erickson RH, Woodley JF, Gulli R, Guan D, Kim YS. Role of rat intestinal brush-border membrane angiotensin-converting enzyme in dietary protein digestion. Am J Physiol 1987;253:G781–6.

93. Fukami H, Okunishi H, Miyazaki M. Chymase: its pathophysiological roles and inhibitors. Curr Pharm Des 1998;4:439–53.

94. Caughey GH, Raymond WW, Wolters PJ. Angiotensin II generation by mast cell alpha- and beta-chymases. Biochim Biophys Acta 2000;1480:245–57.

95. Jaszewski R, Tolia V, Ehrinpreis MN, Bodzin JH, Peleman RR, Korlipara R, Weinstock JV. Increased colonic mucosal angiotensin I and II concentrations in Crohn's colitis. Gastroenterology 1990;98:1543–48.

96. Bailey RW, Bulkley GB, Hamilton SR, Morris JB, Smith GW. Pathogenesis of nonocclusive ischemic colitis. Ann Surg 1986;203:590–99.

97. Levens NR. Control of intestinal absorption by the renin-angiotensin system. Am J Physiol 1985;249:G3–15.

98. Bolton JE, Munday KA, Parsons BJ, York BG. Effects of angiotensin II on fluid transport, transmural potential difference and blood flow by rat jejunum in vivo. J Physiol 1975;253:411–28.

99. Suvannapura A, Levens NR. Norepinephrine uptake by rat jejunum: modulation by angiotensin II. Am J Physiol 1988;254:G135–41.

100. Brown DR, Gillespie MA. Actions of centrally administered neuropeptides on rat intestinal transport: enhancement of ileal absorption by angiotensin II. Eur J Pharmacol 1988;148:411–18.

101. Cooke HJ and Christofi FL. Enteric neural regulation of mucosal secretion. In: Johnson LR, Barrett KE, Ghishan FK, Merchant JL, Said HM, Wood JD, eds. Physiology of the Gastrointesinal Tract 4th ed. San Diego, Elsevier, 2006 (In Press)

102. Andriantsitohaina R, Surprenant A. Acetylcholine released from guinea-pig submucosal neurones dilates arterioles by releasing nitric oxide from endothelium. J Physiol 1992;453:493–02.

103. Bornstein JC, Furness JB. Correlated electrophysiological and histochemical studies of submucous neurons and their contribution to understanding enteric neural circuits. J Auton Nerv Syst 1988;25:1–13.

104. Vanner S, Surprenant A. Neural reflexes controlling intestinal microcirculation. Am J Physiol. 1996;271:G223–30.

105. Liu S, Xia Y, Hu H, Ren J, Gao C, Wood JD. Histamine H3 receptor-mediated suppression of inhibitory synaptic transmission in the submucous plexus of guinea-pig small intestine. Eur J Pharmacol 2000;397:49–54.

106. North RA, Surprenant A. Inhibitory synaptic potentials resulting from alpha 2-adrenoceptor activation in guinea-pig submucous plexus neurones. J Physiol 1985;358:17–33.

107. Wang GD, Wang XY, Hu HZ, Fang XC, Liu S, Gao N, Xia Y, Wood JD. Angiotensin

receptors and actions in guinea pig enteric nervous system. Am J Physiol 2005;289: G614–26.

108. Mayer CJ, Wood JD. Properties of mechanosensitive neurons within Auerbach's plexus of the small intestine of the cat. Pflügers Arch 1975;357:35–49.

109. Lomax AE, Fernandez E, Sharkey KA. Plasticity of the enteric nervous system during intestinal inflammation. Neurogastroenterol Motil 2005;17:4–15.

110. Sharkey KA, Mawe GM. Neuroimmune and epithelial interactions in intestinal inflammation. Curr Opin Pharmacol 2002;2:669–77.

111. Lomax AE, Mawe GM, Sharkey KA. Synaptic facilitation and enhanced neuronal excitability in the submucosal plexus during experimental colitis in guinea-pig. J Physiol 2005;564:863–75.

112. Linden DR, Sharkey KA, Ho W, Mawe GM. Cyclooxygenase-2 contributes to dysmotility and enhanced excitability of myenteric AH neurones in the inflamed guinea pig distal colon. J Physiol 2004;557:191–05.

113. Linden DR, Sharkey KA, Mawe GM. Enhanced excitability of myenteric AH neurones in the inflamed guinea-pig distal colon. J Physiol 2003;547:589–01.

114. Linden DR, Manning BP, Bunnett NW, Mawe GM. Agonists of proteinase-activated receptor 2 excite guinea pig ileal myenteric neurons. Eur J Pharmacol 2001;431: 311–14.

115. Manning BP, Sharkey KA, Mawe GM. Effects of PGE2 in guinea pig colonic myenteric ganglia. Am J Physiol 2002;283:G1388–97.

116. Frieling T, Palmer JM, Cooke HJ, Wood JD. Neuroimmune communication in the submucous plexus of guinea pig colon after infection with Trichinella spiralis. Gastroenterology 1994;107:1602–09.

117. Palmer JM, Wong-Riley M, Sharkey KA. Functional alterations in jejunal myenteric neurons during inflammation in nematode-infected guinea pigs. Am J Physiol 1998;275:G922–35.

118. Frieling T, Cooke HJ, Wood JD. Neuroimmune communication in the submucous plexus of guinea pig colon after sensitization to milk antigen. Am J Physiol 1994;267:G1087–93.

119. Liu S, Hu HZ, Gao N, Gao C, Wang G, Wang X, Peck OC, Kim G, Gao X, Xia Y, Wood JD. Neuroimmune interactions in guinea pig stomach and small intestine. Am J Physiol 2003;284:G154–64.

120. Schemann M, Michel K, Ceregrzyn M, Zeller F, Seidl S, Bischoff, SC. Human mast cell mediator cocktail excites neurons in human and guinea-pig enteric nervous system. Neurogastroenterol Motil 2005;17:281–89.

121. Frieling T, Rupprecht C, Dobreva G, Schemann M. Differential effects of inflammatory mediators on ion secretion in the guinea-pig colon. Comp Biochem Physiol A Physiol 1997;118:341–43.

122. Gwee KA, Leong YL, Graham C, McKendrick MW, Collins SM, Walters SJ, Underwood JE, Read NW. The role of psychological and biological factors in postinfective gut dysfunction. Gut 1999;44:400–06.

123. Wang LH, Fang XC, Pan GZ. Bacillary dysentery as a causative factor of irritable bowel syndrome and its pathogenesis. Gut 2004;53:1096–01.

124. Collins SM, Barbara G. East meets West: infection, nerves, and mast cells in the irritable bowel syndrome. Gut 2004;53:1068–69.

125. Rühl A, Nasser Y, Sharkey KA. Enteric glia. Neurogastroenterol Motil 2004;16 Suppl 1:44–49.

126. Cabarrocas J, Savidge TC, Liblau RS. Role of enteric glial cells in inflammatory bowel disease. Glia 2003;41:81−93.
127. Neunlist M, Toumi F, Oreschkova T, Denis M, Leborgne J, Laboisse CL, Galmiche JP, Jarry A. Human ENS regulates the intestinal epithelial barrier permeability and a tight junction-associated protein ZO-1 via VIPergic pathways. Am J Physiol 2003;285:G1028−36.
128. Flamant M, Sansonetti P, Coron E, Aubert P, Ruehl A, Galmiche JP, Neunlist M. Protective effects of enteric glial cells upon epithelial barrier aggression by *Shigella flexneri*. Gastroenterology 2005;128:A616.
129. Rühl A, Trotter J, Stremmel W. Isolation of enteric glia and establishment of transformed enteroglial cell lines from the myenteric plexus of adult rat. Neurogastroenterol Motil 2001;13:95−106.
130. Tjwa ET, Bradley JM, Keenan CM, Kroese AB, Sharkey KA. Interleukin-1beta activates specific populations of enteric neurons and enteric glia in the guinea pig ileum and colon. Am J Physiol 2003;285:G1268−1276.
131. Sharkey KA, Kroese AB. Consequences of intestinal inflammation on the enteric nervous system: neuronal activation induced by inflammatory mediators. Anat Rec 2001;262:79−90.
132. Rühl A, Franzke S, Collins SM, Stremmel W. Interleukin-6 expression and regulation in rat enteric glial cells. Am J Physiol 2001;280:G1163−71.
133. Rühl A, Hurst S, Collins SM. Synergism between interleukins 1 beta and 6 on noradrenergic nerves in rat myenteric plexus. Gastroenterology 1994;107:993−01.
134. Xia Y, Hu HZ, Liu S, Ren J, Zafirov DH, Wood JD. IL-1beta and IL-6 excite neurons and suppress nicotinic and noradrenergic neurotransmission in guinea pig enteric nervous system. J Clin Invest 1999;103:1309−16.
135. Maudlej N, Hanani M. Modulation of dye coupling among glial cells in the myenteric and submucosal plexuses of the guinea pig. Brain Res 1992;578:94−98.
136. Zhang W, Segura BJ, Lin TR, Hu Y, Mulholland MW. Intercellular calcium waves in cultured enteric glia from neonatal guinea pig. Glia 2003;42:252−62.
137. Bennett MR, Farnell L, Gibson WG. A quantitative model of purinergic junctional transmission of calcium waves in astrocyte networks. Biophys J 2005; (In Press).
138. Kimball BC, Mulholland MW. Enteric glia exhibit P2U receptors that increase cytosolic calcium by a phospholipase C-dependent mechanism. J Neurochem 1996;66:604−12.
139. Garrido R, Segura B, Zhang W, Mulholland M. Presence of functionally active protease-activated receptors 1 and 2 in myenteric glia. J Neurochem 2002;83:556−64.
140. Zhang W, Sarosi GA Jr, Barnhart DC, Mulholland MW. Endothelin-stimulated capacitative calcium entry in enteric glial cells: synergistic effects of protein kinase C activity and nitric oxide. J Neurochem 1998;71:205−12.
141. Barr L, Berger W, Dewey MM. Electrical transmission at the nexus between smooth muscle cells. J Gen Physiol 1968;51:347−68.
142. Prosser CL, Sperlakis N. Transmission in ganglion-free circular muscle from the cat intestine. Am J Physiol 1956;187:536−45.
143. Faussone-Pellegrini MS. Comparative study of interstitial cells of Cajal. Acta Anat (Basel) 1987;130:109−26.
144. Sanders KM, Koh SD, Ward SM. Organization and electrophysiology of interstitial cells of Cajal and smooth muscle cells in the gastrointestinal tract. In: Johnson LR, Barrett KE, Ghishan FK, Merchant JL, Said HM, Wood JD, eds. Physiology of the Gastrointesinal Tract 4th ed. San Diego, Elsevier, 2006 (In Press)

145. Vanderwinden JM. Role of Interstitial Cells of Cajal and their relationship with the enteric nervous system. Eur J Morphol 1999;37:250–6.

146. Burns AJ, Lomax AE, Torihashi S, Sanders KM, Ward SM. Interstitial cells of Cajal mediate inhibitory neurotransmission in the stomach. Proc Natl Acad Sci USA 1996;93:12008–13.

147. Vanderwinden JM, Rumessen JJ. Interstitial cells of Cajal in human gut and gastrointestinal disease. Microsc Res Tech 1999;47:344–60.

148. Daniel EE, Irwin J. Electrical activity of the stomach and upper intestine. Am J Dig Dis 1971;16:602–10.

149. Szurszewski JH. Electrical basis of gastrointestinal motility. In: Johnson LR, Christensen J, Jackson M, Jacobson ED, and Walsh JH, eds. Physiology of the Gastrointestinal Tract. 1st ed. New York: Raven Press, 1981:1435–1466.

150. Sarnelli G, Janssens J, Tack J. Effect of intranasal sumatriptan on gastric tone and sensitivity to distension. Dig Dis Sci 2001;46:1591–5.

151. Janssen P, Tack J, Sifrim D, Meulemans AL, Lefebvre RA. Influence of 5-HT1 receptor agonists on feline stomach relaxation. Eur J Pharmacol 2004;492:259–67.

152. Raybould HE. Visceral perception: sensory transduction in visceral afferents and nutrients. Gut 2002;51 Suppl 1:1–4.

153. Wingate DL. Backwards and forwards with the migrating complex. Dig Dis Sci 1981;26:641–66.

154. Bueno L, Praddaude F, Ruckebusch Y. Propagation of electrical spiking activity along the small intestine: intrinsic versus extrinsic neural influences. J Physiol 1979; 292:15–26.

155. Luiking YC, Akkermans LM, Peeters TL, Cnossen PJ, Nieuwenhuijs VB, Vanberge-Henegouwen GP. Effects of motilin on human interdigestive gastrointestinal and gallbladder motility, and involvement of 5HT3 receptors. Neurogastroenterol Motil 2002;14:151–159.

156. Itoh Z, Takahashi I. Periodic contractions of the canine gallbladder during the interdigestive state. Am J Physiol 1981;240:G183–9.

157. Pimentel M, Soffer EE, Chow EJ, Kong Y, Lin HC. Lower frequency of MMC is found in IBS subjects with abnormal lactulose breath test, suggesting bacterial overgrowth. Dig Dis Sci 2002;47:2639–43.

158. Nieuwenhuijs VB, Verheem A, van Duijvenbode-Beumer H, Visser MR, Verhoef J, Gooszen HG, Akkermans LM. The role of interdigestive small bowel motility in the regulation of gut microflora, bacterial overgrowth, and bacterial translocation in rats. Ann Surg 1998;228:188–93.

159. Lin HC. Small intestinal bacterial overgrowth: a framework for understanding irritable bowel syndrome. JAMA 2004;292:852–858.

160. Pimentel M, Chow EJ, Lin HC. Normalization of lactulose breath testing correlates with symptom improvement in irritable bowel syndrome. a double-blind, randomized, placebo-controlled study. Am J Gastroenterol 2003;98:412–19.

161. Wood JD. Integrative functions of the enteric nervous system. In: Johnson LR, Barrett KE, Ghishan FK, Merchant JL, Said HM, Wood JD, eds. Physiology of the Gastrointesinal Tract 4th ed. San Diego, Elsevier, 2006 (In Press)

162. De Wever I, Eeckhout C, Vantrappen G, Hellemans J. Disruptive effect of test meals on interdigestive motor complex in dogs. Am J Physiol 1978;235:E661–65.

163. Sarr MG, Kelly KA. Myoelectric activity of the autotransplanted canine jejunoileum. Gastroenterology 1981;81:303–10.

164. Chung SA, Rotstein O, Greenberg GR, Diamant NE. Mechanisms coordinating gastric and small intestinal MMC: role of extrinsic innervation rather than motilin. Am J Physiol 1994;267:G800–09.

165. Chung SA, Valdez DT, Diamant NE. Adrenergic blockage does not restore the canine gastric migrating motor complex during vagal blockade. Gastroenterology 1992;103:1491–97.

166. Sarna SK. Giant migrating contractions and their myoelectric correlates in the small intestine. Am J Physiol 1987;253:G697–05.

167. Kamath PS, Phillips SF, O'Connor MK, Brown ML, Zinsmeister AR. Colonic capacitance and transit in man: modulation by luminal contents and drugs. Gut 1990;31:443–49.

168. Krevsky B, Malmud LS, D'Ercole F, Maurer AH, Fisher RS. Colonic transit scintigraphy. A physiologic approach to the quantitative measurement of colonic transit in humans. Gastroenterology 1986;91:1102–12.

169. Wood JD. Neurogasterology and digestive motility. In: Rhoades RA and Tanner GA, eds. Medical Physiology. 2nd ed. Baltimore: Lippincott Williams and Wilkins, 2003. p. 449–480.

170. Connell AM. The motility of the pelvic colon. II. Paradoxical motility in diarrhoea and constipation. Gut 1962;3:342–8.

171. Dubrovsky B, Filipini D. Neurobiological aspects of the pelvic floor muscles involved in defecation. Neurosci Biobehav Rev 1990;14:157–68.

172. Filipini DL, Dubrovsky B. Pelvic floor muscles response to graded rectal distension and cutaneous stimulation. Dig Dis Sci 1991;36:1761–7.

173. Vodušek DB, Enck P. Neural control of pelvic floor muscles. In: Johnson LR, Barrett KE, Ghishan FK, Merchant JL, Said HM, Wood JD, eds. Physiology of the Gastrointestinal Tract 4th ed. San Diego, Elsevier, 2006 (In Press)

174. Laurberg S, Swash M. Effects of aging on the anorectal sphincters and their innervation. Dis Colon Rectum 1989;32:737–42.

175. Miller JM. Criteria for therapeutic use of pelvic floor muscle training in women. J Wound Ostomy Continence Nurs 2002;29:301–11.

176. Brierley SM, Jones RC 3rd, Gebhart GF, Blackshaw LA. Splanchnic and pelvic mechanosensory afferents signal different qualities of colonic stimuli in mice. Gastroenterology 2004;127:166–178.

177. Brierley SM, Carter R, Jones W 3rd, Xu L, Robinson DR, Hicks GA, Gebhart GF, Blackshaw LA. Differential chemosensory function and receptor expression of splanchnic and pelvic colonic afferents in mice. J Physiol 2005;567:267–281.

178. Chey WY, Jin HO, Lee MH, Sun S.W., Lee KY. Colonic motility abnormality in patients with irritable bowel syndrome exhibiting abdominal pain and diarrhea. Am J Gastroenterol 2001;96:1499–1506.

179. Percy JP, Neill ME, Swash M, Parks AG. Electrophysiological study of motor nerve supply of pelvic floor. Lancet 1981;1:16–7.

180. Frenckner B. Function of the anal sphincters in spinal man. Gut 1975;16:638–44.

181. Molander ML, Frenckner B. Electrical activity of the external anal sphincter at different ages in childhood. Gut 1983;24:218–21.

182. Schuster MM. The riddle of the sphincters. Gastroenterology 1975;69:249–62.

183. Yeh CY, Pikarsky A, Wexner SD, Baig MK, Jain A, Weiss EG, Nogueras JJ, Vernava AM 3rd. Electromyographic findings of paradoxical puborectalis contraction correlate poorly with cinedefecography. Tech Coloproctol 2003;7:77–81.

184. Chia YW, Gill KP, Jameson JS, Forti AD, Henry MM, Swash M, Shorvon PJ. Paradoxical puborectalis contraction is a feature of constipation in patients with multiple sclerosis. J Neurol Neurosurg Psychiatry 1996;60:31–5.

185. Mathers SE, Kempster PA, Swash M, Lees AJ. Constipation and paradoxical puborectalis contraction in anismus and Parkinson's disease: a dystonic phenomenon? J Neurol Neurosurg Psychiatry 1988;51:1503–7.

186. Sielezneff I, Sarles JC, Sastre B. Anorectal asynchronism. Clinical, manometric and therapeutic data]. Presse Med 1994;23:1691–4.

187. Kamm MA, van der Sijp JR, Lennard-Jones JE. Colorectal and anal motility during defaecation. Lancet 1992;339:820.

188. Tache Y, Martinez V, Wang L, Million M. CRF1 receptor signaling pathways are involved in stress-related alterations of colonic function and viscerosensitivity: implications for irritable bowel syndrome. Br J Pharmacol 2004;141:1321–30.

189. Enck P, Holtmann G. Stress and gastrointestinal motility in animals: a review of the literature. J Gastrointest Mot 1992;1:83–90.

190. Williams CL, Burks TF. Stress opioids, and gastrointestinal transit. In: Tache Y, Morley J, and Brown MR, eds. Hans Selye Symposia on Neuroendocrinology and Stress: Neuropeptides and Stress. New York: Springer-Verlag, 1989;175–187.

191. Tache Y, Martinez V, Million M, Wang L. Stress and the gastrointestinal tract III. Stress-related alterations of gut motor function: role of brain corticotropin-releasing factor receptors. Am J Physiol 2001;280:G173–7.

192. Tache Y, Perdue MH. Role of peripheral CRF signalling pathways in stress-related alterations of gut motility and mucosal function. Neurogastroenterol Motil 2004;16 Suppl 1:137–42.

193. Velin AK, Ericson AC, Braaf Y, Wallon C, Soderholm JD. Increased antigen and bacterial uptake in follicle associated epithelium induced by chronic psychological stress in rats. Gut 2004;53:494–500.

194. Peck OC and Wood JD. 2000. Brain-gut interactions in ulcerative colitis. Gastroenterology 118:807–8.

195. Wood JD, Peck OC, Tefend KS, Stonerook MJ, Caniano DA, Mutabagani KH, Lhotak S, and Sharma HM. 2000. Evidence that colitis is initiated by environmental stress and sustained by fecal factors in the cotton-top tamarin (*Saguinus oedipus*). Dig Dis Sci 45:385–93.

196. Bradesi S, Eutamene H, Garcia-Villar R, Fioramonti J, Bueno L. Acute and chronic stress differently affect visceral sensitivity to rectal distension in female rats. Neurogastroenterol Motil 2002;14:75–82.

197. Coutinho SV, Plotsky PM, Sablad M, Miller JC, Zhou H, Bayati AI, McRoberts JA, Mayer EA. Neonatal maternal separation alters stress-induced responses to viscerosomatic nociceptive stimuli in rat. Am J Physiol 2002;282:G307–16.

198. La JH, Kim TW, Sung TS, Kang JW, Kim HJ, Yang IS. Visceral hypersensitivity and altered colonic motility after subsidence of inflammation in a rat model of colitis. World J Gastroenterol 2003;9:2791–5.

199. Million M, Wang L, Martinez V, Tache Y. Differential Fos expression in the paraventricular nucleus of the hypothalamus, sacral parasympathetic nucleus and colonic motor response to water avoidance stress in Fischer and Lewis rats. Brain Res 2000;877:345–53.

200. Gunter WD, Shepard JD, Foreman RD, Myers DA, Greenwood-Van Meerveld B. Evidence for visceral hypersensitivity in high-anxiety rats. Physiol Behav 2000;69:379–82.

201. Biggs AM, Aziz Q, Tomenson B, Creed F. Effect of childhood adversity on health related quality of life in patients with upper abdominal or chest pain. Gut 2004;53: 180–6.

202. Barreau F, Ferrier L, Fioramonti J, Bueno L. Neonatal maternal deprivation triggers long term alterations in colonic epithelial barrier and mucosal immunity in rats. Gut 2004; 53:501–6.

203. Solmaz M, Kavuk I, Sayar K. Psychological factors in the irritable bowel syndrome. Eur J Med Res 2003;8:549–56.

204. Spiller RC. Irritable bowel syndrome. Br Med Bull 2004;72:15–29.

205. Halpert A, Dalton CB, Diamant NE, Toner BB, Hu Y, Morris CB, Bangdiwala SI, Whitehead WE, Drossman DA. Clinical response to tricyclic antidepressants in functional bowel disorders is not related to dosage. Am J Gastroenterol 2005; 100:664–71.

206. Cremonini F, Talley NJ. Diagnostic and therapeutic strategies in the irritable bowel syndrome. Minerva Med 2004;95:427–41.

207. Hauger RL, Grigoriadis DE, Dallman MF, Plotsky PM, Vale WW, Dautzenberg FM. International Union of Pharmacology. XXXVI. Current status of the nomenclature for receptors for corticotropin-releasing factor and their ligands. Pharmacol Rev 2003;55:21–6.

208. Turnbull AV, Rivier C. Corticotropin-releasing factor (CRF) and endocrine responses to stress: CRF receptors, binding protein, and related peptides. Proc Soc Exp Biol Med 1997;215:1–10.

209. Bale TL, Vale WW. CRF and CRF receptors: role in stress responsivity and other behaviors. Annu Rev Pharmacol Toxicol 2004;44:525–57.

210. Zobel AW, Nickel T, Kunzel HE, Ackl N, Sonntag A, Ising M, Holsboer F. Effects of the high-affinity corticotropin-releasing hormone receptor 1 antagonist R121919 in major depression: the first 20 patients treated. J Psychiatr Res 2000;34:171–81.

211. Weiss JM, Stout JC, Aaron MF, Quan N, Owens MJ, Butler PD, Nemeroff CB. Depression and anxiety: role of the locus coeruleus and corticotropin-releasing factor. Brain Res Bull 1994;35:561–72.

212. Million M, Grigoriadis DE, Sullivan S, Crowe PD, McRoberts JA, Zhou H, Saunders PR, Maillot C, Mayer EA, Tache Y. A novel water-soluble selective CRF1 receptor antagonist, NBI 35965, blunts stress-induced visceral hyperalgesia and colonic motor function in rats. Brain Res 2003;985:32–42.

213. Lechner SM, Curtis AL, Brons R, Valentino RJ. Locus coeruleus activation by colon distention: role of corticotropin-releasing factor and excitatory amino acids. Brain Res 1997;756:114–24.

214. Lejeune F, Millan MJ. The CRF1 receptor antagonist, DMP695, abolishes activation of locus coeruleus noradrenergic neurones by CRF in anesthetized rats. Eur J Pharmacol 2003;464:127–33.

215. Keck ME, Holsboer F. Hyperactivity of CRH neuronal circuits as a target for therapeutic interventions in affective disorders. Peptides 2001;22:835–44.

Chapter 3

Principles of Applied Neurogastroenterology: Physiology/Motility-Sensation

John E. Kellow, Chair

Fernando Azpiroz, Co-Chair

Michel Delvaux

Gerald F. Gebhart

Howard Mertz

Eamonn M.M. Quigley

André J.P.M. Smout

Introduction

Patients with functional gastrointestinal disorders (FGIDs) often exhibit sensory afferent dysfunction of the digestive tract that is manifested as altered sensitivity to luminal distension or other stimuli, and that selectively affects the visceral territory [1]. Such *visceral hypersensitivity* is regarded as an important pathophysiologic mechanism in the FGIDs [2]. Depending on the specific organ or organs affected, it may underlie common symptoms in the FGIDs such as chest pain, abdominal discomfort, abdominal bloating, and urgency of defecation. In contrast, some symptoms characteristic of the FGIDs, such as constipation and diarrhea, are consistent with altered gut motility (dysmotility) that may include alterations in contractile activity, tone, compliance, and transit in various regions of the digestive tract. While dysmotility has been documented in FGID patients, it is a less reproducible finding than visceral hypersensitivity, at least with current measurement techniques. This chapter provides (1) an overview of the fundamental concepts and terminology of human digestive tract sensorimotor physiology and pathophysiology relevant to the FGIDs, (2) an outline of normal regional sensorimotor physiology along the human digestive tract, (3) a review of currently available techniques for testing sensorimotor function in the FGIDs, (4) a discussion of the putative origins of visceral hypersensitivity and dysmotility in the FGIDs, (5) some examples of the specific symptom correlates of sensorimotor dysfunction in the FGIDs, (6) a description of the current role of sensorimotor testing in the clinical evaluation of patients with FGIDs, and (7) recommendations for future research in this area.

Fundamental Concepts of Human Digestive Tract Sensorimotor Physiology and Pathophysiology

Sensory and motor functions of the gastrointestinal tract are mediated through the enteric nervous system (ENS) and through the extrinsic nerves that connect the gastrointestinal tract to the central nervous system (CNS). A detailed description of the mechano- and chemosensitive receptive endings in the viscera, the central neurons upon which they terminate, and the efferent neural pathways are presented in Chapter 2. Although it is clear that sensation and motility are intimately related, their relevance to the FGIDs will be considered separately in this section because of the historical development of the field.

— Sensation

Most stimuli that activate receptive endings in the gut are not consciously perceived. Sensitivity is a term that has been used to refer to both conscious perception and to activity in visceral sensory afferent pathways, whether related to perception or to reflex responses. For the purposes of this chapter, the term *sensitivity* is restricted to the processes leading to conscious perception. The following discussion will focus on stimuli and mechanisms at the organ level that lead to the subjective experience of *enhanced conscious perception* in the FGIDs, although the role of reflex responses will also be considered where relevant.

Anatomical and Functional Considerations

Mechanical, chemical, and thermal stimuli in the gastrointestinal tract can produce conscious sensations that range from non-noxious to uncomfortable or painful. Unlike other tissues in the body, the viscera are unique in that each organ is innervated by two sets of nerves: vagal and splanchnic spinal nerves or pelvic and splanchnic spinal nerves. (See Chapter 2.) Both systems participate in the reflex control of gut function, but their involvement in conscious sensations differs. Discomfort and pain from the gastrointestinal tract are conveyed to the CNS primarily by spinal afferents. Activation of vagal afferents is not considered to give rise to sensations perceived as painful, although their activation may modulate spinal visceral (and somatic) pain. However, the role of vagal afferents in visceral sensations and in the pathophysiology of the FGIDs may require reconsideration since results from animal experiments suggest that vagal afferents may transmit acute chemonociceptive information to the brainstem [3], sensitize the GI tract to mechanical stimulation [4], and modulate behavioral responses after gastric insult [5].

In addition to mechanosensitive structures (e.g., intraganglionic laminar endings and intramuscular arrays as described in Chapter 2) and polymodal endings, the viscera (like other tissues) are innervated by a group of mechanically insensitive afferent fibers termed "silent" or "sleeping" fibers. Normally, these endings in the viscera are unresponsive to mechanical stimulation, even to distending pressures well above noxious or painful. After organ insult, however, they can acquire spontaneous activity and mechanosensitivity. Such receptor behavior illustrates the plasticity of the nervous system and suggests that mechanosensitivity is not a fixed or invariant property during the life of an individual, either in terms of activation threshold or the relationship between stimulus intensity and firing frequency. There are currently no data available from humans, but animal studies estimate the percentage of silent fibers in the pelvic nerve to be 30–40% in the rat and >80% in the cat [6]. These estimates likely include afferent fibers with chemoselective or chemonociceptive endings in addition to the mechanically in-sensitive endings. Once "awakened," these silent nociceptors have the potential to contribute new and increased input from the periphery to the CNS. Thus altered perceptions associated with the FGIDs are likely due to both increased activity of these nociceptors and sensitized mechano- and chemosensitive receptive endings.

Excitability and Sensitization

In response to tissue insult, the chemical environment at visceral nerve terminals in organs can become extraordinarily rich. In addition to conveying sensory information from the periphery to the CNS, afferent fibers also have efferent functions, particularly when confronted with a local insult. Thus, visceral afferent fibers that release bioactive substances such as substance P, calcitonin gene-related peptide (CGRP), growth factors, and glutamate at their central terminals can also release the same substances from their peripheral terminals resulting in changes in local blood flow and effects on adjacent terminals of intrinsic and/or extrinsic afferent fibers, and other cells. For example, CGRP contributes to local vasodilation and substance P causes mast cells to degranulate. Nearby sympathetic nerve terminals and enterochromaffin cells can contribute substances such as norepi-nephrine, serotonin, histamine, adenosine triphosphate (ATP), adenosine, nerve growth factor, and tryptase to the local environment. Resident leukocytes and other immune competent cells attracted to a site of local insult can contribute substances such as products of cyclooxygenase or lipoxygenase, growth factors, and reactive oxygen species. Many of these bioactive substances either directly activate visceral afferent terminals or sensitize them to other stimuli (e.g., mechanical stimuli) [7, 8].

Sensitization was first used to describe a unique characteristic of cutaneous nociceptors, namely the ability of the receptive ending to display an increased response to a stimulus after acute insult to the skin [9]. In addition to showing an increase in the magnitude of the response, these nociceptors often have a decreased threshold of response (i.e., they become more easily excitable) and develop spontaneous activity. In the gut, sensitization may apply to receptors involved in both conscious sensation and reflex pathways. For example, even those vagal and spinal mechanosensitive afferents with distension response thresholds in the physiologic range (e.g., 2–5 mmHg) can exhibit the property of sensitization. In addition to peripheral sensitization, "central sensitization" can result from the increase in afferent input to the CNS (particularly to the dorsal horn neurons in the spinal cord), and the consequent increased release of bioactive substances. Together, peripheral and central sensitization, which represent increases in neuron excitability both peripherally and centrally, contribute to *visceral hyper-sensitivity,* a characteristic and reproducible feature of the FGIDs. This term refers

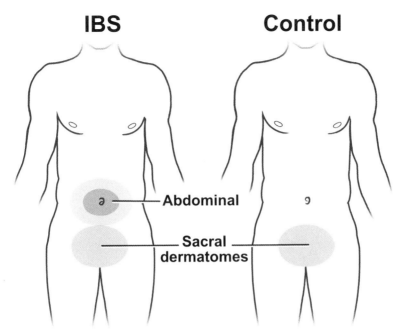

Figure 1. Viscerosomatic referral patterns in irritable bowel syndrome (IBS) patients and healthy (control) subjects. In control subjects (right panel) rectal distension induces sensations in sacral (suprapubic and perianal) dermatomes. Patients with IBS (left panel) report not only suprapubic, but also (66%) abdominal sensation during rectal distension. (Modified from reference 10 with permission from the American Gastroenterological Association.)

to an increased conscious perception of visceral stimuli and it may manifest as abdominal discomfort or pain. Thus, normal nonpainful stimuli and the normal sensations they typically produce (e.g., postprandial fullness, satiety, mild postprandial increase in abdominal girth, signal to defecate, and sensation of complete rectal emptying) can be more intensely perceived in various FGIDs and produce discomfort and even pain (i.e., feelings of excessive postprandial fullness, early satiety, bloating and abdominal distension, urgency to defecate, and sensation of incomplete evacuation). The terms *hyperalgesia* (an increased response to a noxious stimulus) and *allodynia* (pain produced by a normally non-noxious stimulus) have been borrowed from the somatic pain field and applied to visceral pain conditions, including the FGIDs. However, these terms should be avoided in describing the FGIDs given that some stimuli that produce cutaneous pain (e.g., cutting) do not produce visceral pain, and that the mechanisms underlying pain in the skin and in the gut likely differ.

Central Processing

Visceral sensory information is conveyed to supraspinal sites and finally to the cortical areas where conscious perception arises by several pathways. Spinal visceral afferent fibers terminate at second-order neurons in the spinal dorsal horn. A distinguishing characteristic of visceral afferent input to the spinal cord is that the second-order neurons upon which visceral afferents terminate also receive convergent afferent input from somatic structures (*viscerosomatic convergence*) as well as from other viscera (*viscero-visceral convergence*). Thus, increased or exaggerated input from sensitized and awakened visceral afferents leads to expanded areas of referred sensation—a characteristic feature of the FGIDs (Figure 1) [10]. Furthermore, local gut insult may induce hypersensitivity in other visceral and/or somatic sites that are not necessarily contiguous.

In addition to changes in the excitability of spinal neurons following peripheral visceral insult, neurons in supraspinal sites also exhibit increases in excitability, particularly in brain areas associated with descending modulation of spinal sensory transmission. These descending modulatory systems are known to either inhibit or enhance spinal sensory transmission. Animal experiments have verified the ability of descending influences to modulate visceral nociceptive transmission and, conversely, the ability of experimental organ inflammation to increase the excitability of neurons in modulatory circuits. It is thus conceivable that the symptomatic expression of the FGIDs could be sustained via alteration in the normal functioning of the predominantly inhibitory descending modulatory circuits. These modulatory circuits can be influenced in turn by cognitive, affective, and stressful influences, as well as by expectation and prior experience, all of which assume considerable relevance in the setting of the FGIDs.

— Motility

The major functions of human digestive tract motility are to accomplish propulsion along the gut, to mix gut contents with digestive secretions and expose them to the absorptive surface, to facilitate temporary storage in certain regions of the gut, to prevent retrograde movement of contents from one region to another, and to dispose of residues. In the context of the FGIDs, gastrointestinal dysmotility can develop through several mechanisms involving the brain-gut axis. First, various inflammatory, immune, infiltrative, or degenerative processes may directly affect the muscle and/or other elements of the ENS effector system. Dysmotility may also be triggered indirectly in response to excess stimulation by visceral afferent (sensory) fibers that influence local gastrointestinal motor function via modulation of motor neurons in prevertebral ganglia. In addition, activation of visceral afferent fibers induces autonomic changes integrated in the brainstem, such as changes in heart rate, and alterations in colonic tone (e.g., vagally-mediated gastro-colonic motor response) that may be increased in certain FGIDs. Finally, psychosocial stressors can induce profound alterations in gastrointestinal motility. Patients with FGIDs tend to have a greater gastrointestinal motor response to stressful conditions than do controls, which is presumably mediated at a central level.

Anatomical and Functional Considerations

In each region of the gastrointestinal tract, the muscle layers of the gut wall and their innervation are adapted and organized to produce the specific motor patterns which subserve the motor functions of that particular region. The entire gastrointestinal tract interacts with the CNS and communication between various parts of the gut is facilitated by the longitudinal transmission of myogenic and neurogenic signals through the intrinsic neurons, as well as by reflex arcs through autonomic neurons. (See Chapter 2.) The aspects of gut motility that appear most relevant to the FGIDs are contractile activity and tone, compliance and related phenomena, and transit.

Contractile Activity and Tone

Cyclic variations in the transmembrane potential of the smooth muscle cells occur in the stomach, small intestine, and colon. When recorded with extracellular electrodes, this electrical activity is usually referred to as slow-wave activity, electrical control activity, pacesetter potential, or basal electrical rhythm [11]. In the presence of an excitatory neurotransmitter such as acetylcholine, the transmembrane potential depolarizes further and, when the excitation threshold is exceeded, electrical spikes occur that are superimposed on the plateau phase of the slow-wave activity. Phasic (short-duration) contractions originate from these electrical spikes, and thus the frequency of the phasic contractions in the stomach and small intestine is dictated by the slow-wave frequency. Because the slow-wave frequency varies along the length of the gastrointestinal tract, the maximum contractile frequency varies similarly. The maximum contractile frequency in the stomach is 3 per minute, while in the small intestine the frequency declines gradually from 12 per minute in the duodenum to 7 per minute in the terminal ileum. A mixture of slow-wave frequencies are found in the colon and range from 1 to 12 per minute, and the correlation between electrical and contractile activities is much less clear. Whether the gut phasic contractions accomplish mainly mixing or propulsion depends on their temporal (e.g., frequency, duration) and spatial (e.g., spread of propagation) characteristics [11]. In the small intestine, a phasic contraction is usually defined as a contraction whose duration does not exceed the span of a slow-wave cycle. However, some longer lasting motor events are also considered phasic, e.g., "prolonged propagated" or "giant migrating" contractions.

A more prolonged state of contraction referred to as "tone" is not regulated by slow waves and may be clearly recognized in the proximal stomach (accommodation response to a meal) and the colon (response to feeding), as well as in some sphincteric regions. Phasic contractions, such as those regulating lumen occlusion, may be superimposed on tonic activity. Thus, tone can increase the efficiency of phasic contractions by diminishing the diameter of the lumen. The inter-relationships between phasic and tonic activity require further investigation, but it is believed these two types of contractile activity may be independently regulated [12]. Tone also modifies wall tension in response to gut filling, and is therefore one determinant of perception of distension [13, 14].

Compliance and Related Phenomena

Compliance refers to the capability of a region of the gut to adapt to intraluminal distension. It is expressed as the ratio of the change in volume to the change in pressure (dV/dP) and is obtained from the pressure-volume curve. Several factors contribute to compliance including the capacity (diameter) of the organ, the elastic properties of the gut wall (i.e., thickness, fibrotic component, muscular activity), and the elasticity of surrounding organs (that can be influenced by fibrosis, ascites, abdominal masses). Although compliance has sometimes been expressed as the pressure/volume ratio at one distension step, it is more accurately expressed as the entire pressure/volume curve. Compliance can differ markedly in different regions of the gut, and even within an organ; for example the descending colon is less compliant than the ascending colon, while the sigmoid colon is less compliant than the transverse colon. Compliance decreases during contraction and increases during relaxation and in a given organ are determined by the muscular activity of its walls. Hence, short-term changes in compliance reflect the tone of the organ. In that respect, compliance measurements in vivo (volume/pressure relationship) reflect the elongation/tension relationship of the gut wall. However, the interpretation of compliance measurements remains controversial, because the type of distension and the number of distension steps also influence compliance. Consequently, compliance should be compared between studies only when it has been measured in a similar way [15].

A distending intraluminal volume produces a stretch and tension (force) on the gut wall, which determines the intraluminal pressure increment. In any given situation, wall tension, intraluminal pressure and volume are interrelated by Laplace's law: $T = PR/2$ for a sphere; and $T = PR$ for a cylinder, where T refers to wall tension, P transmural pressure (intraluminal minus intra-abdominal pressure), and R radius. However, this equation is influenced by the compliance of the organ. For instance, if the gut contracts (i.e., tone increases), the same intraluminal volume will produce greater wall tension and higher intraluminal pressure than if the gut was not contracted. It has been shown that perception of gut distension is in part determined by wall tension, rather than by intraluminal volume or pressure. Hence, assessment of wall tension may be important in the interpretation of results of tests assessing perception of visceral stimuli, [14, 16–18] but further data are required in each of the various regions of the gut.

Transit

While flow reflects the local movements of intraluminal content, transit refers to the time taken for food or other material to traverse a specified region of the gastrointestinal tract. In clinical terms, transit is one of the most important aspects of motility, as it represents the net interaction of a number of the other parameters discussed above and is a relevant and convenient index of organ function. Most measurements of transit are based on detecting intraluminal movements of an extrinsic marker labeling the luminal content. Transit depends on many factors, such as the physical (e.g., solid, liquid, gas) and chemical (e.g., pH, osmolality, and nutrient composition) nature of both gut contents and the administered marker. Transit measurement is also influenced by the state of gut motility at the time of marker administration (e.g., fasted versus fed motility), and any preparation of the gut (e.g., cleansing of the colon). Summaries of transit measurements commonly employed for solids and liquids include the half time for emptying ($t_{1/2}$) (e.g., of the stomach or colon) and the amount (%) emptied from an organ at a given time after marker administration. In the esophagus, the transit time of the head of a swallowed bolus along the esophageal body is about 2 to 5 seconds. In the stomach, the half-emptying time for the type of light meal commonly used in clinical testing is usually less than 90 minutes. The head of such a meal usually reaches the cecum within 120 minutes. In the colon, the half-emptying time is normally approximately 48 hours but there is wide variability. The half time for organ emptying and other parameters have been shown to be abnormal in some FGIDs.

Regional Sensorimotor Physiology of the Digestive Tract

The motor patterns characteristic of each organ and relevant sensory aspects are discussed in the subsequent organ-specific chapters. However, a general outline of sensorimotor physiology in the various regions of the digestive tract, including the handling of intestinal gas, is useful prior to consideration of the techniques currently available to evaluate sensorimotor physiology. Surprisingly, little scientific data are available regarding the normal conscious perception of physiologic sensations originating from different regions of the gut, such as those related to food ingestion and defecation. Some nonphysiological experimental data are available, however, usually obtained from mechanical distension studies. In each region of the gut, the intensity of perception is stimulus-related, although the character of the sensations can be similar across a range of distensions between the threshold for perception and the threshold for discomfort—when the distension is progressively increased, the nonpainful sensation is replaced by discomfort and then pain.

— Esophagus

The esophagus has relatively simple functions: to enable the passage of swallowed material to the stomach and to prevent reflux of material from the stomach. Normal esophageal motility is dominated by a stereotypic pattern of progressive phasic contractions triggered by swallowing [19]. During basal conditions both the upper and lower esophageal sphincters are contracted. During deglutition, a coordinated action of the tongue, hypopharynx, upper esophageal sphincter, and cervical muscle groups ensures the delivery of the food bolus to the esophagus, while simultaneously protecting the airways. Peristaltic esophageal contractions propagate at a speed of approximately 2 cm per second to the lower esophageal sphincter. The lower esophageal sphincter (LES) relaxes at the initiation of the swallow and remains open until the peristaltic contraction reaches it. Experimental distension of the healthy esophagus normally evokes a sensation of retrosternal fullness or discomfort [20].

— Stomach and Small Intestine

The main functions of gastric motility are to accommodate and store the ingested meal, grind solid particles, and then empty the meal in a regulated fashion into the duodenum. Small intestinal motility mixes the meal with intestinal secretions, propels digesta in an aboral direction (exposing the chyme to the absorptive surface), and clears the residue into the colon. The sphincters at the lower esophageal, pyloric, and ileocecal regions regulate transit across these regions and prevent orad reflux. There are fundamental differences in the patterns of motor activity along the length of the gut during fasting and after feeding. Sensitivity also appears to vary between the fasting and fed states. Thus, during fasting, mechanical (balloon) distension of the stomach is perceived as a sensation of pressure, fullness, or nausea in the epigastric and periumbilical regions [13, 14, 21–23]. Compared to perfusions of protein and mixed nutrients, duodenal perfusion of fat dramatically increases sensations of nausea and fullness in response to gastric barostat distension [24]. Experimental distension of the jejunum is perceived as a sensation of pressure or fullness, or of a colicky or sharp/stinging sensation in the epigastric and periumbilical regions [12, 25]. The conscious perception of distension of the small bowel is also increased by intestinal nutrients, especially fat [26, 27].

Gastric and Small Bowel Motility During Fasting

In the fasted state, motor activity is highly organized into a distinct and cyclically recurring sequence, termed the *migrating motor complex* (MMC) [28]. The MMC consists of three distinct phases of motor activity that migrate slowly along the length of the small intestine. Each sequence begins with a period of motor quiescence (phase 1), followed by a period of apparently random and irregular contractions (phase 2), and culminating in a burst of uninterrupted regular phasic contractions at the maximum contractile frequency (phase 3 or activity front). Individual cycles last between one and two hours and originate in the stomach, duodenum or proximal small intestine, then migrate aborally down to the mid small bowel [29]. The velocity of propagation slows as the activity front progresses distally. MMCs appear between 32 and 35 weeks postconception and are similar to MMCs in older children and adults by the time the child is full-term [30]. Phase 3 of the MMC is believed to have a housekeeping function, sweeping the gut clean once ingestion and digestion are completed.

During gastric phase 3 activity, basal tone in the lower esophageal sphincter is increased and prevents reflux of gastric contents via superimposed phasic contractions. Tone increases in the proximal stomach and superimposed phasic waves can be identified [31]. True rhythmic activity occurs only in the distal antrum where contractions at 3 cycles per minute may be seen at the end of phase 3. As phase 3 progresses, antro-pyloro-duodenal coordination increases and high-amplitude contractions originating in the proximal stomach propagate through the antrum and are associated with transient inhibition of duodenal activity. In the distal ileum, the main features are predominantly irregular contractile activity and clustered contractions. On occasion, a high-amplitude wave sweeps through this region and across the ileocecal sphincter (ICS) into the cecum. This "giant migrating" contraction is thought to clear the ileum of refluxed colonic material. Tone is not a prominent or consistent feature at the ICS and it is believed that coordinated ileal phasic contractions rather than fluctuations in ICS tone regulate the transport of ileal contents into the colon and prevent colo-ileal reflux [32].

Postprandial Gastric and Small Bowel Motility

When food is ingested, the cyclical pattern is abolished, or at least suppressed, and replaced by proximal stomach relaxation, regular antral contractions at a rate of 3 per minute, and by irregular contractions in the small bowel that may be sustained for 2.5 to 8 hours, depending on the size and nature of the meal. Thereafter, the fasted pattern resumes when a substantial part of the meal has emptied from the small bowel [28]. Gastric accommodation is a vagally mediated postprandial reflex that results in reduction of tone and provides a reservoir for the meal [33, 34]. On arrival of a swallow sequence at the esophagogastric junction, the gastric fundus undergoes receptive relaxation, partly mediated by the vagus nerve. As the meal enters the stomach, tonic activity and phasic contractions are inhibited, leading to adaptive relaxation. An important component of normal gastric emptying in response to a meal is the ability of the antropyloric region to discriminate solids by size and to retain solid particles greater than 2 mm in diameter. Emptying of liquids starts immediately, so that by the end of meal ingestion some liquid has already passed into the intestine. By contrast, solid particles are trapped and ground (*triturated*) in the antropyloric mill. When the size of the solids is reduced to 2 mm or less, they are emptied with the liquid phase (Figure 2). Solid emptying does not occur during trituration, resulting in a lag phase that is directly related to the size and consistency of the solid component of the meal. After a typical solid/liquid meal, the lag phase lasts approximately 10–20 minutes. Once the particles are triturated, the emptying phase occurs and typically proceeds in a linear fashion. The content of the meal, however, significantly influences motility and emptying, with liquids, digestible solids, and relatively large undigested solids emptying at different rates.

Gastric emptying of liquids and solids suspended in the liquid phase is ultimately dependent on the interplay between the propulsive force generated by tonic contractions of the proximal stomach and the resistance presented by the antrum, pylorus, and duodenum. Indigestible solids are not emptied during this postprandial stage but are emptied during phase 3 MMC activity. Other factors known to influence the gastric emptying rate of a meal include factors such as the volume, acidity, osmolality, nutrient density, fat, and amino acid composition of the meal, humoral factors such as cholecystokinin and gastrin, and other factors such as the amount of fat present in the ileum and the degree of distension of the rectum and colon. Different food constituents can also significantly affect gastric accommodation reflexes [35]. Certain diets may influence upper gut motility, e.g., consistent exposure to a high fat diet can attenuate the motor response of the pylorus to intraduodenal fat but increase the duodenal motor response to this stimulus [36]. Developmentally, the neuroregulatory mechanisms responsible for the coordination of antropyloric motility and gastric emptying seem to be well-developed by 30 weeks from conception [37].

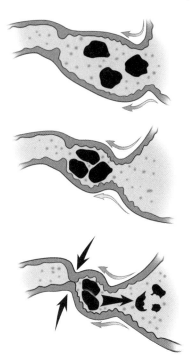

Figure 2. Diagram of normal trituration of solids in the stomach. Solid food particles are trapped and ground in the antropyloric mill until they are reduced to a size of 2 mm or less, when they can be emptied from the stomach.

In the small intestine, detailed studies of the postprandial motor response suggest that there may be considerable organization within the apparently irregular motor activity. Although contractions propagating over long distances are suppressed in the postprandial period, more localized contractile events are common and serve to advance the meal slowly in a caudad direction and promote mixing and digestion. In the terminal ileum, a clear differentiation between fasting and postprandial motor activity may prove difficult. A volume as small as 4 ml/kg of full-strength formula has been found to stimulate a postprandial jejunal motor response in neonates, with intermittent, variable-amplitude contractions and short bursts of clustered contractions [38].

The generation and propagation of the small bowel MMC appear to be intrinsic to the gut and independent of extrinsic nerves. The ability to switch from the fasted to the fed state, however, is largely dependent on the vagus nerve [39]. The postprandial motor response in the stomach is mediated to a large extent through the vagus. While the integration of the gastric component with the small bowel MMC remains incompletely understood, it appears that both extrinsic nerves (especially the vagus) and hormonal factors (in particular motilin) are involved. Thus, phase 3 activity that begins in the stomach is associated with a rise in the serum motilin level. Exogenously administered motilin induces this same activity. However, other activity that begins in the proximal jejunum occurs without a rise in serum motilin [40]. The normal intestinal microflora also provide a stimulatory drive for the initiation and propagation of the small bowel phase 3 activity front [41]. Phase 2 motor activity depends largely on central input, as it is virtually abolished during sleep and after vagotomy.

The act of vomiting encompasses a programmed sequence of events that includes the initiation of retrograde giant contractions that propel the contents of the proximal small bowel into the stomach, the subsequent expulsion of gastric contents by a somatomotor response of diaphragmatic and abdominal muscle contraction, and relaxation of both esophageal sphincters [42].

— Gallbladder and Sphincter of Oddi

A liter of bile is produced daily by the liver and flows preferentially into the gallbladder. In the fasting, state less than one quarter of the bile flows directly through the sphincter of Oddi (SO) into the duodenum. The rate of bile delivery to the duodenum fluctuates with the MMC and is lowest during phase 1 and highest at the end of phase 2 activity. This difference in rate is not only due to variations in the tone of the gallbladder and the SO, but also to variations in the rate of secretion of the bile. After a meal, the gallbladder contracts and empties approximately 50% of the contents of the gallbladder. During postprandial gallbladder emptying the tone of the SO is diminished. In addition, peristaltic contractions occur in the sphincter, which pump bile into the duodenum [43].

— Colon

The motor functions of the colon include propulsion, accommodation or storage, and rapid emptying of a variable portion of the colon during defecation. Propulsion is achieved by a number of motor events including individual contractions, contractile bursts, high-amplitude propagated contractions (HAPCs) and possibly changes in tone. HAPCs propagate rapidly through the colon to propel contents from the ascending or transverse colon to the sigmoid colon or rectum (Figure 3), and correspond to the migrating long-spike bursts described on electromyographic recordings [44]. HAPCs have been correlated, to some extent, with large volume movements of the intraluminal content of the colon that were initially recognized on barium studies as "mass movements." Prolonged recordings of colonic motility have shown that HAPCs occur more often in the morning, during the postprandial period, and preceding defecation [45–47]. HAPCs decrease in frequency from several per hour after a meal in awake toddlers, to only

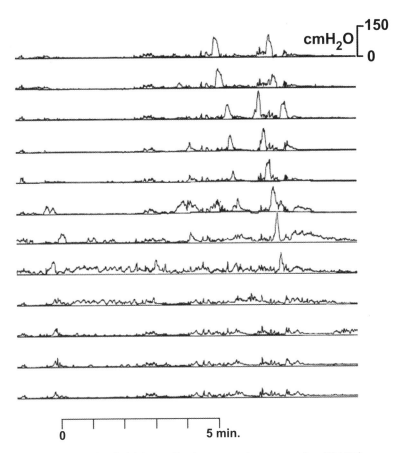

Figure 3. Example of a high-amplitude propagating contraction (HAPC) in the colon. Recording obtained using a 12-channel manometric catheter, positioned to the hepatic flexure and with sensors located at 6-cm intervals along the catheter.

several per day in adults [48]. Other colonic motor events propel contents over short distances in either an orad or an aboral direction, and their primary function appears to be to facilitate mixing. It is likely that regular contractile bursts —colonic motor complexes—do occur, each burst occurring once or twice per hour and lasting approximately six minutes. Periodic or cyclical motor activity is more clearly evident in the rectum, the so-called rectal motor complexes. Although these are also more prominent during sleep, they do not appear to be synchronized with the small intestinal MMC and their precise function and regulation remain unclear. In terms of sensitivity of the colon, experimental distension

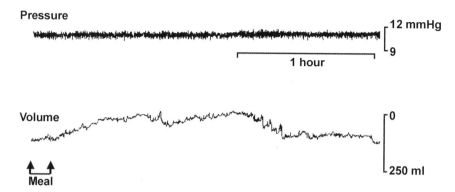

Figure 4. Example of the normal postprandial increase in tone in the descending colon measured using the electronic barostat. Note reduction in volume of colonic balloon (lower tracing) following the meal, which represents an increase in tone.

of the descending or sigmoid colon is perceived as a sensation of cramping, gas, or pressure in the lower abdomen, lower back, or perineum [49].

Accommodation and storage are essential functions of the colon so that fluids, electrolytes, and some products of carbohydrate and fat digestion can be salvaged by bacterial metabolism. However, the mechanisms of such salvage remain unclear. Accommodation and storage are at least partly mediated by colonic tone. Fluctuations in tone (Figure 4) also facilitate distribution of material in the colon. Tone and phasic activity in the colon demonstrate considerable diurnal variation, increasing slowly following a meal, reducing during sleep, and increasing dramatically upon waking [50, 51]. The colonic motor response to eating consists of an increase in phasic and tonic contractile activity that begins within several minutes of ingestion of a meal and continues for a period of up to 3 hours. As in the small bowel, the response is influenced by both the caloric content and composition of the meal. Thus, fat and carbohydrate stimulate colonic motor activity, while amino acids and protein inhibit motor activity. The response of the proximal colon is less substantial than the distal colon [44].

— Anorectum

The anorectum functions in defecation and continence. Defecation is achieved through the integration of a series of motor events and involves both striated and smooth muscle [52, 53]. A sensation of rectal fullness is generated by rectal afferents when colonic contents reach the rectum [17]. Rectal filling also induces the rectoanal inhibitory or rectosphincteric reflex that leads to internal anal sphincter relaxation and external sphincter contractions. At this stage,

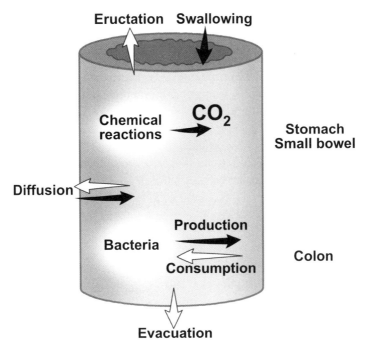

Figure 5. Schematic diagram of intestinal gas metabolism. Gas input results from swallowing, chemical reactions, diffusion from blood, and bacterial fermentation. Gas output is achieved by eructation, absorption, bacterial consumption, and anal evacuation. Gas transit determines the time of exposure for diffusion of gases across the gut-blood barrier, as well as for bacterial consumption, and hence, may influence intestinal gas volume, composition, and tolerance.

the individual can decide to postpone or proceed with defecation. To facilitate the process, the puborectalis muscle and external anal sphincter relax, thereby straightening the rectoanal angle and opening the anal canal. The propulsive force enabling defecation is then generated by contractions of the diaphragm and the muscles of the abdominal wall that propel the rectal contents through the open sphincter. The internal anal sphincter is a continuation of the smooth muscle of the rectum and is under sympathetic control; it provides approximately 80% of normal resting anal tone. The external anal sphincter and pelvic floor muscles are striated muscles that are innervated by sacral roots and the pudendal nerve. The anorectum represents the second site (the first being the upper esophagus) of convergence of the somatic and autonomic nervous systems and is therefore susceptible to disorders of both striated and smooth muscle, as well as to diseases of the central, peripheral, and autonomic nervous systems. Developmentally, the majority of premature infants have normal anorectal pressures and a normal rectoanal inhibitory reflex by 26 weeks of age [54].

— Intestinal Gas

Intestinal gas originates from swallowed air, chemical reactions, diffusion from the blood, and bacterial fermentation. Gas is eliminated from the gut by belching, absorption into the blood, bacterial consumption, and anal evacuation (Figure 5). Under normal conditions, the gut contains only 100–200 ml of gas [55]. The stomach contains a small air bubble introduced by swallowing, and excess gas is eliminated by belching, absorption, or emptying into the intestine. In the proximal small bowel, large quantities of gas are released from neutralization reactions of acids and alkalis. The colon harbors different pools of gas-producing and gas-consuming micro-organisms. Gas-producing bacteria ferment various unabsorbed substrates, releasing hydrogen and carbon dioxide. Gas-consuming micro-organisms metabolize large amounts of gases, particularly hydrogen, and release methane or sulphur-containing gases. Intraluminal gases tend to equilibrate with gases in venous blood depending on diffusibility and the partial pressure of each gas on either side of the gut-blood barrier. Carbon dioxide released in the small bowel is highly diffusible and readily absorbed. A proportion of the gases produced by colonic bacteria undergo diffusion into the blood, and the gases are excreted in the breath, where they can be detected by gas chromatography. The remaining gases are eliminated through the anus. The composition of intraluminal gas varies greatly along the gut, and the gases evacuated in flatus reflect the net balance of the multiple processes within the gut lumen. The propulsion of intestinal gas through both the small and large bowel determines the time available for gas diffusion and for bacterial consumption, and is finely regulated by reflex mechanisms. Gas transit therefore plays a key role in intestinal gas homeostasis [56–59].

Current Techniques to Evaluate Sensorimotor Function of the Digestive Tract

Following the general principles outlined in the previous section, this section will describe the currently available techniques to evaluate digestive tract sensorimotor function, with particular reference to the FGIDs. Both sensory and motor function can be evaluated by provocative testing, depicted schematically in Figure 6. Indeed, most of the sensorimotor alterations documented in the FGIDs have been in response to some form of stimulation. A number of modulatory factors affect the sensorimotor responses elicited to a particular stimulus.

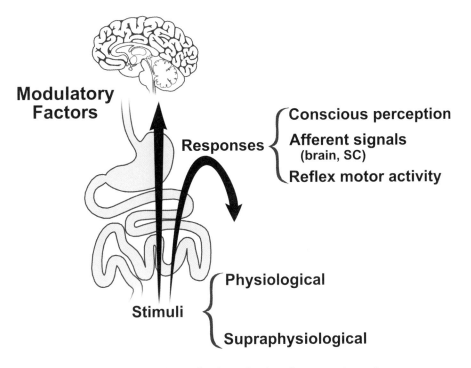

Figure 6. Provocative testing schema for the evaluation of gut sensation and motility in the functional gastrointestinal disorders. See text for further details. SC=spinal cord.

— Stimulation Techniques

The processes of digestion involve numerous stimuli within the gastrointestinal tract. These physiological stimuli induce specific reflexes to accomplish the digestive function, and normally the entire process evolves in an unperceived fashion, as discussed previously. Studies examining visceral sensitivity and enteric dysmotility in FGIDs can be undertaken using different types of physiological or supraphysiological stimulation.

Gastrointestinal Distension

A commonly applied stimulus in studies of FGID patients is gastrointestinal distension. Distension of the gut can be performed by means of a distending device—a balloon or similar device—mounted over a tube. High-compliance latex balloons have relatively low intrinsic pressures, and compliance can be calculated with a reasonably small error by subtracting balloon pressure measured outside the body at equivalent volumes. Flaccid bags with negligible intrinsic pressure require no corrections and may be preferable. However, an oversized bag is required, because if the capacity of the bag is attained during distension, the function of the gut is not reliably recorded. Unfortunately, larger bag size can interfere with delivery, particularly in the upper gut, although ultrathin polyurethane bags can be finely folded and swallowed with minimal discomfort [60]. Standard bags between 40 and 1000 ml are available for distension tests; the size of the bag should be adapted to that of the gut segment under study [15] (e.g., at least 1000 ml for gastric distension and 450 to 600 ml for rectal distension).

Distensions can be produced simply by manual inflation using a syringe, or with more sophisticated methods such as the barostat, which applies fixed intraluminal pressures [15, 31, 60], or the tensostat, which applies fixed tension levels to the gut wall [14]. The barostat is an electronic pump that adapts the volume of air within a distending bag to maintain the desired intrabag pressure. The devices can be conveniently programmed to administer pressure-based or volume-based distensions in a variety of patterns. By analogy, the tensostat is a computerized distension system that, based on intrabag pressure and volume, estimates wall tension and drives an air pump to maintain the desired tension level. As described earlier, it is likely that perception of gut distension relies on stimulation of tension receptors, while intraluminal volume seems not to be a determinant [14, 16, 17]. However, the relationship between wall tension and intraluminal pressure permits the use of barostat devices for most purposes. The major advantages of computerized distension devices over hand-held syringes are standardized inflation rates, maintenance of fixed pressures as the gut accommodates, and the facility to program sequences of distensions. Thus, distension can be applied as graded pressure increments (ascending method of limits) that are administered in phasic (return to baseline pressure between stimuli), stepwise (progressive pressure increases without return to baseline), or ramp fashion (constant gradual increase in pressure) [15, 61]. Alternatively, random or semirandom distension series that make the stimuli less predictable can be performed. Tracking paradigms can be used to test threshold ratings repeatedly (Figure 7) [62]. Assessment of gastric and colonic sensitivity using the barostat can be used to determine the efficacy of novel medications with putative effects on visceral hypersensitivity [63–66].

Other Stimuli

Nutrients

Meal ingestion or intraluminal nutrients infused at physiological concentrations can also serve as provocative stimuli in the FGIDs. Nutrients can be infused into the stomach or duodenum, or more distally into the small intestine.

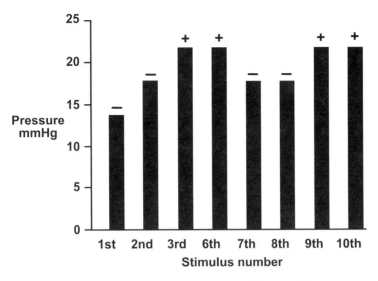

Figure 7. A tracking method for sensory testing is illustrated. Sensory thresholds for a particular sensation can be estimated by allowing the subject to interact with the testing device. In the example above, phasic pressure stimuli increase steadily until the sensation of interest is reported by the subject (+). To reduce the predictability of the testing protocol, the next stimulus is determined randomly by the distention device to be either the same or lower. If that stimulus fails to reach threshold (-), the next stimulus is determined randomly to be the same or higher in intensity. The threshold of interest is thus interrogated. Averaging the pressures (or other measure of intensity) of all stimuli after threshold is first reached, is thought to approximate the sensory threshold of interest.

The composition and nature of nutrients (e.g., proportion of fat, carbohydrate, protein; solid, liquid, or mixed) as well as their route of delivery can be tailored to suit the particular experimental design. The effect of nutrients is exaggerated in functional dyspepsia resulting in aggravation of the hypersensitivity of both the proximal stomach and the antrum [23]. In irritable bowel syndrome (IBS), test meals can evoke more intense small- and large-bowel contractile responses than in health [26, 67].

Load Tests

The main techniques in this category are the so-called drink tests. The general principle of these load techniques is that water or a caloric beverage is ingested until a particular sensory threshold is reached and the volume is recorded.

Alternatively a fixed amount is ingested, followed by a sensory rating [68]. The relative simplicity of this type of testing is attractive, but the drawback of these methods is that the subject is not blinded to the magnitude of the stimulus, and in some circumstances, may be able to vary the rate of intake. Direct infusion into the stomach could theoretically overcome these biases. Intraluminal continuous infusion of gas can also be used to evaluate intestinal handling and tolerance of extrinsic gas loads [59, 69, 70]. In IBS subjects, passage of gas is delayed, and symptoms of bloating are greater than in control subjects [59, 69].

Acid Perfusion

With respect to proximal gut sensation, acid is a relevant stimulus for chemoreceptors and can also affect mechanoreceptors [71]. Thus, acid perfusion of the esophagus leads to cerebral cortical blood flow changes detectable by functional magnetic resonance imaging (fMRI) even in the absence of chest pain or pyrosis [72]. Acid perfusion of the duodenum induces nausea in some normal subjects [73]. Esophageal and duodenal acid perfusion have been used to detect abnormal acid sensitivity in gastro-esophageal reflux disease (GERD) and non-cardiac chest pain [74, 75] and in functional dyspepsia [73] respectively.

Hormonal and Pharmacological Stimulation

A variety of neuropeptides have been applied to FGID patients. Cholecystokinin (CCK) is the best studied of these and has been documented to provoke exaggerated contractile responses of the small and large bowel in patients with IBS when compared to control subjects [67]. Hormonal stimulation has received less attention in recent years, probably because of the difficulty in administering a physiological dose range of the peptide, and studies of visceral hypersensitivity with hormonal stimulation are not available. The potential role of corticotropin-releasing factor (CRF) is discussed later in this chapter. Pharmacological stimulation has also been used in FGID patients, particularly the local administration of laxatives in the colon in patients with functional constipation [76].

Transmucosal Electrical Nerve Stimulation

Testing somatic sensitivity involves a variety of stimuli each activating a specific pathway. For instance, low-threshold mechanoreceptors, which produce a faint tactile sensation at levels near the detection threshold, can be assessed by cotton wisps. Low intensity electrical stimulation activates the same pathways, but does so through direct activation of afferent axons independently from receptors [77]. By analogy to transcutaneous electrical nerve stimulation, transmucosal electrical nerve stimulation can be used as an alternative to mechanical distension for testing visceral sensitivity. Transmucosal electrical stimulation can be produced via intraluminal electrodes mounted over a tube [25]. While this technique has not been widely applied to the FGIDs, it is of interest to note that patients with noncardiac chest pain are hypersensitive to both mechanical and electrical stimulation of the esophagus, whereas IBS patients are hypersensitive only to mechanical stimulation of the small bowel [25] and both mechanical and electrical stimulation of the rectum [78, 79, 80].

— Measurement of the Responses to Stimulation

Gut stimuli may induce a number of responses that can be evaluated in the laboratory, including conscious perception, other measurable cortical responses, specific autonomic responses, and various motor responses.

Measurement of Conscious Perception

There is no "gold standard" with which to measure visceral perception, so a variety of techniques used to measure somatic pain have been adapted to test visceral sensitivity. Assessment of conscious perception encompasses the following aspects: (1) the quality of the perceived sensations (e.g., nausea, fullness, colicky sensation), (2) the intensity of the perceived sensations (e.g., mild to severe), and (3) the affective dimension of the perceived sensations (e.g., pleasant, unpleasant). The intensity of perception can be measured using scales or with threshold detection paradigms (i.e., the magnitude of stimulus required to reach a certain level of perception such as discomfort or pain, see Chapter 15). Scales can introduce verbal descriptors (mild, moderate, severe discomfort, and/or pain) or just allow a rating of intensity or affect associated with the stimulus between none and maximal (e.g., visual analog or Likert scales) [15, 81, 82]. However, it is not clear whether descriptors such as pain or discomfort are related more to the intensity or to the quality of the sensations, and it is important to explain the scales to the subjects prior to testing.

When applying stimuli of increasing magnitude, subjects can be asked to indicate the first stimulus that reaches a certain threshold. One technique to minimize bias while assessing sensory thresholds is the double random staircase stimulation tracking paradigm, a technically complex variant of tracking. This method allows repeated interrogation of the reported threshold in a manner that does not allow anticipation of the next stimulus, thus reducing response bias [82]. With this method, thresholds are defined as the average intensity of stimuli triggering the sensation of interest. In IBS patients, subjective reports of increased visceral sensitivity are reduced by the use of such unbiased sensory testing methods. However, even when the least biased methods of threshold detection are used, many patients may still display response bias, as evidenced by one report that approximately half of IBS patients (n=45) remained "hypersensitive" to rectal distension [82].

The importance of separate collection of data on intensity and affect associated with a stimulus is illustrated by another report that indicated it is the affective dimension of visceral pain that is abnormal in IBS rather than the intensity of the stimulus [83]. In this study, a group of ten IBS patients utilized significantly higher unpleasantness ratings of a rectal distending stimulus compared to healthy subjects, but there were no differences between the two groups in the sensory intensity rating of the stimulus. Various instruments and questionnaires have been used to assess other sensory characteristics, such as the location of the sensation, [15, 81] and altered viscerosomatic referral in the FGIDs. Overall, however, it should be remembered that somatic and visceral sensitivity bear significant differences that are not well defined, and "borrowing" technology from the study of somatic sensation may limit the interpretation of results in the FGIDs. Detailed procedures and protocols for the evaluation of visceral sensitivity using barostat technology are available [15].

Measurement of Central Responses: Detection of Afferent Signals in the Brain

A number of techniques have been developed in the last decade that allow the detection and location of signals within the CNS that result from stimulation of the gastrointestinal tract [84]. These techniques have enabled further investigation of the phenomenon of sensory processing in the FGIDs. In general, the techniques measure either electromagnetic activity of activated brain regions or increases in cerebral blood flow associated with such activation. These methods allow detection of the central representations of visceral stimuli and provide an understanding of the way in which nonpainful and painful visceral sensations are processed in the brain. Such measurements of brain activation associated with a stimulus do not rely on the subjective nature of perception.

Cortical Evoked Potentials (CEP)

This technique is a development of standard techniques used in clinical neurophysiology for the detection of visual and auditory evoked potentials. It involves the repeated high-frequency stimulation of an area of the gastrointestinal tract at a precisely defined interval and the coordinated recording of electroencephalography (EEG) activity from the scalp within a time period of interest. The most robust data come from electrical, rather than mechanical, stimulation. Using averaged signals, extraneous brain activity is reduced in amplitude while the electrical responses of interest become more prominent. Specialized mapping equipment and recording from multiple electrodes attached to the surface of the scalp enables identification of the sites on the somatosensory cortex activated by the upper and lower gut. Furthermore, the latencies associated with pathways can be determined. This provides an estimate of nerve conduction velocities and may imply delays due to central processing of visceral signals. Processing of afferent signals in deeper, noncortical sites cannot be assessed by this technology. Electrical stimulation of the esophagus in patients with noncardiac chest pain provoked lower amplitude and shorter latency CEP than in controls [85]. Two studies of control subjects and patients with IBS indicated concordant findings: patients demonstrated shorter CEP latencies between rectal balloon stimulus and cortical response (in some instances in association with reduced perception thresholds) compared to controls [78, 79]. These findings support the concept of visceral hypersensitivity in the FGIDs by confirming the presence of alterations in the function of neural pathways from the gut to the cortex in FGID patients.

Magnetoencephalography

Magnetoencephalography (MEG) is a sophisticated development of eletroencephalography (see above) involving the use of highly sensitive magnetometers placed over the scalp to detect minute changes in magnetic field induced by cortical afferent nerve activity. This technique has a major advantage over EEG because the magnetic field is not dispersed by overlying tissue (e.g., the skull), enabling the source of the magnetic signal to be localized more accurately. With this technique it is possible to identify the locus for representation of specific gut areas on the primary somatosensory cortex with a resolution of 2 to 3 mm. As with EEG, MEG detects surface projections to the cerebral cortex and cannot be used to assess deeper structures such as the thalamus and limbic system. The technique is not widely available, and has undergone only limited use with respect to gastrointestinal sensory testing [86, 87].

Cerebral Blood Flow

Several techniques are used to assess cerebral blood flow.

Positron Emission Tomography (PET)

This technique involves the use of a sophisticated detecting apparatus capable of recognizing the emission of positrons from the brain. Radio-labeled water produced in a cyclotron is injected intravenously and its concentration within the brain depends upon cerebral blood flow. By comparing regional cerebral blood flow between stimulated and unstimulated conditions, those areas activated by gut stimulation can be identified. Current state-of-the-art equipment is capable of identifying areas of cerebral activation with a spatial resolution of 2–3 mm. Statistically based mapping routines (for example, statistical parametric mapping: SPM, www.fil.ion.ucl.ac.uk/spm) permit a "subtraction" assay to demonstrate focal increases in blood flow over baseline. Such techniques enable comparison between experimental conditions and between groups of subjects. Unlike electrical and magnetic studies, however, the temporal resolution of the technique is relatively low (around 30 to 60 s), so that identification of sequences of activation between brain regions in response to a specific gut stimulus is not possible.

Because FGIDs are frequently associated with depression, neuroimaging data from such patients require controls for the changes observed in depression and other psychiatric disorders [88]. Moreover, the interpretation of the functional significance of differences in CNS blood flow remains problematic due to heterogeneity in individual responses to stimulation, numerous technical variables, and not least our current relatively primitive understanding of brain function. Most FGID studies have to date been limited to rectal distension in IBS. Two such PET studies available in IBS patients both indicate altered brain activation in IBS, particularly in subregions of the anterior cingulate cortex [89, 90]. The anterior cingulate cortex is of interest since visceral stimuli lead to robust activation here, and its subregions are prominently involved in representation of pain and emotions. (See Chapter 2.) Studies of colonic distension in health have revealed similar regions of brain activation as rectal distension [91], but studies in IBS are not available. Differences between cerebral responses to rectal distension in men and women have been reported in a study of healthy subjects and in a study of IBS patients [92, 93]. In both studies, men demonstrated greater activation of the insular cortex than women. Women with IBS had greater activation of the anterior cingulate cortex and amygdala regions—areas typically activated by emotional stimuli—than men. The implications of these gender differences are not fully understood.

Functional Magnetic Resonance Imaging

This technique uses standard magnetic resonance imaging equipment but employs complex data processing to identify areas of regional variation in blood flow induced by gut stimulation. When areas of the brain are activated by neuronal stimulation, the ratio of oxygenated to deoxygenated hemoglobin flowing through the brain region is increased and is associated with an increase in the magnetic signal. This technique has a spatial resolution at least as good as PET, but has greater temporal resolution and can be used repeatedly, both in healthy subjects and in patients, since there is no radiation exposure. A disadvantage of fMRI is susceptibility to artifact around the sinuses and brainstem.

Functional MRI has also been used to study IBS patients. Although there is some heterogeneity among studies, the largest fMRI study of rectal distension in IBS patients and control subjects indicates similar patterns of insula, prefrontal cortex, thalamus, and anterior cingulate activation in both groups. However, the IBS patients demonstrate greater intensity and a larger area of activation in the anterior cingulate cortex than control subjects [94] (Figure 8). These findings have been subsequently confirmed, particularly in the dorsal anterior cingulate [95].

Single Photon Emission Computerized Tomography (SPECT)

SPECT is an adaptation of measured cerebral blood flow using gamma-emitting isotopes. It requires sham and active stimulation studies for comparisons of flow, and since the gamma-emitter (typically ^{99m}TC) has a half-life measured in hours, focal increases in blood flow over background can only be resolved by repeat stud-

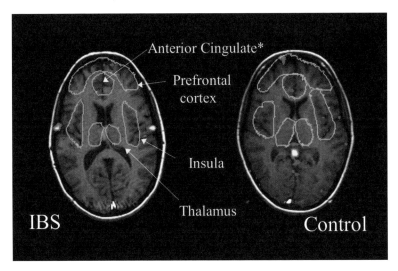

Figure 8. Studies of brain activation in IBS and health using functional magnetic resonance imaging (fMRI). Examples of individual brain responses to painful rectal distension are displayed. Regions of interest with activation in IBS and health are circled, and include the prefrontal cortex, the anterior cingulate cortex, the insula cortex bilaterally, and the thalamus. In IBS patients, greater activation is noted in the anterior cingulate (Reproduced from reference 94 with permission from the American Gastroenterological Association)

ies separated by at least one day [96]. It is possible that the availability of a larger number of appropriate radioligands for SPECT will lead to an increased application of its use to investigate aspects of brain function in the FGIDs.

In summary, data from studies of cerebral blood flow in response to rectal distension in IBS patients indicate altered patterns of cerebral activation and intensities when compared to control subjects. While there is diversity in the literature, the largest studies suggest that IBS patients demonstrate augmented activation in the dorsal portion of the anterior cingulate cortex, which correlates with increased subjective pain reports to the stimuli [90, 94, 95]. These data do not necessarily indicate a cerebral etiology for visceral hypersensitivity; in fact they could reflect a normal cerebral response to a heightened incoming sensory signal. Other studies, however, suggest that brain areas important in descending pain inhibition, namely the perigenual anterior cingulate cortex and the periaqueductal gray region of the brainstem [97] appear to be underactive in IBS [89, 90] and further studies are awaited with interest.

Measurement of Autonomic Responses

In the absence of a widely accepted and convenient test of visceral autonomic integrity, autonomic responses to visceral stimuli are usually measured by using tests of primarily cardiac autonomic innervation; it is not known, however, whether this measurement is representative of other autonomic responses to gut stimuli. Continuous electrocardiograph (ECG) recording before, during and after stimulation allows analysis of the variation in heart rate with the respiratory cycle (heart rate variability). Fourier analysis of this variation can determine the relative amount of high-frequency and low-frequency band power, as indicators of cardiovagal and cardiosympathetic influence respectively; this technique has been widely applied to the study of gastrointestinal phenomena [74]. For example, electrical stimulation of the esophagus in healthy subjects induces an increase in high-frequency power, indicating increased cardiovagal activity [98]. Emmanuel and Kamm [99] have proposed that measurement of rectal mucosal blood flow by laser Doppler flowmetry reflects the level of autonomic innervation specifically to the gut, although other investigators have to date not applied this technique.

The RIII reflex is a polysynaptic reflex that is elicited by electrical stimulation of a sensory nerve via cutaneous electrodes. This stimulation results in a response that is measured at the level of a flexor muscle in the ipsilateral limb. The threshold and amplitude of the RIII reflex are closely related to those of the concomitant cutaneous sensations evoked by electrical stimulation, [100] and such an experimental setup allows an evaluation of somatic perception. The RIII reflex can be inhibited by visceral sensations reaching the level of pain; thus, inhibition of the reflex can be used as a technique to evaluate visceral sensations, and the interaction between somatic and visceral sensitivity [101].

—   Measurement of Gut Motor Responses

Numerous invasive and noninvasive techniques can be employed to measure gastrointestinal motor function; techniques are available to measure each of the phenomena of myoelectrical activity, intraluminal pressure, tone, compliance, wall motion, and transit. Because gut stimuli that induce conscious perception and altered autonomic activity may also induce reflex motor responses in the digestive tract, motility is usually measured during basal conditions and in response to different forms of stimulation (e.g., swallowing, meal ingestion, gut distension). It is less typical to measure other forms of reflex responses such as secretion. The various types of reflex motor responses, particularly in relation to mechanical distension, have been well characterized using animal models and some responses have been used as an indirect index of nociception. However, responses in healthy humans differ from those in acute experiments in anesthetized animals, largely because the magnitude of the stimuli applied in conscious subjects is much smaller. Moreover, since phasic activity is intermittent, it may be difficult to assess contractile responses to brief stimuli, especially since most reflexes induced by distension are inhibitory. In this setting, changes in gut tone, assessed by the barostat, can be useful [60]. For example, in the small bowel, distension of the distal jejunum triggers retrograde mechanosensory reflexes that induce a small and inconstant tonic relaxation in the proximal jejunum a short distance away (5 cm), but a prominent relaxation a long distance away (40 cm). Further, the distal jejunum does not respond to distension of the proximal jejunum, whereas the proximal jejunum responds to both antegrade and retrograde reflexes, with distending stimuli inducing similar relaxation responses at orad and caudad sites. It is important to note that mechanisms mediating perception and reflex motor responses may be different [21]. In the colon, important reflexes include ascending inhibitory reflexes such as the rectocolonic reflex. Thus, irritation of the rectal mucosa by glycerol results in a left colonic reflex marked by a relaxation with superimposed high-amplitude contractions that reach conscious perception, [76] while rectal distension provokes decreased left colonic tone [102]. Gastric emptying [103] and small intestinal contractile activity [104] are also reduced by distension of the rectum. This is consistent with the finding that voluntary suppression of defecation for one week results in delayed gastric emptying [105]. Descending excitatory reflexes include the gastrocolonic, ileocolonic, and colorectal tonic reflexes [106, 107]. These ascending and descending reflexes illustrate the potential for a stimulus at one location to modify sensorimotor function in multiple areas of the gut, and require further investigation in the FGIDs.

Table 1 summarizes some of the techniques to measure motility in the esophagus, stomach, small bowel, gallbladder, sphincter of Oddi, colon, and anorectum, and their relevance to the FGIDs, and these are discussed below. The use of two or more techniques in combination enables a more integrated and comprehensive approach to the assessment of motor function.

Esophagus

Manometry
Manometry is the most widely used technique to evaluate esophageal motility, and the methodology for routine, diagnostic stationary esophageal manometry has been standardized to a large extent [19]. For the evaluation of transient lower esophageal sphincter (LES) relaxations, a key pathogenic mechanism in GERD, prolonged manometry with a sleeve sensor is indicated. Although ambulant (24-hour) esophageal manometry can be used to study phenomena in the tubular esophagus that occur infrequently, such as the peristaltic dysfunction characterized as diffuse

Table I. Measurement of Gastrointestinal Motility (See text for details)

Recording Techniques	Main Applications
I Transit	
radio-opaque markers and X-ray*	gastric emptying, colonic transit
hydrogen breath tests*	orocecal transit
scintigraphy*	esophageal transit
	gastric emptying
	small bowel and colonic transit
	bile flow
	dynamics of defecation
labeled C-substrate breath tests*	gastric emptying
	orocecal transit
magnetic resonance imaging	gastric emptying
pharmacologic markers	
acetaminophen	gastric emptying of liquids
sulfasalazine	orocecal transit time
intraluminal impedance monitoring	esophageal transit
II Reflux	
X-ray	gastroesophageal reflux
scintigraphy	gastroesophageal reflux
pH monitoring	gastroesophageal reflux
bilirubin absorbance monitoring	gastroesophageal reflux
intraluminal impedance monitoring	gastroesophageal reflux
III Wall motion	
ultrasonography	antropyloric contractions
	gastric areas and volume
	gallbladder volume
scintigraphy	antral contractions
magnetic resonance imaging	antral contractions
SPECT	gastric accommodation
IV Intraluminal pressure	
water-perfused manometry*	phasic contractions and sphincter
solid-state transducers	tone at all levels of the digestive tract
V Myoelectrical activity	
electrogastrography	gastric surface electrical activity
intraluminal electromyography	gastric, small intestinal, and colonic electrical activity
needle electromyography	anal sphincter and pelvic floor muscle activity
VI Tone, compliance and wall tension	
barostat	tone and compliance at all levels of the GI tract

*most widely available techniques

Modified from "The Functional Gastrointestinal Disorders," Second Edition, 2000, Ed. Drossman DA with permission esophageal spasm, it is not widely used in clinical practice. The use of high-resolution manometry may enable the identification of clinically important manometric abnormalities not detected by conventional esophageal manometry [108].

Radiography and Scintigraphy

Radiographic and scintigraphic examination of the esophagus can provide information about esophageal transit, at the expense of exposure to ionizing radiation [109]. Although radiographic techniques for the evaluation of esophageal transit are difficult to quantify, for clinical purposes the "timed barium esophagogram" technique may be a reasonable approach [110]. This technique appears to be particularly suitable for the follow-up of patients with achalasia. For the detection of gastroesophageal reflux, radiography and scintigraphy are less suited because of the limited period of observation.

Esophageal pH Monitoring

Although strictly speaking not a test of esophageal motility, ambulatory 24-hour esophageal pH monitoring is a test that provides useful information about the consequences of malfunctioning of the antireflux barrier at the esophageal/gastric junction. Conventional esophageal pH monitoring is carried out with a catheter-mounted pH electrode. Recent developments have made it possible to circumvent the disadvantages of prolonged nasal intubation by using a wireless system with a telemetry capsule [111]. In GERD, esophageal pH monitoring not only allows measurement of the severity of esophageal acid exposure (usually expressed as percentage of time with pH <4), but also allows assessment of the temporal relationship between reflux symptoms and reflux episodes. The latter can be expressed as symptom index [112] or as symptom association probability [113].

Bilirubin Absorbance Monitoring

Theoretical considerations and results of animal experiments suggest that exposure of the distal esophagus to duodenal contents aggravates the deleterious effect of acid exposure. A fiber optic sensor measuring the absorbance of light with the wavelength of bilirubin has been used to study esophageal exposure to duodenal material in humans [114]. The main disadvantage of the technique is that it does not allow the detection of individual, short-lived reflux events [115].

Intraluminal Impedance Monitoring

The technique of intraluminal impedance monitoring [116] using a catheter with an array of closely spaced electrodes has made it possible to monitor esophageal transit [117] and reflux of liquid (including nonacid refluxate) and gaseous material [116] for prolonged periods of time (Figure 9). Intraluminal impedance monitoring may demonstrate the presence of abnormal transit in about 50% of patients with the motor disorder termed ineffective esophageal motility [118]. The imped-

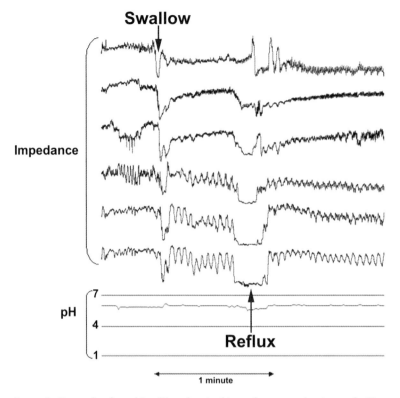

Figure 9. Example of combined intraluminal impedance monitoring and pH recording from the esophagus in an ambulatory subject. The impedance tracings show passage of a liquid bolus in an aboral direction ("swallow") and reflux of liquid material in an oral direction ("reflux"). The concomitant pH tracing shows no drop in pH. The reflux episode should therefore be labeled as "weakly acidic."

ance monitoring technique may provide useful additional information on esophageal motor function, but widespread clinical application is hampered by difficulties with the analysis of the signal.

Stomach

Scintigraphy
Assessment of gastric emptying is often carried out by means of a scintigraphic technique [28]. Various types of meals and isotopes can be used—the important principle being that the isotope should remain totally bound to the solids in the meal during emptying. To assess solid phase emptying [99m]-Technetium-labeled scrambled egg is commonly used; this isotope is not likely to leak into the liquid phase. To achieve standardized results, meals should always be consumed in

the same position and correction for geometric errors should be made by taking anterior and posterior scans and calculating a geometric mean. Because of variations in test substance, methods of scanning, and in calculations, each laboratory should establish its own range of normal values from a control population of adequate size and age- and gender-distribution. However, the use of a standardized low-fat test meal has shown excellent reproducibility and has enabled establishment of international control values [119]. Scintigraphic studies are sensitive and specific for the demonstration of gastric stasis, the sensitivity of the emptying study being related to the nature of the test material.

^{13}C Breath Tests

In recent years, ^{13}C octanoate, ^{13}C acetate, and ^{13}C spirulina breath tests have become increasingly popular to measure solid and liquid emptying [120]. These substances are rapidly digested once they enter the duodenum, releasing labeled carbon dioxide that diffuses into the blood and is excreted in the breath, where it can be measured by gas chromatography. Hence, the level of ^{13}C in the breath reflects gastric emptying. In several studies the ^{13}C octanoic acid breath test has shown reproducibility comparable to standard scintigraphy [121, 122]. Since no radiation is involved, the approach has the potential to become the office-based screening test of gastric emptying in many institutions.

Ultrasonography

This noninvasive method is not only suited to the study of gastric wall movements but to novel 2-dimensional and 3-dimensional methods that allow measurement of cross-sectional areas and volumes [123, 124]. Thus far, more widespread clinical application of ultrasonography is limited by the short observation time feasible, the operator-dependent nature of the results, and the relative paucity of data from studies in disease states.

Electrogastrography (EGG)

Several laboratories have reported the consistent and reliable recording of gastric electrical activity from surface electrodes. Because raw EGG signals are difficult to decipher, their analysis depends on computer-based methods such as fast Fourier transformation and spectral analysis. Abnormal frequencies (bradygastria and tachygastria) can be detected as well as the change in power in relationship to meal ingestion. Though noninvasive and therefore attractive for clinical use, there are numerous pitfalls and the clinical role of EGG remains to be established [125–127].

Magnetic Resonance Imaging

Magnetic resonance imaging (MRI) has been used to assess gastric emptying and to evaluate regional gastric motor function [128, 129]. There is considerable evidence to indicate that this noninvasive technique provides detailed information on gastric function, including the time course of total gastric volume and the intragastric distribution of a meal [130]. It may be possible with MRI to detect abnormal gastric contractile activity, (e.g., patients with gastroparesis) [131]. Fasting gastric volumes determined by 3-dimensional MRI are well correlated with those determined by a gastric barostat [132]. The availability of the technique is limited and the expertise required is considerable—important disadvantages that hinder its use as a clinical tool.

Single Photo Emission Computed Tomography (SPECT)

SPECT can be used as a technique to measure intragastric volumes in addition to its use for evaluating cerebral blood flow discussed previously [133, 134]. Total fasting and postprandial gastric volumes measured by SPECT are larger than intragastric volumes obtained with the gastric barostat. The volumes measured by the two techniques were well correlated in one study [135] but not in another [134]. As with MRI, intragastric volumes do not reflect directly the muscular activity of the gastric wall. The technique remains primarily a research tool since the equipment is not widely available and sophisticated analysis software is required.

Barostat

Although the barostat is an important tool for the assessment of gut sensation, the technique was developed originally to measure gastric tone [31]. The barostat maintains the pressure within an intraluminal bag constant by feedback regulation. Isobaric bag volume changes reflect variations in gut tone: when the gut relaxes (or contracts), the volume increases (or decreases) [60]. The operating pressure in the barostat bag is individually adjusted to 1 to 2 mmHg above intraabdominal pressure. The latter is determined by increasing the pressure slowly, until the barostat captures volume variations associated with respiration [21, 31]. Small differences in the setting of the operating pressure with respect to the intraabdominal pressure may lead to marked differences in the intrabag air volume. Hence, at a constant pressure level the barostat does not measure absolute tone, but only changes in tone. The barostat technique has not become applied widely in clinical practice, as it is invasive and relatively uncomfortable. Nevertheless it remains the reference standard for quantifying gastric accommodation and reflex responses of the stomach to various stimuli [60, 136]. Its reproducibility for intra- or interindividual studies is limited [137].

Small Intestine

Measurement of Intestinal Transit

The radiologic observation of the passage of barium through the gut is difficult to quantify, and in general this technique is not of value for the assessment of transit in clinical practice. Another technique, hydrogen breath testing, relies on the fact that unabsorbed carbohydrates undergo fermentation by the colonic bacterial flora upon arrival in the cecum. The time from ingestion to the onset of rise in breath hydrogen provides an index of the mouth-to-cecum transit time. This technique can be used in clinical practice, using either natural carbohydrate sources such as potatoes, rice or beans, or artificial nonabsorbable compounds such as lactulose and inulin [138]. However, the measured transit time includes not only small intestinal transit but also gastric emptying, and the ingested carbohydrate substrate itself may accelerate small intestinal transit, as was shown for lactulose [139]. Moreover, the test is difficult to interpret when small intestinal bacterial overgrowth is present, as the ingested carbohydrate may then meet bacteria before it has reached the cecum. The early peak in hydrogen excretion measured under these circumstances may lead to the erroneous conclusion that small bowel transit is abnormally rapid. In order to more definitively rule out bacterial overgrowth, a breath hydrogen test with glucose as the substrate can be performed. No rise in hydrogen excretion is expected in the absence of bacterial overgrowth. However, the specificity and sensitivity of breath hydrogen tests to diagnose bacterial overgrowth have not been well defined. More direct tests for the diagnosis of bacterial overgrowth, such as culture or RNA analysis of samples taken from the small intestine, are not widely available and have not been standardized.

Orocecal transit time can also be measured by a ^{13}C-labeled substrate and determination of $^{13}CO_2$ in the expired air [140], while scintigraphic techniques have been used to specifically measure small intestinal transit; these techniques have not found widespread clinical application, however [141]. The transit of gas through the gastrointestinal tract also can be quantified, involving infusion of a gas mixture of nitrogen, oxygen, and carbon dioxide in concentrations as are found in venous blood. By continuous monitoring of the gas evacuated through the rectum, transit, retention and tolerance of intestinal gas can be assessed [56, 57, 142].

Small-Intestinal Manometry
Small-intestinal manometry can be performed with a multilumen perfused catheter with recording sites in the duodenum and proximal jejunum. This technique may be combined with manometry of the antrum, using an array of closely spaced sensors, with or without a pyloric sleeve sensor. High-resolution water-perfused manometry is feasible with silicon microextrusion catheters [143]. Alternatively, a solid-state catheter can be introduced into the small intestine and ambulatory small-intestinal manometry can be done. The assemblies are usually placed under fluoroscopic guidance. The presence and characteristics of the MMC, and its response to stimulation such as nutrient ingestion, are used as markers of enteric motor function [28]. It is important that a sufficiently long recording period in the fasting state is available for analysis [28, 144, 145].

Gallbladder and Sphincter of Oddi (SO)

Scintigraphy

Gallbladder emptying in response to nutrients or hormonal stimulation can be evaluated by means of scintigraphic and ultrasonographic techniques, and an impaired ejection fraction quantified [43]. Following cholecystectomy, bile flow is determined by the rate of bile secretion and the resistance exerted by the SO. By measurement of the rate at which a radiopharmaceutical marker disappears from the biliary tract, in response to stimulation with CCK, an indirect measure of SO tone is obtained. It appears, however, that such scintigraphic results correlate poorly with manometry [146].

SO Manometry

Endoscopic SO manometry is regarded as the most important technique for the assessment of SO motility, but its widespread use is limited because of the risk of acute pancreatitis following the procedure [43, 147]. Because there is significant discordance of basal pressures between the biliary and pancreatic sphincter segments [148, 149] the pancreatic sphincter pressure also should be measured in the case of a normal biliary sphincter pressure. However, the advantages and disadvantages of "dual sphincter" manometry have not been assessed prospectively.

Colon

Scintigraphy, Manometry, and Barostat

These measurement techniques use similar principles as those for the stomach. Scintigraphy with images acquired at long intervals provides an estimate of colonic transit and can identify accelerated or delayed colonic transit. Prolonged stationary multipoint manometry recordings can be obtained in the prepared [45] or in the unprepared [47] colon, while ambulant colonic manometry can also be undertaken in both states [150, 151]. The barostat technique is the reference standard for quantifying colonic and rectal tone [15].

Radiopaque Markers

The radiopaque marker technique is the most widely employed clinical test of colonic motor function. While protocols vary, the essential component of this test is the definition of transit through the colon of orally ingested radio-opaque markers. [152, 153] As well as detecting an overall delay, the pattern of marker distribution can be analyzed as an aid to determining regional colonic transit alterations [153].

Anorectum

Numerous techniques have been applied to assess anal sphincter and pelvic floor function. These include anorectal manometry, defecography (using either radiographic or scintigraphic techniques), balloon expulsion tests, electromyography and tests of rectal tone, compliance, and sensation. Unfortunately, despite their widespread use, these methods have not been completely standardized [52]. Anorectal manometry aims to define resting anal sphincter tone (which primarily reflects the function of the internal anal sphincter and sympathetic innervation), the sphincter pressure during the squeeze maneuver (reflection of external sphincter contraction and parasympathetic innervation), sphincter pressure while straining to defecate (used to detect paradoxical contraction as a cause of outlet dysfunction), the integrity of the rectoanal inhibitory reflex, and rectal sensation. The balloon expulsion test is a simple procedure to identify impaired evacuation (e.g., in patients with functional constipation) [154]. Defecography provides a dynamic evaluation of the function of the pelvic floor during a variety of maneuvers, including attempted evacuation. It may also help to identify such anatomical features as prolapse and rectocele. More commonly, defecography is used to detect the cause of disordered defecation, such as that associated with absent relaxation of the puborectalis, leading to obstructed defecation.

— Modulatory Factors

Many local and extraintestinal factors can modulate visceral perception and therefore require attention in tests of gut sensitivity. For example, perception of gut distension depends not only on gut compliance and tone [13, 14, 155], but also on factors such as the speed of distension [15], and the length of the gut stimulated [156]. Perception may be increased by previous stimulation [49], or simultaneous local stimuli [156]. Ambient blood sugar levels may also influence perception of gastric distension [157] and the menstrual cycle can affect rectal sensitivity in patients with IBS [158]. Extrinsic factors that influence perception include somatovisceral interactions [159], sympathetic arousal [160], and cognitive-affective phenomena [161, 162]. For example, perception of small intestinal distensions is higher during attention than during distraction, and the area of somatic projection is greater during attention [161]. Also, a psychological stress (dichotomous listening) applied during or before rectal distension can induce hypersensitivity to the distension [162], while the same stressor can provoke a moderate increase in the intensity of perception recorded from the sigmoid, but not the transverse, colon [162].

The modulatory factors outlined above as well as the method of measuring the cerebral responses are critical variables that limit direct comparison between studies. For example, anxiety and fear of impending pain can trigger brain activation patterns similar to those evoked by actual stimulation [95]. Similar modulatory factors may also apply to the assessment of motility, including the effects of gut compliance and tone on the responses to gut distension, the phenomenon of spatial and temporal summation, the effects of nutrients and hormones, and cognitive influences, as previously discussed. For example, psychological stress can inhibit postprandial gastric myoelectric activity [163], through both vagal and sympathetic pathway modulation.

Putative Origins of Sensorimotor Dysfunction

As indicated earlier, visceral hypersensitivity and/or enteric dysmotility can be readily documented in the FGIDs and are likely to be important in the pathophysiology of these disorders. This section will focus on the putative underlying causes of this sensorimotor dysfunction, which have been broadly categorized into peripheral or central causes [1] based on our understanding of the organization and control of the brain-gut axis. It is now evident, however, that such factors may potentially play a role at both peripheral and central sites (Figure 10). Moreover, while some factors such as genetics and early life experiences may be regarded as predisposing factors, others such as enteric inflammation and psychosocial stress may be regarded as trigger factors. In some instances, however, the precise role of a given factor, whether predisposing, triggering, or modifying, is unclear.

— Genetic and Early Life Factors

In Chapters 5 and 6, the increasing evidence for the importance of early life experiences and social learning in the pathogenesis of the FGIDs is discussed, and this topic will not be covered here. Genetic factors have also received increasing attention and there is now a body of evidence that supports a likely genetic predisposition to at least some of the FGIDs. This evidence derives from both family and twin studies and is also discussed in Chapters 5 and 6. Some recent genetic studies in postinfectious IBS involving alterations in the frequency of certain phenotypes for specific cytokines, [164] are discussed below, while pharmacogenomic aspects relevant to the FGIDs are discussed in Chapter 4.

Of note in the current context are recent reports in functional dyspepsia (FD) and IBS. In FD, an increased prevalence of a particular G-protein genotype has been documented [165]. This finding raises the possibility that such an underlying second messenger abnormality could explain the variable clinical manifestations of the FGIDs. Thus, G-protein dysfunction potentially could block intracellular signal transduction responses and lead to receptor and consequent sensorimotor dysfunction. Conceivably, precipitation of symptoms could then require additional genetic and/or environmental influences. In IBS, alterations in the synthesis and uptake of secreted serotonin in the gut mucosa have been documented

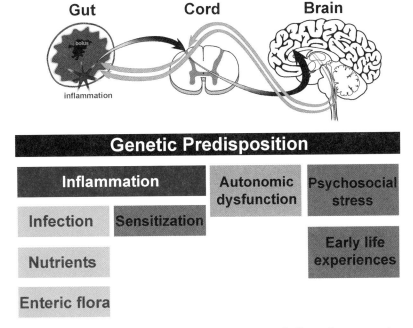

Figure 10. Schematic view of afferent (black arrows) and efferent (grey arrows) signals along the brain-gut axis, and putative factors which may influence these signals (boxes). Afferent signals, particularly consciously perceived ones, are relayed from the gut to the dorsal horn of the spinal cord. Secondary afferents carry these stimuli to the brain. Processing in the brain occurs in several regions, culminating in perception, interpretation, and response. CNS inputs such as psychosocial stress modulate sensory processing and efferent signals to the gut. Efferent signals are generally carried by spinal and vagal/sacral autonomic pathways to the gut. These signals alter motility and secretion in the target organ.

[166], and also alterations in mucosal serotonin turnover and postprandial serotonin release [167]. Given the role of mucosal serotonin in intestinal motility and possibly sensation, it is conceivable that alterations such as those described in the above studies contribute to sensorimotor dysfunction in IBS, but more work needs to be done. Several of the most significant putative environmental factors relevant to the above aspects are discussed in more detail below.

— Enteric Inflammation

The entity of postinfectious IBS (PI-IBS) is well recognized [168], with a prevalence ranging from 7 to 31% following an acute episode of bacterial gastroenteritis [169–178]. Significant risk factors for the development of PI-IBS include female sex, a more prolonged or severe acute episode, and higher scores for anxiety, depression, somatization, and neurosis [169, 171]. Increased numbers of chronic inflammatory cells, rectal mucosal enteroendocrine cells, and T lymphocytes, as well as altered rectal sensorimotor function and altered gut permeability, can be documented in PI-IBS [172, 173, 179, 180]. Indeed, even IBS patients with "normal" conventional histology may also show an increase in intraepithelial lymphocytes and an increase in CD25+ cells in the lamina propria [181]. CD25+ cells are regulatory T cells considered important in the prevention of autoimmunity, as well as in controlling inflammatory responses in the gut. Their increased presence, providing evidence of immune activation, has been postulated to indicate "auto— or exogenous—antigen challenge" in these patients, with these cells preventing the progression to a more florid inflammatory response [182]. In patients with severe IBS, low-grade infiltration of lymphocytes has been demonstrated in the myenteric plexus; in some an associated increase in intraepithelial lymphocytes was present, suggesting a direct, and perhaps causative link, between mucosal inflammation, on the one hand, and inflammation of the ENS, on the other [183]. There was also some evidence of neuronal degeneration, and in most cases, longitudinal muscle hypertrophy and abnormalities in the number and size of interstitial cells of Cajal were also evident. It is conceivable that these patients represent an overlap with chronic idiopathic intestinal pseudo-obstruction, a disorder in which similar neuropathological findings have been described [184].

Prior infection may also explain the increase in terminal ileal and colonic mucosal mast cells documented in IBS [177, 185–189]. The close proximity of mast cells with enteric nerves in IBS raises the possibility of involvement of a neuro-immune axis in the pathophysiology of IBS [187–189]. Mast cells from IBS patients also may be functionally different from those in healthy subjects, spontaneously releasing histamine and tryptase [188]; the number of close nerve-mast cell relationships also correlated well with the presence and severity of abdominal pain (Figure 11). These findings raise the possibility that tryptase may activate specific protease-activated receptors (e.g., PAR-2), shown to be present on sensory nerves, and thus play a role in the development of visceral hypersensitivity in IBS. Histamine also alters neural excitability, and could contribute to altered motility, as well as to altered intestinal barrier function [200].

The persistence of the intestinal inflammatory changes in IBS may arise in response to a relative deficiency of anti-inflammatory cytokines in some individuals [191, 192]. Van der Veek et al. studied single nucleotide polymorphisms of tumor necrosis factor (TNF-α) gene in a large group of IBS patients and healthy subjects, and found a significantly higher frequency of the intermediate producer of TNF genotype in IBS compared to controls [192]. The results were more striking in IBS patients with diarrhea compared to constipated patients or those with alternating bowel habit. A functional correlate of these genomic studies was provided by the demonstration that secretion of cytokines from peripheral blood monocytes

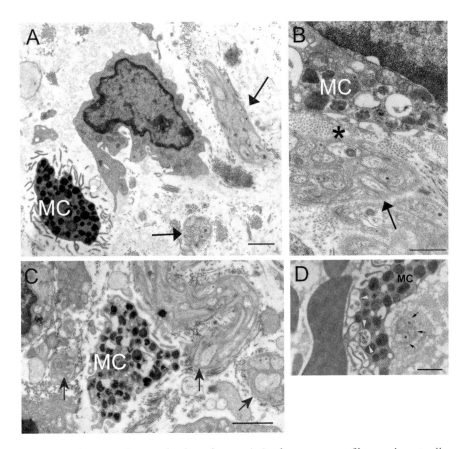

Figure 11. Electron micrographs show the association between nerve fibers and mast cells in the colonic mucosa of a healthy control (A) and IBS patients (B–D). (A) Nerve fibers and a resting mast cell (MC) with characteristic granules in a healthy subject. (B) Electron micrograph obtained from an IBS patient showing membrane-membrane contacts (asterisk) between a degranulating mast cell (MC) and a nerve fiber (arrow). (C) Electron micrograph obtained from an IBS patient showing multiple nerve fibers (arrows) located <5 μm from a degranulating (arrowheads) mast cell (MC). (D) The typical appearance of a degranulating (arrowheads) mast cell (MC) in close vicinity (<5 μm) to a nerve fiber. (bar = 5μm in A,C,D; 2 μm in B). (Reproduced from reference 188 with permission from the American Gastroenterological Association)

of IBS patients differed from controls in a manner predicted by the genetic studies, i.e., the ratio of anti-and pro-inflammatory cytokines was reduced in IBS patients compared to controls [193]. Using interleukin (IL) 1β mRNA as a marker of the inflammatory response to infection, Gwee et al. [194] showed that in patients with acute gastroenteritis, the increase in IL-1β in colonic biopsies was greater in those individuals who went on to develop IBS than those who recovered fully.

This increased expression of the pro-inflammatory cytokine persisted for at least 3 months postinfection. Consistent with this finding is the reduced frequency of the high-producer phenotype for the anti-inflammatory cytokine IL-10 reported in IBS patients [164]. Other evidence for a role of inflammation in IBS comes from reports of an increased prevalence of IBS-type symptoms in patients with inflammatory bowel disease and celiac disease in apparent remission [195].

It should be acknowledged that some studies reporting an association between IBS and immune activation would not be designated as IBS based on current criteria, as they involve the description of pathologic findings indicative of other diagnoses, for example inflammatory bowel disease, celiac disease or microscopic colitis. While these reports reflect the nonspecificity of symptoms of intestinal origin, they also provide avenues for the exploration of the mechanisms whereby inflammation, of any grade, may induce symptoms. However, it must also be stressed that evidence of immune activation has been provided by studies of patients who do not appear to have an alternative diagnosis and who truly appear to suffer from IBS.

Although bacterial gastroenteritis does not appear to be a predisposing factor in functional dyspepsia, [176] upper gut mucosal inflammation and increases in mast cells may play a role in some patients [196, 197]. This is a potentially important area of study, given the high prevalence of infection with *Helicobacter pylori*. Despite this, studies have not generally supported a role for *H. pylori* in the pathogenesis of functional dyspepsia [198–200] and any effect on symptom patterns appears to be minor [201, 202].

Postviral syndromes provide yet another example of infection-provoked dysmotility—a recent review suggested that, among a large group of patients with idiopathic gastroparesis, approximately 25% gave a history that suggested a viral prodrome [203]. Patients with acute and possibly viral-related functional dyspepsia are also more likely to demonstrate impaired fundic accommodation [204] than patients without such an acute onset, and there is evidence for dysfunction at the level of gastric nitrergic neurons in some patients. A major challenge in this area is establishing a definitive diagnosis of the initiating viral insult, since viral infections characteristically leave little imprint. Evidence that specific viruses can profoundly disrupt motor function is provided in a more convincing fashion by the gastroparesis that may accompany cytomegalovirus (CMV) gastritis [205].

— Alterations in Enteric Flora

It is known that bacteria commensal to the gut can influence enteric motor activity, can modulate host immune system development and function, and can enhance epithelial barrier function. It is thus feasible that chronic alterations of the enteric flora may also influence the development of IBS, and there is some evidence that colonic bacteria counts are different in IBS patients compared to healthy subjects [206–208]. More recently, increased bacterial colonization (overgrowth) of the small intestine in IBS has been suggested [209, 210]. Bacterial overgrowth has been associated in IBS and other disorders with a lower frequency of small-intestinal MMCs [211]. This concept is supported by a symptomatic response to the eradication of small-intestinal bacterial overgrowth in IBS, [209, 212] and by the demonstration of overgrowth in disorders commonly associated with IBS, such as fibromyalgia [213]. However, these data are based on lactulose breath testing and have been questioned [214]; further studies in larger populations of IBS are required. An association between antibiotic use and IBS [215] has been reported. It is conceivable that antibiotics may facilitate the enteric effects of potentially immunogenic or pathogenic bacteria by disrupting the normal flora. The use of probiotics as a potential therapy for IBS is currently the subject of intensive research. Preliminary data suggest that IBS patients may respond symptomatically to manipulation of the flora through the use of probiotic bacterial preparations [193, 216–221], but further work is needed before definitive conclusions are made.

— Dietary Components

Patients with both functional dyspepsia and IBS commonly report the exacerbation of their symptoms by food ingestion and assume that this close temporal relationship implies either an allergy or an intolerance to specific food items or constituents [222, 223]. This relationship between eating and symptoms remains poorly understood. The exaggerated sensorimotor effects of certain nutrients (especially fat) in IBS and functional dyspepsia patients have been referred to earlier [23, 26, 59] and could explain symptom provocation without invoking either allergy or intolerance. The nonspecificity of symptoms originating from the GI tract also serves to confound interpretation in this area. For example, while the incomplete absorption in the small intestine of substances such as fructose and sorbitol has been proposed as a trigger for IBS symptoms [224], it is also evident that some of the symptoms of true intolerance to these substances can simulate IBS symptoms.

Relationships between lactose intolerance and IBS also appear quite complex. Thus, while IBS subjects commonly associate milk and milk products with symptom exacerbations [225–227] evidence for an increased prevalence of lactose malabsorption in IBS is lacking [226, 227]. Furthermore, positive lactose breath tests may reflect bacterial overgrowth rather than lactose malabsorption in IBS patients [228]. Although there is some clinical evidence to incriminate other specific foods and chemical substances in the pathogenesis of IBS [222, 225, 229], little substantive evidence exists to link the phenomenon of "food intolerance" to visceral hypersensitivity or dysmotility. Furthermore, trials of elimination diets have provided conflicting and generally disappointing results [225, 226, 229, 230] and there is little evidence for classical forms of food allergy in IBS [224, 229–231]. Some recent studies report some success with elimination diets based on the results of testing for immunoglobin (IG) G (but not IgE) antibodies to foods [232].

The demonstration that intestinal permeability is increased in some patients with PI-IBS, especially those with diarrhea-predominant IBS [180], raises the possibility that luminal antigens may gain more ready access to the mucosal compartment of the gut and enable more prolonged stimulation of the mucosal immune system and the ENS. Other phenomena may also explain the food/symptom link in IBS. For example, abnormal colonic fermentation has been proposed as an important mechanism contributing to food intolerance in IBS on the basis of altered enteric flora due to the effects of gastroenteritis or antibiotic use [233]. In this regard, it is of interest that patients with celiac disease can fulfill symptom criteria for IBS [195, 234–237]. This may simply reflect a significant shift in the presenting symptomatology of celiac disease. Nowadays, this disorder tends to present with "IBS-type" symptoms, such as abdominal pain and bloating, rather than the classical features of malabsorption [238]. At the very least, these observations should prompt screening for celiac disease in patients with IBS [239, 240], especially in areas of high celiac disease prevalence [241, 242]. To further complicate matters, bacterial overgrowth may also complicate celiac disease, and thereby produce IBS-like symptoms [243].

— Autonomic Dysfunction

As outlined earlier, the CNS controls visceral sensorimotor function via the two branches of the autonomic nervous system. An increasing number of studies have documented abnormal autonomic function in the FGIDs, but it remains unclear whether such alterations are a primary phenomenon, are significant modulatory factors, or merely reflect the bidirectional interactions of CNS and ENS dysfunction [244]. As described above, various visceral reflexes have been shown to be abnormal in patients with FGIDs, and although these reflexes are primarily driven by vagal or sympathetic pathways, this does not mean that these patients have a general autonomic dysfunction. Abnormal proximal gastric accommodation in functional dyspepsia may be due to an underlying vagal defect [245], since both functional dyspepsia and postvagotomy patients have a similar impairment of gastric accommodation. Other studies support such a concept [246, 247]. On the other hand, studies of vection-induced nausea and gastric dysrhythmias [248, 249] have raised the possibility of central neurohumoral dysfunction in the pathogenesis of functional dyspepsia. Thus, motion sickness-susceptible and sickness-resistant individuals differed in their central release of vasopressin, rather than displaying a peripheral resistance to its effects. In noncardiac chest pain patients, significantly greater rises in cardiovagal activity in response to esophageal electrical or acid stimulation have been reported [74, 85], while in GERD patients, the perception of heartburn induced by acid infusion was associated with a simultaneous increase in sympathetic modulation [75]. Smart et al. [250] documented abnormal vagal function in IBS, while Aggerwal et al. [251] demonstrated vagal dysfunction to be specifically associated with constipation-predominant IBS, whereas diarrhea-predominant IBS patients displayed evidence of sympathetic adrenergic dysfunction. IBS patients have increased sympathetic activity at rest and impaired suppression of parasympathetic activity during orthostatic stress [252]. Postprandial decreases in cardiovagal tone are observed in diarrhea-predominant IBS patients [253]. Experimental studies indicate that sympathetic activation increases gut perception and may thus contribute to hypersensitivity [160]. In a study of the neuroendocrine and cellular immune responses to a nutrient load [254] it was concluded that IBS patients display an autonomic hyperresponsiveness to visceral stimuli that is independent of acutely perceived gut symptoms and not necessarily associated with hypothalamic-pituitary-adrenocortical activation. These data are preliminary and further studies are required, particularly those that investigate the links between visceral and cardiac autonomic function.

— Psychosocial Stress and Other Cognitive Factors

Factors that influence enteric sensorimotor dysfunction in the FGID include psychological stress and other cognitive aspects [255]. With regard to visceral sensitivity, IBS patients appear to exhibit greater reactivity to mental stress. For example, IBS patients rated rectal distension as more intense when exposed to dichotomous listening compared to relaxing music [256] whereas control subjects did not. Similarly, under conditions of psychological stress, IBS patients displayed increased rectal sensitivity to electrostimulation compared to controls [80]. However, gut-specific efferent autonomic innervation, measured by rectal mucosal blood flow, was not different between IBS and control subjects under stress. Hypervigilance is also a factor that influences symptom reporting by IBS patients during rectal distension testing [82]. Differences between IBS patients and control subjects were not observed with testing methods less subject to bias (e.g., tracking). Cerebral perfusion (prefrontal and anterior cingulate) induced by rectal distension in IBS patients is similar whether a distension was actually administered or merely anticipated [97]. This suggests that psychosocial or cognitive factors may contribute to some of the differences in responses identified in IBS patients. Certainly, anticipatory knowledge increases gut perception [25] and fear of pain (anticipation) or actual pain appear to activate similar cortical networks [95].

With respect to dysmotility, Bennett et al. [257] documented a correlation between delayed gastric emptying in functional dyspepsia and psychological factors, especially suppression of anger, while Haug et al. [258] suggested that reduced vagal activity could be a mediating mechanism by which psychological factors influence gastrointestinal sensorimotor physiology and evoke dyspepsia. Further evidence that cognitive factors contribute to symptom induction in functional dyspepsia was provided by a study demonstrating that both low and high fat foods elicit symptoms if patients perceive the low fat foods as high in fat [259]. In IBS, the effects on small bowel motility of acute psychological stress [260] (produced in a laboratory situation) were not significantly different from controls. These findings contrast with those produced by mental stressors of longer duration, where a pattern similar to clustered contractions was provoked, suggesting that stress of a more chronic nature evokes a different response from that of acute stress [261]. In the colon, the motor response to psychological stress in IBS has been reported as either similar to [262] or higher than [263, 264] that in control subjects. Psychological stress may hasten mouth-to-cecum transit in IBS with diarrhea, but slow transit time in IBS with constipation [265]. Furthermore, a pattern of increasing severity and intensity of psychosocial disturbance was associated with increasing levels of motor and/or sensory dysfunction in IBS [266].

A potential mechanism for the stress-induced responses outlined above is the finding that intestinal permeability can be increased in rats during stress via a cholinergic mechanism [265] and requires the presence of mucosal mast cells [190]. Indeed, chronic psychological stress appears to be an initiating factor in intestinal inflammation in rats by impairing mucosal defenses against luminal bacteria [268]. Other potential mediators of stress-induced gastrointestinal sensorimotor responses include norepinephrine and CRF. CRF has the potential to interact with the entire brain-gut axis as receptors for CRF are diffusely expressed. CRF is known to stimulate release of norepinephrine from the locus ceruleus in the pons. Locus ceruleus activation and subsequent norepinephrine release triggers arousal and attention. There are extensive neural connections from the locus ceruleus to the reticular activating system (which is involved in pain control and arousal) in the brainstem, as well as the parasympathetic motor nuclei of the vagus and sacrum and the sympathetic nuclei of the thoracolumbar spinal cord. Visceral stimulation is known to activate the locus ceruleus, which can be blocked by injection of a CRF antagonist into the CNS [247]. The locus ceruleus therefore has the potential to activate brain responses to visceral stimulation, as well as interact with autonomic effector nuclei in the spinal cord. Hypothalamic CRF release stimulates locus ceruleus norepinephrine release, while locus ceruleus norepinephrine release stimulates hypothalamic CRF release creating a feed-forward loop [247]. Other brain regions such as the amygdala appear able to restrain the release of CRF [269], potentially damping this loop.

In animals, stress is associated with CRF release from the hypothalamus. Two

CRF receptors (1 and 2) have been identified. CRF-1 mediates stress-induced increases in colonic contractility, while CRF-2 mediates stress-induced gastric hypomotility and surgical ileus [270]. Specific antagonists for CRF can block this effect. CRF injected into the fourth ventricle induces similar enteric motor effects in the absence of stress. Of note, the alterations described in response to CRF are similar to those observed in FGID patients: reduced gastric emptying (frequent in functional dyspepsia), and increased colonic contractility (widely described in IBS). Human data suggest that IBS patients are particularly sensitive to CRF effects on colonic motility, showing a greater colonic motor response to CRF infusion than controls [271]. Infusion of CRF into healthy volunteers appears to increase sensitivity to painful rectal distension [272]; studies of sensitivity in IBS patients have yet to be performed. It is conceivable that either heightened release of CRF or heightened sensitivity to CRF contributes to FGID pathophysiology. Other neural and hormonal factors that may play a role in the FGID are CGRP, CCK, serotonin, neurokinins and N-methyl-d-aspartate (NMDA). These substances and their receptors have been variably linked to visceral sensitivity, and in many cases agonists and antagonists are available or are in clinical trials.

Symptom Correlates of Sensorimotor Dysfunction

Ideally, a number of criteria should be satisfied to define a causal relationship between symptoms and sensorimotor dysfunction in the FGIDs, namely: (1) a consistent correlation in time and severity between symptoms and the sensorimotor disorder, followed by (2) an improvement in the sensorimotor disorder associated with clinical improvement, and (3) the production of symptoms by experimental induction of the sensorimotor disorder. None of these criteria has been shown to date to be fulfilled reliably in the FGIDs, and so the clinical relevance of sensorimotor dysfunction in such patients remains unclear. Details on symptom correlates for individual FGIDs can be found in the organ-specific chapters; functional dyspepsia and IBS will be discussed briefly with examples of the difficulties encountered in correlating symptoms with sensorimotor dysfunction, and also to illustrate where progress is being made. Thus, in both functional dyspepsia and IBS, several studies have addressed in detail the relationship between symptoms and sensorimotor dysfunction and some potentially important correlations have emerged.

In functional dyspepsia, although symptoms were generally unhelpful, severe postprandial fullness and vomiting were predictive of gastroparesis [273]. Fock et al. [274] subsequently reported that gastroparesis is associated with the subgroup of "dysmotility-like" functional dyspepsia. In contrast, another study found that functional dyspepsia patients with hypersensitivity to gastric distension were more likely to suffer from epigastric pain, belching, and weight loss, but such visceral hypersensitivity was not associated with gastric motor abnormalities or with *H. pylori* infection [275]. In another large group of functional dyspepsia patients, those with delayed gastric emptying were more likely to suffer from postprandial fullness, nausea, and vomiting [276].

With regard to regional gastric dysmotility, Tack et al. [136] showed that impaired accommodation to a meal is present in 40% of patients with functional dyspepsia. Impaired gastric accommodation was not associated with visceral hypersensitivity, delayed gastric emptying, or the presence of *H. pylori*. The symptom of early satiety was independently associated with impaired gastric accommodation. Weight loss, occurring secondarily to early satiety, was also more prevalent in patients with impaired accommodation. In a group of presumed postinfective functional dyspepsia patients, these same symptoms also were more closely related to impaired accommodation than to other types of sensorimotor dysfunction [204]. A scintigraphic study of the intragastric distribution of a meal in functional dyspepsia has correlated early satiety with early redistribution of liquids to the antrum, and fullness with late proximal retention [277], while in another report [278], a clear relationship between postprandial symptoms and proximal stomach function could not be detected. Administration of the 5-HT1$_P$ receptor agonist sumatriptan was able to restore gastric accommodation in patients with impaired postprandial gastric relaxation and improved early satiety in a double-blind, placebo-controlled, cross-over design [16]. A relationship between antral widening and early postprandial discomfort has also been documented in functional dyspepsia [279, 280]. However, when the relationship between symptoms and ultrasonographic assessments of gastric motor function in functional dyspepsia was examined using glyceryl trinitrate (GTN), an exogenous donor of nitric oxide (NO) [279], it appeared that defective accommodation of the proximal stomach was more likely related to symptom generation than dysmotility of the antrum [16]. In a study of over 400 patients with functional dyspepsia, factor analysis distinguished four main symptom subgroups, and it was possible to relate the groups to different pathophysiological and psychopathological mechanisms, although there remained considerable overlap [282]. Controversy remains, however, as data from another study did not detect differences in symptom patterns in functional dyspepsia patients with and without abnormal accommodation, and with and without delayed gastric emptying of solids [283]. Moreover, Delgado-Aros [284] reported that in tertiary care functional dyspepsia patients, the fasting gastric volume and a rapid initial gastric emptying were associated with reduced maximum tolerated volume, whereas symptoms after meal challenge depended on the volume of meal ingested and increased with faster emptying of nutrients.

Gastric hyporeflexia is another potentially important factor in the reduced tolerance of functional dyspepsia patients to intragastric volume increase, thereby contributing to the generation of clinical symptoms in the absence of major motor dysfunction. Normally, antral filling elicits a reflex relaxation of the proximal stomach that contributes to meal accommodation. Accommodation is then further modulated by enterogastric reflexes depending on the load and composition of intestinal chyme. Impaired gastrogastric and enterogastric reflexes in dyspepsia [23, 159] may result in a defective relaxation of the proximal, but not the distal stomach, with consequent alteration in the intragastric distribution of contents and antral overload. These patients have increased antral perception [23], and overdistension of the hypersensitive antrum may trigger conscious perception and symptoms. Hence, the antrum may represent an important element in the pathophysiology of dyspepsia by playing a dual role: acting as a faulty primer of reflexes and as a symptom-provoking target. Interestingly, antral compliance was found to be greater in patients with dysmotility-like dyspepsia compared to those with ulcer-like dyspepsia, and the replication of the patients' usual symptoms was better with fundic distension in the former and with antral distension in the latter. However, the relevance of these findings remains unclear [23].

In IBS patients, studies of the relationships between motility and sensation show some correlation with symptoms. Steens et al. [285] were able to distinguish IBS patients with diarrhea versus constipation on the basis of rectal sensation, rectal compliance, and rectal tonic responses to a meal. Rectal hypersensitivity is associated with motor hyperactivity in response to gut stimuli [18, 286]; both hypersensitivity and hyper-reactivity could contribute to the perception of rectal tenesmus and fecal urgency in IBS. There is some evidence that postprandial symptoms in IBS are associated with alterations in the colonic motor [287, 288], and sensory [287] response to feeding. Using a 24-hour ambulatory recording of colonic motility, Clemens et al. showed that nonconstipated IBS patients had more segmenting contractions than controls in the sigmoid colon and more high-amplitude contractions [290]. There was a temporal correlation between high-amplitude colonic contractions and pain episodes in nonconstipated IBS patients [290]. However, these high-amplitude contractions were also observed in the absence of pain in IBS patients and did not differ manometrically from those associated with pain. Moreover, only half of the IBS patients in the study showed such contractions. In healthy volunteers, glycerol induces hypersensitivity to rectal distension [291] and triggers giant colonic contractions associated with abdominal pain when infused in the colonic lumen in IBS patients [76]. Although taken together these observations suggest a role for high-amplitude colonic contractions in the pathophysiology of abdominal pain in IBS patients, no evidence has so far been obtained that a pharmacological intervention on these contractions would relieve symptoms.

In the small bowel, the most striking finding supporting the concept of visceral hypersensitivity in IBS patients is the episodes of cramping abdominal pain directly related to the usually nonperceived, intermittent, large-amplitude peristaltic waves in the terminal ileum [67]. These peristaltic waves are more frequent in the postprandial period. Also, IBS patients with jejunal hypersensitivity displayed a higher prevalence of postprandial dysmotility than those without jejunal hypersensitivity [266]. This finding may be relevant to the prominent postprandial symptoms experienced by some IBS patients. In contrast, there was a higher prevalence of fasting dysmotility in the group with normal jejunal sensitivity. Recent studies using a new methodology to evaluate intestinal gas dynamics further substantiate the role of combined sensory and motor disturbances in symptom production. Gas transit studies have provided evidence that patients with bloating have impaired reflex control of gut handling of contents and develop gas retention and symptoms in response to gas loads that are well tolerated by healthy subjects [58, 59]; this dysfunction seems to affect predominantly the small intestine [70]. Segmental pooling, either of gas or alternatively of solid/liquid components, may induce the sensation of bloating, particularly in patients with altered gut perception. Interestingly, symptoms in response to the gas challenge replicate the patients' usual complaints [58, 59, 69]. Recent results suggest that both gas retention and symptoms can be relieved by prokinetic drugs [69]. Furthermore, altered viscerosomatic reflexes may contribute to abdominal wall protrusion and objective distension, even without major intra-abdominal volume increment [292]. Techniques to assess abdominal girth have been developed that are providing a better understanding of the symptoms of abdominal bloating and distension [55, 293, 294].

Role of Sensorimotor Testing in Clinical Practice

Despite the fact that sensorimotor abnormalities can be detected in FGID patients, their diagnostic value in the clinical setting remains limited. This is due to the fact that many of the techniques are not standardized, their indications have not been clearly defined, the correlation between symptoms and abnormalities is poor, and therapeutic options are few. Also, more widespread uptake of many of these procedures in clinical practice has not occurred because they are often either time consuming and relatively expensive (e.g., gastric emptying and colonic transit measurements by isotopic methods), or invasive (e.g., intestinal manometry, barostat recordings). This section will highlight those situations in which these techniques may be helpful in patient management. Further details of testing in relation to specific FGIDs are provided in the organ-specific chapters.

With regard to visceral hypersensitivity, it is clear that the currently available tests to assess digestive tract sensation do not enable a positive diagnosis of an FGID. This is despite the fact that, overall, the presence of visceral hypersensitivity in response to distension can be documented in most of the FGIDs. Specifically in functional dyspepsia and in IBS it appears to be present in about 50–90% of patients [2]. The proportion of patients reported as hypersensitive depends, among other factors, on whether abnormal viscerosomatic referral is included in the definition of hypersensitivity.. In some patients, hypersensitivity may affect more than one region of the gut, while in others it appears likely to be restricted to a specific region. Thus, in IBS without concomitant functional dyspepsia, rectal hypersensitivity alone has been documented, while if functional dyspepsia was also present, gastric hypersensitivity was also documented [295]. The majority of patients with functional dyspepsia alone displayed gastric hypersensitivity, while less than 20% displayed rectal hypersensitivity. The reproducibility of hypersensitivity appears to be greatest with fundic distension in dysmotility-like functional dyspepsia and with antral distension in ulcer-like functional dyspepsia [23].

The lack of clinical utility for sensitivity testing stems largely from the fact that, for both functional dyspepsia and IBS, it is not yet possible to define abnormal values in response to distension that can characterize visceral hypersensitivity, either assessed by conscious perception or by measuring central responses. Based on IBS studies that have included controls, a limit can be proposed of approximately 28 mmHg for the pain threshold during rectal distension to discriminate between IBS patients (who display a threshold lower or equal to 28 mmHg) and controls (threshold usually approximately 32 mmHg or above) [10, 296–297]. These distinctions, however, may not be reliable as sensory thresholds are clearly influenced by a number of factors discussed earlier, and also by the intensity of symptoms at the time of study [10]. Further data on sensitivity testing in clinical practice is provided by a study of IBS patients prospectively screened with a rectal distension test who were compared to controls [298]. At the level of 40 mm Hg, the sensitivity of the rectal barostat to distinguish IBS patients from normal subjects and non-IBS patients was 95% and its specificity was 72%. The positive predictive value was 85%, while the negative predictive value was 90%. However, the lower pressure threshold of 28 mmHg discriminated IBS patients from other subjects, as no control values for pain threshold were under this limit. On the other hand, no IBS patient had a pain threshold above 48 mmHg, but a large number of subjects had pain thresholds between these limits, preventing any conclusions regarding distension tests in those patients from being drawn. Furthermore, given the relatively high prevalence of IBS, the possibility of coexistence of organic disease with a functional disorder remains significant. Tack et al. [275] reported that the lower range of normal (mean ± 2 SD) for the gastric distending pressure inducing discomfort in healthy subjects is 7.1 mmHg above minimal distending pressure; these findings require confirmation in other laboratories. The drinking tests referred to earlier can reveal differences between groups of healthy subjects and functional dyspepsia patients [299–301], but these types of tests require further refinement of abnormal values if they are to enter the clinical realm. With respect to the brain imaging techniques, the current state of the art does not allow the extension of these research techniques into clinical practice.

With regard to dysmotility, several of the techniques to assess digestive tract motility discussed earlier are more standardized and interpretable in the clinical context. These will be briefly discussed by region. The tests of *esophageal function* play an important clinical role in the exclusion of pathology-based motility disorders and gastroesophageal reflux as a cause of the symptoms in patients with suspected esophageal FGID. For instance, in patients with esophageal dysphagia in whom structural esophageal lesions have been ruled out, esophageal manometry will show the characteristic abnormalities of achalasia, or a motor abnormality that does not have a recognized pathological cause, such as ineffective esophageal motility [302], or no abnormalities at all. In the latter cases the diagnosis of functional dysphagia is justified. Likewise, in patients with heartburn, esophageal pH monitoring can be used to exclude gastroesophageal reflux as the cause of the symptoms, thus enabling a diagnosis of functional heartburn. In patients with angina-like chest pain, both esophageal manometry and pH monitoring may be required to arrive at the diagnosis of functional chest pain.

The tests of *gastric motility* have been employed in studies aiming to characterize patients fulfilling the criteria of gastroduodenal FGIDs, in particular functional dyspepsia. As discussed earlier, delayed gastric emptying, antral hypomotility, impaired accommodation of the proximal stomach, abnormal intragastric distribution, and abnormal reflexes have been reported in patients with functional dyspepsia [16, 23, 278, 283, 303]. Overall, despite the fact that 30 to 50% of patients fulfilling the criteria for functional dyspepsia display one or more of these forms of gastric motor dysfunction, none of the above-mentioned tests is useful in the clinical diagnosis of functional dyspepsia because of the poor correlation between symptoms and measured parameters of gastric motor function. Many clinicians would agree, however, that the results of such tests can be helpful in the management of patients with functional gastroduodenal disorders. For instance, when delayed gastric emptying is found in a patient with dyspeptic symptoms, treatment with a prokinetic drug is felt to be more useful than when emptying is found to be normal.

The tests of *small-intestinal motility* are mainly used in research on the pathophysiology of the FGIDs. However, intestinal manometry can be used as an aid to distinguish FGIDs such as IBS and functional dyspepsia from motility disorders with a documented histopathological basis, such as chronic idiopathic intestinal pseudo-obstruction [184, 304, 305]. Thus, episodes of intestinal pseudo-obstruction and erratically-propagating MMCs with normal contraction amplitudes in a patient are highly suggestive of enteric "neuropathy," while normally-propagating MMCs with diminished contraction amplitudes are suggestive of enteric "myopathy." Absence of a prompt interruption of the MMC upon eating is considered indicative of defective afferent vagal innervation of the gut. On the other hand, normal fasting and postprandial small-bowel motor patterns are a strong indication of normal small-bowel function. A subgroup of patients with intractable constipation and a generalized delay in colonic transit display abnormal 24-hour ambulatory jejunal manometry, which indicate more widespread enteric dysmotility [306]. The outcome of colectomy for such patients is poorer than in the subgroup with normal jejunal motor activity [307]. In several of the FGIDs, in particular IBS and functional dyspepsia, more subtle manometric abnormalities of small bowel motility (such as short bursts of clustered contractions) can be seen, but these are not of sufficient sensitivity and specificity to be helpful in the clinical diagnosis of these disorders. Although typical manometric abnormalities have been described in patients with organic obstruction of the bowel, it is obvious that intestinal obstruction should be diagnosed with techniques other than manometry.

With respect to the tests of *gallbladder and SO motility*, there is debate on the definition and clinical significance of gallbladder and SO dysfunction, and the application of these tests for diagnostic purposes varies considerably from center to center. Some reports suggest impaired gall bladder emptying demonstrated with scintigraphy or ultrasonography can provide evidence to support cholecystectomy in the appropriate clinical context [308], while there is some evidence that quantitative scintigraphy can aid in the diagnosis of SO dysfunction after cholecystectomy. SO manometry, on the other hand, does have a more defined role in clinical practice [309], particularly in patients after cholecystectomy. With respect to other FGIDs, there is evidence that gallbladder function may be altered in patients with IBS [310], but further work is required to determine if this finding is clinically relevant.

With respect to the tests of *colonic motility*, measurement of colonic transit, either by radio-opaque markers or scintigraphy, is regarded as clinically useful. Its main use is in the assessment of the severity of the delay in colonic transit in patients with functional constipation, as discussed earlier. Constipated patients with delayed colonic transit may respond differently to treatment than patients with normal transit. Moreover, if transit is delayed, and the pattern of marker distribution is one of retention of the markers throughout the colon, the diagnosis of colonic inertia is suggested. In contrast, if markers are retained in the rectum or rectosigmoid region but have moved in normal fashion through the colon, "outlet" or defecatory dysfunction should be suspected. However, this discriminatory ability of marker studies should not be overemphasized because it has been shown that suppressed defecation, mimicking outlet obstruction, can also lead to retention of markers in the right colon [311]. Colonic manometry and barostat measurements, in some cases together with provocative tests, have also been used to evaluate patients with slow transit constipation, since the disorder does appear to be associated with a lack of response to meal ingestion or to colonic stimulation, including pharmacologic stimulation with bisacodyl [312–314]. Colonic manometry has also revealed abnormal predefecatory motor patterns in patients with "obstructed defecation" [315]. However, the clinical role of colonic manometry is not defined, and it remains primarily a research technique.

As with the esophageal function tests, tests of *anorectal function* are widely used in clinical practice [316]. There is little doubt that manometry is useful in the exclusion of Hirschsprung's disease. However, there are considerable differences in opinion regarding the value of these manometric tests in the diagnostic work-up of patients with (suspected) anorectal FGIDs. For instance, some clinical centers consider manometry pivotal to the diagnosis of pelvic floor dyssynergia whereas others rely mainly on defecography. In patients with pelvic floor dyssynergia, impaired anal sphincter relaxation and paradoxical contraction of the anal sphincter have been shown to be reproducible findings [315], while the balloon expulsion test has been shown to be a useful screening procedure to identify constipated patients who do not have pelvic floor dyssynergia [154]. A recent report suggests that defecography may not provide any additional discriminatory utility to the above tests [317]. Anorectal ultrasound is used in the clinical assessment of patients with fecal incontinence due to focal and potentially surgically correctable defects in the anal sphincter that are detectable on electromyography [318].

Recommendations for Future Research

The concepts of sensory and reflex dysfunction leading to visceral hypersensitivity and enteric dysmotility have provided a conceptual framework for plausible mechanisms of symptom production in FGIDs. Advances in a range of areas are of crucial importance, however, to further clarify the clinical relevance of this sensorimotor dysfunction. Three such areas are:

(1) A greater understanding of the basic origins of gut perception. The key question in comparing animal and human research data is what is important for the encoding of information that ultimately determines the sensation consciously perceived. No data currently are available in this area, but increasingly sophisticated brain imaging techniques as well as spinal recording techniques are required to probe the interactions between cognitive factors and luminal causes of ENS activation in the modulation of cerebral activation patterns. Sensory testing, including evoked brain or spinal cord responses, could be used in the future to categorize FGID patients in order to determine appropriate therapeutics.

(2) More detailed information about the interactions between the ENS and its local environment, such as the presence of low-grade inflammation, luminal contents, hormonal fluctuations, etc. Although the study of an inflammatory basis for IBS is in its infancy, this concept provides a tangible basis for constructing novel animal models enabling investigation of luminal factors, including the enteric flora and dietary constituents that initiate and/or perpetuate gut sensorimotor dysfunction via immune activation. Important data on genetic predisposing factors and the dietary regulation of gene expression, including the effects of different probiotics, are awaited with great interest.

(3) More precise delineation of the relationships between sensorimotor dysfunction, individual symptoms, and individual FGIDs. Conceivably, the clinical manifestations in FGID patients depend on the specific sensory-reflex pathways and territories affected. Improved symptom criteria, together with quantitative data relating to physiological dysfunction (e.g., hypersensitivity, dysmotility, reflex dysfunction), to mucosal inflammation/immune/endocrine activation, to autonomic dysfunction, and in the future to molecular risk factors, should enable better categorization of patient subgroups using techniques such as cluster analysis. More sophisticated techniques to assess compliance, wall tension and accommodation, and flow of luminal content and gas are needed to understand the effects of dietary constituents on sensorimotor function. In this regard, the development of minimally or noninvasive techniques of investigation that can function as true surrogate markers of sensorimotor dysfunction, and that can be repeated in patients after various therapeutic maneuvers, is essential.

Acknowledgements: The authors gratefully acknowledge the contributions of Dr. M. Camilleri, Dr. S. Collins and Dr. C. di Lorenzo in the preparation of this chapter.

References

1. Mayer, EA, Gebhart, GF. Basic and clinical aspects of visceral hyperalgesia. Gastroenterology 1994;107:271–293.
2. Mertz, H. Overview of functional gastrointestinal disorders: dysfunction of the brain-gut axis. In: Functional Disorders of the Gastrointestinal Tract Mertz, H. (ed), Gastroenterol Clin NA Vol 32, No. 2, W.B. Saunders, 2003;463–476.
3. Schuligoi, R, Jocic, M, Heinemann, A, et al. Gastric acid-evoked c-fos messenger RNA expression in rat brainstem is signaled by capsaicin-resistant vagal afferents. Gastroenterology 1998;115:649–660.

4. Kang, Y-M, Bielefeldt, K, Gebhart, GF. Sensitization of mechanosensitive gastric vagal afferent fibers by thermal and chemical stimuli and gastric ulcers. J Neurophysiol 2004;9:1981–1989.

5. Lamb, K, Kang, Y-M, Gebhart, GF, Bielefeldt, K. Gastric inflammation triggers hypersensitivity to acid in awake rats. Gastroenterology 2003;125:1410–1418.

6. Bielefeldt, K, Gebhart, GF. Visceral pain—basic mechanisms. In: Koltzenburg, M, McMahon, S. (eds.), Textbook of Pain, 5th ed, Churchill-Livingstone, in press.

7. Bueno, L, Fioramonti, J, Garcia-Villar, R. Pathobiology of visceral pain: molecular mechanisms and therapeutic implications. III. Visceral afferent pathways: a source of new therapeutic targets for abdominal pain. Am J Physiol 2000;278:G670–G676.

8. Kirkup, AJ, Brunsden, AM., Grundy, D. Receptors and transmission in the brain-gut axis: potential for novel therapies. I. Receptors on visceral afferents. Am J Physiol 2001;280:G787–G794.

9. Perl, ER. Pain and the discovery of nociceptors. In: Belmonte C, Cervero F (ed.), Neurobiology of Nociceptors, Oxford, Oxford University Press, 1996, p. 5–36.

10. Mertz, H, Naliboff, B, Munakata, J et al. Altered rectal perception is a biological marker of patients with irritable bowel syndrome. Gastroenterology 1995;109:40–52.

11. Sarna, SK. Myoelectrical and contractile activities of the gastrointestinal tract. In: Schuster MM, Crowell, MD, Koch, KL (ed) Schuster Atlas of Gastrointestinal Motility in Health and Disease, 2nd ed, BC Decker Inc, Hamilton, 2002, p.1–18.

12. Rouillon, JM, Azpiroz, F, Malagelada, J. Reflex changes in intestinal tone: relationship to perception. Am J Physiol 1991;261:G280–286.

13. Notivol, R, Coffin, B, Azpiroz, F et al. Gastric tone determines the sensitivity of the stomach to distension. Gastroenterology 1995;108:330–336.

14. Distrutti, E, Azpiroz, F, Soldevilla, A, et al. Gastric wall tension determines perception of gastric distension. Gastroenterology 1999;116:1035–1042.

15. Whitehead, WE, Delvaux, M. Standardization of procedures for testing smooth muscle tone and sensory thresholds in the gastrointestinal tract. Dig Dis Sci 1997;42:223–241.

16. Tack, J, Bisschops, R, Sarnelli, G. Pathophysiology and treatment of functional dyspepsia. Gastroenterology 2004;127:1239–1255.

17. Distrutti, E, Salvioli, B, Azpiroz, F, Malagelada, J-R. Rectal function and bowel habit in irritable bowel syndrome. Am J Gastroenterol 2004;99:131–137.

18. Corsetti, M, Cesana, B, Bhoori, S, et al. Rectal hyperreactivity to distension in patients with irritable bowel syndrome: role of distension rate. Clin. Gastroenterol. & Hepatol. 2004;2:49–56.

19. Kahrilas, PJ, Clouse, RE, Hogan, WJ. American Gastroenterological Association technical review on the clinical use of esophageal manometry. Gastroenterology 1994;107:1865–1884.

20. Rao, SSC, Mudipalli, RS, Mujica, VR, et al. Effects of gender and age on esophageal biomechanical properties and sensation. Am J Gastroenterol 2003;98:1688–1695.

21. Azpiroz, F, Malagelada, JR. Perception and reflex relaxation of the stomach in response to gut distension. Gastroenterology 1990;98:1193–1198.

22. Mertz, H, Fullerton, S, Naliboff, B et al. Symptoms and visceral perception in severe functional and organic dyspepsia. Gut 1998;42:814–822.

23. Caldarella, MP, Azpiroz, F, Malagelada, J-R. Antro–fundic dysfunctions in functional dyspepsia. Gastroenterology 2003;124:1220–1229.

24. Feinle, C, Christen, M, Grundy, D, et al. Effects of duodenal fat, protein or mixed-

nutrient infusions on epigastric sensations during sustained gastric distension in healthy humans. Neurogastroenterol Motil 2002;14:205–213.

25. Accarino, AM, Azpiroz, F, Malagelada, J-R. Selective dysfunction of mechanosensitive intestinal afferents in the irritable bowel syndrome. Gastroenterology 1995; 108:636–643.

26. Evans, PR, Kellow, JE. Physiological modulation of jejunal sensitivity in health and in the irritable bowel syndrome. Am J Gastroenterol 1998;93:2191–2196.

27. Accarino, AM, Azpiroz, F, Malagelada, J-R. Modification of small bowel mechanosensitivity by intestinal fat. Gut 2001;48:690–695.

28. Camilleri, M, Hasler, WL, Parkman, HP, et al. Measurement of gastroduodenal motility in the gastrointestinal laboratory. Gastroenterology 1998;115:747–762.

29. Kellow, JE, Borody, TJ, Phillips, SF, et al. Human interdigestive motility: variations in patterns from esophagus to colon. Gastroenterology 1986;91:386–395.

30. Ittman, PI, Amarnath, R, Berseth, CL. Maturation of antroduodenal motor activity in preterm and term infants. Dig Dis Sci 1992;37:14–19.

31. Azpiroz, F, Malagelada, JR. Gastric tone measured by an electronic barostat in health and postsurgical gastroparesis. Gastroenterology 1987;92:934–943.

32. Phillips, SF, Quigley, EMM, Kumar, D, et al. Motility of the ileocolonic junction. Gut 1988;29:390–406.

33. Moragas, G, Azpiroz, F, Pavia, J, et al. Relations among intragastric pressure, postcibal perception and gastric emptying. Am J Physiol 1993;264:G1112–G1117.

34. De Schepper, HV, Cremonini, F, Chittcara, D, et al. Assessment of gastric accommodation: overview and evaluation of current methods. Neutrogastroenterol. Motil. 2004;16:275–285.

35. Feinle-Bisset, C, Vazzo, R, Horowitz, M, et al. Diet, food intake, and disturbed physiology in the pathogenesis of symptoms in functional dyspepsia. Am J Gastroenterol 2004;99:170–181.

36. Boyd, KA, O'Donovan, DG, Doran, S, et al. High fat diet effects on gut motility, hormone and appetite responses to duodenal lipid in healthy man. Am J Physiol 2003; 284:G188–196.

37. Hassan, BB, Butler, R, Davidson, GP, et al. Patterns of antropyloric motlity in fed healthy preterm infants. Arch Dis Child Fetal Neonatal Ed 2002;87:F95–99.

38. Berseth, CL. Gestational evolution of small intestinal motility in preterm and term infants. J Pediatr 1989;115:646–651.

39. Weisbrodt, NW. The regulation of gastrointestinal motility. In: Anuras S, (ed), Motility Disorders of the Gastrointestinal Tract, New York, Raven Press Ltd., 1992, p27–48.

40. Tack, J, Janssens, J, Vantrappen, G, et al. Effect of erythromycin on gastric motility in controls and in diabetic gastroparesis. Gastroenterology 1992;103:72–79.

41. Husebye, E, Hellstrom, PM, Sundler, F, et al. Influence of microbial species on small intestinal myoelectric activity and transit in germ-free rats. Am J Physiol 2001;280: G368–G380.

42. Quigley, EMM, Hassler, CVL, Parkman, HP. AGA technical review on nausea and vomiting Gastroenterology 2001;120:262–286.

43. Prajapati, DN, Hogan, WJ. Sphincter of Oddi dysfunction and other functional biliary disorders: evaluation and treatment. In: Functional Disorders of the Gastrointestinal Tract. Mertz, H (ed) Gastroenterol. Clin. NA. Vol 32, No.2, W.B. Saunders, 2003, p601–618.

44. Scott, SM. Manometric techniques for the evaluation of colonic motor activity: current status. Neurogastroenterol Motil 2003;15:483–513.

45. Bassotti, G, Crowell, MD, Whitehead, WE. Contractile activity of the human colon: lessons from 24-hour studies. Gut 1993;34:129–133.

46. Furukawa, Y, Cook, IJ, Panagopoulos, V, et al. Relationship between sleep patterns and human colonic motor patterns. Gastroenterology 1994;107:1372–1381.

47. Bampton, PA, Dinning, G, Kennedy, ML, et al. Prolonged multipoint recording of colonic manometry in the unprepared human colon. Am J Gastroenterol 2001;96: 1838–1848.

48. Di Lorenzo, C, Flores, AF, Hyman, PE. Age related changes in colon motility. J Pediatr 1995;127:593–6.

49. Ness, TJ, Metcalf, AM, Gebhart, GF. A psychophysical study in humans using phasic colonic distension as a noxious visceral stimulus. Pain 1990;43:377–386.

50. Steadman, CJ, Phillips, SF, Camilleri, M, et al. Variation of muscle tone in the human colon. Gastroenterology 1991;101:373–81.

51. Ford, MJ, Camilleri, M, Wiste, JA, et al. Differences in colonic tone and phasic response to a meal in the transverse and sigmoid human colon. Gut 1995;37:264–269.

52. Diamant, ND, Kamm, MA, Wald, A, et al. AGA technical review on anorectal testing techniques. Gastroenterology 1999;116:735–760.

53. Azpiroz, F, Enck, P, Whitehead, WE. Anorectal functional testing: review of collective experience. Am J Gastroenterol 2002;97:232–240.

54. de Lorijn, F, Omari, TI, Kok, JH, et al. Maturation of the rectoanal inhibitory reflex in very premature infants. J Pediatr 2003;143:630–633.

55. Azpiroz, F, Malagelada, J-R. Abdominal bloating. Gastroenterology, in press.

56. Hernando-Harder, H, Serra, J, Azpiroz, F, et al. Reflex control of intestinal gas dynamics and tolerance in humans. Am J Physiol 2004;286:G89–G94.

57. Hernando-Harder, AC, Serra, J, Azpiroz, F, et al. Sites of symptomatic gas retention during intestinal lipid perfusion in healthy subjects. Gut 2004;53:661–665.

58. Passos, MC, Tremolaterra, F, Serra, J, et al. Impaired reflex control of intestinal gas transit in patients with abdominal bloating. Gut, in press.

59. Serra, J, Salvioli, B, Azpiroz, F, et al. Lipid-induced intestinal gas retention in the irritable bowel syndrome. Gastroenterology 2002;123:700–706.

60. Azpiroz, F, Salvioli, B. Barostat measurements. In: Schuster MM, Crowell MD, Koch KL, ed. Schuster Atlas of Gastrointestinal Motility in Health and Disease. 2nd Edition. Hamilton, Ontario: BC Decker, 2002, p.151–170.

61. Delvaux, M. Role of visceral sensitivity in the pathophysiology of irritable bowel syndrome. Gut 2002;51(suppl 1):i67–i71.

62. Houghton, LA. Evidence of abnormal rectal sensitivity in IBS. In: Camilleri, M, Spiller, RC. (ed), Irritable Bowel Syndrome: diagnosis and treatment. Edinburgh, W.B. Saunders, 2002, p69–76.

63. Delvaux, M, Louvel, D, Mamet, JP, et al. Effect of Alosetron on responses to colonic distension in patients with irritable bowel syndrome. Aliment Pharmacol Ther 1998;12:849–855.

64. Delvaux, M, Louvel, D, Lagier, E, et al. The kappa agonist Fedotozine relieves hypersensitivity to colonic distension in patients with irritable bowel syndrome. Gastroenterology 1999;116:38–45.

65. Delvaux, M, Beck, A, Jacob, J, et al. Asimadoline, a kappa opioid agonist, decreases

pain induced by colonic distension in patients with Irritable Bowel Syndrome. Aliment Pharmacol Ther 2004, in press.

66. Delgado-Aros, S, Chial, HJ, Camilleri, M, et al. Effects of a kappa opioid agonist, asimadolime, on satiation and gastrointestinal motor and sensory functions in humans. Am J Physiol 2003;284:G558–G566.

67. Kellow, JE, Phillips, SF, Miller, LJ, et al. Dysmotility of the small intestine in irritable bowel syndrome. Gut 1988;29:1236–1243.

68. Chial, HJ, Camilleri, C, Delgado-Aros, S, et al. A nutrient drink test to assess maximum tolerated volume and postprandial symptoms: effects of gender, body mass index and age in health. Neurogastroenterol. Motil. 2002;14:249–253.

69. Caldarella, MP, Serra, J, Azpiroz, F, et al. Prokinetic effects in patients with intestinal gas retention. Gastroenterol. 2002;122:1748–1755.

70. Salvioli, B, Serra, J, Azpiroz, F, et al. Origin of gas retention and symptoms in patients with bloating. Gastroenterology, in press.

71. Simren, M, Vos, R, Janssens, J, et al. Acid infusion enhances duodenal mechanosensitivity in healthy subjects. Am J Physiol 2003;285:G309–G315.

72. Kern, M, Birn, R, Jaradeh, S, et al. Identification and characterization of cerebral cortical response to esophageal mucosal acid exposure and distension. Gastroenterology 1998;115:1353–1362.

73. Samsom, M, Verhagen, MA, vanBerge Henegouwen, GP, et al. Abnormal clearance of exogenous acid and increased acid sensitivity of the proximal duodenum in dyspeptic patients. Gastroenterology 1999;116:515–520.

74. Tougas, G, Spaziani, R, Hollerbach, S, et al. Cardiac autonomic function and oesophageal acid sensitivity in patients with non-cardiac chest pain. Gut 2001;49:706–712.

75. Chen, C-L, Orr, WC. Autonomic responses to heartburn induced by esophageal acid infusion. J Gastroenterol Hepatol 2004;19:922–926.

76. Louvel, D, Delvaux, M, Staumont, G, et al. Intracolonic injection of glycerol: A model for abdominal pain in Irritable Bowel Syndrome. Gastroenterology 1996;110:351–361.

77. Gracely, RH. Studies of pain in normal man. In: Wall, PD., Melzack, R (ed), Textbook of Pain, 3rd Ed. Edinburgh, Churchill Livingstone, 1994, p.315–336.

78. Chan, YK, Herkes, GK, Badcock, C, et al. Alterations in cerebral potentials evoked by rectal distension in irritable bowel syndrome. Am J Gastroenterol 2001;96:2413–2417.

79. Sinhamahapatra, P, Saha, SP, Chowdhury, A, et al. Visceral afferent hypersensitivity in irritable bowel syndrome—evaluation by cerebral evoked potential after rectal stimulation. Am J Gastroenterol 2001;96:2150–2157.

80. Murray, CDR, Flynn, J, Ratcliffe, L, et al. Effect of acute physical and psychological stress on gut autonomic innervation in irritable bowel syndrome. Gastroenterology 2004;127:1695–1703.

81. Azpiroz, F. Gastrointestinal perception: pathophysiological implications. Neurogastroenterol Mot. 2002;14:1–11.

82. Naliboff, BD, Munakata, J, Fullerton, S, et al. Evidence for two distinct perceptual alterations in irritable bowel syndrome. Gut 1997;41:505–512.

83. Lembo, T, Naliboff, BD, Matin, K, et al. Irritable bowel syndrome patients show altered sensitivity to exogenous opioids. Pain 2000;87:137–147.

84. Aziz, Q, Thompson, DG. Brain-gut axis in health and disease. Gastroenterology 1998;114:559–578.

85. Hollerbach, S, Bulat, R, May, A, et al. Abnormal cerebral processing of oesophageal stimuli in patients with noncardiac chest pain (NCCP). Neurogastroent Motil 2000; 12:555–565.

86. Schnitzler, A, Volkmann, J, Enck, P, et al. Different cortical organization of visceral and somatic sensation in humans. Eur J Neurosci 1999;11:305–315.

87. Furlong, PL, Aziz, Q, Singh, KD, et al. Cortical localization of magnetic fields evoked by oesophageal distension. Electroencepha. Clin. Neurophysiol 1998;108:234–243.

88. Mayberg, H. Limbic-cortical dysregulation: a proposed model of depression. J Neuropsychiatry Clin Neurosci 1997;9:471–481.

89. Silverman, DHS, Munakata, JA, Ennes, H, et al. Regional cerebral activity in normal and pathological perception of visceral pain. Gastroenterology 1997;112:64–72.

90. Naliboff, BD, Derbyshire, SWG, Munakata, J, et al. Cerebral activation in patients with irritable bowel syndrome and control subjects during rectosigmoid stimulation. Psychosom. Med 2001;63:365–75.

91. Hamaguchi, T, Kano, M, Rikimaru, H. Brain activity during distension of the descending colon in humans. Neurogastroenterol Motil 2004;16:299–309.

92. Kern, MK, Jaradeh S, Arndorter RC, et al. Gender differences in cortical representation of rectal distension in healthy humans. Am J Physiol 2001;281:G1512–G1523.

93. Naliboff, BD, Berman, S, Chang, L, et al. Sex-related differences in IBS patients: central processing of visceral stimuli. Gastroenterology 2003;124:1738–1747.

94. Mertz, H, Morgan, V, Tanner, G, et al. Regional cerebral activation in irritable bowel syndrome and control subjects with painful and non-painful rectal distension. Gastroenterol 2000;118:842–848.

95. Verne, G, Himes, N, Robinson, M, et al. Central representation of visceral and cutaneous hypersensitivity in the irritable bowel syndrome. Pain 2003;103:99–110.

96. Bouras, EP, O'Brien, TJ, Camilleri, M, et al. Cerebral topography of rectal stimulation using single photon emission computed tomography. Am J Physiol 1999;277: G687–G694.

97. Hardy, SGP, Haigler, HJ. Prefrontal influences upon the midbrain: a possible route for pain modulation. Brain Res 1985;339:285–293.

98. Bajwa, A, Hollerbach, S, Kamath, M, et al. Neurocardiac response to esophageal electric stimulation in humans: effects of varying stimulation frequencies. Am J Physiol 1997;272:896–901.

99. Emmanuel, AV, Kamm, MA. Laser Doppler flowmetry as a measure of extrinsic colonic innervation in functional bowel disease. Gut 2000;46:212–217.

100. Willer, JC. Comparative study of perceived pain and nociceptive flexion reflex in man. Pain 1977;3:69–80.

101. Sabate, J-M, Coffin, B, Jian, R, et al. Rectal sensitivity assessed by a reflexologic technique: further evidence for two types of mechanoreceptors. Am J Physiol 2000; 279:G692–G699.

102. Law, N, Bharucha, A, Zinsmeister, A. Rectal and colonic distension elicit viscero-visceral reflexes in humans. Am J Physiol 2002;283:G384–G389.

103. Youle, MS, Read, NW. Effect of painless rectal distension on gastrointestinal transit of solid meal. Dig Dis Sci 1984;29:902–906.

104. Kellow, JE, Gill, RC, Wingate, DL. Modulation of human upper gastrointestinal motility by rectal distension in humans. Gut 1987;28:864–869.

105. Tjeerdsma HC, Smout, AJP, Akkermans, LMA. Voluntary suppression of defecation delays gastric emptying. Dig Dis Sci 1983;38:832–836.

106. Wiley, J, Tatum, D, Kennalt, et al. Participation of gastric mechanoreceptors and intestinal chemoreceptors in the gastro-colonic response. Gastroenterology 1988; 94:1144–1149.

107. Ng, C, Danta, M, Prott, G, Badcock, et al. Modulatory influences on antegrade and retrograde tonic reflexes in the colon and rectum. Am J Physiol 2004;287:G962–G966.

108. Fox, M, Hebbard, G, Janiak, P, et al. High-resolution manometry predicts the success of oesophageal bolus transport and identifies clinically important abnormalities not detected by conventional manometry. Neurogastroentero Motil 2004;16: 533–542.

109. Klein, HA. Esophageal transit scintigraphy. Semin Nucl Med 1995;25:306–317.

110. Kostic, SV, Rice, TW, Baker, ME, et al. Timed barium esophagogram: A simple physiologic assessment for achalasia. J Thorac Cardiovasc Surg 2000;120:935–943.

111. Pandolfino, JE, Richter, JE, Ours, T, et al. Ambulatory esophageal pH monitoring using a wireless system. Am J Gastroenterol 2003;98:740–749.

112. Wiener, GJ, Richter, JE, Copper, JB, Wu, WC, Castell, DO. The symptom index: a clinically important parameter of ambulatory 24-hour esophageal pH monitoring. Am J Gastroenterol 1988;83:358–361.

113. Weusten, BL, Roelofs, JM, Akkermans, LM, et al. The symptom-association probability: an improved method for symptom analysis of 24-hour esophageal pH data. Gastroenterology 1994;107:1741–1745.

114. Koek, GH, Tack, J, Sifrim, D, et al. The role of acid and duodenal gastroesophageal reflux in symptomatic GERD. Am J Gastroenterol 2001;96:2033–2040.

115. Marshall, RE, Anggiansah, A, Owe, WA, et al. The relationship between acid and bile reflux and symptoms in gastro-oesophageal reflux disease. Gut 1997;40:182–187.

116. Sifrim, D., Holloway, R, Silny, J, et al. Acid, non-acid, and gas reflux in patients with gastroesophageal reflux disease during ambulatory 24-hour pH-impedance recordings. Gastroenterology 2001;120:1588–1598.

117. Tutuian, R, Vela, MF, Shay, SS, et al. Multichannel intraluminal impedance in esophageal function testing and gastroesophageal reflux monitoring. J Clin Gastroenterol 2003;37:206–215.

118. Tutuian, R, Castell, DO. Combined multichannel intraluminal impedance and manometry clarifies oesophageal functional abnormalities: study in 350 patients. Am J Gastroenterol 2004;99:1011–1019.

119. Tougas, G, Eaker, EY, Abell, TL, et al. Assessment of gastric emptying using a low fat meal: establishment of international control values. Am J Gastroenterol 2000; 95:1456–1462.

120. Ghoos, YF, Maes, BD, Geypeus, BJ, et al. Measurement of gastric emptying rate of solids by means of a carbon-labelled octanoic acid breath test. Gastroenterology 1993;104:1640–1647.

121. Viramontes, BE, Kim, DY, Cammilleri M, et al. Validation of a stable isotope gastric emptying test for normal, accelerated or delayed gastric emptying. Neurogastroenterol Motil 2001;13:567–574.

122. Bromer, MQ, Kantor, SB, Wagner, DA, et al. Simultaneous measurement of gastric emptying with a simple muffin meal using [13c] octanoate breath test and scintigraphy in normal subjects and patients with dyspeptic symptoms. Dig Dis Sci 2002;47:1657–1663.

123. Berstad, A, Hausken, T, Gilja, OH, et al. Volume measurement of gastric antrum by 3-D ultrasonography and flow measurements through the pylorus by duplex technique. Dig Dis Sci 1994;39:97–108.

124. Tefera, S, Gilja, OH, Olafsdottir, E, et al. Intragastric maldistribution of a liquid meal in patients with reflux oesophagitis assessed by three dimensional ultrasonography. Gut 2002;50:153–158.

125. Mintchev, MP, Kingma, YJ, Bowes, KL. Accuracy of cutaneous recordings of gastric electrical activity. Gastroenterology 1993;104:1273–1280.

126. Verhagen, MAMT, Van Schelven, LJ, Samsom, M, Smout, AJPM. Pitfalls in the analysis of electrogastropgrahic recordings. Gastroenterology 1999;117:453–460.

127. Parkman, HP, Hasler, WL, Barnett, JL, Eaker, EY. Electrogastrography: a document prepared by the gastric section of the American Motility Society Clinical GI motility testing task force. Neurogastroenterol Motil 2003;15:89–102.

128. Evans, DF., Lamont, G, Stehling, MK, et al. Prolonged monitoring of the upper gastrointestinal tract using echo planar magnetic resonance imaging. Gut 1993;34:848–852.

129. Schwizer, W, Fraser, R, Borovicka, J, et al. Measurement of proximal and distal gastric motility with magnetic resonance imaging. Am J Physiol 1996;271:G217–G222.

130. Boulby, P, Gowland, P, Adams, V, et al. Use of echo planar imaging to demonstrate the effect of posture on the intragastric distribution and emptying of an oil-water meal. Neurogastroenterol Motil 1997;9(1):41–47.

131. Ajaj, W, Goedhe, SC, Papanikolau, N, et al. Real time high resolution magnetic resonance imaging for the assessment of gastric motility disorders. Gut 2004;53:1256–1261.

132. De Zwart, IM, Mearadji, B, Lamb, HJ, et al. Gastric motility: comparison of assessment with real time MR imaging or barostat measurement limited experience. Radiology 2002;224(2):592–597.

133. Kim, DY, Delgado-Aros, S, Camilleri, M, et al. Noninvasive measurement of gastric accommodation in patients with idiopathic nonulcer dyspepsia. Am J Gastroenterol 2001;96:3099–3105.

134. Van den Elzen, BD, Bennink, RJ, Wieringa, RE, et al. Fundic accommodation assessed by SPECT scanning: comparison with the gastric barostat. Gut 2003;52:1548–1554.

135. Bouras, EP, Delgado-Aros, S, Camilleri, M, et al. SPECT imaging of the stomach: comparison with barostat, and effects of sex, age, body mass indx and fundoplication. Gut 2002;51:781–786.

136. Tack, J, Piessevaux, H, Coulie, B, et al. Role of impaired gastric accommodation to a meal in functional dyspepsia. Gastroenterology 1998;115:1346–1352.

137. Sarnelli, G, Vos, R, Cuomo, R, et al. Reproducibility of gastric barostat studies in healthy controls and in dyspeptic patients. Am J Gastroenterol 2001;96:1047–1053.

138. Geboes, KP, Luypaerts, A, Rutgeerts, P, et al. Inulin is an ideal substrate for a hydrogen breath test to measure the orocaecal transit time. Aliment Pharmacol Ther 2003;18:721–729.

139. Miller, MA, Parkman, HP, Urbain, JL, et al. Comparison of scintigraphy and lactulose breath hydrogen test for assessment of orocecal transit: lactulose accelerates small bowel transit. Dig Dis Sci 1997;42:10–18.

140. Geypens, B, Bennink, R, Peeters, M, et al. Validation of the lactose-[13C]ureide breath test for determination of orocecal transit time by scintigraphy. J Nucl Med 1999;40:1451–1455.

141. Charles, F, Camilleri, M, Phillips, SF, et al. Scintigraphy of the whole gut: clinical evaluation of transit disorders. Mayo Clin Proc 1995;70:113–118.

142. Serra, J, Azpiroz, F, Malagelada, J-R. Impaired transit and tolerance of intestinal gas in the irritable bowel syndrome. Gut 2001;48:14–19.

143. Andrews, JM, Doran, SM, Hebbard, GS, et al. Nutrient-induced spatial patterning of human duodenal motor function. Am J Physiol 2001;280:G501–G509.

144. Evans, PR, Bak, Y-T, Kellow, JE. Ambulant small bowel manometry in health: comparison of consecutive 24-h recording periods. J Amb Monitoring 1996;9:193–202.

145. Quigley, EMM, Deprez, PH, Hellstrom P, et al. Ambulatory intestinal manometry. A consensus report on its clinical role. Dig Dis Sci 1997;92:2395–2400.

146. Craig, AG, Peter, D, Saccon, GT, et al. Scintigraphy versus manometry in patients with suspected biliary sphincter of Oddi dysfunction. Gut 2003;52:352–357.

147. Wong, GSW, Teoh, N, Dowsett, D, et al. Complications of sphincter of Oddi manometry: biliary-like pain versus acute pancreatitis. Scand J Gastroenterol 2005; 40:1–7.

148. Chan, Y-K, Evans, PR, Dowsett, JF, et al. Discordance of pressure recordings from biliary and pancreatic duct segments in patients with suspected sphincter of Oddi dysfunction. Dig Dis Sci 1997;42:1501–1506.

149. Aymerich, RR, Prakash, C, Aliperti, G. Sphincter of Oddi manometry: is it necessary to measure both biliary and pancreatic sphincter pressure? Gastrointest Endosc 2000;52:183–186.

150. Rao, SS, Sadeghi, P, Beaty, J. Ambulatory 24-hr colonic manometry in healthy humans. Am J Physiol 2001;280:G629–G639.

151. Hagger, R, Kumar, D, Benson, M, et al. Periodic colonic motor activity identified by 24-h pancolonic ambulatory manometry in humans. Neurogastroenterol Motil 2002;14:271–278.

152. Evans RC, Kamm MA, Hinton JM, Lennard-Jones JE. The normal range and a simple diagram for recording whole gut transit time. Int J Colorectal Dis 1992;7:15–17.

153. Metcalf, AM, Phillips, SF, Zinsmeister, AR, et al. Simplified assessment of segmental colonic transit. Gastroenterology 1987;92:40–47.

154. Minguez, M, Herreros, B, Sanchiz, B, et al. Predictive value of the balloon expulsion test for excluding the diagnosis of pelvic floor dyssynergia in constipation. Gastroenterology 2004;126:57–62.

155. Malcolm, A, Phillips, SF, Camilleri, M, et al. Pharmacological modulation of rectal tone alters perception of distension in humans. Gastroenterology 1997;92:2073–2079.

156. Serra, J, Azpiroz, F, Malagelada, J-R. Perception and reflex responses to intestinal distension are modified by simultaneous or previous stimulation. Gastroenterology 1995;109:1742–1749.

157. Rayner, CK, Samsom, M, Jones, KL. Relationships of upper gastrointestinal motor and sensory function with glycemic control. Diabetes Care 2001;24:371–381.

158. Houghton, LA, Lea, R, Jackson, N, et al. The menstrual cycle affects rectal sensitivity in patients with irritable bowel syndrome but not healthy volunteers. Gut 2002;50:471–474.

159. Coffin, B, Azpiroz, F, Malagelada, J-R. Somatic stimulation reduces perception of gut distension. Gastroenterology 1994;107:1636–1642.

160. Iovino, P, Azpiroz, F, Domingo, E, et al. The sympathetic nervous system modulates perception and reflex responses to gut distension in humans. Gastroenterology 1995;108:680–686.

161. Accarino, AM, Azpiroz, F, Malagelada, J-R. Attention and distraction effects on gut perception. Gastroenterology 1997;113:415–422.

162. Ford, MJ, Camilleri, M, Zinsmeister, AR, et al. Psychosensory modulation of colonic sensation in the human transverse and sigmoid colon. Gastroenterology 1995;109:1772–1780.

163. Yin, J, Levanon, D, Chen, JDZ. Inhibitory effects of stress on postprandial gastric myoelectrical activity and vagal tone in healthy subjects. Neurogastroenterol Motil 2004;16:737–744.

164. Gonsalkorale, WM, Perrey, C, Pravica, V, et al. Interleukin 10 genotypes in irritable bowel syndrome; evidence for an inflammatory component. Gut 2003;52:91–93.

165. Holtmann, G, Siffert, W, Haag, S, et al. G-protein B3 825 CC genotype is associated with unexplained (functional) dyspepsia. Gastroenterol. 2004;126:971–979.

166. Coates MD, Mahoney CR, Linden DR, et al. Molecular defects in mucosal serotonin content and decreased serotonin reuptake transporter in ulcerative colitis and irritable bowel syndrome. Gastroenterology 2004;126:1657–1664.

167. Dunlop SP, Coleman NS, Blackshaw E, et al. Abnormalities of 5-hydroxytryptamine metabolism in irritable bowel syndrome. Clinical Gastroenterology & Hepatology 2005;3:349–357.

168. Spiller RC. Postinfectious irritable bowel syndrome. Gastroenterology 203;124:1662–1671.

169. Neal, KR, Hebdon, J, Spiller, R. Prevalence of gastrointestinal symptoms six months after bacterial gastroenteritis and risk factors for development of the irritable bowel syndrome. Br Med J 1997;314:779–782.

170. Garcia Rodriguez, LA, Ruigomez, A. Increased risk of irritable bowel syndrome after bacterial gastroenteritis: cohort study. Brit Med J 1999;318:565–566.

171. Gwee, KA, Graham, JC, McKendrick, MW, et al. Psychometric scores and persistence of irritable bowel after infectious diarrhoea. Lancet 1996;347:150–153.

172. Gwee, K-A, Leong, Y-L, Graham, C, et al. The role of psychological and biological factors in post-infective gut dysfunction. Gut 1999;44:400–406.

173. Spiller, RC, Jenkins, D, Thornley, JP, et al. Increased rectal mucosal enteroendocrine cells, T lymphocytes, and increased gut permeability following acute Campylobacter enteritis and in post-dysenteric irritable bowel syndrome. Gut 2000;47:804–811.

174. Ilnyckyj, A, Balachandra, B, Elliott, L, et al. Post-traveller's diarrhea irritable bowel syndrome: a prospective study. Am J Gastroenterol 2003;98:596–599.

175. Parry, SD, Stansfield, R, Jelley, D, et al. Is irritable bowel syndrome more common in patients presenting with bacterial gastroenteritis? A community-based, case control study. Am J Gastroenterol 2003;98:327–331.

176. Parry, SD, Stansfield, R, Jelley, D, et al. Does bacterial gastroenteritis predispose people to functional gastrointestinal disorders? A prospective, community-based, case control study. Am J Gastroenterol 2003;98:1970–1975.

177. Dunlop, SP, Jenkins, D, Spiller, RC. Distinctive clinical, psychological, and histological features of postinfective irritable bowel syndrome. Am J Gastroenterol 98:2003;1578–1583.

178. Okhuysen PC, Jiang ZD, Carlin L, et al. Post-diarrhea chronic intestinal symptoms and irritable bowel síndrome in North American travellers to Mexico. Am J Gastroenterol 99;2004:1774–1778.

179. Bergin, AJ, Donnelly, TC, McKendrick, MW, et al. Changes in anorectal function in persistent bowel disturbance following salmonella gastroenteritis. Eur J Gastroenterol Hepatol 1993;5:617–620.

180. Dunlop, SP, Jenkins, D, Neal, KR, et al. Relative importance of enterochromaffin cell hyperplasia, anxiety, and depression in postinfectious IBS. Gastroenterology 2003;125:1651–1659.

181. Chadwick, VS, Chen, W, Shu, D, et al. Activation of the mucosal immune system in irritable bowel syndrome. Gastroenterology 2002;122:1778–1783.

182. Collins, SM. A case for an immunological basis for irritable bowel syndrome. Gastroenterology 2002;122:2078–2080.

183. Tornblom, H, Lindberg, G, Nyberg, B, et al. Full-thickness biopsy of the jejunum reveals inflammation and enteric neuropathy in irritable bowel syndrome. Gastroenterology 2002;123:1972–1979.

184. De Giorgio, R, Guerrini, S, Barbara, G, et al. Inflammatory neuropathies of the enteric nervous system. Gastroenterology 2004;126:1872–1883.

185. O'Sullivan, M, Clayton, N, Breslin, NP, et al. Increased mast cells in the irritable bowel syndrome. Neurogastroenterol Motil 2000;12:449–457.

186. Weston, AP, Biddle, WL, Bhatia, PS, et al. Terminal ileal mucosal mast cells in irritable bowel syndrome. Dig Dis Sci 1993;38:1590–1595.

187. Park, CH, Joo, YE, Choi, SK, Few, et al. Activated mast cells infiltrate in close proximity to enteric nerves in diarrhoea-predominant irritable bowel syndrome. J Korean Med Sci 2003;18(2):204–210.

188. Barbara, G, Stanghellini, V, De Giorgio, R, et al. Activated mast cells in proximity to colonic nerves correlate with abdominal pain in irritable bowel syndrome. Gastroenterology 2004;126:693–702.

189. Wang, LH, Fang, XC, Pan, GZ. Bacillary dysentery as a causative factor of irritable bowel syndrome and its pathogenesis. Gut 2004;53:1096–1101.

190. Santos, J, Yang, PC, Soderholm, JD, et al. Role of mast cells in chronic stress induced colonic epithelial barrier dysfunction in the rat. Gut 2001;48:630–636.

191. Spiller, RC. Neuropathology of IBS? Gastroenterology 2002;123:2144–2147.

192. Van der Veek, P, de Kroon, Y, Van den Berg, M, et al. Tumour necrosis factor alpha and interleukin 10 gene polymorphisms in irritable bowel syndrome. Gastroenterology 2004;126(Suppl.2), A52.

193. O'Mahony, L, McCarthy, J, Kelly P, et al. A randomized, placebo-controlled, double-blind comparison of the probiotic bacteria lactobacillus and bifidobacterium in irritable bowel syndrome (IBS): symptom responses and relationship to cytokine profiles. Gastroenterology 2005;128:541–551.

194. Gwee, K-A, Collins, SM, Read, NW, et al. Increased rectal mucosal expression of interleukin 1B in recently acquired post-infectious irritable bowel syndrome. Gut 2003;52:523–526.

195. O'Leary, C, Wieneke, P, Buckley, S, et al. Celiac disease and irritable bowel-type symptoms. Am J Gastroenterol 2002;97:1463–1467.

196. Collins, JS, Hamilton, PW, Watt, PC, et al. Quantitative histological study of mucosal inflammatory cell densities in endoscopic duodenal biopsy specimens from dyspeptic patients using computer-linked image analysis. Gut 1990;31: 858–861.

197. Matter, SE, Bhatia, PS, Miner PB, Jr. Evaluation of antral mast cells in nonulcer dyspepsia. Dig Dis Sci 1990;35:1358–1363.

198. Mearin, F, Ribot X, Balboa, A, et al. Does Helicobacter pylori infection increase gastric sensitivity in functional dyspepsia. Gut 1995;37:47–51.

199. Klatt, S., Pieramico, O., Guethner, C., et al. Gastric hypersensitivity in nonulcer dyspepsia: an inconsistent finding. Dig Dis Sci 1997;92:720–723.

200. Sarnelli, G, Cuomo, R, Janssens, J, et al. Symptom patterns and pathophysiological mechanisms in dyspeptic patients with and without Helicobacter pylori. Dig Dis Sci 2003;48:2229–2236.

201. Moayyedi, P, Deeks, J, Tally, NJ, et al. An update of the cochrane systemic review of Helicobacter pylori eradication therapy in nonulcer dyspepsia: resolving the discrepancy between systemic reviews. Am J Gastroenterol 2003;98:2621–2626.

202. McNamara, D, Buckley, G, Gilvarry, J, et al. Does Helicobacter pylori eradication affect symptoms in nonulcer dyspepsia: a 5-year follow-up study. Helicobacter 2002;7:317–321.

203. Soykan, I, Sivri, B, Sarosiek, I, et al. Demography, clinical characteristics, psychological and abuse profiles, treatment and long-term follow-up of patients with gastroparesis. Dig Dis Sci 1998;43:2398–2404.

204. Tack, J, Demedts, I, Dehondt, G, et al. Clinical and pathophysiogical characteristics of acute-onset functional dyspepsia. Gastroenterology 2002;122:1738–1747.

205. Quigley, EMM. Enteric neuropathology: recent advances and implications for clinical practice. The Gastroenterologist 1997;5:233–241.

206. Balsari, A, Ceccarelli, A, Dubini, F, et al. The fecal microbial population in the irritable bowel syndrome. Microbiologica 1982;5:185–194.

207. Madden JA, Hunter JO. A review of the role of the gut microflora in irritable bowel syndrome and the effects of probiotics. Br J Nutr 2002;88(suppl 1):S67–S72.

208. Si JM, Yu YC, Fan YJ, et al. Intestinal microecology and quality of life in irritable bowel syndrome patients. World J Gastroenterol 2004;10:1802–1805.

209. Pimentel, M, Chow, EJ, Lin, HC. Eradication of small bowel bacterial overgrowth reduces symptoms of irritable bowel syndrome. Am J Gastroenterol 2000;95:3503–3506.

210. Lin HC. Small intestinal bacterial overgrowth: a framework for understanding irritable bowel syndrome. JAMA 2004;292:852–858.

211. Pimentel M, Soffer EE, Chow EJ, et al. Lower frequency of MMC is found in IBS subjects with abnormal lactulose breath test, suggesting bacterial overgrowth. Dig Dis Sci 2002:2639–2643.

212. Pimentel, M, Chow, E, Lin, H. Normalization of lactulose breath testing correlates with symptom improvement in irritable bowel syndrome: a double-blind, randomized, placebo-controlled study. Am J Gastroenterol 2003;98:412–419.

213. Pimentel M, Wallace D, Hallegua D, et al. A link between irritable bowel syndrome and fibromyalgia may be related to findings on lactulose breath testing. Ann Rheum Dis 2004;63:450–452.

214. Hasler, W. Lactulose breath testing, bacterial overgrowth, and IBS: just a lot of hot air? Gastroenterology 2003;125:1898–1900.

215. Maxwell, PR, Rink, E, Kumar, D, Mendall, MA. Antibiotics increase functional abdominal symptoms. Am J Gastroenterol 2002;97:104–108.

216. Nobaek, S, Johansson, M-L, Molin, G. et al. Alteration of intestinal microflora is as-

sociated with reduction in abdominal bloating and pain in patients with irritable bowel syndrome. Am J Gastroenterol 2000;95:1231–1238.

217. O'Sullivan, MA, O'Morain, CA. Bacterial supplementation in the irritable bowel syndrome. A randomized double-blind placebo-controlled crossover study. Dig Liver Dis 2000;32:294–301.

218. Niedzielin K, Kordecki H, Birkenfeld B. A controlled, double-blind, randomized study on the efficacy of Lactobacillus plantarum 299V in patients with irritable bowel syndrome. Eur J Gastroenterol Hepatol 2001;13:1143–1147.

219. Bazzocchi G, Gionchetti P, Almergigi PF, et al. Intestinal microflora and oral bacteriotherapy in irritable bowel syndrome. Dig Liver Dis 2002;34(suppl 2):S48–S53.

220. Kim, HJ, Camilleri, M, McKinzie, S, et al. A randomised controlled trial of probiotic, VSLNo.3, on gut transit and symptoms in diarrhoea-predominant irritable bowel syndrome. Aliment Pharmacol Ther 2003;17:895.

221. Saggioro A. Probiotics in the treatment of irritable bowel syndrome. J Clin Gastroenterol 2004;38(suppl 6):S104–S106.

222. Locke GR, Zinsmeister AR, Talley NJ, et al. Risk factors for irritable bowel syndrome: role of analgesics and food sensitivities. Am J Gastroenterol 2000;95:157–165.

223. Simren M, Mansson A, Langkilde AM, et al. Food-related gastrointestinal symptoms in the irritable bowel syndrome. Digestion 2001;63:108–115.

224. Choi, YK, Johlin, FC, Summers, RW, et al. Fructose intolerance: an under-recognized problem. Am J Gastroenterol 2003;98:1348–1353.

225. Niec AM, Frankum B, Talley NJ, et al. Are adverse reactions to food linked to irritable bowel syndrome? Am J Gastroenterol 1998;93:2184–2190.

226. Vesa TH, Seppo LM, Marteau PR, et al. Role of irritable bowel syndrome in subjective lactose intolerance. Am J Clin Nutr 1998;67:710–715.

227. Parker TJ, Woolner JT, Prevost AT, et al. Irritable bowel syndrome: is the search for lactose intolerance justified? Eur J Gastroenterol Hepatol 2001;13:219–225.

228. Pimentel M, Kong Y, Park S. Breath testing to evaluate lactose intolerance in irritable bowel syndrome correlates with lactulose testing and may not reflect true lactose malabsorption. Am J Gastroenterol 2003;98:2700–2704.

229. Jones, A, Shorthouse, M, McLaughlan, P, et al. Food intolerance: a major factor in the pathogenesis of the irritable bowel syndrome. Lancet 1982;2:1115–1117.

230. Bentley SJ, Pearson DJ, Rix KJB. Food hypersensitivity in irritable bowel syndrome. Lancet 1983;2:295–297.

231. Roussos A, Koursarakos P, Patsopoulos D, et al. Increased prevalence of irritable bowel syndrome in patients with bronchial asthma. Respir Med 2003;97:75–79.

232. Atkinson W, Sheldon TA, Shaath N, et al. Food elimination based on IgG antibodies in irritable bowel syndrome: a randomized controlled trial. Gut 2004;53:1459–1464.

233. King, TS, Elia, M, Hunter, JO. Abnormal colonic fermentation in irritable bowel syndrome. Lancet 1998;352:1187–1189.

234. Sanders DS, Carter MJ, Hurlstone DP, et al. Association of adult coeliac disease with irritable bowel syndrome: a case-control study in patients fulfilling Rome II criteria referred to secondary care. Lancet 2001;358:1504–1508.

235. Wahnschaffe U, Ullrich R, riecken EO, Schulzke JD. Celiac disease-like abnormali-

ties in a subgroup of patients with irritable bowel syndrome. Gastroenterology 2001; 121:1329–1338.

236. Sanders DS, Patel D, Stephenson TJ, et al. A primary care cross-sectional study of undiagnosed adult coeliac disease. Eur J Gastroenterol Hepatol 2003;15:407–413.

237. Shahbazkhani B, Forootan M, Merat S, et al. Coeliac disease presenting with symptoms of irritable bowel syndrome. Aliment Phramacol Ther 2003;18:231–235.

238. Zipser RD, Patel S, Yahya KZ, et al. Presentations of adult celiac disease in a nationwide patient support group. Dig Dis Sci 2003;48:761–764.

239. Brandt LJ, Bjorkman D, Fennerty MB, et al. Systematic review on the management of irritable bowel syndrome in North America. Am J Gastroenterol 2002;97(Suppl): S7–S26.

240. Cash BD, Schonfeld P, Chey WD. The utility of diagnostic tests in irritable bowel syndrome patients: a systematic review. Am J Gastroenterol 2002;97:2812–2819.

241. Spiegel BM, DeRosa VP, Gralnek IM, et al. Testing for celiac sprue in irritable bowel syndrome with predominant diarrhea: a cost-effectiveness analysis. Gastroenterology 2004;126:1721–1732.

242. Mein SM, Ladabaum U. Serological testing for celiac disease in patients with symptoms of irritable bowel syndrome: a cost effectiveness analysis. Aliment Pharmacol Ther 2004;19:1199–1210.

243. O'Leary, C, Quigley EM. Small bowel bacterial overgrowth, celiac disease, and IBS: what are the real associations? Am J Gastroenterol 2003;98:720–722.

244. Tougas, G. The autonomic nervous system in functional bowel disorders. Gut 2000;47:iv78–81.

245. Troncon, LE, Thompson, DG, Ahuwalia, NK, et al. Relations between upper abdominal symptoms and gastric distension abnormalities in dysmotility like functional dyspepsia and after vagotomy. Gut 1995;37:17–22.

246. Greydanus, MP, Vassallo, M, Camilleri, M, et al. Neurohormonal factors in functional dyspepsia: insights on pathophysiological mechanisms. Gastroenterology 1991;100:1311–1318.

247. Mayer, EA. The neurobiology of stress and gastrointestinal disease. Gut 2000;4:861–869.

248. Muth, ER, Stern, RM, Koch, KL. Effects of vection-induced motor sickness on gastric myoelectric activity and oral-caecal transit time. Dig Dis Sci 1996;41:330–334.

249. Kim, MS, Chey, WD, Owyang, C, et al. Role of plasma vasopressin as a mediator of nausea and gastric slow wave dysrhythmias in motion sickness. Am J Physiol 1997;35:G853–G862.

250. Smart, HL, Atkinson, M. Abnormal vagal function in irritable bowel syndrome. Lancet 1987;2:475–478.

251. Aggarwal, A, Cutts, TF, Abell, TL, et al. Predominant symptoms in irritable bowel syndrome correlate with specific autonomic nervous system abnormalities. Gastroenterology 1996;110:393–404.

252. Adeyemi, EO, Desai, KD, Towsey, M, Ghista, D. Characterisation of autonomic dysfunction in patients with the irritable bowel syndrome by means of heart rate variability studies. Am J Gastroenterol 1999;94:816–823.

253. Elsenbruch, S, Orr, W. Diarrhea- and constipation-predominant IBS patients differ in postprandial autonomic and cortisol responses. Am J Gastroenterol 2001;96:460–466.

254. Elsenbruch, S, Holtmann, G, Oezcan, D, et al. Are there alterations of neuroendo-

crine and cellular immune responses to nutrients in women with irritable bowel syndrome? Am.J.Gastroenterol. 2004;99:703–710.

255. Whitehead, WE, Palsson, OS. Is rectal pain sensitivity a biological marker for irritable bowel syndrome: psychological influences on pain perception. Gastroenterology 1998;115:1263–1271.

256. Dickhaus, B, Mayer, EA, Firooz, N, et al. Irritable bowel syndrome patients show enhanced modulation of visceral perception by auditory stress. Am J Gastroenterol 2003;98:135–143.

257. Bennett, EJ, Kellow, JE, Cowan, H, et al. Suppression of anger and gastric emptying in patients with functional dyspepsia. Scand J Gastroenterol 1992;27:869–874.

258. Haug, TT, Svebak, S, Hausken, T, et al. Low vagal activity as mediating mechanism for the relationship between personality factors and gastric symptoms in functional dyspepsia. Psychosom Med 1994;56:181–186.

259. Feinle-Bisset, C, Meier, B, Fried, M, et al. Role of cognitive factors in symptom induction following high and low fat meals in patients with functional dyspepsia. Gut 2003;52:1414–1418.

260. Kellow, JE, Langeluddecke, PM, Eckersley, GM, et al. Effects of acute psychologic stress on small-intestinal motility in health and the irritable bowel syndrome. Scand J Gastroenterol 1992;27:53–58.

261. Kumar, D, Wingate, DL. The irritable bowel syndrome: A paroxysmal motor disorder. Lancet 1985;2:973–977.

262. Latimer, PR, Sarna, SK, Campbell, D, et al. Colonic motor and myoelectrical activity: a comparative study of normal patients, psychoneurotic patients and patients with irritable bowel syndrome (IBS). Gastroenterology 1981;80:893–901.

263. Welgan, P, Meshkinpour, H, Hoehler, F. The effect of stress on colon motor and electrical activity in irritable bowel syndrome. Psychosom Med 1985;47:139–149.

264. Welgan, P, Meshkinpour, H, Beeler, M. Effect of anger on colon motor and myoelectric activity in irritable bowe syndrome. Gastroenterology 1988;94:1150–1156.

265. Cann, PA, Read, NW, Brown, C, et al. Irritable bowel syndrome: relationship of disorders in the transit of a single solid meal to symptom patterns. Gut 1983;24:405–411.

266. Evans, PR, Bennet, EJ, Bak, Y-T, et al. Jejunal sensorimotor dysfunction in irritable bowel syndrome—Clinical and psychosocial features. Gastroenterology 1996;110:393–404.

267. Saunders, PR, Koseck, V, McKay, DM, et al. Acute stressors stimulate ion secretion and increase epithelial permeability in rat intestine. Am.J.Physiol. 1994;267:G794–G799.

268. Soderholm, JD, Yan P-C, Ceponis, P, et al. Chronic stress induces mast cell-dependent bacterial adherence and initiates mucosal inflammation in rat intestine. Gastroenterology 2002;123:1099–1108.

269. Gue, M, Tekamp, A, Tabis, N, et al. Cholecystokinin blockade of emotional stress- and CRF-induced colonic motor alterations in rats: role of the amygdala. Brain Res 1994;658:232–238.

270. Tache, Y, Martinez, V, Million, M, et al. Stress and the gastrointestinal tract III. Stress-related alterations of gut motor function: role of brain corticotropin-releasing factor receptors. Am J Physiol 2001;280:G173–G177.

271. Fukudo, S, Suzuki, J. Colonic motility, autonomic function, and gastrointestinal hormones under psychological stress on IBS. J Exp Med 1987;151:373–385.

272. Lembo, T, Plourde, V, Shui, Z, et al. Effects of the corticotrophin-releasing factor (CRF) on rectal afferent nerves in humans. Neurogastroenterol Motil 1996;8:9–19.

273. Stanghellini, V, Tosetti, C, Patermico, A, et al. Risk indicators of delayed gastric emptying of solids in patients with functional dyspepsia. Gastroenterology 1996; 110:1036–1042.

274. Fock, KM, Khoo, TK, Chia, KS, et al. Helicobacter pylori infection and gastric emptying of indigestible solids in patients with dysmotility-like dyspepsia. Scand J Gastroenterol 1997;32:676–680.

275. Tack, J, Caenepeel, P, Fischler, B, et al. Symptoms associated with hypersensitivity to gastric distension in functional dyspepsia. Gastroenterology 2001;121:526–535.

276. Sarnelli, G, Caenepeel, P, Geypens, B, et al. Symptoms associated with impaired gastric emptying of solids and liquids in functional dyspepsia. Am J Gastroenterol 2003;98:783–788.

277. Piessevaux, H, Tack, H, Walrand, S, et al. Intragastric distribution of a standardized meal in health and functional dyspepsia; correlation with specific symptoms. Neurogastroenterol Motil 2003;124:903–910.

278. Boeckxstaens, GE, Hirsch, DP, Kuiken, SD, et al. The proximal stomach and postprandial symptoms in functional dyspeptics. Am J Gastroenterol 2002;97:40–48.

279. Hausken, T, Berstad, A. Wide gastric antrum in patients with non-ulcer dyspepsia. Effect of cisapride. Scand J Gastroenterol 1992;27:427–432.

280. Hveem, K, Jones, KL, Chatterton, BE, et al. Scintigraphic measurement of gastric emptying and ultrasonographic assessment of antral area: relation to appetite. Gut 1996;38:816–821.

281. Gilja, OH, Hausken, T, Barg, CJ, et al. Effect of glyceryl trinitrate on gastric accommodation and symptoms in functional dyspepsia. Dig Dis Sci 1997;42:2124–2131.

282. Fischler, B, Tack, J, de Gucht, V, et al. Heterogeneity of symptom pattern, psychosocial factors, and pathophysiological mechanisms in severe functional dyspepsia. Gastroenterol 2003;124:903–910.

283. Bredenoord, AJ, Chial, HJ, Camilleri, M, et al. Gastric accommodation and emptying in evaluation of patients with upper gastrointestinal symptoms. Clin Gastroenterol Hepatol 2003;1:264–272.

284. Delgado-Aros, S, Camilleri, M, Cremonini, F, et al. Contributions of gastric volumes and gastric emptying to meal size and postmeal symptoms in functional dyspepsia. Gastroenterology 2004;127:1685–1694.

285. Steens, J, Van der Schaar, PJ, Penning, C, et al. Compliance, tone and sensitivity of the rectum in different subtypes of irritable bowel syndrome. Neurogastroenterol Motil 2002;14:241–247.

286. Whitehead, WE, Holtkotter, B, Enck, P, et al. Tolerance for rectosigmoid distension in irritable bowel syndrome. Gastroenterology 1990;98:1187–1192.

287. Snape, WJ, Carlson, GM, Cohen, S. Colonic myoelectric activity in the irritable bowel syndrome. Gastroenterolgoy 1976;70:326–330.

288. Bazzocchi, G, Ellis, J, Villanueva-Meyer, J, et al. Effect of eating on colonic motility and transit in patients with functional diarrhea. Gastroenterology 1991;101:1298–1306.

289. Simren, M, Abrahamsson, H, Bjornsson, ES. An exaggerated sensory component of the gastrocolonic response in patients with irritable bowel syndrome. Gut 2001; 48:20–27.

290. Clemens, CH, Samsom, M, Roelofs, JM, et al. Association between pain episodes and high amplitude propagated pressure waves in patients with irritable bowel syndrome. Am J Gastroenterol 2003;98:1838–1843.

291. Bouin, M, Delvaux, M, Blanc, C, et al. Intrarectal injection of glycerol induces hypersensitivity to rectal distension in healthy subjects without modifying rectal compliance. Euro J Gastroenterol 2001;13:573–580.

292. Tremolaterra, F, Serra, J, Azpiroz, F, Villoria, A. Bloating and abdominal wall dystony. Gastroenterology 2004;126:A53.

293. Lewis, MJ, Reilly, B, Houghton, LA, et al. Ambulatory abdominal inductance plethysmography: towards objective assessment of abdominal distension in irritable bowel syndrome. Gut 2001;48:2126–220.

294. Basilisco, G, Marino, B, Passerini, L, et al. Abdominal distension after colonic lactulose fermentation recorded by a new extensometer. Neurogastroenterol Motil 2003;15:427–433.

295. Bouin, M, Lupien, F, Riberdy, M, et al. Intolerance to visceral distension in functional dyspepsia or irritable bowel syndrome: an organ-specific defect or a panintestinal dysregulation? Neurogastroenterol Motil 2004;16:311–314.

296. Lembo, T, Munakata, J, Mertz, H, et al. Evidence for the hypersensitivity of lumbar splanchnic afferents in irritable bowel syndrome. Gastroenterology 1994;107:1686–1696.

297. Bradette, M, Delvaux, M, Staumont, G, et al. Evaluation of colonic sensory thresholds in IBS patients using a barostat. Definition of optimal conditions and comparisons with healthy subjects. Dig Dis Sci 1994;39:449–457.

298. Bouin, M, Plourde, V, Boivin, M, et al. Rectal distension testing in patients with the irritable bowel syndrome: sensitivity, specificity, and predictive values of pain sensory thresholds. Gastroenterology 2002;122:1771–1777.

299. Tack, J, Caenepeel, P, Piessevaux, H. et al. Assessment of meal induced gastric accommodation by a satiety drinking test in health and in severe functional dyspepsia. Gut 2003;52:1271–1277.

300. Jones, MP, Hoffman, S, Shah, D, et al. The water load test: observations from healthy controls and patients with functional dyspepsia. Am J Physiol 2003;284:G896–G904.

301. Boeckxstans, G, Hirsch, D, Van den Elzen, BJ, et al. Impaired drinking capacity in patients with functional dyspepsia: relationship with proximal stomach function. Gastroenterology 2001;121:1054–1063.

302. Spechler, SJ, Castell, DO. Classification of esophageal motility abnormalities. Gut 2001;49:145–151.

303. Coffin, B, Azpiroz, F, Guarner, F, et al. Selective gastric hypersensitivity and reflex hyporeactivity in functional dyspepsia. Gastroenterology 1994;101:1345–1351.

304. Soffer, E, Thonsgawat, S. Clinical value of duodenojejunal manometry. Its usefulness in diagnosis and management of patients with gastrointestinal symptoms. Dig Dis Sci 1996;41:859–863.

305. Verhagen, MA, Samsom, M, Jebbink, RJ, Smout, AJPM. Clinical relevance of antroduodenal manometry. Eur J Gastroenterol Hepatol 1999;11:523–528.

306. Scott, SM, Picon, L, Knowles, CH, et al. Automated quantitative analysis of nocturnal jejunal motor activity identifies abnormalities in individuals and subgroups of patients with slow transit constipation. Am J Gastroenterol 2003;98:1123–1134.

307. Glia, A, Akerlund, JE, Lindberg, G. Outcome of colectomy for slow-transit constipation in relation to presence of small-bowel dysmotility. Dis Colon Rectum 204; 47:96–102.

308. DiBaise, JK, Oleynikov, D. Does gallbladder ejection fraction predict outcome after cholecystectomy for suspected chronic acalculous gallbladder dysfunction? A systematic review. Am J Gastroenterol 2003;98:2605–2611.

309. Toouli, J, Robers-Thomson, IC, Kellow J, et al. Manometry based randomised trial of endoscopic sphincterotomy for sphincter of Oddi dysfunction. Gut 2000;46:98–102.

310. Kellow, JE, Miller, LJ, Phillips, SF, et al. Altered sensitivity of the gallbladder to cholecystokinin octapeptide in irritable bowel syndrome. Am J Physiol 1987;253:G650–G655.

311. Klauser, AG, Voderholzer, WA, Heinrich, CA, et al. Behavorial modification of colonic function. Can constipation be learned? Dig Dis Sci 1990;35:1271–1275.

312. Bassotti, G, Chiarioni, G, Imbimbo, BP, et al. Impaired colonic motor response to cholinergic stimulation in patients with severe chronic idiopathic (slow transit type) constipation. Dig Dis Sci 1992;30:1040–1045.

313. De Schryver, AM, Samsom, M, Smout, AJ. Effects of a meal and bisacodyl on colonic motility in healthy volunteers and patients with slow transit constipation. Dig Dis Sci 2003;48:1206–1212.

314. Herve, S, Savoye, G, Behbahani, A, et al. Results of 24h manometric recording of colinic motor activity with endoluminal instillation of bisacodyl in patients with severe chronic slow transit constipation. Neurogastroenterol Motil 2004;16:397–402.

315. Dinning, PG, Bampton, PA, Andre, J, et al. Abnormal predefecatory colonic motor patterns define constipation in obstructed defecations. Gastroenterol 2004;127:49–56.

316. Rao, SSC, Azpiroz, F, Diamant, N, et al. Minimum standards of anorectal manometry. Neurogastroenterol Motil 2002;14:553–559.

317. Rao, SSC, Mudipalli, RS, Stessman, M, et al. Investigation of the utility of colorectal function tests and Rome II criteria in dyssynergic defecation (anismus). Neurogastroenterol Motil 2004;16:589–596.

318. Bharucha, AE. Outcome measures for fecal incontinence: anorectal structure and function. Gastroenterology 2004;126:S90–S98.

Chapter 4

Pharmacological and Pharmacokinetic Aspects of Functional Gastrointestinal Disorders

Michael Camilleri, Chair

Lionel Bueno, Co-Chair

Fabrizio De Ponti

Jean Fioramonti

R. Bruce Lydiard

Jan Tack

Introduction

The goals of this new chapter are to review the following: animal pharmacology and models that have been validated for the study of sensation and motility; preclinical pharmacology, pharmacokinetics and toxicology that are usually required for introduction of novel therapeutic agents; validated biomarkers for sensation and motility endpoints in experimental medicine; pharmacology of medications that are applied or have potential for the treatment of functional gastrointestinal disorders (FGIDs) in humans, including psychopharmacology; and pharmacogenomics applied to these medications and disorders.

Animal Pharmacology: Models Validated for the Study of Sensation and Motility

Development of new drugs for treatment of FGIDs is facilitated by preclinical animal models that must reproduce, as closely as possible, the alterations of FGIDs. Assessment of gastrointestinal (GI) motility in animals produces data comparable to that obtained in humans. However, because alterations of motility in FGIDs are not well defined and their etiology not established, there is no absolute model of altered motility in animals. Evaluation of sensation is not easy in humans. In animals, the term "sensation" cannot be used, and only surrogates of "pain" or "nociception" can be measured. Many models have been developed to assess somatic [1] and visceral [2] pain in animals. Since FGIDs are characterized by hypersensitivity to visceral stimuli, models of visceral allodynia and hyperalgesia have been proposed in animals. This section reviews the most commonly used animal models of visceral pain and hyperalgesia or disturbed GI motility (Figure 1).

— Visceral Pain

Mechanical Stimuli

Experiments are performed in awake or anesthetized rats, and the most often used stimulus of pain is latex balloon distension of a gut segment. The balloon is generally made from the tip of a condom that is then mounted on a polyethylene catheter and connected to a barostat to measure simultaneously the compliance of the gut and the noxious response. For example, a tachykinin neurokinin 3 (NK_3) receptor antagonist has antinociceptive action on colorectal distension

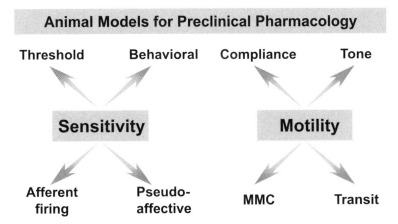

Figure 1. Summary of endpoints in experimental animal models.
MMC = migrating motor complex

in rats without modifying the balloon volume, regardless of the pressure applied [3]. A balloon can also be chronically implanted in the gut [4–6], although variability in balloon construction and unfolding influences reproducibility of experiments. Arterial embolectomy probes [7] have a very reproducible diameter, but do not permit measurement of pressure-volume relationships. All of the distension procedures commonly used in humans [8] can be used in animals; the currently favored approach is a step-wise increase in pressure or volume.

Chemical Stimuli

In the rat, infusion of glycerol into the colon through a chronically implanted catheter induces abdominal cramps that are attenuated by 5-hydroxytriptamine type 3 (5-HT$_3$) receptor antagonists [9]. This model is considered clinically relevant since intracolonic glycerol induces abdominal pain in humans, and interestingly, mimics pain in irritable bowel syndrome (IBS) patients [10]. The mechanisms involve local mucosal irritation since pain can be abolished after mucosal application of lidocaine [10]. Intracolonic irritants, such as mustard oil and capsaicin, have also been used to evoke spontaneous visceral pain [11].

Other Stimuli

Other stimuli have been used to investigate visceral pain modulation in animal models, including other chemical irritants (such as trinitrobenzene sulfuric acid, dioctyl sodium sulfonylceinate, zyprogen) and parasite infestations (such as *Nippostrongylus brasiliensis* or *Trichinella spiralis*). The "writhing test," consisting of an intraperitoneal injection of an irritant compound such as acetic acid

[12], is used for pharmacological studies of analgesic compounds, but it reflects peritoneal irritation rather than visceral pain. Traction of the mesentery in the anesthetized rat may be relevant for pharmacological studies aimed to reduce autonomic reactions in patients undergoing abdominal surgery, but not for visceral pain. Stimulation of the splanchnic nerves or electrical stimulation of the stomach or the small intestine by mucosal electrodes [13] also induce painful responses [13, 14]. At present, there is no consensus as to the best model to study visceral pain.

Endpoints

In animals, nociceptive responses to stimuli, named "pseudo-affective" responses, were first characterized by Sherrington and coworkers in 1904 [14]. These responses are brain stem or spinal reflexes and include flexion/withdrawal, head turning, grimacing, vocalization, cardiovascular changes, respiratory changes, and regional or generalized muscle contraction. Pseudo-affective responses characteristically cease when the noxious stimulus is terminated.

The most commonly used endpoint in the rat is the contraction of abdominal muscles induced by rectal or colorectal distension, typically recorded by electromyography (EMG) [7, 14] with bipolar electrodes chronically implanted in the abdominal oblique musculature and exteriorized on the back of the neck. The number of spike bursts or integrated signals correspond to abdominal contractions over the period of distension, and they are correlated with the number of contractions and the intensity of the stimulus applied [7, 15].

The pressure threshold is the first distending pressure inducing a number of abdominal contractions significantly different from the number of contractions in the absence of distension. Distending threshold in rabbits is the pressure of a balloon in the distal colon that triggers a sudden contraction of the abdominal and hind leg muscles [16]. In mice, colorectal distension triggers only one sustained contraction at the onset of the distension [17, 18]. Recording EMG activity through telemetry permits performance of distension studies in freely moving rats, but there are signal artifacts due to animal movements [6]. An alternative to EMG of the striated abdominal muscle is to directly record the contraction by suturing a strain gauge transducer to the abdominal muscle [19] and counting the number of contractions during distension. Abdominal contractions are induced by colorectal distension. Gastric distension in rats does not induce abdominal contractions, but stretching of the body or raising of the head, and EMG of neck (acromiotrapezius) muscles have been used as nociceptive response to gastric distension [4, 5]. This technique demonstrated a role of central serotinergic 5-HT$_{1A}$ receptor in the nociceptive response to gastric distension [20]. It is, however, also possible that the EMG recording may reflect contractions associated with a distension-induced defecation reflex rather than being a measure of pain.

Visceral distension also induces viscero-visceral reflexes, such as relaxation of anal sphincters [15], rectocolonic inhibition, or inhibition of gastric empty-ing [21]. Such upstream inhibitory reflexes are enhanced in IBS patients [22, 23]. Different pathways are involved in visceral and somatic responses; for example, a tachykinin NK_2 receptor antagonist reduces the abdominal contractions induced by colorectal distension, but does not modify the concomitant inhibition of the motility of the proximal colon [24].

Change in blood pressure is a pseudo-affective response widely used to as-sess visceral pain. In anesthetized rats, visceral distension increases arterial blood pressure with tachycardia, while in deeply anesthetized rats there is a depressor response with bradycardia [15]. The depressor response depends upon the anes-thetic compound used; a very weak response occurs under ketamine, and a pow-erful response under pentobarbital. Mechanisms of the differences in responses to distension are unclear. Heart rate response is also a reliable pseudo-affective re-sponse. In anesthetized rats, gastric distension induces bradycardia, with intensity related to the volume of distension [25]. Cardiovascular and muscular responses act via brainstem reflexes; both are vigorous in decerebrated, but not spinalized rats [15]. However, the significances of the responses are different, particularly under inflammatory conditions [26].

Electrophysiological recordings from sensory neurons or second-order neurons in the spinal cord may provide the most direct evidence that a pharmacological agent alters afferent function [27, 28]. Measurements of the effect of the medica-tion on viscus compliance are essential to differentiate effects on volume thresh-olds to activate sensory fibers from drug-induced contraction or relaxation [29].

Several behavioral endpoints have been used. They involve brain centers higher than the brain stem and responses do not cease when the noxious stimulus is ter-minated. Therefore, they are not pseudo-affective responses [14]. A simple be-havioral response in the rat during colorectal distension [26] is to score 0 for an absence of response, 1 for a brief head movement followed by immobility, 2 for contraction of abdominal muscles, 3 for lifting of abdomen, and 4 for body arch-ing and lifting of pelvic structures. In mice, pain related behaviors, such as licking the abdomen, stretching, squashing of the abdomen against the floor, and abdom-inal retractions have been evaluated after colonic administration of mustard oil [11]. Referred somatic hyperalgesia is evaluated in mice by application of von Frey hairs with forces from 1 to 32 mN on the abdomen and scoring the subsequent be-havioral response that is videotaped as (1) sharp reaction of the abdomen, (2) es-cape reaction accompanied by immediate licking of the site of application of hair, and (3) jumping with all four paws off the floor.

In a passive avoidance behavioral paradigm [15], rats are placed on a platform and the latency of step-down is measured (normal around 10 seconds). When the rat is submitted to colorectal distension after each trial, the latency increases and correlates with the distending pressure. Another behavioral test measures the per-formance of rats in an aversive light stimulus avoidance experimental device during colitis induced by trinitrobenzene sulphonic acid (TNBS) [30]. Intestinal or colonic distension in rats affects feeding behavior and elicits taste aversion [31]. These behavioral models are difficult to quantify and not easy to use for pharmacological purposes. However, they cannot be neglected, as they may be relevant for FGIDs given the high incidence of psychopathology [32], including alterations of feeding behavior seen in these disorders [33].

Direct Afferent Recordings

The most direct approach is measurement of neuronal activity of afferent neurons in anesthetized animals. For example, neurons in the superficial spinal dorsal horn of the T13-L2 spinal segments respond to colorectal distension in the rat [34] and are suppressed by morphine [35]. Recordings of pelvic nerve afferent fibers have also been used to evaluate the visceral antinociceptive effect of various compounds such as the κ-opioid receptor agonist fedotozine, which reduces the activity [36] and the number of abdominal contractions induced by colorectal distension in awake rats [3]. Long-term neuronal responses can be evaluated from the expression of immediate early gene-encoded proteins such as c-Fos in different areas of the spinal cord, including the dorsal horn [37]. The tachykinin NK_2 receptor antagonist, nepadutant, reduces c-Fos expression evoked in the spinal dorsal horn by TNBS-induced colitis, but not by colorectal distension [38]. The N-methyl-d-aspartate (NMDA) receptor antagonist MK-801 reduces c-Fos expression induced in the spinal cord by a noxious (80 mmHg) or an innocuous (20 mmHg) colorectal distension [39].

Allodynia and Hyperalgesia

Several animal models have been proposed in an attempt to reproduce the visceral hypersensitivity to mechanical stimulus in FGID. However, they are not fully predictive of activity in patients, although it is believed that the probability of these animal models predicting efficacy of a new FGID agent increases with the number of positive effects in multiple animal models.

Esophagus: No validated experimental models of esophageal sensitivity in gastroesophageal reflux (GER) were developed in animals. One study evaluated the nociceptive response to esophageal distension by measuring the EMG of the spinotrapezius muscles [40].

Stomach: In the few models available, hypersensitivity to distension has been induced by inflammation. Acetic acid (20%) or iodoacetamide (0.1%) in drinking water for several days induces hyperalgesia to gastric distension in rats, assessed by neck muscle contraction [5]. Because of the presence of ulcers, the acetic acid model is questionable as a relevant model for FGIDs. The iodoacetamide model seems more relevant since it induces no macroscopic damage and only a moderate increase in myeloperoxidase activity (leucocytes) and minor microscopic lesions (edema in the submucosa, mild inflammatory cell infiltrate) [41]. Another rat model of gastric hyperalgesia (demonstrable by fall in arterial blood pressure after distension) results from the ingestion for three weeks of very low doses of the herbicide diquat, a food contaminant [42]. Hyperalgesia is clearly observed for distending pressures from 10 to 40 mmHg and is not associated with macroscopic gastric lesions but with a moderate increase in myeloperoxidase activity and hyperplasia of mast cells. However, not all food contaminants induce gastric hyperalgesia. Ingestion of nitrate, which is a tap water contaminant, reduces gastric sensitivity to distension after nitrate metabolism to nitric oxide in the stomach [43].

Small intestine: Hypersensitivity to distensions assessed by the fall in blood pressure occurs after infection with the nematode *Nippostrongylus brasiliensis* [44], which induces a jejunal inflammation peaking at two weeks and resolving two weeks later when hypersensitivity is associated with normal myeloperoxidase activity but persistent mast cell hyperplasia. The latter seems clinically relevant given the increased number of mucosal mast cells in IBS patients [45]. Postinfective hyperalgesia is blocked by mast cell stabilizers, and tachykinin NK_2 receptor antagonists are more effective to reduce the fall in arterial pressure induced by jejunal distension in the postinfective period than in control animals [46]. Not all nematode infections are associated with hypersensitivity. For example, *Trichinella spiralis*-induced intestinal inflammation in rats is associated with decreased sensitivity to gastric distension [47].

Colon-rectum: More models of hyperalgesia or allodynia are available for large intestines than for the upper gastrointestinal tract. In acute restraint stress in rats, wrapping forelimbs and the thoracic trunk induces both allodynia and hyperalgesia to colorectal distension [48]. Repeated acute stress sessions only trigger hypersensitivity to the largest volumes of distension [49]. Both allodynia and hyperalgesia after stress involve corticotropin releasing factor (CRF) and mast cell degranulation. A greater stress-induced hypersensitivity has been observed in female rats than in males and is estrogen-dependent [50] or linked to differences in mast cell sensitization under stress that requires the expression of NK_1 receptors under the influence of estrogens [51].

In rats, administration of lipopolysaccharide (LPS, bacterial endotoxin) induces allodynia that appears 3 hours and 9 to 12 hours after administration [52], though the central and peripheral release of cytokines like interleukin 1beta (IL-1β) and tumor necrosis factor (TNF) is consistent with mast cell degranulation. Vagotomy enhances the effects of LPS, suggesting a primary peripheral site of action and a role of the vagus in the control of the local immune response that triggers allodynia. Activation of the proteinase-activated receptor-2 (PAR-2) by the cleavage of its N-terminal domain by proteinases such as trypsin with unmasking of a tethered ligand can also be considered as a model of visceral hyperalgesia. In rats, intracolonic trypsin or the tethered ligand of PAR-2 induces a delayed

(24-hour) hyperalgesia to rectal distension [53] via activation of local receptors on epithelial cells, leading to increased paracellular permeability, mucosal inflammatory reaction, and sensitization of primary afferent neurons [54].

A classical method to induce hyperalgesia to colorectal distension is a previous induction of inflammation, such as by TNBS [7], zymosan [55], turpentine [56], or acetic acid [26]. The relevance of inflammatory models of hyperalgesia for therapeutics of functional bowel disorders may be questionable, since these disorders are not inflammatory diseases even though local immune activation has been described. However, some common mechanisms are involved in inflammatory and noninflammatory models of hyperalgesia. For example, tachykinin NK_3 receptor antagonists similarly reduce hyperalgesia induced by restraint stress and colonic inflammation [3].

Two long-term models of colonic hyperalgesia are available. In the first model [57], colonic inflammation is induced in young rats (intracolonic injections of mustard oil daily between the ages of 8 and 21 days), and the sensitivity to rectal distension is tested when the rats are 3-month old adults. Hypersensitivity is demonstrable with behavioral parameters and neuronal recordings in the spinal cord. Another long-term model results from maternal separation (3 hours per day) from postnatal days 2 to 14 [58]. This stressor induces hypersensitivity to rectal distension in 2-month old rats, as shown by the amplitude of abdominal muscle electromyogram. An acute or chronic stress model is shown by the increase in the response to colorectal distension induced by an acute stress in maternally deprived rats, in comparison with untouched rats [59]. Hypersensitivity of the adult rat depends on the experimental protocol of maternal separation [60]. Separation of all the pups from the mother induces greater hyperalgesia to rectal distension than separation of only half of the littermates, indicating that stress experienced by the mother also plays a role. Hypersensitivity induced by maternal separation is associated with alterations in colonic epithelial barrier and mucosal immunity [58].

— Motility

The techniques used to record motility or measure GI transit in animals may differ from techniques used in humans. However, the endpoints are identical. For example, the motility index calculated from manometric records in humans or strain gauge records in animals, which corresponds to the area under the contractile curve, has the same meaning in both humans and animals. In animals, gamma camera studies of gastric emptying have not been fully validated. Thus, gastric emptying is most often determined at only one time point after meal ingestion. Gastric emptying of solid and liquid phases of the meal can be discriminated in animals by using specific markers. Intestinal and colonic transit in larger animals are performed as in humans [61]. For smaller animals, the geometric center of tracer (radioactive markers or phenol red) is determined after sacrifice of the animals. Stable isotope measurements can be used in small or large animals to measure gastric emptying [62, 63] or orocecal transit [64].

Animal models available for pharmacological purposes in the scope of functional bowel disorders are mainly models of delayed gastric emptying and altered colonic motility and transit. However, GER is associated with transient relaxation of the lower esophageal sphincter (LES) and models of altered LES openings have been developed in animals.

Techniques for examining fundic/gastric tone in larger animals [65] have been scaled down to smaller animals [66].

Transient Relaxation of the LES

A dog model has been developed for the study of transient lower esophageal sphincter relaxations (TLESRs) [67] by monitoring esophageal, LES, and gastric pressure during continuous air insufflation into the stomach. Several pharmacological agents have been tested in dogs, and results with cholecystokinin (CCK_1) receptor antagonists [68], gamma-aminobutyric acid B (GABA-B) receptor agonists [69] and nitric oxide (NO) synthase inhibitors [70] have been reproduced in humans. TLESRs have been also measured and inhibited by GABA-B receptor agonists in ferrets [71].

Delayed Gastric Emptying

Stress is the most commonly used perturbation to inhibit gastric emptying in animals [72] and humans. Numerous stressors have been proposed to inhibit gastric emptying: restraint [73], acoustic [74], cold [74], combined acoustic and cold [75], passive avoidance in rats [76], and transport to an unknown environment in dogs [77]. The effect depends on the stressor applied and the nature of the test meal. In mice, acoustic or cold stress accelerates gastric emptying of a nutritive test meal, with no effect on emptying of a nonnutritive meal (methylcellulose) [74].

Prolonged colonic distension [21] inhibits gastric emptying in dogs, and this is considered relevant since voluntary suppression of defecation for four days inhibits gastric emptying in humans [78]. This inhibition of gastric emptying by colonic distension in dogs is reversed by the κ-opioid receptor agonist fedotozine [21] and by the 5-HT_3 receptor antagonist granisetron.

In a model of gastroparesis, gastric emptying can be pharmacologically delayed. This is a questionable model for testing compounds for future development in treatment of functional bowel disorders, since the pharmacological perturbation may not reflect the pathophysiology in FGIDs and this test compound may interfere with the drug used to inhibit gastric emptying.

An elegant experimental method to inhibit gastric emptying is the duodenal infusion of lipids in humans or animals. This has been done in rats fitted with a duodenal cannula [79] and is relevant to the FGIDs.

Gastric Compliance, Fasting, and Postprandial Gastric Tone

Placement of strain gauges on the fundic gastric wall or the barostatically-controlled balloon have been used successfully to evaluate the influence of drugs on gastric functions [80]. This model has been scaled down for use in rats and mice [66].

Altered Duodenojejunal Migrating Motor Complex Pattern

Stress affects migrating motor complex (MMC) patterns and may be important in maintaining a gradient in intestinal microflora and gut absorptive functions. However, very few animal models of altered MMC pattern have been developed. Acoustic stress in dogs alters the duodenojejunal MMC pattern and increases the duration of postprandial MMC disruption [81].

Altered Colonic Motility and Transit

Colonic motility can be inhibited by several pharmacological compounds. α_2- adrenoceptor agonists such as clonidine are very potent inhibitors of colonic and small intestine motility in rats [82], and this effect is centrally mediated [83]. μ-opioid receptor agonists, such as morphine, also strongly inhibit colonic motility in rats [84]. There are important differences between animal species regarding the effects of morphine. As for gastric motility and emptying, pharmacological inhibition of colonic motility is also a questionable model.

Stress is probably the most often used model to stimulate colonic motility [85], colonic transit, and fecal excretion in rats [86]. Effects are centrally mediated in part by the release of CRF, since they are blocked by an intracerebroventricular administration of a CRF receptor antagonist and reproduced by administration of CRF [85, 86]. Interestingly, the effects of stress on colonic motility in rats and humans share some common features. For example, habituation reduces the stress-related increase in colonic motility in rats and humans [85, 87].

In summary, present knowledge of the physiopathology of FGIDs is limited and does not permit a definitive selection of one or more relevant animal models of visceral hyperalgesia. It is difficult, based on a single animal model, to predict efficacy of a compound in clinical trials. Using more than one animal model may enhance the probability of selecting effective drugs for further development. To date, only two medications (tegaserod and cilansetron) have had a track record of both proven efficacy in animal models (for both transit and sensation) and proven clinical efficacy. In addition, pain is not the only FGID symptom affecting quality of life, and animal models of altered motility may be relevant to the assessment of new compounds.

Preclinical Pharmacology, Pharmacokinetics, and Toxicology Required for Novel Therapeutic Agents

Despite exponential growth in the number of compounds of potential interest for the treatment of FGIDs, few have received marketing authorization and we cannot ignore the regulatory problems that have led to restriction on use (or even withdrawal) of some new drugs.

Nevertheless, significant opportunities for the development of new drugs are provided by the increasing understanding of basic neuroenteric science and by the recent advances in clinical trial design and the use of clinically significant endpoints to assess drug efficacy. New medications (e.g., serotonergic, tachykininergic, opioid, and cannabinoid modulators) are now in the clinical development pipeline and are being carefully appraised as potential drugs for the use in FGIDs.

This section will outline some general pharmacodynamic, pharmacokinetic and safety aspects that are important for the development of new drugs for functional gut disorders.

— The Pharmacodynamic Target

Increased understanding of gastrointestinal pharmacology and the significant change in the efficacy endpoints used in clinical trials have revolutionized the current approach to drug development.

Drug Selectivity

Selectivity refers to the ability of a compound to interact with only one receptor subtype, leaving other receptors unaffected at concentrations achieved at clinically used doses and avoiding side effects. This was often considered the key to finding the "magic bullet." There are several important pitfalls to this approach (Table 1).

Table 1. The Issue of Drug Selectivity

- The drug should preferentially target a whole pathophysiological mechanism rather than a single receptor, unless this single receptor is proved to play a key role in the pathophysiology of the disorder.

- The classification of drugs as agonists or antagonists at a given receptor subtype is often an oversimplification because each compound has a complex spectrum of actions.

- "Selective" ligands may actually have multiple effects: (a) because of the many possible locations of the receptor subtype being considered as a target, (b) because of the potential of the "selective" ligand to act through more than one receptor subtype.

Table 2. Protean Nature of Pharmacodynamics of Some Compounds

Cisapride	5-HT$_4$ receptor agonist
	5-HT$_3$ receptor antagonist
	HERG K [+] channel blocker
Sumatriptan	5-HT$_{1B/D}$ receptor agonist
	5-HT$_{1F}$ receptor agonist
	5-HT$_7$ receptor agonist (weak)
Tegaserod	5-HT$_4$ receptor agonist
	5-HT$_{2B}$ receptor antagonist
Buspirone	5-HT$_{1A}$ receptor agonist
	D$_2$ dopamine receptor antagonist
	one metabolite is an α_2-adrenoceptor antagonist
Erythromycin	antibacterial macrolide
	potent motilin receptor agonist
	potent CYP3A4 inhibitor

5-HT = 5-hydroxytryptamine

First, drug selectivity is a relative concept, and the tendency to label a drug as a "selective" ligand for a given receptor subtype often leads us to ignore that a single molecule, at therapeutic doses, may have several, sometimes disparate, biological targets (Table 2). There are instances where the pharmacological properties responsible for the therapeutic effect of a compound are clarified only after the compound has undergone clinical trials (e.g., cisapride was found to be a partial 5-HT$_4$ receptor agonist [88], a 5-HT$_3$ receptor antagonist, and a fairly potent human ether-a-go-go related gene (HERG) K [+] channel blocker [89]). HERG K [+] channels are expressed in cardiac cells, gut smooth muscle, and interstitial cells of Cajal [90, 91].

Increasing Degree of Overlap of Two Pharmacophores

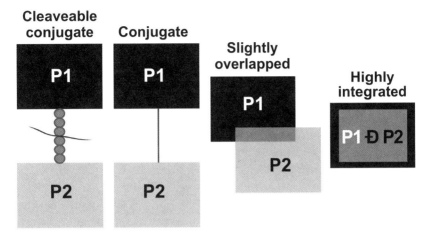

Figure 2. The degree of pharmacophore overlap varies significantly among "designed" multiple ligands. There is a continuum from conjugates where the pharmacophores are well separated by a linker group to ligands where the pharmacophores are highly intermingled. P = pharmacophore. Reproduced with permission from Morphy et al. 2004 [92].

The second pitfall is that, because of the multifactorial pathophysiology of FGIDs, single receptor modulating drugs may be less likely to achieve a substantial therapeutic gain. In several fields [92], evidence suggests that a balanced modulation of multiple targets can provide a superior therapeutic effect and side effect profile compared to the action of a selective ligand. Rational approaches in which structural features from selective ligands are combined have produced *designed* multiple ligands that span a large variety of targets (Figure 2) [92]. A key challenge in the design of multiple ligands is attaining a balanced activity at each target of interest while simultaneously achieving a wider selectivity and a suitable pharmacokinetic profile. The less selective a ligand is the harder it is to predict toxicity, and once toxicity occurs it becomes even more difficult to provide a mechanistic explanation for it. This may jeopardize the development and regulatory approval of less selective ligands.

Third, it is likely that the mechanisms underlying symptoms in FGIDs may differ from one patient to another and, hence, require using multiple therapies or "designed" multiple ligands. With the selective approach, primary clinical endpoints were achieved in less than 70% of patients with the approved agents such as tegaserod or alosetron [93–95], and phase II studies did not suggest that a higher dose would increase the response. When treating medical conditions such as hypertension or asthma, if monotherapy does not provide an adequate response, combination therapy is the rule. Given the redundancy of mechanisms controlling neurosensory and neuromuscular functions in the gut, it is conceivable that effective treatment of functional gut disorders may require combination therapy or designed multiple ligands.

One example is provided by the possible combination of a $5\text{-}HT_3$ receptor antagonist with a $5\text{-}HT_4$ receptor agonist to modulate visceral sensitivity, peristalsis and fluid absorption. However, $5\text{-}HT_3$ receptor antagonists slow transit, and 30% of patients treated with alosetron in trials developed constipation [93, 95, 96]. Since $5\text{-}HT_4$ receptors stimulate prokinesia [97], compounds with mixed properties (i.e., a $5\text{-}HT_3$ receptor antagonist with partial agonist action at $5\text{-}HT_4$ receptors) may improve the therapeutic gain obtained with pure $5\text{-}HT_3$ receptor antagonists. This hypothesis must undergo formal testing in clinical trials.

Another example is provided by tachykinin receptor antagonists: it has been suggested that the analgesic efficacy and motility inhibition of multi- or pantachykinin receptor antagonists are superior to those of monoreceptor antagonists [98, 99].

Uncertainties of Determining the Pharmacodynamic Target In Vivo

It is not uncommon to discover new actions of a compound serendipitously, without an understanding of the mechanism of action or the receptor(s) involved. This might be more likely to occur because of the complexities in the possible targets in vivo (different receptor systems, different locations of the same receptor, possibility of peripheral and central sites of action). In these cases, it is difficult to use the compound as a model to develop new drugs.

For example, sumatriptan is reported to improve gastric accommodation to a meal and reduce perception of gastric distension, hence relieving epigastric symptoms in dyspepsia [100]. However, different receptor subtypes seem to be responsible for the gastric relaxing effect of sumatriptan depending on the species [80, 101], and the precise site of action of sumatriptan in humans is unknown. Moreover, sumatriptan delays emptying of solids and liquids, may increase transient lower esophageal sphincter relaxations, and has the potential to induce esophageal and coronary spasm. Thus, sumatriptan per se is an unlikely contender in the therapeutic arena and developing new drugs using sumatriptan as a model drug is, at present, a difficult task.

Pharmacodynamic vs. Pathophysiological Target

When drugs address a single mechanism, heterogeneity in pathophysiology (e.g., dysmotility vs. hypersensitivity) has a negative impact on the therapeutic gain if patients are not selected on the basis of the specific disorder. Indeed, some of the disappointing results of the past decade can be ascribed to the heterogeneity of functional disorders, lack of understanding of pathophysiology, and lack of short-term mechanistic studies that can predict clinical outcome.

New drugs should target the entire pathophysiological mechanism(s) contributing to the functional disorder rather than only an individual part or a specific receptor. Thus, nonselective agents designed to modulate multiple targets of the whole pathophysiological process (e.g., dysmotility, sensory disorder, inflammation) would be advantageous over highly selective medications addressing a single mechanism. Appropriate patient subgroups should be recruited to show the therapeutic properties of a medication but this may reduce the generalizability of the results of the trial.

Mechanistic (pathophysiological) studies provide a rationale for drug development, but do not generally predict symptomatic success and do not necessarily identify the most appropriate dose for clinical trials. An important goal is to develop noninvasive tests that identify important pathophysiological mechanisms and assess symptom pattern in short-term therapeutic trials. This is addressed in the section on pharmacodynamic endpoints.

Finally, clinical efficacy should assess clinical endpoints or the perspective of the patient (e.g., global assessment of multiple symptoms).

Pharmacokinetics

The ideal pharmacokinetic characteristics of a drug are summarized in Table 3. Pharmacokinetics may help to achieve GI selectivity. This approach may be attempted when there are potential actions outside the GI tract. The typical example is provided by opioid receptor ligands. Loperamide is an antidiarrheal agent with no central effects because of its poor penetration of the blood-brain barrier. More recently, the prokinetic potential of peripherally restricted opioid receptor antagonists such as methylnatrexone and alvimopan has been investigated [102, 103]. These compounds do not cross the blood-brain barrier and, in addition, have very low oral bioavailability, thus, their action seems to be restricted to the gut.

Targeted drug delivery to the colon with pH- or time-dependent release [104, 105] or bacterial activation of prodrugs offers potential new approaches for FGIDs.

Another important pharmacokinetic property is the lack of significant interactions with other drugs. CYP2D6 (10% slow metabolizers in the community), CYP3A4, and CYP2C19 are important isoenzymes because of their involvement in the metabolism of many drugs and drug-drug interactions. Avoiding potent inhibitory interactions with both of these enzymes is highly desirable in early drug discovery, long before entering clinical trials. This may be achieved by computa-

Table 3. Ideal Drug for Treatment of Functional Gastrointestinal Disorders

1. *Pharmacodynamics*
   a. Targets important pathophysiological mechanism(s) (rather than receptor)
   b. No tachyphylaxis (the effect is maintained over time)

2. *Pharmacokinetics*
   a. Good oral bioavailability
   b. Half-life suitable for once daily administration
   c. Not a cytochrome P (CYP) substrate (lack of drug interactions)
   d. No metabolites with different or unwanted pharmacological actions
   e. No interactions with food

3. *Safety*
   a. High therapeutic index (maximum tolerated dose/effective dose$_{50}$)
   b. No interference with HERG K [$^+$] channels (no QT prolongation)

tional prediction with cost savings by decreased molecule synthesis and in vitro screening [106, 107]. Specifically, it is important to distinguish between pharmacokinetic modification resulting from drug metabolism by one of the enzymes versus drug interactions at one of the enzymes, which may be inhibition or induction. In both situations, drug-drug interactions may occur if inhibition or induction occurs at clinically relevant doses.

Safety Aspects

Apart from those aspects involved in the safety evaluation of every new medicinal product, there are three issues that deserve special attention because of the recent regulatory cases of cisapride (QT prolongation) and alosetron or cilansetron (ischemic colitis). Only these three will be discussed in detail here because of their strong bearing on the risk benefit/profile of drugs that are designed for functional disorders that are not life threatening.

— QT Prolongation

Prolongation of the QT interval of the electrocardiogram is a typical effect of class III anti-arrhythmic drugs. These agents prolong cardiac repolarization (hence the QT interval) due to blockade of potassium channels. Several classes of drugs used for noncardiovascular indications may prolong the QT interval as a side effect [108] and cause ventricular tachyarrhythmias, namely torsades de pointes (TdP), that may cause syncope and degenerate into ventricular fibrillation and sudden death [109]. Although a rare event (less than 1 in 100,000), even a low risk is not justified for those drugs providing only symptomatic improvement of a benign disease.

Second, approximately 2–3% of all drug prescriptions involve medications that may unintentionally cause the long QT syndrome (LQTS) [110]. Only some agents within a therapeutic class share the ability to significantly affect cardiac repolarization [111–113]. Thus, the drug development process should identify as early as possible compounds with this undesired effect [114].

Third, potentially fatal arrhythmias such as TdP are uncommon and are unlikely to occur during the course of phase I–III studies when relatively small numbers of subjects are exposed to the investigational drug. On the other hand, several of these adverse reactions might have been preventable had the drug development program been conducted according to recent standards. QT prolongation has become a surrogate marker of cardiotoxicity and has received increasing regulatory attention [90]. The standards for the early detection of an undesirable effect on cardiac repolarization are currently under review by regulatory agencies.

— Ischemic Colitis

Because it has been speculated that some drugs, such as those used to treat IBS, may cause ischemic colitis [115–117], it is worthwhile to determine whether there is any increase in the incidence of ischemic colitis in patients with specific illnesses. This issue is debated [118, 119] and most of the data are available only in abstract form. The incidence of ischemic colitis in the general population in published studies ranges from 4.5 to 44 cases per 100,000 person-years [118]. Compared with the general population, the relative risk for ischemic colitis in IBS patients is reported to increase approximately threefold, as measured in retrospective studies of health care databases [118]. These data, however, have been questioned [119]. Constipation is another comorbidity that appears to be a risk factor for ischemic colitis. Constipation is believed to promote ischemia by increasing intraluminal pressure and compressing the mucosal vessels [120]. However, reports in patients receiving tegaserod question this interpretation [119]. Older age and female sex also seem to increase the risk of ischemic colitis, although statistical comparisons are not available. Overall, low risk of these adverse effects or minor adverse events may be acceptable in patients when FGIDs are severe and affect daily living.

The pathophysiology of ischemic colitis associated with the use of alosetron is still unclear. It is also unknown whether this is a class effect of 5-HT$_3$ receptor antagonists when used in patients with IBS (notably, ischemic colitis is not an issue when 5-HT$_3$ receptor antagonists are used for chemotherapy-induced emesis). A preliminary account of a study carried out in rats [121] reports a decrease of mesenteric blood flow and vascular conductance with alosetron and cilansetron (but not with tegaserod). However, the predictive value of this experimental model for ischemic colitis is unknown, and reports of ischemic colitis in patients treated with tegaserod also question the relevance of the animal model.

— Drug Interactions

A third issue of particular relevance in FGIDs is the potential for drug interactions, given the problem of polypharmacy and the frequent use of psychotropic agents (which often depend on CYP2D6 metabolism).

Human Pharmacology

Table 4 reports a synopsis of the pharmacological approaches for the treatment of FGIDs. The most important of these will also be reviewed in this section. However, it is important to recognize two other classes of agents that are commonly used in FGIDs, that is, laxatives in the treatment of constipation (alone or in association with IBS), and probiotics.

The range of treatments for constipation have been reviewed extensively elsewhere [112]. Probiotics were initially shown to relieve bloating in patients with IBS [123, 124]. More recent data suggest that there is benefit for the treatment of overall symptoms of IBS with *Bifidobacteria* rather than *Lactobacillus*-based probiotics; this appears related to the reversal of IL10/IL12 mucosal cytokine relationships, suggesting an anti-inflammatory effect [125].

A meta-analysis of pharmacological treatments for IBS has been published recently [126]. The pharmacology of agents directed to amine receptors (Table 4A) or peptides (Table 4B) is summarized.

— Serotonergic Agents

Presence of 5-HT in the Gastrointestinal Tract

Serotonin, or 5-HT, is a neurotransmitter in the central nervous system (CNS). The gastrointestinal tract is by far the largest 5-HT storage depot in the body [127]. In most species, the bulk of 5-HT of the gut is contained within the enterochromaffin cells in the epithelial layer of the mucosa. 5-HT can be released from the enterochromaffin cells to initiate peristalsis by pressure applied to the mucosa [128–130], vagal stimulation [131], chemotherapeutic agents, and cholera toxin [132]. The remainder is found within neurons in the myenteric plexus of the stomach, the small intestine, and the colon of several species, including humans [133–139]. These neurons resemble 5-HT neurons in the CNS, for example, in their response to selective or nonselective 5-HT reuptake inhibitors. A 5-HT reuptake system is also present in the gastrointestinal tract. Selective serotonin reuptake inhibitors (SSRIs) enhance the availability of physiologically released 5-HT [140]. This review will briefly address the available data on human pharmacology and clinical therapeutics.

5-HT Reuptake Inhibitors

SSRIs prolong the availability of released 5-HT at the level of the enteric nervous system (ENS), allowing an indirect assessment of the role of 5-HT in the control of gastrointestinal functions. In the long term, they may lead to desensitization of 5-HT receptors.

In humans, an SSRI reduced the periodicity of the migrating motor complex in the jejunum [141] and accelerated small-intestinal, but not whole-gut transit [142]. Short-term administration of the SSRI paroxetine was shown to enhance gastric accommodation to a meal [143–144]; another SSRI, citalopram, increased colonic compliance and inhibited the colonic response to feeding [145].

Kuiken et al. found no beneficial effect of fluoxetine on symptoms and on rectal sensitivity in IBS [146]. Symptomatic benefit of citalopram in IBS was reported, possibly through its central action since there was no significant change in colonic sensorimotor function [145].

—   5-HT Receptors in the Gastrointestinal Tract

Smooth muscle is variably responsive to 5-HT [147, 148] while neural effects to 5-HT are much more consistent. 5-HT acts on enteric ganglia to activate neurons that release acetylcholine and cause contraction of longitudinal and circular muscle [149–152]. 5-HT also activates nonadrenergic noncholinergic inhibitory neurons and can therefore relax the gut if excitatory neurotransmission is blocked [147, 148, 151]. Several 5-HT receptor subtypes are present on both nerves and smooth muscle and mediate a number of different actions (Table 4) [97].

5-HT$_{1A}$ Receptors

The 5-HT$_1$ receptor group can be subdivided into several subtypes, of which only the 5-HT$_{1A}$ receptor subtype has been consistently found to be pres-

Table 4. Pharmacological Approaches in Functional Gastrointestinal Disorders

A. Agents Directed to Amines/Receptors

Target receptor	Type of ligand (Examples)	Distribution of receptors	Pharmacological action in animals	Pharmacological action in humans
5-HT	5-HT_3-receptor antagonists (e.g., alosetron, cilansetron)	Intrinsic and extrinsic neurons	Inhibits visceral sensitivity, absorption/secretion, motility	Slows transit, increases colonic compliance
	5-HT_4 receptor agonists (e.g., tegaserod, renzapride, prucalopride)	Enteric neurons, smooth muscle cells	Enhances secretion, and motility, reduces visceral sensitivity	Accelerates transit, increases colonic HAPC, and gastric accommodation, reduces inhibition of RIII reflex during rectal distension
	5-HT_{1A} receptor agonists (e.g., buspirone)	Enteric neurons, extrinsic afferent neurons	Inhibits motility and enhance compliance	Increases accommodation
ACh (Muscarinic)	M_3 receptor antagonists	Smooth muscle cells	Increases smooth muscle relaxation, compliance	No published data
	M_1 and M_2 receptor antagonists	Enteric neurons, smooth muscle cells	Increases gastric emptying	May enhance accommodation
Adreno-ceptors	β_3-adrenoceptor agonists	Smooth muscle cells	Inhibits motility	No published data
	α_2-adrenoceptor agonists	Enteric neurons, enterocytes	Reduces secretion, enhances compliance and reduces motility and tone	Reduces secretion, enhances compliance and reduces motility and tone and sensation
Dopamine	D_2 receptor antagonists (e.g., domperidone, levosulpiride, metoclopramide)	Area postrema, smooth muscle cells, enteric neurons	Contracts muscle	Antiemetic, prokinetic, reduced sensation?

B. Agents Directed to Peptides

Target receptor	Type of ligand (Examples)	Distribution of receptors	Pharmacological action in animals	Pharmacological action in humans
Motilin	Motilides	Smooth muscle cells, enteric neurons	Motility stimulation	Motility and transit stimulation
Opioid	μ-receptor agonists (e.g., loperamide)	Enterocytes, enteric neurons, afferent neurons, inflammation	Reduces intestinal secretion and transit	Slows colonic transit, antidiarrheal, increases resting anal tone
	μ-receptor antagonists (e.g., naloxone, methyl-naltrexone, alvimopan)	Enteric neurons, afferent neurons, inflammation	Reverses opioid effects on motility	Accelerates colonic transit, reverses effect of opiates on bowel dysfunction, reduces duration of postoperative ileus
	κ-receptor agonists (e.g., fedotozine, asimadoline)	Enteric neurons, afferent neurons	Reduces sensation, variable effects on motility	Reduces sensation
Somatostatin	SSR-2 receptor agonists (e.g., octreotide, lanreotide)	Enterocytes, submucosal neurons, Myenteric neurons	Retards transit, reduces afferent firing and sensation	Retards transit, reduces sensitivity, enhances absorption
Tachykinin	NK$_1$ receptor antagonists (e.g., aprepitant)	Enteric neurons, ICC, smooth muscle cells, immune cells	Inhibits motility, fluid secretion, vagal afferent sensation, and inflammation	Antiemetic
	NK$_2$ receptor antagonists (e.g., nepadutant)	Enteric neurons, smooth muscle cells, extrinsic afferents	Inhibits motility, fluid secretion, sensation, and inflammation	Inhibits NKA-induced motility
	NK$_3$ receptor antagonists (e.g., talnetant)	Enteric neurons, extrinsic afferents	Inhibits motility and sensation	No published data
CCK	CCK$_1$ receptor antagonists (e.g., dexloxiglumide)	Afferent vagal nerves, enteric neurons	Accelerates gastric emptying, inhibits TLESR	Inhibits lipid-induced gastric motor effects, inhibits TLESR

CCK = cholecystokinin   5-HT = 5 hydroxytryptamine   NKA = neurokinin A   ICC = interstitial cells of Cajal   TLESR = transient lower
ACh = acetylcholine   HAPC = high-amplitude propogated contractions   NK = neurokinin   SSR = somatosensory response   esophageal sphincter relaxations

ent in the ENS. Activation of 5-HT_{1A} receptors inhibits the release of acetylcholine [153]. The physiological role of 5-HT_{1A} receptors is unclear. Extrinsic afferents also express inhibitory 5-HT_{1A} receptors [154].

In humans, buspirone, a 5-HT_{1A} receptor agonist, increases LES tone, relaxes the proximal stomach, slows gastric emptying and induces a premature small bowel activity front [155]. Buspirone significantly decreased symptom scores after a liquid nutrient meal challenge [156]. Buspirone decreased rectal tone and significantly increased the volume thresholds during rectal distension, but failed to alter colonic sensorimotor function [156, 157].

A preliminary placebo-controlled, cross-over study reported that buspirone reduced symptoms and enhanced gastric accommodation in patients with functional dyspepsia [158]. A four-week multicenter placebo-controlled study with the 5-HT_{1A} receptor agonist R-137696 in functional dyspepsia failed to show any benefit [159]. However, repeat gastric barostat studies failed to show any effect of the drug on gastric compliance and accommodation after 4 weeks of treatment, suggesting that desensitization had occurred.

5-HT₃ Receptors

5-HT_3 receptors are found on enteric neurons, sympathetic nerves, and the vagus and the area postrema of the vomiting center. The receptor is a ligand-gated cation channel [160] that mediates a short-lived depolarizing response [161, 162]. The physiological role of the 5-HT_3 receptor in gastrointestinal functions has only been incompletely elucidated. 5-HT_3 receptors have been implicated in both arms of the peristaltic reflex, but data are equivocal [163–165].

Potent 5-HT_3 receptor antagonists have no prokinetic effect [166–168] and do not alter postprandial gastric volumes [169]. Studies have demonstrated that 5-HT_3 receptor antagonists delay orocecal and colonic transit times and reduce the tonic gastrocolonic response to feeding [170–173].

5-HT, acting through 5-HT_3-receptors, is a putative excitatory mediator in visceral sensory pathways, and some 5-HT_3 antagonists may reduce perception of visceral distension in animals [174]. Human studies have been less convincing. Gastric sensation was not altered by 5-HT_3 antagonists [175, 176]. Thresholds for rectal balloon distension were not significantly altered by ondansetron or alosetron [175, 177]. Alosetron was shown to alter colonic compliance, but not colonic sensitivity to isobaric distension [178].

Clinical trials show that the 5-HT_3 receptor antagonist alosetron improves stool pattern and provides relief of pain/discomfort in diarrhea-predominant IBS [93]. A meta-analysis of published studies confirmed the efficacy of alosetron in IBS with diarrhea [95]. Preliminary data suggest a similar potential for the 5-HT_3 receptor antagonist cilansetron [179], though there is also potential for ischemic colitis [180]. Shortly after its introduction to the American market, alosetron was withdrawn due to suspected side-effects of ischemic colitis/colonic ischemia [181] and it is now available only for restricted use in the U.S.

A dose-finding study suggested a potential modest effect of alosetron on symptoms of fullness and satiety in functional dyspepsia [182], but no further clinical development has occurred.

5-HT₄ Receptors

5-HT$_4$ receptors are present on intrinsic neurons and on smooth muscle cells, secretory cells, and enterochromaffin cells in the guinea pig ileum [183–185]. The 5-HT$_4$ receptor is involved in the initiation of the peristaltic reflex and enhances cholinergic neurotransmission [186–189]. In humans, there is only a modest effect of 5-HT$_4$ receptor antagonism on colonic transit [190], suggesting that the physiological role of 5-HT$_4$ receptors in the control of colonic function requires further study.

5-HT$_4$ receptor agonists stimulate gastric, small bowel, and colonic transit [191–193]. Tegaserod enhances small bowel transit and right colonic emptying in constipation-predominant IBS patients [194], and prucalopride increases gastrointestinal and colonic transit in constipation [195, 196]. A manometric study revealed stimulation of colonic high-amplitude propagated contractions by prucalopride [197]. A stimulatory effect on transit by benzamides (which are 5-HT$_4$ receptor agonists) is often limited by additional 5-HT$_3$ receptor antagonism [198]. Thus, the pharmacological effect on transit needs to be specifically tested—for example, renzapride accelerates colonic transit in IBS with constipation [199].

Both cisapride and tegaserod were found to enhance (postprandial) proximal gastric volumes in health, but they did not decrease sensitivity to gastric distension [144, 200]. In animals, tegaserod may decrease sensitivity to colonic distension [201]. In healthy subjects, tegaserod did not alter volumes, pressure thresholds or sensory ratings during rectal distension, but administration of tegaserod was associated with inhibition of the RIII reflex caused by slow-ramp colorectal distension, which was proposed as a surrogate marker of visceral pain [202, 203]. Tegaserod improved constipation and provided relief of pain/discomfort and bloating for women with constipation-predominant IBS and for men and women below 65 years of age with chronic constipation [94, 204, 205]. Prucalopride and tegaserod were shown to be effective in the treatment of constipation [206, 207].

5-HT$_{1P}$ Receptors

An atypical 5-HT receptor on enteric neurons termed 5-HT$_{1P}$ (P for "peripheral") mediates a slow depolarizing response to 5-HT, thus mimicking slow excitatory synaptic transmission [208]. Data on the full characterization and physiologic role of 5-HT$_{1P}$ receptors and therapeutic potential are unclear.

5-HT$_{1B/D}$ Receptors

The 5-HT$_{1B/D}$ receptor agonist sumatriptan induced a premature activity front in the small bowel, increased the amplitude and duration of esophageal contractions, relaxed the proximal stomach, and slowed gastric emptying in humans [209–213]. The underlying pathways are incompletely elucidated. The gastric relaxatory effect of sumatriptan in cats and in humans seems to involve the release of nitric oxide [214, 215]. No studies have convincingly shown expression of 5-HT$_{1B/D}$ receptors in the gastrointestinal tract.

— Muscarinic Receptors

Muscarinic receptor antagonists are relatively selective to the gut for pharmacokinetic reasons and they inhibit contractile responses in the gastrointestinal tract largely by M$_3$ muscarinic receptors, although this receptor subtype accounts for only 20% of the total muscarinic receptor population in the smooth muscle [216]. The mixed M$_1$ and M$_2$ receptor antagonist Z-338 is currently under investigation for FGIDs.

— Motilin Receptors

Motilin is a 22 amino acid gut peptide that stimulates contractility of gastrointestinal smooth muscle [217]. Motilin is present in mucosal endocrine cells, which are abundant in the duodenum [218]. In dogs and humans, motilin plasma levels fluctuate in synchrony with changes in interdigestive motility in the stomach and the small bowel [219–221], and exogenous motilin induces phase III of the MMC [222, 223].

Motilin contracts muscle by a direct muscular effect and through the release of acetylcholine from enteric nerves, depending on the species and region studied [224]. This also applies to humans based on observations of the effects of the macrolide antibiotic erythromycin on antral contractility in healthy human subjects [225], and on expression studies of the human motilin receptor [226] in the human gastric wall [227].

Macrolide antibacterials act as motilin receptor agonists [228]. Several nonpeptide motilin receptor agonists have been developed [229]. Erythromycin and motilin increase fasting and postprandial fundic tone in humans [230–232] through an atropine-resistant mechanism [232]. Motilin, erythromycin, and the macrolide prokinetic ABT-229 stimulate antral contractility in humans [233, 234].

The strong gastroprokinetic actions of erythromycin were demonstrated in diabetic gastroparesis [233], and beneficial effects of treatment with erythromycin in gastroparesis [235, 236] have been confirmed. A systematic review questioned the quality of available studies and the clinical significance of the overall efficacy of erythromycin in gastroparesis [237].

Different macrolide prokinetics, devoid of antibiotic properties, were developed and one of these, ABT-229, was studied in large clinical trials [238, 239]. There is tachyphylaxis with macrolide prokinetics and especially with ABT-229 [234, 240], which did not change symptom severity in gastroparesis or dyspepsia. Although macrolides enhance esophageal motor function in health and gastroesophageal reflux disease (GERD) [241–243], clinical studies failed to reduce esophageal acid exposure or heartburn [244–246].

Motilin has a 47% homology with ghrelin, a 28-amino acid motilin-related peptide [247], and their respective receptors display a remarkable 52% homology [226, 248]. Animal studies revealed that ghrelin has stimulatory effects on gastrointestinal motility that can be mediated through receptors on cholinergic neurons, on myenteric neurons, and on the vagus nerve [249–252]. Preliminary human studies report that intravenous ghrelin induced a premature activity front in humans [253] and enhanced gastric emptying in gastroparesis [254].

— Tachykinin Receptors

Three distinct receptors mediate the biological effects of endogenous tachykinins in the gastrointestinal tract. They are known as tachykinin neurokinin $(NK)_1$, NK_2, and NK_3 receptors that have some preferential (though sometimes negligible) affinity for substance P, NKA, and NKB ligands, respectively. The pharmacological characterization of tachykinin receptors was made possible by the development of potent and selective peptide-derived agonists or nonpeptide antagonists [255, 256].

NK_1 Receptor Antagonists

NK_1 receptor antagonists include aprepitant, which is used as an antiemetic in the relief of chemotherapy-induced delayed emesis [257–259], which suggests significant inhibition of vagal afferents. Other selective NK_1 receptor antagonists inhibit colonic propulsive activity induced by NK_1 receptor agonists in vitro [260].

Their potential application in FGIDs is based on their ability to block the target NK1 receptors for substance P in myenteric neurons and afferent pathways. NK_1 receptor blockade may also inhibit peristalsis, an effect probably mediated by the inhibition of postjunctional (muscular) NK_1 receptors. Preliminary data suggest that the IBS patients were less angered by the distension of a balloon in the rectum after treatment with the NK_1 receptor antagonist CJ-11974 [261]. These antagonists may also have other beneficial effects in IBS. For example, they have effects on bowel inflammation [262] and an antisecretory action [263].

NK₂ Receptor Antagonists

Experimental data indicate a role for NK_2 receptors in the regulation of intestinal motor functions (both excitatory and inhibitory), secretions, inflammation, and visceral sensitivity. NK_2 receptor antagonists include nepadutant and saredutant [257, 264].

Lördal et al. [265] conducted a randomized double-blind study to investigate the importance of NK_2 receptors for the regulation of intestinal motility in humans. They showed that nepadutant is capable of alleviating intestinal motor responses and symptoms in humans evoked by infusion of NKA, but had no effect on baseline motility.

NK₃ Receptor Antagonists

NK_3 receptor antagonists include osanetant and talnetant [257] that block receptors on sensory neurons. NK_3 receptors are present on spinal terminals of capsaicin-sensitive neurons and within neurons of the spinal cord. Intrathecal NK_3 receptor antagonist SR 142,801 reduced rat behavioral response to noxious colorectal distension.

A peripheral role for the NK_3 receptor in the mechanisms of intestinal nociception is also possible [3]. Thus, both talnetant (which crosses the rat blood–brain barrier) and SB-235375 (which does not) reduce colonic sensation (assessed by abdominal contractions in response to colorectal distension) without altering colonic compliance [3].

— Opioid Receptors

The opioid peptides are involved in reducing somatic and visceral pain. They reduce gut sensitivity by exerting an effect on peripheral (spinal afferents) or central (spinocerebral pathways and anterior cingulate cortex) sites involved in the perception of pain and the unpleasantness associated with visceral pain.

Three types of receptors for opioid peptides have been identified as having effects on human gastrointestinal function: μ-, δ- and κ-receptors. μ opioid receptors are located in the enteric nervous system as well as on nociceptive pathways conducting pain to the CNS (reviewed in De Luca and Coupar [266]). They reduce neuronal excitability and inhibit acetylcholine release.

The μ- opioid receptor agonist loperamide inhibits secretion, reduces colonic transit, and increases resting anal sphincter tone [267]. Opioid receptor antagonists may also display a prokinetic effect. The peripherally restricted μ-opioid receptor antagonists, such as N-methylnaltrexone and alvimopan, make it possible to normalize bowel function in opiate-treated patients without compromising central opioid analgesia [103].

In IBS with constipation, antagonism of gut μ-opioid receptors has been tested based on the rationale that endogenous opiates may play a role in motility disorders. A study compared naloxone vs. placebo, and showed no significant improvement in the scores for pain, bloating, straining and urgency in the naloxone group [268]. However, larger clinical trials are needed to evaluate the usefulness of opioid antagonism in constipation-predominant IBS.

κ-opioid Receptors

The κ-receptors also mediate analgesia, are more abundant in peripheral nerves than in central nerves, and are thought to induce fewer central side effects. Recently, κ-opioid receptor agonists have been proposed as a pharmacological approach to the treatment of FGIDs on the basis that κ-opioid receptors are thought to be located on vagal and nonvagal afferent pathways [269].

Fedotozine has been shown to suppress afferent visceral activity in several animal models [269]. In healthy humans, fedotozine decreased gastric sensitivity to distension [270] without modifying gastric compliance or somatic sensitivity. More importantly, oral fedotozine (30 mg t.i.d.) was reported to reduce dyspeptic symptoms and epigastric pain in functional dyspepsia and abdominal pain in patients with IBS [271, 272]. In the latter study, fedotozine also improved the quality of life. Delvaux et al. showed that fedotozine reduced colonic sensitivity [273]. However, additional studies with fedotozine in IBS have been disappointing.

Asimadoline is another κ-opioid receptor agonist proposed as an antinociceptive with predominantly peripheral action [274, 275]. The data suggest that its action may be at least partly through blockade of sodium channels. Two pharmacodynamic studies have been published suggesting that it can reduce colonic sensation at subnoxious levels of distension and it also reduces gastric sensation after a satiating meal [276, 277]. A study conducted in patients with constipation-predominant IBS, in which pharmacodynamic end points of colonic compliance, tone, and sensory thresholds were investigated showed that there was a reduction of colonic sensation in response to colonic distensions [278].

— Adrenoceptors

β-adrenoceptor Agonists

β-adrenoceptor agonists administered in vivo usually inhibit gut motility [279]. Theoretically, in patients with IBS and high colonic motility indices, the spasmolytic effect of β-adrenoceptor agonists may be beneficial. Indeed terbutaline has been reported to reduce sigmoid motility in patients with IBS [280]. The use of a β-adrenoceptor agonist might even have an advantage over antimuscarinic agents, since the former compounds directly relax smooth muscle cells, while the latter can only counteract an excessive cholinergic tone. However, symptomatic improvement with β-adrenoceptor agonists still needs to be documented by appropriate studies. Important cardiovascular side effects may constitute a significant limitation, although they can be attenuated by resorting to GI-selective compounds: for instance, in dogs, the $β_3$-adrenoceptor agonist SR 58611A inhibited colonic motility at doses having only minor cardiovascular effect [281].

Functional in vitro and expression studies detected $β_3$-adrenoceptors in the human colon, suggesting further studies are needed on the potential use of $β_3$-adrenoceptor agonists as antispasmodics [282, 283].

$α_2$-adrenoceptor Agonists

Clonidine was shown to reduce colonic pain sensation in response to distension and colonic tone [284–286]. A preliminary study of clonidine in IBS with diarrhea suggests that 0.1 mg clonidine twice daily may be associated with an improvement in the proportion of patients achieving satisfactory relief of IBS and an improvement in overall bowel function [287]. However, it is clear that excessive somnolence or postural hypotension is dose-limiting and more GI selectivity is a prerequisite to further develop this class of medications.

— Dopamine Receptors

Antidopaminergic gastrointestinal prokinetics are used clinically for the management of motor disorders of the upper gastrointestinal tract, including functional dyspepsia, gastric stasis of various origin, and emesis. Their prokinetic effect is claimed to be mediated through blockade of enteric (neuronal and muscular) inhibitory D_2 receptors [288]. From a physiological and pharmacological standpoint, the functional significance of dopamine receptors in relation to motility is a matter of controversy. Although serotonergic compounds may be superior to antidopaminergic agents with respect to prokinetic activity, antidopaminergic compounds also have central antiemetic action resulting in suppression of nausea and vomiting.

The pharmacological profile of marketed compounds differs in terms of molecular structure, affinity at D_2 receptors, ability to interact with other receptor systems (e.g., $5\text{-}HT_3$ and $5\text{-}HT_4$ receptors for metoclopramide and $5\text{-}HT_4$ receptors for levosulpiride) and to permeate the blood-brain barrier (compared with other compounds, domperidone does not easily cross the barrier). It has been suggested that the serotonergic (via $5\text{-}HT_4$ receptors) component of some antidopaminergic prokinetics may enhance their therapeutic efficacy in GI disorders such as functional dyspepsia and diabetic gastroparesis [288]. Recently, there has been renewed interest in some antidopaminergic compounds such as levosulpiride [289]. This compound, at the dose of 25 mg three times a day is marketed in some countries in the treatment of functional dyspepsia. Itopride is a mixed D_2 receptor antagonist and acetyl cholinesterase inhibitor of possible value in functional dyspepsia [290]. It is currently approved in Japan.

Antagonism of central D_2 receptors may lead to both therapeutic (e.g., antiemetic effect due to D_2 receptor blockade in the area postrema) and adverse effects, including hyperprolactinemia and extrapyramidal dystonic reactions.

It must be pointed out that only rarely have meta-analyses and systematic reviews on the effectiveness of prokinetics in treating gastrointestinal disorders included antidopaminergics, because of the poor quality of existing clinical trials. For the use of antidopaminergics in dyspepsia, Moayyedi et al. [291] suggested further research to conclusively establish their place in therapy. Veldhuyzen van Zanten et al. [292] performed a meta-analysis to determine the efficacy of domperidone in functional dyspepsia. Efficacy analysis was based on global assessment of improvement by the investigator. An odds ratio of 7.0 (95% confidence interval: 3.6–16) favored domperidone versus placebo. Thus, domperidone seems to be efficacious in functional dyspepsia, although this conclusion is largely based on global assessment by the investigator, which is not an optimal outcome measure.

— Cannabinoid Receptors

The target for cannabis and endocannabinoids is the CB_1 receptor, which is present mainly in the central and the peripheral nervous system, and the CB_2 receptor, which is expressed in the immune system [293, 294]. The endogenous ligands are anandamide (which also activates transient receptor potential ion channel of the vanilloid type 1 (TRPV1) receptors), 2-arachidonoylglycerol, and 2-arachidonyl glycerol ether.

CB_1 receptors are expressed on nociceptive afferents in dorsal root ganglia [295] and enteric nervous system (ENS) neurons. When CB1 receptors on ENS neurons are activated, there is inhibition of the release of acetylcholine from cholinergic nerves [296–298]. CB_1 receptor ligands inhibit GI transit in animals. In the rat gastric fundus, CB_1 receptor activation modulates release of inhibitory neurotransmitters [299]. Activation of the CB_1 receptor in the brain stem was shown to inhibit triggering of transient LES relaxations by gastric distension [300–301].

Delta-9-tetrahydrocannabinol has strong antiemetic properties and is used in the treatment of chemotherapy-induced vomiting [302]. Delta-9-tetrahydrocannabinol (DHC) may delay gastric emptying of solids in humans [303]. It is unclear whether CB_1 agonists' potential for abuse would preclude their regulatory approval. Inverse CB_1 agonists (which function as antagonists at constitutively active CB_1 receptors) [304] are being developed for treatment of obesity, since they may induce nausea and vomiting. The effects on stomach function are unclear. On the other hand, agonists at the nonneuronal CB_2 receptors have no abuse potential and exert antinociceptive effects in pain associated with inflammation [305].

— Transient Receptor Potential Ion Channel of the Vanilloid Type I (TRPVI)

The TRPV1 is expressed by primary afferent neurons innervating the gut and other organs and is viewed as a trigger for chemonociception [306, 307]. TRPV1 is activated not only by vanilloids such as capsaicin, but also by noxious heat, acidosis and intracellular lipid mediators such as anandamide and lipoxygenase products, and activation of various proalgesic pathways. Upregulation of TRPV1 in inflammatory bowel disease and the beneficial effect of TRPV1 downregulation in functional dyspepsia and irritable bladder make this polymodal nociceptor a potential therapeutic target in chronic abdominal pain. In patients with fecal urgency and rectal hypersensitivity, increased numbers of nerve fibers expressing TRPV1 have been reported [308].

A recent study showed that long-term administration of red pepper was more effective than placebo in decreasing the intensity of dyspeptic symptoms in patients with functional dyspepsia [309]. Studies of the effect of capsaicin on gastric sensitivity in humans showed acute sensitization followed by decreased perception of epigastric symptoms [310].

— CCK₁ Receptors

CCK has a large number of biological actions that involve the gut (e.g., stimulation of gallbladder contraction, stimulation of pancreatic enzyme secretion, inhibition of gastric emptying and gastric acid secretion, initiation of satiety, a wide spectrum of direct and neurally mediated effects on intestinal smooth muscle, etc.) as well as antianalgesic and behavioral activities [311].

Although evidence points to a central role of CCK in food intake, or a role in stimulation of the vagal afferent pathway originating from the gastroduodenal mucosa, it is possible that CCK may alter the function of the stomach during the postprandial period by acting on peripheral CCK receptors, thereby influencing postprandial symptoms, including satiation. It is unclear whether CCK also plays a role in control of gastric functions in the fasting period.

CCK_1 receptor antagonists are usually classified among GI prokinetics since they antagonize the effects of CCK, which is known to delay gastric emptying. CCK_1 receptor antagonists are also inhibitors of gallbladder contraction and can accelerate colonic transit time in healthy volunteers and patients with IBS. These drugs are therefore of potential value in the treatment of motility disorders such as constipation and constipation-predominant IBS [312]. It should be noted, however, that in spite of many mechanistic studies exploring the effects of CCK_1 receptor antagonists on gastrointestinal motility and their ability to antagonize the effects of CCK, their place in therapy remains uncertain, partly because of some discrepancies among studies. An important aspect is the species-dependent expression of CCK receptors and responses to CCK_1 receptor antagonists.

In addition to their potential prokinetic action, CCK_1/CCK_2 receptor antagonists may be putative modulators of visceral afferent information [313].

— Smooth Muscle Relaxants

These have mixed pharmacological actions working on calcium channels in intestinal smooth muscle. Cimetropium, otilonium, pinaverium, and mebeverine are examples and they are used in some countries for the treatment of IBS. Meta-analyses suggest they are superior to placebo in IBS-related pain [314], though the quality of trials has been questioned.

— Somatostatin Analogs

Somatostatin and its stable analogs such as octreotide have antinociceptive effects in various animal models and have been shown to induce analgesia in humans (for a review, see De Ponti and Malagelada [279]). This observation raised the question as to whether somatostatin and its analogs also affect intestinal visceral perception. However, it should be kept in mind that somatostatin has a large number of well known effects in several districts and can profoundly affect gut motility as well as absorption/secretion.

Several reports suggest an inhibitory effect of octreotide on rectal sensation [315–317]. In patients with IBS, octreotide increased thresholds of colonic visceral perception without modifying muscle tone or compliance [318] and seems to exert primarily an antihyperalgesic effect [319]. In the stomach, conflicting results are reported in healthy humans. In one study [320] octreotide increased the threshold for fullness during distension, while Bourgeois et al. [321] found no effect of octreotide on either perception or discomfort thresholds. The need for multiple subcutaneous injections, high cost, and potential side effects (e.g., severe dumping syndrome) limit its present use.

Table 5. Strategies for Development of Medications
                for Functional Gastrointestinal Disorders

1. Target an important mechanism or transmitter.

2. Develop a strong clinical pharmacology portfolio of the medication.

3. Be aware of, but beware of the Rome criteria.

4. Recruit appropriate patient subgroups for the medication and its properties or actions.

5. Use the study run-in phase to consolidate the diagnosis or subgroup of interest.

6. Do not enter phase III prematurely.

7. Recruit patients in quality GI offices with experience in conduct of trials.

8. Use a global, threshold-based primary endpoint that requires the patient to adjudicate clinical significance. Secondary endpoints address specific symptoms.

9. Use a strong experimental design: placebo-controlled, parallel group, sufficient power to identify a clinically meaningful change in endpoints.

10. An effective medication!

Pharmacodynamics: Biomarkers for Sensation and Motility Endpoints in Experimental Medicine

Sensorimotor disorders of the stomach, small intestine, and colon have a limited repertoire of clinical manifestations, and there is the potential for more than one mechanism to lead to symptoms. In many clinical trial programs of novel agents in neurogastroenterology, the emphasis has been placed primarily on symptom assessment of broad groups of patients identified by the Rome criteria. Drugs of potential value have fallen by the wayside with this approach. Certain biomarkers can be used to predict the success of an experimental medicine in some FGIDs, including IBS and functional dyspepsia. These studies may be incorporated in the recommended steps for drug development (Table 5).

   This section reviews the application of currently established physiological tests as potential biomarkers for clinically relevant endpoints in FGIDs.

— Radiopaque Markers for Colonic Transit

   The radiopaque marker test for colonic transit is a commonly performed and widely available test. Studies with loperamide for diarrhea and fiber for constipation used radiopaque markers to assess whole gut transit time [322, 323]. These studies suggest that overall effects of these therapies were predicted by the marker transit test. However, other studies addressing more specific endpoints suggest that the colonic marker transit time (< 15 or > 60 hours) accurately predicts the extremes of stool consistency, with a great deal of overlap in the range of transit times between those extremes [193].

— Radioscintigraphic Markers for Colonic Transit in IBS

Several examples from the literature support the use of detailed colonic transit measurement in the development of medications for IBS-associated changes in bowel function. First, alosetron (a 5-HT$_3$ receptor antagonist) slows overall colonic transit and, on average, increases the time for emptying the ascending colon by 50% [324]. Clinical trials have demonstrated the efficacy of alosetron in patients with diarrhea-predominant IBS [95], and the medication improved quality of life vs. placebo in women with IBS [325]. Second, tegaserod (a 5-HT$_4$ receptor agonist) accelerates overall colonic transit and, on average, halves the time for emptying the ascending colons [194]. Several studies show that this medication is effective in the treatment of IBS with constipation [94, 204, 205]. On the other hand, piboserod (a 5-HT$_4$ receptor antagonist) was ineffective on the same transit measurements [190] and has not been efficacious in clinical trials [326].

— Intraluminal Measurements of Rectal or Colonic Motility and Sensations

Intraluminal measurements may serve as biomarkers for motor or sensory modulation in lower FGIDs. Thus, intracolonic measurements of postprandial tone in healthy subjects [173] showed the potential of 5-HT$_3$ receptor antagonists to prevent diarrhea and other postprandial symptoms in diseases including IBS and carcinoid diarrhea [327]. This information suggests that the intraluminal measurement of tone is a useful biomarker justifying subsequent trial for clinical efficacy.

Measurement of rectal sensation has also been associated with responsiveness to octreotide [315–318] and opiates [328]. The application of these observations on visceral sensitivity testing may assist in the testing of novel medications. On the other hand, pressure or volume thresholds for rectal balloon distension do not seem to be significantly altered by tegaserod, at least when using rapid distension [203]. Alosetron was shown to alter colonic compliance, but not colonic sensitivity to isobaric distension [178]. Previously, the κ opioid receptor agonist fedotozine was shown to decrease sensitivity to colonic distension, but the therapeutic gain in placebo-controlled studies in IBS was found to be of insufficient magnitude for further development [33, 272, 273].

The sample size required to avoid a type 2 error while assessing clinically meaningful effect sizes is larger with testing of sensation biomarkers [329] than with transit endpoints in healthy volunteers; in patients, the variability may even be higher. Nevertheless, these sample sizes (12 to 20 per treatment arm) are still more practical than testing symptom endpoints, which require much larger samples [277]. Thus, a 25% to 30% effect size can be demonstrated with ~20 subjects per treatment arm in sensation-based studies and ~12 per treatment arm in studies of transit and gastric accommodation, based on the published variability [277, 330].

— Do Gastric Biomarkers "Predict" Symptom Response to Therapy in Dyspepsia?

There are four approaches that appear promising because they are applicable to relatively large numbers of patients in experimental medicine studies. First, scintigraphic gastric emptying has been a classical investigation for drug development for gastroparesis [331]; however, the prediction of clinical efficacy even with medications such as erythromycin is unclear [237]. This analysis is also complicated by tachyphylaxis to some medications, as with the macrolide prokinetic ABT-229 [234, 238, 239]. Another important pitfall is that the gastric emptying also changes with placebo (and a coefficient of variation of at least 12% can be expected with scintigraphic gastric emptying [332]). This questions the effectiveness of gastric emptying as a predictive biomarker.

A second approach is to use the intragastric balloon linked to a barostat to measure gastric compliance, tone, and sensitivity. The κ-opioid receptor agonist fedotozine was shown to decrease gastric sensitivity to distension [270], but the therapeutic gain in placebo-controlled studies of oral administration for several weeks in functional dyspepsia was found to be of insufficient magnitude for further development [271, 333]. Acute studies in healthy volunteers established that the 5-HT$_{1A}$ receptor agonist R-137696 had a dose-dependent relaxatory effect on the proximal stomach, but a four-week multicenter placebo-controlled study failed to show any benefit [159]. Interpretation of predictive value is also complicated by potential tachyphylaxis. Moreover, barostat studies seem an impractical biomarker for a trial because multicenter studies are difficult to standardize and the test is invasive.

A third and potentially promising approach in evaluating symptoms in dyspepsia has used the symptoms induced by a standardized meal. The symptoms have been recorded 30 minutes after a maximum tolerated volume of water or a nutrient drink [334], or after a solid meal [335]. Both nutrient or water load tests and barostat-based pressure sensation are capable of differentiating healthy controls from dyspeptics. However, they were insufficiently specific to differentiate patients with impaired gastric accommodation, gastric hypersensitivity, or combined pathophysiology. It is still unclear whether the provocative meal tests will prove effective predictors of clinical efficacy.

Fourth, the combined use of the nutrient drink test with assessment of symptoms and measurement of gastric volume and emptying, as with single-photon emission computed tomography (SPECT), ultrasonography, or magnetic resonance imaging (MRI) may be useful since several potential biomarkers are measured simultaneously [336, 337]. For example, in an experimental study in healthy individuals, alosetron reduced the aggregate symptom score without altering gastric volume [169]. A subsequent multicenter, 12-week study demonstrated that alosetron was superior to placebo in inducing adequate relief of dyspepsia symptoms [182].

In summary, transit biomarkers used in the lower functional gastrointestinal disorders provide a strategy for development of surrogate markers for clinical trials. Further validation is needed for transit markers in the upper gut, and for sensation at all levels. Pharmacological modulation of validated endpoints may help to predict success or failure of new medications in therapeutic trials.

Principles of Pharmacogenomics in FGIDs

Pharmacogenetics refers to the study of individual variations in DNA sequence related to drug response. Pharmacogenomics is the study of the variability of the expression of individual genes relevant to disease susceptibility as well as drug response at the cellular, tissue, individual, or population level. There is a growing appreciation that "one size does not fit all" and that individual genetic variations may impact on the pharmacokinetics and pharmacodynamics of medications that ultimately determine efficacy or adverse effects [338, 339]. Two issues will be briefly addressed in relation to FGIDs: First, is there a genetic predisposition to FGIDs? Second, are there genetic variations that influence response to medication [340]?

— Are Polymorphisms Biomarkers of Disease?

Polymorphisms may be markers associated with an FGID-related phenotype. Examples in the literature include:

a. IBS patients with significantly reduced frequencies of the high producer genotype for IL-10 than controls (21% v 32%; p=0.003), suggesting that some IBS patients may be genetically predisposed to produce lower amounts of the anti-inflammatory cytokine IL-10. This lends some support to the hypothesis that there may be an inflammatory or genetic component in some cases of IBS [341].

   b. There are contradictory data in the literature suggesting an association of IBS subgroups with polymorphisms of SLC6A4 [342].

   c. A polymorphism (C825T) in the gene controlling G-protein synthesis has been described in functional dyspepsia and IBS [343].

Clearly, more studies are needed to confirm or refute the genotype associations for IL-10 and GNß3.

— Pharmacogenomic Considerations in FGID

Genetic polymorphisms in drug metabolism, transporters and drug targets are three classes of genetic variations [344] to be considered.

Genetic Polymorphism in Drug Metabolism

The number of functional CYP450 2D6 genes determines the pharmacokinetics and plasma levels of the commonly used tricyclic agent nortryptiline [345], or the action of codeine (which has to be converted by the 2D6 isoenzyme to morphine to be effective). Note also that several antidepressants are metabolized by these enzymes and their clinical efficacy is affected. (See the next section on psychopharmacology.)

Genetic Polymorphism in Transporters

Genetic polymorphism in transporters [346] may influence the response to medications. Two examples of pharmacodynamic variation are provided from the study of FGIDs.

5-HT undergoes re-uptake by a serotonin transporter protein (SERT). Variations in the promoter for synthesis of SERT (SERT-P) influence response to serotonergic medications in depressed individuals. SERT polymorphisms were associated with a greater colonic transit response in those with long homozygous than those with heterozygous polymorphisms in diarrhea-predominant IBS [347]. These data suggest that pharmacogenomic studies may serve to identify patients who are more likely to respond to therapy based on the genotypic variations.

A second example is provided by the observation that the response of patients with functional dyspepsia to a variety of medications may be influenced by the genetic variation in GNß3 translation. Holtmann et al. demonstrated that G-protein polymorphisms were predictors of symptom outcome in functional dyspepsia, based on the rationale that G proteins functionally act as second messengers and may influence multiple control mechanisms [343]. These results require confirmation, but suggest that genetic variation may be one key explanation of the heterogeneity of response seen in the IBS and functional dyspepsia.

Genetic Polymorphism in Drug Targets

No examples are available to date in FGIDs.

In summary, pharmacogenetics may explain important variations in both pharmacokinetic and pharmacodynamic aspects of drug response and needs to be considered in drug development programs and clinical therapeutics. It also may provide new insights on the mechanisms or pathophysiology of FGIDs.

Psychopharmacology of Functional Gastrointestinal Disorders

Psychotropic agents are used to treat patients with IBS and other FGIDs [348]. The commonly observed overlap of IBS with other FGIDs and reported benefits from psychotropics are presumed to reflect some degree of shared pathophysiology, and since psychotropics have been most studied in IBS, it will be used as a representative model. This section will compare and contrast two recent summaries of the literature addressing the efficacy of antidepressants in IBS and will highlight more recent studies. The importance of coexisting anxiety and depression as key targets in the medical evaluation and treatment planning for patients with FGIDs will be discussed, as will the implications of psychiatric disorders for long-term health outcome. Psychotropics may have basic actions that normalize some of the gastrointestinal pathophysiology of FGIDs independent of psychiatric disorders.

— Pharmacology of Psychotropic Agents

The acute effects of various psychotropics are shown in Table 6. 5-HT_{1a} and α_2 receptors are both pre- and postsynaptic as well as heteroreceptors (i.e., they modulate norepinephrine (NE) and 5-HT neurotransmission respectively via presynaptic somatodendritic receptors). Chronic antidepressants all enhance glucocorticoid signaling and inhibit CRF overactivity in the brain and presumably in the periphery. Each class affects several transmitters via reciprocal actions between amine and neuropeptide systems, and reduces excessive cytokine release associated with various conditions in which inflammatory cytokines play a role.

Table 6. Pharmacological Actions of Psychotropic Drugs on Monoamine Reuptake and Receptors

	Neurotransmitter Reuptake Blockade			Receptor Blockade					
	5-HT	NE	DA	α_1	α_2	H_1	ACh	5-HT$_{1a}$	5-HT$_2$
TCAs									
Amitriptyline	+++++	+++	-	+++	+	++++	+++	+	+++
Imipramine	++++	+++++	-	++	+	++++	++	++	++
Desipramine	+++	+++++	-	++	+	++	++	-	-
Clomipramine	+++++	+++	-	++		+++	++	-	-
SSRIs									
Fluoxetine	+++++	++	-	-	-	-	-	-	-
Paroxetine	+++++	+++	+-		-	0	++	_	_
Sertraline	+++++	+	+++	++	+	0	+	-	-
Citalopram	+++++	-	0	+	+	+	0	-	-
SNRIs									
Venlafaxine	++++	+	-	0	0	0	0	0	0
Duloxetine	+++++	++++	+	-	-	-	-	-	-
Atypical Agents									
Bupropion	0	+	+	-	-	-	0	-	-
Nefazodone	++	++	++	+++	-	++	-		+++
Mirtazapine*	-	0	0	+		++++	+		+++
Azapirones									
Buspirone	0	0	0	0	0	0	0	++	0

*Mirtazapine also blocks 5-HT$_3$ receptors (+++), which reduces nausea and has acute anxiolytic effects in humans.

5-HT = serotonin
α = alpha-adrenergic
Ach = muscarine acetylcholine
DA = dopamine
H = histamine

NE = norepinephrine
SNRI = serotonin noradrenoline reuptake inhibitor
SSRI = selective serotonin reuptake inhibitor
TCA = tricyclic antidepressant

Symbols: + to +++++ = increasing levels of potency, - = weak, 0= no effect.

Clinical correlates of monoamine reuptake inhibition are as follows:

- 5-HT: antidepressant, anxiolytic and antiobsessive, transient jitteriness, insomnia, nausea/GI distress, delayed sexual dysfunction, possible delayed weight gain;
- NE: tremor, diaphoresis, transient nausea, slight increase in blood pressure, possible delayed sexual dysfunction;
- Dopamine (DA): antidepressant, enhanced motivation, improved cognition, antiparkinsonian, psychomotor activation, aggravation of psychosis, possible enhanced sexual function.

Clinical correlates of receptor blockade are as follows:

- α_1: sedation and postural hypotension/dizziness, potentiation of the antihypertensive effects of prazosin, terazosin, doxazosin, tamsulosin, and labetalol, reflex tachycardia;
- α_2: antidepressant, anxiolytic jitteriness, psychomotor activation, enhanced erectile function;
- H_1: potentiation of CNS depressants, drowsiness and weight gain;
- Cholinoceptors: antidepressant, dry mouth, constipation, drowsiness, blurry vision, urinary retention, precipitate or worsen closed-angle glaucoma, sinus tachycardia, memory dysfunction, delirium at high concentrations;
- 5-HT_{1A}: anxiolytic, antidepressant, nausea and dizziness;
- 5-HT_2 (postsynaptic): anxiolytic, antidepressant, sleep-promoting, weight gain.

Chronic treatment with any antidepressant alters receptor sensitivity, which in all cases is thought to result in enhanced 5-HT neurotransmission. Tricyclic antidepressants (TCAs), but not selective seratonin reuptake inhibitors (SSRIs) or serotonin-norepinephrine reuptake inhibitors (SNRIs) increase the sensitivity of postsynaptic 5-HT receptors, and down-regulate α_2 presynaptic and heteroreceptors. The analgesic effect of TCAs is also mediated by blockage of a class of voltage-dependent sodium channels in extrinsic sensory neurons. SSRIs and SNRIs reduce the sensitivity of 5-HT_{1A} auto- and heteroreceptors. Buspirone (not an antidepressant) down-regulates 5-HT_{1A} somatodendritic autoreceptors to produce anxiolysis. Down-regulation of 5-HT_{1A} receptors is thought to play the most important role in antidepressant, anxiolytic, and analgesic effects of antidepressants.

Benzodiazepines enhance the inhibitory effects of GABA via potentiation at the GABA A receptors, and indirectly enhance 5-HT and diminish NE neurotransmission, and antagonize the effects of CCK in brain and gut, which result in immediate anxiolytic activity.

— Evidence for Efficacy of Psychotropic Treatments in FGID

For over 30 years clinical reports and randomized controlled trials (RCTs) have suggested that psychotropic medications—most frequently antidepressants—are clinically useful tools for treating some patients with FGID. The majority of clinical and research reports have focused on the TCAs for the treatment of IBS [348].

Two groups that recently examined the accrued evidence for efficacy of antidepressants for IBS reached remarkably different conclusions! Jackson et al. [349] conducted a meta-analysis of RCTs published in English between 1966 and 1988 and focused on the effectiveness of antidepressants for FGIDs. Most studies included exclusively IBS samples and a few included nonulcer dyspepsia patients. Of 90 studies meeting a priori criteria, 11 were chosen for the analysis. Two studies included employed mianserin (not available in the US), and the others utilized TCAs. Where possible, response versus nonresponse and pain were assessed. The meta-analysis indicated that antidepressants were as effective for IBS than other commonly prescribed treatments, such as antispasmodics and antidiarrheals (3.2 number needed to treat (NTT); confidence interval (CI) 2.1–6.5). However, there is justifiable debate over the conclusions drawn due to the inclusion of one study showing an unusually large treatment effect, without which the findings would have been less conclusive.

Brandt et al. [350] undertook an equally ambitious assessment of RCTs for all studies published between 1980 and 2001 that examined the efficacy of different IBS treatments, including TCAs. Using somewhat different a priori criteria and different methodology (i.e., not meta-analysis), these authors assigned quality ratings for each study. The potential for Type 1 (false negative) and 2 errors (false positive) in all studies was included in the quality ratings. Five of the six TCA studies, conducted between 1978 and 1987, were of poor scientific quality; none were sufficiently long or employed sufficiently large sample sizes to assure a high probability of excluding Type 1 or 2 errors. In five of six TCA studies, treatment arms contained 30 or fewer subjects. One study employed sample sizes of 60 to 80 per treatment sample, but statistical significance of treatment differences could still not be discerned in the five different treatment arms. Brandt et al. [350] concluded that TCAs are not superior to placebo for global IBS symptoms, but added that there was "limited evidence that TCAs may decrease abdominal pain." In the studies cited, there were a total of nine active treatment arms. Statistically significant drug-placebo differences were found via posthoc analyses in one of four doses of trimipramine versus placebo, and in diarrhea-predominant subjects in one of two desipramine studies. Positive descriptions of pain relief in two others were noted. TCAs are clearly useful for some, but not all, patients.

Based on the available literature, the hypothesis that TCAs are effective in overall core IBS symptoms or any other FGIDs has not yet been adequately tested. Likewise, the empirical evidence that low doses of TCAs are effective for abdominal pain has not been unequivocally established. Since low doses of TCAs are broadly used in GI patients, it seems important to test the hypotheses and bring the state of the art into the realm of evidence-based medicine via adequately designed RCTs.

— Newer Studies of Psychotropics in FGID

Tricyclic Antidepressants (TCAs)

Drossman et al. [351] employed methodology consistent with Rome standards to compare the efficacy of the TCA desipramine (DES) (dosage range 50–150, average~100 mg/day) with placebo in women with moderate to severe FGID. This was part of a larger study design which also examined psychosocial treatment. This NIH-funded study included only women to maximize the feasibility of recruiting adequate sample sizes at each of two participating sites. The comparison groups had comparable demographics, including abuse history (~60%) and diagnosis (~ 80% IBS). Some information on psychiatric status was gathered. In the intent-to-treat (ITT) analysis, DES treatment showed a trend toward statistical superiority over placebo (60% DES vs. 47% placebo responders; NNT 8.1; p=0.16) in the overall sample. Posthoc completers analysis and an analysis excluding subjects with undetectable DES levels were both statistically significant and favored DES over placebo on the main outcome measure. The patients benefiting most from DES were those with moderate (versus severe) GI illness, prior abuse, minimal depression, and diarrhea-predominant bowel symptoms. There were statistical trends favoring DES over placebo on quality of life and pain measures (p=0.09 each). Interestingly, the outcome variable most sensitive to DES treatment was a patient-rated 'satisfaction with treatment' measure (DES > placebo; p=0.011).

Tolerability of DES treatment ultimately limited the statistical power of this study. Twenty-six of the 29 patients who dropped out for adverse effects were DES recipients; an additional 12 had nondetectable DES levels. Interpatient variation in hepatic metabolism may have contributed to one extremely high (> 800 ng/ml) DES level, and possibly to undetectable levels (< 10 ng/ml) in the rare patient. "Unblinding" of some patients due to side effects may also have been a factor, as noted by the authors. The average DES dose of 100 mg daily was higher than in most prior TCA studies, but may have been too low to treat some subjects with anxiety and mood disorders.

Selective Serotonin Reuptake Inhibitors (SSRIs)

In clinical gastroenterology, SSRIs appear to be useful for some patients with IBS and other FGIDs [351]. Kuiken et al. [146] reported that 6 weeks of fluoxetine treatment (20 mg/day) daily was not superior to placebo overall, but did reduce abdominal pain in the subgroup with low prestudy rectal distension discomfort thresholds. These findings should be interpreted cautiously in light of the small sample sizes (about 20 each) and relatively short observation period. Tack et al. [352] reported that a single intravenous dose of citalopram did not affect colonic sensitivity in normals. In a pediatric population with recurrent abdominal pain, Campo et al. [353] reported responses in 21 of 24 subjects (ages 7–18) after 12 weeks' flexible dose citalopram treatment. If this finding is replicated in a placebo-controlled study, RCTs using this agent or its active isomer escitalopram in adults with functional abdominal pain or other FGIDs may be informative.

In the only placebo-controlled RCT of the SSRI paroxetine to date, Tabas et al. [354] compared 12 weeks' flexible dose treatment with paroxetine (10–40 mg/

day) versus placebo in 81 Rome I IBS patients (paroxetine n = 38; placebo n = 43). The sample was drawn from a group of IBS patients who were unimproved after consuming a high fiber diet ($\geq$ 25 g/day) for at least seven weeks. At study end, 23% of the patients were taking 10 mg paroxetine per day, 43% were taking 20 mg per day, and 33% were taking 40 mg per day. While relevant outcome variables were chosen, the method of determining response differed from all other IBS treatment studies, making it impossible to compare the results with other published studies.

The authors made overly optimistic assumptions in calculating the necessary sample size. This included an estimated 20% placebo response rate, which was exceeded in most outcome variables (for example, 50% for placebo vs. 32.6% paroxetine responders on pain ratings). Compliance was not reported, nor were statistical corrections for multiple comparisons. This study included important features, such as flexible dosing and selection of patients unresponsive to initial treatment with high dietary fiber. Like nearly every study to date, the design was inadequate for testing the hypothesis. Perhaps the most useful clinical information provided was that prior to unblinding the study, 84% of paroxetine recipients vs. 34% of placebo recipients would have chosen to continue the study medication. Had the study been larger, analysis by dosage might have provided some useful information for planning future studies. One controlled study in healthy normals showed that paroxetine had beneficial effects on upper GI symptoms [355].

Two open label treatment studies that employed paroxetine in IBS have been recently published [356, 357]. As part of a larger study, Creed et al. [356] treated 86 patients with severe Rome I IBS with 12 weeks' paroxetine (20 mg per day). Validated assessment and outcome measures were employed for IBS and psychiatric disorders. A little less than 50% of the patients had current anxiety disorders or major depression; 12% had prior sexual abuse. Twenty-nine of the 86 patients discontinued paroxetine due to side effects, most during the first 6 weeks. Subjective physical and mental well-being, pain days, and global severity improved from baseline in the total group (ITT analysis) with paroxetine treatment. In the 42 completers, visual analogue scale (VAS) subjective pain severity also significantly improved during the 12-week treatment. IBS subtype, gender, initial pain severity, and psychiatric status did not predict outcome. At follow-up one year later, 36/42 completers had continued paroxetine. Inclusion of both sexes in a relatively large sample and "real world" evidence of unsatisfactory initial treatment response were strengths of this study.

Masand et al. [357] treated 20 Rome I IBS patients, half of whom had a lifetime history of anxiety disorders, with paroxetine (mean dose 31 mg, range 20–40 mg) for 12 weeks. All 20 patients completed the treatment. Greater than 50% improvement in overall pain (13 patients), pain severity (14 patients), and frequency (11 patients) were observed in those with and without anxiety histories. Similar findings were reported for most other IBS measures in patients with or without anxiety history. A trend toward greater degrees of improvement in pain measures in patients with anxiety disorders versus those without was noted. The 100% completion rate versus about 70% in the Creed et al. study may reflect differences in patient samples [356]. Conclusions regarding efficacy are not possible due to the open-label design of these two studies.

Serotonin-Norepinephrine Reuptake Inhibitors (SNRIs)

There have been no reports of the SNRI venlafaxine treatment of patients with FGIDs. Chial and colleagues [355] reported that venlafaxine (75 mg daily for 11 days) produced modest, but significantly greater reductions in colonic sensation, response to feeding and compliance in healthy normals than placebo. Both SSRIs and venlafaxine have been associated with transient nausea early in treatment, and concern over the tolerability of therapeutic doses of these agents is a clinical concern.

Three clinically relevant issues were raised in the newer studies. It appears that response to the SSRI paroxetine did not depend on the presence of a psychiatric disorder, and also that all subtypes of IBS benefited from paroxetine treatment [356, 357]. The third point is that anxious patients with high levels of GI distress appear to tolerate the SNRI venlafaxine as well as those with lower levels of GI distress. There is a substantial need for IBS treatments that are effective for IBS subtypes, benefit those with or without psychiatric disorder, and are adequately tolerated by most patients. Examination of the efficacy of SSRIs and SNRIs in IBS patients with adequate methodology is clearly warranted.

— Practical Use of Psychotropics for Functional Gastrointestinal Disorders

Psychotropic agents are indicated in the presence of significant psychiatric symptoms. In this section, the goal is to achieve both relief of gastrointestinal and psychosocial distress. This will obviously not be the case for all patients. Patients with a history of worrisome or unstable behavior should be referred promptly for assessment by a mental health specialist who can work as a consultant with the practitioner.

The Therapeutic Trial

In clinical practice, a critical part of psychotropic treatment is to assure an adequate dose for a minimum of at least 6, and preferably 8 weeks. Inadequate intensity of treatment is by far the most common cause of psychotropic treatment failure. An important aspect of patient education in those for whom psychotropic treatment is being considered should include discussion of the need to complete

Table 7. Comparative Efficacy of Psychotropic Agents across Anxiety Disorders and Depression*

Diagnosis	Panic Disorder	PTSD	GAD	Social Anxiety Disorder	Major Depression
TCAs	+	+	+	0	+
SSRIs**	+	+	+	+	+
SNRIs***	+	+	+	+	+
Mirtazapine	0	0	0	0	+
Trazodone	0	0	+	0	+
Bupropion	0	0	0	0	+
Benzodiazepines	+	0	+	+	0
Buspirone	0	0	+	0	0

GAD = generalized anxiety disorder
PTSD = post-traumatic stress disorder
RCT = randomized clinical trial

SNRI = serotonin noradrenoline reuptake inhibitor
SSRI = selective serotonin reuptake inhibitor

0 = not effective via at least one RCT
+ = evidence via at least one RCTs

* Not all compounds within each class have received approval for each indication, but all have been approved for major depression and at least one anxiety disorder; paroxetine and sertraline are approved for all indications.

** SSRIs are consistently superior to TCAs for patients with atypical features (hyperphagia, weight gain, hypersomnia, carbohydrate craving, extreme fatigue, and interpersonal sensitivity)

*** Venlafaxine is reflected in the table; Duloxetine is a new SNRI that was been FDA-approved for major depression and diabetes-related neuropathic pain.

the therapeutic trial before switching agents. Using an analogy to antibiotics for an infection sometimes helps in this process. Patients hoping for rapid relief will often ask clinicians to try other treatments well before it is clear that the current treatment has failed. Clinicians who are similarly eager to achieve help for distressed patients may succumb to these requests prematurely.

Choice of Agent

All the antidepressant classes and the anxiolytics shown in Table 7 had efficacy in placebo-controlled RCTs for the disorders shown. As can be seen, not all antidepressants are broadly effective anxiolytics. For example, bupropion is ineffective for panic disorder and social anxiety disorder, and TCAs are ineffective for social anxiety disorder and obsessive-compulsive disorder. Neither the benzodiazepines nor buspirone produce reliable antidepressant effects. When used effectively, agents that are effective both as antidepressants and anxiolytics as a first-line approach may protect against the accrual of additional psychiatric disorders (i.e., depression and/or anxiety disorders).

Table 8. Dosing Guidelines for Treating Major Psychiatric Disorders
with Antidepressants and Anxiolytics*

	Treatment (6–8 weeks)	Starting Dose	CYP Properties/ Comments (Inhibits) [Substrate]
Antidepressants			
Sertraline	≥ 150 mg	12.5–25 mg	(± 2D6) [3A4]
Paroxetine	≥ 40 mg	5–10 mg	(2D6) [2D6]
Fluoxetine	≥ 40 mg	2–5 mg	(2D6,3A4) [2D6, 3A4]
Escitalopram	≥ 30 mg	5 mg	(none) [3A4,2C19]
Citalopram	≥ 40 mg	10 mg	(none) [3A4,2C19]
Fluvoxamine	≥ 150 mg	25 mg	(1A2,2C9,3A4) [?]
Venlafaxine	≥ 225 mg	18.75 mg	(none) [2D6]
High-Potency Benzodiazepines**			
Alprazolam	≥ 4 mg	0.5–1 mg tid	1 mg oral ~10 ng/ml (NA) [3A4]
Clonazepam	≥ 2 mg	0.25–0.5 mg bid	1 mg oral ~12 ng/ml (NA) [3A4]
TCAs			
Imipramine	≥ 200 mg	10 mg	[IMI + DMI] ≥ 225 ng/ml ≥ 1.5–3mg/kg oral (2D6)
Desipramine	≥ 200 mg	10 mg	≥ 125 ng/ml for panic and depression (2D6)
Clomipramine	≥ 150 mg	2.5–10 mg	Both TCA and SSRI (2D6)

* The usual dose needed for treatment of functional gastrointestinal disorders is typically one half of the dose required for psychiatric treatment

**Not useful as antidepressants

CYP = cytochrome P; DMI = desipramine; IMI = imipramine; SSRI = selective serotonin reuptake inhibitor; TCA = tricyclic antidepressant

Table 8 lists the dosing guidelines for antidepressants and anxiolytics for major psychiatric disorders. For the treatment of patients without psychiatric symptoms, about half of the dosage shown is usually sufficient. If the clinician is considering combining a low dose of a TCA with a newer antidepressant, there is probably some advantage to venlafaxine due to its low drug-drug interaction potential, while fluoxetine and paroxetine may increase TCA levels by inhibiting microsomal metabolism of the TCA (Table 8). Obtaining TCA plasma levels (8–12 hours after the last dose) prior to and after initiating the combination can help assure continued patient safety.

Other Antidepressants

Mirtazapine is a novel antidepressant that causes inhibition of reuptake of both 5-HT and NE via pre- and postsynaptic autoreceptors and heteroreceptors. It is also a 5-HT_3 and 5-HT_{2C} antagonist, thereby minimizing initial activation/jitteriness and nausea during initiation of treatment in anxious patients. Unfortunately, it can cause significant sedation, and weight gain is problematic for many patients with long-term use. Some clinicians combine mirtazapine with an SSRI or SNRI during initiation of treatment to reduce unpleasant nausea and promote sleep. To date, mirtazapine has not been studied in RCTs of the FGIDs.

Bupropion is an effective antidepressant, but appears to be ineffective in panic disorder. It has not been studied in the FGIDs. It can be combined with SSRIs or SNRIs to improve treatment-related sexual dysfunction which occurs in 30% to 40% of patients with long-term use.

The triazolopiperazine trazodone is the only marketed agent in this class available in the U.S. Trazodone has been shown to be effective for generalized anxiety disorder (GAD) and beneficial in some esophageal disorders. Sedation is a major limiting adverse effect and trazodone is currently used more often as a hypnotic in primary care than for psychiatric conditions.

Nefazodone, the other antidepressant in this class, was recently withdrawn from the market due to hepatitis in a small but significant number of individuals receiving it.

Benzodiazepines

Some patients are simply intolerant of antidepressants. Many of these patients have prominent anxiety and can justifiably be treated with benzodiazepines, which are useful anxiolytic agents. However, long-term use in the FGID patient is discouraged due to a number of factors. These include the risk of physical dependence with chronic usage (> 2 weeks), the tendency of benzodiazepines to produce sedation, and even cognitive impairment. Finally, benzodiazepines can increase pain sensitivity in some patients.

Azapirones

Buspirone is a nonbenzodiazepine partial 5-HT_{1A} receptor agonist, and is the only marketed compound in its class. It has been shown to have some potentially beneficial effects on upper GI symptoms in healthy subjects [355]. In clinical practice, its efficacy appears to be limited to GAD. Buspirone has clinical utility for psychiatric treatment of a few selected patients, but may be more beneficial in some patients with FGIDs.

The Treatment Process

An algorithm for the use of psychotropic agents for psychiatric symptoms is outlined in Figure 3. In general, any given antidepressant prescribed at sufficient dosage should begin to show benefits within the first 6 weeks of treatment. If a patient has shown a partial response to treatment, it is prudent to continue increasing the dose of that agent gradually, then reassess response and tolerability after an additional 4 to 6 weeks until no further treatment benefit is apparent. Some patients benefit from doses lower than those shown in Table 8. For patients who receive effective treatment over a sufficient period of time, it is possible to achieve complete remission of anxiety and depression (e.g., no bothersome symptoms or illness-related impairment, as though the patient had never been ill) as well as improvement in GI symptoms in many patients. If there is no response at 6 weeks, and compliance and treatment intensity appears to be adequate, referral for psychiatric consultation is indicated.

In summary, the presence of clinically significant psychiatric symptoms in patients with FGIDs is clearly an indication for aggressive treatment with psychotropic agents. Enthusiasm for scientific examination of the potential utility of newer antidepressants for treating FGIDs is based on their broad efficacy in the relevant psychiatric conditions and clinical observations suggesting efficacy on core IBS symptoms and in IBS subtypes. Confirmation of existing practices via RCTs would similarly be informative. Building on the recent advances in our understanding of the neurobiology of the brain-gut axis, information from scientifically sound studies of the psychotropic agents in the treatment of FGID may be fruitful.

— Conclusion

Clinician and basic investigators involved in the treatment or investigation of functional gastrointestinal disorders or disease models need to have a comprehensive understanding of a vast range of medications. It is anticipated that the interaction between investigators of basic science, basic and applied pharmacology, and clinical trials will lead to better treatment of these disorders.

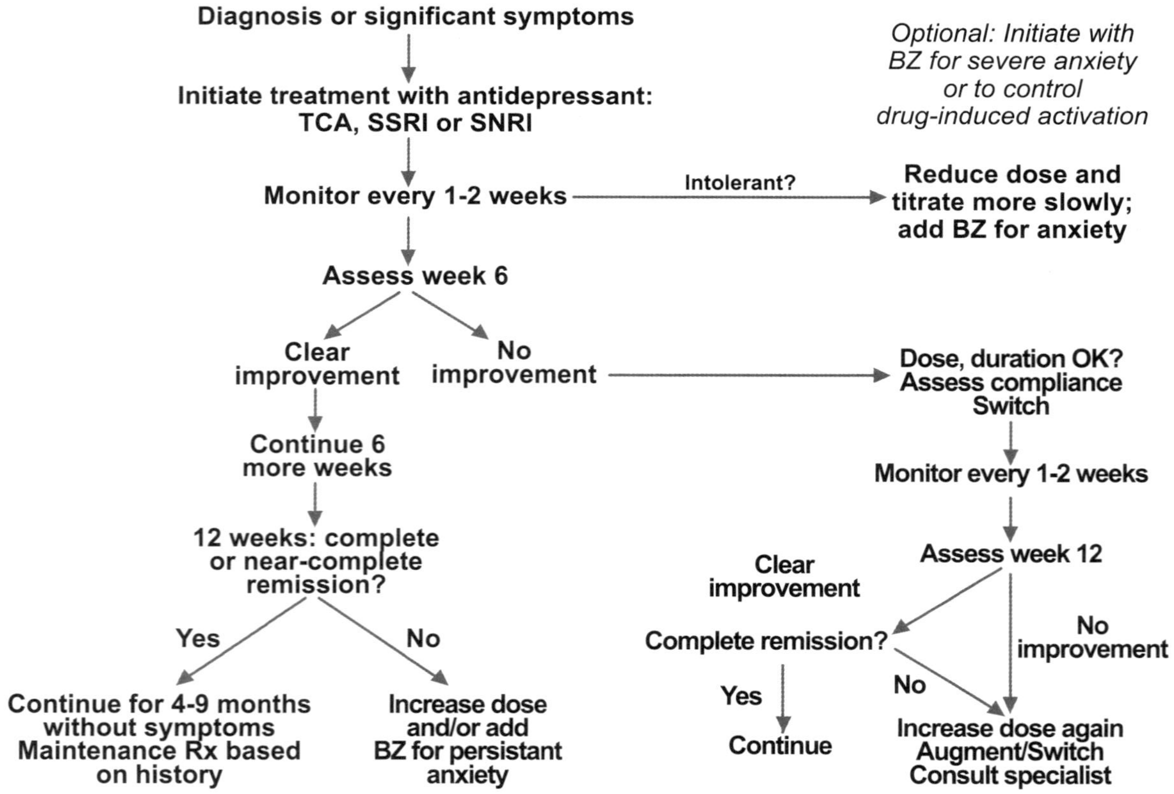

Figure 3. Algorithm for use of antidepressants for treating psychiatric symptoms in FGID patients in clinical practice.

References

1. Le Bars D, Gozariu M, Cadden SW. Animal models of nociception. Pharmacol Rev 2001;53:597–652.
2. Ness TJ, Gebhart GF. Visceral pain: a review of experimental studies. Pain 1990;41: 167–234.
3. Fioramonti J, Gaultier E, Toulouse M, Sanger GJ, Bueno L. Intestinal anti-nociceptive behaviour of NK3 receptor antagonism in conscious rats: evidence to support a peripheral mechanism of action. Neurogastroenterol Motil 2003;15:363–369.
4. Rouzade ML, Fioramonti J, Bueno L. A model for evaluation of gastric sensitivity in awake rats. Neurogastroenterol Motil 1998;10:157–163.
5. Ozaki N, Bielefeldt K, Sengupta JN, Gebhart GF. Models of gastric hyperalgesia in the rat. Am J Physiol 2002;283:G666–G676.
6. Nijsen MJ, Ongenae NG, Coulie B, Meulemans AL. Telemetric animal model to evaluate visceral pain in the freely moving rat. Pain 2003;105:115–123.
7. Morteau O, Hachet T, Caussette M, Bueno L. Experimental colitis alters visceromotor response to colorectal distension in awake rats. Dig Dis Sci 1994;39:1239–1248.
8. Whitehead WE, Delvaux M. Standardization of barostat procedures for testing smooth muscle tone and sensory thresholds in the gastrointestinal tract. The Working Team of Glaxo-Wellcome Research, UK. Dig Dis Sci 1997;42:223–241.
9. Botella A, Fioramonti J, Eeckhout C, Bueno L. Intracolonic glycerol induces abdominal contractions in rats: role of 5-HT3 receptors. Fundam Clin Pharmacol 1998;12:619–623.
10. Louvel D, Delvaux M, Staumont G, Camman F, Fioramonti J, Bueno L, Frexinos J. Intracolonic injection of glycerol: a model for abdominal pain in irritable bowel syndrome? Gastroenterology 1996;110:351–361.
11. Laird JM, Martinez-Caro L, Garcia-Nicas E, Cervero F. A new model of visceral pain and referred hyperalgesia in the mouse. Pain 2001;92:335–342.
12. Blumberg H, Wolf PS, Dayton HB. Use of writhing test for evaluating analgesic activity of narcotic antagonists. Proc Soc Exp Biol Med 1965;118:763–766.
13. Bardos G, Nagy J, Adam G. Thresholds of behavioral reactions evoked by intestinal and skin stimuli in rats. Physiol Behav 1980;24:661–665.
14. Woodsworth RS, Sherrington CS. A pseudo affective reflex and its spinal path. J Physiol 1904;31:234–243.
15. Ness TJ, Gebhart GF. Colorectal distension as a noxious visceral stimulus: physiologic and pharmacologic characterization of pseudo affective reflexes in the rat. Brain Res 1988;450:153–169.
16. Borgbjerg FM, Frigast C, Madsen JB. Tonic endogenous opioid inhibition of visceral noxious information in rabbits. Gastroenterology 1996;111:78–84.
17. Kamp EH, Jones RC, III, Tillman SR, Gebhart GF. Quantitative assessment and characterization of visceral nociception and hyperalgesia in mice. Am J Physiol 2003;284: G434–G444.
18. Larsson M, Arvidsson S, Ekman C, Bayati A. A model for chronic quantitative studies of colorectal sensitivity using balloon distension in conscious mice—effects of opioid receptor agonists. Neurogastroenterol Motil 2003;15:371–381.

19. Plourde V, St Pierre S, Quirion R. Calcitonin gene-related peptide in viscerosensitive response to colorectal distension in rats. Am J Physiol 1997;273:G191–G196.

20. Rouzade ML, Fioramonti J, Bueno L. Decrease in gastric sensitivity to distension by 5-HT1A receptor agonists in rats. Dig Dis Sci 1998;43:2048–2054.

21. Gue M, Junien JL, Bueno L. The kappa agonist fedotozine modulates colonic distention-induced inhibition of gastric motility and emptying in dogs. Gastroenterology 1994;107:1327–1334.

22. Youle MS, Read NW. Effect of painless rectal distension on gastrointestinal transit of solid meal. Dig Dis Sci 1984;29:902–906.

23. Law NM, Bharucha AE, Zinsmeister AR. Rectal and colonic distension elicit viscerovisceral reflexes in humans. Am J Physiol 2002;283:G384–G389.

24. Julia V, Morteau O, Bueno L. Involvement of neurokinin 1 and 2 receptors in viscerosensitive response to rectal distension in rats. Gastroenterology 1994;107:94–102.

25. Tougas G, Wang L. Pseudo affective cardioautonomic responses to gastric distension in rats. Am J Physiol 1999;277:R272–R278.

26. Burton MB, Gebhart GF. Effects of intracolonic acetic acid on responses to colorectal distension in the rat. Brain Res 1995;672:77–82.

27. Su X, Julia V, Gebhart GF. Effects of intracolonic opioid receptor agonists on polymodal pelvic nerve afferent fibers in the rat. J Neurophysiol 2000;83:963–970.

28. Booth CE, Kirkup AJ, Hicks GA, Humphrey PP, Grundy D. Somatostatin sst(2) receptor-mediated inhibition of mesenteric afferent nerves of the jejunum in the anesthetized rat. Gastroenterology 2001;121:358–369.

29. Fioramonti J, Gaultier E, Toulouse M, Sanger GJ, Bueno L. Intestinal anti-nociceptive behaviour of NK3 receptor antagonism in conscious rats: evidence to support a peripheral mechanism of action. Neurogastroenterol Motil 2003;15:363–369.

30. Messaoudi M, Desor D, Grasmuck V, Joyeux M, Langlois A, Roman FJ. Behavioral evaluation of visceral pain in a rat model of colonic inflammation. Neuroreport 1999;10:1137–1141.

31. Bardos G. Conditioned taste aversion to gut distension in rats. Physiol Behav 2001; 74:407–413.

32. Ringel Y, Sperber AD, Drossman DA. Irritable bowel syndrome. Annu Rev Med 2001;52:319–338.

33. Dapoigny M, Stockbrugger RW, Azpiroz F, Collins S, Coremans G, Muller-Lissner S, Oberndorff A, Pace F, Smout A, Vatn M, Whorwell P. Role of alimentation in irritable bowel syndrome. Digestion 2003;67:225–233.

34. Ness TJ, Gebhart GF. Characterization of superficial T13-L2 dorsal horn neurons encoding for colorectal distension in the rat: comparison with neurons in deep laminae. Brain Res 1989;486:301–309.

35. Omote K, Kawamata M, Iwasaki H, Namiki A. Effects of morphine on neuronal and behavioural responses to visceral and somatic nociception at the level of spinal cord. Acta Anaesthesiol Scand 1994;38:514–517.

36. Ness TJ. Kappa opioid receptor agonists differentially inhibit two classes of rat spinal neurons excited by colorectal distention. Gastroenterology 1999;117:388–394.

37. Lanteri-Minet M, Isnardon P, de Pommery J, Menetrey D. Spinal and hindbrain structures involved in visceroception and visceronociception as revealed by the expression of Fos, Jun and Krox-24 proteins. Neuroscience 1993;55:737–753.

38. Birder LA, Kiss S, de Groat WC, Lecci A, Maggi CA. Effect of nepadutant, a neurokinin 2 tachykinin receptor antagonist, on immediate-early gene expression after

trinitrobenzenesulfonic acid-induced colitis in the rat. J Pharmacol Exp Ther 2003;
304:272–276.

39. Traub RJ, Zhai Q, Ji Y, Kovalenko M. NMDA receptor antagonists attenuate noxious
and nonnoxious colorectal distention-induced Fos expression in the spinal cord and
the visceromotor reflex. Neuroscience 2002;113:205–211.

40. Jou CJ, Farber JP, Qin C, Foreman RD. Convergent pathways for cardiac- and esoph-
ageal-somatic motor reflexes in rats. Auton Neurosci 2002;99:70–77.

41. Larauche M, Anton PM, Garcia-Villar R, Theodorou V, Frexinos J, Bueno L, Fioramonti J. Protective effect of dietary nitrate on experimental gastritis in rats. Br J
Nutr 2003;89:777–786.

42. Anton PM, Theodorou V, Fioramonti J, Bueno L. Chronic low-level administration
of diquat increases the nociceptive response to gastric distension in rats: role of mast
cells and tachykinin receptor activation. Pain 2001;92:219–227.

43. Rouzade ML, Anton P, Fioramonti J, Garcia-Villar R, Theodorou V, Bueno L. Reduction of the nociceptive response to gastric distension by nitrate ingestion in rats.
Aliment Pharmacol Ther 1999;13:1235–1241.

44. McLean PG, Picard C, Garcia-Villar R, Ducos dL, More J, Fioramonti J, Bueno L.
Role of kinin B1 and B2 receptors and mast cells in post intestinal infection-induced
hypersensitivity to distension. Neurogastroenterol Motil 1998;10:499–508.

45. O'Sullivan M, Clayton N, Breslin NP, Harman I, Bountra C, McLaren A, O'Morain
CA. Increased mast cells in the irritable bowel syndrome. Neurogastroenterol Motil
2000;12:449–457.

46. McLean PG, Picard C, Garcia-Villar R, More J, Fioramonti J, Bueno L. Effects of
nematode infection on sensitivity to intestinal distension: role of tachykinin NK2
receptors. Eur J Pharmacol 1997;337:279–282.

47. De Giorgio R, Barbara G, Blennerhassett P, Wang L, Stanghellini V, Corinaldesi R,
Collins SM, Tougas G. Intestinal inflammation and activation of sensory nerve
pathways: a functional and morphological study in the nematode infected rat. Gut
2001;49:822–827.

48. Gue M, Rio-Lacheze C, Eutamene H, Theodorou V, Fioramonti J, Bueno L. Stress-
induced visceral hypersensitivity to rectal distension in rats: role of CRF and mast
cells. Neurogastroenterol Motil 1997;9:271–279.

49. Bradesi S, Eutamene H, Garcia-Villar R, Fioramonti J, Bueno L. Acute and chronic
stress differently affect visceral sensitivity to rectal distension in female rats. Neurogastroenterol Motil 2002;14:75–82.

50. Bradesi S, Eutamene H, Garcia-Villar R, Fioramonti J, Bueno L. Stress-induced visceral hypersensitivity in female rats is estrogen-dependent and involves tachykinin
NK1 receptors. Pain 2003;102:227–234.

51. Bradesi S, Eutamene H, Fioramonti J, Bueno L. Acute restraint stress activates
functional NK1 receptor in the colon of female rats: involvement of steroids. Gut
2002;50:349–354.

52. Coelho AM, Fioramonti J, Bueno L. Systemic lipopolysaccharide influences rectal sensitivity in rats: role of mast cells, cytokines, and vagus nerve. Am J Physiol
2000;279:G781–G790.

53. Coelho AM, Vergnolle N, Guiard B, Fioramonti J, Bueno L. Proteinases and proteinase-activated receptor 2: a possible role to promote visceral hyperalgesia in rats.
Gastroenterology 2002;122:1035–1047.

54. Cenac N, Garcia-Villar R, Ferrier L, Larauche M, Vergnolle N, Bunnett NW, Coelho

AM, Fioramonti J, Bueno L. Proteinase-activated receptor-2-induced colonic inflammation in mice: possible involvement of afferent neurons, nitric oxide, and paracellular permeability. J Immunol 2003;170:4296–4300.

55. Coutinho SV, Meller ST, Gebhart GF. Intracolonic zymosan produces visceral hyperalgesia in the rat that is mediated by spinal NMDA and non-NMDA receptors. Brain Res 1996;736:7–15.

56. Ness TJ, Gebhart GF. Inflammation enhances reflex and spinal neuron responses to noxious visceral stimulation in rats. Am J Physiol 2001;280:G649–G657.

57. Al Chaer ED, Kawasaki M, Pasricha PJ. A new model of chronic visceral hypersensitivity in adult rats induced by colon irritation during postnatal development. Gastroenterology 2000;119:1276–1285.

58. Barreau F, Ferrier L, Fioramonti J, Bueno L. Neonatal maternal deprivation triggers long term alterations in colonic epithelial barrier and mucosal immunity in rats. Gut 2004;53:501–506.

59. Coutinho SV, Plotsky P, Sablad M, Miller JC, Zhou H, Bayati AI, McRoberts JA, Mayer EA. Neonatal maternal separation alters stress-induced responses to viscerosomatic nociceptive stimuli in rat. Am J Physiol 2002;282:G307–G316.

60. Rosztoczy A, Fioramonti J, Jarmay K, Barreau F, Wittmann T, Bueno L. Influence of sex and experimental protocol on the effect of maternal deprivation on rectal sensitivity to distension in the adult rat. Neurogastroenterol Motil 2003;15:679–686.

61. Iwanaga Y, Wen J, Thollander MS, Kost LJ, Thomforde GM, Allen RG, Phillips SF. Scintigraphic measurement of regional gastrointestinal transit in the dog. Am J Physiol 1998;275:G904–G910.

62. Schoonjans R, Van Vlem B, Van Heddeghem N, Vandamme W, Vanholder R, Lameire N, Lefebvre R, De Vos M. The 13C-octanoic acid breath test: validation of a new noninvasive method of measuring gastric emptying in rats. Neurogastroenterol Motil 2002;14:287–293.

63. Sutton DG, Bahr A, Preston T, Christley RM, Love S, Roussel AJ. Validation of the ^{13}C-octanoic acid breath test for measurement of equine gastric emptying rate of solids using radioscintigraphy. Equine Vet J 2003;35:27–33.

64. Brown NJ, Rumsey RD, Read NW. Adaptation of hydrogen analysis to measure stomach to caecum transit time in the rat. Gut 1987;28:849–854.

65. Azpiroz F, Malagelada JR. Physiological variations in canine gastric tone measured by an electronic barostat. Am J Physiol 1985;248:G229–G237.

66. Monroe MJ, Hornby PJ, Partosoedarso ER. Central vagal stimulation evokes gastric volume changes in mice: a novel technique using a miniaturized barostat. Neurogastroenterol Motil 2004;16:5–11.

67. Patrikios J, Martin CJ, Dent J. Relationship of transient lower esophageal sphincter relaxation to postprandial gastroesophageal reflux and belching in dogs. Gastroenterology 1986;90:545–551.

68. Boulant J, Mathieu S, D'Amato M, Abergel A, Dapoigny M, Bommelaer G. Cholecystokinin in transient lower oesophageal sphincter relaxation due to gastric distension in humans. Gut 1997;40:575–581.

69. Zhang Q, Lehmann A, Rigda R, Dent J, Holloway RH. Control of transient lower oesophageal sphincter relaxations and reflux by the GABA(B) agonist baclofen in patients with gastro-oesophageal reflux disease. Gut 2002;50:19–24.

70. Hirsch DP, Tiel-Van Buul MM, Tytgat GN, Boeckxstaens GE. Effect of L-NMMA on

postprandial transient lower esophageal sphincter relaxations in healthy volunteers. Dig Dis Sci 2000;45:2069–2075.

71. Blackshaw LA, Staunton E, Lehmann A, Dent J. Inhibition of transient LES relaxations and reflux in ferrets by GABA receptor agonists. Am J Physiol 1999;277:G867–G874.

72. Lenz HJ, Raedler A, Greten H, Vale WW, Rivier JE. Stress-induced gastrointestinal secretory and motor responses in rats are mediated by endogenous corticotropin-releasing factor. Gastroenterology 1988;95:1510–1517.

73. Dumas J, Peres G. The mechanism of action of restraint on gastric emptying in the rat. Role of the adrenal glands. C R Seances Soc Biol Fil 1974;168:47–50.

74. Gue M, Fioramonti J, Bueno L. Influence of stress on gastric emptying depends on the nature of meals, stressors, and animal species. J Gastroint Mot 1990;2 :18–22.

75. Ferrier L, Mazelin L, Cenac N, Desreumaux P, Janin A, Emilie D, Colombel JF, Garcia-Villar R, Fioramonti J, Bueno L. Stress-induced disruption of colonic epithelial barrier: role of interferon-gamma and myosin light chain kinase in mice. Gastroenterology 2003;125:795–804.

76. Enck P, Merlin V, Erckenbrecht JF, Wienbeck M. Stress effects on gastrointestinal transit in the rat. Gut 1989;30:455–459.

77. Mistiaen W, Blockx P, Van Hee R, Bortier H, Harrisson F. The effect of stress on gastric emptying rate measured with a radionuclide tracer. Hepatogastroenterology 2002; 49:1457–1460.

78. Tjeerdsma HC, Smout AJ, Akkermans LM. Voluntary suppression of defecation delays gastric emptying. Dig Dis Sci 1993;38:832–836.

79. Holzer HH, Turkelson CM, Solomon TE, Raybould HE. Intestinal lipid inhibits gastric emptying via CCK and a vagal capsaicin-sensitive afferent pathway in rats. Am J Physiol 1994;267:G625–G629.

80. De Ponti F, Crema F, Moro E, Nardelli G, Frigo G, CREMA A. Role of 5-HT1B/D receptors in canine gastric accommodation: effect of sumatriptan and 5-HT1B/D receptor antagonists. Am J Physiol 2003;285:G96–104.

81. Gue M, Peeters T, Depoortere I, Vantrappen G, Bueno L. Stress-induced changes in gastric emptying, postprandial motility, and plasma gut hormone levels in dogs. Gastroenterology 1989;97:1101–1107.

82. Fargeas MJ, Fioramonti J, Bueno L. Central alpha 2-adrenergic control of the pattern of small intestinal motility in rats. Gastroenterology 1986;91:1470–1475.

83. Umezawa T, Guo S, Jiao Y, Hisamitsu T. Effect of clonidine on colonic motility in rats. Auton Neurosci 2003;107:32–36.

84. Primi MP, Bueno L. Effects of centrally administered naloxone on gastrointestinal myoelectrical activity in morphine-dependent rats. J Pharmacol Exp Ther 1987; 240:320–326.

85. Gue M, Junien JL, Bueno L. Conditioned emotional response in rats enhances colonic motility through the central release of corticotropin-releasing factor. Gastroenterology 1991;100:964–970.

86. Williams CL, Peterson JM, Villar RG, Burks TF. Corticotropin-releasing factor directly mediates colonic responses to stress. Am J Physiol 1987;253:G582–G586.

87. Narducci F, Snape WJ, Jr., Battle WM, London RL, Cohen S. Increased colonic motility during exposure to a stressful situation. Dig Dis Sci 1985;30:40–44.

88. Briejer MR, Veen GJ, Akkermans LM, Lefebvre RA, Schuurkes JA. Cisapride and

structural analogs selectively enhance 5-hydroxytryptamine (5-HT)-induced purinergic neurotransmission in the guinea pig proximal colon. J Pharmacol ExpTher
1995;274:641–648.

89. Tonini M, De Ponti F, Di Nucci A, Crema F. Review article: cardiac adverse effects
of gastrointestinal prokinetics. Aliment Pharmacol Ther 1999;13:1585–1591.

90. Recanatini M, Poluzzi E, Masetti M, Cavalli A, De Ponti F. QT prolongation
through hERG K+ channel blockade: Current knowledge and strategies for the
early prediction during drug development. Med Res Rev 2005;in press.

91. Farrelly AM, Ro S, Callaghan BP, Khoyi MA, Fleming N, Horowitz B, Sanders KM,
Keef KD. Expression and function of KCNH2 (HERG) in the human jejunum. Am
J Physiol 2003;284:G883–G895.

92. Morphy R, Kay C, Rankovic Z. From magic bullets to designed multiple ligands.
Drug Discov Today 2004;9:641–651.

93. Camilleri M, Northcutt AR, Kong S, Dukes GE, McSorley D, Mangel AW. Efficacy
and safety of alosetron in women with irritable bowel syndrome: A randomised,
placebo-controlled trial. Lancet 2000;355:1035–1040.

94. Muller-Lissner SA, Fumagalli I, Bardhan KD, Pace F, Pecher E, Nault B, Ruegg P.
Tegaserod, a 5-HT4 receptor partial agonist, relieves symptoms in irritable bowel
syndrome patients with abdominal pain, bloating and constipation. Aliment Pharmacol Ther 2001;15:1655–1666.

95. Cremonini F, Delgado-Aros S, Camilleri M. Efficacy of alosetron in irritable bowel
syndrome: a meta-analysis of randomized controlled trials. Neurogastroenterol
Motil 2003;15:79–86.

96. Lembo AJ, Olden KW, Ameen VZ, Gordon SL, Heath AT, Carter EG. Effect of
alosetron on bowel urgency and global symptoms in women with severe, diarrhea-
predominant irritable bowel syndrome: analysis of two controlled trials. Clin Gastroenterol Hepatol 2004;2:675–682.

97. De Ponti F. Pharmacology of serotonin: what a clinician should know. Gut 2004;
53:1520–1535.

98. Holzer P. Tachykinin receptor antagonists: silencing neuropeptides with a role in
the disturbed gut. In: Spiller R and Grundy D, eds. Pathophysiology of the Enteric
Nervous System. London: Blackwell, 2004:212–227.

99. Tonini M, Spelta V, De Ponti F, De Giorgio R, D'Agostino G, Stanghellini V, Corinaldesi R, Sternini C, Crema F. Tachykinin-dependent and -independent components of peristalsis in the guinea pig isolated distal colon. Gastroenterology 2001;
120:938–945.

100. Tack J, Piessevaux H, Coulie B, Caenepeel P, Janssens J. Role of impaired gastric accommodation to a meal in functional dyspepsia. Gastroenterology 1998;115:1346–
1352.

101. Janssen P, Tack J, Sifrim D, Meulemans AL, Lefebvre RA. Influence of 5-HT1 receptor agonists on feline stomach relaxation. Eur J Pharmacol 2004;492:259–267.

102. De Ponti F. Methylnaltrexone Progenics. Curr Opin Investig Drugs 2002;3:614–
620.

103. Holzer P. Opioids and opioid receptors in the enteric nervous system: from a problem in opioid analgesia to a possible new prokinetic therapy in humans. Neurosci
Lett 2004;361:192–195.

104. Bott C, Rudolph MW, Schneider AR, Schirrmacher S, Skalsky B, Petereit HU,

Langguth P, Dressman JB, Stein J. In vivo evaluation of a novel pH- and time-based multiunit colonic drug delivery system. Aliment Pharmacol Ther 2004;20:347–353.

105. Nugent SG, Kumar D, Rampton DS, Evans DF. Intestinal luminal pH in inflammatory bowel disease: possible determinants and implications for therapy with aminosalicylates and other drugs. Gut 2001;48:571–577.

106. Ekins S, Berbaum J, Harrison RK. Generation and validation of rapid computational filters for CYP2D6 and CYP3A4. Drug Metab Dispos 2003;31:1077–1080.

107. Lewis DF. Molecular modeling of human cytochrome P450-substrate interactions. Drug Metab Rev 2002;34:55–67.

108. De Ponti F, Poluzzi E, Montanaro N. Organising evidence on QT prolongation and occurrence of Torsades de Pointes with non-antiarrhythmic drugs: a call for consensus. Eur J Clin Pharmacol 2001;57:185–209.

109. Ray WA, Murray KT, Meredith S, Narasimhulu SS, Hall K, Stein CM. Oral erythromycin and the risk of sudden death from cardiac causes. N Engl J Med 2004; 351:1089–1096.

110. De Ponti F, Poluzzi E, Montanaro N, Ferguson J. QTc and psychotropic drugs. Lancet 2000;356:75–76.

111. Potet F, Bouyssou T, Escande D, Baro I. Gastrointestinal prokinetic drugs have different affinity for the human cardiac human ether-a-gogo K(+) channel. J Pharmacol Exp Ther 2001;299:1007–1012.

112. Kang J, Wang L, Chen XL, Triggle DJ, Rampe D. Interactions of a series of fluoroquinolone antibacterial drugs with the human cardiac K+ channel HERG. Mol Pharmacol 2001;59:122–126.

113. Redfern WS, Carlsson L, Davis AS, Lynch WG, MacKenzie I, Palethorpe S, Siegl PK, Strang I, Sullivan AT, Wallis R, Camm AJ, Hammond TG. Relationships between preclinical cardiac electrophysiology, clinical QT interval prolongation and torsade de pointes for a broad range of drugs: evidence for a provisional safety margin in drug development. Cardiovasc Res 2003;58:32–45.

114. De Ponti F, Poluzzi E, Cavalli A, Recanatini M, Montanaro N. Safety of non-antiarrhythmic drugs that prolong the QT interval or induce torsade de pointes: an overview. Drug Safety 2002;25:263–286.

115. Friedel D, Thomas R, Fisher RS. Ischemic colitis during treatment with alosetron. Gastroenterology 2001;120:557–560.

116. Wooltorton E. Tegaserod (Zelnorm) for irritable bowel syndrome: reports of serious diarrhea and intestinal ischemia. CMAJ 2004;170:1908.

117. Moynihan R. Alosetron: a case study in regulatory capture, or a victory for patients' rights? BMJ 2002;325:592–595.

118. Higgins PD, Davis KJ, Laine L. Systematic review: the epidemiology of ischemic colitis. Aliment Pharmacol Ther 2004;19:729–738.

119. Brinker A, Avigan M. Epidemiology of ischemic colitis. Aliment Pharmacol Ther 2004;20:697–698.

120. Beck IT. Possible mechanisms for ischemic colitis during alosetron therapy. Gastroenterology 2001;121:231–232.

121. Holzer P, Painsipp E, Weber E, Pfannkuche HJ. 5-HT$_3$ receptor antagonists, alosetron and cilansetron, impair mesenteric blood flow in rats. Gastroenterology 2003;124 (Suppl 1):A148–A149.

122. Lembo A, Camilleri M. Chronic constipation. N Engl J Med 2003;349:1360–1368.
123. Nobaek S, Johansson ML, Molin G, Ahrne S, Jeppsson B. Alteration of intestinal microflora is associated with reduction in abdominal bloating and pain in patients with irritable bowel syndrome. Am J Gastroenterol 2000;95:1231–1238.
124. Kim HJ, Camilleri M, McKinzie S, Lempke MB, Burton DD, Thomforde GM, Zinsmeister AR. A randomized controlled trial of a probiotic, VSL#3, on gut transit and symptoms in diarrhoea-predominant irritable bowel syndrome. Aliment Pharmacol Ther 2003;17:895–904.
125. O'Mahony L, McCarthy J, Kelly P, Hurley G, Luo F, Chen K, O'Sullivan GC, Kiely B, Collins JK, Shanahan F, Quigley EMM. A randomized, placebo-controlled, double-blind comparison of the probiotic bacteria lactobacillus and bifidobacterium in irritable bowel syndrome (IBS): symptom responses and relationship to cytokine profiles. Gastroenterology 2005;128:541–51.
126. Lesbros-Pantoflickova D, Michetti P, Fried M, Beglinger C, Blum AL. Meta-analysis: the treatment of irritable bowel syndrome. Aliment Pharmacol Ther 2004;20:1253–1269.
127. Erspamer V. Occurrence of indolealkylamines in nature. Handbook of Experimental Pharmacology. Vol 19 ed. New York: Springer Verlag, 1966:132–181.
128. Bülbring E, LIN RC. The effect of intraluminal application of 5-hydroxytryptamine and 5-hydroxytryptophan on peristalsis; the local production of 5-HT and its release in relation to intraluminal pressure and propulsive activity. J Physiol (Lond) 1958;140:381–407.
129. Bülbring E, CREMA A. Observations concerning the action of 5-hydroxytryptamine on the peristaltic reflex. Br J Pharmacol 1958;13:444–457.
130. Bülbring E, CREMA A. The release of 5-hydroxytryptamine in relation to pressure exerted on the intestinal mucosa. J Physiol (Lond) 1959;146:18–28.
131. Gronstad KO, DeMagistris L, Dahlstrom A, Nilsson O, Price B, Zinner MJ, Jaffe BM, Ahlman H. The effects of vagal nerve stimulation on endoluminal release of serotonin and substance P into the feline small intestine. Scand J Gastroenterol 1985;20:163–169.
132. Beubler E, Horina G. 5-HT2 and 5-HT3 receptor subtypes mediate cholera toxin-induced intestinal fluid secretion in the rat. Gastroenterology 1990;99:83–89.
133. Furness JB, Costa M. Neurons with 5-hydroxytryptamine-like immunoreactivity in the enteric nervous system: their projections in the guinea-pig small intestine. Neuroscience 1982;7:341–349.
134. Costa M, Furness JB, Cuello AC, Verhofstad AA, Steinbusch HW, Elde RP. Neurons with 5-hydroxytryptamine-like immunoreactivity in the enteric nervous system: their visualization and reactions to drug treatment. Neuroscience 1982;7:351–363.
135. Dahlstrom A, Ahlman H. Immunocytochemical evidence for the presence of tryptaminergic nerves of blood vessels, smooth muscle and myenteric plexus in the rat small intestine. Acta Physiol Scand 1983;117:589–591.
136. Griffith SG, Burnstock G. Serotoninergic neurons in human fetal intestine: an immunohistochemical study. Gastroenterology 1983;85:929–937.
137. Kurian SS, Ferri GL, De Mey J, Polak JM. Immunocytochemistry of serotonin-containing nerves in the human gut. Histochemistry 1983;78:523–529.
138. Legay C, Saffrey MJ, Burnstock G. Coexistence of immunoreactive substance P and serotonin in neurones of the gut. Brain Res 1984;302:379–382.

139. Mawe GM, Schemann M, Wood JD, Gershon MD. Immunocytochemical analysis of potential neurotransmitters present in the myenteric plexus and muscular layers of the corpus of the guinea pig stomach. Anat Rec 1989;224:431–442.

140. Gershon MD, Jonakait GM. Uptake and release of 5-hydroxytryptamine by enteric 5-hydroxytryptaminergic neurones: effects of fluoxetine (Lilly 110140) and chlorimipramine. Br J Pharmacol 1979;66:7–9.

141. Gorard DA, Libby GW, Farthing MJ. 5-Hydroxytryptamine and human small intestinal motility: effect of inhibiting 5-hydroxytryptamine reuptake. Gut 1994;35:496–500.

142. Gorard DA, Libby GW, Farthing MJ. Influence of antidepressants on whole gut and orocaecal transit times in health and irritable bowel syndrome. Aliment Pharmacol Ther 1994;8:159–166.

143. Tack J, Broekaert D, Coulie B, Fischler B, Janssens J. Influence of the selective serotonin re-uptake inhibitor, paroxetine, on gastric sensorimotor function in humans. Aliment Pharmacol Ther 2003;17:603–608.

144. Tack J, Vos R, Janssens J, Salter J, Jauffret S, Vandeplassche G. Influence of tegaserod on proximal gastric tone and on the perception of gastric distension. Aliment Pharmacol Ther 2003;18:1031–1037.

145. Tack J, Broekaert D, Fischler B, Gevers AM, Vandenberghe J, Janssens J. A placebo-controlled cross-over study of citalopram, a selective serotonin reuptake inhibitor, in the irritable bowel syndrome. Gut. 2006 Jan 9; [Epub ahead of print] PMID: 16401691.

146. Kuiken SD, Tytgat GN, Boeckxstaens GE. The selective serotonin reuptake inhibitor fluoxetine does not change rectal sensitivity and symptoms in patients with irritable bowel syndrome: a double blind, randomized, placebo-controlled study. Clin Gastroenterol Hepatol 2003;1:219–228.

147. Bülbring E, Gershon MD. 5-hydroxytryptamine participation in the vagal inhibitory innervation of the stomach. J Physiol (Lond) 1967;192:823–846.

148. Costa M, Furness JB. The sites of action of 5-hydroxytryptamine in nerve-muscle preparations from the guinea-pig small intestine and colon. Br J Pharmacol 1979; 65:237–248.

149. Gaddum JH, Picarelli ZP. Two kinds of tryptamine receptor. Br J Pharmacol 1957; 12:323–328.

150. Brownlee G, Johnson ES. The site of the 5-hydroxytryptamine receptor on the intramural nervous plexus of the guinea-pig isolated ileum. Br J Pharmacol 1963;21:306–322.

151. Drakontides AB, Gershon MD. 5-hydroxytryptamine receptors in the mouse duodenum. Br J Pharmacol 1968;33:480–492.

152. Vizzi F, De Rocco R. Biliary ileus. Minerva Gastroenterol 1977;23:5–10.

153. Galligan JJ, Surprenant A, Tonini M, North RA. Differential localization of 5-HT1 receptors on myenteric and submucosal neurons. Am J Physiol 1988;255:G603–G611.

154. Todorovic S, Anderson EG. Serotonin preferentially hyperpolarizes capsaicin-sensitive C type sensory neurons by activating 5-HT1A receptors. Brain Res 1992; 585:212–218.

155. Di Stefano M, Vos R, Sifrim D, Janssens J, Tack J. Effect of buspirone, a 5HT1A receptor agonist on oesophageal peristalsis and lower oesophageal sphincter function in healthy volunteers. Gastroenterology 126 (Suppl. 2), A638. 2004.

156. Chial HJ, Camilleri M, Ferber I, Delgado-Aros S, Burton D, McKinzie S, Zinsmeister AR. Effects of venlafaxine, buspirone, and placebo on colonic sensorimotor functions in healthy humans. Clin Gastroenterol Hepatol 2003;1:211–218.

157. Tack J, Piessevaux H, Coulie B, et al. A placebo-controlled trial of buspirone, a fundus-relaxing drug, in functional dyspepsia: Effect on symptoms and gastric sensory and motor function. Gastroenterology 1999;116,part2:G1423.

158. Coulie B, Tack J, Janssens J. Influence of buspirone-induced fundus relaxation on the perception of gastric distention in man. Gastroenterology 112 [4], A715. 1997.

159. Tack J, Van Elzen B, Tytgat G, Wajs E, Van Nueten L, De Ridder F, Boeckxstaens G. A placebo-controlled trial of the 5-HT1A agonist R-137696 on symptoms, visceral hypersensitivity and on impaired accommodation in functional dyspepsia. Gastroenterology 2004;126 (Suppl. 2):A70.

160. Derkach V, Surprenant A, North RA. 5-HT3 receptors are membrane ion channels. Nature 1989;339:706–709.

161. Wood JD, Mayer CJ. Serotonergic activation of tonic-type enteric neurons in guinea pig small bowel. J Neurophysiol 1979;42:582–593.

162. Surprenant A, Crist J. Electrophysiological characterization of functionally distinct 5-hydroxytryptamine receptors on guinea-pig submucous plexus. Neuroscience 1988;24:283–295.

163. Neya T, Mizutani M, Yamasato T. Role of 5-HT3 receptors in peristaltic reflex elicited by stroking the mucosa in the canine jejunum. J Physiol (Lond) 1993;471:159–173.

164. Tonini M, Candura SM, Onori L, Coccini T, Manzo L, Rizzi CA. 5-hydroxytryptamine4 receptor agonists facilitate cholinergic transmission in the circular muscle of guinea pig ileum: antagonism by tropisetron and DAU 6285. Life Sci 1992;50:L173–L178.

165. Yuan SY, Bornstein JC, Furness JB. Investigation of the role of 5-HT3 and 5-HT4 receptors in ascending and descending reflexes to the circular muscle of guinea-pig small intestine. Br J Pharmacol 1994;112:1095–1100.

166. Talley NJ, Phillips SF, Haddad A, Miller LJ, Twomey C, Zinsmeister AR, Ciociola A. Effect of selective 5HT3 antagonist (GR 38032F) on small intestinal transit and release of gastrointestinal peptides. Dig Dis Sci 1989;34:1511–1515.

167. Nielsen OH, Hvid-Jacobsen K, Lund P, Langholz E. Gastric emptying and subjective symptoms of nausea: lack of effects of a 5-hydroxytryptamine-3 antagonist ondansetron on gastric emptying in patients with gastric stasis syndrome. Digestion 1990;46:89–96.

168. Schiavone A, Volonte M, Micheletti R. The gastrointestinal motor effect of benzamide derivatives is unrelated to 5-HT3 receptor blockade. Eur J Pharmacol 1990;187:323–329.

169. Kuo B, Camilleri M, Burton D, Viramontes B, McKinzie S, Thomforde G, O'Connor MK, Brinkmann BH. Effects of 5-HT(3) antagonism on postprandial gastric volume and symptoms in humans. Aliment Pharmacol Ther 2002;16:225–233.

170. Talley NJ, Phillips SF, Haddad A, Miller LJ, Twomey C, Zinsmeister AR, MacCarty RL, Ciociola A. GR 38032F (ondansetron), a selective 5HT3 receptor antagonist, slows colonic transit in healthy man. Dig Dis Sci 1990;35:477–480.

171. Gore S, Gilmore IT, Haigh CG, Brownless SM, Stockdale H, Morris AI. Colonic transit in man is slowed by ondansetron (GR38032F), a selective 5-hydroxytryptamine receptor (type 3) antagonist. Aliment Pharmacol Ther 1990;4:139–144.

172. Scolapio JS, Camilleri M, der Ohe MR, Hanson RB. Ascending colon response to feeding: evidence for a 5-hydroxytryptamine-3 mechanism. Scand J Gastroenterol 1995;30:562–567.

173. von der Ohe MR, Hanson RB, Camilleri M. Serotonergic mediation of postprandial colonic tonic and phasic responses in humans. Gut 1994;35:536–541.

174. Moss HE, Sanger GJ. The effects of granisetron, ICS 205–930 and ondansetron on the visceral pain reflex induced by duodenal distension. Br J Pharmacol 1990;100:497–501.

175. Zighelboim J, Talley NJ, Phillips SF, Harmsen WS, Zinsmeister AR. Visceral perception in irritable bowel syndrome. Rectal and gastric responses to distension and serotonin type 3 antagonism. Dig Dis Sci 1995;40:819–827.

176. Zerbib F, Bruley d, V, Oriola RC, McDonald J, Isal JP, Galmiche JP. Alosetron does not affect the visceral perception of gastric distension in healthy subjects. Aliment Pharmacol Ther 1994;8:403–407.

177. Hammer J, Phillips SF, Talley NJ, Camilleri M. Effect of a 5HT3-antagonist (ondansetron) on rectal sensitivity and compliance in health and the irritable bowel syndrome. Aliment Pharmacol Ther 1993;7:543–551.

178. Delvaux M, Louvel D, Mamet JP, Campos-Oriola R, Frexinos J. Effect of alosetron on responses to colonic distension in patients with irritable bowel syndrome. Aliment Pharmacol Ther 1998;12:849–855.

179. Caras S, Krause G, Biesheuvel E, Steinborn C. Cilansetron shows efficacy in male and female non-constipated patients with irritable bowel syndrome in a United States study. Gastroenterology 2001;120 (Suppl 1):A217.

180. Chey WD, Cash BD. Cilansetron: a new serotonergic agent for the irritable bowel syndrome with diarrhea. Expert Opin Investig Drugs 2005;14:185–193.

181. Thompson CA. Alosetron withdrawn from market. Am J Health Syst Pharm 2001; 58:13.

182. Talley NJ, Van Zanten SV, Saez LR, Dukes G, Perschy T, Heath M, Kleoudis C, Mangel AW. A dose-ranging, placebo-controlled, randomized trial of alosetron in patients with functional dyspepsia. Aliment Pharmacol Ther 2001;15:525–537.

183. Baxter GS, Craig DA, Clarke DE. 5-Hydroxytryptamine4 receptors mediate relaxation of the rat oesophageal tunica muscularis mucosae. Naunyn Schmiedeberg's Arch Pharmacol 1991;343:439–446.

184. Gebauer A, Merger M, Kilbinger H. Modulation by 5-HT3 and 5-HT4 receptors of the release of 5-hydroxytryptamine from the guinea-pig small intestine. Naunyn Schmiedeberg's Arch Pharmacol 1993;347:137–140.

185. Kuemmerle JF, Murthy KS, Grider JR, Martin DC, Makhlouf GM. Coexpression of 5-HT2A and 5-HT4 receptors coupled to distinct signaling pathways in human intestinal muscle cells. Gastroenterology 1995;109:1791–1800.

186. Buchheit KH, Buhl T. 5-HT receptor subtypes involved in the stimulatory effect of 5-HT on their peristaltic reflex in vitro. J Gastroint Mot 1993;5:49–55.

187. Grider JR, Kuemmerle JF, Jin JG. 5-HT released by mucosal stimuli initiates peristalsis by activating 5-HT4/5-HT1p receptors on sensory CGRP neurons. Am J Physiol 1996;270:G778–G782.

188. Tonini M, Coccini T, Onori L, Candura SM, Rizzi CA, Manzo L. The influence of neuronal 5-hydroxytryptamine receptor antagonists on non-cholinergic ganglionic transmission in the guinea-pig enteric excitatory reflex. Br J Pharmacol 1992;107: 5–7.

189. Pan H, Galligan JJ. 5-HT1A and 5-HT4 receptors mediate inhibition and facilitation of fast synaptic transmission in enteric neurons. Am J Physiol 1994;266:G230–G238.

190. Bharucha AE, Camilleri M, Haydock S, Ferber I, Burton D, Cooper S, Tompson D, Fitzpatrick K, Higgins R, Zinsmeister AR. Effects of a serotonin 5-HT(4) receptor antagonist SB-207266 on gastrointestinal motor and sensory function in humans. Gut 2000;47:667–674.

191. Bouras EP, Camilleri M, Burton DD, McKinzie S. Selective stimulation of colonic transit by the benzofuran 5HT4 agonist, prucalopride, in healthy humans. Gut 1999; 44:682–686.

192. Poen AC, Felt-Bersma RJ, Van Dongen PA, Meuwissen SG. Effect of prucalopride, a new enterokinetic agent, on gastrointestinal transit and anorectal function in healthy volunteers. Aliment Pharmacol Ther 1999;13:1493–1497.

193. Degen L, Matzinger D, Merz M, Appel-Dingemanse S, Osborne S, Luchinger S, Bertold R, Maecke H, Beglinger C. Tegaserod, a 5-HT4 receptor partial agonist, accelerates gastric emptying and gastrointestinal transit in healthy male subjects. Aliment Pharmacol Ther 2001;15:1745–1751.

194. Prather CM, Camilleri M, Zinsmeister AR, McKinzie S, Thomforde G. Tegaserod accelerates orocecal transit in patients with constipation-predominant irritable bowel syndrome. Gastroenterology 2000;118:463–468.

195. Bouras EP, Camilleri M, Burton DD, Thomforde G, McKinzie S, Zinsmeister AR. Prucalopride accelerates gastrointestinal and colonic transit in patients with constipation without a rectal evacuation disorder. Gastroenterology 2001;120:354–360.

196. Sloots CE, Poen AC, Kerstens R, Stevens M, De Pauw M, Van Oene JC, Meuwissen SG, Felt-Bersma RJ. Effects of prucalopride on colonic transit, anorectal function and bowel habits in patients with chronic constipation. Aliment Pharmacol Ther 2002;16:759–767.

197. De Schryver AM, Andriesse GI, Samsom M, Smout AJ, Gooszen HG, Akkermans LM. The effects of the specific 5HT4 receptor agonist, prucalopride, on colonic motility in healthy volunteers. Aliment Pharmacol Ther 2002;16:603–612.

198. Mine Y, Yoshikawa T, Oku S, Nagai R, Yoshida N, Hosoki K. Comparison of effect of mosapride citrate and existing 5-HT4 receptor agonists on gastrointestinal motility in vivo and in vitro. J Pharmacol Exp Ther 1997;283:1000–1008.

199. Camilleri M, McKinzie S, Fox J, Foxx-Orenstein A, Burton D, Thomforde G, Baxter K, Zinsmeister AR. Effect of renzapride on transit in constipation-predominant irritable bowel syndrome. Clin Gastroenterol Hepatol 2004;2:895–904.

200. Tack J, Broeckaert D, Coulie B, Janssens J. The influence of cisapride on gastric tone and the perception of gastric distension. Aliment Pharmacol Ther 1998;12:761–766.

201. Schikowski A, Thewissen M, Mathis C, Ross HG, Enck P. Serotonin type-4 receptors modulate the sensitivity of intramural mechanoreceptive afferents of the cat rectum. Neurogastroenterol Motil 2002;14:221–227.

202. Bouhassira D, Chollet R, Coffin B, Lemann M, Le Bars D, Willer JC, Jian R. Inhibition of a somatic nociceptive reflex by gastric distention in humans. Gastroenterology 1994;107:985–992.

203. Coffin B, Farmachidi JP, Rueegg P, Bastie A, Bouhassira D. Tegaserod, a 5-HT4 receptor partial agonist, decreases sensitivity to rectal distension in healthy subjects. Aliment Pharmacol Ther 2003;17:577–585.

204. Novick J, Miner P, Krause R, Glebas K, Bliesath H, Ligozio G, Ruegg P, Lefkowitz

M. A randomized, double-blind, placebo-controlled trial of tegaserod in female patients suffering from irritable bowel syndrome with constipation. Aliment Pharmacol Ther 2002;16:1877–1888.

205. Kellow J, Lee OY, Chang FY, Thongsawat S, Mazlam MZ, Yuen H, Gwee KA, Bak YT, Jones J, Wagner A. An Asia-Pacific, double blind, placebo controlled, randomised study to evaluate the efficacy, safety, and tolerability of tegaserod in patients with irritable bowel syndrome. Gut 2003;52:671–676.

206. Emmanuel AV, Roy AJ, Nicholls TJ, Kamm MA. Prucalopride, a systemic enterokinetic, for the treatment of constipation. Aliment Pharmacol Ther 2002;16:1347–1356.

207. Johanson JF, Wald A, Tougas G, Chey WD, Novick JS, Lembo AJ, Fordham F, Guella M, Nault B. Effect of tegaserod in chronic constipation: a randomized, double-blind, controlled trial. Clin Gastroenterol Hepatol 2004;2:796–805.

208. Gershon MD, Wade PR, Kirchgessner AL, Tamir H. 5-HT receptor subtypes outside the central nervous system. Roles in the physiology of the gut. Neuropsychopharmacology 1990;3:385–395.

209. Houghton LA, Foster JM, Whorwell PJ, Morris J, Fowler P. Is chest pain after sumatriptan oesophageal in origin? Lancet 1994;344:985–986.

210. Coulie B, Tack J, Maes B, Geypens B, De Roo M, Janssens J. Sumatriptan, a selective 5-HT1 receptor agonist, induces a lag phase for gastric emptying of liquids in humans. Am J Physiol 1997;272:G902–G908.

211. Tack J, Coulie B, Wilmer A, Peeters T, Janssens J. Actions of the 5-hydroxytryptamine 1 receptor agonist sumatriptan on interdigestive gastrointestinal motility in man. Gut 1998;42:36–41.

212. Tack J, Coulie B, Wilmer A, Andrioli A, Janssens J. Influence of sumatriptan on gastric fundus tone and on the perception of gastric distension in man. Gut 2000;46:468–473.

213. Sifrim D, Holloway RH, Tack J, Zelter A, Missotten T, Coulie B, Janssens J. Effect of sumatriptan, a 5HT1 agonist, on the frequency of transient lower esophageal sphincter relaxations and gastroesophageal reflux in healthy subjects. Am J Gastroenterol 1999;94:3158–3164.

214. Coulie B, Tack J, Sifrim D, Andrioli A, Janssens J. Role of nitric oxide in fasting gastric fundus tone and in 5-HT1 receptor-mediated relaxation of gastric fundus. Am J Physiol 1999;276:G373–G377.

215. Tack J, Demedts I, Dehondt G, Caenepeel P, Fischler B, Zandecki M, Janssens J. Clinical and pathophysiological characteristics of acute-onset functional dyspepsia. Gastroenterology 2002;122:1738–1747.

216. Giraldo E, Monferini E, Ladinsky H, Hammer R. Muscarinic receptor heterogeneity in guinea pig intestinal smooth muscle: binding studies with AF-DX 116. Eur J Pharmacol 1987;141:475–477.

217. Brown JC, Cook MA, Dryburgh JR. Motilin, a gastric motor activity stimulating polypeptide: the complete amino acid sequence. Can J Biochem 1973;51:533–537.

218. Pearse AG, Polak JM, Bloom SR, Adams C, Dryburgh JR, Brown JC. Enterochromaffin cells of the mammalian small intestine as the source of motilin. Virchows Arch B Cell Pathol 1974;16:111–120.

219. Itoh Z, Takeuchi S, Aizawa I, Mori K, Taminato T, Seino Y, Imura H, Yanaihara N. Changes in plasma motilin concentration and gastrointestinal contractile activity in conscious dogs. Am J Dig Dis 1978;23:929–935.

220. Peeters TL, Vantrappen G, Janssens J. Fasting plasma motilin levels are related to the interdigestive motility complex. Gastroenterology 1980;79:716–719.

221. Bormans V, Peeters TL, Janssens J, Pearce D, Vandeweerd M, Vantrappen G. In man, only activity fronts that originate in the stomach correlate with motilin peaks. Scand J Gastroenterol 1987;22:781–784.

222. Itoh Z, Honda R, Hiwatashi K, Takeuchi S, Aizawa I, Takayanagi R, Couch EF. Motilin-induced mechanical activity in the canine alimentary tract. Scand J Gastroenterol Suppl 1976;39:93–110.

223. Vantrappen G, Janssens J, Peeters TL, Bloom SR, Christofides ND, Hellemans J. Motilin and the interdigestive migrating motor complex in man. Dig Dis Sci 1979; 24:497–500.

224. Itoh Z. Motilin and clinical application. Peptides 1997;18:593–608.

225. Coulie B, Tack J, Peeters T, Janssens J. Involvement of two different pathways in the motor effects of erythromycin on the gastric antrum in humans. Gut 1998;43: 395–400.

226. Feighner SD, Tan CP, McKee KK, Palyha OC, Hreniuk DL, Pong SS, Austin CP, Figueroa D, MacNeil D, Cascieri MA, Nargund R, Bakshi R, Abramovitz M, Stocco R, Kargman S, O'Neill G, Van Der Ploeg LH, Evans J, Patchett AA, Smith RG, Howard AD. Receptor for motilin identified in the human gastrointestinal system. Science 1999;284:2184–2188.

227. Miller P, Roy A, St Pierre S, Dagenais M, Lapointe R, Poitras P. Motilin receptors in the human antrum. Am J Physiol 2000;278:G18–G23.

228. Peeters T, Matthijs G, Depoortere I, Cachet T, Hoogmartens J, Vantrappen G. Erythromycin is a motilin receptor agonist. Am J Physiol 1989;257:G470–G474.

229. Peeters TL, Muls E, Janssens J, Urbain JL, Bex M, Van Cutsem E, Depoortere I, De Roo M, Vantrappen G, Bouillon R. Effect of motilin on gastric emptying in patients with diabetic gastroparesis. Gastroenterology 1992;102:97–101.

230. Bruley d, V, Parys V, Ropert A, Chayvialle JA, Roze C, Galmiche JP. Erythromycin enhances fasting and postprandial proximal gastric tone in humans. Gastroenterology 1995;109:32–39.

231. Piessevaux H, Tack J, Wilmer A, Coulie B, Geubel A, Janssens J. Perception of changes in wall tension of the proximal stomach in humans. Gut 2001;49:203–208.

232. Cuomo R, Tack J, Van Daele P, Coulie B, Peeters T, Depoortere I, Janssens J. Influence of motilin on gastric fundus tone and on meal-induced satiety in man. Submitted for publication. 2004.

233. Annese V, Janssens J, Vantrappen G, Tack J, Peeters TL, Willemse P, Van Cutsem E. Erythromycin accelerates gastric emptying by inducing antral contractions and improved gastroduodenal coordination. Gastroenterology 1992;102:823–828.

234. Verhagen MA, Samsom M, Maes B, Geypens BJ, Ghoos YF, Smout AJ. Effects of a new motilide, ABT-229, on gastric emptying and postprandial antroduodenal motility in healthy volunteers. Aliment Pharmacol Ther 1997;11:1077–1086.

235. Richards RD, Davenport K, McCallum RW. The treatment of idiopathic and diabetic gastroparesis with acute intravenous and chronic oral erythromycin. Am J Gastroenterol 1993;88:203–207.

236. DiBaise JK, Quigley EM. Efficacy of prolonged administration of intravenous erythromycin in an ambulatory setting as treatment of severe gastroparesis: one center's experience. J Clin Gastroenterol 1999;28:131–134.

237. Maganti K, Onyemere K, Jones MP. Oral erythromycin and symptomatic relief of gastroparesis: a systematic review. Am J Gastroenterol 2003;98:259–263.

238. Talley NJ, Verlinden M, Snape W, Beker JA, Ducrotte P, Dettmer A, Brinkhoff H, Eaker E, Ohning G, Miner PB, Mathias JR, Fumagalli I, Staessen D, Mack RJ. Failure of a motilin receptor agonist (ABT-229) to relieve the symptoms of functional dyspepsia in patients with and without delayed gastric emptying: a randomized double-blind placebo-controlled trial. Aliment Pharmacol Ther 2000;14:1653–1661.

239. Talley NJ, Verlinden M, Geenen DJ, Hogan RB, Riff D, McCallum RW, Mack RJ. Effects of a motilin receptor agonist (ABT-229) on upper gastrointestinal symptoms in type 1 diabetes mellitus: a randomised, double blind, placebo controlled trial. Gut 2001;49:395–401.

240. Bologna SD, Hasler WL, Owyang C. Down-regulation of motilin receptors on rabbit colon myocytes by chronic oral erythromycin. J Pharmacol Exp Ther 1993; 266:852–856.

241. Chaussade S, Michopoulos S, Sogni P, Guerre J, Couturier D. Motilin agonist erythromycin increases human lower esophageal sphincter pressure by stimulation of cholinergic nerves. Dig Dis Sci 1994;39:381–384.

242. Pennathur A, Tran A, Cioppi M, Fayad J, Sieren GL, Little AG. Erythromycin strengthens the defective lower esophageal sphincter in patients with gastroesophageal reflux disease. Am J Surg 1994;167:169–172.

243. Chrysos E, Tzovaras G, Epanomeritakis E, Tsiaoussis J, Vrachasotakis N, Vassilakis JS, Xynos E. Erythromycin enhances oesophageal motility in patients with gastro-oesophageal reflux. ANZ J Surg 2001;71:98–102.

244. Champion G, Richter JE, Singh S, Schan C, Nellans H. Effects of oral erythromycin on esophageal pH and pressure profiles in patients with gastroesophageal reflux disease. Dig Dis Sci 1994;39:129–137.

245. Netzer P, Schmitt B, Inauen W. Effects of ABT-229, a motilin agonist, on acid reflux, oesophageal motility and gastric emptying in patients with gastro-oesophageal reflux disease. Aliment Pharmacol Ther 2002;16:1481–1490.

246. Chen CL, Orr WC, Verlinden MH, Dettmer A, Brinkhoff H, Riff D, Schwartz S, Soloway RD, Krause R, Lanza F, Mack RJ. Efficacy of a motilin receptor agonist (ABT-229) for the treatment of gastro-oesophageal reflux disease. Aliment Pharmacol Ther 2002;16:749–757.

247. Tomasetto C, Karam SM, Ribieras S, Masson R, Lefebvre O, Staub A, Alexander G, Chenard MP, Rio MC. Identification and characterization of a novel gastric peptide hormone: the motilin-related peptide. Gastroenterology 2000;119:395–405.

248. McKee KK, Tan CP, Palyha OC, Liu J, Feighner SD, Hreniuk DL, Smith RG, Howard AD, Van Der Ploeg LH. Cloning and characterization of two human G protein-coupled receptor genes (GPR38 and GPR39) related to the growth hormone secretagogue and neurotensin receptors. Genomics 1997;46:426–434.

249. Trudel L, Tomasetto C, Rio MC, Bouin M, Plourde V, Eberling P, Poitras P. Ghrelin/motilin-related peptide is a potent prokinetic to reverse gastric postoperative ileus in rat. Am J Physiol 2002;282:G948–G952.

250. Fujino K, Inui A, Asakawa A, Kihara N, Fujimura M, Fujimiya M. Ghrelin induces fasted motor activity of the gastrointestinal tract in conscious fed rats. J Physiol (Lond) 2003;550:227–240.

251. Edholm T, Schmidt. Ghrelin stimulates interdigestive migrating myoelectrical complex in the rat small intestine: involvement of cholinergic neurons. Neurogastroenterol Motil 15, 575. 2003.

252. Kitamura S, Yokota I, Hosoda H, Kotani Y, Matsuda J, Naito E, Ito M, Kangawa K, Kuroda Y. Ghrelin concentration in cord and neonatal blood: relation to fetal growth and energy balance. J Clin Endocrinol Metab 2003;88:5473–5477.

253. Tack J, Depoortere I, Bisschops R, Coulie B, Meulemans A, Janssens J, Peeters TL. Influence of ghrelin on interdigestive gastrointestinal motility in man. Submitted for publication 2004.

254. Tack J, Depoortere I, Bisschops R, Verbeke K, Janssens J, Peeters TL. Influence of ghrelin on gastric emptying and meal-related symptoms in gastroparesis. Aliment Pharmacol Ther 2005;22:847–53.

255. Holzer P, Holzer-Petsche U. Tachykinins in the gut. Part II. Roles in neural excitation, secretion and inflammation. Pharmacol Ther 1997;73:219–263.

256. Holzer P, Holzer-Petsche U. Tachykinins in the gut. Part I. Expression, release and motor function. Pharmacol Ther 1997;73:173–217.

257. Giardina GA, Gagliardi S, Martinelli M. Antagonists at the neurokinin receptors— recent patent literature. IDrugs 2003;6:758–772.

258. Chawla SP, Grunberg SM, Gralla RJ, Hesketh PJ, Rittenberg C, Elmer ME, Schmidt C, Taylor A, Carides AD, Evans JK, Horgan KJ. Establishing the dose of the oral NK1 antagonist aprepitant for the prevention of chemotherapy-induced nausea and vomiting. Cancer 2003;97:2290–2300.

259. Poli-Bigelli S, Rodrigues-Pereira J, Carides AD, Julie MG, Eldridge K, Hipple A, Evans JK, Horgan KJ, Lawson F. Addition of the neurokinin 1 receptor antagonist aprepitant to standard antiemetic therapy improves control of chemotherapy-induced nausea and vomiting. Results from a randomized, double-blind, placebo-controlled trial in Latin America. Cancer 2003;97:3090–3098.

260. Onori L, Aggio A, Taddei G, Loreto MF, Ciccocioppo R, Vicini R, Tonini M. Peristalsis regulation by tachykinin NK1 receptors in the rabbit isolated distal colon. Am J Physiol 2003;285:G325–G331.

261. Lee OY, Munakata J, Naliboff B, Chang L, Mayer EA. A double blind parallel group pilot study of the effects of CJ-11,974 and placebo on perception and emotional responses to rectosigmoid distension in IBS patients. Gastroenterology 118, A846. 2000.

262. Stucchi AF, Shofer S, Leeman S, Materne O, Beer E, McClung J, Shebani K, Moore F, O'Brien M, Becker JM. NK-1 antagonist reduces colonic inflammation and oxidative stress in dextran sulfate-induced colitis in rats. Am J Physiol 2000;279: G1298–G1306.

263. Moriarty D, Goldhill J, Selve N, O'Donoghue DP, Baird AW. Human colonic anti-secretory activity of the potent NK(1) antagonist, SR140333: assessment of potential anti-diarrhoeal activity in food allergy and inflammatory bowel disease. Br J Pharmacol 2001;133:1346–1354.

264. Lecci A, Capriati A, Maggi CA. Tachykinin NK2 receptor antagonists for the treatment of irritable bowel syndrome. Br J Pharmacol 2004;141:1249–1263.

265. Lördal M, Navalesi G, Theodorsson E, Maggi CA, Hellstrom PM. A novel tachykinin NK2 receptor antagonist prevents motility-stimulating effects of neurokinin A in small intestine. Br J Pharmacol 2001;134:215–223.

266. De Luca A, Coupar IM. Insights into opioid action in the intestinal tract. Pharmacol Ther 1996;69:103–115.

267. Corazziari E. Role of opioid ligands in the irritable bowel syndrome. Can J Gastroenterol 1999;13 Suppl A:71A-75A.
268. Hawkes ND, Rhodes J, Evans BK, Rhodes P, Hawthorne AB, Thomas GA. Naloxone treatment for irritable bowel syndrome—a randomized controlled trial with an oral formulation. Aliment Pharmacol Ther 2002;16:1649–1654.
269. Rivière PJ. Peripheral kappa-opioid agonists for visceral pain. Br J Pharmacol 2004; 141:1331–1334.
270. Coffin B, Bouhassira D, Chollet R, Fraitag B, De Meynard C, Geneve J, Lemann M, Willer JC, Jian R. Effect of the kappa agonist fedotozine on perception of gastric distension in healthy humans. Aliment Pharmacol Ther 1996;10:919–925.
271. Fraitag B, Homerin M, Hecketsweiler P. Double-blind dose-response multicenter comparison of fedotozine and placebo in treatment of nonulcer dyspepsia. Dig Dis Sci 1994;39:1072–1077.
272. Dapoigny M, Abitbol JL, Fraitag B. Efficacy of peripheral kappa agonist fedotozine versus placebo in treatment of irritable bowel syndrome: A multicenter dose-response study. Dig Dis Sci 1995;40:2244–2248.
273. Delvaux M, Louvel D, Lagier E, Scherrer B, Abitbol JL, Frexinos J. The κ-agonist fedotozine relieves hypersensitivity to colonic distention in patients with irritable bowel syndrome. Gastroenterology 1999;116:38–45.
274. Ozaki N, Sengupta JN, Gebhart GF. Differential effects of mu-, delta-, and kappa-opioid receptor agonists on mechanosensitive gastric vagal afferent fibers in the rat. J Neurophysiol 2000;83:2209–2216.
275. Su X, Julia V, Gebhart GF. Effects of intracolonic opioid receptor agonists on polymodal pelvic nerve afferent fibers in the rat. J Neurophysiol 2000;83:963–970.
276. Delgado-Aros S, Chial HJ, Cremonini F, Ferber I, McKinzie S, Burton DD, Camilleri M. Effects of asimadoline, a kappa-opioid agonist, on satiation and postprandial symptoms in health. Aliment Pharmacol Ther 2003;18:507–514.
277. Delgado-Aros S, Chial HJ, Camilleri M, Szarka LA, Weber FT, Jacob J, Ferber I, McKinzie S, Burton DD, Zinsmeister AR. Effects of a kappa-opioid agonist, asimadoline, on satiation and GI motor and sensory functions in humans. Am J Physiol 2003;284:G558–G566.
278. Delvaux M, Jacob J, Beck A, Bouzamondo H, Weber FT, Frexinos J. Effect of asimadoline, a new agonist of kappa opiate receptors on pain induced by rectal distension in IBS patients. Gastroenterology 122, A221. 2002.
279. De Ponti F, Malagelada JR. Functional gut disorders: from motility to sensitivity disorders. A review of current and investigational drugs for their management. Pharmacol Ther 1998;80:49–88.
280. Lyrënas E, Abrahamsson H, Dotevall G. Rectosigmoid motility response to beta-adrenoceptor stimulation in patients with the irritable bowel syndrome. Scand J Gastroenterol 1985;20:1163–1168.
281. De Ponti F, Cosentino M, Costa A, Girani M, Gibelli G, D'Angelo L, Frigo G, CREMA A. Inhibitory effects of SR 58611A on canine colonic motility: evidence for a role of β3-adrenoceptors. Br J Pharmacol 1995;114:1447–1453.
282. De Ponti F, Gibelli G, Croci T, Arcidiaco M, Crema F, Manara L. Functional evidence of atypical β3-adrenoceptors in the human colon using the β3-selective adrenoceptor antagonist, SR59230A. Br J Pharmacol 1996;117:1374–1376.
283. Roberts SJ, Papaioannou M, Evans BA, Summers RJ. Functional and molecular evidence for beta 1-, beta 2- and beta 3- adrenoceptors in human colon. Br J Pharmacol 1997;120:1527–1535.

284. Bharucha AE, Camilleri M, Zinsmeister AR, Hanson RB. Adrenergic modulation of human colonic motor and sensory function. Am J Physiol 1997;273:G997–1006.

285. Viramontes BE, Malcolm A, Camilleri M, Szarka LA, McKinzie S, Burton DD, Zinsmeister AR. Effects of an α2-adrenergic agonist on gastrointestinal transit, colonic motility, and sensation in humans. Am J Physiol 2001;281:G1468–G1476.

286. Malcolm A, Camilleri M, Kost L, Burton DD, Fett SL, Zinsmeister AR. Towards identifying optimal doses for alpha-2 adrenergic modulation of colonic and rectal motor and sensory function. Aliment Pharmacol Ther 2000;14:783–793.

287. Camilleri M, Kim DY, McKinzie S, Kim HJ, Thomforde GM, Burton DD, Low PA, Zinsmeister AR. A randomized, controlled exploratory study of clonidine in diarrhea-predominant irritable bowel syndrome. Clin Gastroenterol Hepatol 2003;1:111–121.

288. Tonini M, Cipollina L, Poluzzi E, Crema F, Corazza GR, De Ponti F. Review article: clinical implications of enteric and central D2 receptor blockade by antidopaminergic gastrointestinal prokinetics. Aliment Pharmacol Ther 2004;19:379–390.

289. Corazza GR, Biagi F, Albano O, Porro GB, Cheli R, Mazzacca G, Miglio F, Naccarato R, Quaglino D, Surrenti C, Verme G, Gasbarrini G. Levosulpiride in functional dyspepsia: a multicentric, double-blind, controlled trial. Ital J Gastroenterol 1996;28:317–323.

290. Holtmann G, Schnittker J, Boos G, Matiba B, Talley NJ. A randomized, double-blind, placebo-controlled dose finding study of itopride for the treatment of patients with functional dyspepsia. Gastroenterology 2004;126:A100.

291. Moayyedi P, Soo S, Deeks J, Delaney B, Innes M, Forman D. Pharmacological interventions for non-ulcer dyspepsia. Cochrane Database Syst Rev 2004;CD001960.

292. Veldhuyzen van Zanten SJ, Jones MJ, Verlinden M, Talley NJ. Efficacy of cisapride and domperidone in functional (nonulcer) dyspepsia: a meta-analysis. Am J Gastroenterol 2001;96:689–696.

293. Munro S, Thomas KL, Abu-Shaar M. Molecular characterization of a peripheral receptor for cannabinoids. Nature 1993;365:61–65.

294. Matsuda LA, Lolait SJ, Brownstein MJ, Young AC, Bonner TI. Structure of a cannabinoid receptor and functional expression of the cloned cDNA. Nature 1990;346:561–564.

295. Ahluwalia J, Urban L, Capogna M, Bevan S, Nagy I. Cannabinoid 1 receptors are expressed in nociceptive primary sensory neurons. Neuroscience 2000;100:685–688.

296. Pertwee RG, Fernando SR, Nash JE, Coutts AA. Further evidence for the presence of cannabinoid CB1 receptors in guinea-pig small intestine. Br J Pharmacol 1996;118:2199–2205.

297. Coutts AA, Pertwee RG. Inhibition by cannabinoid receptor agonists of acetylcholine release from the guinea-pig myenteric plexus. Br J Pharmacol 1997;121:1557–1566.

298. Croci T, Manara L, Aureggi G, Guagnini F, Rinaldi-Carmona M, Maffrand JP, Le Fur G, Mukenge S, Ferla G. In vitro functional evidence of neuronal cannabinoid CB1 receptors in human ileum. Br J Pharmacol 1998;125:1393–1395.

299. Storr M, Gaffal E, Saur D, Schusdziarra V, Allescher HD. Effect of cannabinoids on neural transmission in rat gastric fundus. Can J Physiol Pharmacol 2002;80:67–76.

300. Lehmann A, Blackshaw LA, Branden L, Carlsson A, Jensen J, Nygren E, Smid SD. Cannabinoid receptor agonism inhibits transient lower esophageal sphincter relaxations and reflux in dogs. Gastroenterology 2002;123:1129–1134.

301. Partosoedarso ER, Abrahams TP, Scullion RT, Moerschbaecher JM, Hornby PJ. Cannabinoid1 receptor in the dorsal vagal complex modulates lower oesophageal sphincter relaxation in ferrets. J Physiol (Lond) 2003;550:149–158.

302. Frytak S, Moertel CG, O'Fallon JR, Rubin J, Creagan ET, O'Connell MJ, Schutt AJ, Schwartau NW. Delta-9-tetrahydrocannabinol as an antiemetic for patients receiving cancer chemotherapy. A comparison with prochlorperazine and a placebo. Ann Intern Med 1979;91:825–830.

303. McCallum RW, Soykan I, Sridhar KR, Ricci DA, Lange RC, Plankey MW. Delta-9-tetrahydrocannabinol delays the gastric emptying of solid food in humans: a double-blind, randomized study. Aliment Pharmacol Ther 1999;13:77–80.

304. Van Gaal LF, Rissanen AM, Scheen AJ, Ziegler O, Rossner S, RIO-Europe Study Group. Effects of the cannabinoid-1 receptor blocker rimonabant on weight reduction and cardiovascular risk factors in overweight patients: 1-year experience from the RIO-Europe study. Lancet 2005;365:1389–1397.

305. Valenzano KJ, Tafesse L, Lee G, Harrison JE, Boulet JM, Gottshall SL, Mark L, Pearson MS, Miller W, Shan S, Rabadi L, Rotshteyn Y, Chaffer SM, Turchin PI, Elsemore DA, Toth M, Koetzner L, Whiteside GT. Pharmacological and pharmacokinetic characterization of the cannabinoid receptor 2 agonist, GW405833, utilizing rodent models of acute and chronic pain, anxiety, ataxia and catalepsy. Neuropharmacology 2005;48:658–672.

306. Holzer P. TRPV1 and the gut: from a tasty receptor for a painful vanilloid to a key player in hyperalgesia. Eur J Pharmacol 2004;500:231–241.

307. Schmidt B, Hammer J, Holzer P, Hammer HF. Chemical nociception in the jejunum induced by capsaicin. Gut 2004;53:1109–1116.

308. Chan CL, Facer P, Davis JB, Smith GD, Egerton J, Bountra C, Williams NS, Anand P. Sensory fibres expressing capsaicin receptor TRPV1 in patients with rectal hypersensitivity and faecal urgency. Lancet 2003;361:385–391.

309. Bortolotti M, Coccia G, Grossi G, Miglioli M. The treatment of functional dyspepsia with red pepper. Aliment Pharmacol Ther 2002;16:1075–1082.

310. Lee KJ, Vos R, Tack J. Effects of capsaicin on the sensorimotor function of the proximal stomach in humans. Aliment Pharmacol Ther 2004;19:415–425.

311. Walsh JH. Gastrointestinal hormones. Physiology of the Gastrointestinal Tract. New York: Raven, 1994:1–128.

312. Varga G, Balint A, Burghardt B, D'Amato M. Involvement of endogenous CCK and CCK1 receptors in colonic motor function. Br J Pharmacol 2004;141:1275–1284.

313. Bueno L, Fioramonti J, Delvaux M, Frexinos J. Mediators and pharmacology of visceral sensitivity: from basic to clinical investigations. Gastroenterology 1997;112: 1714–1743.

314. Poynard T, Regimbeau C, Benhamou Y. Meta-analysis of smooth muscle relaxants in the treatment of irritable bowel syndrome. Aliment Pharmacol Ther 2001;15:355–361.

315. Plourde V, Lembo T, Shui Z, Parker J, Mertz H, Tache Y, Sytnik B, Mayer EA. Effects of the somatostatin analogue octreotide on rectal afferent nerves in human. Am J Physiol 1993;265:G751.

316. Hasler W, Soudah HC, Owyang C. Somatostatin analog inhibits afferent response to rectal distention in diarrhea-predominant irritable bowel patients. J Pharmacol Exp Ther 1994;268:1206–1211.

317. Hasler WL, Soudah HC, Owyang C. A somatostatin analogue inhibits afferent path-

ways mediating perception of rectal distention. Gastroenterology 1993;104:1390–1397.

318. Bradette M, Delvaux M, Staumont G, Fioramonti J, Bueno L, Frexinos J. Octreotide increases thresholds of colonic visceral perception in IBS patients without modifying muscle tone. Dig Dis Sci 1994;39:1171–1178.

319. Schwetz I, Naliboff B, Munakata J, Lembo T, Chang L, Matin K, Ohning G, Mayer EA. Anti-hyperalgesic effect of octreotide in patients with irritable bowel syndrome. Aliment Pharmacol Ther 2004;19:123–131.

320. Mertz H, Walsh JH, Sytnik B, Mayer EA. The effect of octreotide on human gastric compliance and sensory perception. Neurogastroenterol Motil 1995;7:175–185.

321. Bourgeois S, Coulie B, Tack J, Janssens J. The somatostatin-analogue octreotide does not affect visceral perception of the fundus in man. Gastroenterology 112, A1134. 1997.

322. Cann PA, Read NW, Holdsworth CO. What is the benefit of coarse wheat bran in patients with irritable bowel syndrome? Gut 1984;25:168–173.

323. Cann PA, Read NW, Holdsworth CD, Barends D. Role of loperamide and placebo in management of irritable bowel syndrome. Dig Dis Sci 1984;29:239–247.

324. Viramontes B, Camilleri M, McKinzie S, Pardi DS, Burton D, Thomforde GM. Gender-related differences in slowing colonic transit by a 5-HT3 antagonist in subjects with diarrhea-predominant irritable bowel syndrome. Am J Gastroenterol 2001;96:2671–2676.

325. Watson ME, Lacey L, Kong S, Northcutt AR, McSorley D, Hahn B, Mangel AW. Alosetron improves quality of life in women with diarrhea-predominant irritable bowel syndrome. Am J Gastroenterol 2001;96:455–459.

326. Talley NJ. Pharmacologic therapy for the irritable bowel syndrome. Am J Gastroenterol 2003;98:750–758.

327. von der Ohe MR, Camilleri M, Kvols LK, Thomforde GM. Motor dysfunction of the small bowel and colon in patients with the carcinoid syndrome and diarrhea. N Engl J Med 1993;329:1073–1078.

328. Lembo T, Naliboff BD, Matin K, Munakata J, Parker RA, Gracely RH, Mayer EA. Irritable bowel syndrome patients show altered sensitivity to exogenous opioids. Pain 2000;87:137–147.

329. Hammer HF, Phillips SF, Camilleri M, Hanson RB. Rectal tone, distensibility, and perception: reproducibility and response to different distensions. Am J Physiol 1998; 274:G584–G590.

330. Sarnelli G, Vos R, Cuomo R, Janssens J, Tack J. Reproducibility of gastric barostat studies in healthy controls and in dyspeptic patients. Am J Gastroenterol 2001; 96:1047–1053.

331. Sturm A, Holtmann G, Goebell H, Gerken G. Prokinetics in patients with gastroparesis: a systematic analysis. Digestion 1999;60:422–427.

332. Cremonini F, Mullan BP, Camilleri M, Burton DD, Rank MR. Performance characteristics of scintigraphic transit measurements for studies of experimental therapies. Aliment Pharmacol Ther 2002;16:1781–1790.

333. Read NW, Abitbol JL, Bardhan KD, Whorwell PJ, Fraitag B. Efficacy and safety of the peripheral kappa agonist fedotozine versus placebo in the treatment of functional dyspepsia. Gut 1997;41:664–668.

334. Chial HJ, Camilleri C, Delgado-Aros S, Burton D, Thomforde G, Ferber I, Camilleri M. A nutrient drink test to assess maximum tolerated volume and postpran-

dial symptoms: effects of gender, body mass index and age in health. Neurogastro-enterol Motil 2002;14:249–253.

335. Arts, J., Caenepeel, P., Verbeke, K., and Tack, J. Influence of erythromycin on gastric emptying and meal related symptoms in functional dyspepsia with delayed gastric emptying. Gut 2005;in press.

336. Simonian HP, Maurer AH, Knight LC, Kantor S, Kontos D, Megalooikonomou V, Fisher RS, Parkman HP. Simultaneous assessment of gastric accommodation and emptying: studies with liquid and solid meals. J Nucl Med 2004;45:1155–1160.

337. Bouras EP, Delgado-Aros S, Camilleri M, Castillo EJ, Burton DD, Thomforde GM, Chial HJ. SPECT imaging of the stomach: comparison with barostat, and effects of sex, age, body mass index, and fundoplication. Single photon emission computed tomography. Gut 2002;51:781–786.

338. Evans WE, Relling MV. Pharmacogenomics: Translating functional genomics into rational therapeutics. Science 1999;286:487–491.

339. McLeod HL, Evans WE. Pharmacogenomics: unlocking the human genome for better drug therapy. Annu Rev Pharmacol Toxicol 2001;41:101–121.

340. Committee for Proprietary Medicinal Products. Position paper on terminology in pharmacogenetics (EMEA/CPMP/3070/01). 2002. European Medicines Evaluation Agency.

341. Gonsalkorale WM, Perrey C, Pravica V, Whorwell PJ, Hutchinson IV. Interleukin 10 genotypes in irritable bowel syndrome: evidence for an inflammatory component? Gut 2003;52:91–93.

342. Camilleri M. Is there a SERT-ain association with IBS? Gut 2004;53:1396–1399.

343. Holtmann G, Siffert W, Haag S, Mueller N, Langkafel M, Senf W, Zotz R, Talley NJ. G-protein beta 3 subunit 825 CC genotype is associated with unexplained (functional) dyspepsia. Gastroenterology 2004;126:971–979.

344. Weinshilboum R. Inheritance and drug response. N Engl J Med 2003;348:529–537.

345. Dalen P, Dahl ML, Ruiz ML, Nordin J, Bertilsson L. 10-Hydroxylation of nortriptyline in white persons with 0, 1, 2, 3, and 13 functional CYP2D6 genes. Clin Pharmacol Ther 1998;63:444–452.

346. Glatt CE, Reus VI. Pharmacogenetics of monoamine transporters. Pharmacogenomics 2003;4:583–596.

347. Camilleri M, Atanasova E, Carlson PJ, Ahmad U, Kim HJ, Viramontes BE, McKinzie S, Urrutia R. Serotonin-transporter polymorphism pharmacogenetics in diarrhea-predominant irritable bowel syndrome. Gastroenterology 2002;123:425–432.

348. Drossman DA, Camilleri M, Mayer EA, Whitehead WE. AGA Technical Review on Irritable Bowel Syndrome. Gastroenterology 2002;123:2108–2131.

349. Jackson JL, O'Malley PG, Tomkins G, Balden E, Santoro J, Kroenke K. Treatment of functional gastrointestinal disorders with anti-depressants: A meta-analysis. Am J Med 2000;108:65–72.

350. Brandt LJ, Bjorkman D, Fennerty MB, Locke GR, Olden K, Peterson W, Quigley E, Schoenfeld P, Schuster M, Talley N. Systematic review on the management of irritable bowel syndrome in North America. Am J Gastroenterol 2002;97:S7–S26.

351. Drossman DA, Toner BB, Whitehead WE, Diamant NE, Dalton CB, Duncan S, Emmott S, Proffitt V, Akman D, Frusciante K, Le T, Meyer K, Bradshaw B, Mikula K, Morris CB, Blackman CJ, Hu Y, Jia H, Li JZ, Koch GG, Bangdiwala SI. Cognitive-

behavioral therapy versus education and desipramine versus placebo for moderate to severe functional bowel disorders. Gastroenterology 2003;125:19–31.

352. Tack J, Broekaert D, Fischler B, Corsetti M, Janssens J. Influence of the selective serotonin reuptake inhibitor citalopram on colonic sensorimotor function in man. Aliment Parmacol Ther 2006;23:265–74.

353. Campo JV, Perel J, Lucas A, Bridge J, Ehmann M, Kalas C, Monk K, Axelson D, Birmaher B, Ryan N, Di Lorenzo C, Brent DA. Citalopram Treatment of Pediatric Recurrent Abdominal Pain and Comorbid Internalizing Disorders: An Exploratory Study. J Am Acad Child Adolesc Psych 2004;43:1234–1242.

354. Tabas G, Beaves M, Wang J, Friday P, Mardini H, Arnold G. Paroxetine to treat irritable bowel syndrome not responding to high-fiber diet: a double-blind, placebo-controlled trial. Am J Gastroenterol 2004;99:914–920.

355. Chial HJ, Camilleri M, Burton D, Thomforde G, Olden KW, Stephens D. Selective effects of serotonergic psychoactive agents on gastrointestinal functions in health. Am J Physiol 2003;284:G130–G137.

356. Creed F, Fernandes L, Guthrie E, Palmer S, Ratcliffe J, Read N, Rigby C, Thompson D, Tomenson B. The cost-effectiveness of psychotherapy and paroxetine for severe irritable bowel syndrome. Gastroenterology 2003;124 :303–317.

357. Masand PS, Gupta S, Schwartz TL, Kaplan D, Virk S, Hameed A, Lockwood K. Does a preexisting anxiety disorder predict response to paroxetine in irritable bowel syndrome? Psychosomatics 2002;43:451–455.

Chapter 5

Gender, Age, Society, Culture, and the Patient's Perspective

Brenda B. Toner, Chair

Lin Chang, Co-Chair

Shin Fukudo

Elspeth Guthrie

G. Richard Locke

Nancy Norton

Ami D. Sperber

Introduction

This new chapter has been developed to discuss important variables that have been largely overlooked in the study of the functional gastrointestinal disorders (FGIDs), namely gender, age, society, culture, and the patient's perspective. These variables should be included in the design of research protocols in order to provide a more comprehensive understanding of these disorders from both a theoretical and methodological perspective. Failure to consider these variables may result in an overly simplistic and incomplete interpretation of research data.

This chapter was developed and written by a multinational team consisting of a psychologist, a psychiatrist, the founder and chair of an international patient support group, and four gastroenterologists. All participants have expertise in the FGIDs.

Although more has been written about gender than the other factors, most of these variables have received little attention in the published literature on FGIDs. Accordingly, more space has been devoted to issues associated with gender. The discussion of gender is followed by sections on age, society, culture, methodological issues, and conclusions. The majority of studies mentioned in this chapter focus on irritable bowel syndrome (IBS) because it is the most studied of the FGIDs. Traditionally, knowledge generation and transfer have been the domain of the "expert," who is usually a scientist or clinician rather than the person who has the specific condition under study. In order to acknowledge the importance of understanding the experience of persons living with FGIDs for effective clinical management, this chapter will begin with the patient's perspective.

The Patient's Perspective

Living with an FGID means living with chronic illness. Chronic illnesses are characterized by long-term courses, unpredictable symptom episodes, and disabling effects that are often accompanied by minimally effective treatments, social stigma, and isolation [1]. Symptoms of chronic illness place demands on families as well as patients, and impair functioning while placing perpetual demands on the individual patient [2]. The experience of persons living with IBS illustrates the challenges frequently faced by those with FGIDs. People with IBS are often confronted with seeking care, social, and professional support for a condition that lacks the specificity of an acute illness with a known etiology and is often viewed as having an "ambiguous identity" [2, 3]. They will likely discontinue seeing a physician despite the persistence of their symptoms and struggle to manage their own symptoms over the long-term course of the disorder [2].

— The IBS Patient

Most studies examine the illness experience from the point of view of the physician observer, not the patient. The IBS illness experience is one that impairs physiologic as well as sociologic functioning of the affected individual. In one quantitative survey of 277 women and 73 men who reported a diagnosis of IBS, most patients described living for years with IBS and experiencing episodic symptoms that occurred weekly or more frequently [3]. The majority of respondents described major interferences with daily life due to symptoms. Disruptions of work were common, but more common were missed leisure or social activities indicating personal sacrifices while trying to battle their symptoms. Patients consulted primary care physicians more frequently than gastroenterologists, and reported high health care utilization. IBS sufferers reported using 281 different medical treatments for symptom relief, including prescription drugs, over-the-counter (OTC) medications, and herbal and dietary supplements. Yet less than one third reported satisfaction with the drugs and remedies used to treat their symptoms. In another study conducted in IBS patients belonging to a health maintenance organization, overall 57% of patients reported satisfactory relief of their bowel symptoms after 6 months of usual medical care, which included education, dietary and lifestyle advice, and medications. However, only 22% reported that symptom severity was reduced by half [4].

A qualitative survey using focus groups that included 43 women and 8 men also found that patients perceived IBS as a frustrating and isolating chronic condition with adverse effects on quality of life, particularly social and sexual functioning [2]. Symptoms were most often perceived as severe. Anticipation, worry, and frustration about the unpredictability of symptom onset and lack of consistency of trigger factors imposed limitations on planning and daily life. Frustration, isolation, a perceived lack of validation for the disorder, and a lack of understanding from family, coworkers, and physicians were major problems. A sense of isolation arises from the embarrassing nature of symptoms, inability to share or discuss them with their social network, and a feeling of being alone with the disorder.

— Living with IBS

While articles have been written on the health care-seeking behavior of IBS patients, few explore the health living behavior of this population. What matters to most patients with chronic illness are how well they are able to function and how they feel about their day-to-day lives. Living with IBS means living with (1) unpredictable symptom onset, severity, and triggers, and an unexplained etiology; (2) the stigma of a potentially disabling condition that is invisible to and misunderstood by others, embarrassing to talk about, and often equated with psychological problems; and (3) resulting social isolation.

Health care providers describe moderate IBS symptoms as "intermittent disruptions in activities, for example, missing social functions, work, or school" [5]. What does this mean from the patient's perspective? "Intermittent" would be experienced as long-term, repetitive, unpredictable, and uncontrollable, while "disruptions in activities" would be experienced as painful spasms, uncontrollable diarrhea, and loss of bowel control to solids, liquids, or gas. Finally, "for example, missing social functions, work, or school" would be experienced as losses—of dignity, freedom and spontaneity, potential and productivity, social contact, intimacy, and belief of being in control of one's own destiny [6]. As Royer eloquently explains, "Two generalizations can be made about the consequences of chronic illnesses: (1) the person with a chronic illness experiences impaired functioning in more than one, often multiple, body, mind, and spirit systems; (2) the illness-related demands on the individual are never completely eliminated" [1].

The uncertainty of living with IBS results from the lack of a definitive biological marker in the diagnosis, lack of adequate treatment for the global symptoms, and the lack of certainty surrounding symptom onset and severity [7]. This also makes it difficult for others to comprehend and provide empathy towards affected individuals [2]. Inability to control symptoms leads to loss of control over daily living.

Patients find the symptoms of IBS embarrassing or difficult to talk about. There is no socially acceptable way to discuss personal bowel habits. The general public is neither well informed nor accurately informed about digestive health and disease [8]. In 1999 when the International Foundation for Functional Gastrointestinal Disorders (IFFGD) produced an educational public service announcement about IBS for television, one half of the major media outlets surveyed prior to distribution said they would not air the video if the word "bowel" was used. Having a stigmatized condition or diagnosis raises the possibility that the person with the disorder will be devalued by others [9]. In response, individuals may develop strategies to cope such as avoidance, withdrawal, vigilance, and concealment. The degree to which these strategies are applied may vary from person to person, but each has its own associated cost that further contributes to the social isolation or frustration felt by IBS patients. More recently, there has been increased public awareness and education of FGIDs that will hopefully break down the myths and misconceptions and improve the understanding, management, and overall experience of living with these conditions.

— The Patient-Physician Encounter

The patient-physician encounter in IBS is challenging and often frustrating to both parties. While the term "patient-physician" is generally used, it refers to all health care providers. Patients who seek diagnosis and treatment often report an unsatisfactory or unhelpful experience with health care professionals. Lack of empathy, adequate treatment, and adequate medical explanation, and the perception that their illness experience is not fully appreciated or taken seriously have been reported [2]. Physicians share frustration with patients over the poorly understood nature of IBS as a disease as well as a lack of treatments [10]. IBS patients are often not provided with a convincing or adequate explanation of the condition, possibly due to a lack of time or lack of understanding [11]. However, adequate explanation is a critical factor to alleviate alarm about symptoms (e.g., Do I have a life-threatening disease?) and address concerns about the disruptive impact symptoms have on daily activities and interpersonal relationships.

To the patient, unsatisfactory explanations may be experienced as a denial of the legitimacy of their reported symptoms, an implication that negative test results imply an absence of cause, and a lack of understanding or belief in their suffering [12]. To patients, whose primary source of health education comes from social contacts and the media, discussion of the role of stress, mind, and body take on meanings that may be at odds with medical interpretations. Words like "biopsychosocial" or "stress" become problematic because they involve concepts that are either not well understood or not explained in a common language that patients can embrace. Rather, they tend to impart meanings having to do with personality characteristics and psychological or emotional problems that then become a part of both the physician's and patient's IBS framework.

In general, patients are not health experts and do not necessarily know how or what to ask their physician. They tend to give inconsistent accounts of their symptom experience and bodily functions [13]. There are no universally applied diagnostic criteria. Although the means to make a positive diagnosis is available through the Rome diagnostic criteria, most primary care physicians and some gastroenterologists are unaware of the criteria and only a portion of those use them in clinical practice [14]. The application of experiential clinical understanding then varies depending on physician experience and biases. Thus patients seeking clear explanations may encounter uncertain or even conflicting views [10, 11].

FGID symptoms are often equated with psychological associations with neurosis and a trivialization of the very real physical symptoms they are experiencing. Psychological equates with "all in the mind." The lack of a clear medical explanation is transformed into a personal failing on the patient's part. Many patients thus feel stigmatized and let down [10].

— The Patient and Physician Working Together

Patients are not generally taught *how* to care for their own illnesses [15] and knowing how to manage a chronic illness experience is not an innate quality. It must be taught. This process best begins at the time of diagnosis with a clear, understandable, and legitimizing explanation of the condition. Patients need information relevant to their ongoing daily lives, not only about what is wrong, but also about concerns over what the condition means and how it will influence their lives [13]. They need clear explanations about treatment choices and management issues. Until better treatments with more universal and consistent efficacy (and low side-effect profiles) are available, the individual with IBS needs self-management tools as they try to adapt and live as normal a life as possible. Physicians can initiate this self-management process by eliciting patient concerns and addressing them in ways that are individually relevant and affirming [16]. Self-care is integral to coping with chronic IBS in daily life [10]. "The psychological construct of helplessness (the belief that one is unable to exert some control over his or her symptoms) appears to be as important as disease severity in how patients assess their own health status" [17].

Mabeck describes how patients embody medical explanation: "It is generally accepted that a fundamental distinction exists between a patient's everyday notion of illness and the medical conception of disease. What the patient comprehends is based on lived experiences, while medical understanding essentially rests on conceptions of the human body and its functioning as 'an object within a scientific framework:' a framework that represents an abstraction from lived experience. Patients who seek medical help experience their problems in terms of illness—this is radically different from the physician's interest in discernible "symptoms and signs" [13]. Illness can be defined as a subjective state of feeling unwell that may include impairment of normal physiological and social function. Though IBS symptoms are episodic, their unpredictability means they nevertheless impact daily upon the lives of those affected. In addition to effective treatments, the desire of the individual is to become better informed so that they can better cope and manage their daily lives.

A strong doctor-patient relationship is fundamental to successful management. For the patient, this process should begin immediately at the time of diagnosis. Patients' understanding of their own health problems are influenced by everyday experiences as well as cultural, social, and media interactions. Physician recognition of this and of the patient's individual illness experience will help improve the doctor-patient interaction [2]. Patients need convincing explanations about the diagnosis and nature of their symptoms that encourages the view of IBS as a legitimate disorder for which a clear pathogenesis has not yet been found [10, 13]. An empowering doctor-patient relationship can be remarkably affirming and valuable [12]. Empowerment provides the patient with a framework in which to understand and legitimize their symptoms, remove self-doubt or blame, and identify internal or external factors that may contribute to symptoms that the patient can influence or control within the context of their own experiences. The physician and patient thus become allies in the management of the condition. "Self-management support involves collaboratively helping patients and their families acquire the skills and confidence to manage their chronic illness, providing self-management tools and routinely assessing problems and accomplishments" [18].

— Summary of the Patient's Perspective

IBS can be challenging to both the physician and the patient. Though many people with IBS in the community do not seek medical advice for the condition, IBS patients place significant demands on health services both in terms of numbers of consultations and the challenges of diagnosis and treatment. Patients must learn to self-manage the condition, which is either not well understood or is misunderstood within the general community in which they must function.

Physicians can help by eliciting and addressing patient concerns, by offering a positive diagnosis and clear, understandable, and legitimizing explanations of the disorder, and by helping identify factors that influence symptoms. By helping patients and their families find the most effective ways to manage the profound impact IBS has on everyday living, physicians can enter into a meaningful partnership that helps individuals replace feelings of helplessness with means of empowerment.

Gender

Like other medical conditions, the FGIDs exist within a larger socially constructed context beyond the individual, with factors such as gender, society, culture, and age that impact upon the patient. Gender is discussed in the following content areas: (a) definitions of sex, gender, and gender role, (b) epidemiology, (c) biological factors, (d) psychological factors, (e) social factors, and (f) treatment response.

— Sex, Gender, and Gender Role

The term *sex* is generally used to refer to a person's biological femaleness or maleness. *Gender* is generally used to refer to the nonbiological aspects of being female or male such as the social or cultural expectations associated with femininity or masculinity [19]. However, we know that most differences between males and females are a function of the interaction between biology and environment [19]. In this chapter, gender will be used as a more inclusive term. Sex will be used for the classification of individuals based on their reproductive organs and functions assigned by chromosomal complement. *Gender roles* are based on sex stereotypes, which are socially shared beliefs that biological sex determines certain qualities. For example, masculinity has been thought of as being instrumental and competency-oriented, including such characteristics as independence, rationality, competitiveness, providing, and objectivity. Femininity, on the other hand, has been thought of as being expressive and relationship-oriented, including such characteristics as dependence, intuition, submissiveness, nurturing, and emotionality [19].

— Gender and Epidemiology

FGIDs are extremely common conditions [20, 21]. Many people with FGIDs do not seek care and the decision to seek care introduces bias in research [22]. For this reason, population-based research has been used to fully evaluate the epidemiology and clinical symptoms in individuals with FGIDs. This section will review the epidemiology of FGID with a focus on gender. Additional information on these FGIDs, including their definitions, is provided in the other chapters.

Functional Esophageal Disorders

Functional esophageal disorders include globus, functional chest pain, functional heartburn, and functional dysphagia. Studies have shown that these functional esophageal disorders are all quite common [20, 23]. Globus sensation is reported by 7% to 12.5% of the population [20, 23] and is more common in women. Rumination syndrome, considered for Rome III a gastroduodenal disorder, is reported by 10.9% of the population [20] and no difference in gender has been reported. The prevalence estimates of functional chest pain vary between 12.5% to 23.1% [20, 23, 24] and have relied on the individual's self report of not having cardiac disease. Patients with functional chest pain of esophageal origin comprise a subgroup of those with noncardiac chest pain, which has an equal gender prevalence in the general population [20, 23, 24] but a higher female-to-male ratio in tertiary care referral centers [25]. The rest of the conditions are equally common in women and men. Many of the symptoms of functional esophageal disorders are experienced by people with gastroesophageal reflux disease (GERD) [23]. The challenge in research studies of functional esophageal disorders is identifying those individuals who predominantly have a functional esophageal disorder rather than GERD, which is not associated with gender differences in prevalence rates or reflux symptoms [23, 26–28]. The prevalence of heartburn does not vary by gender [23]. Dysphagia is reported by 7%–13% of the population [20, 23] and it is unclear whether dysphagia is associated with gender. One study found a difference of 6.3% in men and 8.5% in women to be statistically significant [20], whereas in another study, the difference of 12.4% of men and 14.6% of women was not statistically significant [23].

Functional Gastroduodenal Disorders

The prevalence of dyspepsia does not vary by gender [20, 29]. Distinct subgroups of dyspepsia have been defined: ulcer-like dyspepsia, dysmotility-like dyspepsia, and unspecified dyspepsia [30]. The prevalence of the ulcer-like and dysmotility-like dyspepsia subgroups also do not vary by gender. However, a recent multicenter, nontreatment study conducted in Denmark and Sweden demonstrated that female gender was a significant predictor of functional dyspepsia compared with organic causes of dyspepsia. Female gender has also been associated with delayed gastric emptying [31, 32] and lower tolerance of the water-loading test in functional dyspepsia [33]. In the latter study, gender differences were seen in both the healthy controls and functional dyspepsia patients, and therefore may not be specific to functional dyspepsia. Nonetheless, there seems to be little relationship between these physiologic measures and symptom severity. In addition, there is little evidence that symptoms of functional dyspepsia are influenced by menstrual cycle phase or menopausal status.

The prevalence of aerophagia has been estimated to be 23.4% to 29% [20, 34]. Men are slightly more likely to report aerophagia than women.

The overall prevalence of functional vomiting is 2.3% and there is no association with gender. In general, although more men than women report vomiting, the difference is not statistically significant [29, 35].

Functional Bowel Disorders

IBS is the best studied of all the FGIDs. Population-based studies have varied in their results regarding sex-specific prevalence rates. While some studies report that the prevalence of IBS in the United States is equal between men and women [36], the majority have reported female-to-male ratios of 2–3:1 [20, 37]. Possible explanations for the gender differences are discussed further in other sections in this chapter. Tables 1 & 2 show the gender-specific prevalence rates across studies. In a study of 1264 patients in a health maintenance organization (HMO), 68% of those with IBS symptoms were female. In those with mild symptoms (< 3 Manning criteria), 65% were female, and in those with more severe symptoms (≥ 3 Manning criteria), 80% were female [38]. In another study, symptom severity (composite of frequency of abdominal complaints, interference with daily activities, and avoidance behavior) was compared in 109 IBS patients from primary care clinics and 86 patients from university internal medicine outpatient clinics [39].

Table I. Prevalence of IBS in a Sample of Western Countries, by Sex, with Varying Diagnostic Criteria (M=Manning, RI=Rome I, RII=Rome II).

Source	Year	Population	N	Country	Diagnostic criteria	% IBS		
						Women	Men	All
(36)	1991	Olmstead county, white=99%	835	USA	≥ 3 M	13.6	12.1	12.8
(253)	1992	English urban, white=99%	1,896	UK	≥ 3 M	13.0	5.0	9.5
(254)	1992	English, mostly white	1,620	UK	≥ 2 M	24.3	18.7	21.6
(20)	1993	US householder, mostly white		USA	Rome I	14.5	7.7	9.4
(255)	1994	Population	3,608	Denmark	Symptom criteria	7.7	5.6	6.6
(224)	1995	Hispanic=64% White=36%		USA Whites Hispanics	Drossman criteria	26.5 21.7	13.9 7.1	21.8 16.9
(256)	2000	Population	2,707	Sweden	RI	13.3	7.4	10.6
(257)	2000	Population	2,910	Australia	M RI RII	17.2 6.4 9.2	9.8 2.2 4.6	13.6 4.4 6.9
(258)	2001	Birth cohort	890	New Zealand	≥ 2 M	14.6	10.8	12.7
(259)	2002	Random national telephone survey	1,149	Canada	RI Mod. RII	18.1 15.2	8.5 8.7	13.5 12.1
(260)	2002	National survey	11,131	France	RI	5.3	2.5	4.0
(261)	2003	Olmstead county	643	USA	RI RII	8.0 4.5	4.5 4.9	6.8 4.7
(262)	2004	National survey	20,000	France	RII	5.7	3.7	4.7
(263)	2004	National survey	3,650	Finland	≥ 2 M ≥ 3 M RI RII	19.2 11.2 6.1 5.3	13.1 8.3 5.1 5.1	16.2 9.7 5.5 5.1
(264)	2004	Clinic-based	4,807	UK	RII	14.0	6.6	10.5
(265)	2004	National survey	8,221	France	M RI RII M/RI/RII	3.1 2.8 1.3 3.2	1.7 1.4 0.9 1.8	2.5 2.1 1.1 2.6

Table 2. Prevalence of IBS in a Sample of Non-Western Countries, by Sex, with Varying Diagnostic Criteria (M=Manning, RI=Rome I, RII=Rome II).

Source	Year	Population	N	Country	Diagnostic criteria	% IBS		
						Women	Men	All
(247)	2001	Two villages	2,426	Bangaladesh	M	27.7	20.6	24.4
					RI	10.7	5.8	8.5
(200))	2001	Guangzhou City, random sample and clinics	4,393	China	RII	F:M - 1.51:1		5.6
(266)	2002	2 housing blocks	1,300	China	RII	3.8	3.6	
(267)	2002	Random telephone numbers	1,000	Hong Kong	RII	F:M - 1.3:1		6.6
(268)	2003	Medical students	533	Malaysia	RI	18.8	11.8	15.8
(269)	2003	Hospital check-up	2,018	Taiwan	RII	22.8	21.8	22.1
(270)	2004	Random cluster-sampling	4,178	China	RII	F:M - 1.25:1		5.6
(271)	2004	Random households	2,276	Singapore	M	12.6	9.5	11.0
					RI	11.7	9.0	10.4
					RII	9.4	7.8	8.6
(272)	2004	Urban	1,776	Turkey	RII	7.4	5.0	6.3
(273)	2004	West Malaysia, households	949	Malaysia	RII	F:M - 1.4:1		14.0
(274)	2004	Household interviews	1,617	Western Nicaragua	RII	16	9	13
(275)	2005	Population	981	Israel (Jews)	RII	3.7	1.8	2.9
(238)	2005	Clinic-based	1,755	Israel Nomad Bedouins	RII	6.6	4.7	5.8
				Settled Bedouins		11.0	7.3	9.4

Women attending the outpatient clinics had a higher severity score than men attending the same clinics, but severity scores for women and men attending the primary care clinics were similar.

Increasing evidence from a small number of studies support similar prevalence rates for pain-related symptoms in men and women with IBS [40] but a greater female predominance in nonpain associated symptoms of constipation, bloating, and extraintestinal manifestations. Several studies report similar abdominal pain scores for men and women with IBS; however, men report more diarrhea and women report more constipation [41–43]. In addition, women with IBS were more likely to report bloating and nausea as well as extraintestinal symptoms compared to men [44]. There appears to be a gender difference with regard to bowel habit predominance with a greater female preponderance for IBS with constipation compared to the other two bowel habit subgroups [45, 46].

The menstrual cycle appears to influence IBS symptom reports with an amplification of symptoms during the late luteal and early menses phases [44, 47–50]. In many women with and without IBS, symptoms closely associated with menstrual cycle function (e.g., breast tenderness, sense of bloating, affective changes) increase in the luteal phase and decrease after the start of menstrual flow [49]. Heitkemper and colleagues [50] found that gastrointestinal (GI) symptoms tend to be elevated across all cycle phases in women with IBS and increase in severity immediately prior to or at the onset of menses.

In contrast to IBS, much less is known about the epidemiology of functional abdominal bloating. One study found that women were more likely than men to report bloating or abdominal distention. The prevalence in women was 19% vs. 10% in men [51]. However, another study found that men were more likely than women to report bloating (34% vs. 27%) [20].

Studies evaluating gender differences in the prevalence of functional constipation and functional diarrhea have reported a female predominance in functional constipation, but similar rates in men and women with functional diarrhea [20, 35, 36, 52, 53]. Chronic constipation is a common condition, which has been self-reported in 20.8% of women and 8.0% of men [52]. A more recent study that conducted nationwide telephone interview surveys of more than 10,000 individuals reported the prevalence of constipation in 16% of women and 12% of men [52]. The female-to-male ratio was elevated for both the "outlet" type (1.65) and the combined "IBS-outlet" type (2.27) of functional constipation. While at least 50% of the men and women included in this study may have had IBS with constipation, there were no significant gender differences in the reporting of the specific constipation-associated symptoms of decreased bowel movement frequency, incomplete bowel movement, unsuccessful bowel movement, abdominal bloating, and trouble relaxing muscles to let stool come out. Pare et al. reported that women with functional constipation were more likely to seek medical care compared to men (35.6% vs. 19.5%) at all ages except for 50 to 64 years, where probability rates were similar [54].

The studies of functional diarrhea relied on self-report. The prevalence estimates vary from 1.6% to 27% [20, 35, 36]. However, some people with functional diarrhea do not always have symptoms, and individual diarrhea symptoms do not correlate well to an overall self-report of diarrhea. Thus, these numbers must be considered with caution [55].

The prevalence of functional abdominal pain has been estimated to be 1.7% [20]. The rate was higher in women.

Functional Disorders of the Biliary Tract and Pancreas

A single study estimated the prevalence of sphincter of Oddi dyskinesia to be 0.8%. The rate was much higher in women (2.3% vs. 0.6%) [20].

Functional Anorectal Disorders

Prevalence rates of fecal incontinence vary from 3% to 11% [20, 56–58] and the role of gender has varied by study. Among nursing home residents, incontinence has been reported to be more common in men [59]; whereas, among older people living at home, the reported rates are higher in women [60]. Men are more likely to report soiling of underclothes [61].

There is relatively little data on functional anorectal pain. The estimated prevalence is 11.3% with no difference in gender [20].

Pelvic floor dysfunction is a recognized cause of constipation. The prevalence of outlet delay has varied from 4.6% [53] and 11% [62] and is more common in women. In the one study that attempted to estimate the prevalence of dyschezia, the rate was 13% with higher rates in women [20].

Summary

Symptoms of FGIDs are quite prevalent in the community. In general, women report these symptoms more than men (Table 3). Women are more likely to report globus, IBS, bloating, constipation, chronic functional abdominal pain, sphincter of Oddi dysfunction, fecal incontinence and pelvic floor dysfunction. In contrast, women and men report similar rates of functional esophageal symptoms and dyspepsia. Clinical symptoms of IBS appear to be influenced by the menstrual cycle, with increased symptoms just prior to and at the onset of menses. Most of the high-quality epidemiologic studies have been conducted in Western populations with IBS, constipation, heartburn, and dyspepsia but not the other FGIDs. In general, very little is known about the prevalence of FGIDs in other parts of the world.

Table 3. Prevalence by Sex and Change with Age, for the Various FGID.

FGID	Prevalence by sex	Change with age
Esophageal		
Globus	F>M	↓
Rumination	F=M	↓
Functional chest pain	F=M	↓
Functional heartburn	F=M	=
Dysphagia	F>M	↑
Gastroduodenal		
Dyspepsia	F=M	↓
Aerophagia	M>F	↓
Functional vomiting	F=M	↓
Biliary tract	F	↑
Lower GI tract		
IBS	F	↓
Functional constipation	F	↑
Functional diarrhea	M>F	↓
Functional bloating	Discordant studies	Discordant studies
FAPS	F>M	↓
Fecal incontinence	F>M (at home)	↑
	M>F (nursing homes)	
Functional anorectal pain	F>M	↓
Outlet delay	F	=

Some of the data in this table are based on single studies or multiple small-scale studies and should be interpreted with caution.

FAPS = functional abdominal pain syndrome; FGID = functional gastrointestinal disorder; GI = gastrointestinal; IBS = irritable bowel syndrome; F = female; M = male.

— Gender and Biological Factors

FGIDs are best viewed as biopsychosocial disorders with dysregulation of the brain-gut axis [63]. (See Chapters 1, 2, and 3) This results in alterations in visceral pain perception, autonomic function, and central processing of visceral stimuli. Gender differences in these mechanisms have been evaluated primarily in IBS and will be discussed in this section. In addition, the potential underlying mechanisms of these physiologic alterations, including sexually dimorphic pain pathways and the effect of female sex hormones on GI function, will be highlighted.

Visceral Pain Perception

Healthy men and women   Gender differences in responses to experimental pain have been studied in human and animal studies. These differences have been more extensively studied for somatic pain than visceral pain. In a review of human studies, Berkeley summarized that women have lower pain thresholds, higher pain ratings, and less tolerance for intense stimuli under controlled experimental conditions, but these findings are relatively small and inconsistently observed [64]. However, a recently published meta-analysis of more than 20 experimental pain studies showed that women have a moderate degree of greater pain sensitivity and less pain tolerance than men [65]. Visceral pain sensitivity of the upper and lower GI tract has been compared in healthy men and women in a few studies but sample sizes have been relatively small. Two studies measured esophageal thresholds to balloon distension in healthy men and women [66, 67]. Volume, but not pressure, thresholds to pain in the esophagus from distension were lower in women than men, although compliance comparisons between men and women were not reported [66]. In another study, Rao et al. [67] compared esophageal pressure thresholds for discomfort and pain using graded balloon distension at the striated and smooth muscle segments of the esophagus in healthy younger and older men and women, however, both age groups were comprised of only 5 men and 6 women. There were no significant gender differences in esophageal sensory perception.

Two studies have compared colorectal distension in healthy women and men [68]. Soffer et al. found that women appeared to have higher perceptual ratings (i.e., increased perception) compared to men at the higher distension pressures of the descending colon, but there were no significant differences before or after a meal [68]. Most of the women were postmenopausal. The second study compared visceral perception to rectosigmoid distension in healthy men and women, and men and women with IBS. The healthy women had reduced perceptual responses (i.e. higher discomfort thresholds) to rectosigmoid stimuli compared to the other three groups [69]. No attempt to control for menstrual cycle was made in either study.

Men and women with FGID   While there have been multiple studies showing enhanced visceral perception in some FGID patients, including those with atypical chest pain [70], functional dyspepsia [71], and IBS [72–76] relative to healthy control subjects, few have compared visceral perception in male and female patient populations. In a study of 39 women and 13 men, Ragnarsson et al. [77] found a significant decrease in postprandial rectal thresholds (mmHg) of maximal tolerated distension (i.e., increased perception) in 50% of women compared to 25% of men. Another study assessed the presence of gender differences in rectal discomfort thresholds before and after noxious sigmoid distensions in 26 healthy individuals (9 men, 17 women) and 58 IBS patients (34 men and 24 women) [78]. They found that rectal discomfort thresholds were significantly lower in women with IBS, consistent with increased perception, compared to men with IBS. In addition, healthy women had higher rectal discomfort thresholds than women with IBS. Both female groups were more likely to demonstrate a decrease in thresholds after a sensitizing noxious stimulus (i.e., repetitive sigmoid distensions) than the male groups. Holtmann et al. [79] measured duodenal perceptual thresholds to distension in 22 patients with functional dyspepsia alone (n = 9), functional dyspepsia and IBS (n = 8), and IBS alone (n = 5) and in 22 healthy controls. While the patient group had significantly lower thresholds to first perception and pain compared the control group, no significant differences between male and female subjects were found.

In summary, healthy men and women have similar visceral perception except for possible decreased sensitivity in the rectosigmoid colon. However, women with IBS have enhanced rectosigmoid sensitivity compared to men with IBS. Studies with relatively larger sample sizes are needed to further characterize sex differences in visceral perception in health and in FGID. These studies should control for menstrual cycle and assess any regional differences in sensitivity as suggested by previous studies (e.g., increased visceral sensitivity in women with IBS to pelvic but not upper GI stimuli).

GI Motility

Overall, healthy men have shorter intestinal and total GI transit times than healthy women. Teff et al. [80] found that women had delayed gastric emptying of liquids and solids relative to men. Three studies found that mean colon transit times were shorter in men than women, particularly in the right colon [81–83]. However, two studies found no difference in transit times [84, 85]. With regard to colonic motility, there have been two studies that compared motility patterns in healthy women and men [68, 86]. Using standard colonic motility and barostat testing, Soffer et al. compared left colonic motility and compliance in a relatively small sample of healthy women and men [68]. There were no gender differences in fasting, postprandial frequency of contractions, motility index, or compliance. However, in a second study by Rao et al., who utilized ambulatory 24-hour colonic manometry in 25 age-matched healthy men and women, healthy women showed significantly less pressure activity in the colon than men, and this difference was particularly significant in the transverse/descending colon and during the day [86]. There was no attempt to control for phase of menstrual cycle in either of these studies. There are no published nondrug studies comparing colonic motility in women and men with IBS.

Comparison of anorectal function in 15 healthy men (mean age 41 ± 3 years) and 20 women (mean age 43 ± 2 years, 5 nulliparous) was performed by Sun and Read [87]. Healthy men had higher minimum and maximal basal anal sphincter pressures, higher anal pressures during maximum conscious sphincter contraction, lower rectal volumes required to cause an anal relaxation and higher volumes to induce a desire to defecate. In addition, significantly fewer men experienced pain during a one-minute 100-ml rectal distension (using syringe inflation) compared to women (13% vs. 55%). These results suggest that healthy men have stronger anal sphincter pressures and that women have either lower rectal compliance or increased rectal sensitivity.

Cardioautonomic Tone

There are very little data evaluating gender differences in other measures of autonomic function other than GI motility between men and women with IBS. Heart rate variability that measures cardioautonomic tone is becoming an increasingly frequent noninvasive technique of assessing autonomic function. One study demonstrated that men with IBS have greater cardiosympathetic and lower cardiovagal tone in response to rectosigmoid distention than women with IBS [88]. Several studies have compared cardiosympathetic and vagal tone in female patients with constipation or diarrhea [35, 42]. Women with severe IBS with constipation had lower cardiovagal tone than those with IBS with diarrhea [35]. In women having IBS with diarrhea, an increase in postprandial cardiosympathetic relative to cardiovagal tone and greater postprandial salivary cortisol levels were reported [42].

Central Processing of Visceral Stimuli

Altered brain-gut interactions play a central role in the pathophysiology of functional bowel disorders. These proposed alterations in the brain-gut axis have been supported by recent findings in functional neuroimaging studies performed to assess the regional cerebral blood flow (rCBF) to various visceral stimuli. However, only a few studies have addressed gender differences in health and GI disease. Gender differences in the structure and function of the brain have been described [89–91].

Studies comparing rCBF in response to visceral stimuli between men and women who are healthy or have FGIDs are limited. Kern et al. [92] compared brain activation patterns using functional magnetic resonance imaging (fMRI) in response to rectal distension in healthy men and women. While men showed activation in sensory and parieto-occipital areas, women showed greater activation in the anterior cingulate and insular cortices, which are regions associated with greater sensory and affective responses to noxious stimuli.

While there have been published studies reporting altered brain activation responses to colorectal distension in IBS patients compared to healthy controls [93–97], there are only two neuroimaging studies that have examined gender differences in IBS. Unlike the findings in healthy women and men, Berman et al. reported significantly greater activation of the insula bilaterally in men with IBS compared to women with IBS [99, 100]. Men and women with IBS had a significant difference in brain response to aversive pelvic visceral stimuli. Even though both groups of patients showed activation of the expected pain regions, compared to women with IBS, men with IBS had greater activation of regions (including the lateral prefrontal cortex, dorsal anterior cingulate cortex (ACC) and dorsal pons/periaqueductal grey) that may be involved in endogenous pain inhibition. In contrast, women with IBS showed greater activation of limbic and paralimbic regions (including the amygdala, ACC, and infragenual cingulate cortex) that may be part of a pain facilitation circuit.

In summary, these findings suggest that men and women with IBS may process aversive information originating from the pelvic viscera differently. Further studies are needed to clearly determine if gender differences in the central nervous system (CNS) processing of visceral information exist and how these differences are altered and influence the clinical and physiologic responses in FGIDs.

Potential Mechanisms of Gender Differences in FGIDs

Gender related factors that may explain the differences in pain responses include type of stimulus, sex of the experimenter, willingness to report, and attitudes towards pain [64]. However, gender differences in FGIDs may be due to several biologic factors that differ in males and females, including differences in biobehavioral responses to stress, pain modulatory pathways, and sex hormone effects on GI function. Taylor [98] proposes that gender differences in IBS may at least be in part due to the different biobehavioral responses to stress in females and males. Females respond to stress by building on attachment/caregiving processes that have evolved with a behavioral pattern referred to as "tend and befriend." These behavioral responses may be linked to physiologic responses such as down-regulation of the sympathetic nervous system and hypothalamic-pituitary-adrenal axis. In contrast, males respond to stress with the more aggressive prototypic "fight-or-flight" response thought to be mediated through androgens and the sympathetic nervous system. However, it remains to be shown whether these behavioral responses to laboratory stress models are applicable to humans, and in particular to those with FGIDs.

Sex-related biological differences in the integration, processing and, modulation of pain may also be key mechanisms responsible for the greater female prevalence of many chronic pain disorders and the gender differences in the clinical symptoms and physiologic responses reported in FGIDs. Potential mechanisms of gender differences include sex differences in pain modulatory pathways mediated by serotonin [99], calcitonin gene-related peptide (CGRP) [100], μ- and κ-opioid agonists [101–103], and α-adrenergic agonists [104, 105], and estrogen-dependent pain modulatory pathways via neurokinin (NK1) receptors [106, 107], and the estrogen-oxytocin-opioid antinociceptive pathway [108, 109].

Sex hormones may affect pain perception and GI motility. Rectal sensitivity was compared across the four phases of the menstrual cycle (menses, follicular phase, luteal phase, and premenstrual phase) in healthy women and women with IBS. In healthy female volunteers, no differences were found in measures of rectal sensitivity, distension-induced rectal motility, and rectal compliance across the different phases of the menstrual cycle [110]. In contrast, perceptual thresholds were lower during menses compared to other menstrual cycle phases in women with IBS [111]. While these findings were not accounted for by psychological factors, an ascending series of distensions was used in this study that may reflect a hormonal influence on hypervigilance. Similar results were found in an experimental animal model of visceral pain. Giamberdino et al. [112] found enhanced ureteral pain sensitivity during metestrus/diestrus in female rats (equivalent to the perimenstrual period in women).

Somatic but not visceral pain thresholds have been studied during pregnancy in animals and humans. Somatic pain thresholds are increased during pregnancy in rats [113] and humans [114]. Administration of 17-β-estradiol and progesterone also elevates pain thresholds in pseudopregnant rats [115]. This phenomenon is also observed in women. During the luteal phase, in which plasma levels of both estrogen and progesterone are increased, somatic pain thresholds increase [116].

Although effects of estrogen and progesterone on visceral pain thresholds need to be better understood, several empirical studies have been reported. The effect of estrogen and progesterone on nociception may be dependent on noradrenergic and/or serotonergic neurotransmission [117, 118]. There is some evidence that estrogen alone induces visceral hypersensitivity in rats. Oophorectomy decreases the magnitude of the visceromotor neuron and abrupt neuron response to colorectal distention compared with cycling rats [119]. After estrogen injection, the magnitude of the visceromotor neuron and abrupt neuron response to colorectal distention returned to the level or greater than that of cycling rats [119]. The response to innocuous colorectal distention is sensitized in estrogen-treated rats but not ovariectomized or cycling rats [119].

Estrogen and progesterone also affect GI motility. Women usually show delayed gastrointestinal transit [120, 121] and a tendency for constipation [120, 122] during the luteal phase, during which plasma levels of estrogen and progesterone rise. Moreover, estrogen and progesterone pretreatment of ovariectomized rats resulted in a decrease in the geometric center of colonic transit compared with the untreated ovariectomized rats [123]. Sex-related differences in GI motility may be due to several mechanisms that include the effects of female sex hormones on gastrointestinal smooth muscle function [124], NO neurons in the myenteric plexus [125], mast cells of the gastrointestinal mucosa [126], and/or motilin concentration [127]. Distinct estrogen receptors are present in the gastrointestinal tract in humans [124]. Expression of progesterone receptor B has been demonstrated in

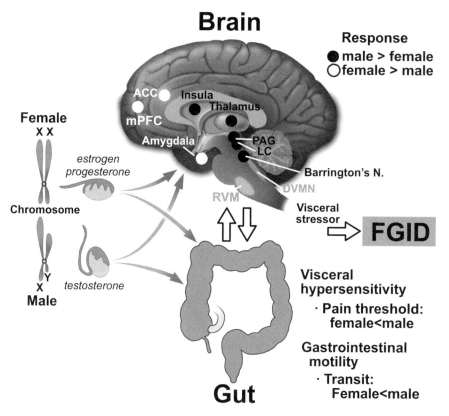

Figure 1. Sex-related Effects on Brain-Gut Interactions in FGID.

Differences in brain-gut function between women and men with IBS have been reported, including GI motility and transit, perception, and brain activation patterns in response to rectosigmoid stimulation. Gonadal hormones appear to exert effects on both brain and gut function, however the effects of testosterone have not been well studied. Also, it should be noted that the gender difference in GI transit in IBS have been studied in diarrhea-predominant IBS patients treated with alosetron. The gender differences shown apply to IBS and not necessarily healthy controls. See the text for the detail. The brain schema was modified from Naliboff BD, Berman S, Chang L, Derbyshire SWG, Suyenobu B, Vogt BA, Mandelkern MA, Mayer EA. Sex-related differences in IBS patients: central processing of visceral stimuli. Gastroenterology 124:1738–1747, 2003.

ACC = anterior cingulate cortex
mPFC = medial prefrontal cortex
PAG = periaqueductal grey
DVMN = dorsal vagal motor nucleus

MCC = mid cingulate cortex
DLPFC = dorsolateral prefrontal cortex
LC = locus ceruleus
RVM = rostral ventromedial medulla

the colonic smooth muscle [128]. Progesterone reduces the contraction amplitude of the circular and longitudinal muscle and contraction frequency, and may exert its inhibitory effect on colonic smooth muscle via changes in the cytoplasmic calcium concentration [129].

Summary

Women and men with IBS differ in visceral pain perception, GI transit and motility, and brain activation patterns to visceral stimuli. Female sex hormones appear to influence gut function and pain perception. Evidence also supports sexually dimorphic pain modulatory pathways between males and females. The role of male sex hormones in FGIDs is largely unknown. These findings are summarized in Figure 1. Future studies are needed to more completely understand how sex differences in biologic factors play a role in the greater vulnerability of women to develop chronic pain disorders such as IBS and the differences in symptom presentation and physiologic responses in FGIDs.

— Gender and Psychological Factors

There are clear gender role differences in the reporting and experiencing of psychological symptoms in the general population. Both men and women experience stress, but the psychological manifestation and presentation may be different. In epidemiological surveys, women are more likely to report symptoms of anxiety and depression than men [130, 131], whereas men have higher rates of antisocial behavior such as alcohol and drug abuse [132, 133] and violence [134]. Women are more likely to recognize psychological and emotional problems in themselves [135], and are more likely to consult doctors than men [136]. The reason for these marked gender role differences is unclear, but it involves a complex mix of biological, genetic, and culturally determined factors. Any consideration of gender role differences in psychological symptoms in FGIDs, should take into account the marked differences between men and women that are already apparent in the general population.

Although there are many studies of psychological functioning in FGIDs, relatively few investigators have examined gender differences. Most studies have not been powered to undertake this analysis, and study populations are predominantly female. This reflects the larger proportion of women to men with FGIDs, particularly those who are seen in a treatment setting.

A small number of studies in FGIDs have chosen to focus exclusively on women. To our knowledge, there are no studies that have included only men. Women-only studies have examined a number of psychological aspects of FGIDs that may be particularly relevant to women rather than men. One aspect that has been studied is the relationship between the menstrual cycle, stress, and gastrointestinal symptoms. This is covered in more detail in the previous section on biological aspects of gender in FGIDs.

Women-only studies have also been carried out to examine the role of eating disorder symptoms in FGIDs. Female outpatients with IBS are more likely to report difficulties or problems with eating than normal controls or patients with organic gastrointestinal disease [137, 138], although only a small number of women with IBS (5%) are likely to meet diagnostic criteria for an eating disorder such as bulimia nervosa or anorexia nervosa. There is also an association between bowel symptom severity and certain subscales of the Eating Disorder Inventory (perfectionism and ineffectiveness) [139].

There is obviously some overlap between symptoms of FGIDs and eating disorders. In both conditions, bloating and feelings of fullness after eating are common. Diarrhea is also common in patients who use laxatives to control weight, and there is some evidence that individuals with IBS may have problems with obesity [140], possibly prompting a greater preoccupation with methods of dietary control.

In the following sections, studies that have considered gender issues in relation to psychological symptomatology in FGID will be discussed. The sections are divided into clinic-based, primary care-based and population-based studies.

Clinic-Based Studies

The majority of studies on FGIDs that have included a psychological evaluation have been carried out in gastrointestinal outpatient clinics. In general, the findings of most studies suggest that FGID patients seen in GI outpatient clinics have high rates of psychiatric disorder and psychological distress (between 40%–60%). The ratio of women to men in these studies has varied from 1:1 to 4:1 (Table 4), although most have recruited a larger proportion of women than men, and some investigators have chosen to exclusively study women.

Many studies that have included measures of psychological symptoms in outpatients with FGIDs have not examined gender differences. These include studies by Hislop [141], Bouchier [142], MacDonald and Bouchier [143], Craig and Brown, Latimer et al. [144], Ford et al. [145], Colgan et al. [146, 147], Toner et al. [148], Yadav et al. [149], Dinan et al. [150], Masand et al. [151], Gomborone et al. [152], and Van der Horst et al. [39].

In studies that have examined gender differences in FGID, or reported on certain aspects of gender, relatively few studies have reported differences in psychological symptom scores between men and women (Table 4). Blewett and colleagues [153] found no difference in the prevalence of psychiatric disorder, using a semi-structured interview, between male and female outpatients with IBS. In a large study using the Symptom Check List (SCL)-90R in 714 patients with IBS, Lee and colleagues [44] also found no difference between men and women in terms of psychological symptoms. Of note, some psychological tests have different norms for men vs. women and this could affect the interpretation of these studies.

Blanchard and colleagues [154] compared gender differences in patients seeking psychological treatment for IBS. They assessed individuals using both self-report measures and a semistructured psychiatric diagnostic interview. On the self-report measures, women reported more symptoms of depression and trait anxiety than men (albeit the differences were small in magnitude), but on the diagnostic interview, carried out by psychologists, the prevalence rates of psychiatric disorder for the two sexes were similar. One reason for the apparent discrepancy between the two forms of tests may be that women with IBS are more likely to volunteer symptoms of psychological distress, whereas men may need to be asked specifically about symptoms before acknowledging them. The rates of psychiatric disorder were relatively high in both men and women, but this may reflect the self-selective nature of the population since all patients were seeking psychological treatment for their IBS.

Two small studies, one from the UK and one from Singapore, have reported differences between men and women with IBS [43, 155]. Corney and Stanton [43] found that women with IBS had higher scores on both a psychological self-report measure (the General Health Questionnaire) and a semistructured interview than men with IBS. In the second study [155], the investigators did not report a direct comparison between men and women with IBS, but instead analyzed data for a small number of men and women separately. They used the Eysenck Personality Questionnaire and found that women with IBS had higher rates of psychiatric disorder than patients with organic bowel disease (63% vs. 18%); whereas there were no differences for men between these two groups.

Creed and colleagues [156] examined the relationship between health-related quality of life, health care costs, and psychological factors in patients with severe, refractory IBS. Approximately one fifth of the 257 patients they studied were male (n=52), and one quarter were unemployed because of illness. Although specific gender comparisons were not reported in this paper, gender was one of five variables to be selected into a logistic regression model to predict unemployment due to ill health, with men more likely than women to report their condition interfered with working. Three of the other variables were psychological factors, and the final variable was "years of education." No physical symptom factors were selected into the model.

Primary Care-Based Studies

Few studies of IBS or other FGIDs in primary care have been published. However, a recent Swedish study by Simren and colleagues [41] compared patients with IBS referred to a hospital center and those seen in primary care. Ap-

Table 4. Studies in FGIDs That Assessed Gender Differences on Psychological Measures

Study	Number	% Women	Setting and recruitment	FGID/Criteria	Measures	Findings
Corney and Stanton, 1990	42	74%	GI outpatient clinic—UK	IBS-Abd pain & alteration in bowel habit for six months	GHQ- (SR) CIS- (SSI)	Women reported more psychological distress than men and were more likely to have psychiatric diagnosis.
Blewett et al, 1996	76	66%	GI outpatient clinic—UK	IBS-Manning criteria	HAD (SR) CIDI (SSI)	No difference in prevalence of psychiatric disorder between men and women
Simren et al, 2001	343	73%	(209 outpatients/134 primary care patients via advertisement)—Sweden	IBS-Rome I	HAD (SR) STAI (SR) PGWB (SR)	Women > men for fatigue, depression, and anxiety—differences more marked for outpatients than primary care
Fock et al, 2001	43	63%	GI outpatients—Singapore	Manning criteria	EPI (SR) Psychiatric diagnosis established by a psychiatrist	62% of women had psychiatric diagnoses compared to 17% of women with organic GI illness. Women with IBS also had higher scores on the EPI than organic controls. No difference between men with IBS or organic disease on psychological measures.
Lee et al, 2001	714	67%	(315 specialist referrals/399 subjects via advertisement) GI outpatient clinic—USA	IBS-Rome I	SCL-90R (SR)	No difference in psychological symptoms

Study	Number	% Women	Setting and recruitment	DGIF/Criteria	Measures	Findings
Blanchard et al, 2001	341	70%	(IBS subjects who sought nondrug treatment)—USA	IBS-Rome I (retrospective)	BDI (SR) STAI (SR) MMPI (SR) ADIS (SSI)	Women were more depressed than men (mean BDI 12.4 (8.0) vs 9.9 (6.7)) and showed greater trait anxiety. No difference on state anxiety. % of patients with an Axis I psychiatric disorder—women 65%, men 68%.
Creed et al, 2001	257	80%	Outpatients with severe and refractory symptoms—UK GI outpatient clinic	IBS-Rome I	SCL-90-R (SR) Hamilton Depression Inventory (SSI) SF-36 (SR)	No direct comparison between men and women, but psychological symptoms, years of education, and gender independently predicted unemployment due to illness.
Westbrook et al, 2002	748	53.6%	Population based—Australia	Dyspepsia –Rome I	SF-12 (Mental well-being summary score)	Women had poorer mental well being than men.

HAD Scale= Hospital Anxiety and Depression Scale
STAI= Spielberger State Trait Anxiety Inventory
PGWB= Psychological General Well-Being Index
SCL-90-R= Symptom Checklist Revised
BDI= Beck Depression Inventory
EPI= Eysenck Personality Inventory
GHQ = General Health Questionnaire

CIDI= Composite International Diagnostic Interview
ADIS= Anxiety Disorders Interview Schedule
MMPI= Minnesota Multiphasic Personality Inventory
SF-12= Short Form 12
SF-36= Short Form 36
Abd = abdominal
CSI = Creative Imagination Scale

proximately 25% of the study population was male, and a careful analysis of the effects of gender on both psychological symptoms and health-related quality of life (HRQoL) was carried out. Regardless of practice type, women with IBS (n=343) reported reduced HRQoL and had more symptoms of depression and anxiety compared with men. Female outpatients reported a poorer HRQoL than female primary care patients, and had greater psychological distress on some quality of life measures. These differences depending on practice type were not seen in men.

The higher prevalence of anxiety and depression in female IBS patients in comparison with men is not surprising and may be a reflection of the observation that women in general report more symptoms of anxiety and depression than men. However, the study suggests that IBS female patients seen in referral centers may be psychologically different from those who are seen in primary care. This does not seem to apply to men with IBS.

Population-Based Studies

Population-based studies have usually included roughly equal numbers of men and women, from which individuals with symptoms suggestive of FGIDs have been identified. As FGIDs are more common in women than men, this gender difference is reflected in the community samples identified in such studies. Most population-based studies that have included a psychological evaluation have not reported direct comparisons between men and women with FGIDs [157–159].

One recent population-based study of dyspepsia by Westbrook and colleagues [160] did not include a psychological symptom measure, but did include a measure of mental health well being (the mental health component score of the SF-12). The general levels of mental well being for dyspeptics were low, and women had poorer mental well being than men.

Another large population-based study has examined the relationship between functional abdominal symptoms, psychological distress, and health care contacts over a 12-month period [161]. A random sample of 361 community subjects (67% female) who reported having unexplained abdominal pain was sequentially assessed every 4 months for 1 year and compared with a sample of 120 community controls. Although the principle aim of the study was not to compare men and women, investigators found that being female and having greater psychological distress were both independently associated with persistent bloating over time, while more worry and anxiety about bowel symptoms, greater psychological distress, and being female were associated with having persistent constipation-type symptoms over time.

Summary

At present, there is no convincing evidence of any major differences between men and women with FGIDs in terms of psychological profile. Those differences that have been reported are most likely to reflect the differences between men and women in the general population with respect to psychological symptom reporting rather than any specific GI-related phenomenon. Few studies have included sufficient numbers of men to be able to make valid comparisons between the sexes, and there are no studies that have specifically focused upon the psychological well being of men with FGIDs.

— Gender and Social Factors

It is important to acknowledge that health and illness occur within a larger social context. The meaning and expression of illness occur against a complex backdrop of a multitude of social determinants of health. While there have been many studies evaluating the role of stress and abuse in FGIDs, there has been relatively little effort to date directed toward identifying other social factors that have been associated with FGIDs. Several social determinants of health need to be incorporated into our understanding of health and health-related illnesses. These include the social gradient (including socioeconomic status), stress, early life, social exclusion, work, unemployment, social support, addiction, food, and transportation. The few social determinants that have been investigated in FGID include: life stressors, including history of sexual, physical, and emotional abuse, early life experiences, including gender role socialization, social support, and social factors that have been assessed by quality of life scales. This section will focus on the association between gender and social factors in FGIDs. For a general review of social factors in gastrointestinal disorders, the reader is referred to the Psychosocial Aspects of FGIDs chapter in this book (Chapter 6).

Life Stress

Several studies found that IBS patients report more lifetime and daily stressors compared with medical control groups or healthy controls [150, 162–168]. While stress affects the gut in most people, patients with IBS appear to experience greater reactivity to a variety of stressors, including social stressors. Stress has been found to be associated with both symptom onset and severity in patients with IBS [167–170]. Moreover, stressful life events and chronic social stress have been shown to adversely affect health status and clinical outcome in patients with IBS [166, 169, 171]. However, there are no studies to date that have assessed gender differences in life stress related to FGIDs. While the data support a significant role for life stress in IBS, future studies will need to determine whether there are similarities and differences in the relationship between stress and FGIDs in women and men.

History of Sexual, Physical, and Emotional Abuse

One form of social stress or oppression that has received increased attention in the past decade in the study of FGIDs is sexual, physical, or emotional abuse. However, most work in this area has included only women. In the few studies investigating abuse histories that have included men, significant differences are not statistically quantified due to insufficient numbers of men in the sample. Talley and colleagues [172] found no differences between male and female IBS patients with regard to a history of sexual, physical, emotional or verbal abuse. In contrast, Walker et al. [173], found that all of the IBS patients that reported a history of sexual abuse were female. In a primary care sample, Longstreth and Wold-Isadik [38] found that a history of sexual abuse was more common in women than in men but the authors did not differentiate between patients with or without IBS. Clearly, further research is needed to determine whether there are gender differences in history of abuse in FGIDs.

Gender Role Socialization

One important social factor that impacts on health and well-being, begins in early life, and continues throughout life is gender role socialization. The literature suggests that many of the physical and mental health concerns experienced by women are influenced by socialization into the female gender role. Despite postulated links between health problems such as eating disorders, depression, anxiety disorders, and functional somatic disorders including FGIDs, there have been few empirical investigations. Toner and colleagues [174] identified several common gender role concerns or themes that have been highly salient and meaningful to women with functional bowel disorders. These themes have been incorporated into a cognitive behavioral treatment (CBT) protocol for women. Results from a randomized trial indicated that the composite outcome score that included ratings of satisfaction, HRQoL, global well-being and pain improved for women with functional bowel disorders receiving CBT compared to those in a control group who received education only [175]. While further research will need to dismantle which components in the CBT treatment protocol were responsible for improvement at the end of treatment, the following gender role themes were identified and integrated into a manualized CBT treatment protocol [174]. Several of these issues have also been discussed in the previous section, "The Patient's Perspective," in this chapter.

Shame and Bodily Functions

One central theme that women with IBS commonly reported was feelings of shame associated with losing control of bodily functions. Women receive different social messages than men. Women are taught that bodily functions are something to be kept private and secret as compared to men. One important implication of such teachings is that for women, bowel functioning becomes a source of shame and embarrassment more so than it does for men. The sanction against public admission and/or display of bodily functioning in women can be seen as part of the socialization process that encourages girls and women to be always clean, neat, fresh, and in control [176]. This same socialization process permits boys and men to be more unrestrained, messy, and dirty, and even to view their bodily functions as a source of amusement and pleasure. For example, while belching and passing gas are not usually desirable in public for either sex, girls and women are socialized into believing that they are especially not ladylike. Belching and farting contests are traditionally less frequent among female than male adolescents.

Bloating and Physical Appearance

The finding that women often score higher on indices of bloating and constipation can also be discussed as a gender-related theme. Society's focus on how women look, and its perpetuation of thinness as a necessary standard of attractiveness [19, 176], may lead women to experience bloating not only as a source of physical discomfort, but of psychological distress as well. For many women, the sensation of being overweight, with or without an increase in the size of their abdomen, may evoke worry and shame about their body, and therefore about themselves. To the degree that women are subjected to being valued and/or devalued for their physical attractiveness (i.e., thinness), they will be attentive to and concerned by those IBS symptoms that have an impact on how they experience their bodies. The physical and psychological distress that women may experience with abdominal discomfort, coupled with the perception that their pain is being minimized or trivialized by health care professionals, may lead women to respond by becoming more hypervigilant to any sign of pain or discomfort. This increased attention to bodily symptoms may lead to increased pain in some women with IBS.

Pleasing Others, Assertion, and Anger

Women, as compared with men, are socialized to please others, often at the expense of their own needs [176, 177]. To some degree, this may contribute to women's higher rates of doctor visits and multiple consultations, since female patients who believe that their physician does not understand their experience may seek help elsewhere, rather than expecting satisfaction from their current physician. This would hold true as well for those patients who feel unable to be assertive or angry with their physician, because of the socialized ideal of women as compliant, understanding, and never overtly angry. Women who express anger, make demands, or question authority are often given the label "hysteric," have their complaints dismissed, or have their femininity called into question [176]. These potential repercussions for women who express their own wants and needs are often sufficient to keep women silent. Self-silencing is a helpful construct developed by Jack [177] to describe this socially constructed experience. According to Jack, women are socialized to behave in certain ways to maintain safe, intimate relationships. These social expectations of women can lead to the silencing of certain thoughts, feelings, and behaviors rather than jeopardize relationships that are in place. A study by Ali et al. [178] points to the relevance of this construct for IBS patients. These authors compared female IBS patients with female inflammatory bowel disease (IBD) patients, and found that IBS patients score higher on measures of self-silencing than IBD patients. Future research will need to identify themes that are salient for men with IBS to determine similarities and differences between women and men with IBS.

Health-Related Quality of Life (HRQoL)

Several studies have found that patients with IBS and functional dyspepsia have impaired HRQoL compared to other chronic conditions. Few studies have investigated whether women and men with FGIDs differ on HRQoL measures. In a study of referral center and primary care patients, Simren et al. [41] found that women with IBS reported a lower quality of life compared to men with IBS. In another study, Lee et al. [179] also found that women with IBS reported lower scores on quality of life measures. However, after these authors controlled for gender differences in the general population, most of the gender effects disappeared. The only remaining gender effect was greater bodily pain scores in female patients with IBS.

Dancey et al [180] found that men and women with IBS reported similar HRQoL scores as well as similar levels of symptom severity, perceived stigma, and illness intrusiveness. However, these authors also found significant gender differences in the relationship among these variables. For example, among women, IBS symptom severity exerted a significant impact on quality of life. For men, the psychosocial impact illness intrusiveness was greater in every domain except sexual relations. The authors suggest that these results have implications for how gender socialization shapes IBS-related sex differences.

Summary

It is important to acknowledge that the meaning and expression of illness occurs within a complex network of social determinants of health. This section has reviewed the limited theoretical and empirical work that has been published in the area of gender and social factors in FGIDs. These include life stress, history of sexual, physical, and emotional abuse, gender role socialization, and health-related quality of life. In general, these factors are thought to influence the experience of FGIDs. Most of the work in this area, however, has included women-only samples or did not test for gender effects due to small numbers of men in the study.

— Gender and Treatment Response

Psychological Treatment

There is a small, but growing body of evidence for the beneficial effects of psychological treatment in FGIDs. (See Chapter 6 on psychosocial aspects of FGIDs.) Most randomized controlled trials of psychological treatment in FGIDs have not included subanalyses to determine whether or not there is a differential response to treatment for men and women. Psychological treatment studies have not been powered to examine different response patterns between men and women, and many studies have recruited more women than men, reflecting gender differences in health treatment settings.

Blanchard and colleagues [154] and Corney and colleagues [43] examined differences between men and women in two small studies investigating the efficacy of cognitive behavioral treatments for IBS. They reported similar response patterns, but the studies were not powered to detect gender differences. Guthrie and colleagues [181] reported advantages for women in response to therapy compared to men, but gender was not selected into the final analysis model. In an earlier study by Svedlund and colleagues [182] in IBS, no direct comparison between men and women was made in relation to outcome, but the investigators reported that gender was not selected into a predictive model of treatment response.

A recent large evaluation of hypnotherapy, carried out in Manchester, UK, has reported different response patterns for men and women with respect to this form of psychological treatment. The study was not a randomized controlled trial, but a before-and-after evaluation of 250 patients with IBS who had had symptoms for at least 2 years and had been unresponsive to previous treatments. The age ranges of the men (n = 50) and women (n = 200) in the study were similar. There was greater overall improvement in treatment response to 12 sessions of hypnotherapy in women compared to men (52% in women and 33% in men, p<0.001). The poor response with men was largely seen in those with IBS with diarrhea (20% improvement), while men with IBS with constipation appeared to have a good response to hypnotherapy (78% improvement), but the numbers in this group were very small (n = 8). For women, responses were similar regardless of IBS subtype. Further work by Whorwell and colleagues has shown that men have a poorer long-term outcome following hypnotherapy than women (42% vs. 25%)

[183]. The reason for the poor response to hypnotherapy of men with diarrhea symptoms is unclear. Men with diarrhea may have underlying pathophysiological processes that are less amenable to modification by hypnotherapy. While men in general are less responsive to hypnotherapy than women, men with IBS with constipation appeared to respond well to hypnotherapy, which argues against a simple gender bias in treatment response.

Psychotropic Agents

The efficacy of antidepressants and other psychotropic agents in FGIDs is covered in the chapter on psychosocial aspects of FGIDs. A systematic review of pharmacotherapy in IBS [184] included seven trials of psychotropic agents, of which only one was found to be of good quality. The systematic review did not include a separate analysis by gender, and excluded most of the trials of psychotropic drug treatment from a meta-analysis because of poor quality. A meta-analysis of antidepressant treatment medication in FGIDs [185] was published in the same year. The meta-analysis was conducted on 11 studies but did not include a separate gender analysis. The authors commented that many of the trials of psychotropic drug treatment in FGID have been small (approximate number of subjects 40) and most of the participants were women. It is not possible at this stage to determine whether there are any gender differences in response to psychotropic agents in FGIDs.

Pharmacologic Treatment

There is evidence to suggest that gender-related differences may exist with respect to response to pharmacologic therapy. Alosetron is a 5-HT$_3$ antagonist currently indicated only for women with severe, chronic IBS with diarrhea who have failed conventional therapy, since serious gastrointestinal events, including colonic ischemia and bowel motor dysfunction, have been reported with alosetron use. An initial dose-ranging study evaluating the efficacy of the alosetron in men and women with IBS demonstrated a significant improvement in adequate relief of abdominal pain and discomfort, stool frequency, stool consistency and urgency in women but not men [186]. However, the lack of effect in men may have been due to the fact that relatively few men enrolled in the study compared to women. A subsequent dose-ranging study with alosetron which enrolled 662 men with IBS with diarrhea showed significant improvement of adequate relief of IBS pain and discomfort and reduction of stool consistency at the usual dose of 1 mg twice daily [187]. However, no significant effects of alosetron were seen with regard to urgency, number of bowel movements, bloating, and incomplete evacuation. One factor that may contribute to the greater efficacy in women than men is that alosetron has been shown to be more effective in slowing overall colonic transit in women than men [188].

Cilansetron is a novel 5-HT$_3$ receptor antagonist in development for the treatment of IBS with diarrhea. It has been shown to be efficacious in treating the symptoms of IBS with diarrhea in men and women [189–191]. Analyses by gender demonstrated that the response rates for adequate relief of IBS symptoms, abdominal pain/discomfort, and abnormal bowel habits were higher for women receiving cilansetron versus placebo. While there was an overall significant improvement in men, the treatment difference for men was smaller relative to women.

Tegaserod is a 5-HT$_4$ agonist that is currently indicated only for women with IBS with constipation [192–194] and for men and women under the age of 65 for chronic constipation [195]. Because of the small numbers of men with IBS in these studies, it was not possible to permit any conclusions concerning the efficacy of tegaserod in men, although there was an up-to-10% therapeutic gain noted that was not statistically significant. Tegaserod has been more recently shown to be effective in improving symptoms in patients with chronic constipation [195]. Since chronic constipation is more common in women, and women are more likely to enroll in a clinical trial, there were relatively few men who participated in the treatment study. Women, but not men, treated with tegaserod were found to have a significantly higher responder rate of ≥ 1 complete spontaneous bowel movement/week compared with placebo, which was the primary efficacy endpoint. However, further analysis demonstrated that tegaserod was associated with significantly higher responder rates for ≥ 3 complete spontaneous bowel movements/week in both women and men. Thus, tegaserod has been recently approved by the U.S. Federal Drug Administration (FDA) for the treatment of chronic constipation in women and men. Further studies are needed to more completely evaluate gender differences in pharmacologic treatments (both serotonergic and nonserotonergic agents) and to determine the mechanisms that may be responsible for the differences in symptom responses to these treatments in men and women with FGIDs.

Summary

In summary, there is little evidence to suggest that men and women have a differential response to psychological treatments. However, most studies were not powered to detect efficacy in subgroups and therefore were not powered to determine whether there are different response patterns for men and women, and further study is required. While women with FGIDs appear to respond well to psychological treatment, many studies have included such small numbers of men that relatively little is known about how men with FGIDs respond to psychological treatment interventions. For women with chronic and severe symptoms, the greatest impact of psychological treatment may be on satisfaction, quality of life, and costs. Patients who have been sexually abused, particularly women, may do well with psychological treatments. With regard to pharmacologic treatment, gender differences have only been addressed with the newer serotonergic agents. Similar to psychological treatment studies, relatively few men have been studied compared to women. Women and men with FGIDs both seem to respond to 5-HT$_3$ antagonists and a 5-HT$_4$ agonist, although there is a more robust response in women than men.

Age

The FGIDs affect people across the spectrum of age. Extensive epidemiological data exist for IBS, dyspepsia, heartburn, constipation and fecal incontinence, but less is known about the other FGIDs (see Table 3). For many FGIDs such as globus, rumination, and sphincter of Oddi dysfunction, the only data on prevalence by age come from a single study [20]. To date, the epidemiological studies have been conducted primarily in Western populations; data from other areas of the world are limited.

In regard to the functional esophageal disorders, the confounding influence of GERD is as much of an issue in evaluating age effects as it is with gender differences. The prevalence of most of these disorders decreases with age. Specifically, globus, rumination syndrome, and self-reported functional chest pain are all more common in younger people [20, 23, 24]. As mentioned earlier, functional heartburn cannot be identified by a symptom survey in the community because of the need for diagnostic testing to exclude GERD. The prevalence of heartburn overall is similar among people ages 25 to 74 [23]. The prevalence of dysphagia in one study increased with age, most notably in participants in the 65–74 year category [23]. The proportion of these people who have functional dysphagia versus another esophageal disorder (e.g., esophageal obstruction or a motility disorder) is not known.

Multiple studies have evaluated the prevalence of dyspepsia in the community. As noted previously, community studies typically do not include endoscopy and thus the diagnosis of functional dyspepsia can only be assumed. Some studies have suggested that the prevalence of dyspepsia decreases with age [35, 196, 197] although the distribution of subtypes (ulcer-like and dysmotility-like) does not vary by age. Young people are slightly more likely to report aerophagia than older people [20, 34]. Vomiting decreases with age [29, 35].

In general, the prevalence of IBS gradually decreases with age [20, 46, 198]. However, among the elderly, the prevalence of IBS was found to increase with age from 8% among those 65 to 74 years to over 12% for those over 85. As opposed to

IBS, much less is known about the epidemiology of bloating. The existing literature is discordant in regard to the changes in the estimates of bloating by age [20, 51].

The prevalence of constipation has been shown to increase with advancing age [56, 199, 200], although one study found that it affects the young and elderly with similar frequency [54]. Less is known regarding functional diarrhea, although one study identified decreasing rates of diarrhea with age [35].

Only one study has assessed the prevalence of chronic functional abdominal pain and sphincter of Oddi dysfunction. The prevalence of chronic functional abdominal pain decreased slightly with age and sphincter of Oddi dysfunction increased with age [20]. Fecal incontinence has been extensively studied and increases with age [26, 56–58]. Functional anorectal pain has decreasing rates with age [20]. The prevalence of rectal outlet delay does not vary by age [62] and outlet delay is more common in women. Finally, prevalence of dyschezia has been reported to be similar by age.

The epidemiologic data are summarized in Table 3. Some FGIDs increase with age and others decrease. The challenge is that these studies do not include diagnostic tests. Thus, they measure symptom reporting rather than being true estimates of the prevalence of the FGIDs. Exclusions are often done based upon self-report, but this is not entirely accurate.

Most of the studies have been of middle-aged populations. However, recent studies have focused on patients at the two extremes of age, children and the elderly. For example, fecal incontinence in particular has been evaluated in the elderly. In general, GI symptoms increase in age from 65 to greater than 85 years [198]. Constipation is the most common symptom. In one report, constipation affected 40% of participants greater than 65 years of age [201]. Certainly investigation would appear warranted before assuming that symptoms in the elderly are due to FGIDs. Surprisingly, elderly participants with these symptoms were not very likely to seek care [29] and thus the exact proportion with a functional disorder is uncertain.

The presence of FGIDs in children is well recognized. For example, rumination syndrome is classically reported in children with decreased mental faculties. However, only recently have studies begun to examine the relationship between GI symptoms in children and adults. The exact age of onset of FGIDs remains to be determined. More information is provided in the chapters specific to pediatric FGIDs.

This section briefly explores how societal stigma and myths may serve to add further stress in individuals suffering from FGIDs in general and IBS in particular. Unless referenced with a specific study, this section is mainly based on theoretical and clinical speculation. Further research will be needed to demonstrate empirical support for these theories.

Functional somatic syndromes have been identified in most medical specialties. These syndromes have been traditionally defined by physical symptoms that have no identified organic cause. In Western societies, there is often a "moral" and pejorative connotation attributed to a functional disorder. It is often contrasted with organic disease and thought to be less legitimate or real. The stigma associated with a functional disorder may lead patients to believe that their problems are treated as "artificial" and due to a psychological or moral defect or weakness [202].

In spite of our growing understanding of "so-called functional somatic disorders" in general and disorders associated with FGID such as IBS in particular, several societal myths persist today. A sampling of these myths associated with IBS include the following: symptoms are trivial or unimportant; symptoms are all in the person's head; IBS is simply caused by stress; IBS is a psychiatric disorder; nothing can help persons with IBS; if pain is severe, there must be an organic cause; patients with IBS may "benefit" from the "sick role;" and people with IBS are difficult patients [203]. The reader is referred to the section on The Patient's Perspective earlier in this chapter for a discussion of how several of these myths affect patients' life experiences along many social domains.

We need to recognize that these societal myths and the stigma associated with IBS in our health care system in particular and society in general can cause further frustration and stress in patients who suffer from IBS. In one study, Letson and Dancey [204] found that nurses held negative attitudes toward people with IBS. The authors reported that if these were communicated to patients with IBS, even in a subtle manner, some patients would feel stigmatized. Since there is no medical explanation for IBS, people in our society who are unaffected by this condition may mistakenly feel that people with IBS are malingerers and hold negative attitudes (204). Social labels may function as an indicator of what is expected of a person as well as influencing self-evaluations [180]. If labels are negative and stigmatizing, self-esteem and self-efficacy (i.e. belief in one's own ability to cope with situations) can be affected [205]. According to Dancey and Backhouse (1997), the social undesirability associated with bowel habits leads people with FGIDs to hide their condition from others because of shame and embarrassment. This may lead to restriction of life experiences including leisure, travel, diet, employment, social life, and sex [206], due in part to the stigma associated with their condition.

In summary, a multitude of social factors may impact the meaning, expression, and course of illnesses. These factors are applicable not only to FGIDs but to functional syndromes in general and are often overlooked by health care providers. Acknowledging and incorporating them into clinical practice will increase the quality of patient care, patient-physician relationship, and health outcomes.

Culture

Health disparities, rooted in race, ethnicity, culture, socioeconomic status, and other factors (including genetics), may develop within society. The interaction between culture and health affects the interpretation and meaning of symptoms, the type of health care, and health outcomes. Cultural/ethnic factors may affect pathophysiology, the patient-physician relationship, the diagnostic process, therapy, and health outcomes. Some population subgroups, including ethnic and racial groups, are more likely to receive suboptimal health care than others and [3] have worse health care outcomes. The concept of health literacy has been coined to describe the skills required to function in the health care environment [207]. Many individuals in cultural subgroups do not have these skills and function with a handicap within the health care system.

Often the importance of cultural factors goes unrecognized. In clinical practice, this can result in poor health outcomes. In research, it can cause methodological shortcomings that lead to biased conclusions and the inappropriate application of research results. In the absence of a substantial body of research and literature on the association between culture and FGIDs, we will review the relationship of culture and health, followed by a discussion of those studies that have been published, and ending with recommendations for further research in the field and the application of appropriate culture-related research methodology to accomplish this objective.

— Definitions

Culture has been defined as a shared system of values, beliefs, and learned patterns of behavior [208] of a particular group that guide thinking, decisions, and actions in a patterned way [209]. Two components have been delineated for cultural processes, heritage and adaptation [210]. Heritage represents the formal and informal transfer of culture from generation to generation. Adaptation is the behavior patterns and coping styles that cultural groups develop collectively in response to the social and physical environment in which they exist, which is not necessarily their native environment.

The terms culture, ethnicity, and race are often used interchangeably. Ethnicity can be thought of as a measure of cultural heritage in contrast to race, which is based more on phenotype (e.g., skin color) [211]. Thus, ethnicity refers more to shared cultural and linguistic characteristics, whereas race refers to a group with a common gene pool in the past [212]. These differences have gray areas of interaction that affect research in the field.

— The Patient's Perspective

From the perspective of the patient the effect of culture can be expressed in illness beliefs [213], perceptions relating to disease and illness, symptom expression, illness behavior including assumption of the sick role, learned coping patterns, and the role of the family in health decisions. Cultural/ethnic factors may also effect pathophysiology, the patient-physician relationship, the diagnostic process [214], therapy [214], and health outcomes [216]. These aspects will be discussed below.

Patients' explanatory models are a useful way to approach their perspective of the health care encounter [217]. Patients have symptom- or disease-related beliefs that affect their concerns, anxieties, and expectations from the health care process. This set of beliefs has been called the explanatory model [218]. Cultural background, socioeconomic status, educational level, and gender are major factors that interact in the development of explanatory models [219].

The explanatory model is particularly important in the treatment of patients with FGIDs in which the physician-patient relationship is a critical part of the therapy. Thus it is very important to elicit the patient's explanatory model, to understand the cultural background in which it developed, and to negotiate a treatment partnership that will be effective within the context of the patient's and the medical team's beliefs and attitudes [220].

— Effect of Culture on Health Outcomes

Studies have shown that the cultural/ethnic background can affect the diagnostic process and health outcomes. In a series of studies, Dimsdale found that patient ethnicity exerts an enormous influence on doctors' behavior in ordering diagnostic studies as well as on the medications prescribed [214]. He states that the social circumstances of the doctor and patient cast a large shadow on treatment. Doctors apparently have preconceived notions about patients' needs for medication that are tied to ethnicity and not to the illness per se [214, 215].

Some population subgroups, including ethnic groups, are more likely to receive suboptimal health care than others [216]. Many individuals in cultural subgroups do not have the skills required to function in the health care environment. Limited literacy skills, particularly in a second language, may lead to difficulty understanding diagnoses, discharge instructions, and treatment recommendations. These difficulties may put patients at risk for noncompliance with treatment regimes and for adverse reactions [221, 222] that lead to poor health outcomes.

— The Health Care Providers' Perspective

From the health care providers' perspective, an important culture-related factor is cultural competence. This concept relates to the ability of the medical staff to function optimally under cross-cultural circumstances. This skill is gaining in importance because of the multicultural background of patients in many medical practices, both community and hospital-based. Cultural competence includes overcoming any language barrier (linguistic competence) and an understanding of the cultural background from which the patient comes and within which he/she develops explanatory models of illness. Thus knowledge of the language and of the cultural background is essential for the development of cultural competence [223]. All physician-patient encounters have the potential for cross-cultural misunderstanding. Issues that may lead to these misunderstandings and their unwanted consequences include differing or even conflicting attitudes relating to authority, physical contact, communication style, gender, sexuality, and family, among other sensitive subjects [220]. The development of cultural competence should have high priority in medical education and in the training of the medical and allied teams.

— The Research Perspective

In discussing cross-cultural research, two relevant, but different, settings should be considered. One is cross-cultural comparison among individuals in two or more cultural groups, all in their native surroundings. For example, a comparative study of the epidemiology of IBS in different countries would be in this category. The second is the study of cultural minorities and immigrant populations who are not living in their native surroundings. In this case the component of adaptation mentioned above comes into play alongside that of heritage. An example of this might be the comparison of bowel habits and health care-seeking behavior related to bowel habits conducted in Texas between Hispanic and non-Hispanic adults [224, 225].

Selection bias is a serious problem in studies of ethnic minorities that are frequently under-represented in clinical trials [226] because of difficulties in sampling and in recruiting sufficient numbers of subjects [227]. Selection bias is made more complex by the possibility that some sections of the population may change their ethnic affiliation. A study conducted in 1971–1972 found that one third of the U.S. population reported a different racial or ethnic status one year after their initial interview [228]. Another issue is mixed parentage. What ethnic status should be assigned to these individuals? This question is very significant in countries where ethnic or racial intermarriage is common (e.g., Sephardim and Ashkenazim among Jews, blacks and whites in many places in the world).

Even when a cross-cultural study is well designed to compare population subgroups, some groups may be more difficult to recruit and/or more difficult to survey in a representative population sample than others. For example, in a comparative study of the epidemiology of IBS among Israeli Jews, Israeli Bedouins, and Israeli non-Bedouin Arabs, it was much more difficult to obtain a representative sample of the non-Jewish subpopulations. Another problem is that even when participation rates among subgroups are reasonable, individuals who agree to participate in studies are likely to be more literate and more fluent in the study language than those who do not [227]. It has been shown, for example, that patients who do not speak English are typically excluded, either explicitly or implicitly, from English-language studies in which patient reported data are collected on forms [229].

The term cross-cultural research competence can be used to describe the skill required to conduct research involving population subgroups of differing cultural and ethnic backgrounds. This includes culturally appropriate research design and methods and culturally suitable study instruments that have been appropriately translated into and validated in other languages [230, 231]. Since cross-cultural studies are increasing in number it is imperative that investigators gain cross-cultural research competence. In drug trials one should keep in mind potential differences between ethnic groups in terms of response to drugs, metabolism of drugs, concurrent diseases, and contraindications [232].

It is often difficult to distinguish between effects of culture and social class, a potential confounder, since large proportions of some ethnic groups may belong to specific social strata, often of low socioeconomic status. An example of this is seen in studies of cultural differences between Sephardic and Ashkenazi Jews in Israel. Sephardim have been found to have increased expression of stress in physical terms [233] and are more likely to seek medical help in stressful times [234]. However, these subgroups are also distinguished on socioeconomic terms with Sephardim representing a lower status than Ashkenazim, so the cultural differences may be confounded by socioeconomic ones [235, 236]. Since there is a strong association between social class and race/ethnicity, studies of ethnic/racial differences should control for socioeconomic status [237].

— Cross-Cultural Studies of Functional GI Disorders

There is an area of overlap between epidemiological and cross-cultural studies on IBS in two respects: (1) prevalence rates can be compared across ethnic groups provided that the methodology is similar enough to make the results comparable, and (2) many studies also look at health behavior, health-related beliefs, and health care-seeking behavior, all of which may be affected by cultural affiliation. Thus most of the studies reviewed below are epidemiological by design.

The majority of published studies on IBS, particularly in relation to health-related behavior and health care seeking, are ethnocentric in that they concentrate on predominantly white populations, usually from the United States and Europe. However, some studies have focused on ethnic comparisons assessing the effects of culture-related factors. A major difficulty in reviewing and comparing the results of these studies is the lack of uniformity in research methodology, composition of study population, sampling methods, and diagnostic criteria (from no specific criteria for IBS in early studies to variations of the Manning criteria and through to Rome I and Rome II).

Zuckerman et al. conducted a comparative study of IBS among Hispanic and non-Hispanic whites in Texas, USA in which they studied prevalence rates and investigated ethnic differences such as health care-seeking patterns and health-related behaviors [224, 225]. The difference between the two groups in IBS prevalence, using Manning and Rome I criteria, was not statistically significant after the investigators controlled for factors such as gender, age, socioeconomic status, diet, and use of laxatives. Significant differences were found in relation to dietary habits (intake of coffee, beans, and chili) and laxative use. Hispanics also tended to self-medicate with folk remedies for relief of their bowel problems rather than turning to the health care system [225]. They also had a poorer perception of their general health condition and expressed greater concern about their health in general and about their bowel problems in particular. The investigators concluded that ethnicity determines, in part, the perception of health and bowel function and affects health care behavior in relation to these perceptions [225].

A newly published study compared rates of IBS between Israeli Bedouins still living under rural conditions with those who resettled in permanent towns [238]. Half of Israeli Bedouin society has undergone this transition over the last 35 years, causing cultural and social upheaval. Integration of the Bedouin population into the general Israeli society has been a prolonged, painful process. It is affected by cultural and socioeconomic factors, government policy, and Bedouin heritage. Many Bedouin values and norms have been upset by the transition, which has associated increases in poverty, substance abuse and crime, and has led to stress at the individual and societal levels and, in some cases, to an identity crisis. The prevalence of IBS among Bedouins who resettled in permanent towns was found to be significantly higher than those still living in traditional rural settings (9.4% vs.

5.8%, p<0.01). Although it is tempting to attribute these differences to the stressful circumstances of the transition, such a conclusion cannot be fully based on the data from the study. Other possible explanations include changes in nutrition and other lifestyle variables, such as differences in health care-seeking behavior.

Few studies have been conducted on IBS in Africa. Reports of IBS prevalence from Kenya and Nigeria highlight some of the problems in making comparisons and drawing conclusions among studies. The Kenyan study, which reported a prevalence of IBS of 8%, was a retrospective review of files of consecutive patients presenting with abdominal pain with normal investigations, and the diagnosis of IBS was based on the Manning criteria [239]. The study population was highly selected. In this study more men had IBS than women. The Nigerian study, which was also based on the Manning criteria, reported a prevalence rate of 30%. However the study population, comprised of native African medical students, was highly selected and unrepresentative of the general population [240].

Information on the prevalence of IBS and sociocultural factors associated with it in Asian countries has also been scant. A study was conducted in Singapore among the Chinese, Malay, and Indian subgroups, to assess the prevalence of IBS and any ethnic differences [241]. The overall prevalence of IBS was 2.3%, much lower than most estimates in Western countries. Also in contrast to most reports from the West, the majority of respondents went to physicians for their symptoms. No ethnic differences were found among the three ethnic subgroups. A similar rate of IBS was found in a study conducted in Hong Kong among ethnic Chinese subjects [242] that reported a prevalence of 4.1% using the Rome I criteria. Similar to reports from the West, IBS was associated with anxiety, depression, medical consultation, sick leave, and impaired quality of life. Similarly low prevalence rates were reported in a study from Thailand [243] among rural villagers and hotel employees, and among Asian Americans in a US study [38]. In the latter study using the Manning criteria, Asian ethnicity was a negative predictor of IBS in the overall study population of HMO members. In contrast, a Chinese study [244] reported a prevalence rate of 23% for IBS. However, that study was conducted among a highly selected population of hospital employees and elderly patients. A study conducted in China tested the possibility that Chinese differ from Westerners in physiological factors associated with IBS [245]. The rationale behind the study was that since there are differences in terms of culture, diet, and physical environment, there might also be differences in pathophysiological findings. To test this hypothesis the investigators evaluated psychological profiles and tested autonomic nervous system function in Chinese IBS patients. Similar to reports from the West, they found that patients with IBS with constipation had abnormal vagal cholinergic function. However, in contrast with the West, their diarrhea-predominant patients did not have abnormal adrenergic function and they found no associations between autonomic dysfunction and psychological variables. The authors proposed that cultural differences could account for some of these findings, but clearly further studies are required. A study from Iran [246] compared IBS in male rural nomads and industrial workers. The rates were 3.1% and 3.6%, respectively. A study from Bangadalesh [247] with a large representative population of rural residents showed that the prevalence of IBS, the gender distribution, and the pattern of health care seeking for individuals meeting the Rome I criteria for IBS were similar to those reported from the West.

In contrast, often quoted early studies of the epidemiology of IBS from India [248, 249] highlight some of the potential problems associated with the cultural interpretation applied to study results. In these studies the prevalence of IBS was found to be higher among men than women. This result has been interpreted to be representative of a significant cultural difference in health care-seeking behavior between Indians and others. However, these studies were based on clinic populations that are not necessarily representative of the Indian population at large, so such broad-ranging conclusions are probably unwarranted in this case.

A cross-cultural study of response to occupational stressors in relation to gender and nationality was conducted among Brazilian and American professionals [250]. One of the disorders assessed was IBS, in which the investigators report a higher incidence among Americans compared to Brazilians.

Taub et al. [40] conducted a factor analysis among male and female African-American and Caucasian psychology students to assess whether the three core Manning criteria have equal applicability to both genders and races. They reported that African Americans had more constipation, straining, and milk intolerance, while Caucasians had more diarrhea, nausea, and vomiting. However the Manning criteria were similar in both races and race made no difference in the criteria for IBS (16.9% for African Americans and 15.0% for Caucasians). The authors state that the differences found could reflect unmeasured confounders such as socioeconomic status and diet.

A recent study was designed to assess possible racial differences among IBS patients. White and nonwhite IBS patients were compared using the generic Short Form (SF)-36 HRQoL assessment [257]. Patients who were unable to read or understand English were excluded (see comment above). The nonwhite population was mixed (African American, Hispanic, Asian American and a few native Americans and others), which could also bias the results, especially since the study was underpowered for subgroup comparisons. The whites may also have been a heterogeneous group (socioeconomic status, religion, etc.), but this information is not provided. Interestingly, differences that were initially found between the races disappeared when the data were adjusted for age, gender, income, and education. These results not only shed light on potential racial differences among IBS patients, but highlight the importance of taking other confounders into careful consideration before drawing conclusions.

Summary

The prevalence of IBS appears to be lower in non-Western countries. This difference may reflect a true cultural or biological phenomenon or stem from methodological differences such as the difficulties in carrying out population studies in some of these countries. Recognition and understanding of the association between culture and health is important for the treatment of FGID patients as well as for research in the field. In order to integrate this factor into clinical and research practices it is necessary to develop clinical cultural competence and cross-cultural research competence. These skills should enable clinicians and researchers to make greater advances in their respective areas of interest.

Methodological Issues in FGIDs

Due to methodological issues limiting interpretation of studies, there remain many unanswered questions concerning gender, age, society, culture, and patient's perspective in FGIDs. Due to the female predominance and greater likelihood of women to participate in research studies, there are insufficient numbers of male participants to make meaningful interpretations and adequately assess gender differences in psychological, physiological, and treatment studies. Another major methodological concern is that most studies have involved a cross-sectional design, which limits the more comprehensive understanding of the pathogenesis, development, course, and impact of these disorders in men and women.

— Epidemiological Studies

While much is known about IBS, abdominal pain, and bowel habits in the Western world, epidemiologic data regarding differences in men and women in several of the other FGIDs in the various patient (primary care, secondary, and tertiary care centers) and nonpatient (community) populations is lacking. Furthermore, there are several methodological factors in those studies which may affect their uniformity and validity. For example, the population setting, sociocultural influences, sample sizes of age, sex, and ethnic subgroups, response rates, the study instruments used (linguistically and culturally sensitive), the method of administration (interview vs. mailed questionnaires, etc.), the diagnostic criteria used (e.g., Manning, Rome I, Rome II, Rome III), and the validity and applicability of these criteria can all have an effect.

— Physiological Studies

Many of the issues raised for epidemiological studies are also applicable to physiologic studies. For example, patient populations are heterogeneous but many physiologic studies include relatively small sample sizes and do not account for psychosocial variables, overlapping FGIDs, or comorbidities, and therefore may not apply to the general patient population. Furthermore, the results of these studies may be influenced by the selection bias of participants who are willing to undergo invasive research protocols.

Before determining if there are sex-based differences in both physiological and psychosocial studies in FGIDs, comparison studies in the healthy population need to be performed. Some of the reported differences in patients with FGIDs may be due mainly to sex differences in health that carry over into the patient population. Another methodological issue involves the assessment of physiologic responses at basal conditions as compared to a stress-induced state. Stress is believed to play a major role in the pathophysiology and clinical presentation of FGIDs and is associated with symptom onset, exacerbation, and severity [63]. Sex differences may not be present at baseline, but may only be measurable following a stressor.

Translating the various mechanisms of pain and GI function from animal studies to humans can be a challenging task. Differences in the type and strain of the animal model and type of stressor, if used, need to be taken into account when interpreting these studies. In addition, studying female animals is especially daunting because the estrus cycle (i.e., proestrus, oestrus, metestrus, and diestrus phases) needs to be controlled for. Furthermore, in order to evaluate the roles of estrogen and progesterone, females are often studied postoophorectomy and following the administration of estrogen and/or progesterone.

Similarly, for women, the menstrual cycle needs to be considered in studies. In most studies, menstrual phase is frequently not determined, or is assessed by the count forward/backward method and not by measuring the leutinizing hormone surge to more accurately assess the follicular and luteal phases. Other confounding methodological issues which may affect outcome measures and therefore need to be considered when conducting and/or interpreting data in women include the use of oral contraceptive agents, hormonal replacement therapy, and pre- vs. postmenopausal women. The impact of the transition from a premenopausal to perimenopausal state to menopause on GI function and FGID symptoms remains unknown.

— Psychological and Sociological Studies

Most studies examining psychological factors have focused on anxiety and depression and, to a lesser extent, on personality traits. Other aspects of psychological functioning such as quality of relationships, social support, health perceptions, traumatic and stressful events, and effects of childhood experience other than abuse have been largely ignored in studies comparing men and women. Other sociological determinants of health that have not been systematically investigated include HRQoL, socialization, social exclusion, work and unemployment, and socioeconomic status. Very little work has been examined in FGIDs to understand the role of the patient-physician relationship in influencing outcome. Most studies have examined illness experience from the perspective of the health care provider and not the patient.

— Treatment Responses

Adequate sample sizes of each sex, particularly men, and comparable treatment doses must be obtained to determine if men and women respond similarly to treatment. There may be gender and/or cultural differences in placebo response. Complete dose-response studies should be performed in clinical trials where gender differences are observed or expected, since the optimal doses of these medications may differ in men and women. Patients for clinical trials are generally recruited from specialty practices where women are more likely to be referred than men [251], thus compounding problems of selection bias.

— Gender Role versus Biological Sex of Study Participants

Studies investigating differences and similarities between men and women with IBS have focused on distinctions based on the biological sex of study participants. An alternate way of approaching gender differences research is to distinguish the impact of gender role from biological sex [19]. Future studies will need to have adequate numbers of men with gender-related variables such as history of abuse, anxiety, or depression [252]. In those studies, the sex differences could possibly disappear as research identifies more gender-related variables.

Conclusion

This chapter has reviewed the literature regarding the relationship between gender, age, society, and culture and FGIDs. Particular emphasis has been placed on the patient's perspective. A conceptual model for the interaction of these factors is shown in Figure 2. The model is adapted from the one discussed in the Psychosocial Aspects of FGIDs chapter. As demonstrated in the modified model, this chapter emphasizes: (1) the importance of the patient's experience and perspective, (2) the influence of society, culture, gender, and age on all aspects of the individual's experience, (3) the influential role of an individual's sex on the biologic and physiologic processes of brain-gut interactions, and (4) the potential of the health care provider in influencing patient outcome.

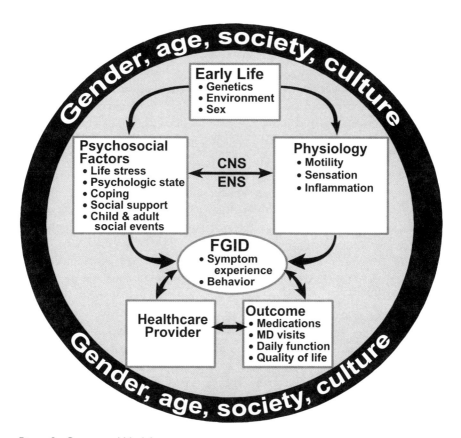

Figure 2. Conceptual Model
Expanded model for the development of functional gastrointestinal disorders that incorporates cultural and biopsychosocial factors.
CNS = central nervous system   ENS = enteric nervous system

To advance the field of FGIDs, the following are suggested:

From a research perspective
1. Studies using quantitative and qualitative methods to better understand the patient's illness experience and their views of the health care system.
2. Studies of varied populations around the world with appropriate tools to measure cultural and societal influences.
3. Studies evaluating sufficient numbers of men with IBS and comparing healthy men and women to determine if gender differences in FGIDs are disease-specific.
4. Studies to identify positive aspects of patient-provider interactions that improve outcome—including recognition of patient's perspective, cultural and gender sensitivity—and implementation of them in patient care programs.

From a clinical practice perspective
1. Recognize that FGID patients view their conditions as illnesses associated with uncertainty, stigma, and social isolation. Physicians can help patients manage their condition by eliciting and addressing patient concerns, offering a positive diagnosis, providing clear, understandable, and legitimizing explanations of the disorder, and by helping to identify factors within the context of the patient's own illness that they can influence and control.
2. A number of sex- and gender-related factors may impact the clinical symptoms and response to treatment of IBS and should be considered (e.g., gender role, sociocultural differences, hormonal effects such as menstrual cycle variation, and biologic differences influencing gut function and treatment response).
3. Both men and women in clinical settings have psychological issues that may need to be addressed. There is a possibility that men may not do as well with psychological treatment in comparison with women.
4. Recognition and understanding of the association between culture and health are also important for patient care. It may be helpful to discuss with patients any cultural issues that may have an impact on their clinical presentation or management of their condition. In addition, medical training and continuing medical education should include and emphasize cross-cultural competencies.

References

1. Royer A. Life with chronic illness: social and psychological dimensions. Westport, CT: Praeger Publishers, 1998.
2. Bertram S, Kurland M, Lydick E, Locke GR, III, Yawn BP. The patient's perspective of irritable bowel syndrome. J Fam Pract 2001;50:521–525.
3. IFFGD. IBS in the real world survey. 2002. Milwaukee, WI, IFFGD.
4. Whitehead WE, Levy RL, Von Korff M, Feld AD, Palsson OS, Turner M, Drossman DA. The usual medical care for irritable bowel syndrome. Aliment Pharmacol Ther 2004;20:1305–1315.
5. Drossman DA. The functional gastrointestinal disorders and the Rome II process. In: Drossman DA, Corazziari E, Talley NJ, and et al, eds. Rome II. The Functional Gastrointestinal Disorders, Pathophysiology and Treatment: A Multinational Consensus. 2nd ed. McLean, VA: Degnon Associates, 2000:1–30.
6. The patient perspective (Internet) Milwaukee, WI. IFFGD (U.S.). 2003.
7. Brashers DE, Neidig JL, Reynolds NR, Haas SM. Uncertainty in illness across the HIV/AIDS trajectory. J Assoc Nurses AIDS Care 1998;9:66–77.
8. Kreps GL, Ruben BD, Baker MW, Rosenthal SR. Survey of public knowledge about digestive health and diseases: implications for health education. Public Health Rep 1987;102:270–277.
9. Crocker J, Major B, Steele C. Social Stigma. In: Gilbert D, Fiske ST, and Lindzey G, eds. Handbook of social psychology. 4th ed. Boston: McGraw Hill, 1998:504–553.
10. Dixon-Woods M, Critchley S. Medical and lay views of irritable bowel syndrome. Fam Pract 2000;17:108–113.
11. Thompson WG, Heaton KW, Smyth GT, Smyth C. Irritable bowel syndrome in general practice: prevalence, characteristics, and referral. Gut 2000;46:78–82.
12. Salmon P, Peters S, Stanley I. Patients' perceptions of medical explanations for somatisation disorders: qualitative analysis. BMJ 1999;318:372–376.
13. Mabeck CE, Olesen F. Metaphorically transmitted diseases. How do patients embody medical explanations? Fam Pract 1997;14:271–278.
14. Gladman LM, Gorard DA. General practitioner and hospital specialist attitudes to functional gastrointestinal disorders. Aliment Pharmacol Ther 2003;17:651–654.
15. Bodenheimer T, Wagner EH, Grumbach K. Improving primary care for patients with chronic illness: the chronic care model, Part 2. JAMA 2002;288:1909–1914.
16. Kennedy A, Robinson A, Rogers A. Incorporating patients' views and experiences of life with IBS in the development of an evidence based self-help guidebook. Patient Educ Couns 2003;50:303–310.
17. Weyland CM, Wortmann R, Weyland C, Klippel J. Primer on the Rheumatic Diseases: An Official Publication of the Arthritis Foundation. 1998. Longstreet Press.
18. Bodenheimer T, Lorig K, Holman H, Grumbach K. Patient self-management of chronic disease in primary care. JAMA 2002;288:2469–2475.
19. Lips H. Sex and Gender. Mountainview, CA: Mayfield Publishing, 1997.
20. Drossman DA, Li Z, Andruzzi E, Temple RD, Talley NJ, Thompson WG, Whitehead WE, Janssens J, Funch-Jensen P, Corazziari E. U.S. householder survey of functional gastrointestinal disorders. Prevalence, sociodemography, and health impact. Dig Dis Sci 1993;38:1569–1580.

21. Locke GR, III. The epidemiology of functional gastrointestinal disorders in North America. Gastroenterol Clin North Am 1996;25:1–19.

22. Koloski NA, Talley NJ, Boyce PM. Does psychological distress modulate functional gastrointestinal symptoms and health care seeking? A prospective, community Cohort study. Am J Gastroenterol 2003;98:789–797.

23. Locke GR, III, Talley NJ, Fett SL, Zinsmeister AR, Melton LJ, III. Prevalence and clinical spectrum of gastroesophageal reflux: a population-based study in Olmsted County, Minnesota. Gastroenterology 1997;112:1448–1456.

24. Eslick GD, Jones MP, Talley NJ. Non-cardiac chest pain: prevalence, risk factors, impact and consulting—a population-based study. Aliment Pharmacol Ther 2003; 17:1115–1124.

25. Cormier LE, Katon W, Russo J, Hollifield M, Hall ML, Vitaliano PP. Chest pain with negative cardiac diagnostic studies. Relationship to psychiatric illness. J Nerv Ment Dis 1988;176:351–358.

26. Ter RB. Gender differences in gastroesophageal reflux disease. J Gend Specif Med 2000;3:42–44.

27. Ter RB, Johnston BT, Castell DO. Influence of age and gender on gastroesophageal reflux in symptomatic patients. Dis Esophagus 1998;11:106–108.

28. Fass R, Sampliner RE, Mackel C, McGee D, Rappaport W. Age- and gender-related differences in 24-hour esophageal pH monitoring of normal subjects. Dig Dis Sci 1993;38:1926–1928.

29. Talley NJ, Zinsmeister AR, Schleck CD, Melton LJ, III. Dyspepsia and dyspepsia subgroups: a population-based study. Gastroenterology 1992;102:1259–1268.

30. Talley NJ, Stanghellini V, Heading RC, Koch KL, Malagelada JR, Tytgat GN. Functional gastroduodenal disorders. Gut 1999;45 Suppl 2:II37–II42.

31. Talley NJ, Verlinden M, Jones M. Can symptoms discriminate among those with delayed or normal gastric emptying in dysmotility-like dyspepsia? Am J Gastroenterol 2001;96:1422–1428.

32. Stanghellini V, Tosetti C, Paternic inverted question mA, Barbara G, Morselli-Labate AM, Monetti N, Marengo M, Corinaldesi R. Risk indicators of delayed gastric emptying of solids in patients with functional dyspepsia. Gastroenterology 1996; 110:1036–1042.

33. Strid H, Norstrom M, Sjoberg J, Simren M, Svedlund J, Abrahamsson H, Bjornsson ES. Impact of sex and psychological factors on the water loading test in functional dyspepsia. Scand J Gastroenterol 2001;36:725–730.

34. Frexinos J, Denis P, Allemand H, Allouche S, Los F, Bonnelye G. [Descriptive study of digestive functional symptoms in the French general population]. Gastroenterol Clin Biol 1998;22:785–791.

35. Agreus L, Svardsudd K, Nyren O, Tibblin G. The epidemiology of abdominal symptoms: prevalence and demographic characteristics in a Swedish adult population. A report from the Abdominal Symptom Study. Scand J Gastroenterol 1994;29:102–109.

36. Talley NJ, Zinsmeister AR, Van Dyke C, Melton LJ, III. Epidemiology of colonic symptoms and the irritable bowel syndrome. Gastroenterology 1991;101:927–934.

37. Sandler RS. Epidemiology of irritable bowel syndrome in the United States. Gastroenterology 1990;99:409–415.

38. Longstreth GF, Wolde-Tsadik G. Irritable bowel-type symptoms in HMO examinees. Prevalence, demographics, and clinical correlates. Dig Dis Sci 1993;38:1581–1589.

39. van der Horst HE, van Dulmen AM, Schellevis FG, van Eijk JT, Fennis JF, Bleijenberg G. Do patients with irritable bowel syndrome in primary care really differ from outpatients with irritable bowel syndrome? Gut 1997;41:669–674.

40. Taub E, Cuevas JL, Cook EW, III, Crowell M, Whitehead WE. Irritable bowel syndrome defined by factor analysis. Gender and race comparisons. Dig Dis Sci 1995;40:2647–2655.

41. Simren M, Abrahamsson H, Svedlund J, Bjornsson ES. Quality of life in patients with irritable bowel syndrome seen in referral centers versus primary care: the impact of gender and predominant bowel pattern. Scand J Gastroenterol 2001;36:545–552.

42. Talley NJ, Boyce P, Jones M. Identification of distinct upper and lower gastrointestinal symptom groupings in an urban population. Gut 1998;42:690–695.

43. Corney RH, Stanton R. Physical symptom severity, psychological and social dysfunction in a series of outpatients with irritable bowel syndrome. J Psychosom Res 1990;34:483–491.

44. Lee OY, Mayer EA, Schmulson M, Chang L, Naliboff B. Gender-related differences in IBS symptoms. Am J Gastroenterol 2001;96:2184–2193.

45. Camilleri M. Management of the irritable bowel syndrome. Gastroenterology 2001; 120:652–668.

46. Talley NJ, Zinsmeister AR, Melton LJ, III. Irritable bowel syndrome in a community: symptom subgroups, risk factors, and health care utilization. Am J Epidemiol 1995;142:76–83.

47. Whitehead WE, Cheskin LJ, Heller BR, Robinson JC, Crowell MD, Benjamin C, Schuster MM. Evidence for exacerbation of irritable bowel syndrome during menses. Gastroenterology 1990;98:1485–1489.

48. Crowell MD, Dubin NH, Robinson JC, Cheskin LJ, Schuster MM, Heller BR, Whitehead WE. Functional bowel disorders in women with dysmenorrhea. Am J Gastroenterol 1994;89:1973–1977.

49. Heitkemper MM, Jarrett M, Cain KC, Shaver J, Walker E, Lewis L. Daily gastrointestinal symptoms in women with and without a diagnosis of IBS. Dig Dis Sci 1995; 40:1511–1519.

50. Heitkemper MM, Cain KC, Jarrett ME, Burr RL, Hertig V, Bond EF. Symptoms across the menstrual cycle in women with irritable bowel syndrome. Am J Gastroenterol 2003;98:420–430.

51. Sandler RS, Stewart WF, Liberman JN, Ricci JA, Zorich NL. Abdominal pain, bloating, and diarrhea in the United States: prevalence and impact. Dig Dis Sci 2000; 45:1166–1171.

52. Everhart JE, Go VL, Johannes RS, Fitzsimmons SC, Roth HP, White LR. A longitudinal survey of self-reported bowel habits in the United States. Dig Dis Sci 1989;34:1153–1162.

53. Stewart WF, Liberman JN, Sandler RS, Woods MS, Stemhagen A, Chee E, Lipton RB, Farup CE. Epidemiology of constipation (EPOC) study in the United States: relation of clinical subtypes to sociodemographic features. Am J Gastroenterol 1999;94:3530–3540.

54. Pare P, Ferrazzi S, Thompson WG, Irvine EJ, Rance L. An epidemiological survey of constipation in canada: definitions, rates, demographics, and predictors of health care seeking. Am J Gastroenterol 2001;96:3130–3137.

55. Talley NJ, Weaver AL, Zinsmeister AR, Melton LJ, III. Self-reported diarrhea: what does it mean? Am J Gastroenterol 1994;89:1160–1164.

56. Chen GD, Hu SW, Chen YC, Lin TL, Lin LY. Prevalence and correlations of anal incontinence and constipation in Taiwanese women. Neurourol Urodyn 2003;22:664–669.

57. Lynch AC, Dobbs BR, Keating J, Frizelle FA. The prevalence of faecal incontinence and constipation in a general New Zealand population; a postal survey. N Z Med J 2001;114:474–477.

58. Rizk DE, Hassan MY, Shaheen H, Cherian JV, Micallef R, Dunn E. The prevalence and determinants of health care-seeking behavior for fecal incontinence in multiparous United Arab Emirates females. Dis Colon Rectum 2001;44:1850–1856.

59. Nelson R, Furner S, Jesudason V. Fecal incontinence in Wisconsin nursing homes: prevalence and associations. Dis Colon Rectum 1998;41:1226–1229.

60. Edwards NI, Jones D. The prevalence of faecal incontinence in older people living at home. Age Ageing 2001;30:503–507.

61. Walter S, Hallbook O, Gotthard R, Bergmark M, Sjodahl R. A population-based study on bowel habits in a Swedish community: prevalence of faecal incontinence and constipation. Scand J Gastroenterol 2002;37:911–916.

62. Talley NJ, Weaver AL, Zinsmeister AR, Melton LJ, III. Functional constipation and outlet delay: a population-based study. Gastroenterology 1993;105:781–790.

63. Mayer EA, Naliboff BD, Chang L, Coutinho SV. V. Stress and irritable bowel syndrome. Am J Physiol Gastrointest Liver Physiol 2001;280:G519–G524.

64. Berkley KJ. Sex differences in pain. Behav Brain Sci 1997;20:371–380.

65. Riley JL, III, Robinson ME, Wise EA, Myers CD, Fillingim RB. Sex differences in the perception of noxious experimental stimuli: a meta-analysis. Pain 1998;74:181–187.

66. Nguyen P, Lee SD, Castell DO. Evidence of gender differences in esophageal pain threshold. Am J Gastroenterol 1995;90:901–905.

67. Rao SS, Mudipalli RS, Mujica VR, Patel RS, Zimmerman B. Effects of gender and age on esophageal biomechanical properties and sensation. Am J Gastroenterol 2003; 98:1688–1695.

68. Soffer EE, Kongara K, Achkar JP, Gannon J. Colonic motor function in humans is not affected by gender. Dig Dis Sci 2000;45:1281–1284.

69. Chang L, Mayer EA, Labus J, Schmulson M, Lee OY, Olivas TI, Stains J, Naliboff BD. Effect of sex on perception of rectosigmoid stimuli in irritable bowel syndrome. Am J Physiol—Regul Integr Comp Physiol 2006; in press.

70. Paterson WG, Wang H, Vanner SJ. Increasing pain sensation to repeated esophageal balloon distension in patients with chest pain of undetermined etiology. Dig Dis Sci 1995;40:1325–1331.

71. Tack J, Caenepeel P, Fischler B, Piessevaux H, Janssens J. Symptoms associated with hypersensitivity to gastric distention in functional dyspepsia. Gastroenterology 2001;121:526–535.

72. Whitehead WE, Holtkotter B, Enck P, Hoelzl R, Holmes KD, Anthony J, Shabsin HS, Schuster MM. Tolerance for rectosigmoid distention in irritable bowel syndrome. Gastroenterology 1990;98:1187–1192.

73. Ritchie J. Pain from distension of the pelvic colon by inflating a balloon in the irritable colon syndrome. Gut 1973;14:125–132.

74. Munakata J, Naliboff B, Harraf F, Kodner A, Lembo T, Chang L, Silverman DH, Mayer EA. Repetitive sigmoid stimulation induces rectal hyperalgesia in patients with irritable bowel syndrome. Gastroenterology 1997;112:55–63.

75. Naliboff BD, Munakata J, Fullerton S, Gracely RH, Kodner A, Harraf F, Mayer EA.

Evidence for two distinct perceptual alterations in irritable bowel syndrome. Gut 1997;41:505–512.

76. Bouin M, Plourde V, Boivin M, Riberdy M, Lupien F, Laganiere M, Verrier P, Poitras P. Rectal distention testing in patients with irritable bowel syndrome: sensitivity, specificity, and predictive values of pain sensory thresholds. Gastroenterology 2002;122:1771–1777.

77. Ragnarsson G, Hallbook O, Bodemar G. Abdominal symptoms are not related to anorectal function in the irritable bowel syndrome. Scand J Gastroenterol 1999;34:250–258.

78. Chang L, Naliboff B, Schmulson M, Lee OY, Olivas TI, Mayer EA. The role of gender and bowel habit predominance on visceral perception in IBS. Gastroenterology 120 [A755]. 2001. Ref Type: Abstract

79. Holtmann G, Goebell H, Talley NJ. Functional dyspepsia and irritable bowel syndrome: is there a common pathophysiological basis? Am J Gastroenterol 1997;92: 954–959.

80. Teff KL, Alavi A, Chen J, Pourdehnad M, Townsend RR. Muscarinic blockade inhibits gastric emptying of mixed-nutrient meal: effects of weight and gender. Am J Physiol 1999;276:R707–R714.

81. Metcalf AM, Phillips SF, Zinsmeister AR, MacCarty RL, Beart RW, Wolff BG. Simplified assessment of segmental colonic transit. Gastroenterology 1987;92:40–47.

82. Meier R, Beglinger C, Dederding JP, Meyer-Wyss B, Fumagalli M, Rowedder A, Turberg Y, Brignoli R. Influence of age, gender, hormonal status and smoking habits on colonic transit time. Neurogastroenterol Motil 1995;7:235–238.

83. Lampe JW, Fredstrom SB, Slavin JL, Potter JD. Sex differences in colonic function: a randomised trial. Gut 1993;34:531–536.

84. Hinds JP, Stoney B, Wald A. Does gender or the menstrual cycle affect colonic transit? Am J Gastroenterol 1989;84:123–126.

85. Cremonini F, Mullan BP, Camilleri M, Burton DD, Rank MR. Performance characteristics of scintigraphic transit measurements for studies of experimental therapies. Aliment Pharmacol Ther 2002;16:1781–1790.

86. Rao SS, Sadeghi P, Beaty J, Kavlock R, Ackerson K. Ambulatory 24-h colonic manometry in healthy humans. Am J Physiol Gastrointest Liver Physiol 2001;280: G629–G639.

87. Sun WM, Read NW. Anorectal function in normal human subjects: effect of gender. Int J Colorectal Dis 1989;4:188–196.

88. Tillisch K, Mayer EA, Labus JS, Stains J, Chang L, Naliboff B. Gender-specific alterations in autonomic function among patients with irritable bowel syndrome. Gut 2005;54:1396–1401.

89. Rabinowicz T, Petetot JM, Gartside PS, Sheyn D, Sheyn T, de CM. Structure of the cerebral cortex in men and women. J Neuropathol Exp Neurol 2002;61:46–57.

90. Van Laere KJ, Dierckx RA. Brain perfusion SPECT: age- and sex-related effects correlated with voxel-based morphometric findings in healthy adults. Radiology 2001; 221:810–817.

91. Killgore WD, Yurgelun-Todd DA. Sex differences in amygdala activation during the perception of facial affect. Neuroreport 2001;12:2543–2547.

92. Kern MK, Jaradeh S, Arndorfer RC, Jesmanowicz A, Hyde J, Shaker R. Gender differences in cortical representation of rectal distension in healthy humans. Am J Physiol Gastrointest Liver Physiol 2001;281:G1512–G1523.

93. Silverman DH, Munakata JA, Ennes H, Mandelkern MA, Hoh CK, Mayer EA. Regional cerebral activity in normal and pathological perception of visceral pain. Gastroenterology 1997;112:64–72.

94. Naliboff BD, Derbyshire SW, Munakata J, Berman S, Mandelkern M, Chang L, Mayer EA. Cerebral activation in patients with irritable bowel syndrome and control subjects during rectosigmoid stimulation. Psychosom Med 2001;63:365–375.

95. Mertz H, Morgan V, Tanner G, Pickens D, Price R, Shyr Y, Kessler R. Regional cerebral activation in irritable bowel syndrome and control subjects with painful and nonpainful rectal distention. Gastroenterology 2000;118:842–848.

96. Bernstein CN, Frankenstein UN, Rawsthorne P, Pitz M, Summers R, McIntyre MC. Cortical mapping of visceral pain in patients with GI disorders using functional magnetic resonance imaging. Am J Gastroenterol 2002;97:319–327.

97. Bonaz B, Baciu M, Papillon E, Bost R, Gueddah N, Le Bas JF, Fournet J, Segebarth C. Central processing of rectal pain in patients with irritable bowel syndrome: an fMRI study. Am J Gastroenterol 2002;97:654–661.

98. Taylor SE, Klein LC, Lewis BP, Gruenewald TL, Gurung RA, Updegraff JA. Biobehavioral responses to stress in females: tend-and-befriend, not fight-or-flight. Psychol Rev 2000;107:411–429.

99. Nishizawa S, Benkelfat C, Young SN, Leyton M, Mzengeza S, de Montigny C, Blier P, Diksic M. Differences between males and females in rates of serotonin synthesis in human brain. Proc Natl Acad Sci U S A 1997;94:5308–5313.

100. Rosztoczy A, Fioramonti J, Jarmay K, Barreau F, Wittmann T, Bueno L. Influence of sex and experimental protocol on the effect of maternal deprivation on rectal sensitivity to distension in the adult rat. Neurogastroenterol Motil 2003;15:679–686.

101. Mogil JS. Interactions between sex and genotype in the mediation and modulation of nociception in rodents. In: Fillingim RB, ed. Sex, Gender and Pain. Seatle: ISAP Press, 2000:25–40.

102. Zubieta JK, Smith YR, Bueller JA, Xu Y, Kilbourn MR, Jewett DM, Meyer CR, Koeppe RA, Stohler CS. mu-opioid receptor-mediated antinociceptive responses differ in men and women. J Neurosci 2002;22:5100–5107.

103. Gear RW, Miaskowski C, Gordon NC, Paul SM, Heller PH, Levine JD. Kappa-opioids produce significantly greater analgesia in women than in men. Nat Med 1996;2:1248–1250.

104. Mitrovic I, Margeta-Mitrovic M, Bader S, Stoffel M, Jan LY, Basbaum AI. Contribution of GIRK2-mediated postsynaptic signaling to opiate and alpha 2-adrenergic analgesia and analgesic sex differences. Proc Natl Acad Sci U S A 2003;100:271–276.

105. Mogil JS, Wilson SG, Chesler EJ, Rankin AL, Nemmani KV, Lariviere WR, Groce MK, Wallace MR, Kaplan L, Staud R, Ness TJ, Glover TL, Stankova M, Mayorov A, Hruby VJ, Grisel JE, Fillingim RB. The melanocortin-1 receptor gene mediates female-specific mechanisms of analgesia in mice and humans. Proc Natl Acad Sci U S A 2003;100:4867–4872.

106. Bradesi S, Eutamene H, Garcia-Villar R, Fioramonti J, Bueno L. Stress-induced visceral hypersensitivity in female rats is estrogen-dependent and involves tachykinin NK1 receptors. Pain 2003;102:227–234.

107. Bradesi S, Eutamene H, Fioramonti J, Bueno L. Acute restraint stress activates

functional NK1 receptor in the colon of female rats: involvement of steroids. Gut 2002;50:349–354.

108. Uvnas-Moberg K. Oxytocin may mediate the benefits of positive social interaction and emotions. Psychoneuroendocrinology 1998;23:819–835.

109. Louvel D, Delvaux M, Felez A, Fioramonti J, Bueno L, Lazorthes Y, Frexinos J. Oxytocin increases thresholds of colonic visceral perception in patients with irritable bowel syndrome. Gut 1996;39:741–747.

110. Jackson NA, Houghton LA, Whorwell PJ, Currer B. Does the menstrual cycle affect anorectal physiology? Dig Dis Sci 1994;39:2607–2611.

111. Houghton LA, Lea R, Jackson N, Whorwell PJ. The menstrual cycle affects rectal sensitivity in patients with irritable bowel syndrome but not healthy volunteers. Gut 2002;50:471–474.

112. Giamberardino MA, Affaitati G, Valente R, Iezzi S, Vecchiet L. Changes in visceral pain reactivity as a function of estrous cycle in female rats with artificial ureteral calculosis. Brain Res 1997;774:234–238.

113. Gintzler AR. Endorphin-mediated increases in pain threshold during pregnancy. Science 1980;210:193–195.

114. Cogan R, Spinnato JA. Pain and discomfort thresholds in late pregnancy. Pain 1986;27:63–68.

115. Dawson-Basoa MB, Gintzler AR. 17-Beta-estradiol and progesterone modulate an intrinsic opioid analgesic system. Brain Res 1993;601:241–245.

116. Giamberardino MA, Berkley KJ, Iezzi S, de Bigontina P, Vecchiet L. Pain threshold variations in somatic wall tissues as a function of menstrual cycle, segmental site and tissue depth in non-dysmenorrheic women, dysmenorrheic women and men. Pain 1997;71:187–197.

117. Liu NJ, Gintzler AR. Gestational and ovarian sex steroid antinociception: relevance of uterine afferent and spinal alpha(2)-noradrenergic activity. Pain 1999;83:359–368.

118. Danzebrink RM, Gebhart GF. Antinociceptive effects of intrathecal adrenoceptor agonists in a rat model of visceral nociception. J Pharmacol Exp Ther 1990;253:698–705.

119. Ji Y, Murphy AZ, Traub RJ. Estrogen modulates the visceromotor reflex and responses of spinal dorsal horn neurons to colorectal stimulation in the rat. J Neurosci 2003;23:3908–3915.

120. Davies GJ, Crowder M, Reid B, Dickerson JW. Bowel function measurements of individuals with different eating patterns. Gut 1986;27:164–169.

121. Wald A, Van Thiel DH, Hoechstetter L, Gavaler JS, Egler KM, Verm R, Scott L, Lester R. Gastrointestinal transit: the effect of the menstrual cycle. Gastroenterology 1981;80:1497–1500.

122. Rees WD, Rhodes J. Altered bowel habit and menstruation. Lancet 1976;1:475.

123. Ryan JP, Bhojwani A. Colonic transit in rats: effect of ovariectomy, sex steroid hormones, and pregnancy. Am J Physiol 1986;251:G46–G50.

124. Winborn WB, Sheridan PJ, McGill HC, Jr. Sex steroid receptors in the stomach, liver, pancreas, and gastrointestinal tract of the baboon. Gastroenterology 1987;92:23–32.

125. Shah S, Nathan L, Singh R, Fu YS, Chaudhuri G. E2 and not P4 increases NO release from NANC nerves of the gastrointestinal tract: implications in pregnancy. Am J Physiol Regul Integr Comp Physiol 2001;280:R1546–R1554.

126. Bradesi S, Eutamene H, Theodorou V, Fioramonti J, Bueno L. Effect of ovarian hormones on intestinal mast cell reactivity to substance P. Life Sci 2001;68:1047–1056.

127. Christofirdes ND, Ghatei MA, Bloom SR, Borberg C, Gillmer MD. Decreased plasma motilin concentrations in pregnancy. Br Med J 1982;285:1453–1454.

128. Salomaa S, Pekki A, Sannisto T, Ylikomi T, Tuohimaa P. Progesterone receptor is constitutively expressed in chicken intestinal mesothelium and smooth muscle. J Steroid Biochem 1989;34:345–349.

129. Gill RC, Bowes KL, Kingma YJ. Effect of progesterone on canine colonic smooth muscle. Gastroenterology 1985;88:1941–1947.

130. Alonso J, Angermeyer MC, Bernert S, Bruffaerts R, Brugha TS, Bryson H, et al. Prevalence of mental disorders in Europe: results from the European Study of the Epidemiology of Mental Disorders (ESEMeD) project. Acta Psychiatr Scand Suppl 2004;21–27.

131. Ustun TB. Cross-national epidemiology of depression and gender. J Gend Specif Med 2000;3:54–58.

132. Anthony JC, Warner LA, Kessler R. Comparative epidemiology of dependence on tobacco, alcohol, controlled substances, and inhalants: Basic findings from the National Comorbidity Survey. In: Marlatt G and VandenBos GR, eds. Addictive behaviors: Readings on etiology, prevention and treatment. Washington, DC: American Psychological Association, 1997:3–39.

133. Zilberman M, Tavares H, el Guebaly N. Gender similarities and differences: the prevalence and course of alcohol- and other substance-related disorders. J Addict Dis 2003;22:61–74.

134. Chiswick D, Thomson LDG. The relationship between crime and psyciatry. In: Johnstone EC, Cunningham DC, Owens SM, Lawrie SM, Sharpe M, and Freeman CPL, eds. In Companion to Psychiatric Studies. 7 ed. Edinburgh: Churchill, Livingstone, 2005:701–727.

135. Horwitz A. The pathways into psychiatric treatment: some differences between men and women. J Health Soc Behav 1977;18:169–178.

136. Corney RH. Sex differences in general practice attendance and help seeking for minor illness. J Psychosom Res 1990;34:525–534.

137. Guthrie E, Creed F, Whorwell PJ. Eating disorders in pateints with the irritable bowel syndrome: A comparison with inflammatory bowel disease and peptic ulceration. Eur J of Gastroenterology and Hepatology 1990;2:471–473.

138. Sullivan G, Blewett AE, Jenkins PL, Allison MC. Eating attitudes and the irritable bowel syndrome. Gen Hosp Psychiatry 1997;19:62–64.

139. Tang TN, Toner BB, Stuckless N, Dion KL, Kaplan AS, Ali A. Features of eating disorders in patients with irritable bowel syndrome. J Psychosom Res 1998;45:171–178.

140. Svedberg P, Johansson S, Wallander MA, Hamelin B, Pedersen NL. Extra-intestinal manifestations associated with irritable bowel syndrome: a twin study. Aliment Pharmacol Ther 2002;16:975–983.

141. Hislop IG. Psychological significance of the irritable colon syndrome. Gut 1971;12:452–457.

142. Fava GA, Pavan L. Large bowel disorders. II. Psychopathology and alexithymia. Psychother Psychosom 1976;27:100–105.

143. MacDonald AJ, Bouchier IA. Non-organic gastrointestinal illness: a medical and psychiatric study. Br J Psychiatry 1980;136:276–283.

144. Latimer P, Sarna S, Campbell D, Latimer M, Waterfall W, Daniel EE. Colonic motor and myoelectrical activity: a comparative study of normal subjects, psychoneurotic patients, and patients with irritable bowel syndrome. Gastroenterology 1981; 80:893–901.
145. Ford MJ, Miller PM, Eastwood J, Eastwood MA. Life events, psychiatric illness and the irritable bowel syndrome. Gut 1987;28:160–165.
146. Colgan S, Creed F, Klass H. Symptom complaints, psychiatric disorder and abnormal illness behaviour in patients with upper abdominal pain. Psychol Med 1988; 18:887–892.
147. Walker EA, Roy-Byrne PP, Katon WJ. Irritable bowel syndrome and psychiatric illness. Am J Psychiatry 1990;147:565–572.
148. Toner BB, Garfinkel PE, Jeejeebhoy KN. Psychological factors in irritable bowel syndrome. Can J Psychiatry 1990;35:158–161.
149. Yadav SK, Jain AK, Bahre PB, Gupta JP. Neuroticism in patients with irritable bowel syndrome. Indian J Gastroenterol 1990;9:29–31.
150. Dinan TG, O'Keane V, O'Boyle C, Chua A, Keeling PW. A comparison of the mental status, personality profiles and life events of patients with irritable bowel syndrome and peptic ulcer disease. Acta Psychiatr Scand 1991;84:26–28.
151. Masand PS, Kaplan DS, Gupta S, Bhandary AN, Nasra GS, Kline MD, Margo KL. Major depression and irritable bowel syndrome: is there a relationship? J Clin Psychiatry 1995;56:363–367.
152. Gomborone J, Dewsnap P, Libby G, Farthing M. Abnormal illness attitudes in patients with irritable bowel syndrome. J Psychosom Res 1995;39:227–230.
153. Blewett A, Allison M, Calcraft B, Moore R, Jenkins P, Sullivan G. Psychiatric disorder and outcome in irritable bowel syndrome. Psychosomatics 1996;37:155–160.
154. Blanchard EB, Keefer L, Galovski TE, Taylor AE, Turner SM. Gender differences in psychological distress among patients with irritable bowel syndrome. J Psychosom Res 2001;50:271–275.
155. Fock KM, Chew CN, Tay LK, Peh LH, Chan S, Pang EP. Psychiatric illness, personality traits and the irritable bowel syndrome. Ann Acad Med Singapore 2001;30:611–614.
156. Creed F, Ratcliffe J, Fernandez L, Tomenson B, Palmer S, Rigby C, Guthrie E, Read N, Thompson D. Health-related quality of life and health care costs in severe, refractory irritable bowel syndrome. Ann Intern Med 2001;134:860–868.
157. Talley NJ, Phillips SF, Wiltgen CM, Zinsmeister AR, Melton LJ, III. Assessment of functional gastrointestinal disease: the bowel disease questionnaire. Mayo Clin Proc 1990;65:1456–1479.
158. Herschbach P, Henrich G, von Rad M. Psychological factors in functional gastrointestinal disorders: characteristics of the disorder or of the illness behavior? Psychosom Med 1999;61:148–153.
159. Weinryb RM, Osterberg E, Blomquist L, Hultcrantz R, Krakau I, Asberg M. Psychological factors in irritable bowel syndrome: a population-based study of patients, non-patients and controls. Scand J Gastroenterol 2003;38:503–510.
160. Westbrook JI, Talley NJ. Empiric clustering of dyspepsia into symptom subgroups: a population-based study. Scand J Gastroenterol 2002;37:917–923.
161. Koloski NA, Talley NJ, Boyce PM. Does psychological distress modulate functional gastrointestinal symptoms and health care seeking? A prospective, community Cohort study. Am J Gastroenterol 2003;98:789–797.

162. Drossman DA, Sandler RS, McKee DC, Lovitz AJ. Bowel patterns among subjects not seeking health care. Use of a questionnaire to identify a population with bowel dysfunction. Gastroenterology 1982;83:529–534.

163. Drossman DA, McKee DC, Sandler RS, Mitchell CM, Cramer EM, Lowman BC, Burger AL. Psychosocial factors in the irritable bowel syndrome. A multivariate study of patients and nonpatients with irritable bowel syndrome. Gastroenterology 1988;95:701–708.

164. Mendeloff AI, Monk M, Siegel CI, Lilienfeld A. Illness experience and life stresses in patients with irritable colon and with ulcerative colitis. An epidemiologic study of ulcerative colitis and regional enteritis in Baltimore, 1960–1964. N Engl J Med 1970; 282:14–17.

165. Fava GA, Pavan L. Large bowel disorders. I. Illness configuration and life events. Psychother Psychosom 1976;27:93–99.

166. Whitehead WE, Crowell MD, Robinson JC, Heller BR, Schuster MM. Effects of stressful life events on bowel symptoms: subjects with irritable bowel syndrome compared with subjects without bowel dysfunction. Gut 1992;33:825–830.

167. Walker LS, Garber J, Smith CA, Van Slyke DA, Claar RL. The relation of daily stressors to somatic and emotional symptoms in children with and without recurrent abdominal pain. J Consult Clin Psychol 2001;69:85–91.

168. Levy RL, Cain KC, Jarrett M, Heitkemper MM. The relationship between daily life stress and gastrointestinal symptoms in women with irritable bowel syndrome. J Behav Med 1997;20:177–193.

169. Drossman DA, Li Z, Leserman J, Toomey TC, Hu YJ. Health status by gastrointestinal diagnosis and abuse history. Gastroenterology 1996;110:999–1007.

170. Creed F, Craig T, Farmer R. Functional abdominal pain, psychiatric illness, and life events. Gut 1988;29:235–242.

171. Bennett EJ, Tennant CC, Piesse C, Badcock CA, Kellow JE. Level of chronic life stress predicts clinical outcome in irritable bowel syndrome. Gut 1998;43:256–261.

172. Talley NJ, Boyce P, Owen BK. Psychological distress and seasonal symptom changes in irritable bowel syndrome. Am J Gastroenterol 1995;90:2115–2119.

173. Walker EA, Katon WJ, Roy-Byrne PP, Jemelka RP, Russo J. Histories of sexual victimization in patients with irritable bowel syndrome or inflammatory bowel disease. Am J Psychiatry 1993;150:1502–1506.

174. Toner B, Segal Z, Emmott S, Myran D. Cognitive-behavioral treatment of irritable bowel syndrome: The brain-gut connection. London/NewYork: Guilford Press, 2000.

175. Drossman DA, Toner BB, Whitehead WE, Diamant NE, Dalton CB, Duncan S, Emmott S, Proffitt V, Akman D, Frusciante K, Le T, Meyer K, Bradshaw B, Mikula K, Morris CB, Blackman CJ, Hu Y, Jia H, Li JZ, Koch GG, Bangdiwala SI. Cognitive-behavioral therapy versus education and desipramine versus placebo for moderate to severe functional bowel disorders. Gastroenterology 2003;125:19–31.

176. Bepko C, Krestan J. Too good for her own good. New York, NY: Harper and Row, 1990.

177. Jack DC. Silencing the self: Inner dialogues and outer realities. In: Joiner T and Coyne J, eds. The interactional nature of depression. Washington, D.C.: American Psychological Association, 1999:221–246.

178. Ali A, Toner BB, Stuckless N, Gallop R, Diamant NE, Gould MI, Vidins EI. Emo-

tional abuse, self-blame, and self-silencing in women with irritable bowel syndrome. Psychosom Med 2000;62:76–82.

179. Lee OY, Mayer EA, Schmulson M, Chang L, Naliboff B. Gender-related differences in IBS symptoms. Am J Gastroenterol 2001;96:2184–2193.

180. Dancey CP, Hutton-Young A, Moyle S, Devins GM. Perceived stigma, illness intrusiveness and quality of life in men and women with irritable bowel syndrome. Psychology, Health & Medicine 2002;7:381–395.

181. Guthrie E, Creed F, Dawson D, Tomenson B. A controlled trial of psychological treatment for the irritable bowel syndrome. Gastroenterology 1991;100:450–457.

182. Svedlund J, Sjodin I, Ottosson JO, Dotevall G. Controlled study of psychotherapy in irritable bowel syndrome. Lancet 1983;2:589–592.

183. Gonsalkorale WM, Miller V, Afzal A, Whorwell PJ. Long term benefits of hypnotherapy for irritable bowel syndrome. Gut 2003;52:1623–1629.

184. Jailwala J, Imperiale TF, Kroenke K. Pharmacologic treatment of the irritable bowel syndrome: a systematic review of randomized, controlled trials. Ann Intern Med 2000;133:136–147.

185. Jackson JL, O'Malley PG, Tomkins G, Balden E, Santoro J, Kroenke K. Treatment of functional gastrointestinal disorders with antidepressant medications: a meta-analysis. Am J Med 2000;108:65–72.

186. Camilleri M, Mayer EA, Drossman DA, Heath A, Dukes GE, McSorley D, Kong S, Mangel AW, Northcutt AR. Improvement in pain and bowel function in female irritable bowel patients with alosetron, a 5-HT3 receptor antagonist. Aliment Pharmacol Ther 1999;13:1149–1159.

187. Chang L, Ameen VZ, Dukes GE, McSorley D, Mayer EA. A dose-ranging, phase II study of the efficacy and safety of alosetron hydrochloride (Lotronex®) in men with diarrhea-predominant IBS. Am.J.Gastroenterol 2005;100:115–23.

188. Viramontes BE, Camilleri M, McKinzie S, Pardi DS, Burton D, Thomforde GM. Gender-related differences in slowing colonic transit by a 5-HT3 antagonist in subjects with diarrhea-predominant irritable bowel syndrome. Am J Gastroenterol 2001;96:2671–2676.

189. Bradette M, Moennikes H, Carter F, et al. Cilansetron in irritable bowel syndrome-with diarrhea predominance (IBS-D). Efficacy and safety in a 6 month study. Gastroenterology 126:A-42. 2004. Ref Type: Abstract

190. Coremans G, Clouse RE, Carter F, et al. Cilansetron, a novel 5-HT3 antagonist, demonstrated efficacy in males with irritable bowel syndrome with diarrhea-predominance (IBS-D). Gastroenterology 126:A-643. 2004. Ref Type: Abstract

191. Miner P, Stanton DB, Carter C, Caras S, Krause G, Steinborn C. Cilansetron in irritable bowel syndrome with diarrhea predominance (IBS-): efficacy and safety in a 3 month US study. Am.J Gastroenterol 99[S277]. 2004. Ref Type: Abstract

192. Muller-Lissner SA, Fumagalli I, Bardhan KD, Pace F, Pecher E, Nault B, Ruegg P. Tegaserod, a 5-HT(4) receptor partial agonist, relieves symptoms in irritable bowel syndrome patients with abdominal pain, bloating and constipation. Aliment Pharmacol Ther 2001;15:1655–1666.

193. Kellow J, Lee OY, Chang FY, Thongsawat S, Mazlam MZ, Yuen H, Gwee KA, Bak YT, Jones J, Wagner A. An Asia-Pacific, double blind, placebo controlled, randomised study to evaluate the efficacy, safety, and tolerability of tegaserod in patients with irritable bowel syndrome. Gut 2003;52:671–676.

194. Nyhlin H, Bang C, Elsborg L, Silvennoinen J, Holme I, Ruegg P, Jones J, Wagner A. A double-blind, placebo-controlled, randomized study to evaluate the efficacy, safety and tolerability of tegaserod in patients with irritable bowel syndrome. Scand J Gastroenterol 2004;39:119–126.

195. Johanson JF, Wald A, Tougas G, Chey WD, Novick JS, Lembo AJ, Fordham F, Guella M, Nault B. Effect of tegaserod in chronic constipation: a randomized, double-blind, controlled trial. Clin Gastroenterol Hepatol 2004;2:796–805.

196. Jones LA, Chin LT, Longo DL, Kruisbeek AM. Peripheral clonal elimination of functional T cells. Science 1990;250:1726–1729.

197. Kay L, Jorgensen T. Epidemiology of upper dyspepsia in a random population. Prevalence, incidence, natural history, and risk factors. Scand J Gastroenterol 1994; 29:2–6.

198. Bennett G, Talley NJ. Irritable bowel syndrome in the elderly. Best Pract Res Clin Gastroenterol 2002;16:63–76.

199. Wong ML, Wee S, Pin CH, Gan GL, Ye HC. Sociodemographic and lifestyle factors associated with constipation in an elderly Asian community. Am J Gastroenterol 1999;94:1283–1291.

200. Wei X, Chen M, Wang J. The epidemiology of irritable bowel syndrome and functional constipation of Guangzhou residents. Zhonghua Nei Ke Za Zhi 2001;40:517–520.

201. Talley NJ, Fleming KC, Evans JM, O'Keefe EA, Weaver AL, Zinsmeister AR, Melton LJ, III. Constipation in an elderly community: a study of prevalence and potential risk factors. Am J Gastroenterol 1996;91:19–25.

202. Drossman DA. Functional GI disorders: what's in a name? Gastroenterology 2005; 128:1771–1772.

203. Toner B, Casati J. Diseases of the digestive system. In: Perry N, Johnson SB, and Rozensky R, eds. Medical Disorders and behviroal applications. Volume 1. Washington, DC: American Psychological Association, 2002:283–305.

204. Letson S, Dancey CP. Nurses' perceptions of irritable bowel syndrome (IBS) and sufferers of IBS. J Adv Nurs 1996;23:969–974.

205. Link BG, Struening EL, Rahav M, Phelan JC, Nuttbrock L. On stigma and its consequences: evidence from a longitudinal study of men with dual diagnoses of mental illness and substance abuse. J Health Soc Behav 1997;38:177–190.

206. Dancey CP, Blackhouse S. A complete guide to relief from Irritable Bowel Syndrome. London: Constable Robinson, 1997.

207. Health literacy: report of the Council on Scientific Affairs. Ad Hoc Committee on Health Literacy for the Council on Scientific Affairs, American Medical Association. JAMA 1999;281:552–557.

208. Low SM. The cultural basis of health, illness and disease. Soc Work Health Care 1984;9:13–23.

209. Leininger M. Qualitative Research Methods in Nursing. Orlando, FL: Grune & Stratton, 1985.

210. Whaley AL. Ethnicity/race, ethics, and epidemiology. J Natl Med Assoc 2003;95:736–742.

211. Jones CP. Invited commentary: "race," racism, and the practice of epidemiology. Am J Epidemiol 2001;154:299–304.

212. Cooper R. A note on the biologic concept of race and its application in epidemiologic research. Am Heart J 1984;108:715–722.

213. Rothschild SK. Cross-cultural issues in primary care medicine. Dis Mon 1998;44: 293–319.
214. Dimsdale JE. Stalked by the past: the influence of ethnicity on health. Psychosom Med 2000;62:161–170.
215. Ng B, Dimsdale JE, Rollnik JD, Shapiro H. The effect of ethnicity on prescriptions for patient-controlled analgesia for post-operative pain. Pain 1996;66:9–12.
216. Quality first: Better health care for all Americans. Final report of the President's Advisory Commission on Concumer Protection and Quality in the Health Care Industry. 1998. Washington, DC, U.S. Government Printing Office. Ref Type: Report
217. Helman CG. Communication in primary care: the role of patient and practitioner explanatory models. Soc Sci Med 1985;20:923–931.
218. Eisenberg L. Disease and illness. Distinctions between professional and popular ideas of sickness. Cult Med Psychiatry 1977;1:9–23.
219. Ware NC, Kleinman A. Culture and somatic experience: the social course of illness in neurasthenia and chronic fatigue syndrome. Psychosom Med 1992;54:546–560.
220. Carrillo JE, Green AR, Betancourt JR. Cross-cultural primary care: a patient-based approach. Ann Intern Med 1999;130:829–834.
221. Baker DW, Parker RM, Williams MV, Pitkin K, Parikh NS, Coates W, Imara M. The health care experience of patients with low literacy. Arch Fam Med 1996;5:329–334.
222. Spandorfer JM, Karras DJ, Hughes LA, Caputo C. Comprehension of discharge instructions by patients in an urban emergency department. Ann Emerg Med 1995;25:71–74.
223. Luna I. Diversity issues in the delivery of healthcare. Lippincotts Case Manag 2002;7:138–143.
224. Zuckerman MJ, Guerra LG, Drossman DA, Foland JA, Gregory GG. Comparison of bowel patterns in Hispanics and non-Hispanic whites. Dig Dis Sci 1995;40:1763–1769.
225. Zuckerman MJ, Guerra LG, Drossman DA, Foland JA, Gregory GG. Health-care-seeking behaviors related to bowel complaints. Hispanics versus non-Hispanic whites. Dig Dis Sci 1996;41:77–82.
226. Heiat A, Gross CP, Krumholz HM. Representation of the elderly, women, and minorities in heart failure clinical trials. Arch Intern Med 2002;162:1682–1688.
227. Chaturvedi N, McKeigue PM. Methods for epidemiological surveys of ethnic minority groups. J Epidemiol Community Health 1994;48:107–111.
228. Johnson CE. Consistency of reporting ethnic origin in the current population survey. U.S. Department of Commerce Technical Report No. 31. 1974. Washington, DC, Bureau of the Census. Ref Type: Report
229. Hahn EA, Cella D. Health outcomes assessment in vulnerable populations: measurement challenges and recommendations. Arch Phys Med Rehabil 2003;84:S35–S42.
230. Sperber AD, De Vellis RF, Bochlecke B. Cross-cultural translation: methodology and validation. J Cross-Cult Psychol 1994;25:501–524.
231. Sperber AD. Translation and validation of study instruments for cross-cultural research. Gastroenterology 2004;126:S124–S128.
232. Krecic-Shepard ME, Park K, Barnas C, Slimko J, Kerwin DR, Schwartz JB. Race and sex influence clearance of nifedipine: results of a population study. Clin Pharmacol Ther 2000;68:130–142.

233. Datan N, Aaron A, Benjamin MA. A Time to Reap: The Middle Age of Women in Five Israeli Subcultures. Baltimore, MD: The John Hopkins University Press, 1981.

234. Carmel S, Anson O, Levin M. Emergency department utilization by two subcultures in the same geographical region. Soc Sci Med 1990;31:557–563.

235. Carmel S, Koren I, Ilia R. Coping with the Gulf war: subculture differences among ischemic heart disease patients in Israel. Soc Sci Med 1993;37:1481–1488.

236. Carmel S, Barnoon S, Zalcman T. Social class differences in coping with a physicians' strike in Israel. J Community Health 1990;15:45–57.

237. Williams DR. Race/ethnicity and socioeconomic status: measurement and methodological issues. Int J Health Serv 1996;26:483–505.

238. Sperber AD, Friger M, Shvartzman P, Abu-Rabia M, Abu-Rabia R, Aborshed M, et al. Rates of functional bowel disorders among Israeli Bedouins in rural areas compared to those who moved to permanent towns. Clin Gastroenterol Hepatol 2005;3:342–8.

239. Lule GN, Amayo EO. Irritable bowel syndrome in Kenyans. East Afr Med J 2002; 79:360–363.

240. Olubuyide IO, Olawuyi F, Fasanmade AA. A study of irritable bowel syndrome diagnosed by Manning criteria in an African population. Dig Dis Sci 1995;40: 983–985.

241. Ho KY, Kang JY, Seow A. Prevalence of gastrointestinal symptoms in a multiracial Asian population, with particular reference to reflux-type symptoms. Am J Gastroenterol 1998;93:1816–1822.

242. Hu WH, Wong WM, Lam CL, Lam KF, Hui WM, Lai KC, Xia HX, Lam SK, Wong BC. Anxiety but not depression determines health care-seeking behaviour in Chinese patients with dyspepsia and irritable bowel syndrome: a population-based study. Aliment Pharmacol Ther 2002;16:2081–2088.

243. Danivat D, Tankeyoon M, Sriratanaban A. Prevalence of irritable bowel syndrome in a non-Western population. Br Med J (Clin Res Ed) 1988;296:1710.

244. Bi-Zhen W, Qi-Ying P. Functional bowel disorders in apparently healthy Chinese people. Chin J Epid 1998;9:345–349.

245. Lee CT, Chuang TY, Lu CL, Chen CY, Chang FY, Lee SD. Abnormal vagal cholinergic function and psychological behaviors in irritable bowel syndrome patients: a hospital-based Oriental study. Dig Dis Sci 1998;43:1794–1799.

246. Massarrat S, Saberi-Firoozi M, Soleimani A, Himmelmann GW, Hitzges M, Keshavarz H. Peptic ulcer disease, irritable bowel syndrome and constipation in two populations in Iran. Eur J Gastroenterol Hepatol 1995;7:427–433.

247. Masud MA, Hasan M, Khan AK. Irritable bowel syndrome in a rural community in Bangladesh: prevalence, symptoms pattern, and health care seeking behavior. Am J Gastroenterol 2001;96:1547–1552.

248. Kapoor KK, Nigam P, Rastogi CK, Kumar A, Gupta AK. Clinical profile of irritable bowel syndrome. Indian J Gastroenterol 1985;4:15–16.

249. Pimparkar BD. Irritable colon syndrome. J Indian Med Assoc 1970;54:95–103.

250. Sime WE, Rossi AM, Lubbers CA. Incidence of stress-related disorders among American and Brazilian men and women. Int J Psychosom 1990;37:62–67.

251. Yawn BP, Locke GR, III, Lydick E, Wollan PC, Bertram SL, Kurland MJ. Diagnosis and care of irritable bowel syndrome in a community-based population. Am J Manag Care 2001;7:585–592.

252. Toner BB, Akman D. Gender role and irritable bowel syndrome: literature review and hypothesis. Am J Gastroenterol 2000;95:11–16.

253. Heaton KW, O'Donnell LJ, Braddon FE, Mountford RA, Hughes AO, Cripps PJ. Symptoms of irritable bowel syndrome in a British urban community: consulters and nonconsulters. Gastroenterology 1992;102:1962–1967.

254. Jones R, Lydeard S. Irritable bowel syndrome in the general population. BMJ 1992;304:87–90.

255. Kay L, Jorgensen T, Jensen KH. The epidemiology of irritable bowel syndrome in a random population: prevalence, incidence, natural history and risk factors. J Intern Med 1994;236:23–30.

256. Osterberg E, Blomquist L, Krakau I, Weinryb RM, Asberg M, Hultcrantz R. A population study on irritable bowel syndrome and mental health. Scand J Gastroenterol 2000;35:264–268.

257. Boyce PM, Koloski NA, Talley NJ. Irritable bowel syndrome according to varying diagnostic criteria: are the new Rome II criteria unnecessarily restrictive for research and practice? Am J Gastroenterol 2000;95:3176–3183.

258. Talley NJ, Howell S, Poulton R. The irritable bowel syndrome and psychiatric disorders in the community: is there a link? Am J Gastroenterol 2001;96:1072–1079.

259. Thompson WG, Irvine EJ, Pare P, Ferrazzi S, Rance L. Functional gastrointestinal disorders in Canada: first population-based survey using Rome II criteria with suggestions for improving the questionnaire. Dig Dis Sci 2002;47:225–235.

260. Bommelaer G, Dorval E, Denis P, Czernichow P, Frexinos J, Pelc A, Slama A, El Hasnaoui A. Prevalence of irritable bowel syndrome in the French population according to the Rome I criteria. Gastroenterol Clin Biol 2002;26:1118–1123.

261. Saito YA, Talley NJ, Melton J, Fett S, Zinsmeister AR, Locke GR. The effect of new diagnostic criteria for irritable bowel syndrome on community prevalence estimates. Neurogastroenterol Motil 2003;15:687–694.

262. Dapoigny M, Bellanger J, Bonaz B, Bruley d, V, Bueno L, Coffin B, Ducrotte P, Flourie B, Lemann M, Lepicard A, Reigneau O. Irritable bowel syndrome in France: a common, debilitating and costly disorder. Eur J Gastroenterol Hepatol 2004;16:995–1001.

263. Hillila MT, Farkkila MA. Prevalence of irritable bowel syndrome according to different diagnostic criteria in a non-selected adult population. Aliment Pharmacol Ther 2004;20:339–345.

264. Wilson S, Roberts L, Roalfe A, Bridge P, Singh S. Prevalence of irritable bowel syndrome: a community survey. Br J Gen Pract 2004;54:495–502.

265. Bommelaer G, Poynard T, Le Pen C, Gaudin AF, Maurel F, Priol G, Amouretti M, Frexinos J, Ruszniewski P, El Hasnaoui A. Prevalence of irritable bowel syndrome (IBS) and variability of diagnostic criteria. Gastroenterol Clin Biol 2004;28:554–561.

266. Lau EM, Chan FK, Ziea ET, Chan CS, Wu JC, Sung JJ. Epidemiology of irritable bowel syndrome in Chinese. Dig Dis Sci 2002;47:2621–2624.

267. Kwan AC, Hu WH, Chan YK, Yeung YW, Lai TS, Yuen H. Prevalence of irritable bowel syndrome in Hong Kong. J Gastroenterol Hepatol 2002;17:1180–1186.

268. Tan YM, Goh KL, Muhidayah R, Ooi CL, Salem O. Prevalence of irritable bowel syndrome in young adult Malaysians: a survey among medical students. J Gastroenterol Hepatol 2003;18:1412–1416.

269. Lu CL, Chen CY, Lang HC, Luo JC, Wang SS, Chang FY, Lee SD. Current patterns of irritable bowel syndrome in Taiwan: the Rome II questionnaire on a Chinese population. Aliment Pharmacol Ther 2003;18:1159–1169.

270. Xiong LS, Chen MH, Chen HX, Xu AG, Wang WA, Hu PJ. A population-based epidemiologic study of irritable bowel syndrome in Guangdong province. Zhonghua Yi Xue Za Zhi 2004;84:278–281.

271. Gwee KA, Wee S, Wong ML, Png DJ. The prevalence, symptom characteristics, and impact of irritable bowel syndrome in an asian urban community. Am J Gastroenterol 2004;99:924–931.

272. Celebi S, Acik Y, Deveci SE, Bahcecioglu IH, Ayar A, Demir A, Durukan P. Epidemiological features of irritable bowel syndrome in a Turkish urban society. J Gastroenterol Hepatol 2004;19:738–743.

273. Rajendra S, Alahuddin S. Prevalence of irritable bowel syndrome in a multi-ethnic Asian population. Aliment Pharmacol Ther 2004;19:704–706.

274. Morgan D, Cortez L, Pena R, Morales J, Torres M, Heidt P. A population-based prevalence study of Irritable Bowel Syndrome and the functional gastrointestinal disorders in Latin America. Am J Gastroenterol 2004;99:S283–S284.

275. Sperber AD, Shvartzman P, Friger M, Fich A. Unexpectedly low prevalence rates of IBS among adult Israeli Jews. Neurogastroenterol.Motil 2005. In Press

Chapter 6

Psychosocial Aspects of Functional Gastrointestinal Disorders

Francis Creed, Chair
Rona L. Levy, Co-Chair
Laurence A. Bradley
Carlos Francisconi
Douglas A. Drossman
Bruce D. Naliboff
Kevin W. Olden

Introduction: A Model for How Psychological and Social Factors Can Affect Gut Function

In functional gastrointestinal disorders (FGIDs) psychological and social influences may affect gut function, the experience of pain, health-related quality of life, work absenteeism, health care use and medical and societal costs [1–4]. This chapter critically examines the evidence for these statements and explores the mechanisms by which psychological and social variables influence physiological functions and outcomes of these disorders. Many of the mechanisms described in this chapter are not specific to FGIDs; they can be observed in other medical conditions also. They are particularly important and visible in FGIDs because of the close connections between brain and gut.

In this chapter, a multinational panel of gastroenterologists, psychiatrists, psychologists, physiologists, and health service investigators review the clinical implications of recent research, and provide a treatment algorithm for the treatment of the psychosocial aspect of FGIDs. It is important to recognize that any psychosocial influences must be understood within the wider social and cultural environment outside the individual, which may affect the experiences of pain and other symptoms and the expression of illness.

— Historical Aspects

Beliefs about the interaction between mind and body have been expressed in two competing concepts: *dualism*, which separates, and *holism*, which unifies these two entities [5, 6]. The former is associated with the philosopher Descartes, who proposed the separation of the thinking mind (*res cogitans*) from the body (*res extensa*). Pasteur's discovery of microorganisms and Koch's development of the germ theory of disease moved medicine further in the direction of duality and biologic reductionism. Consistent with dualism is the concept of psychogenesis: if mind and body are separate, then psychological processes (as an external factor) can cause (rather than be a part of) medical disease.

The alternative view holds that mind and body are inseparable, and a change in one is associated with simultaneous changes in the other. This was exemplified in early studies reporting the immediate effect of emotions such as anger and fear on the activity of the gastric mucosa [7]. This concept, developed from the Greek concept of *holos*, or whole, suggests that the study of medical disease must take into account the whole person rather than merely the diseased part; such an approach is referred to as "holistic" or "whole person medicine."

Psychosomatic Medicine

The theoretical basis of classical psychosomatic medicine in the 1950s came from observations made in small clinical studies. Patients helped by psychoanalytic therapy reported improvement in various diseases, including inflammatory bowel disease and peptic ulcer, from which it was wrongly deduced that the prime causative agent lay in emotional conflicts. Larger studies demonstrated that these disorders could exist without such emotional conflicts, though they might be exacerbated by anxiety or depression, and the full range of etiological factors was established.

The Biopsychosocial Model

Partly as a reaction to such erroneous "psychosomatic" ideas, research into FGIDs moved firmly towards the biological aspects with studies of gut motility and specific physiological abnormalities, raising hopes that a set of "biological markers" for FGID could be found. When it became clear that any such marker did not correlate well with symptoms, a broader and more comprehensive approach to understanding illness and disease was needed. Concurrently, in the late 1970's George Engel proposed a more holistic view of illness that integrated psychological, social, and biological variables: the "biopsychosocial model" [8]. In this model biological and psychosocial influences could be integrated not only into disease conceptualization but also applied to medical care and provide a multidisciplinary model for research. Such research became a reality with the advent of improved tools to measure psychological and social variables relevant to FGIDs, as well as the introduction of modern epidemiologic study techniques and laboratory methods that allow investigators to examine the effects of psychosocial variables, such as conditioning, on psychophysiologic responses.

During the 1980s and 90s the reliable assessment of psychological distress, psychiatric disorders, personality, recent stressful life events, childhood abuse, social support, and coping style meant that the relationship of psychological and social factors to the onset and outcome of FGIDs could be established. Furthermore, population-based studies demonstrated that many people with the symptoms of FGIDs do not visit doctors; psychological and social factors may determine treatment-seeking as well as influence reports of symptom severity [9, 10]. These relationships are not specific to FGIDs as they are found in related syndromes such as chronic fatigue syndrome and fibromyalgia as well as for conditions in which pathological processes contribute to their symptoms (e.g., inflammatory bowel disease, gastroesophageal reflux disease).

In the late 1960's, Fordyce began to study the effects of classical and operant conditioning on the responses of patients with chronic pain. Fordyce's early work demonstrated how the alteration of environmental/social contingencies through operant conditioning could be used to decrease the frequency of overt pain behaviors and increase the frequency of relatively healthy behaviors [11]. Other work has shown that autonomic or other physiological functions (e.g., gastrointestinal secretion and motility) may be modified through conditioning, or through relaxation training. Conditioning experiences might also contribute to the development of a psychophysiological disorder such as irritable bowel syndrome (IBS) [12].

Current Status of the Biopsychosocial Model

Increased effort has been devoted recently to biopsychosocial-based studies that more fully integrate the biological and psychosocial aspects of FGIDs [5]. For example, it has been shown that psychological and social variables in people with gastroenteritis can predict later inflammation of the gut mucosa and symptoms of IBS [13]. Psychological influences have been studied also in relation to rectal distension in IBS [14, 15]. Studies using positron emission tomography (PET) have shown that psychological distress as well as bowel symptoms are associated with increased central nervous system (CNS) activation in brain regions that process the sensory, affective, and cognitive dimensions of pain in response to rectal distension [16].

— Proposed Model

The conceptual model used as the basis of this chapter is shown in Figure 1. This is consistent with the biopsychosocial model as it presents potential interactions among genetic, environmental, psychological, and physiologic factors that contribute to the outcomes associated with the FGIDs. From the environmental (i.e., social) perspective there are important early life experiences that may shape future responses to stress and to abdominal symptoms and stressors, such as divorce or bereavement, that may occur at any stage in life. An individual's response to such stressors may be shaped by a variety of influences including genetic background and childhood experience as well as the individual's personality, constitution, and degree of social support from family members or other individuals who are close. Exposure to stressors may lead to anxiety or depressive disorders in vulnerable individuals as well as produce physiological and psychological changes. Psychological changes may include altered perception of bodily sensations—innocent bodily sensations might be regarded as indicators of severe disease. These may become persistent and lead to frequent medical help-seeking by people who may be difficult to reassure even after a normal investigation result.

The gut is sensitive to environmental stressors and psychological changes and

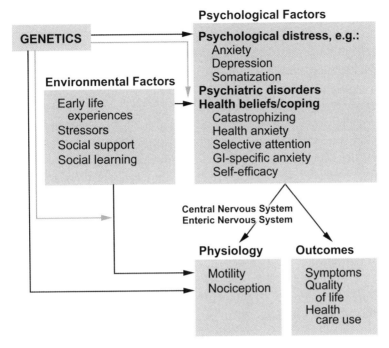

Figure 1. Conceptual model illustrating potential interactions among genetic, environmental, psychological, and physiologic factors that contribute to the outcomes associated with the FGIDs.

may be affected directly by them so there are two-way interactions along the "brain-gut" axis. (See Chapter 1.) Thus the experience of pain has many influences both internal and external, central and peripheral. These different components all influence the enteric nervous system (ENS). In addition, psychological factors affect the outcome of FGIDs by mechanisms which are discussed in the section below on psychophysiology.

— Childhood and Genetic Factors Related to Gut Function

This section outlines the growing body of evidence supporting genetic influences and learning process mechanisms that occur in childhood and contribute to the development of the FGIDs. The latter are important for prevention and treatment of childhood FGIDs as well as prevention of disorders in adulthood. For example, one third to one half of children with recurrent abdominal pain (RAP) continue to report abdominal pain and related symptoms as adults [17].

— Genetic Influences

There has been a substantial increase in studies of family aggregation of IBS and related disorders since 2000 [18]. Recognition of the role of genetics contributes to this increase. There is evidence that gene polymorphisms associated with pain sensitivity and affective or anxiety disorders are associated with disorders that frequently co-occur with IBS, such as fibromyalgia and temporomandibular dysfunction (TMD). These include a polymorphism in the regulatory region of the 5-HT transporter gene [19, 20] and the val[158] met polymorphism of the catechol-O-methyltransferase (COMT) gene [21]. The former is also associated with diarrhea-predominant IBS [22], although negative findings regarding this relationship also have been reported [23]. Moreover, COMT haplotypes associated with pain sensitivity, in combination with high levels of somatization, predict the onset of TMD in young adult women and may be relevant to the experience of pain in FGIDs [21, 24].

— Environmental Influences

In addition to important genetic influences, there is clear evidence that what children learn from parents with IBS may make an even stronger contribution to the risk of developing an FGID, independent of genetic contribution [25]. Thus the observed aggregation of FGIDs in families [18] may have both a genetic and an environmental origin. The children of adult IBS patients make more health care visits than the children of non-IBS parents, but this pattern is not confined to gastrointestinal (GI) complaints [26].

Children with RAP have higher levels of anxiety and depression than healthy children [27] and high levels of depression predict persistent symptoms over a five-year period [28]. Depressed children with RAP report numerous bodily symptoms in response to daily stressors, suggesting that stress reactivity is important in these children [29]. They also show low academic competence and are at particular risk of avoiding school in response to abdominal pain. This may become an established pattern that persists into adulthood [30].

Numerous somatic complaints and more prolonged symptoms in children with RAP are also associated with high levels of stress, anxiety, depression, and somatization in the child's parents [31]. This pattern [32] holds for both maternal and paternal symptoms, suggesting that a child may learn illness behaviors from either parent [31].

Two population-based studies argue powerfully that social learning helps mediate the intergenerational transmission of medically unexplained symptoms. In German and UK cohorts, RAP in children was associated with a family pattern of gastrointestinal problems [33], mothers with high neuroticism scores [34], and numerous bodily symptoms in adulthood [35].

— Mechanisms of Social Learning

The social learning influences on RAP in children could be explained by a number of social learning phenomena, including modeling, in which children observe and learn to display the illness behavior of their parents. Evidence also suggests that positive reinforcement contributes to RAP. Children whose mothers strongly reinforce illness behavior experience more severe stomachaches and more school absences than other children [36]. Further supporting this mechanism, recent studies have demonstrated that when parents of children with RAP are taught to reduce positive or sympathetic responses to their children's pain complaints, the frequency of these complaints decreased.

Environmental Stressors in Childhood and Adult Life

This section describes how the stress components of the model outlined in Figure 1 relate to the presentation and outcome of FGIDs. Most research has focused on IBS and it is not clear whether all of the findings can be extrapolated to other FGIDs. Although childhood abuse has been most widely studied, it may be a marker of wider family disturbance and associated with other difficulties in the environment during childhood.

— Sexual and Physical Abuse

Although an association between sexual and physical abuse and FGIDs has been generally accepted in the medical community [37], methodological issues have precluded a full characterization of the relationship of abuse to GI illness relative to other psychosocial factors. The various definitions of abuse (exhibitionism, fondling or contact abuse, battering or physical abuse, and penetration or rape) and the different measurement methods have led to a wide range of estimated prevalence of abuse (from 6% to 62%) [38]. Another issue is that of serious under-recognition of abuse in clinical practice, which may be as low as 17% of women who have had an abuse history [39]. Finally, it is not clear whether abuse is found in a higher proportion of people with functional relative to organic disorders, though in clinic samples more severe abuse is found in a higher proportion of patients with IBS relative to patients with organic GI diagnoses [9, 40]. Population-based studies have led to conflicting results with regard to the association between self-reported FGIDs and abuse history in the general population [41, 42]. Similar differences exist in the association between abuse history and visiting a physician for IBS [41, 43]. Most, but not all national population studies have shown that abuse is associated with increased risk of abdominal pain and functional GI disorders [44, 45].

Despite these contentious issues there are several conclusions that are well supported by the literature. Firstly, high frequency rates of abuse (30%–56%) have been reported from many different referral centers in the U.S. and Europe [40, 46–50], and these figures are significantly higher than healthy control groups (Table 1). These tend to be higher in specialist or secondary care clinics than in primary care [39, 51]. Secondly, high frequencies of childhood abuse (approaching 50%) are not unique to patients with functional GI disorders—they are also reported by patients with non-GI chronic or recurrent painful functional conditions (e.g., pelvic pain, headaches, fibromyalgia) as well as many other physical and psychological disorders in adult life [52–54]. Thirdly, abusive experiences affect health outcomes, so GI patients with abuse histories report more severe pain, greater psychological distress, greater impairment of functioning in their daily lives, and more frequent visits to the doctor than GI patients without an abuse history [9, 37, 39, 55, 56]. Finally, it should be noted that these findings relate to severe abuse such as rape (penetration), repeated or multiple abuses, and life-threatening physical abuse, rather than other forms of abuse [57]. Therefore, the comprehensive assessment of patients with severe FGIDs should include an abuse history.

— Environmental Stressors in Adult Life

Studies using the Life Events and Difficulties Schedule (LEDS) [58, 59], have shown that the onset of FGIDs is associated with the experience of severely threatening events, such as the breakup of an intimate relationship. In these studies, two thirds of patients had experienced such a severe life event compared to a quarter of healthy controls, indicating the strength of the association between stress and onset of FGIDs [58].

Prospective studies have demonstrated that the experience of stressful life events is associated with symptom exacerbation among adults with IBS [60], heartburn [61], RAP in children, and frequent health care-seeking for IBS [29, 60, 62]. Chronic life stress has been reported as the main predictor of IBS symptom intensity over 16 months even after controlling for relevant confounders (severity of IBS, anxiety, and demographic features) [59].

Table I. The Prevalence of Abuse History in Clinic Samples of FGIDs and Comparison Groups

Study	Subjects	Prevalence of sexual abuse history	Comments
Drossman 1990 [39]	206 female tertiary referral center	Rape—31% functional GI 18% organic diagnoses. All abuse—53% functional, 27% organic diagnoses	Low response rate Low detection rate by physicians
Drossman 1996 [9]	506 female tertiary referral center	Severe sexual abuse = 33% FGIDs v 20% of organic GI diseases. (37% v 23% for life-threatening physical abuse)	Detailed abuse history interview. Abuse very strong predictor of adverse health outcome.
Talley 1995 [40]	440 FGID 557 organic GI	22% FGID 16% Organic GI	Patients with history of abuse more likely to report IBS-type symptoms
Walker 1993 [46]	28 IBS 19 IBD	32% IBS 0% IBD	Number of medically unexplained symptoms, depression and anxiety differentiate abused and nonabused.
Delvaux 1997 [47]	196 IBS 135 organic diseases 200 ophthalmic clinic patients	20% IBS 10% organic GI 5% opthalmic	
Scarinici [311]	13 GERD 26 NCCP 11 IBS	GERD 92% IBS 82% NCCP 27%	Abused patients had lower pain thresholds and more functional disability, psychiatric disorders, and other pain disorders.
Heitkemper 2001 [48]	167 IBS 86 controls Community advert/ HMO	Two samples: 46% IBS v 21% controls & 26% IBS v 10% controls	Abuse not associated with GI or physiological arousal index. Psychological symptoms only increased in those with both child and adult abuse.
Ali 2000 [49]	25 IBS 25 IBD in tertiary care setting	Touch: 44% IBS 18% IBD Rape: 34% IBS, 14% IBD	No association of abuse with depression
Longstreth 1993 [51]	1264 HMO enrollees	51% severe IBS symptoms 25% less severe IBS symptoms 12% healthy	Nongastrointestinal symptoms, previous surgery. Common in abused.

FGID = functional gastrointestinal disorders; GERD = gastroesophageal reflux disease; GI = gastrointestinal; HMO = health maintenance organization; IBD = inflammatory bowel disease; IBS = irritable bowel syndrome; NCCP = noncardiac chest pain

Psychological States and Traits Shown to be Related to Gut Function

This section reviews evidence concerning the common forms of psychological distress that are seen in the GI clinic and that, if modified, lead to improved well-being and daily functioning. The more severe forms of distress that merit a psychiatric diagnosis and the less common personality factors are reviewed below.

— Psychological State

Anxiety and Depression

IBS patients, like patients with other chronic medical disorders, record scores of depression and anxiety that are intermediate between psychiatric populations and healthy controls [9, 63–66]. These findings are not confined to high-income countries [67, 68]. The severity of psychological distress relates to health care-seeking status [67, 69, 70], but is also observed in IBS and functional dyspepsia nonconsulters compared to healthy controls [70, 71]. Psychological distress in IBS patients can usually be reversed with appropriate treatment, whereas patients with IBS who have marked personality difficulties (see below) are much less amenable to treatment. Prospective studies have found that anxiety and depression are significant and independent predictors of postinfective IBS [72, 73]. Anxiety and depression also predict a poor outcome of IBS, including a poor response to treatment [74].

Somatization

There are two very different conceptualizations of somatization. The term is sometimes used as shorthand for the somatoform psychiatric disorders, which are discussed in the next section. More commonly, the term "somatization" is used for people who report a large number of bodily symptoms that are associated with impairment of function and increased demand for health care [75]. This process of somatization involves increased awareness of and concern about normal bodily sensations.

This common form of somatization, represented by high scores on somatization questionnaires, has been reported in clinic patients with FGIDs [76, 77] and also in population-based studies of FGIDs [71]. Somatization might represent a separate dimension of somatic distress, which is partly genetically determined and which also overlaps with anxiety and depression [78]. Somatization

Table 2. Prevalence of Psychiatric Disorder in Functional Bowel Disorder/Irritable Bowel Syndrome using Standardised Research Psychiatric Interviews

| | | | % with anxiety and depressive disorder | | |
| | | | | Comparison groups | |
	Subjects	Psychiatric interview	Patients with functional bowel disorders	Organic gastrointestinal disorder	Healthy controls
McDonald & Boucher 1980 [312]	FBD[1]	CIS[3]	53% (n=35)	20% (n=32)	-
Colgan 1988 [144]	FBD	CIS	57% (n=37)	6%	-
Corney & Stanton 1990 [313]	IBS	CIS	48% (n=42)	-	-
Craig & Brown 1984 [314]	FBD	PSE[4]	42% (n=79)	18% (n=56)	8% (n=135)
Ford 1987 [315]	IBS[2]	PSE	42% (n=48)	6% (n=16)	
Toner 1990 [316]	IBS	DIS[5]	61% (n=44)	-	14%
Blanchard 1990 [317]	IBS	DIS	56% (n=68)	25% (n=44)	18% (n=38)

[1] FBD = Functional bowel disorder (i.e. consecutive nonorganic gastrointestinal disorders in the clinic);
[2] IBS = Irritable bowel syndrome patients; [3] CIS = Clinical Interview Schedule;
[4] PSE = Present State Examination; [5] DIS = Diagnostic Interview Schedule.

has been associated also with a history of abuse or a rejecting parenting style during childhood, environmental stress, and concurrent anxiety and depression. The high prevalence of somatization in FGIDs explains the frequent "extragastrointestinal symptoms" of IBS [79], and the high co-occurrence of those syndromes (e.g., chronic fatigue syndrome, fibromyalgia, multiple chemical sensitivity syndrome) that are defined by unexplained bodily symptoms [80]. The degree of somatization is directly correlated with severity of FGID symptoms and degree of impairment [81]. Somatization is associated with poor health-related quality of life in clinic and population-based samples [82, 83]; it predicts a poor response to treatment [84, 85] and high health care costs [86].

— Comorbid Psychiatric Disorders

When the symptoms of anxiety, depression, or somatization are sufficiently marked and persistent, they may fulfill the criteria for a psychiatric diagnosis. Anxiety and depressive disorders, for example, are more common (40%–60%) in clinic patients with some FGIDs (notably IBS) compared to patients with similar abdominal symptoms explained by underlying organic GI disease (<25%) and healthy controls (<20%) (Table 2) [87]. This finding has been confirmed in a recent meta-analysis and a systematic review [69, 80]. The meta-analysis also found that anxiety, but not depressive symptoms, were associated with consulting for abdominal symptoms [69].

Among IBS patients studied at medical centers, the most frequent diagnostic categories are (1) anxiety disorders [panic, generalized anxiety and post-traumatic stress disorder (PTSD), (2) mood disorders (major depression and dysthymic disorder), and (3) somatoform disorders (hypochondriasis and somatization disorder) [46, 50, 88] (for definitions see [89]).

No single psychiatric disorder is uniquely associated with the FGIDs although specific attention has been paid to panic disorder, which has been linked to IBS [88], functional chest pain [90], and functional vomiting [91] with a prevalence of approximately 30% (range 15%–41%) [80]. In IBS accompanied by panic disorder, the GI symptoms improve when the panic is successfully treated [92], suggesting that diarrhea is directly attributable to the panic disorder. However, panic disorder only occurs in a minority of people with IBS and cannot be regarded as a common explanation for diarrhea in FGIDs.

Anxiety or depressive disorders often predate or coincide with the onset of the FGID [93, 94], indicating that the psychiatric disorder cannot be regarded as a response to the FGID. Like abuse history, psychiatric disorder is greater among IBS patients seen in referral centers (up to 94% may report lifetime psychiatric disorder), which compares to about 18% of IBS patients seen in the community [95].

The somatoform psychiatric disorders include: *somatization disorder, undifferentiated somatoform disorder, conversion disorder, pain disorder, hypochondriasis,* and *body dysmorphic disorder* (BDD) [96]. All involve a focus on bodily/somatic complaints that cannot be explained fully by a general medical condition, substance use, another mental disorder (e.g., depressive disorder), or intentional self-infliction (factitious disorders). High rates of somatization disorder have been reported for FGID patients recruited from GI or tertiary populations [97, 98] and these are associated with more psychiatric symptoms and abnormal illness behaviors. *Somatization disorder* is defined as (1) a history of many physical complaints beginning before 30 years of age that are persistent and lead to treatment-seeking and/or significant impairment in social, occupational, or other areas of functioning, and (2) presence of all of the following at some time during the course of the disturbance: (i) four pain symptoms, (ii) two gastrointestinal tract symptoms, (iii) one sexual symptom, and (iv) one pseudoneurological symptom (e.g., weakness). This definition comes from studies in specialized clinic settings. In primary care or population-based samples the disorder is very rare with a lifetime prevalence of 0.1% to 0.2%, so a less stringent definition is used in most studies [75]. *Neurasthenia* is a psychiatric diagnosis made when there is persistent and distressing fatigue after mental or minor physical effort associated with muscular aches or pains, dizziness, sleep disturbance, irritability, dyspepsia and mild depressive symptoms [99]. It is, therefore, very similar to chronic fatigue syndrome, which commonly co-occurs with IBS [80, 100]. When the two conditions occur together there is greater impairment of health-related quality of life and poorer outcome than when the syndromes occur singly [100–102].

— Psychological Traits

Personality

Personality traits refer to enduring traits that are evident in early adult life and are stable throughout life. The concept is usually concerned with the way an individual relates to other people and responds to environmental changes. Personality traits may underlie the high level of anxiety seen in some patients with FGIDs attending GI clinics, and such anxiety is difficult to treat. This is less common than the anxiety state, which is a reversible condition that can be modified frequently with treatment.

As shown in controlled studies, IBS patients have recorded higher neuroticism scores and a greater tendency to be anxious than people without health problems or a nonclinical population with similar GI complaints [62, 64, 66, 103–106]. This association may reflect the self-selection of individuals into health care facilities [62, 70, 107] and similar findings are found in clinic patients with other medical disorders. Thus, there is no support for a specific personality profile that is unique to IBS or other FGIDs [108]. The experience of chronic symptoms of pain and bodily dysfunction can lead to raised scores on personality measures [109] and reduction of these scores when symptoms resolve [110]. This makes it difficult to determine causality without prospective studies. Two such studies suggest that new episodes of IBS can be predicted by neuroticism and "psychological vulnerability," but further studies are needed to define the personality traits associated with later onset of IBS [72, 111]. Neuroticism is a personality characteristic that may act as a mediator between prior abuse and presence of IBS [112]; it may also predict a poor response to treatment [113].

Psychophysiology: Affect and Stress Modulation of GI Function

It is well recognized that environmental stress and related mood changes alter GI function and symptom perception in persons with GI diseases such as gastroesophageal reflux disease (GERD), as well as in those with FGIDs such as IBS. Common experiences include stress-related increases in reflux symptoms in the absence of alterations in esophageal acid exposure, as well as the perceptions of a "nervous stomach," stress-evoked episodes of diarrhea, and the feeling of being "kicked in the gut" following acute stressors among persons with IBS. The relationship of stressors to GI function is viewed as a direct consequence of the critical and exquisite modulation of GI function by the CNS, including motor responses, pain modulation, and even immune function [114, 115]. In addition, there is growing evidence that the relationship is bidirectional, with the GI system providing important modulatory input into the CNS [116].

These interactive relationships are important since they provide the foundation for hypotheses of CNS dysregulation as causative in FGID symptom onset and maintenance. This section briefly reviews laboratory-based studies of the effects of acute laboratory stressors on alterations in GI function and symptoms, then examines alterations in CNS systems that may help mediate the relationships between stressors and GI function and symptoms. These include the autonomic nervous system (ANS), neuroendocrine pathways, and sleep.

— Experimental Studies of Stress Influences on GI Function

Several recent articles have reviewed this literature for both the upper and lower GI tract [114, 115, 117, 118].

Esophagus and Stomach

Laboratory studies have shown that stressors increase esophageal contraction amplitude but not tertiary contractions (i.e., nonpropulsive contractions) in normal subjects. Perhaps more important for heartburn, stressors evoke increases in acid sensitivity and symptoms of heartburn in patients with relatively high levels of anxiety but do not alter measures of esophageal acid [119]. Stressors are associated with increased swallowing and some FGID symptoms may be related to stress-induced increased air swallowing (aerophagia) and the associated increase in gas. It has been reported that exposure to stressors delays gastric emptying of solids, probably through an inhibition of antral motility [120].

Small Intestine and Colon

There is evidence that patients with IBS show altered motility [121] and increased pain response to giant contractions in the small intestine (> 75 mmHg). They may also show increased contractions to a visceral stimulus [122]. Therefore, several investigators have examined the extent to which stressors influence motility and symptom reports. With regard to small intestine motility, it has been found that a variety of stressors disrupt the cyclic pattern of motility normally seen during fasting as well as decreasing the overall amount of contractions [123–125]. Cann et al. [126] reported that stressors significantly speeded mouth to cecum transit time in diarrhea-predominant IBS and slowed transit in constipation-predominant patients.

With respect to colon function, IBS patients show exaggerated motility to psychological stress, balloon distension, eating, and injection of cholecystokinin. The contractions observed following stressors are principally nonperistaltic contractions that could contribute to IBS symptoms by retarding the movement of gas and stool or by altering tension in the gut wall leading to pain. Laboratory stressors also produce increased smooth muscle tone in the rectum [127], which has been associated with IBS [15]. However, a critical role for motility disturbance in producing symptoms in a majority of IBS patients has not been clearly demonstrated.

With regard to perception, several studies of the effects of stressors on perception of colorectal distention have produced inconsistent findings [128]. It is likely that the variations among the stressors or the subject samples used in these studies contribute to the inconsistent findings. For example, some stressors may have reduced symptom perception because they distracted the subjects from the rating task. A recent study that controlled for distraction demonstrated that patients with IBS, but not healthy subjects, produced higher ratings of rectal stimulus intensity and unpleasantness during a dichotomous listening stress compared to a relaxation condition. In addition, only the patients reported higher ratings of stress, anger, and anxiety during the task compared to the relaxing condition [129]. Similar findings have been reported for response to acid exposure among patients with heartburn.

— Altered Autonomic Nervous System (ANS) Responses in FGIDs

The ANS is the primary link between the brain and the GI tract and is responsible for homeostatic regulation of gut function [130]. Studies using primarily cardiovascular measures of ANS sympathetic and parasympathetic function (e.g., heart rate, blood pressure, heart rate variability) have indicated the presence of altered ANS function in persons with IBS and other functional GI populations under both resting state conditions and during exposure to stressors [130]. IBS studies have shown diarrhea-predominant subjects with sympathetic increases and constipation-predominant subjects with parasympathetic dysfunction [131]. In addition, altered ANS responses (particularly increased sympathetic or decreased parasympathetic tone) are associated with increased sensitivity and symptoms among some persons with IBS and heartburn [132].

ANS alterations may also vary as a function of symptom severity and sex. One investigation, for example, found that women with severe constipation displayed reduced vagal (parasympathetic) tone while those with severe pain unrelated to meals showed increased vagal tone [133]. Although the literature on ANS function suggests that abnormalities exist among patients with FGIDs, the prevalence of these abnormalities and their role in the pathophysiology of functional symptom generation or exacerbation is unclear. Most studies are of small samples with mixed symptom features and poor control of potentially confounding variables such as menstrual cycle in women, psychological status, and comorbid conditions [134]. In addition, it is not known to what extent the cardiovascular ANS measures in these studies represent reliable and sensitive markers for GI ANS function. GI-specific measures have not been reliably identified, although two candidate measures include pancreatic polypeptide levels (acting via abdominal vagal activation) [135] and mucosal blood flow.

— Neuroendocrine Stress Responses

A variety of neuroendocrine pathways have been implicated in stress-induced alterations in GI function [118]. Activation of CNS circuits that include the emotional motor system lead to neuroendocrine responses such as the release of corticotrophin-releasing factor (CRF), cortisol, as well as norepinephrine and epinephrine.

Endogenous CRF may have a particularly significant role in CNS mediation of stress-induced inhibition of upper GI and stimulation of lower GI motor function through activation of brain CRF receptors [118]. The inhibition of gastric emptying by CRF may be mediated by interaction with the CRF-2 receptor, while CRF-1 receptors are involved in the colonic and anxiogenic responses to stress. Endogenous serotonin (5-HT), peripherally released in response to stress, appears to be involved in both stress and central CRF induced stimulation of colonic motility through its effects on 5-HT$_3$ receptors.

Studies of catecholamines and cortisol levels in IBS patients have produced mixed results. Several studies have reported higher levels of cortisol in patients with IBS [136, 137] and increased postprandial cortisol in patients with diarrhea-predominant IBS [138] Other studies, however, have failed to find IBS-related differences in catecholamine or cortisol levels [129, 138].

— Sleep Abnormalities in FGIDs

Subjective reports of fatigue and sleep disturbance are common in IBS and other FGIDs [139, 140] and there is a positive correlation between subjective sleep disturbances and GI symptoms [141]. Conversely, restful sleep is associated with improved IBS symptoms [141] and IBS patients report lower symptom levels in the morning after awakening than the evening [140].

Data on objective measures of sleep physiology are less consistent. Increased rapid eye movement activity has been found in persons with IBS but other studies have not found any sleep abnormalities in IBS patients compared to controls [142, 143]. These differences may be due to the heterogeneity of IBS subgroups in the various studies in terms of both bowel habit and symptom severity [139].

Health Beliefs and Coping

This section describes the beliefs that many patients hold about the causes of their symptoms (e.g., that gut symptoms indicate cancer or other serious illness) and how these beliefs may lead to particular behaviors, such as adopting a limited lifestyle (e.g., always staying close to a toilet when this is not really necessary) [70, 74]. Sometimes the beliefs regarding GI symptoms may be catastrophic, for example, "I cannot live another day like this, my life is ruined." When catastrophic beliefs are accompanied by excessive worry about the illness and lifestyle consequences, there is poor coping with the illness. These marked concerns about the disorder and marked impairment of functioning are often associated with general psychological distress or depression, as discussed earlier in this chapter [144].

Patients' behaviors may become understandable when we also appreciate their underlying beliefs. Thus beliefs, or *cognitions,* about the likely cause of symptoms and concerns that they indicate serious disease may explain certain *behaviors* such as dietary modification and seeking medical treatment. This *cognitive-behavioral* model applies to a wide range of clinical presentations and is not specific to FGIDs [145, 146], but specific cognitions may occur in specific medical conditions. For example, fear of sudden death may accompany symptoms referable to the heart, whereas fears of cancer are more common in people with FGIDs.

— GI-Specific Cognitions

There are certain cognitions that appear to be common in GI conditions. Recent research has focused on two related constructs: "catastrophizing" and "GI symptom-specific anxiety" as potential markers of psychological processes that mediate GI symptoms and illness impact.

Catastrophizing refers to the tendency to exaggerate the threat of certain symptoms [147]. Thus, everyone experiences abdominal pain and diarrhea from time to time, but to interpret such symptoms as indicating cancer when there is no other evidence to support such a conclusion may be regarded as catastrophizing.

Pain-related catastrophizing includes at least three components: helplessness (perceived difficulty in coping effectively with pain), magnification (a tendency to consistently anticipate that pain will produce highly negative consequences) and rumination (perceived difficulty in distracting oneself from pain) [148]. People who report a high degree of catastrophizing display great difficulty in shifting their attention from the unpleasant emotional aspects of a brief, painful stimulus in the laboratory to the less threatening, sensory aspects of the stimulus [149]. It is not surprising, then, that catastrophizing has been shown to mediate in part the relationship between depression and pain severity [150] and is associated with poor outcome among persons with IBS [55].

GI-specific anxiety is heightened sensitivity to, and fear of, anxiety-related GI sensations (such as palpitations or "butterflies in the stomach") and is an important predictor of anxiety reactions such as panic attacks and panic disorder [151]. This hypersensitivity to anxiety-related bodily sensations is based upon beliefs that they have harmful somatic, psychological, or social consequences [151]. Both anxiety sensitivity and general trait anxiety are conceptualized as stable personality traits indicating persistent, lifelong tendencies. Whereas the latter indicates a general tendency to respond anxiously to a wide range of external stressors, anxiety sensitivity represents a specific tendency to respond fearfully to bodily sensations of anxiety (i.e. these bodily sensations act as the stressful stimulus). This construct of anxiety sensitivity has been shown to be an important predictive variable in somatic pain [152] and to be significantly associated with IBS even after controlling for general anxiety [153].

Health anxiety reflects a constitutional tendency to worry about bodily symptoms and deny psychological problems and may precede the development of IBS [13]. Compared to depressed patients seeing a psychiatrist, IBS patients record higher scores on hypochondriacal beliefs, disease phobia, and bodily preoccupation scales of the Illness Attitude Scale [155]. These patients are also wary of the negative stigma and moral connotations associated with a psychological explanation for their symptoms [156].

These worries about illness can be modified. A satisfactory consultation with the gastroenterologist leads to a reduction of overall anxiety, less fear that the symptoms represent cancer and a reduction in the patient's preoccupation and helplessness in relation to the pain [157]. Such worries may also resolve when results of clinical evaluation are normal [158]. They may not resolve, however, if there is a very high level of health anxiety prior to the investigation [158] and/or there is concurrent anxiety or depressive disorder [144]. Marked worries about serious illness predict a poor outcome and underlie the repeated visits to GI specialists or use of alternative treatments.

Selective attention to thoughts and perceptions that confirm their understanding of GI symptoms may occur in people who worry about bodily symptoms. Patients with IBS are more likely to selectively recall GI words relative to words from other categories [159]. They may selectively dismiss information or sensory input that is inconsistent with their beliefs regarding the seriousness of their bowel disorder [160] and ignore, or even deny, the role of other contributing factors such as life stressors, psychological distress, overwork, interpersonal conflict, or loss [62]. It is important for physicians to be aware of these beliefs in order to elicit each patient's level of concern about their symptoms and implement effective treatment strategies when these concerns are high [161].

These constructs of specific GI-related health anxiety, catastrophizing, and selective attention are different aspects of poor coping observed in patients with FGIDs and are all amenable to treatment by cognitive-behavior means.

Influence of Psychological Factors on Outcomes in Patients with FGIDs

The effect of psychological factors on outcomes in FGID patients is seen clearly in relation to health-related quality of life and medical treatment-seeking/health care use.

— Health-Related Quality of Life

It is well-recognized that patients with IBS and other FGIDs experience considerable impairment of health-related quality of life [2–4]. Several recent studies have shown that only some of this impairment can be accounted for by the symptoms of FGIDs; psychological factors have a major and unique, negative impact on health-related quality of life, which is reversible with appropriate psychological treatment (Table 3) [86, 100, 162–165].

— Health Care-Seeking

The two aspects of health care-seeking that have been studied in FGIDs are (a) the factors that distinguish people in the general population who seek

Table 3. Influence of Psychological Distress /Psychiatric Disorders on Health-Related Quality of Life (HRQoL) in IBS and Other Disorders

	No. and type of subjects	Measures of psychological distress & HRQoL	Findings of multivariate analysis
Naliboff 1998 [162]	337 patients in a clinical trial referred from a tertiary center and from community advertisements	SCL-90 & SF36	In multiple regression, somatization/distress independently contributed to HRQoL
Spiegel 2004 [163]	770 IBS patients at a university center	SCL-90 & SF36	Psychological factors predicted both physical and mental aspects of HRQoL.
Halder 2004 [83]	112 (dyspepsia and IBS) and 110 controls in population-based study	SCL-90 & SF-36	Association between IBS and HRQoL was mediated by SCL somatization score.
Creed [86, 100]	257 patients with severe IBS	SCL-90 and SCAN & SF36	After adjustment for abdominal pain and other IBS symptom severity, severity of depression, depressive disorder, panic and neurasthenia associated with impaired HRQoL. Depression and neurasthenia predict continued impairment over 1 year; improvement of depression was associated with improved role functioning.
Drossman 2004 [165]	397 female patients with IBS entering a treatment trial	SCL-90 and CSQ & IBS-QOL and SIP	Impaired HRQoL was associated with low SCL score, low catastrophizing score, and psychiatric diagnosis after adjustment for severity of IBS symptoms.

SCL-90 = Symptom Check List -90; SF-36 = Short Form 36; SCAN = Schedule for Clinical Assessment in Neuropsychiatry; CSQ= Coping Strategies Questionnaire; SIP = Sickness Impact Profile; IBS = irritable bowel syndrome; IBS-QOL = IBS Quality of Life.

treatment for FGIDs from those who report symptoms but who do not seek treatment and (b) the correlation between degree of psychological distress and amount of health care use, including number of physician visits, prior surgery, and medication.

The primary factors observed in IBS patients who seek treatment (IBS consulters) compared to people in the community with IBS symptoms who do not consult (IBS nonconsulters) are greater pain severity, greater duration of pain, increased concern about illness, and greater anxiety and depression [56, 74] (Table

Table 4. IBS Severity Indicators and Psychological Variables that Independently Predict Consultation for IBS

Author	Severity of IBS symptoms	Psychological variables
Heaton 1991 [318]	Bowel suffering score	Anxiety and depression
Drossman 1988 [62]	Diarrhea severity Pain severity	Depression score (MMPI) Illness behavior score (IBQ)
Kettell 1992 [319]	Pain severity Abdominal distension	Health concerns Anxiety & depression
Talley 1991 [320]	Pain severity/frequency Daily activities interrupted	—
Van den Horst [321]	Pain severity Daily activities interrupted	Somatic attribution Health concerns
Talley 1997 [43]	Severity and duration of pain	—
Herschbach 1999 [70]	Duration & seriousness of symptoms	Depression Symptoms unrelated to stress
Koloski 2003 [322]		Anxiety about abdominal pain Psychological distress

MMPI =Minnesota Multiphasic Personality Inventory, IBQ = Illness Behaviour Questionnaire; IBS = irritable bowel syndrome.

4). Thompson, et. al. [166] found that the subgroup of primary care IBS patients who choose to further consult specialists were less likely to see a link between stress and their IBS symptoms.

Compared to comparison groups, patients with FGIDs make 2 to 3 times as many visits to physicians for nongastrointestinal complaints [1], and have increased hospitalizations and surgical procedures [9], including hysterectomy [167]. Medical consultations, tests, and medications lead to very high costs in some patients with FGIDs, but some of these costs are attributable directly to somatization and other psychosocial factors in addition to those attributable to the functional GI disorder itself [86, 168]. In a UK study comparing IBS and control subjects' health care use, attendance at primary care was increased by 43%, prescriptions by 85%, and gastroenterology appointments by 68% in the IBS group [2]. These data are comparable to other studies [169], but the costs are highly skewed. Half of a population-based sample of IBS sufferers incur costs comparable to the general population and 14% incur costs five times that of the general population [170]— the latter is comparable to patients with severe IBS seen in a gastroenterology clinic [100]. Only 20% to 30% of the total cost difference between IBS patients and population controls can be attributed to lower GI-related services, indicating the generally increased demand for health care of some patients with IBS [171]. High health care use is partly attributable to psychosocial factors such as depression and somatization, in addition to symptoms related to the FGID itself, and may be reduced by at least 25% following psychological treatment [172].

Maladaptive Illness Behavior and Health Care-Seeking

Excessive medical help-seeking may be regarded as abnormal "illness behavior." This occurs at two ends of a continuum: denial of illness may lead to delay in seeking help for chest pain or similar alarming symptom. At the other extreme are people who repeatedly seek treatment for symptoms that are misperceived as serious and who cannot be reassured. In the latter situation normal bodily sensations are misinterpreted as evidence of disease. This type of illness behavior may elicit negative feelings in the physician that can adversely affect the patient-physician interaction.

— Mechanisms by which Psychological Factors Influence Outcomes in FGIDs

Psychiatric disorders in patients with FGID influence outcomes [86, 162] because of increased number of bodily symptoms, greater concern about the seriousness of such symptoms, and the negative effect of depression on daily functioning [173]. The environmental stressors and psychological factors that lead to a poor outcome of FGIDs (Figure 1) should not be regarded as specific etiological factors for these disorders, but rather as factors that lead to a poor outcome through a variety of mechanisms, including:

1. Genetic Factors
   a. There may be genetic factors that are shared by FGIDs and anxiety, depression, somatization, and pain sensitivity.
2. Life Events
   a. Abuse and stressful life events associated with impaired adult relationships [174] increase the chance of subsequent psychological distress and psychiatric disorders that can increase the chance of FGIDs with poor outcomes [37, 63, 175, 176].
   b. Poor coping, catastrophizing, selective attention to bodily symptoms, and dissociation may also link early abuse and FGID in adult life [55, 177].
   c. The improvement following cognitive-behavioral treatment [178] and psychodynamic (interpersonal) psychotherapy [172] in IBS patients who have an abuse history may be understood in terms of better coping, less

preoccupation with abdominal and other bodily symptoms, and reduced anxiety or depression.

d. Stressful life events may lead to exacerbation and perpetuation of symptoms because of acute effects on gut function.

3. Physiological Factors

a. Visceral hypersensitivity (see Chapter 1) may be explained by alterations in processing of visceral sensation in patients with FGIDs who also have concomitant psychiatric disorders [16, 179–182].

b. Patients with FGIDs who have a concomitant psychiatric diagnosis may manifest alterations in autonomic nervous system function, particularly diminished parasympathetic tone [183]. These changes may mediate altered gut motility and sensation.

c. Cross-sectional studies suggest no direct association between lowered tolerance to rectal distension and sexual abuse history [15, 184], but the marked beneficial effect of psychotherapy is accompanied by increased tolerance to rectal distension [181], suggesting altered pain perception [14, 185] similar to that found in fibromyalgia and back pain [186].

d. Increased autonomic function and/or intestinal motility may be due to hyperarousal [187].

e. Recent studies suggest that the affective pain experience may be mediated through alterations in the region of the anterior cingulate cortex and associated areas [16, 188]. However, it remains uncertain how or whether these alterations are related to associated psychological changes.

Assessment: Interviews and Self-Report Instruments

In view of the importance of physiological, social, and psychological factors in determining outcomes of FGID we suggest that physicians include a brief psychosocial assessment of each patient with FGID in addition to a full clinical assessment of the presenting symptoms. This requires a satisfactory patient-doctor relationship, established during the early part of the consultation, and a few specific questions about key psychosocial variables integrated into the routine history-taking. A more detailed psychosocial assessment is particularly useful for severe symptoms, previous treatment failure, poor adherence to a treatment regimen, and marked disability. This will usually be performed by a psychologist, psychiatrist, or a specially trained gastroenterologist. Such a stepped approach is used frequently in other medical disciplines, such as rheumatology, in which (a) patients require medical management over extended time periods and (b) psychosocial variables are associated with long-term outcomes [189].

Table 5. Brief Clinical Assessment of Important Psychological
         and Social Influences on FGID

Area of assessment	
Depression	Over the last 2 weeks how often have you been bothered by any of the following problems:
	a. Little interest or pleasure in doing things?
	b. Feeling down, depressed, or hopeless?
	Score for each question: not at all = 0, several days = 1, more than half the days = 2, nearly every day = 3. A total score of 3 or more indicates an 83% chance of depressive disorder
	And/or ask about sleep, appetite, libido, and concentration within routine symptoms review.
	And/or administer Hospital Anxiety and Depression Scale (HADS)
Anxiety	Have you been anxious or feeling tense recently?
	And/or administer Hospital Anxiety and Depression Scale (HADS)
Somatization	In the systems review include questions about headaches, chest pains, palpitations, limb and joint pains, fatigue, tightness of throat, difficulty with swallowing, with micturition, dysmenorrhoea, dyspareunia.
	And/or administer a somatization scale.
Attribution of symptoms/ worry about illness	What do you think causes these symptoms?
	How worried are you about these symptoms?
	Have you worried that they might indicate a serious illness such as cancer?
	And/or administer a health anxiety questionnaire
Illness impact and quality of life	How much do these symptoms interfere with your daily life?
	And/or administer a quality of life questionnaire (See the section on Reliable and Valid Questionnaires below.)

— Assessments Performed by Physicians

Due to the demands of busy clinic schedules, many physicians feel that they do not have sufficient time to perform adequate psychosocial assessments. We suggest, however, that psychological and social variables are too important in the FGIDs to be overlooked. In primary care, up to three quarters of marked psychological problems are missed, which leads to needless continued disability and excessive health care utilization [190]. Our recommendation is designed to avoid this situation in FGID patients.

Psychosocial assessment should encompass the following (suggested screening instruments are included for each): (a) *depression and anxiety* (Hospital Anxiety

Table 6. Reliability and Validity of Self-administered Questionnaires

	Acceptable measure
Reliability represents the stability of a measure when used in a variety of different conditions, e.g., (a) by different people; (b) on different occasions; or (c) in different places.	The minimum correlation coefficient required in tests of reliability is generally considered to be 0.75 to 0.80.
Validity is the extent to which an instrument actually measures the construct (e.g., anxiety about bowel symptoms) it is intended to assess. This depends in part on its reliability, but high reliability does not guarantee acceptable validity.	In the comparison between a new and a well-recognized standardized instrument, acceptable correlation coefficients generally range between 0.30 and 0.70.
Response bias is the tendency of some people to score the questionnaire in a way that minimizes distress (socially desirable responses) or maximizes symptoms through high anxiety.	

and Depression Scale) [191, 192], (b) *somatization* (Patient Health Questionnaire) [193], (c) *health beliefs and coping* (Cognitive Strategies Questionnaire—Catastrophizing or Visceral Sensitivity Index) [194, 195], and (d) *illness impact and health-related quality of life* (IBS-Quality of Life) [196].

Suggested questions that may be used in routine consultations are listed in Table 5 and additional standardized self-report questionnaires are listed in the Appendix. In addition to asking the relevant questions, the psychosocial assessment will only be satisfactory if the patient is able to speak freely, which requires privacy and sufficient time. Sensitive areas of discussion include depressed mood, possible suicidal thoughts, and the nature of close relationships. Sometime these require a second appointment directed towards this area of assessment.

Questions about psychosocial issues fit neatly into the clinician's routine questions about how the FGID impacts on the person's life. If the patient queries the relevance of these questions the physician may then truthfully respond by saying: "I always ask my patients these questions as part of my initial assessment—it helps me work out the best way to help. The items may, or may not apply to you." In addition, the physician should provide feedback regarding the results of the entire evaluation and discuss treatment plans, which may involve both medical and psychosocial treatment strategies. If questionnaires are used, they should be valid and reliable (Table 6). The physician should be acquainted with the significance of the results of such questionnaires and a close working relationship with a mental health professional is helpful in this respect.

— Reliable and Valid Questionnaires

Standardized self-report questionnaires are available to enhance the information obtained at clinical interview. Such questionnaires only provide meaningful information if they are reliable and valid and the clinician is aware of potential response biases. The reliability and validity of the majority of self-report measures described below have been established in multiple investigations. Details of each are given in the Appendix.

Anxiety, Depression, and Somatization

Most measures of anxiety and depression include items that focus primarily on somatic (bodily) symptoms. This means that a patient who experiences medical symptoms may record a high score that inappropriately suggests depression [197]. The *Hospital Anxiety and Depression Scale (HADS)*, however, has been specifically designed to overcome this difficulty by omitting bodily symptoms. It has been widely used [191, 192], but experience suggests that the published cut-off points may be too low [198]. The *Symptom Check List (SCL-90)* [199] includes a useful subscale of somatization. The shorter versions (53-items *Brief Symptom Inventory (BSI)* [200], and the *BSI 18*), have not been used extensively in patients with FGID. The *Patient Health Questionnaire-15 (PHQ-15)* [201] is derived from the PRIME-MD diagnostic instrument for common mental disorders [193]. The total symptom counts on the PHQ-15 correlate strongly with psychological distress, functional impairment, and health care use [202].

Health Beliefs and Coping

Measures include the brief *Whitely Index (WI)* [203] and the longer *Illness Behavior Assessment Schedule* [204]. Both are reliably associated with other measures of hypochondriasis (illness worry) [205], but the subscales represent one primary factor similar to neuroticism [205]. The *Catastrophizing and Control scales* from the *Coping Strategies Questionnaire (CSQ)* measure coping responses of individuals with persistent pain [194].

The *Cognitive Scale for Functional Bowel Disorders (CS-FBD)* [206] has been used as an outcome measure in studies of psychosocial interventions for patients with IBS [178].

Health-Related Quality of Life

The most widely used generic measure is the *Medical Outcomes Study Short-Form Health Survey (SF-36)* [207]. This and its shortened version, the SF-12, are both highly sensitive and specific in IBS [208–210]. *Illness-specific QOL* measures for IBS include the well-validated *Irritable Bowel Syndrome Quality of*

Life measurement (IBS-QOL) [196], which also shows sensitivity to change [211], making it useful for inclusion in IBS treatment trials [212]. It has moderate construct validity with the SF-36 and differentiates between individuals with high and low symptom severity and frequency [213]. The *Functional Digestive Disorders Quality of Life (FDDQL)* questionnaire measures health-related QOL in patients with functional dyspepsia as well as IBS [214]. There are also QOL measures for heartburn and GERD [215].

Stressful Life Events

Divorce, unemployment, financial problems, and other stressful life events are measured by the *Life Experiences Survey* [216] and the *Life Events and Difficulties Schedule* [217], while everyday stressors are measured with other instruments [218]. Self-report measures may often suffice as they are easy to administer and inexpensive [219], but the responses are influenced by the respondent's personality traits and current mental state, which can produce selective or distorted recall of stressful events. To overcome these problems the detailed interview-based method of the *Life Events and Difficulties Schedule (LEDS)* [217] is used. Self-administered questionnaires cannot assess whether stressors preceded or followed a FGID [220, 221].

Sexual/Physical Abuse

The optimal method of eliciting data relating to sexual, physical, or emotional abuse is not clear. Self-administered questionnaires preserve the anonymity of the respondent but do not control for the effect of selective recall or disclosure [222], which can lead to over-reporting of certain abusive experiences [223]. For research purposes, accurate data collection requires a confidential assessment with a trained investigator in a supportive environment, free of coercion and using operational definitions [37]. In clinical practice, the patients' disclosure of an abusive experience should be considered truthful unless the data suggest otherwise [37]. The most frequently used instrument for rapid clinic-based assessment of abuse is the interview-based measure developed by Drossman, Leserman and colleagues [39, 224].

— Structured Interviews Used by Psychologists or Psychiatrists

Structured Psychiatric Interviews

When compared to self-administered questionnaires, the use of validated psychiatric diagnostic criteria such as the International Classification of Disease

(ICD-10) [99] and the American Diagnostic and Statistical Manual of Mental Disorders (DSM-IV) [225] enables trained researchers to diagnose depression and other psychiatric disorders independent of the bodily symptoms that occur in FGIDs. These research interviews are not used in routine clinical practice.

The *Diagnostic Interview Schedule (DIS)* [226] is a highly structured interview that requires specialized training, but inexperienced clinicians can be trained. The *Structured Clinical Interview for DSM (SCID)* [227] was designed for use by experienced clinicians who may supplement the structured interview with additional data [228]. The *Schedule of Clinical Assessment in Neuropsychiatry (SCAN 99)* and *Composite International Diagnostic Interview (CIDI)* [229] are essentially similar to the SCID [230].

Personality measures often include GI symptoms that may lead to spuriously high scores, so studies of FGIDs should include a comparison group of patients with organic GI disorders who also seek medical treatment [231]. Alternatively, the results can be reanalyzed after excluding the "somatic" items relevant to FGIDs [232]. Some IBS patients adopt a "response style" of socially desirable characteristics that alter the accuracy of certain psychological tests [156].

— Recommendations for Assessment Batteries

For screening purposes a questionnaire for mood (e.g., HADS) and a measure of somatization (e.g., PHQ-15) would be satisfactory; patients with elevated scores on either of these measures may require further attention and assessment. A more detailed evaluation by a psychologist or psychiatrist is likely to include measures of (a) health-related cognitions, (b) quality of life, and (c) psychological distress (e.g., SCL-90, DIS, or SCID).

With regard to research, choice of instruments is determined by the specific hypotheses of the study. However, most studies of patients with FGIDs should include at least one measure each of mood, cognition, and health-related quality of life. In addition, assessment to meet inclusion criteria of a trial might require standardized assessment of psychiatric disorders by use of the SCID or DIS.

Treatment

— General Principles of Treatment with Regard to the Psychosocial Aspects of FGIDs

Approach to the Patient

Success in treating patients with FGIDs starts with an effective doctor-patient relationship in which questions arise and information is passed from the physician to the patient and vice versa [233]. An "active listening" approach greatly improves both the quality of the physician-patient relationship and adherence to the proposed treatment regimen [234]. An enthusiastic, positive, and encouraging attitude on the part of the dispensing physician can be helpful in promoting a therapeutic response to all treatments for IBS [235].

1. Different interview styles: The doctor's style of interviewing may determine the amount and quality of information obtained. Although closed questions (e.g., "Have you experienced a change in bowel habit?" [*yes or no?*], "Do you experience nausea?" [*yes or no?*]) enable the physician to elicit symptoms rapidly, such an approach discourages the patient to talk spontaneously. A profoundly different approach is the *patient-centered approach,* in which the doctor encourages spontaneous expression of the patient's reasons for attending—their symptoms, thoughts, and feelings. Patients report high satisfaction with consultations that allow good communication between the doctor and patient, and a partnership in which patients' questions arising from information obtained from the internet, patient advocacy organizations, and other literature can be openly discussed.

2. The patient's view of their illness—addressing fears of cancer: Many patients fear that cancer or other serious disease might be the cause of their symptoms and such fears need to be addressed directly [157, 166]. Since patients have unique health beliefs concerning causation, these must be elicited by the doctor before reassurance is given. Premature or inappropriate reassurance is perceived by the patient as insincere, or as a lack of thoroughness by the physician. When the physician can confidently reject a diagnosis of cancer or similar serious disease, (s)he must also be prepared to provide an alternative explanation. This explanation should include the relationship to stress and distress, the postulated mechanisms of pain production, and emphasis on the overall favorable prognosis for the FGIDs. The patient should be helped to understand and accept the nature of the illness as a set of troublesome symptoms rather than an indication of underlying pathology. Patients feel enabled to cope with their illness when the doctor shows a specific interest in the effect of the illness on the patient's life and uses a positive approach [237]. Reassurance is more effective if accompanied by some written material to reinforce the points made by the doctor during the consultation, as anxious patients may remember little of what the doctor says during the consultation.

3. Feed back the results of negative investigations: Some physicians review the psychosocial aspects of a patient's illness only when investigation results are reported as normal. This is far from ideal as patients may be left feeling: "Does the doctor not believe that I really suffer severe pain?" or "Does the doctor mean that it is all in my mind?" While doctors may be surprised by such responses, they are consistent with points covered earlier in this chapter that many patients with FGIDs may hold excessive concerns about their health yet have particular worries about being regarded as neurotic.

We recommend that physicians explain fully why an investigation is being performed and, when appropriate, warn the patient beforehand that the result is likely to be normal. This will be helpful as it adds weight to the physician's working diagnosis of FGID. An essential aspect of feeding back negative results is the ascertainment beforehand of the patient's belief regarding the cause of the symptom.

4. Address psychosocial factors: Establishing the relationship between the FGID and anxiety or depression can be achieved with a brief list of relevant questions (Table 5) [89], which help also to demonstrate that the physician is interested in all aspect of illness—physical and psychological. If it becomes clear that stress is related to exacerbations and the person has catastrophic thoughts (e.g., "It is so bad that I must go to bed."), strategies are needed that will help the person to respond with less negative cognitions and less maladaptive coping strategies—an essential part of cognitive-behavioral therapy.

Some patients may be unwilling to accept a role for psychosocial factors in the illness even when it is evident to others. In this case, it is *not* helpful to discuss psychosocial and biological factors in terms of causation (e.g., "It's due to stress.") or as being separate ("The work-up is negative; it must be psychiatric.") [238]. Rather the physician should help the patient to understand the effects of the illness on their emotions, quality of life, and family and social dynamics and work to change these.

5. Accept the adaptations of chronic illness: For a small number of patients who have chronic and disabling symptoms a "care" rather than a "cure" approach may be more appropriate—this been shown to be much more effective in eliciting a positive outcome for the patient [233]. The "care" model requires that the physician (1) elicits and acknowledges the patient's beliefs, concerns and expectations, (2) offers empathy when needed, (3) clarifies misunderstandings, (4) provides education, and (5) negotiates the plan of treatment with the patient [238]. Use of self-care and support services (particularly support groups) with sustained followup by the principal care provider can maximize outcomes [239]. Caution should be exercised when using this approach, however, that this strategy does not lead to reinforcement of excessive illness behavior, rewarded by attention from others, release from usual responsibilities, and possibly social and financial compensation.

6. Reinforce healthy behaviors: If the physician focuses on symptoms rather than a broader psychosocial agenda the patient will assume that the physician's interest is contingent on continued illness. The challenge for the physician is to reinforce positive coping behaviors, such as a determination to lead a normal life in spite

Table 7. "Red Flags" that Indicate the Need to Consider Early Referral to a Mental Health Professional

- Severe depression, which may be accompanied by suicidal ideas
- Chronic refractory pain
- Severe disability
- Maladaptive illness behavior
- Difficulties in physician-patient interaction
- Idiosyncratic health beliefs
- Other identifiable psychiatric difficulties [somatization disorder, post-traumatic stress disorder, severe anxiety]
- History of abuse that leads to continuing distress and/or marked distress

of the symptoms. This involves moving the patient gently away from focusing on physical symptoms to a discussion of daily activities that encourage the patient out of "the sick role." Involvement of the patient in the choice of treatment can help give back to the patient more responsibility for their care and their health. When the doctor shows interest and praise in relation to increased activity, even in spite of continued pain, the patient feels valued because of health-promoting behavior [240].

Referral to a Mental Health Professional

It is preferable for gastroenterologists and primary care doctors to work closely with one or more mental health professional, if available. This facilitates referral of individual patients but also provides the gastroenterologist with advice about specific treatments (e.g., antidepressant dose regimes) and management strategies for the psychosocial aspect of illness. Referral to a mental health professional is appropriate when

a. Brief education and reassurance by the physician is unsuccessful and a more in-depth assessment is needed to assess whether psychological or antidepressant treatment is required;

b. Psychiatric disorders (e.g., major depression, panic disorder) are suspected that require specific treatments (e.g., antidepressants, cognitive-behavior or other psychotherapy);

c. A history of abuse or other significant trauma is present that has a significant negative impact on the patient's life;

d. The patient has persistent pain and/or serious impairment in daily function that requires specific treatment;

e. The patient has a history of multiple unexplained symptoms, with numerous consultations across specialties;

f. The patient asks for such a referral;

g. Any of the reasons to consider early referral to a mental health professional listed as "red flags" in Table 7 exist.

Preparing for a Referral to a Mental Health Professional

Many patients seeing a physician with a FGID are reluctant to be referred to a psychologist, psychiatrist, or other mental health professional for fear of being stigmatized. The patient may view the problem as "physical," and would prefer to visit a medical physician, protesting that "I am not crazy" when referral to a mental health professional is suggested. If the referral is made at the end of a medical evaluation, the patient may see it as a rejection ("The work up is negative, it must be nerves."). Furthermore, the patient may not be aware of the potential benefits of psychological evaluation and treatment.

The major goal in preparing the patient for a referral to the mental health professional is for the physician to define the patient's complaints in terms of a biopsychosocial disorder rather than a "physical" illness alone, and to get the patient motivated to further address all relevant biopsychosocial factors. It is usually not effective, to "turn over" the care to the mental health professional, since the patient will view this as a dismissal by the physician. Continued involvement of the physician, in line with the biopsychosocial model, provides the best model of "shared care" between mental health professional and physician.

Making the Referral

The physician should clearly explain to the patient why referral to a mental health professional is recommended. Ideally the latter should be seen as a member of the team involved in the patient's overall care: "I have a colleague, Dr _____, who sees many of my patients with these symptoms and we find that his/her treatment can help us with your care."

The mental health professional will require a detailed referral letter from the physician that states the nature of the presenting complaint, its duration and any psychosocial factors that have been identified or suspected (e.g., a history of major loss, abuse, interpersonal difficulties) including concerns about cancer (e.g., previous experience of a relative with bowel symptoms who later developed cancer).

The Role of the Consultant Mental Health Professional

If the patient has reservations about the referral, the mental health professional should explore them before attempting any psychological or psychopharmacologic treatment. Sometimes the first consultation is taken up with this task. Patients will not attend any subsequent appointments unless they feel that their view of the illness has been understood. Time spent reviewing the patient's

GI symptoms as well as types of psychological treatment relevant to them will be rewarded by the patient's increased interest and adherence to recommended treatment.

The mental health professional should review the problem in detail, while keeping an open mind regarding the relative importance of its physical and psychological aspects. He or she should explain that, in a multidisciplinary approach to treatment, psychological treatments can be helpful in addition to the usual medical treatments and psychological treatments (antidepressants and psychotherapy) may even be combined [241].

— Overview of Treatment Aimed at Psychosocial Aspects of FGID

Various treatment approaches have been found to be successful in FGIDs. Our knowledge of the mechanisms by which these interventions help patients is far from complete. For treatment to be effective, however, it is important to have the patient's acceptance of the need for treatment and his/her engagement in the change process. A patient's belief in the providers' competence and concern for her/him is likely to be a key requirement for this acceptance and engagement to occur. Close collaboration between physicians and mental health providers should support this process.

Algorithm of Treatment for Psychological Aspects of the FGIDs

There is a range of intensity of psychological approaches to treatment (Figure 2). The appropriate intensity of treatment needs to be matched to the severity of the FGID. This can be conceptualized as a series of steps.

Step 1 In the initial assessment the physician has three tasks: developing a satisfactory patient-doctor relationship, making a diagnosis of the FGID, and identifying any "red flag" indications that require consideration of an early referral to a mental health professional (Table 7 and Figure 2).

Step 2 In terms of psychosocial management, the next step is to facilitate the patient's understanding of the disorder.

Step 3 The next step in management of patients with FGIDs may include symptomatic medication and/or simple behavioral/lifestyle changes. The former includes dietary manipulation, laxatives, bulking agents, antidiarrheals, antispasmodics, serotonergic drugs such as alosetron, cilansetron and tegaserod, prokinetics, H_2 blockers, and proton pump inhibitors (PPIs). Detailed discussions of the situation(s) in which the patient's symptoms deteriorate can lead to suggestions for behavioral and lifestyle changes. Treatment may, for example, lead to different ways of handling

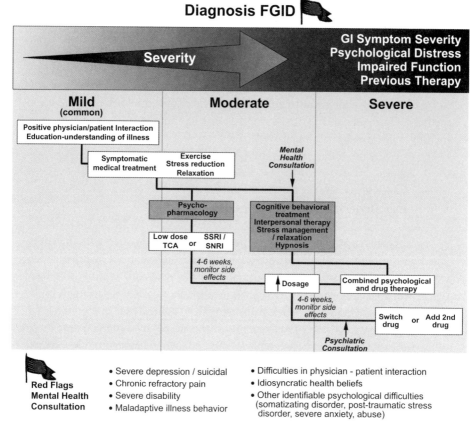

Figure 2. Treatment algorithm for patients with FGIDs. "Red flags" are indications for consideration of early referral to a mental health professional. TCA = tricyclic antidepressants; SSRI = selective serotonin reuptake inhibitor; SNRI = serotonin norepinephrine reuptake inhibitor; GI = gastrointestinal; FGID = functional gastrointestinal disorder.

excessive demands at work or difficult interpersonal conflicts. In addition, the physician may recommend those forms of relaxation (yoga, relaxation classes, and meditation) which are generally available.

Step 4 requires a decision to use an antidepressant or psychological/behavioral management. There is evidence to support both psychopharmacological and psychological forms of treatment, but the choice may be determined by availability of a psychologist or other professional who can perform the relevant psychological treatment described below. Other determinants may include time or cost constraints (of medications and testing), health insurance, and referral physician assumptions. If the psychological route is chosen, this will mean that a detailed psychosocial assessment is performed by the psychologist and that the physician should be prepared to prescribe and monitor an antidepressant. (See Chapter 4 for more details.)

Step 5 involves two possibilities. One is to add the second form of treatment (psychopharmacological or psychological/behavioral) to the first. There is clear evidence that this strategy is helpful for depressive and anxiety disorders and chronic pain [241–244], but there have been no trials to formally establish the efficacy of combined treatments in FGIDs. Clinical practice suggests combined behavioral and antidepressant treatment is helpful for patients who have not responded to either treatment alone. There are good theoretical grounds for combined treatment as antidepressants have some direct action on pain, anxiety, and depression and can increase the patient's motivation to engage in therapy. Psychological treatments are effective in modifying health anxiety, selective attention, catastrophizing, and other aspects of poor coping and can also increase adherence to psychopharmacological treatments. Another strategy is to further adjust the antidepressant medication, probably with the help of a psychiatrist.

— Psychological Treatments

Psychological treatments are helpful to patients with functional GI disorders as (a) there are high levels of anxiety and depression, (b) many have experienced traumatic life events, (c) the close relationship between daily stress or hassles and gut symptoms must be managed, and (d) the effects of health beliefs and learned behaviors may adversely affect outcome.

The term "psychological therapy" covers a variety of different therapies that need to be accurately defined for research purposes (usually with a "manual," which allows another researcher at another center to replicate the therapy exactly). In clinical practice a combination of more than one psychological therapy is used, making it difficult for researchers to identify the effects of each component of treatment. Until recently studies of psychological therapies have tended to be small and to use symptom monitoring, waiting list, or conventional medical therapy as the "control" condition but these do not provide an equivalent expectation of improvement (placebo response). There is convincing evidence from a systematic review and meta-analysis of rigorously executed trials in IBS that psychological treatments as a whole are effective in IBS [245]; there is inadequate evidence to say whether psychological treatments are effective in functional dyspepsia [246].

Cognitive-Behavioral Therapy (CBT)

Cognitive-behavioral approaches include a wide array of techniques, and recently women's issues have been integrated into cognitive behavioral practice [247, 248]. The main theoretical basis of cognitive-behavioral therapy (CBT) is social learning theory, which recognizes that behavior is shaped as a result of its social consequences (e.g., increased attention from others, escape from unpleasant tasks). The theory focuses on ways to increase or decrease a particular behavior. CBT interventions address the thoughts, behaviors, and responses that result from patients' daily interactions.

CBT may be particularly valuable for IBS patients because it helps patients recognize the role played by illness beliefs and behavior in chronic pain [249]. In addition, anxiety and depression, assertion difficulties, and perfectionist attitudes are all amenable to CBT [87]. Relaxation/stress management is often incorporated into CBT packages because of its effect in reducing autonomic arousal and anxiety in IBS [250].

Empirical Support for CBT

Small studies have shown that cognitive behavior therapy delivered in individual or group therapy situations leads to greater GI symptom reduction for IBS patients than symptom monitoring or a self-help support group [250, 251]. Since these studies recruited patients by advertisement it is not clear whether the results are generalizable to clinic patients.

In a recent large study based on that of Toner [252], CBT was found to be more effective than an educational intervention in terms of satisfaction, overall symptom relief and global well-being after 3 months, but there was little or no difference in pain scores or of health-related quality of life [178]. Often patients reported that "the pain is still there but I'm managing it better," indicating improved coping. These findings mirror much of the material presented in this chapter—psychological aspects are important in the global well-being of patients with FGIDs rather than in the specific etiology of the pain. Improvement of this global well-being is important as it may be associated with less time off work and less treatment-seeking. The CBT was effective regardless of the severity of the IBS, or whether an abuse history or current depression were present [178].

Small studies of children with RAP included self-monitoring of pain, parent training in reinforcement of nonillness behaviors, distraction, relaxation, imagery, and self-instruction such as coping self-statements. These led to significantly more pain-free days at followup compared to standard medical care or symptom monitoring [254]. The strongest predictor of reduction of children's pain diary scores after treatment was the parental response category of ignoring pain complaints and encouraging independence.

Relaxation Training

Relaxation or arousal reduction techniques use different methods to teach patients to counteract the physiological sequelae of stress or anxiety. The most widely used arousal reduction techniques include (a) progressive muscle relaxation training [255], (b) biofeedback for striated muscle tension, skin temperature, or electrodermal activity [256], (c) autogenic training [257], and (d) transcendental or Yoga meditation [258]. Progressive muscle relaxation training and electromyograph (EMG) biofeedback reduce skeletal muscle tension, as this leads to decreased autonomic arousal and subjective tension or anxiety. Skin temperature and electrodermal biofeedback training attempt to reduce autonomic arousal directly and autogenic training attempts to reduce smooth muscle activity through imagery in a technique closely resembling hypnosis. Transcendental meditation and yoga aim to modify both skeletal muscle tension and autonomic arousal indirectly through cognitive focusing techniques, also similar to hypnosis.

Empirical Support for Relaxation Training

There have been only two studies that examined relaxation/autogenic training alone (i.e., not combined with psychotherapy or CBT). Both showed that the relaxation led to a significant reduction in gastrointestinal symptoms [255, 259]. In one study the improvement was comparable to that achieved with the combined treatment of CBT and relaxation. Currently there are insufficient data to identify which characteristics predict a good response to relaxation training.

Combined Psychotherapies

Nine studies have shown combined progressive muscle relaxation training with CBT to be superior to a waiting list control group or conventional medical therapy [6]. Of the two studies that used an active placebo control, one found the combination of CBT and relaxation to be superior to an educational control treatment and the other found no difference. Relaxation training combined with psychodrama [260] was no better than standard therapy for bowel symptoms, but was more effective for anxiety reduction. A combination of different behavioral techniques (exposure, education, and bowel retraining) was no better than standard medical treatment [260].

Multicomponent behavioral therapy has included IBS information and education, progressive muscle relaxation, training in illness-related cognitive coping strategies, problem-solving, and assertiveness training. This multicomponent treatment showed significantly greater IBS symptom reduction than patients receiving standardized symptom-oriented medical treatment [261]. Overall wellbeing, control of health, and quality of life significantly improved in the multicomponent group but remained unchanged in the standardized medical treatment group. Rectovisceral perception remained unchanged in both groups.

A recent study excluded patients with "resistant" IBS and found no significant differences between CBT or relaxation and standard care in a range of outcomes, but this study had such a low response rate at followup no firm conclusions can be drawn [262].

Dynamic Psychotherapy

This form of therapy (similar to brief interpersonal psychotherapy [263, 264]) requires a close relationship between the patient and therapist. By far the most important practical aspect of treatment is engaging the patient in this type of treatment. This may require a very long first interview that starts with a detailed discussion of bowel symptoms. In this context, phrases such as "I feel all churned up inside" and "I fear losing control" made in relation to bowel symptoms can be reflected back to the patient who might apply them to broader aspects of their lives.

The theoretical basis for the treatment lies in the interpersonal problems experienced by many patients with FGIDs. These may be associated with childhood adversity so the person has difficulty in trusting other adults in close relationships. Within the therapy, these difficulties are mirrored or recur, leading the patient to experience increased anxiety or distress, often accompanied by abdominal discomfort. In this way the link is made between stress, distress, and abdominal symptoms.

As the patient comes to understand the problems in his/her relationships, he or she may act upon these insights, which may lead to a reduction in psychological symptoms, and generally improved bowel symptoms. The treatment may be performed in groups [265], although such treatment requires further evaluation.

Empirical Support for Dynamic Psychotherapy

Psychodynamic therapy has been shown to be superior to routine medical care in IBS and functional dyspepsia in terms of improved bowel dysfunction, abdominal pain, and psychological symptoms at one year after the end of therapy [266–269]. One critical review found all studies to be methodologically deficient [270], whereas others found support for psychological therapies in IBS [245, 271].

A recent, large study demonstrated that brief psychodynamic therapy is widely acceptable in routine clinical practice for patients with IBS who have not responded to routine treatments. Such treatment is cost-effective [172]. Both psychodynamic interpersonal therapy and the selective serotonin reuptake inhibitor (SSRI) antidepressant paroxetine led to a marked improvement in health-related quality of life in the long term, compared to treatment as usual [172]. This result was achieved, like that of the Drossman trial [253], without significantly greater improvement in pain and could not be accounted for solely by improved psychological status.

There were preliminary data from this study to suggest that patients with a history of sexual abuse did particularly well with psychotherapy [172, 272] and a subanalysis suggests that the improvement occurring with dynamic psychotherapy is associated with improved rectal tolerance to distension, probably reflecting a reduction of hypervigilance [181]. One other study, however, found no change in rectal distension threshold after psychotherapy [273].

On the basis of these results we conclude that psychodynamic interpersonal therapy is a useful and cost-effective treatment in patients with IBS who have not responded to usual treatment.

Hypnotherapy

Hypnotherapy has become increasingly popular in England principally for IBS and functional dyspepsia [274–280]. The hypnotic "state" is a state of unusual concentration on the suggestion of the therapist and depends on the willingness of the subject to follow the therapist's requests. Following induction, the hypnotherapist uses progressive muscular relaxation with "gut-directed" imagery and suggestions to relax gastrointestinal smooth muscle. Patients are requested to place their hand on the abdomen and to sense both a positive feeling of abdominal warmth and increased control over gut function. This is accompanied by visualization of the gut as gentle flowing river. Patients are also asked to practice autohypnosis at home with an audiotape with the goal of being able to self-administer suggestions of relaxation.

Empirical Support for Hypnotherapy

Controlled trials of hypnotherapy in IBS and functional dyspepsia have shown this to be an effective treatment with persistent benefit over time [276, 281]. Little is known about the applicability in a wide range of patients as most studies have been performed on patients seeking this type of treatment at selected centers. Older people with marked anxiety and atypical symptoms respond less well to hypnotherapy. Uncontrolled studies support the efficacy of group hypnotherapy [275].

The mechanisms underlying improvement following hypnotherapy are not clear. Some work has shown that hypnotherapy reduced contractile activity in the gut and is associated with normalization of pain threshold from distension of a balloon in the rectum [282], but others have not confirmed this [283]. Other studies have shown improvement to be associated with cognitive changes similar to those found following cognitive therapy [284] and reduction of anxiety and somatization scores without change in rectal pain threshold, autonomic activity, or rectal smooth muscle tone [283].

We would like to add a caveat to the interpretation of many studies described above. Many used waiting list or "treatment as usual" as control conditions (thus not controlling for potentially confounding and powerful affects of attention and support), studies often included very small numbers, and participants were recruited by advertisement from the general population (raising questions of their generalizability to clinic populations). However, the use of increased methodologic rigor in some of the recent trials discussed above does permit greater confidence in their conclusions, and we expect further information will become available as additional studies are conducted.

— Pharmacological Treatment

The use of psychopharmacologic agents in functional bowel disorders is based on the following: (a) antidepressants have analgesic effects, particularly for neuropathic pain, (b) FGIDs are frequently associated with psychiatric disorders, which could favorably respond to treatment with antidepressant medications, (c) antidepressant agents tend to improve a sense of "global well-being" in patients suffering from functional bowel disorders [285]. In this section, recommendations will be made on ideal usage of these medications in the setting of treating functional bowel patients with particular attention to side effects. Further details of the actions of psychotropic drugs in FGIDs are discussed in the Pharmacology chapter (chapter 4).

Antidepressants as Analgesics

Antidepressants, particularly tricyclic antidepressants (TCA) can be used to treat chronic neuropathic pain, including diabetic and other peripheral neuropathies, migraine headaches, and other neuropathic pain syndromes [286, 287]. A number of recent meta-analyses [288, 289] support the use of antidepressant agents when used in doses lower than those for major depressive disorder. The analgesic effect of TCA may be due to a common biochemical pathway for both pain and depression, or to the influence of neurogenic amines on the activity of endorphins and enkephalins [290]. Animal studies suggest that the analgesic effect of the TCAs may be due to their effect on opioid receptors [291] and, possibly, by regulating the activity of the N-methyl-D-aspartate (NMDA) receptor producing a sensation of analgesia in the brain [291]. SSRI antidepressants may have a similar action as they also have an analgesic effect on neuropathic pain [292]. Because of the narrower dose ranges associated with SSRIs, the doses used for the treatment of neuropathic pain are closer to the doses used to treat major depressive disorder and anxiety disorders [293].

In FGIDs the findings are conflicting. Imipramine increased the pain threshold (tested by balloon distension of the gut) in normal subjects, suggesting the presence of a primary visceral analgesic effect for imipramine [294]. On the other hand amitriptyline did not differ from placebo in its effect on perception of rectal or esophageal distention or alterations in luminal compliance [295], even though it increased the threshold for cutaneous electrical stimulation compared to placebo. Duloxetine is a new serotonin/noradrenaline reuptake inhibitor (SNRI) that has been studied both for the treatment of major depressive disorder and peripheral neuropathy. To date there have been no published studies of duloxetine in the treatment of FGID. On theoretical grounds, however, this agent, which has proven efficacy for neuropathic pain and fibromyalgia [296], may find a role in the treatment of FGIDs. Venlafaxine, the other currently available SNRI, has limited usefulness in FGIDs due to its tendency to produce gastrointestinal distress, particularly nausea and vomiting.

Systematic Reviews of the Efficacy of Antidepressants in FGIDs

Early case reports and small controlled trials supported the efficacy of TCAs in FGIDs [297], and one study showed that the improvement in GI symptoms after desipramine could not be attributed to its anticholinergic effects [298]. In the first systematic review the authors concluded that psychotropic agents in IBS showed a tendency to improved abdominal pains and diarrhea, but not constipation, probably reflecting the predominance of studies using TCAs, which can produce constipation [299].

The more recent meta-analysis [300] identified 11 randomized placebo-controlled trials of acceptable quality, eight concerned IBS, two concerned nonulcer dyspepsia and one studied both. Most studies used pain severity as the outcome measure. The antidepressants included in this review were amitriptyline, clomipramine, desipramine, doxepin, trimipramine, and mianserin. The summary odds ratio for improvement of functional bowel disorders using antidepressants compared with placebo was 4.2 (95% confidence interval 2.3 to 7.9) (number needed to treat was 3.2 on average), demonstrating that antidepressant treatment of functional gastrointestinal disorders is effective. The study was not able to differentiate whether the effect was independent of the antidepressant effect of these drugs.

Another systematic review included six randomized control trials conducted in the United States of antidepressant therapy in FGIDs [297]. All trials were of "low quality" based on the Rome working team recommendations. These authors concluded that TCAs were not more effective than placebo for relieving global IBS symptoms, but there was limited evidence that they lead to improved abdominal pain. The review could not draw any clear conclusions regarding the utility of SSRIs in the treatment of IBS.

The more recent antidepressant treatment trials for functional bowel disorders with satisfactory trial design have shown that both desipramine and paroxetine have significant general beneficial effects, at least in those patients who complied fully with the treatment to which they were randomized [172, 178]. In both studies there was a serious problem of dropouts with both antidepressants. This reflects the impact of side effects from these medications, but also reflects reluctance among patients to use these drugs.

The trial that used paroxetine included patients with moderate or severe IBS who had not responded to usual treatment, and only 50% complied fully with paroxetine that was prescribed by the gastroenterologist or general practitioner. In spite of this poor compliance, paroxetine was superior to treatment as usual in significantly improving health-related quality of life [172]. Among the patients who were fully compliant with 3 months of antidepressant treatment, paroxetine had a significantly beneficial effect on pain, though this finding was not placebo-controlled. The study suggests that paroxetine is superior to routine medical treatment for IBS.

A further study assessed the benefits of paroxetine (10 mg daily) given over 12 weeks to IBS patients who had not responded to a high fiber diet [301]. Compared to placebo, the paroxetine group showed significant improvements in overall well-being, quality of life scores, reduction in problems with stool passage, and IBS-related anxiety, but there was no significant improvement in abdominal pain between the two groups.

In the other recent large trial [178], the TCA desipramine given for 12 weeks showed no significant benefit over placebo in an intention-to-treat analysis, but did show statistically significant benefit in the per protocol analysis, especially when participants with nondetectable blood levels of desipramine (indicating lack of treatment compliance) were excluded.

Taken together these three studies provide strong evidence that SSRIs and TCAs lead to benefit for patients with moderate or severe IBS, provided patients adhere to the prescribed medication. All studies used a small dose and further research is needed to clarify the role and mechanism of action of antidepressants in IBS and other FGIDs. We conclude that these drugs do generally lead to an improvement in global well-being and health-related quality of life and this appears to be a beneficial long term effect. They do appear to have some effect on pain but their beneficial effect is not confined to patients who have concurrent depressive disorder. Lastly, patients are unlikely to take antidepressants unless the gastroenterologist takes particular care in discussing this treatment with them.

Psychiatric Consultation for Psychopharmacological Treatment

Since patients with FGIDs often display particularly troublesome side effects from antidepressants it is important that the gastroenterologist or primary care physician encourages adherence from the outset and encourages the patient to continue with the drug, since side effects decrease with time and the beneficial effect becomes more prominent. If a patient cannot tolerate an antidepressant, it is reasonable to change to another drug in the same class; this has been shown to be effective in psychopharmacological practice [302]. If (s)he still does not improve, then referral to a psychiatrist is warranted. A psychiatrist can be particularly helpful in optimizing selection of drugs and dosage regimens. Likewise a psychiatrist can help determine if multicomponent treatment, including behavioral intervention, may be indicated or whether there are specific indications for psychological treatment. In people with a history of abuse and chronic depression, for example, the response to psychological treatment may be so pronounced that antidepressants may add relatively little further improvement [303]; the same appears to be true of patients with severe IBS and an abuse history [272].

Anxiolytics

Anxiolytic agents, most often represented by the benzodiazepines, can be used in certain situations, including treating patients with comorbid generalized anxiety and panic disorders. Benzodiazepines are excellent antipanic agents, but the CNS depressant effect of these agents is synergistic with other CNS depressants such as alcohol or barbiturates, and they need to be used with caution in these settings. Alprazolam has been successfully used in the treatment of IBS associated with panic disorder [305]. However, the risk of addiction with the benzodiazepines, and their tendency to produce mild transient cognitive dysfunction, mean that they have very limited use in the gastrointestinal setting. Benzodiazepine dependence is not common, but we recommend that a psychiatrist be consulted to evaluate patients in order to firmly establish the presence of a psychiatric diagnosis that may make prescribing benzodiazepines reasonable. Prescribing benzodiazepines on a chronic basis is unwise and alternative strategies for the treatment of anxiety should be utilized.

A newer class of anti-anxiety agents, the azapirones, act by serotonin agonist activity at presynaptic $5\text{-}HT_{1A}$ receptors [259]. Buspirone is the best known member of this class. Buspirone has no antipanic activity but has been used as an adjunctive treatment to potentiate the action of antidepressants. Buspirone is well tolerated, displaying only occasional serotonergic-related side effects. It has no addictive potential and is a reasonable alternative in treating anxious patients who cannot tolerate benzodiazepines [306]. Buspirone, although not a particularly potent anxiolytic, may act via its $5\text{-}HT_{1A}$ agonist activity to reduce visceral sensation.

Anticonvulsants

A number of studies demonstrate the usefulness of anticonvulsants in the treatment of neuropathic pain syndromes including trigeminal neuralgia, postherpetic neuralgia, diabetic peripheral neuropathy, migraine prophylaxis, and poststroke pain. A wide variety of anticonvulsants, including older drugs such as carbamazepine, phenytoin, valproic acid, as well as newer agents such as felbamate, gabapentin, and lamotrigine, have been used successfully in this setting. However, to date there have been no trials to suggest a role for anticonvulsant agents in the treatment of visceral pain. This lack of data in combination with the significant toxicity that can be associated with some of these agents preclude recommending their use as first line agents for the treatment of FGIDs at this time [307].

Opiates

The use of opiates in the treatment of FGIDs is to be discouraged for a number of reasons and have been discussed in detail elsewhere. (See Chapter 4.)

— Conclusions Concerning Efficacy and Effectiveness of Psychologic and Pharmacologic Treatment

Our overall conclusion regarding psychological treatments is that many different types of psychological treatments appear to be effective in IBS but insufficient research has been performed in other FGIDs. In line with other studies of chronic pain [308], psychological treatments lead to improvements in health-related quality of life, global well-being and, possibly, reduced health care use. Findings are more equivocal in relation to pain reduction and there is relatively little evidence of normalization of rectal tolerance to distension following psychological treatment, except possibly in selected groups (e.g., receiving hypnotherapy, abuse history). There may be general as well as specific elements of psychological treatment that are responsible for their effect [309].

The most stringent reviews of psychological treatment studies found very few trials that met criteria of high quality [245, 271] and many came from a single center. These studies included very small numbers, the control condition was a wait list or similar inactive treatment (thus not controlling for potentially confounding and powerful affects of attention and support), and participants were recruited by advertisement from the general population, raising questions of their generalizability to clinic populations. Both reviews indicated superiority of psychological treatments over the control conditions in terms of abdominal pain, bowel dysfunction, depression, and anxiety but the quality of the trials was questioned [245, 310]. Of studies graded as of reasonable quality with more than 30 patients in each arm, one showed no advantage of multicomponent treatment over the attention-placebo condition but the other two studies (each with more than 100 patients) did show superiority of interpersonal psychotherapy over supportive listening or medical treatment alone.

Our conclusions are the same as these two major reviews, namely that the evidence is still inadequate to determine definitively which, if any, psychological treatments are effective in reducing IBS symptoms. The recent large trials are methodologically superior but focus on different questions; one shows that CBT is superior to attentional control in a global rating of outcome [178] and the other showed the cost benefits of dynamic psychotherapy [172].

With regard to antidepressants there is more evidence of their efficacy in relation to pain reduction, probably as a result of their direct, primarily central analgesic action with additional benefit from their antidepressant action. The latter may be responsible for their benefit in relation to global well-being. However, some antidepressants are not well tolerated (though this may be similar to the tolerability of these drugs for depressive disorder in routine primary care) and compliance with treatment needs to be monitored closely.

Very few studies have examined effectiveness of these treatments in routine clinical practice, but one study shows fairly good acceptability of psychological treatment among people with severe IBS [172].

Recommended Training Curriculum of Psychosocial Aspects of FGIDs for Gastroenterologists and Primary Care Physicians

The next step in improving the psychological care of people with FGIDs is to ensure that the current effective psychological and antidepressant drug treatments are used more widely. This requires that more training is made available for gastroenterologists and primary care physicians who are likely to treat people with FGIDs. We suggest training in the following areas to help these physicians be ready to follow the recommendations for assessment and treatment proposed in this paper:

- Interviewing skills:
    Establishing rapport and empathy
    Providing education and reassurance
    Facilitating patient disclosure of psychosocial information
    Facilitating patient involvement in care
    Eliciting patient disclosure of thoughts and feelings
- Application of biopsychosocial principles in assessment and treatment
- Ability to screen for anxiety, depression, somatization within a clinical interview
- Ability to use appropriate psychotropic drugs in clinical practice
- Skills in working within a multidisciplinary team

- Knowledge and skills concerning when and how to refer to a mental health professional
- Providing continuity of care, especially for patients with persistent FGIDs
- Awareness of physician's personal reactions and appropriate response to difficulties in doctor-patient relationships

Recommendations for Future Research

This review suggests a number of areas for future research. Some of these areas have been partially addressed, but below we have grouped by categories questions or areas in which further research is needed.

Epidemiology: Large, population-based studies are required to elucidate further the outstanding questions regarding the relationship between childhood experiences, adult stressors, and psychiatric disorder and the onset, course, and outcome of a wide range of FGIDs.

Laboratory studies need to include measures of psychological distress so that we can determine whether abnormalities are associated directly with FGIDs or whether the abnormalities are really a result of accompanying psychological distress or concurrent psychiatric disorders or environmental stressors.

Health services research: Much is already known about the importance of psychosocial factors in FGIDs but further work is needed to understand how we can best integrate this knowledge into improved routine clinical practice. The problem is not confined to gastroenterological practice; the problem of underdetection and undertreatment of depression and anxiety is well recognized in primary care also [190]. Further research is needed to determine whether screening for the psychosocial factors is effective and which forms of physician education make a difference, especially the evaluation of clinical guidelines and treatment algorithms. With one exception [172], there is very little work evaluating the cost-effectiveness of different interventions in real-life clinical settings.

Clinical questions: No treatment is universally effective in clinical medicine. We need to determine which treatments are effective for which subgroups of patients (based on characteristics, cultural groups, etc.) and whether there are differential responses based on severity of pain, presence of marked anxiety, depression, or somatization. We are ignorant of the relative efficacy of tricyclic, SSRI, and SNRI antidepressants in treating the FGIDs. We need to consider whether it is possible to identify preventative strategies for development of FGIDs in high risk populations, similar to strategies for post-traumatic stress disorder (PTSD). As treatments for PTSD (e.g., exposure-type therapies) address only whether symptoms improve, we need to determine whether FGIDs (and other associated health problems) are also helped by this treatment.

Transcultural aspects of psychosocial issues: Current knowledge tends to be limited to Western cultures and specific gender or ethnic groups. Future work needs to translate and validate questionnaires across different cultures and examine the relationship between psychosocial factors and the FGIDs and the effectiveness of relevant treatments transculturally. The reader is also referred to Chapter 5, on "Gender, Age, Society, Culture, and the Patient's Perspective," for further information about current knowledge on culture and FGIDs.

Mechanism questions: The outstanding research questions that have been highlighted by this review include questions concerning the mechanisms linking psychosocial factors to symptom expression and outcomes in FGIDs. Neurobiological and psychosocial mechanisms need to be studied simultaneously, not separately. The mechanisms involved in coping, the treatment response in psychological and pharmacological interventions, and the mechanisms involved in the pain experience need to be studied. The mechanisms involved in the relationship between psychological and social variables and gut function need to be understood more fully.

Conclusions

This review of recent research concerning the psychosocial aspects of the FGIDs concludes that there is strong evidence of the association between psychological distress, childhood trauma and recent environmental stress, and several of the functional gastrointestinal disorders, most notably IBS. There is also strong evidence that psychosocial variables are important determinants of the outcomes of global well-being, health-related quality of life, and health care-seeking in FGID patients. Much of the evidence relates specifically to IBS but it is likely that the relationships hold across most of the FGIDs; further research is needed to clarify this. This association between psychosocial variables and outcome is not unique to FGIDS, though it is pronounced in these disorders because of the close association between psychological and social variables and gut function.

In line with these descriptive findings, there is now increasing evidence that a number of psychological treatments and antidepressants are helpful in reducing symptoms and other consequences of the FGIDs. Again, most of the evidence relates to IBS or functional dyspepsia but may relate also to other FGIDs.

Some of the psychological mediators of the association between psychosocial variables and outcome have now been defined (e.g., catastrophizing cognitions, GI-specific anxiety) and these are useful pointers to more focused psychological treatments. The physiological pathways that mediate these relationships are less clear, however, and more work is needed in this field.

As these are investigated further, the complex interactions between biological, psychological, and social variables that occur in FGIDs will become clearer and facilitate further development of psychological and psychotropic treatments for these disorders. At present, the psychological and antidepressant treatments that are currently available could be much more widely used if gastroenterologists and primary care physicians were appropriately trained and more confident in their use. We would therefore particularly like to encourage training in psychosocial assessment as part of GI fellowship training and perhaps even recertification, since we believe this chapter has demonstrated that the ability to take a psychosocial history is as important and as frequently used as most typically taught GI procedures.

Appendix. Commonly Used Measures of Psychosocial Domains

Psychosocial Domain	Measure	Description	Comments
I. Current Mood	Hospital Anxiety and Depression Scale (HAD Scale) [191, 192]	Designed for medical populations. Consists of 14 items with subscales for anxiety and depression graded for severity.	Population-based studies provide evidence of good internal reliability coefficients [0.76–0.80] and construct validity. Has clinical "cutoff" scores for both anxiety and depression and is easy to use.
	Hopkins Symptom Checklist (SCL-90) [199]	Consists of 90 items grouped in 9 subscales and 3 global measures of psychological distress (e.g., Global Severity Index) found primarily among psychiatric and medical patients including somatization, obsessive-compulsive, interpersonal sensitivity, depression, anxiety, hostility, phobic anxiety, paranoid ideation, and psychoticism.	Widely used as both a screening device and an outcome measure in a broad spectrum of clinical research. Internal and test-retest reliability coefficients range from 0.76 to 0.90. Multiple studies show good evidence of predictive and construct validity. However, the subscales and global measures of distress tend to be highly correlated with one another. The Brief Symptom Inventory is a shortened version (53 items) of the SCL-90, but there are far fewer studies of the reliability and validity of this instrument.
	Millon Behavioral Health Inventory (MBHI) [154]	Comprised of 20 subscales grouped into broad categories such as coping styles, psychosocial problems, and prognostic indices. Norms are based on responses of patients with medical illnesses or disorders.	Internal and test-retest reliability coefficients range from 0.66 to 0.90. Content and construct validity have been established by examining associations between MBHI subscales and established instruments such as the SCL-90, Life Events Survey, Minnesota Multiphasic Personality Inventory, etc. The MBHI Somatic Anxiety and Gastrointestinal Susceptibility scales have been shown to be useful in research involving patients with gastrointestinal reflux disease and hypotonic lower esophageal sphincter.
II. Health-Related Cognition	Visceral Sensitivity Index [323]	Fifteen item scale of symptom-specific anxiety in IBS. Includes items for fear, worry, vigilance, and avoidance related to visceral sensations.	Internal reliability coefficient of 0.93. Factor analysis yielded a single dimension and validity study demonstrated unique relationship with IBS symptoms over general anxiety. May be useful as both assessment and outcome measure of symptom-specific anxiety in IBS and related conditions.

Appendix Continued. Commonly Used Measures of Psychosocial Domains

Psychosocial Domain	Measure	Description	Comments
II. Health-Related Cognition, *continued*	Pain Anxiety Symptoms Scale (PASS) [324]	Includes 53 items that are grouped into 3 subscales that assess the cognitive, behavioral, and physiological dimensions of anxiety about pain.	Internal reliability coefficients range from 0.81 to 0.94. Evidence for construct validity was established by associations between PASS scores and scores on other established measures of anxiety and functional ability. This measure has not been widely used in studies of patients with FGID. However, it has been shown to be very useful in studies of patients with fibromyalgia and other chronic pain syndromes that frequently overlap with FGID. It may be especially useful in studies of individuals who tend to anticipate or experience increased pain during exposure to modest levels of sensory input.
	Fear of Pain Questionnaire-III (FPQ-III) [325]	This instrument consists of 30 items designed to evaluate fear of pain in both healthy persons as well as in those with painful conditions.	Internal reliability coefficients range from 0.87 to 0.92. Test-retest reliability over a 3-week period ranges from 0.60 to 0.76. Construct validity studies suggest the presence of 3 content dimensions: fear of minor pain, fear of severe pain, and fear of medical pain. These studies indicate that high scores on this measure are associated with high scores on established measures of anxiety and depression. Similar to the PASS, this measure has been used primarily in studies of patients with musculo-skeletal pain. Nevertheless, it contains fewer items than the PASS and thus may be useful for rapid screening or clinical studies of patients with FGID.

Appendix Continued. Commonly Used Measures of Psychosocial Domains

Psychosocial Domain	Measure	Description	Comments
II. Health-Related Cognition, *continued*	Coping Strategies Questionnaire [236]	The 6 subscales of this instrument include 53 items that relate to coping with painful conditions. In studies of patients with a wide array of chronic pain syndromes, catastrophizing shows the most reliable relationships with the negative sequelae of chronic pain such as disability and psychological distress.	Internal reliability coefficients for all but one of the CSQ subscales range from 0.71 to 0.85. Only "Increasing Pain Behaviors" shows low reliability [0.28] and is rarely used for research or clinical purposes. With regard to predictive validity, only the subscales that assess catastrophizing and perceived control and ability to decrease pain are associated with adverse health outcomes in patients with gastrointestinal disorders.
	Pain Catastrophizing Scale (PCS) [148]	This scale includes 13 items that assess 3 dimensions of catastrophizing: magnification, rumination, and helplessness. The latter subscale is identical to the catastrophizing subscale of the Coping Strategies Questionnaire.	Test-retest reliability coefficient over a 6-week period is 0.75. Evidence of construct validity established in studies indicate that PCS scores are associated with patients' ratings of pain or pain unpleasantness during exposure to noxious sensory stimulation as well as with scores on the FPQ-III.
III. Somatization	Cognitive Scale for Functional Bowel Disorders (CS-FBD) [206]	This 7-point scale indicates the extent to which respondents agree or disagree with statements relating to personal attributions about the condition. The scale is reliable and achieves psychometric validation.	Reliability was established by Cronbach's alpha = 0.93 and criterion validity established by its correlation with the interference scale r = .71, p < 0.001 and the DAS r = .38, p < 0.01.
	Whitely Index [203]	This instrument is a binary 14-item questionnaire to measure 3 interrelated constructs: bodily preoccupation, disease phobia, and disease conviction.	The internal reliability coefficient for the total score has been reported between .76 and .80. Initial factor analysis suggested 3 separate factors, interpreted as bodily preoccupation, disease phobia, and disease conviction, however this has not been replicated in more recent studies. A 7-item single dimension version has recently shown good sensitivity and specificity for detection of somatization disorder [Fink et al. 1999].

Appendix Continued. Commonly Used Measures of Psychosocial Domains

Psychosocial Domain	Measure	Description	Comments
III. Somatization, *continued*	Illness Behavior Questionnaire [253]	This instruments consists of 52 items that comprise 7 subscales including 2 on hypochondriasis (disease phobia, disease conviction), 3 affect scales (affective inhibition, affective disturbance, and irritability), a denial scale, and a scale measuring psychological vs. somatic perception of illness.	The original papers describing the development of this instrument did not provide data on the internal or test-retest reliability of the 7 subscales. However, when presented in an interview format, there is good inter-rater agreement [88%). Factor analytic studies suggest that neuroticism underlies responses to all 7 subscales. It is not surprising, then, that the instrument is not well accepted by patients presenting with a medical complaint because the items primarily focus on negative affective states.
	Patient Health Questionnaire-15 (PHQ-15) [201]	This 15-item scale assesses 14 of the 15 most prevalent symptoms of somatization included in the DSM-IV diagnostic criteria.	The internal reliability coefficient for the instrument is 0.80. Evidence for the construct validity of the instrument shows that PHQ-15 scores are correlated with ratings of functional disability and number of physician visits.
IV. Illness Impact and Quality of Life	Medical Outcomes Short-Form Health Survey (SF-36) [207]	The 36 items that comprise this instrument assess 8 domains including physical limitations, physical and mental role limitations, social activities, pain, general health perception, mental health, and vitality. There also are 2 composite subscales of Physical and Psychosocial function.	The SF-36 is one of the most widely used means of HRQoL for health conditions. Internal and test-retest reliability coefficients are consistently above 0.70 across numerous studies and most of the coefficients exceed 0.80. Studies of the construct validity and predictive validity of the SF-36 consistently show that both the individual scales and composite subscales are associated with independent measures of similar constructs as well as with utilization of health care services, the clinical course of depression, loss of job within 1 year, and 5-year survival.

Appendix Continued. Commonly Used Measures of Psychosocial Domains

Psychosocial Domain	Measure	Description	Comments
IV. Illness Impact and Quality of Life, *continued*	Quality of Life with IBS (IBS-QOL) [196]	Thirty-four-item self-report questions with 8 subscales: dysphoria, interference with activity, body image, health worry, food avoidance, social reaction, and sexual relationship	Developed from focus groups of IBS patients at two institutions. Has achieved good psychometric validation. Responsiveness testing is underway.
	IBSQOL [304]	Thirty-item self-report questionnaire with 9 subscales: emotional, mental health, sleep, energy, physical functioning, diet, social role, physical role, and sexual relations	Items developed based on review of literature and interviews with physicians which were then modified by a sample of patients. Has achieved psychometric validation.
	Functional Digestive Disorders Quality of Life (FDDQOL) [214]	Forty-three-item questionnaire with 8 subscales including activities, anxiety, diet, sleep, discomfort, coping, control and stress	The global Cronbach's α coefficient was 0.94, and scale coefficients ranged from 0.69 to 0.89. Validated for IBS and FD with moderate associations with SF-36 and symptoms. Developed cross-culturally. Needs further validation but potentially useful instrument for IBS and FD.
V. Stressful Life Events and Sexual/Physical Abuse	Life Experiences Survey (LES) [216]	This instrument is a 57-item scale that assesses the positive or negative impact of major life events defined by the investigators as well as those chosen by the subject.	Over a 5-week period, test-retest reliability coefficients range from 0.19 to 0.53 for positive change scores and 0.56 to 0.88 for negative change scores. Evidence of construct validity of the instrument includes positive correlations between the LES and measures of anxiety as well as a near-zero correlation between LES scores and a measure of social desirability.

Appendix Continued. Commonly Used Measures of Psychosocial Domains

Psychosocial Domain	Measure	Description	Comments
V. Stressful Life Events and Sexual/Physical Abuse, *continued*	Life Events and Difficulties Schedule (LEDS) [217]	This is the most widely used interview-based measure for stressful life events. It consists of an interview (approximately 1 to 2 hours in length) concerning stressful events that may have occurred over the past 12 months. Once an event is mentioned, the interviewer asks objective questions surrounding the event ("What led up to the event?", "What followed it?") as well as the severity of the identified event.	Inter-rater reliability may be low unless interviewers undergo training in administration of this instrument. However, among trained interviewers, reliability coefficients as high as 0.93 have been reported. Another potential disadvantage of this instrument is its length and the possibility that respondents may be reluctant to reveal stressful events in the interview format. Nevertheless, validity studies have shown that scores on the Life Events and Difficulties Schedule differentiate patients with globus and other functional bowel disorders from healthy controls, contribute to the prediction of depression and antidepressant response, and are associated with measures of adrenergic physiology in caregivers of patients with Alzheimer's disease, as well as exacerbations of multiple sclerosis activity.
	Daily Hassles Scale [326]	This instrument is a 117-item scale that assesses the frequency and intensity of minor stressful events that have occurred over the past month.	Mean test-retest reliability, calculated each month over a 9-month period, is 0.79 for frequency and 0.48 for intensity. Evidence for the construct validity of the instrument includes positive correlations between Daily Hassles scores over the 9-month period and scores on the Hopkins Symptoms Checklist in healthy persons, as well as self-reports of health status and functional ability among patient samples.

Psychosocial Domain	Measure	Description	Comments
V. Stressful Life Events and Sexual/Physical Abuse, *continued*	Daily Stress Inventory [337]	This 60-item instrument was designed as a relatively brief, alternate measure to the Daily Hassles Scale. Respondents report the frequency and impact (i.e., amount of stress) produced by each of 58 minor stressful events that have occurred over the past 24 hours. Respondents also may identify 2 additional minor stressful events that have occurred during this time period.	Internal reliability of the frequency and impact scores of this instrument are 0.83 and 0.87, respectively. Studies of the construct validity of this measure indicate that respondents' impact scores on this measure are significantly associated with their global ratings of daily stress (0.35–0.49). Similarly, respondents' frequency and impact scores are significantly associated with their Daily Hassles Scale reports of frequency [0.33] and intensity [0.53–0.57] of stressful events.
	Schedule of Recent Life Events [328]	This 51-item instrument represents another alternate measure to the Daily Hassles Scale. Similar to the former instrument, the items that comprise the Schedule of Recent Life Events represent minor stressful events, but none of these events include content regarding physical or mental health or perceptions of "being stressed."	The internal reliability coefficient of the instrument is 0.92. Evidence for the construct validity of the instrument includes associations of 0.57 to 0.60 between the Schedule of Recent Life Events scores and scores on the Perceived Stress Scale.
VI. Psychiatric Disorders	Diagnostic Interview Schedule (DIS) [226]	Structured interview from which psychiatric diagnoses (DSM-IV Axis I) may be systematically obtained. It can be administered by a trained technician either in interview format or through a computerized software program.	Test-retest studies have produced median kappa coefficients (agreement independent-of-chance factors) of 0.37 to 0.59. The validity of the DIS was established by assessing agreement on diagnoses produced by psychiatrists and lay interviewers, both of whom used the DIS protocol. The kappa coefficients for these analyses range from 0.47 to 1.0.
	Structured Clinical Interview for DSM-III-R (SCID) [227]	This a semistructured interview for making DSM-IV Axis I and Axis II diagnoses. It is designed for use by experienced psychiatrists or other clinicians who may supplement the interview by using additional records, interviews with family members, or follow-up questions. There is a computerized version of the screening version of the SCID.	Reliability was evaluated by examining the consistency with which trained clinicians assigned lifetime diagnoses to large samples of psychiatric patients and healthy controls. The mean kappa coefficients for these analyses were 0.68 for the patients and 0.51 for the controls. Validity studies have compared the diagnoses made by the SCID interview and those made by experienced clinicians. The kappa coefficients were 0.85 for Axis I diagnoses and 0.65 for Axis II conditions.

References

1. Drossman DA, Li Z, Andruzzi E, Temple R, Talley NJ, Thompson WG, Whitehead WE, Janssens J, Funch-Jensen P, Corazziari E, Richter JE, Koch GG. U.S. Householder Survey of Functional Gastrointestinal Disorders: Prevalence, Sociodemography and Health Impact. Dig Dis Sci 1993;38:1569–1580.
2. Akehurst RL, Brazier JE, Mathers N, O'Keefe C, Kaltenthaler E, Morgan A, Platts M, Walters SJ. Health-related quality of life and cost impact of irritable bowel syndrome in a UK primary care setting. Pharmacoeconomics 2002;20:455–462.
3. El Serag HB, Olden K, Bjorkman D. Health-related quality of life among persons with irritable bowel syndrome: a systematic review. Aliment Pharmacol Ther 2002; 16:1171–1185.
4. Luscombe FA. Health-related quality of life and associated psychosocial factors in irritable bowel syndrome: a review. Qual Life Res 2000;9:161–176.
5. Drossman DA. Presidential Address: Gastrointestinal Illness and Biopsychosocial Model. Psychosom Med 1998;60:258–267.
6. Drossman DA, Creed FH, Olden KW, Svedlund J, Toner BB, Whitehead WE. Psychosocial aspects of the functional gastrointestinal disorders. In: Drossman DA, Corazziari E, Talley NJ, Thompson WG, and Whitehead WE, eds. Rome II. The functional gastrointestinal disorders: Diagnosis, pathophysiology and treatment; A multinational consensus. 2 ed. Degnon and Associates, 2000:157–245.
7. Almy TP, Kern FJr, Tulin M. Alteration in colonic function in man under stress: II. Experimental production of sigmoid spasm in healthy persons. Gastroenterology 1949;12:425–436.
8. Engel GL. The need for a new medical model: A challenge for biomedicine. Science 1977;196:129–136.
9. Drossman DA, Li Z, Leserman J, Toomey TC, Hu Y. Health status by gastrointestinal diagnosis and abuse history. Gastroenterology 1996;110:999–1007.
10. Sandler RS, Drossman DA, Nathan HP, McKee DC. Symptom complaints and health care seeking behavior in subjects with bowel dysfunction. Gastroenterology 1984; 87:314–318.
11. Fordyce WE, Fowler RS, Delateur B. Case histories and shorter communications: An application of behavior modification technique to a problem of chronic pain. Behavior Res Ther 1968;6:105–107.
12. Whitehead WE, Crowell MD, Heller BR, Robinson JC, Schuster MM, Horn S. Modeling and reinforcement of the sick role during childhood predicts adult illness behavior. Psychosom Med 1994;56:541–550.
13. Gwee KA, Leong YL, Graham C, McKendrick MW, Collins SM, Walters SJ, Underwood JE, Read NW. The role of psychological and biological factors in post-infective gut dysfunction. Gut 1999;44:400–406.
14. Naliboff BD, Munakata J, Fullerton S, Gracely RH, Kodner A, Harraf F, Mayer EA. Evidence for two distinct perceptual alterations in irritable bowel syndrome. Gut 1997;41:505–512.
15. Whitehead WE, Crowell MD, Davidoff AL, Palsson OS, Schuster MM. Pain from rectal distension in women with irritable bowel syndrome: Relationship to sexual abuse. Dig Dis Sci 1997;42:796–804.
16. Drossman DA, Ringel Y, Vogt B, Leserman J, Lin W, Smith JK, Whitehead W. Altera-

tions of brain activity associated with resolution of emotional distress and pain in a case of severe IBS. Gastroenterology 2003;124:754–761.

17. Walker LS, Guite JW, Duke M, Barnard JA, Greene JW. Recurrent abdominal pain: a potential precursor of irritable bowel syndrome in adolescents and young adults. J Pediatr 1998;132:1010–1015.

18. Locke GR, III, Zinsmeister A, Talley NJ, Fett SL, Melton J. Familial association in adults with functional gastrointestinal disorders. Mayo Clin Proc 2000;75:907–912.

19. Offenbaecher M, Bondy B, de Jonge S, Glatzeder K, Kruger M, Schoeps P, Ackenheil M. Possible association of fibromyalgia with a polymorphism in the serotonin transporter gene regulatory region. Arthritis Rheum 1999;42:2482–2488.

20. Caspi A, Sugden K, Moffitt TE, Taylor A, Craig IW, Harrington H, McClay J, Mill J, Martin J, Braithwaite A, Poulton R. Influence of life stress on depression: moderation by a polymorphism in the 5-HTT gene. Science 2003;301:386–9.

21. Zubieta JK, Heitzeg MM, Smith YR, Bueller JA, Xu K, Xu Y, Koeppe RA, Stohler CS, Goldman D. COMT val158met genotype affects mu-opioid neurotransmitter responses to a pain stressor. Science 2003;299:1240–1243.

22. Yeo A, Boyd P, Lumsden S, Saunders T, Handley A, Stubbins M, Knaggs A, Asquith S, Taylor I, Bahari B, Crocker N, Rallan R, Varsani S, Montgomery D, Alpers DH, Dukes GE, Purvis I, Hicks GA. Association between a functional polymorphism in the serotonin transporter gene and diarrhoea predominant irritable bowel syndrome in women. Gut 2004;53:1452–1458.

23. Camilleri M. Is there a SERT-ain association with IBS? Gut 2004;53:1396–1399.

24. Diatchenko L, Slade GD, Nackley AG, Bhalang K, Sigurdsson A, Belfer I, Goldman D, Xu K, Shabalina SA, Shagin D, Max MB, Makarov SS, Maixner W. Genetic basis for individual variations in pain perception and the development of a chronic pain condition. Hum Mol Genet 2005;14,135–143.

25. Levy RL, Jones KR, Whitehead WE, Feld SI, Talley NJ, Corey LA. Irritable bowel syndrome in twins: Heredity and social learning both contribute to etiology. Gastroenterology 2001;121:799–804.

26. Levy RL, Whitehead WE, Von Korff MR, Saunders KW, Feld AD. Intergenerational transmission of gastrointestinal illness behavior. Am J Gastroenterol 2000;95:451–456.

27. Walker LS, Garber J, Greene JW. Psychosocial correlates of recurrent childhood pain: a comparison of pediatric patients with recurrent abdominal pain, organic illness, and psychiatric disorders. J Abnorm Psychol 1993;102:248–258.

28. Walker LS, Heflinger C.A. Qulaity of life predictors in paediatric abdominal pain patients: Findings at initial assessment and five year follow-up. In: Drotar D.D., ed. Measuring health-related quality of life in children and adolescents: Implications for reearch and practice. Mahwah, NJ: Lawrence Eribaum, 1998:237–252.

29. Walker LS, Garber J, Smith CA, Van Slyke DA, Claar RL. The relation of daily stressors to somatic and emotional symptoms in children with and without recurrent abdominal pain. J Consult Clin Psychol 2001;69:85–91.

30. Walker LS, Claar RL, Garber J. Social consequences of children's pain: when do they encourage symptom maintenance? J Pediatr Psychol 2002;27:689–698.

31. Walker LS, Garber J, Greene JW. Somatic complaints in pediatric patients: A prospective study of the role of negative life events, child social and academic competence, and parental somatic symptoms. J Consult Clin Psych 1994;62:1213–1221.

32. Walker LS, Garber J, Greene JW. Somatization symptoms in pediatric abdominal

pain patients: relation to chronicity of abdominal pain and parent somatization. J Abnormal Child Psychol 1991;19:379–394.

33. Bode G, Brenner H, Adler G, Rothenbacher D. Recurrent abdominal pain in children: evidence from a population-based study that social and familial factors play a major role but not Helicobacter pylori infection. J Psychosom Res 2003;54:417–421.

34. Hotopf M, Carr S, Mayou R, Wadsworth M, Wessely S. Why do children have chronic abdominal pain, and what happens to them when they grow up? Population based cohort study. BMJ 1998;316:1196–1200.

35. Hotopf M, Mayou R, Wadsworth M, Wessely S. Childhood risk factors for adults with medically unexplained symptoms: results from a national birth cohort study. Am J Psychiatry 1999;156:1796–1800.

36. Levy RL, Whitehead WE, Walker LS, Von Korff M, Feld AD, Garner M, Christie D. Increased somatic complaints and health-care utilization in children: effects of parent IBS status and parent response to gastrointestinal symptoms. Am J Gastroenterol 2004;99:2442–2451.

37. Drossman DA, Talley NJ, Olden KW, Leserman J, Barreiro MA. Sexual and physical abuse and gastrointestinal illness: Review and recommendations. Ann Intern Med 1995;123:782–794.

38. Peters SD, Wyatt GE, Finkelhor D. Prevalence. In: Finkelhor D, ed. A sourcebook on child sexual abuse. 1 ed. Beverly Hills: Sage Publications, 1986:15–59.

39. Drossman DA, Leserman J, Nachman G, Li Z, Gluck H, Toomey TC, Mitchell CM. Sexual and physical abuse in women with functional or organic gastrointestinal disorders. Ann Intern Med 1990;113:828–833.

40. Talley NJ, Fett SL, Zinsmeister AR. Self-reported abuse and gastrointestinal disease in outpatients: Association with irritable bowel-type symptoms. Amer J Gastroenterol 1995;90:366–371.

41. Talley NJ, Fett SL, Zinsmeister AR, Melton LJ. Gastrointestinal tract symptoms and self-reported abuse: A population-based study. Gastroenterology 1994;107:1040–1049.

42. Romans S, Belaise C, Martin J, Morris E, Raffi A. Childhood abuse and later medical disorders in women. An epidemiological study. Psychother Psychosomat 2002;71:141–150.

43. Talley NJ, Boyce PM, Jones M. Predictors of health care seeking for irritable bowel syndrome: a population based study. Gut 1997;41:394–398.

44. McCauley J, Kern DE, Kolodner K, Dill L, Schroeder AF, DeChant HK, Ryden J, Derogatis LR, Bass EB. Clinical characteristics of women with a history of childhood abuse: Unhealed wounds. JAMA 1997;277:1362–1368.

45. Walker EA, Gelfand A, Katon WJ, Koss MP, Von Korff M, Bernstein D, Russo J. Adult health status of women with histories of childhood abuse and neglect. Am J Med 1999;107:332–339.

46. Walker EA, Katon WJ, Roy-Byrne PP, Jemelka RP, Russo J. Histories of sexual victimization in patients with irritable bowel syndrome or inflammatory bowel disease. Am J Psychiatry 1993;150:1502–1506.

47. Delvaux M, Denis P, Allemand H, French Club of Digestive Motility. Sexual and physical abuses are more frequently reported by IBS patients than by patients with organic digestive diseases or controls. Results of a multicenter inquiry. Euro J Gastroenterol Hepat 1997;9:345–352.

48. Heitkemper M, Jarrett M, Walker E, Landenburger K, Bond EF. Effect of sexual and

physical abuse on symptom experiences in women with Irritable Bowel Syndrome. Nursing Res 2001;50:1–9.

49. Ali A, Toner BB, Stuckless N, Gallop R, Diamant NE, Gould M, Vidins E. Emotional abuse, self-blame and self-silencing in women with irritable bowel syndrome. Psychosom Med 2000;62:76–82.

50. Irwin C, Falsetti SA, Lydiard RB, Ballenger JC, Brock CD, Brener W. Comorbidity of posttraumatic stress disorder and irritable bowel syndrome. J Clin Psychiatry 1996;57:576–578.

51. Longstreth GF, Wolde-Tsadik G. Irritable bowel-type symptoms in HMO examinees. Prevalence, demographics, and clinical correlates. Dig Dis Sci 1993;38:1581–1589.

52. Leserman J, Toomey TC, Drossman DA. Medical consequences of sexual and physical abuse in women. Humane Med 1995;11:23–28.

53. Johnson CF. Child sexual abuse. Lancet 2004;364:462–470.

54. Laws A. Does a History of Sexual Abuse in Childhood Play a Role in Women's Medical Problems? A Review. J Women's Health 1993;2:165–172.

55. Drossman DA, Li Z, Leserman J, Keefe FJ, Hu YJ, Toomey TC. Effects of coping on health outcome among female patients with gastrointestinal disorders. Psychosom Med 2000;62:309–317.

56. Koloski NA, Talley NJ, Boyce PM. Predictors of health care seeking for irritable bowel syndrome and nonulcer dyspepsia: A critical review of the literature on symptom and psychosocial factors. Am J Gastroenterol 2001;96:1340–1349.

57. Leserman J, Drossman DA, Li Z, Toomey TC, Nachman G, Glogau L. Sexual and physical abuse in gastroenterology practice: How types of abuse impact health status. Psychosom Med 1996;58:4–15.

58. Creed FH, Craig T, Farmer RG. Functional abdominal pain, psychiatric illness and life events. Gut 1988;29:235–242.

59. Bennett EJ, Tennant CC, Piesse C, Badcock CA, Kellow JE. Level of chronic life stress predicts clinical outcome in irritable bowel syndrome. Gut 1998;43:256–261.

60. Whitehead WE, Crowell MD, Robinson JC, Heller BR, Schuster MM. Effects of stressful life events on bowel symptoms: Subjects with irritable bowel syndrome compared to subjects without bowel dysfunction. Gut 1992;33:825–830.

61. Naliboff BD, Mayer M, Fass R, FitzGerald LZ, Chang L, Bolus R, Mayer EA. The effect of life stress on symptoms of heartburn. Psychosom Med 2004;66:426–434.

62. Drossman DA, McKee DC, Sandler RS, Mitchell CM, Cramer EM, Lowman BC, Burger AL. Psychosocial factors in the irritable bowel syndrome. A multivariate study of patients and nonpatients with irritable bowel syndrome. Gastroenterology 1988;95:701–708.

63. Walker EA, Katon W, Roy-Byrne PP, Li L, Amos D. Psychiatric illness and irritable bowel syndrome: a comparison with inflammatory bowel disease. Am J Psychiatry 1990;147:1656–1661.

64. Whitehead WE, Holtkotter B, Enck P, Hoelzl R, Holmes KD, Anthony J, Shabsin HS, Schuster MM. Tolerance for rectosigmoid distention in irritable bowel syndrome. Gastroenterology 1990;98:1187–1192.

65. Smith RC, Greenbaum DS, Vancouver JB, Henry RC, Reinhart MA, Greenbaum RB, Dean HA, Mayle JE. Psychosocial factors are associated with health care seeking rather than diagnosis in irritable bowel syndrome. Gastroenterology 1990;98:293-301.

66. Blanchard EB, Radnitz CL, Evans DD, Schwartz SP, Neff DF, Gerardi MA. Psychological comparisons of irritable bowel syndrome to chronic tension and migraine headache and nonpatient controls. Biofeedback Self Reg 1986;11:221–230.

67. Cheng C. Seeking medical consultation: Perceptual and behavioral characteristics distinguishing consulters and nonconsulters with functional dyspepsia. Psychosom Med 2000;62:844–852.

68. Chakraborti SK, Dey BK, Ghosh N, Chaudhury AN, Guha Mazumder DN. Objective evaluation of psychological abnormality in irritable bowel syndrome. Indian J Gastroenterol 1996;15:43–45.

69. Henningsen P, Zimmermann T, Sattel H. Medically unexplained physical symptoms, anxiety, and depression: a meta-analytic review. Psychosom Med 2003;65:528–533.

70. Herschbach P, Henrich G, von Rad M. Psychological factors in functional gastrointestinal disorders: Characteristics of the disorder or of the illness behavior? Psychosom Med 1999;61:148–153.

71. Locke GR, III, Weaver AL, Melton LJ, III, Talley NJ. Psychosocial factors are linked to functional gastrointestinal disorders: a population based nested case-control study. Am J Gastroenterol 2004;99:350–357.

72. Gwee KA, Graham JC, McKendrick MW, Collins SM, Marshall JS, Walters SJ, Read NW. Psychometric scores and persistence of irritable bowel after infectious diarrhoea. Lancet 1996;347:150–153.

73. Neal KR, Barker L, Spiller RC. Prognosis in post-infective irritable bowel syndrome: a six year follow up study. Gut 2002;51:410–413.

74. Creed F. The relationship between psychosocial parameters and outcome in irritable bowel syndrome. Am J Med 1999;107:74S–80S.

75. Creed F, Barsky A. A systematic review of the epidemiology of somatisation disorder and hypochondriasis. J Psychosom Res 2004;56:391–408.

76. Wilhelmsen I, Haug TT, Ursin H, Berstad A. Discriminant analysis of factors distinguishing patients with functional dyspepsia from patients with duodenal ulcer. Significance of somatization. Dig Dis Sci 1995;40:1105–1111.

77. Haug TT, Svebak S, Wilhelmsen I, Berstad A, Ursin H. Psychological factors and somatic symptoms in functional dyspepsia. A comparison with duodenal ulcer and healthy controls. J Psychosom Res 1994;38:281–291.

78. Gillespie NA, Zhu G, Heath AC, Hickie IB, Martin NG. The genetic aetiology of somatic distress. Psychol Med 2000;30:1051–1061.

79. Zaman MS, Chavez NF, Krueger R, Talley NJ, Lembo T. Extra-intestinal symptoms in patients with irritable bowel syndrome (IBS). Gastroenterology 2001;120[5(1)], A636.

80. Whitehead WE, Palsson O, Jones KR. Systematic review of the comorbidity of irritable bowel syndrome with other disorders: What are the causes and implications? Gastroenterology 2002;122:1140–1156.

81. Katon W, Lin E, Von Korff M, Russo J, Lipscomb P, Bush T. Somatization: a spectrum of severity. Am J Psychiatry 1991;148:34–40.

82. Talley NJ, Dennis EH, Schettler-Duncan VA, Lacy BE, Olden KW, Crowell MD. Overlapping upper and lower gastrointestinal symptoms in irritable bowel syndrome patients with constipation or diarrhea. Am J Gastroenterol 2003;98:2454–2459.

83. Halder SL, Locke GR, III, Talley NJ, Fett SL, Zinsmeister AR, Melton LJ, III. Impact of functional gastrointestinal disorders on health-related quality of life: a population-based case-control study. Aliment Pharmacol Ther 2004;19:233–242.

84. Holtmann G, Kutscher SU, Haag S, Langkafel M, Heuft G, Neufang-Hueber J, Goebell H, Senf W, Talley NJ. Clinical presentation and personality factors are predictors

of the response to treatment in patients with functional dyspepsia; a randomized, double-blind placebo-controlled crossover study. Dig Dis Sci 2004;49:672–679.

85. Porcelli P. Psychological abnormalities in patients with irritable bowel syndrome. Indian J Gastroenterol 2004;23:63–69.

86. Creed F, Ratcliffe J, Fernandez L, Tomenson B, Palmer S, Rigby C, Guthrie E, Read N, Thompson D. Health-related quality of life and health care costs in severe, refractory irritable bowel syndrome. Ann Intern Med 2001;134:860–868.

87. Drossman DA, Camilleri M, Mayer EA, Whitehead WE. AGA Technical Review on Irritable Bowel Syndrome. Gastroenterology 2002;123:2108–2131.

88. Lydiard RB, Fossey MD, Marsh W, Ballenger JC. Prevalence of psychiatric disorders in patients with irritable bowel syndrome. Psychosomatics 1993;34:229–234.

89. Creed FH. Relationship between IBS and psychiatric disorder. In: Camilleri M and Spiller R, eds. Irritable Bowel Syndrome: Diagnosis and Treatment. W.B.Saunders, 2002:45–54.

90. Zaubler TS, Katon W. Panic disorder and medical comorbidity: a review of the medical and psychiatric literature. Bulletin Menninger Clinic 1996;60:A12–38.

91. Olden KW. Panic Attack Induced Vomiting: Clinical and Behavioral Characteristics. Am J Gastroenterol 1999;94:2614.

92. Lydiard RB, Greenwald S, Weissman MM, Johnson J, Drossman DA, Ballenger JC. Panic disorder and gastrointestinal symptoms: Findings from the NIMH Epidemiologic Catchment Area project. Am J Psychiatry 1994;151:64–70.

93. Craig T.K.J. Abdominal pain. In: Brown G.W. and Harris T.O., eds. Life Events and Illness. New York: Guildford, 1989:233–259.

94. Sykes MA, Blanchard EB, Lackner J, Keefer L, Krasner S. Psychopathology in irritable bowel syndrome: support for a psychophysiological model. J Behav Med 2003;26:361–372.

95. Walker EA, Katon WJ, Jemelka RP, Roy Bryne PP. Comorbidity of gastrointestinal complaints, depression, and anxiety in the Epidemiologic Catchment Area (ECA) Study. Am J Med 1992;92:26S-30S.

96. American Psychiatric Association. Somatoform Disorders. Diagnostic and Statistical Manual of Mental Disorders—revised. 3 ed. Washington, D.C.: American Psychiatric Association, 1987:255–267.

97. Miller AR, North CS, Clouse RE, Wetzel RD, Spitznagel EL, Alpers DH. The association of irritable bowel syndrome and somatization disorder. Ann Clin Psychiatry 2001;13:25–30.

98. North CS, Downs D, Clouse RE, Alrakawi A, Dokucu ME, Cox J, Spitznagel EL, Alpers DH. The presentation of irritable bowel syndrome in the context of somatization disorder. Clin Gastroenterol Hepatol 2004;2:787–795.

99. Anonymous. World Health Organization Schedules for Clinical Assessment in Neuropsychiatry. 1994. American Psychiatric Association Press, Inc.

100. Creed FH, Ratcliffe J, Fernandes L, Palmer S, Rigby C, Tomenson B, Guthrie E, Read N, Thompson DG. Outcome in severe irritable bowel syndrome with and without depressive, panic and neurasthenic disorders. Br J Psychiatry 2005;186:507–515.

101. Simren M, Abrahamsson H, Svedlund J, Bjornsson ES. Quality of life in patients with irritable bowel syndrome seen in referral centers versus primary care: the impact of gender and predominant bowel pattern. Scand J Gastroenterol 2001;36:545–552.

102. Sperber AD, Carmel S, Atzmon Y, Weisberg I, Shalit Y, Neumann L, Fich A, Friger M, Buskila D. Use of the Functional Bowel Disorder Severity Index (FBDSI) in a study of patients with the Irritable bowel syndrome and fibromyalgia. Am J Gastroenterol 2000;95:995–998.

103. Esler MD, Goulston KJ. Levels of anxiety in colonic disorders. New Engl J Med 1973;288:16–20.

104. Cook IJ, van Eeden A, Collins SM. Patients with irritable bowel syndrome have greater pain tolerance than normal subjects. Gastroenterology 1987;93:727–733.

105. Talley NJ, Phillips SF, Bruce B, Twomey CK, Zinsmeister AR, Melton LJ. Relation among personality and symptoms in nonulcer dyspepsia and the irritable bowel syndrome. Gastroenterology 1990;99 [2]:327–333.

106. Heaton KW. What makes people with abdominal pain consult their doctor. In: Creed FH, Mayou R, and Hopkins A, eds. Medical symptoms Not Explained by Organic Disease. London: Royal Colleges of Physicians and Psychiatrists, 1992:1–8.

107. Whitehead WE, Bosmajian L, Zonderman AB, Costa PTJr, Schuster MM. Symptoms of psychologic distress associated with irritable bowel syndrome. Comparison of community and medical clinic samples. Gastroenterology 1988;95:709–714.

108. Sjodin I, Svedlund J. Psychological aspects of non-ulcer dyspepsia: a psychosomatic view focusing on a comparison between the irritable bowel syndrome and peptic ulcer disease. Scand J Gastroenterol 1985;109:51–58.

109. Creed F, Guthrie E. Relation among personality and symptoms in nonulcer dyspepsia and the irritable bowel syndrome. Gastroenterology 1991;100:1154–1155.

110. Abell TL, Cutts TF, Cooper T. Effect of cisapride therapy for severe dyspepsia on gastrointestinal symptoms and quality of life. Scand J Gastroenterol 1995;195:60–64.

111. Kay L, Jorgensen T, Jensen KH. The epidemiology of irritable bowel syndrome in a random population: prevalence, incidence, natural history and risk factors. J Intern Med 1994;236:23–30.

112. Talley NJ, Boyce PM, Jones M. Is the association between irritable bowel syndrome and abuse explained by neuroticism? A population based study. Gut 1998;42:47–53.

113. Tanum L, Malt UF. Personality traits predict treatment outcome with an antidepressant in patients with functional gastrointestinal disorder. Scand J Gastroenterol 2000;35:935–941.

114. Mulak A, Bonaz B. Irritable bowel syndrome: a model of the brain-gut interactions. Medical Science Monitor 2004;10:RA55–RA62.

115. Mayer EA, Naliboff BD, Chang L, Coutinho SV. Stress and the gastrointestinal tract v. stress and irritable bowel syndrome. Am J Physiol Gastrointest Liver Physiol 2001;280:G519–G524.

116. Damasio A R. The Feeling of What Happens: Body and Emotion in the Making of Consciousness. New York: Harcourt Brace, 1999.

117. Monnikes H, Tebbe JJ, Hildebrandt M, Arck P, Osmanoglou E, Rose M, Klapp B, Wiedenmann B, Heymann-Monnikes I. Role of stress in functional gastrointestinal disorders. Evidence for stress-induced alterations in gastrointestinal motility and sensitivity. Dig Dis 2001;19:201–211.

118. Tache Y, Martinez V, Million M, Wang L. Stress and the gastrointestinal tract: III. Stress-related alterations of gut motor function: Role of brain-corticotropin-releasing factor receptors. Am J Physiol Gastrointest Liver Physiol 2001;280:G173–G177.

119. Bradley LA, Richter JE, Pulliam TJ, Haile JM, Scarinci IC, Schan CA, Dalton CB, Salley AN. The relationship between stress and symptoms of gastroesophageal reflux: the influence of psychological factors. Am J Gastroenterol 1993;88:11–19.

120. Stanghellini V, Malagelada JR, Zinsmeister AR, Go VLW, Kao PC. Stress-induced gastroduodenal motor disturbances in man: Possible humoral mechanisms. Gastroenterology 1983;85:83–91.

121. Kellow JE, Eckersley GM, Jones M. Enteric and central contributions to intestinal dysmotility in irritable bowel syndrome. Dig Dis Sci 1992;37:168–174.

122. Kellow JE, Phillips SF, Miller LJ, Zinsmeister AR. Dysmotility of the small intestine in irritable bowel syndrome. Gut 1988;29:1236–1243.

123. Kumar D, Wingate DL. The irritable bowel syndrome: A paraxysmal motor disorder. Lancet 1985;2:973–977.

124. Kellow JE, Langeluddecke PM, Eckersley GM, Jones MP, Tennant CC. Effects of acute psychologic stress on small-intestinal motility in health and the irritable bowel syndrome. Scand J Gastroenterol 1992;27:53–58.

125. Evans PR, Bennett EJ, Bak Y-T, Tennant CC, Kellow JE. Jejunal sensorimotor dysfunction in irritable bowel syndrome: Clinical and psychosocial features. Gastroenterology 1996;110:393–404.

126. Cann PA, Read NW, Brown C, Hobson N, Holdsworth CG. Irritable bowel syndrome: relationship of disorders in the transit of a single solid meal to symptom patterns. Gut 1983;24:405–411.

127. Bell AM, Pemberton JH, Camilleri M, Hanson RB, Zinsmeister AR. The effect of acute stress on rectal tone and anal sphincter pressure. Gastroenterology 1989;96:A38.

128. Simren M, Castedal M, Svedlund J, Abrahamsson H, Bjornsson E. Abnormal propagation pattern of duodenal pressure waves in the irritable bowel syndrome (IBD). Dig Dis Sci 2000;45:2151–2161.

129. Dickhaus B, Mayer EA, Firooz N, Stains J, Conde F, Olivas TI, Fass R, Chang L, Mayer M, Naliboff BD. Irritable bowel syndrome patients show enhanced modulation of visceral perception by auditory stress. Am J Gastroenterol 2003;98:135–143.

130. Tougas G. The autonomic nervous system in functional bowel disorders. Gut 2000;47 Suppl 4:iv78–iv80.

131. Elsenbruch S, Orr WC. Diarrhea-and constipation-predominant IBS patients differ in postprandial autonomic and cortisol responses. Am J Gastroenterol 2001;96:460–466.

132. Gupta V, Sheffield D, Verne GN. Evidence for autonomic dysregulation in the irritable bowel syndrome. Dig Dis Sci 2002;47:1716–1722.

133. Burr RL, Heitkemper M, Jarrett M, Cain KC. Comparison of autonomic nervous system indices based on abdominal pain reports in women with irritable bowel syndrome. Biol Res Nursing 2000;2:97–106.

134. Chang L, Heitkemper MM. Gender differences in irritable bowel syndrome. Gastroenterology 2002;123:1686–1701.

135. Mearadji B, Straathof JW, Naaykens C, Frolich M, Lamers CB, Masclee AA. Effect of modified sham feeding and insulin-induced hypoglycemia on function of the proximal stomach. Digestion 2000;62:110–115.

136. Patacchioli FR, Angelucci L, Dellerba G, Monnazzi P, Leri O. Actual stress, psychopathology and salivary cortisol levels in the irritable bowel syndrome (IBS). J Endocrinological Inv 2001;24:173–177.

137. Heitkemper M, Jarrett M, Cain K, Shaver J, Bond E, Woods NF, Walker E. Increased urine catecholamines and cortisol in women with irritable bowel syndrome. Am J Gastroenterol 1996;91:906–913.

138. Elsenbruch S, Lovallo WR, Orr WC. Psychological and physiological responses to postprandial mental stress in women with the irritable bowel syndrome. Psychosom Med 2001;63:805–813.

139. Heitkemper M, Jarrett M, Cain KC, Burr R, Levy RL, Feld A, Hertig V. Autonomic nervous system function in women with irritable bowel syndrome. Dig Dis Sci 2001;46:1276–1284.

140. Elsenbruch S, Thompson JJ, Hamish MJ, Exton MS, Orr WC. Behavioral and physiological sleep characteristics in women with irritable bowel syndrome. Am J Gastroenterol 2002;97:2306–2314.

141. Jarrett M, Heitkemper M, Cain KC, Burr RL, Hertig V. Sleep disturbance influences gastrointestinal symptoms in women with irritable bowel syndrome. Dig Dis Sci 2000;45:952–959.

142. Orr WC, Elsenbruch S, Harnish MJ. Autonomic regulation of cardiac function during sleep in patients with irritable bowel syndrome. Am J Gastroenterol 2000; 95:2865–2871.

143. Thompson JJ, Elsenbruch S, Harnish MJ, Orr WC. Autonomic functioning during REM sleep differentiates IBS symptom subgroups. Am J Gastroenterol 2002; 97:3147–3153.

144. Colgan S, Creed FH, Klass SH. Psychiatric disorder and abnormal illness behaviour in patients with upper abdominal pain. Psychol Med 1988;18:887–892.

145. Beck AT, Emery G, Greenberg R. Anxiety Disorders and Phobias: A Cognitive Perspective. New York: Basic Books, 1985.

146. Warwick HM, Salkovskis P. Hypochondriasis. Behav Res Ther 1990;28:105–117.

147. Sullivan MJ, Thorn B, Haythornthwaite JA, Keefe F, Martin M, Bradley LA, Lefebvre JC. Theoretical perspectives on the relation between catastrophizing and pain. Clinical Journal of Pain 2001;17:52–64.

148. Sullivan MJL, Bishop S. The Pain Catastrophizing Scale: Development and validation. Psychological Assessment 1995;7:524–532.

149. Michaels ES BJW. Catastrophizing and pain sensitivity among chronic pain patients: moderating effects of sensory and affect focus. Ann Behavioral Med 27, 185–194. 2004.

150. Lackner JM, Quigley BM, Blanchard EB. Depression and Abdominal Pain in IBS Patients: The Mediating Role of Catastrophizing. Psychosom Med 2004;66:435–441.

151. Taylor S, Cox B.J. Anxiety sensitivity: Multiple dimensions and hierarchic structure. Behaviour Res Ther 1998;36:Jan-51.

152. Asmundson GJ, Norton P. Beyond pain: The role of fear and avoidance in chronicity. Clin Psychiatry Rev Kingdom;19:Jan-119.

153. Hazlett-Stevens H, Craske MG, Mayer EA, Chang L, Naliboff BD. Prevalence of irritable bowel syndrome among university students: the roles of worry, neuroticism, anxiety sensitivity and visceral anxiety. J Psychosom Res 2003;55:501–505.

154. Millon T, Green CJ, Meagher RB. Millon Behavioral Health Inventory Manual, 3rd ed. Minneapolis: Natural Computer Systems, 1982.

155. Gombrone J, Dewsnap P, Libby G, Farthing M. Abnormal illness attitudes in patients with irritable bowel syndrome. J Psychosom Res 1995;39:227–230.

156. Toner BB, Koyama E, Garfinkel PE, Jeejeebhoy KN, Gasbarro I. Social desirability and irritable bowel syndrome. Int J Psychiatry Med 1992;22:99–103.

157. Van Dulmen AM, Fennis JFM, Mokkink HGA, Van Der Velden HGM, Bleijenberg G. Doctor-dependent changes in complaint-related cognitions and anxiety during medical consultations in functional abdominal complaints. Psychol Med 1995; 25:1011–1018.

158. Lucock MP, Morley S, White C, Peake MD. Responses of consecutive patients to reassurance after gastroscopy: results of self administered questionnaire survey. BMJ 1997;315:572–575.

159. Gibbs-Gallagher N, Palsson OS, Levy RL, Meyer K, Drossman DA, Whitehead WE. Selective recall of gastrointestinal-sensation words: Evidence for a cognitive-behavioral contribution to irritable bowel syndrome. Am J Gastroenterol 2001;96:1133–1138.

160. Barsky AJ, Geringer E, Wool CA. A cognitive-educational treatment for hypochondriasis. Gen Hosp Psychiatry 1988;10:322–327.

161. Drossman DA. Challenges in the physician-patient relationship: Feeling "drained". Gastroenterology 2001;121:1037–1038.

162. Naliboff BD, Balice G, Mayer EA. Psychosocial moderators of quality of life in irritable bowel syndrome. Eur J Surg Suppl 1998;57–59.

163. Spiegel BM, Gralnek IM, Bolus R, Chang L, Dulai GS, Mayer EA, Naliboff B. Clinical determinants of health-related quality of life in patients with irritable bowel syndrome. Arch Int Med 2004;164:1773–1780.

164. Halder SL, Locle GR 3rd, Talley NJ, Fett SL, Zinmaster AR, Melton LJ 3rd. Impact of functional gastrointestinal disorder on health-related quality of liofe: a population-based case-control study. Aliment Pharmacol Ther2004;19:233–242.

165. Drossman DA, Morris CB, Hu Y, Blackman C, Toner BB, Diamant N, Whitehead WE, Leserman J, Bangdiwala SI. What factors explain health related quality of life (HRQOL) in functional bowel disorders. Gastroenterology 2004;126(S2):A477.

166. Thompson WG, Heaton KW, Smyth T, Smyth C. Irritable bowel syndrome in general practice: prevalence, characteristics, and referral. Gut 2000;46:78–82.

167. Prior A, Whorwell PJ. Gynaecological consultation in patients with the irritable bowel syndrome. Gut 1989;30:996–998.

168. Sandler RS, Everhart JE, Donowitz M, Adams E, Cronin K, Goodman C, Gemmen E, Shah S, Avdic A, Rubin R. The burden of selected digestive diseases in the United States. Gastroenterology 2002;122:1500–1511.

169. Camilleri M, Williams DE. Economic burden of irritable bowel syndrome reappraised with strategies to control expenditures. PharmacoEconomics 2000;17:331–338.

170. Le Pen C, Ruszniewski P, Gaudin AF, Amouretti M, Bommelaer G, Frexinos J, Poynard T, Maurel F, Priol G, Bertin C. The burden cost of French patients suffering from irritable bowel syndrome. Scand J Gastroenterol 2004;39:336–343.

171. Levy RL, Von Korff M, Whitehead WE, Stang P, Saunders K, Jhingran P, Barghout V, Feld AD. Costs of care for irritable bowel syndrome patients in a health maintenance organization. Am J Gastoenterology 2001;96:3122–3129.

172. Creed F, Fernandes L, Guthrie E, Palmer S, Ratcliffe J, Read N, Rigby C, Thompson D, Tomenson B. The cost-effectiveness of psychotherapy and paroxetine for severe irritable bowel syndrome. Gastroenterology 2003;124 :303–317.

173. Rutter CL, Rutter DR. Illness representation, coping and outcome in irritable bowel

syndrome (IBS). [References]. British Journal of Health Psychology 2002;7:Nov-392.

174. Biggs AM, Aziz Q, Tomenson B, Creed F. Effect of childhood adversity on health related quality of life in patients with upper abdominal or chest pain. Gut 2004;53:180–186.

175. Drossman DA. Physical and sexual abuse and gastrointestinal illness: What is the link? Am J Med 1994;97:105–107.

176. Blanchard EB, Keefer L, Payne A, Turner SM, Galovski TE. Early abuse, psychiatric diagnoses and irritable bowel syndrome. Behav Res Ther 2002;40:289–298.

177. Salmon P, Skaife K, Rhodes J. Abuse, dissociation, and somatization in irritable bowel syndrome: towards an explanatory model. J Behav Med 2003;26:1–18.

178. Drossman DA, Toner BB, Whitehead WE, Diamant NE, Dalton CB, Duncan S, Emmott S, Proffitt V, Akman D, Frusciante K, Le T, Meyer K, Bradshaw B, Mikula K, Morris CB, Blackman CJ, Hu Y, Jia H, Li Z, Koch GG, Bangdiwala SI. Cognitive-Behavioral Therapy vs. education and Desipramine vs. Placebo for Moderate to Severe Functional Bowel Disorders. Gastroenterology 2003;125:19–31.

179. Mertz H, Morgan V, Tanner G, Pickens D, Price R, Shyr Y, Kessler R. Regional cerebral activation in irritable bowel syndrome and control subjects with painful and nonpainful rectal distension. Gastroenterology 2000;118:842–848.

180. Naliboff BD, Derbyshire SWG, Munakata J, Berman S, Mandelkern M, Chang L, Mayer EA. Cerebral activation in irritable bowel syndrome patients and control subjects during rectosigmoid stimulation. Psychosom Med 2001;63:365–375.

181. Guthrie E, Barlow J, Fernandes L, Ratcliffe J, Read N, Thompson DG, Tomenson B, Creed F, North of England IBS Research Group. Changes in tolerance to rectal distension correlate with changes in psychological state in patients with severe irritable bowel syndrome. Psychosom Med 2004;66:578–582.

182. Blomhoff S, Spetalen S, Jacobsen MB, Malt UF. Phobic anxiety changes the function of brain-gut axis in irritable bowel syndrome. Psychosom Med 2001;63:959–965.

183. Jarrett ME, Burr RL, Cain KC, Hertig V, Weisman P, Heitkemper MM. Anxiety and depression are related to autonomic nervous system function in women with irritable bowel syndrome. Dig Dis Sci 2003;48:386–394.

184. Ringel Y, Whitehead WE, Toner BB, Diamant NE, Hu Y, Jia H, Bangdiwala SI, Drossman DA. Sexual and Physical Abuse are Not Associated with Rectal Hypersensitivity in Patients with Irritable Bowel Syndrome. Gut 2004;53:838–842.

185. Whitehead WE, Palsson OS. Is rectal pain sensitivity a biological marker for irritable bowel syndrome: psychological influences on pain perception. Gastroenterology 1998;115:1263–1271.

186. Linton SJ. A prospective study of the effects of sexual or physical abuse on back pain. Pain 2002;96:347–351.

187. Kendall-Tackett KA. Physiological correlates of childhood abuse: Chronic hyperarousal in PTSD, depression, and irritable bowel syndrome. Child Abuse Neglect 2000;24:799–810.

188. Ringel Y, Drossman DA, Turkington TG, Hawk TC, Bradshaw B, Coleman RE, Whitehead WE. Regional Brain Activation in Response to Rectal Distention in Patients with Irritable Bowel Syndrome and the Effect of a History of Abuse. Dig Dis Sci 2003;48:1774–1781.

189. Von Korff M, Moore JC. Stepped care for back pain: activating approaches for primary care. Ann Intern Med 2001;134:911–917.

190. Gelenberg A. Depression is still underrecognized and undertreated.[comment]. Arch Intern Med 1999;159:1657–1658.

191. Bjelland I, Dahl AA, Haug TT, Neckelmann D. The validity of the Hospital Anxiety and Depression Scale. An updated literature review. J Psychosom Res 2002;52:69–77.

192. Zigmond AS, Snaith RP. The Hospital Anxiety and Depression Scale. Acta Psychiatr Scand 1983;67:361–370.

193. Spitzer RL, Williams JB, Kroenke K, Linzer M, deGruy FV, III, Hahn SR, Brody D, Johnson JG. Utility of a new procedure for diagnosing mental disorders in primary care. The PRIME-MD 1000 study. JAMA 1994;272:1749–1756.

194. Keefe FJ, Brown GK, Wallston KA, Caldwell DS. Coping with rheumatoid arthritis pain: catastrophizing as a maladaptive strategy. Pain 1989;37:51–56.

195. Labus JS, Bolus R, Chang L, Wiklund I, Naesdal J, Mayer EA, et al. The Visceral Sensitivity Index: development and validation of a gastrointestinal symptom-specific anxiety scale. Aliment Pharmacol Ther 2004;20:89–97.

196. Patrick DL, Drossman DA, Frederick IO, DiCesare J, Puder KL. Quality of life in persons with irritable bowel syndrome: Development of a new measure. Dig Dis Sci 1998;43:400–411.

197. Pincus T, Callahan LF, Bradley LA, Vaughn WK, Wolfe F. Elevated MMPI scores for hypochondriasis, depression, and hysteria in patients with rheumatoid arthritis reflect disease rather than psychological status. Arthritis Rheum 1986;29:1456–1466.

198. Lowe B, Grafe K, Kroenke K, Zipfel S, Quenter A, Wild B, Fiehn C, Herzog W. Predictors of psychiatric comorbidity in medical outpatients. Psychosom Med 2003;65:764–770.

199. Derogatis LR. SCL-90-R: Administration, Scoring, and Procedures Manual II—For the R (evised) Version. 1 ed. Towson: Clinical Psychometric Research, 1983.

200. Derogatis L, Spencer P. BSI manual I: Adminstration and procedures. Baltimore: John Hopkins University School of Medicine, Clinical Psychometirc Unit, 1983.

201. Kroenke K, Spitzer RL, Williams JB. The PHQ-15: validity of a new measure for evaluating the severity of somatic symptoms. Psychosom Med 2002;64:258–266.

202. Kroenke K, Spitzer RL, Williams JB, Linzer M, Hahn SR, deGruy FV, III, Brody D. Physical symptoms in primary care. Predictors of psychiatric disorders and functional impairment. Arch Fam Med1994;3:774–779.

203. Pilowsky I. Dimensions of hypochondriasis. Br J Psychiatry 1967;113:89–93.

204. Pilowsky I, Bassett D, Barrett R, Petrovic L, Minniti R. The Illness Behavior Assessment Schedule: reliability and validity. Int J Psychiatry Med 1983;13:11–28.

205. Speckens AE, Spinhoven P, Sloekers PP, Bolk JH, van Hemert AM. A validation study of the Whitely Index, the Illness Attitude Scales, and the Somatosensory Amplification Scale in general medical and general practice patients. J Psychosom Res 1996;40:95–104.

206. Toner BB, Stuckless N, Ali A, Downie FP, Emmott SD, Akman DE. The development of a cognitive scale for functional bowel disorders. Psychosom Med 1998;60:492–497.

207. Ware JE, Sherbourne CD. The MOS 36-item short form Health Survey (SF-36): I. Conceptual framework and item selection. Med Care 1992;30:473–483.

208. Eisen GM, Locke GR, Provenzale D. Health-related quality of life: A primer for gastroenterologists. Am J Gastroenterol 1999;94:2017–2021.

209. Whitehead WE, Burnett CK, Cook E, III, Taub E. Impact of irritable bowel syndrome on quality of life. Dig Dis Sci 1996;41:2248–2253.

210. Hahn BA, Kirchdoerfer LJ, Fullerton S, Mayer E. Patient-perceived severity of irritable bowel syndrome in relation to symptoms, health resource utilization and quality of life. Aliment Pharmacol Ther 1997;11:553–559.

211. Bijkerk CJ, de Wit NJ, Muris JW, Jones RH, Knottnerus JA, Hoes AW. Outcome measures in irritable bowel syndrome: comparison of psychometric and methodological characteristics. Am J Gastroenterol 2003;98:122–127.

212. Irvine EJ. Measuring quality of life: a review. Scand J Gastroenterol—Supplement 1996;221:5–7.

213. Drossman DA, Patrick DL, Whitehead WE, Toner BB, Diamant NE, Hu YJB, Jia H, Bangdiwala SI. Further validation of the IBS-QOL: A disease specific quality of life questionnaire. Am J Gastoenterology 2000;95:999–1007.

214. Chassany O, Marquis P, Scherrer B, Read NW, Finger T, Bergmann JF, Fraitag B, Geneve J, Caulin C. Validation of a specific quality of life questionnaire for functional digestive disorders. Gut 1999;44:527–533.

215. Talley NJ, Fullerton S, Junghard O, Wiklund I. Quality of life in patients with endoscopy-negative heartburn: Reliability and sensitivity of disease-specific in. Am J Gastroenterol 2001;96:1998–2004.

216. Sarason IG, Johnson JH, Siegel JM. Assessing the impact of life changes: development of the life experiences survey. J Consult Clin Psychol 1978;46:932–946.

217. Brown GW, Harris TO. Social origins of depression: A study of psychiatric disorder in women. London: Tavistock, 1978.

218. Kohn PM, Lafreniere K, Gurevich M. Hassles, health, and personality. J Pers Soc Psychol 1991;61:478–482.

219. Garrett VD, Brantley PJ, Jones GN, McKnight GT. The relation between daily stress and crohn's disease. J Behav Med 1991;14:87.

220. Jenkins CD, Hurst MW, Rose RM. Life changes: Do people really remember? Arch Gen Psychiatry 1979;36:379–384.

221. Klein DN, Rubovits DR. The reliability of subjects' reports on stressful life events inventories: a longitudinal study. J Behav Med 1987;10:501–512.

222. Friedman S. On the "true-false" memory syndrome: the problem of clinical evidence. Am J Psychother 1997;51:102–122.

223. Talley NJ, Owen B, Bai J, Boyce P. Does psychological distress account for the apparent association between abuse and irritable bowel syndrome? A population-based study. Gastroenterology 110, A767. 1995.

224. Leserman J, Li Z, Drossman DA, Toomey TC, Nachman G, Glogau L. Impact of sexual and physical abuse dimensions on health status: Development of an abuse severity measure. Psychosom Med 1997;59:152–160.

225. American Psychiatric Association. Diagnostic and Statistical Manual of Mental Disorders—DSM-IV. 4 ed. Washington, D.C.: American Psychiatric Association, 1994.

226. Helzer JE, Robins LN. The diagnostic interview schedule: its development, evolution, and use. Soc Psychiatry Psychiatr Epidemiol 1988;23:6–16.

227. Spitzer RL, Williams JBW, Gibbon M, First MB. The Structured Clinical Interview for DSM-III-R (SCID). I: History, Rationale, and Description. Arch Gen Psychiatry 1992;49:624–629.

228. First M.B., Spitzer R.L., Gibbon M, Williams J.B.W. User's guide for the Structured Clinical Interview for DSM-IV Axis I Disorders: SCID-I clinican version. Washington DC: American Psychioatric Press, 1997.

229. Wittchen HU. Reliability and validity studies of the WHO—Composite International Diagnostic Interview (CIDI): a critical review. J Psychiatr Res 1994;28:57–84.

230. Andrews G, Peters L, Guzman AM, Bird K. A comparison of two structured diagnostic interviews: CIDI and SCAN. Aust N Z J Psychiatry 1995;29:124–132.

231. Guthrie E, Creed FH. Severe sexual dysfunctioning in women with IBS: comparison with IBD and duodenal ulceration. Br Med J 1987;2:577–578.

232. Hurwicz ML, Berkanovic E. The stress process in rheumatoid arthritis. J Rheumatol 1993;20:1836–1844.

233. Ong LM, de Haes JC, Hoos AM, Lammes FB. Doctor-patient communication: a review of the literature. Soc Sci Med 1995;40:903–918.

234. Brown JB, Boles M, Mullooly JP, Levinson W. Effect of clinician communication skills training on patient satisfaction. Ann Intern Med 1999;131:822–828.

235. Owens DM, Nelson DK, Talley NJ. The irritable bowel syndrome: Long term prognosis and the physician-patient interaction. Ann Intern Med 1995;122:107–112.

236. Rosenstiel AF, Keefe FJ. The use of coping strategies in chronic low back pain patients: relationship to patient characteristics and current adjustment. Pain 1983;17:33–40.

237. Little P, Everitt H, Williamson I, Warner G, Moore M, Gould C, Ferrier K, Payne S. Observational study of effect of patient centredness and positive approach on outcomes of general practice consultations. BMJ 2001;323:908–911.

238. Drossman DA. Psychosocial Sound Bites: Exercises in the patient-doctor relationship. Am J Gastroenterol 1997;92:1418–1423.

239. Von Korff M, Gruman J, Schaefer J. Collaborative management of chronic illness. Ann Intern Med 1997;127:1097–1102.

240. Barsky AJ. Hypochondriasis. Medical management and psychiatric treatment. Psychosomatics 1996;37:48–56.

241. Pilowsky I, Barrow CG. A controlled study of psychotherapy and amitriptyline used individually and in combination in the treatment of chronic intractable, 'psychogenic' pain. Pain 1990;40:3–19.

242. Keller MB, McCullough JP, Klein DN, Arnow B, Dunner DL, Gelenberg AJ, Markowitz JC, Nemeroff CB, Russell JM, Thase ME, Trivedi MH, Zajecka J. A comparison of nefazodone, the cognitive behavioral-analysis system of psychotherapy, and their combination for the treatment of chronic depression. N Engl J Med 2000;342:1462–1470.

243. Barlow DH, Gorman JM, Shear MK, Woods SW. Cognitive-behavioral therapy, imipramine, or their combination for panic disorder: A randomized controlled trial. JAMA 2000;283:2529–2536.

244. March J, Silva S, Petrycki S, Curry J, Wells K, Fairbank J, Burns B, Domino M, McNulty S, Vitiello B, Severe J, Treatment for Adolescents With Depression Study (TADS) Team. Fluoxetine, cognitive-behavioral therapy, and their combination for adolescents with depression: Treatment for Adolescents With Depression Study (TADS) randomized controlled trial. JAMA 2004;292:807–820.

245. Lackner JM. Psychological treatments for irritable bowel syndrome: a systematic review and meta-analysis. J Consult Clin Psychol 72, 1100–1113. 2004.

246. Soo S, Forman D, Delaney BC, Moayyedi P. A systemativ review of psychological therapies for nonulcer dyspepsia. Am J Gastroenterol 2004;99:1817–22.

247. Greenberger D. Mind over mood: A cognitive therapy treatment manual for clients. New York, NY, US: Guilford Press 215.

248. Toner BB. Cognitive-behavioral treatment of functional somatic syndromes: Integrating gender issues. Cogn Behav Pract 1994;1:157–178.

249. Toner BB, Segal ZV, Emmott S, Myran D, Ali A, DiGasbarro I, Stuckless N. Cognitive behavior group therapy for patients with irritable bowel syndrome. Int J Group Psychother 1998;48:215–243.

250. Payne A, Blanchard EB. A controlled comparison of cognitive therapy and self-help support groups in the treatment of irritable bowel syndrome. J Consult Clin Psychol 1995;63:779–786.

251. Greene B, Blanchard EB. Cognitive therapy for irritable bowel syndrome. J Consult Clin Psychol 1994;62:576–582.

252. Toner BB, Segal ZV, Emmott SD, Myran D. Cognitive-behavioral treatment of irritable bowel syndrome: The brain-gut connection. London/New York: Guilford Press, 2000.

253. Pilowsky IS. Manual for the Illness Behavior Questionnaire (IBQ), 2nd ed. Adelaide: University of Adelaide Press, 1983.

254. Weydert JA, Ball TM, Davis MF. Systematic review of treatments for recurrent abdominal pain. Pediatrics 2003;111:e1–11.

255. Blanchard EB, Greene B, Scharff L, Schwarz-McMorris SP. Relaxation training as a treatment for irritable bowel syndrome. Biofeedback Self Reg 1993;18:125–132.

256. Bernstein DA, Borkovec TD. Progressive relaxation training. Champaign: Champaign Illinois Research Press, 1973.

257. Blanchard EB, Schwarz SP, Suls JM, Gerardi MA, Scharff L, Greene B, Taylor AE, Berreman C, Malamood HS. Two controlled evaluations of multicomponent psychological treatment of irritable bowel syndrome. Behav Res Ther 1992;30:175–189.

258. Benson H. The relaxation response. 1 ed. New York: William Morrow, 1975.

259. Voirol MW, Hipolito J. Anthropo-analytical relaxation in irritable bowel syndrome: results 40 months later. Schweiz Med Wochenschr 1987;117:1117–1119.

260. Arn I, Theorell T, Uvnas-Moberg K, Jonsson C-O. Psychodrama group therapy for patients with functional gastrointestinal disorders. Psychother Psychosom 1989;51: 113–119.

261. Heymann-Mönnikes I, Arnold R, Florin I, Herda C, Melfsen S, Mönnikes H. The combination of medical treatment plus multicomponent behavioral therapy is superior to medical treatment alone in the therapy of irritable bowel syndrome. Am J G astroenterol 2000;95:981–994.

262. Boyce PM, Talley NJ, Balaam B, Koloski NA, Truman G. A randomized controlled trial of cognitive behavior therapy, relaxation training, and routine clinical care for the irritable bowel syndrome. Am J Gastroenterol 2003;98:2209–2218.

263. Guthrie E, Creed F, Dawson D, Tomenson B. A randomised controlled trial of psychotherapy in patients with refractory irritable bowel syndrome. Br J Psychiatry 1993;163:315–321.

264. Klerman GL, Weissman MM, Rounsaville BJ, Chevron ES. Interpersonal Psychotherapy of Depression. New York, NY: Basic Book Inc. Publishers, 1984.

265. Poitras M, Verrier P, So C, Paquet S, Bouin M, Poitras P. Group counseling psy-

chotherapy for patients with functional gastrointestinal disorders Development of new measures for symptom severity and quality of life. Dig Dis Sci 2002;47:1297–1307.

266. Svedlund J, Sjodin I, Ottosson JO, Dotevall G. Controlled study of psychotherapy in irritable bowel syndrome. Lancet 1983;2:589–591.

267. Guthrie E, Creed F, Dawson D, Tomenson B. A controlled trial of psychological treatment for the irritable bowel syndrome. Gastroenterology 1991;100:450–457.

268. Hamilton J, Guthrie E, Creed F, Thompson D, Tomenson B, Bennet R, Moriary K, Stephens W, Liston R. A randomized controlled trial of psychotherapy in patients with chronic functional dyspepsia. Gastroenterology 2000;119:661–669.

269. Svedlund J. Psychotherapy in irritable bowel syndrome: A controlled outcome study. Acta Psychiatr Scand 1983;67, Suppl 306:1–86.

270. Talley NJ, Owen BK, Boyce P, Paterson K. Psychological treatments for irritable bowel syndrome: A critique of controlled treatment trials. Am J Gastroenterol 1996; 91:277–286.

271. Spanier JA, Howden CW, Jones MP. A systematic review of alternative therapies in the irritable bowel syndrome. Arch Intern Med 2003;163:265–274.

272. Creed F, Guthrie E, Ratcliffe J, Fernandes L, Rigby C, Tomenson B, Read N, Thompson DG. Reported sexual abuse predicts impaired functioning but a good response to psychological treatments in patients with severe irritable bowel syndrome. Psychosom Med 2005;67:490–499.

273. Poitras P, Riberdy PM, Plourde V, Boivin M, Verrier P. Evolution of visceral sensitivity in patients with irritable bowel syndrome. Dig Dis Sci 2002;47:914–920.

274. Whorwell PJ, Prior A, Faragher EB. Controlled trial of hypnotherapy in the treatment of severe refractory irritable bowel syndrome. Lancet 1984;2:1232–1233.

275. Harvey RF, Hinton RA, Gunary RM, Barry RE. Individual and group hypnotherapy in treatment of refractory irritable bowel syndrome. Lancet 1989;1:424–425.

276. Calvert EL, Houghton LA, Cooper P, Morris J, Whorwell PJ. Long-term improvement in functional dyspepsia using hypnotherapy. Gastroenterology 2002;123:1778–1785.

277. Forbes A, MacAuley S, Chiotakakou-Faliakou E. Hypnotherapy and therapeutic audiotape: effective in previously unsuccessfully treated irritable bowel syndrome? Int J Colorectal Dis 2000;15:328–334.

278. Galovski TE, Blanchard EB. The treatment of irritable bowel syndrome with hypnotherapy. Applied Psychophysiology and Biofeedback 1998;23:219–232.

279. Gonsalkorale WM, Houghton LA, Whorwell PJ. Hypnotherapy in irritable bowel syndrome: A large-scale audit of a clinical service with examination of factors influencing responsiveness. Am J Gastroenterol 2002;97:954–961.

280. Whorwell PJ, Prior A, Colgan SM. Hypnotherapy in severe irritable bowel syndrome: further experience. Gut 1987;28:423–425.

281. Gonsalkorale WM, Miller V, Afzal A, Whorwell PJ. Long term benefits of hypnotherapy for irritable bowel syndrome. Gut 2003;52:1623–1629.

282. Lea R, Houghton LA, Calvert EL, Larder S, Gonsalkorale WM, Whelan V, Randles J, Cooper P, Cruickshanks P, Miller V, Whorwell PJ. Gut-focused hypnotherapy normalizes disordered rectal sensitivity in patients with irritable bowel syndrome. Aliment Pharmacol Ther 2003;17:635–642.

283. Palsson OS, Turner MJ, Johnson DA, Burnelt CK, Whitehead WE. Hypnosis treat-

ment for severe irritable bowel syndrome: investigation of mechanism and effects on symptoms. Dig Dis Sci 2002;47:2605–2614.

284. Gonsalkorale WM, Toner BB, Whorwell PJ. Cognitive change in patients undergoing hypnotherapy for irritable bowel syndrome. J Psychosom Res 2004;56:271–278.

285. Gruber AJ, Hudson JI, Pope HG, Jr. The management of treatment-resistant depression in disorders on the interface of psychiatry and medicine. Fibromyalgia, chronic fatigue syndrome, migraine, irritable bowel syndrome, atypical facial pain, and premenstrual dysphoric disorder. Psychiatr Clin North Am 1996;19:351–369.

286. Salerno SM, Browning R, Jackson JL. The effect of antidepressant treatment on chronic back pain: a meta-analysis. Arch Intern Med 2002;162:19–24.

287. O'Malley PG, Jackson JL, Santoro J, Tomkins G, Balden E, Kroenke K. Antidepressant therapy for unexplained symptoms and symptom syndromes. J Fam Pract 1999;48:980–990.

288. Lynch ME. Antidepressants as analgesics: a review of randomized controlled trials. J Psychiatry Neurosci 2001;26:30–36.

289. Onghena P, Houdenhove BV. Antidepressant-induced analgesia in chronic non-malignant pain: A meta-analysis of 39 placebo-controlled studies. Pain 1992;49:205–219.

290. Feinmann C. Pain relief by antidepressants: possible modes of action. Pain 1985; 23:1–8.

291. Su X, Gebhart GF. Effects of tricyclic antidepressants on mechanosensitive pelvic nerve afferent fibers innervating the rat colon. Pain 1998;76:105–114.

292. Singh VP, Jain NK, Kulkarni SK. On the antinociceptive effect of fluoxetine, a selective serotonin reuptake inhibitor. Brain Res 2001;915:218–226.

293. Tabas G, Beaves M, Wang J, Friday P, Mardini H, Arnold G. Paroxetine to treat irritable bowel syndrome not responding to high-fiber diet: a double-blind, placebo-controlled trial. Am J Gastroenterol 2004;99:914–920.

294. Peghini PL, Katz PO, Castell DO. Imipramine decreases oesophageal pain perception in human male volunteers. Gut 1998;42:807–813.

295. Gorelick AB, Koshy SS, Hooper FG, Bennett TC, Chey WD, Hasler WL. Differential effects of amitriptyline on perception of somatic and visceral stimulation in healthy humans. Am J Physiol 1998;275:G460–G466.

296. Arnold LM, Lu Y, Crofford LJ, Wohlreich M, Detke MJ, Iyengar S, Goldstein DJ. A double-blind, multicenter trial comparing duloxetine with placebo in the treatment of fibromyalgia patients with or without major depressive disorder. Arthritis Rheum 2004;50:2974–2984.

297. Brandt LJ, Bjorkman D, Fennerty MB, Locke GR, Olden K, Peterson W, Quigley E, Schoenfeld P, Schuster M, Talley N. Systematic review on the management of irritable bowel syndrome in North America. Am J Gastroenterol 2002;97:S7–S26.

298. Greenbaum DS, Mayle JE, Vanegeren LE, Jerome JA, Mayor JW, Greenbaum RB, Matson RW, Stein GE, Dean HA, Halvorsen NA, Rosen LW. The effects of desipramine on IBS compared with atropine and placebo. Dig Dis Sci 1987;32:257–266.

299. Jailwala J, Imperiale TF, Kroenke K. Pharmacologic treatment of the irritable bowel syndrome: A systematic review of randomized, controlled trials. Ann Intern Med 2000;133:136–147.

300. Jackson JL, O'Malley PG, Tomkins G, Balden E, Santoro J, Kroenke K. Treatment of functional gastrointestinal disorders with antidepressant medications: a meta-analysis. Am J Med 2000;108:65–72.

301. Tabas G, Beaves M, Wang J, Friday P, Mardini H, Arnold G. Paroxetine to treat ir-

ritable bowel syndrome not responding to high-fiber diet: a double-blind, placebo-controlled trial. Am J Gastroenterol 2004;99:914–920.

302. Brown WA, Harrison W. Are patients who are intolerant to one serotonin selective reuptake inhibitor intolerant to another? J Clin Psychiatry 1995;56:30–34.

303. Nemeroff CB, Heim CM, Thase ME, Klein DN, Rush AJ, Schatzberg AF, Ninan PT, McCullough JP, Jr., Weiss PM, Dunner DL, Rothbaum BO, Kornstein S, Keitner G, Keller MB. Differential responses to psychotherapy versus pharmacotherapy in patients with chronic forms of major depression and childhood trauma. Proc Natl Acad Sci U S A 2003;100:14293–14296.

304. Hahn BA, Kirchdoerfer LJ, Fullerton S, Mayer E. Evaluation of a new quality of life questionnaire for patients with irritable bowel syndrome. Aliment Pharmacol Ther 1997;11:547–52.

305. Noyes RJr, Cook B, Garvey M, Summers R. Reduction of gastrointestinal symptoms following treatment for panic disorder. Psychosomatics 1990;31:75–79.

306. Blier P, Bergeron R, DeMontigny C. Selective activation of postsynaptic 5-HT1a receptors produces a rapid antidepressant response. Neuropsychopharm 1997;16:333–338.

307. Covington EC. Anticonvulsants for neuropathic pain and detoxification. Cleve Clin J Med 1998;65 Suppl 1:SI21–SI29.

308. Turk DC. Clinical effectiveness and cost-effectiveness of treatments for patients with chronic pain. Clin J Pain 2002;18:355–365.

309. Guthrie E, Thompson D. Abdominal pain and functional gastrointestinal disorders. BMJ 2002;325:701–703.

310. Spanier JA, Howden CW, Jones MP. A systematic review of alternative therapies in the irritable bowel syndrome. Arch Intern Med 2003;163:265–274.

311. Scarinci IC, Haile JM, Bradley LA, Schan CA, Richter JE. Pain perception and psychosocial correlates of sexual/physical abuse among patients with gastrointestinal disorders. Gastroenterology 102, A509. 1992.

312. MacDonald AJ, Bouchier IAD. Non-organic gastrointestinal illness: A medical and psychiatric study. Br J Psychiatry 1980;136:276–283.

313. Corney RH, Stanton R. Physical symptom severity, psychological and social dysfunction in a series of outpatients with irritable bowel syndrome. J Psychosom Res 1990;34:483–491.

314. Craig TKJ, Brown GW. Goal frustration and life events in the aetiology of painful gastrointestinal disorder. J Psychosom Res 1984;28:411–421.

315. Ford MJ, Miller PM, Eastwood J, Eastwood MA. Life events, psychiatric illness and the irritable bowel syndrome. Gut 1987;28:160–165.

316. Toner BB, Garfinkel PE, Jeejeebhoy KN. Psychological factors in irritable bowel syndrome. Can J Psychiatry 1990;35:158–161.

317. Blanchard EB, Scharff L, Schwartz SP, Suls JM, Barlow DH. The role of anxiety and depression in the irritable bowel syndrome. Behav Res Ther 1990;28:401–405.

318. Heaton KW, Ghosh S, Braddon FEM. How bad are the symptoms and bowel dysfunction of patients with the irritable bowel syndrome? a prospective, controlled study with emphasis on stool form. Gut 1991;32:73–79.

319. Kettell J, Jones R, Lydeard S. Reasons for consultation in irritable bowel syndrome: symptoms and patient characteristics. Br J Gen Pract 1992;42:459–461.

320. Talley NJ, Zinsmeister AR, Van Dyke C, Melton III LJ. Epidemiology of colonic symptoms and the irritable bowel syndrome. Gastroenterology 1991;101:927–934.

321. van der Horst HE, Van Dulmen AM, Schellevis FG, van Eijk JT, Fennis JF, Bleijenberg G. Do patients with irritable bowel syndrome in primary care really differ from outpatients with irritable bowel syndrome? Gut 1997;41:669–674.

322. Koloski NA, Talley NJ, Boyce PM. Does psychological distress modulate functional gastrointestinal symptoms and health care seeking? A prospective, community Cohort study. Am J Gastroenterol 2003;98:789–797.

323. Labus JS, Bolus R, Chang L, Wiklund I, Naesdal J, Mayer EA, Naliboff BD. The Visceral Sensitivity Index: development and validation of a gastrointestinal symptom-specific anxiety scale. Aliment Pharacol Ther 2004;20:89–97.

324. McCracken LM, Zayfert C, Gross RT. The Pain Anxiety Symptoms Scale: development and validation of a scale to measure fear of pain. Pain 1992;50:67–73.

325. McNeil DW, Rainwater AJ 3rd. Development of the Fear of Pain Questionnaire—III. J Behav Med 1998;21:389–410.

326. Kanner AD, Coyne JC, Schaefer C, Lazarus RS. Comparison of two modes of stress measurement: daily hassles and uplifts versus major life events. J Behav Med 1981;4:1–39.

327. Brantley PJ, Waggoner CD, Jones GN, Rappaport NBA. Daily Stress Inventory: development, reliability, and validity. J Behav Med 1987;10:61–74.

328. Holmes TH, Rahe RH. The social readjustment rating scale. J Psychosomatic Research 1967;11:213–218.

Chapter 7

Functional
Esophageal
Disorders

Jean Paul Galmiche, Chair

Ray E. Clouse, Co-Chair

András Bálint

Ian J. Cook

Peter J. Kahrilas

William G. Paterson

André J.P.M. Smout

Introduction

Functional esophageal disorders are represented by chronic symptoms typifying esophageal disease that have no readily identified structural or metabolic basis (Table 1). These disorders are most commonly encountered in adults and collectively represent a major strain on health care resources. Similar to functional gastrointestinal disorders (FGIDs) in other anatomical regions, the symptoms of the individual esophageal disorders often overlap and are frequently associated with psychosocial factors that contribute to the clinical presentation. The physiological mechanisms responsible for these disorders remain poorly understood. (A diagram of the esophagus is shown in Figure 1). Combinations of physiological and psychosocial factors likely escalate the symptoms to a level requiring medical attention; most available information arises from studies of patients who have sought medical care. Consequently, basic mechanisms responsible for symptoms remain poorly understood in all the functional esophageal disorders.

The symptom overlap in patients presenting with the functional symptoms of heartburn, chest pain, dysphagia, and globus in conjunction with the observation that each can be produced by specific distal esophageal diseases [e.g., gastroesophageal reflux disease (GERD)] suggest that these syndromes may not in fact be independent functional disorders. However, the disorders and their criteria remain separate since distinctions appear relevant for the exclusion of struc-

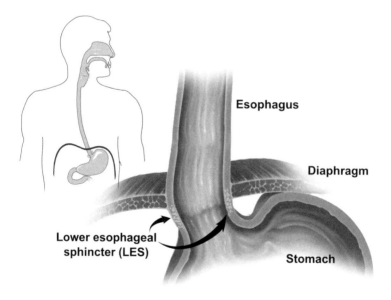

Figure 1. Structure of the esophagus showing the location of the lower esophageal sphincter relative to the stomach and diaphragm.

Table I. Functional Gastrointestinal Disorders

A. Functional Esophageal Disorders

A1. Functional heartburn
A2. Functional chest pain of presumed esophageal origin
A3. Functional dysphagia
A4. Globus

B. Functional Gastroduodenal Disorders

B1. Functional dyspepsia
   B1a. Postprandial distress syndrome (PDS)
   B1b. Epigastric pain syndrome (EPS)
B2. Belching disorders
   B2a. Aerophagia
   B2b. Unspecified excessive belching
B3. Nausea and vomiting disorders
   B3a. Chronic idiopathic nausea (CIN)
   B3b. Functional vomiting
   B3c. Cyclic vomiting syndrome (CVS)
B4. Rumination syndrome in adults

C. Functional Bowel Disorders

C1. Irritable bowel syndrome (IBS)
C2. Functional bloating
C3. Functional constipation
C4. Functional diarrhea
C5. Unspecified functional bowel disorder

D. Functional Abdominal Pain Syndrome (FAPS)

E. Functional Gallbladder and Sphincter of Oddi (SO) Disorders

E1. Functional gallbladder disorder
E2. Functional biliary SO disorder
E3. Functional pancreatic SO disorder

F. Functional Anorectal Disorders

F1. Functional fecal incontinence
F2. Functional anorectal pain
   F2a. Chronic proctalgia
      F2a1. Levator ani syndrome
      F2a2. Unspecified functional anorectal pain
   F2b. Proctalgia fugax
F3. Functional defecation disorders
   F3a. Dyssynergic defecation
   F3b. Inadequate defecatory propulsion

G. Functional Disorders: Neonates and Toddlers

G1. Infant regurgitation
G2. Infant rumination syndrome
G3. Cyclic vomiting syndrome
G4. Infant colic
G5. Functional diarrhea
G6. Infant dyschezia
G7. Functional constipation

H. Functional Disorders: Children and Adolescents

H1. Vomiting and aerophagia
   H1a. Adolescent rumination syndrome
   H1b. Cyclic vomiting syndrome
   H1c. Aerophagia
H2. Abdominal pain-related FGIDs
   H2a. Functional dyspepsia
   H2b. Irritable bowel syndrome
   H2c. Abdominal migraine
H2d. Childhood functional abdominal pain
   H2d1. Childhood functional abdominal pain syndrome
H3. Constipation and incontinence
   H3a. Functional constipation
   H3b. Nonretentive fecal incontinence

tural diseases that might present with similar symptoms—cardiac disease, for example, in the case of chest pain, eosinophilic esophagitis in the case of dysphagia, and neck or pharyngeal diseases in the case of globus. In this third edition of the Rome Criteria, rumination syndrome, which has important distinctions from functional esophageal disorders, is now treated in another chapter. (See Chapter 8, "Functional Gastroduodenal Disorders.")

Several diagnostic requirements are uniform across the functional esophageal disorders:

1. Exclusion of structural or metabolic disorders that might be producing the symptoms is essential and is a principal criterion for all FGIDs [1]. Careful consideration and investigation of otolaryngological, pulmonary and cardiac causes may be needed. In the case of dysphagia, an exclusion of structural lesions is necessary.

2. A requirement of at least 3 months of symptoms with onset occurring at least 6 months before diagnosis is applied to each diagnosis to establish chronicity. Since evidence-based research supporting an adjustment in this time constraint is lacking, this criterion is arbitrary. However, in the case of the functional esophageal disorders, this limit decreases the risk of overlooking a structural lesion.

3. Gastroesophageal reflux disease (GERD) must be excluded as an explanation for symptoms.

4. Finally, the primary symptom source must not be indicative of motor disorders with known histopathological bases (e.g., achalasia, scleroderma esophagus).

The final two diagnostic requirements require a degree of definition, as both reflux and motor events are potential contributors to symptoms in several functional esophageal disorders. An important modification in threshold for the third uniform requirement has occurred in this re-evaluation of the functional esophageal disorders [1]. Satisfactory evidence of a symptom relationship with acid reflux events, either by analytical determination from an ambulatory pH study or through subjective outcome from therapeutic antireflux trials—even in the absence of objective GERD evidence—now is sufficient to indicate GERD (Figure 2). Indeed, recent studies using prolonged observation of symptoms, quality of life measures, and treatment requirements failed to clearly discriminate patients with reflux-related symptoms in the absence of excess acid exposure by pH monitoring from patients with more typical GERD, especially the endoscopy-negative subset [2, 3]. As a consequence, the so-called "acid-sensitive esophagus," previously classified within the functional domain, now is excluded from the group of functional esophageal disorders, even if some physiological data strongly suggest that

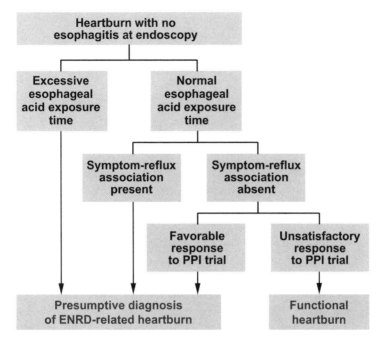

Figure 2. Further classification of patients with heartburn and no evidence of esophagitis at endoscopy using ambulatory pH monitoring and response to a therapeutic trial of proton pump inhibitors (PPI). The subset with functional heartburn has no findings that would support a presumptive diagnosis of endoscopy-negative reflux disease (ENRD). The precise thresholds for separation of subjects at each step remain uncertain. The figure demonstrates classification categories by findings and is not meant to suggest a diagnostic management algorithm for use in clinical practice.

hypersensitivity of the esophagus may encompass other stimuli than simply acid. In contrast to previous editions, the term "pathological gastroesophageal reflux" is no longer used to describe the clinical condition of patients with evidence of esophagitis or abnormal acid exposure time on an ambulatory pH study. The degree of investigation required for GERD exclusion (e.g., ambulatory pH monitoring, trial of acid suppression) is not specified in the criteria and may vary depending on the setting. This should be specified in research reports. The purpose of this modification is to preferentially diagnose GERD over a functional disorder in the initial evaluation so that effective GERD treatments are not overlooked in management. Presumably, symptoms that persist despite GERD interventions or that do not correlate with the GERD findings ultimately would be re-evaluated for a functional diagnosis. The role of weakly acidic reflux events (reflux events with pH values between 4 and 7) remains unclear, and technological advances (e.g., applications of multichannel intraluminal impedance monitoring) are expected to further define the small proportion of patients with functional heartburn truly meeting all stated criteria (see below).

Esophageal motor dysfunction of the type and severity found in histopathology-based disorders (e.g., achalasia, scleroderma involvement of the esophagus) remains an exclusionary criterion. In contrast, high-amplitude peristaltic contractions (e.g., nutcracker esophagus and other spastic disorders) do not preclude a functional diagnosis. The distinction is based on (a) observations that fail to establish a disease basis for this type of motor dysfunction, (b) the indirect relationship of motor events with symptoms in the average case, and (c) the unsatisfactory response to treatments directed solely at abnormal motility.

The criteria remain guidelines for the categorization and investigation of patients. Summary information for each disorder is discussed under the headings of epidemiology, diagnostic criteria and justification for changes, clinical evaluation, physiological features, psychological features, and treatment. With respect to epidemiology, prevalence rates of the functional esophageal disorders have not been well-documented in some cultures and regions, especially in the Asia-Pacific region, Africa, and South America. The information in this chapter should be of benefit to the investigator and clinician interested in the functional esophageal disorders, and hopefully will stimulate further investigations in this field and in a broad range of populations. Important focuses for future research work were identified by the subcommittee and are outlined in the final section of the chapter.

A1. Functional Heartburn

— Definition

Functional heartburn is defined as episodic retrosternal burning in the absence of GERD, histopathology-based motility disorders, or structural explanations. Symptoms related to acid reflux events in the absence of abnormal esophageal acid exposure [2, 4, 5] are now excluded from the diagnosis of functional heartburn (Figure 2). This diagnosis is constrained, however, by difficulties in the recognition of the symptom of heartburn, lack of specificity [6, 7] of therapeutic response to a short course of strong acid suppression with a proton pump inhibitor (PPI), and artifacts and errors associated with ambulatory pH monitoring [8,

9]. The fact that a majority of individuals who experience heartburn never seek medical attention nor require specific investigation limits our current knowledge of this quite heterogeneous and perhaps artificially chracterized entity. With the development of new technologies such as esophageal bilirubin monitoring (Bilitec) and multichannel intraluminal impedance monitoring, both acid and non-acid reflux episodes can be identified [9]. Altogether, these novel technologies may change our current classification of patients with esophageal symptoms and ultimately reduce the proportion of those with so-called "functional heartburn."

— Epidemiology

Twenty to forty percent of subjects in Western populations claim to suffer from heartburn, depending on the thresholds for a positive response [1, 10, 11]. Heartburn occurring at least once per week is reported by 15% to 20% of individuals irrespective of sex and age (in the range of 20–70 years). A minority of individuals with heartburn seek medical attention. Allowing for variations in the definition of heartburn, consultation rates are approximately 20%–40%. Consequently, most information about the relationship between heartburn and diagnostic tests of reflux is obtained from this minority. Additionally, a high proportion of patients with reflux symptoms continue prior treatment that may heal esophagitis before index evaluation. In a recent study by Martinez et al. [5], 71 of 149 consecutive patients seen for classic heartburn were found to have nonerosive disease at endoscopy. According to the respective values of esophageal acid exposure and symptom index (SI) determined during ambulatory pH monitoring, these patients were classified by esophageal acid exposure (above or below 4.2%) and SI (association of heartburn and acid reflux episodes $\geq$ 50% or <50%). In the final categorization, 7 and 12 patients with normal acid exposure had positive or negative symptom/reflux associations, respectively. Although that study did not further investigate the therapeutic response to acid suppression, it is assumed that those with normal acid exposure and poor association on the SI had "functional heartburn," according to our present definition. Considering potential caveats in any type of estimation, functional heartburn probably accounts for less than 10% of patients complaining of heartburn to gastroenterologists. However, the figure may be somewhat different in a primary care setting where the proportion of endoscopy-negative patients is higher and where anxiety, stress, and worry are among the most frequently reported aggravating factors in patients having symptoms suggestive of GERD [12].

AI. Diagnostic Criteria* for Functional Heartburn

Must include *all* of the following:
1. **Burning retrosternal discomfort or pain**
2. **Absence of evidence that gastroesophageal acid reflux is the cause of the symptom**
3. **Absence of histopathology-based esophageal motility disorders**

***Criteria fulfilled for the last 3 months with symptom onset at least 6 months prior to diagnosis**

— Justification for Change in Criteria

The threshold for the second criteria has been revised to exclude patients with normal esophageal acid exposure and acid-related symptom events on ambulatory pH monitoring (sometimes described in the literature as the acid-sensitive esophagus). These patients are now considered to be part of the GERD spectrum because of the difficulties in discriminating this group from GERD in terms of (a) initial clinical presentation, (b) manometric findings, (c) impact on quality of life, and (d) natural history. These subjects frequently respond, at least in the short term, to a course of PPI therapy, although higher daily doses may be necessary to alleviate symptoms [13]. Some subjects improve with antireflux surgery, although the outcomes in this group tend to be poorer than in patients having elevated preoperative acid exposure times [14] or erosive esophagitis [15].

— Clinical Evaluation

Clarification of the nature of the symptom is an essential first step. Heartburn is characterized by pain or discomfort of burning quality that originates high in the epigastrium with intermittent cephalad retrosternal radiation. The feeling may be associated with salivation, voluntary swallowing, and regurgitation of sour-tasting fluid. The symptom is often exacerbated by meals, certain foods, and postural changes. There are no evidence-based data to determine the specific symptom features of functional heartburn, including diurnal characteristics, exacerbating factors, and ameliorating maneuvers. The benefit of structured questionnaires to better identify and categorize patients suffering from heartburn in a primary care setting remains controversial [16].

Functional heartburn usually occurs during the day and, like the heartburn of GERD, may be elicited or exacerbated by certain foods and by lying down or bending over. However, it is difficult to extrapolate from data representing the whole "heartburn spectrum" to that of functional heartburn. Finally, and irrespective of the clinical setting (i.e., primary care or specialty practice), functional heartburn frequently occurs in association with symptoms usually considered components of the dyspeptic syndrome such as nausea, bloating, or early satiety [4, 12, 17]. In GERD, two or more days weekly of mild heartburn are sufficient to influence quality of life, but similar thresholds for symptom frequency or severity have not been determined for functional heartburn [18].

Little in the way of formal diagnostic work-up is required for heartburn subjects with episodic, short-lasting, typical symptoms that are responsive to antacids, alginates or a short course of PPI therapy. Patients with longer lasting, troublesome symptoms that have a limited response to medication require assessment, and the investigative sequence is straightforward [19, 20]. Clinical history, upper gastrointestinal endoscopy, and ambulatory esophageal pH monitoring with symptom analysis provide the most relevant information. However, endoscopy that reveals no evidence of esophagitis is insufficient, especially in those subjects who are evaluated while remaining on, or shortly after discontinuing, antireflux therapy. Ambulatory pH monitoring can better classify patients who have negative endoscopic evaluations, including those whose symptoms persist despite therapy. While the magnitude of acid exposure measured by ambulatory pH monitoring discriminates patients with erosive esophagitis from normal healthy individuals reasonably well, the diagnostic performance of the test is far less sound in endoscopy-negative patients [8]. A recent study using a pH probe with its tip located at the gastroesophageal junction suggested that the role of acid reflux may be underestimated, particularly for reflux events providing limited exposure to the very distal esophagus [21]. A careful analysis of the temporal relationship between symptom events and acid reflux episodes, conveniently expressed as an SI or even better as a Symptom Association Probability (SAP) [22], can increase the diagnostic yield of the examination, and is required to recognize subjects who have normal acid exposure yet have meaningful associations of reflux events with symptoms. In routine practice, it is likely that many investigators do not perform such statistical analyses.

Whether the GERD exclusionary criteria should also require negative outcome from a therapeutic trial with a PPI remains controversial. The PPI test, as initially described, consists of monitoring the symptomatic response to a PPI given in a large dose for a short period [23]. The test is considered positive when a 50% to 75% improvement in symptoms is observed. For practical reasons, this non-invasive approach usually is taken by general practitioners before performing pH monitoring or even endoscopy. Although a positive outcome from a trial with a PPI is not specific for the diagnosis of GERD [7], a lack of response probably has a high negative predictive value. However, it is now established that the proportion of nonresponders to a PPI is higher in nonerosive than in erosive GERD (For review see [24, 25]). Whether patients with normal endoscopy, a negative pH test (including symptom analysis), and no clear response to a short PPI course truly represent an entity distinct from GERD or overlap with a nonacid reflux group is unknown [26]. Recently developed investigations such as esophageal bilirubin monitoring (Bilitec) and impedance monitoring [27, 28] may help to clarify these issues and lead to reconsidering the definition of functional heartburn.

Finally, other esophageal (e.g., achalasia) and nonesophageal sources (e.g., coronary artery disease) should be considered and appropriately evaluated when atypical esophageal symptoms, unusual symptom characteristics (e.g., exercise exacerbations), or a paucity of typical characteristics are present.

— Physiological Features

Although, by definition GERD is excluded, reflux of gastric material into the esophagus may still play a role in the genesis of functional heartburn (Figure 3). Furthermore it should be remembered that the threshold of pH 4 used for the detection of acid reflux during pH monitoring, even if clinically and therapeutically relevant, is an arbitrary choice with no true physiological basis. For example, a recent working team report proposed new definitions of acid reflux including weakly acid and weakly alkaline reflux episodes [9]. Further investigation is needed to determine if these mechanisms are involved in patients with functional heartburn.

The prevailing view is to consider visceral perception as a major factor involved in the pathogenesis of functional disorders in general, including functional heartburn in particular. Indeed, several pieces of evidence suggest some degree of hypersensitivity to one or several intraluminal stimuli, including chemical and mechanical stimuli. For example, Rodriguez-Stanley et al., [29] showed that approximately 30% of individuals chronically using antacids for heartburn had esophageal sensitivity to mechanical (balloon distention) or chemical stimuli (Bernstein test). Approximately half of the individuals with normal esophageal acid exposure perceived balloon distension as painful. Similar data have been reported by others (for review see [30]) suggesting that some patients with typical heartburn have a low threshold for esophageal sensation and pain. Interestingly, in the study of Martinez et al. [5], patients in the endoscopy-negative group with normal acid exposure and a negative SI reported having heartburn at pH<4 only 12.7% of the time compared to 70.7% of the time in those with a positive SI. In contrast, the percentages of heartburn complaints that occurred at pH>6 were 42.2% in the former group versus 12.9% in the latter. Therefore, among patients with classic heartburn symptoms, normal endoscopy, and no increased acid exposure, the reflux characteristics

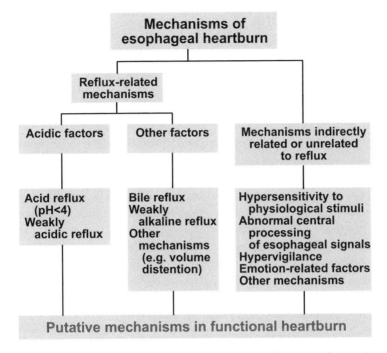

Figure 3. Reflux-related and unrelated factors involved in the pathogenesis of heartburn with particular attention to putative mechanisms for functional heartburn.

associated with symptom occurrence suggest a heterogeneous group of esophageal disorders.

Different factors may affect the perception of an esophageal stimulus either at the central or peripheral levels. For example, duodenal fat infusion has been shown to reduce the latency for onset and increase the intensity of acid-induced heartburn [31].The summation of short-lasting or weakly-acidic reflux episodes also may trigger the perception of esophageal pain, including heartburn sensation when a certain "acid burden" has been reached. Functional imaging techniques [32] promise to provide insights into the role that cognitive and emotional factors could play in modulating the brain processing of esophageal sensations. Using functional magnetic resonance imaging analysis of simultaneous phasic visual and esophageal nonpainful balloon distension stimuli, Gregory et al. [33] recently provided evidence that cognitive factors such as attention can influence the cerebral processing of visceral sensation in healthy volunteers. Neuroimaging will likely prove useful in studying all patients with FGIDs.

— Psychological Features

Psychological determinants have been reported in several studies of reflux symptoms. For example, a recent survey conducted in Hong Kong [34] showed that patients with symptoms of reflux had higher anxiety and depression scores than those without. However, these scores were not significantly different between consulters and non-consulters. Certainly, psychological factors may influence symptom perception in functional heartburn patients, as they do in other functional and organic GI disorders. Acute experimental stress has been reported to enhance perception of esophageal acid in GERD patients, without promoting increased reflux [35, 36, 37]. This enhanced perception appears to be influenced by the patient's underlying psychological status [36]. Some studies comparing endoscopy-negative heartburn patients with abnormal esophageal acid exposure on ambulatory pH recordings to heartburn patients with a normal pH study have failed to demonstrate differences in psychological profiles [38, 39]. However, Johnston et al. [40] reported that patients with heartburn that did not correlate well with acid reflux events on pH monitoring displayed higher anxiety and hysteria scores as well as lower social support structures than patients whose heartburn episodes correlated with acid reflux events.

— Treatment

Based on current evidence, empirical acid suppressant therapy for all patients with heartburn and no alarm symptoms seems reasonable [19, 25]. Acid suppression with a PPI or H_2 receptor antagonist has unequivocal benefit in patients with reflux esophagitis, endoscopy-negative heartburn but abnormal acid exposure on ambulatory pH recording, and endoscopy-negative patients with normal acid exposure but a positive symptom association [13, 41, 42]. Unfortunately, it appears that as a group, functional heartburn patients will not respond to acid suppression [13], because in most of these patients acid reflux is not the cause of the symptoms. Indeed, the diagnosis of functional heartburn usually is first considered when a patient with heartburn fails to improve on PPI therapy. However, some of these patients may be sensitive to small amounts of acid or acidic fluid with a pH>4 [5, 30]. Therefore a trial of more vigorous acid suppressant therapy should be considered.

Treatment of functional heartburn patients who have failed to respond to twice-daily PPI therapy is problematic, and at present is largely empirical. Because the pathophysiology may be similar to noncardiac chest pain and involve heightened visceral sensation, use of low dose tricyclic antidepressants and possibly selective serotonin reuptake inhibitors is reasonable. Similarly, psychological approaches such as behavioral modification or relaxation therapy [37] may be beneficial. However, to date no published controlled trials demonstrate efficacy of any of these interventions in functional heartburn patients.

Newer techniques (e.g., intraluminal impedance and bilirubin recording) are emerging to define the role of non-acid reflux events in these patients [28, 43]. If such non-acid reflux events are convincingly demonstrated as a cause of symptoms in functional heartburn patients, then therapy directed at reducing reflux events, rather than acid suppression, would be appropriate. In a recent open labeled study, Koek et al. [44] reported that the GABA(B) agonist baclofen normalized esophageal bilirubin exposure and improved symptoms in a group of patients with persisting reflux symptoms and abnormal bile reflux while on PPI therapy. This drug has been shown to decrease reflux events by inhibiting transient lower esophageal sphincter relaxations [45–47]. Antireflux surgery in patients with functional heartburn and non-acid reflux events has not been fully evaluated, but surgical management would not be expected to be as beneficial as in GERD.

A2. Functional Chest Pain of Presumed Esophageal Origin

— Definition

Functional chest pain of presumed esophageal origin is characterized by episodes of unexplained midline chest pain of visceral quality, and therefore potentially of esophageal origin. The pain easily is confused with cardiac angina or pain from other esophageal disorders including achalasia and GERD. Exclusion of these esophageal and non-esophageal disorders is required to establish the diagnosis.

— Epidemiology

The prevalence of functional chest pain of presumed esophageal origin is not known precisely. However, inferential data suggest that this is a common disorder. Between 15% and 30% of coronary angiograms performed in chest pain patients are normal and coronary spasm rarely explains the symptom [48]. An exclusionary criterion subsequently is detected in no more than a third of patients with negative cardiac evaluations [49]. Considering that at least 500,000 coronary angiograms are performed in the United States yearly for chest pain of recent onset, a functional disorder may be present in 75,000 to 150,000 per year. However, these figures underestimate the total number of subjects with a functional disorder because many patients under 40 years of age do not undergo cardiac catheterization.

Although once considered most common in elderly women, chest pain without specific diagnosis was reported in a household survey twice as commonly by subjects 15–34 years of age than by subjects more than 45 years old with equal gender representation [50]. Using survey responses to estimate rates of functional chest pain and other functional esophageal disorders, however, is confounded by the fact that the diagnoses depend heavily on medical exclusionary criteria. Patients with functional chest pain of presumed esophageal origin have a favorable prognosis from the standpoint of morbid cardiac events—very low rates of myocardial infarction and death from cardiac causes (less than 1% for each) are found over 10 years of observation once the diagnosis is established [51–55].

A2. Diagnostic Criteria* for Functional Chest Pain of Presumed Esophageal Origin

Must include *all* of the following:
1. **Midline chest pain or discomfort that is not of burning quality**
2. **Absence of evidence that gastroesophageal reflux is the cause of the symptom**
3. **Absence of histopathology-based esophageal motility disorders**

*Criteria fulfilled for the last 3 months with symptom onset at least 6 months prior to diagnosis

— Justification for Change in Criteria

As for other functional esophageal disorders, pain episodes linked to reflux events are now considered to fall within the spectrum of symptomatic GERD. It is widely recognized that a subset of patients with GERD experience acid reflux events as angina-like chest pain rather than as heartburn or odynophagia. The relationship between chest pain episodes and acid reflux events in an individual patient can be assessed by ambulatory pH monitoring with symptom analysis. Several studies have shown that a positive relationship between symptoms and acid reflux can occur in the absence of abnormal acid exposure [22]. The committee felt therefore that patients with a positive reflux-pain association should be excluded from the diagnosis of functional chest pain, irrespective of the presence or absence of abnormal acid exposure. This criteria change is analogous to the change in the criteria for functional heartburn.

— Clinical Evaluation

In the case of functional chest pain, exclusion of cardiac diseases is of pivotal importance. The history and clinical presentation are inaccurate in predicting the presence of coronary artery disease [56] and the extent of the investigations typically is determined by the patient's age, family history and risk factors. Self-attribution of chest pain to the heart differs by race: African American patients with chest pain are more likely to attribute their symptoms to a gastrointestinal source than white patients [57]. In most cases an exercise electrocardiogram with or without a Thallium scan will be included in the work-up. Older patients frequently will undergo coronary angiography. Some patients with cardiac disease have pain that is poorly explained by the cardiac findings [58], but making a concurrent diagnosis of functional chest pain requires extremely careful consideration. The diagnosis of "microvascular angina", characterized by small vessel coronary artery disease and increased coronary artery resistance, is no longer considered a tenable explanation for chest pain in patients without other cardiac findings [59, 60].

After the exclusion of cardiac disease, identifying GERD as the cause of the symptoms is of primary importance, because this disease is easily treated. On average, endoscopy is abnormal in less than 20% of patients [61–63], and esophagitis provides only inferential evidence that reflux disease is the cause of pain. Other studies can better define the relationship of reflux events to pain. The acid perfusion (Bernstein) test has been popular but is insensitive compared to ambulatory pH monitoring. For example, in a study in 75 patients with noncardiac chest pain who underwent an acid perfusion test and experienced chest pain during ambulatory monitoring, the acid perfusion test was found to be specific (90%), but poorly sensitive (36%) for acid-related pain using the ambulatory study as the standard [64]. Moreover, even the specificity of the Bernstein test has not been confirmed in other studies [65, 66]. Indeed, these authors found that only a minority of patients with noncardiac chest pain whose symptoms were reproduced with acid perfusion had good correlation between spontaneous pain episodes and acid reflux events during ambulatory pH/motility recording. Ambulatory pH monitoring with numerical analysis of the relationship between symptoms and reflux (SI or SAP testing) is the most sensitive test for identifying acid reflux as the likely cause of chest pain [4, 67, 68]. This test also helps to identify acid-related pain in the subset of patients without abnormal acid exposure [4, 68]. When combining subjects with and without abnormal acid exposure, 40% of patients with normal coronary angiograms may have acid-related pain [56, 64–66, 69–78]. Treadmill testing during ambulatory pH monitoring may be further revealing if the pain is associated with exertion [78].

Symptom relief during antireflux therapy with a PPI may be the ultimate method of proving a clinically relevant association of reflux and chest pain. For this reason a therapeutic trial with a PPI has also been proposed for chest pain evaluation (e.g., omeprazole of 40–80 mg daily or equivalent). Studies on the clinical value of such a trial in chest pain subjects have mainly focused on cost-effectiveness [79–81]. The specificity and sensitivity for acid-induced chest pain have not yet been determined adequately. There is a statistically significant relationship between esophageal acid exposure, as measured by ambulatory pH monitoring, and the response to a brief PPI trial [82]. Primary treatment strategies are more cost effective than test-and-treat approaches in excluding GERD considering all who are referred for gastroenterological evaluation of otherwise unexplained chest pain [80].

Other diagnostic tests rarely provide results that exclude the diagnosis of functional chest pain. Conventional manometric testing of the esophagus has a low yield for significant motor disorders that mandate specific intervention [83]. Ambulatory esophageal pressure monitoring, acid perfusion test (Bernstein test), and balloon distention studies may support that the symptoms are of esophageal origin rather than the heart and may thus provide reassurance [84]. However, since such tests have little effect on diagnosis or treatment they are described in the following section as physiological features of the disorder.

— Physiological Features

Abnormal responses to esophageal sensory stimuli and alterations in esophageal motor behavior are common in patients with functional chest pain. Historically, motility abnormalities were considered to be primary contributing factors. A shift in thinking has attributed greater pathophysiological relevance to sensory features, including central processing of afferent signals. Subjects with reflux esophagitis or elevations in acid exposure time demonstrated by pH monitoring typically have been excluded from mechanistic studies. In contrast, investigators seldom segregated subjects in whom chest pain can be reproduced with acid instillation from subjects who are insensitive to acid. Consequently, previous findings may not fully be applicable to functional chest pain as presently defined.

Sensory Findings

Richter et al. first demonstrated differences between patients with unexplained chest pain and asymptomatic control subjects in chest pain production with an intra-esophageal balloon distention stimulus [85]. Fifty percent of the patients, all of whom lacked overt evidence of reflux disease, developed pain at balloon volumes of 8 ml or less, while control subjects first reported pain only at greater volumes. Subsequent studies have shown that mechanosensitivity also predicts sensitivity to other provocative agents such as intraluminal acid, and some patients with symptomatic reflux disease may have been included in the studied group [86]. More recently, Rao et al. used impedance planimetry to study unexplained chest pain and monitored cross-sectional luminal area and balloon pressure rather than volume in relation to provoked discomfort or pain [87]. These authors demonstrated that chest pain patients could be completely segregated from control subjects by pressure thresholds. The studied subjects had no evidence of esophagitis at endoscopy and normal acid exposure time on ambulatory pH monitoring, but some subjects likely had acid sensitivity. Thus, balloon distention sensitivity is considered a shared feature of chest pain subjects with or without a relationship between acid sensitivity and symptoms who have no other evidence of reflux disease.

Interrelationships of balloon distention and acid sensitivity reveal the potential role of reflux events in the pathophysiological cascade. Acute acid instillation in the distal esophagus in normal subjects reduces sensation thresholds to a barostat-driven balloon distention stimulus [88]. Sarkar et al. demonstrated that distal acid instillation further reduces the threshold required for pain reproduction with esophageal electrical stimulation, another stimulus that is perceived at low stimulus intensity by chest pain patients [89]. Thus, acid appears to be a sensitizing factor in susceptible subjects and induces hypersensitivity to other esophageal stimuli (e.g., balloon distention and electrical stimulation) that characterize functional chest pain. The effect is not present in all subjects and cannot be generalized to reflux disease. Fass et al. did not find that tissue damage from chronic acid exposure induced mechanosensitivity and assumed that other susceptibility factors must be required [90].

Taken together, these observations help explain the high likelihood of detecting a reflux-symptom association during ambulatory pH monitoring in chest pain patients. On average, nearly 40% of subjects with unexplained chest pain and normal endoscopy will have reflux-related pain, a finding that is not restricted to the group with elevated acid exposure times [8]. Subjects with acid as the dominant factor responsible for mechanosensitivity or sensitivity to other provocative agents are now classified as having reflux disease as the principle underlying process; a therapeutic antireflux trial may be required for proof. In contrast, reflux does not appear to have this role in patients with functional chest pain, and distention stimuli assume primary importance in diagnosis.

How subjects with functional chest pain reach the hypersensitivity state is not clear. Intermittent stimulation by physiological acid reflux may be involved. Spontaneous distention events with swallowing or belching may also be relevant in this regard [91]. Dysfunction of the belch reflex with belching against a closed upper esophageal sphincter has been described in association with chest pain [92]. Recent data suggest that bolus entrapment in the proximal esophagus during repeated swallows in patients with unexplained esophageal symptoms and poor peristaltic inhibition produces segmental elevations in intra-bolus pressure that might serve as spontaneous pain stimuli [93]. Balloon distention sensitivity also serves as a marker for sensitivity to other provocative maneuvers that have been invoked in chest pain production, such as ingestion of hot and cold liquids or a solid food bolus, or those that reflect the hypersensitive state (e.g., infusion of pentagastrin, vasopressin, ergonovine, bethanecol, and edrophonium) [94]. Despite the conspicuous relevance of stimulus sensitivity in the pathophysiology of functional chest pain, no single provocative test has surfaced for routine diagnostic use.

Central Signal Processing

Alterations in central nervous system (CNS) processing of afferent signals in chest pain patients were first detected using balloon distention paradigms. Bradley and colleagues applied sensory decision theory to determine whether reduced pain thresholds from esophageal balloon distention were related to heightened neurosensory perception or tendencies to alter standards for reporting pain (response bias) [95, 96]. Patients with unexplained pain were compared to control groups consisting of healthy individuals, patients with GERD (reflux esophagitis or elevated acid exposure time), coronary artery disease patients, and patients with irritable bowel syndrome (IBS). Perceptual discrimination was similar among groups but chest pain patients tended to set lower standards for judging esophageal distention stimuli as painful (response bias). Both acid-sensitive and acid-insensitive patients with no evidence of reflux disease were represented, and other than the primary peripheral trigger, CNS mechanisms are likely similar between these two subsets. The findings suggest that an error in central interpretation of afferent signals rather than an increase in peripheral sensitivity is the relevant pathophysiological feature of functional chest pain. Similar alterations in central signal processing have been demonstrated using balloon distention in other painful gastrointestinal functional disorders [97].

Hollerbach et al. further studied central signal processing in chest pain patients using electrical stimulation and cortical evoked potentials [98]. Thresholds to pain production with electrical stimulation were reduced in patients compared with controls, but cortical representations of the peripheral signals were not augmented. The authors concluded that increased perception of the esophageal stimulus resulted from enhanced cerebral processing of visceral sensory input rather than a hyperalgesic response in afferent pathways [98]. The same investigators used heart rate variability to measure autonomic activity before, during and after esophageal stimulation, as heart rate variability can reflect autonomic output in response to esophageal sensory signals [99]. Electrical or mechanical esophageal stimulation appeared to increase reflex vagal efferent activity. For patients with acid sensitive symptoms, acid instillation also produced a vagally mediated esophagocardiac reflex alteration in heart rate variability if chest pain was reproduced by the stimulus [100].

Collectively these studies indicate that chest pain reproduced by esophageal mechanical or electrical stimulation is accompanied by errors in central signal processing and an autonomic response. In acid sensitive subjects, the findings are further provoked by acid instillation. Central sensitization has been shown to extend hypersensitivity to esophageal and chest locations remote from the acid stimulus, and this finding further supports the importance of central mechanisms in the chest pain response [89]. Changes in pain threshold were exaggerated and of longer duration in pain patients compared with control subjects suggesting that a shift in the way peripheral sensory input is handled centrally is of pathophysiological importance [89].

Motility Findings

Up to half of subjects with unexplained chest pain who have no evidence of esophagitis or elevated acid exposure times will have motility abnormalities on conventional esophageal manometry [49, 83, 101]. The principal findings are those of the spastic disorders, including nonspecific spastic disorders (such as nutcracker esophagus) and diffuse esophageal spasm. A causal relationship of motility events to pain has been difficult to establish. Ambulatory motility studies suggest that, (a) on average, pain could conceivably be attributed to motor events in no more than 15% of episodes, (b) pain rarely accompanies even marked dysmotility at the time of conventional manometry, and (c) correction of abnormalities (such as correction of abnormal amplitudes using smooth muscle relaxants) has an unreliable effect on pain reporting [94, 101, 102]. These observations support the nonspecific nature of most of the detected motor abnormalities and have helped shift attention away from dysmotility as being an important pathophysiological factor in pain production.

Balaban et al. have shown that an abrupt increase in distal esophageal wall thickness precedes episodes of unexplained chest pain, a recent finding that challenges the limited relevance of motor activity [103]. This thickening, detected using high frequency intraluminal ultrasound, represents sustained contraction of esophageal longitudinal muscle and is not measured by conventional intraluminal manometry. Although these observations again draw attention to esophageal motor activity as a potential pain explanation, neither the specificity of these sustained esophageal contractions for pain nor their relationship to sensory phenomena has been determined.

At a minimum, abnormal motor activity may serve as a marker for other mechanisms more directly related to pain production. For example, esophageal contraction amplitudes show at least modest correlation with sensitivity to balloon distention, a finding supporting a relationship between hypersensitivity and hypermotility [104]. Likewise, impedance planimetry has confirmed that hypersensitivity to balloon distention is present in nearly all patients with the nutcracker esophagus, and represents one extreme within the spectrum of spastic disorders [105]. Impedance planimetry also demonstrates that the esophagus is stiff, noncompliant, and hyper reactive to distending stimuli in chest pain patients in general [87, 105]. Atropine relaxes the esophagus yet fails to abolish balloon distention hypersensitivity [106]. Autonomic activity represents an important contributor to esophageal tone, and it is possible that abnormalities in autonomic tone and reactivity participate in the production of the motor abnormalities observed in chest pain subjects [107]. Further studies incorporating all relevant physiological domains (sensory activity, CNS processing and autonomic reactivity, and motility findings) may ascertain the relative contributions of each toward pain production in functional chest pain and may also help define specific subgroups.

— Psychological Features

Psychiatric comorbidity is common in patients with chest pain who are referred for further gastroenterological evaluation and lack conspicuous evidence of reflux disease. Psychological symptoms of anxiety and neuroticism are more common in community samples with no cardiac pain explanation [108]. At least 60% of patients meet criteria for psychiatric diagnoses with the most common being anxiety disorders, depression, and somatization disorder [109–112]. They are particularly fearful of cardiopulmonary sensations [113], and attacks consistent with panic are reported by approximately one-third of patients [114]. Chest pain associated with panic attacks may account for 25% of visits for chest pain seen in the emergency room [115]. The validity of a panic disorder diagnosis in patients with functional chest pain is supported by high rates of panic disorder and major depression in first-degree relatives [114]. Inhalation of carbon dioxide, an agent known to trigger panic attacks, also precipitates pain episodes in many chest pain patients with or without known diagnoses of panic disorder [116].

Specific psychiatric diagnoses have not segregated well with physiological abnormalities, such as balloon distention sensitivity or the presence of esophageal motor disorders, and their relationships remain unclear. Psychiatric comorbidity appears important in spastic motor disorders. In two studies, more than 75% of patients with these manometric findings and unexplained esophageal symptoms had psychiatric diagnoses—rates at least 2–3 times higher than those expected in the general population or in symptomatic patients with achalasia [109, 117]. Recent work by Ringel et al. combining psychological and physiological measures in patients with chest pain and other functional esophageal symptoms has demonstrated strong correlations between psychological variables (global distress, anxiety) and esophageal sensation and tone [118].

The relevance of psychiatric comorbidity and psychological symptoms in the clinical presentation is uncertain, but a role in mediating chest pain occurrence or severity is likely. This notion is supported by a large-scale investigation of psychological symptoms in symptomatic patients referred for esophageal manometry; psychological ratings rather than manometric features were the best predictors of pain reporting [119]. Interactions of psychological factors with provocative esophageal stimuli are plausible. Indeed, the response bias discovered by Bradley et al. when using a balloon distention stimulus and sensory decision theory generally is thought to reflect cultural and emotional influences on standards for reporting pain [95, 96]. Some of the psychological factors detected in that study that possibly contributed to the response bias included greater use of negative pain coping strategies, less ability to perform specific behaviors to decrease pain, and reinforcement of pain behavior by spouses or significant others.

Additional data demonstrate the potential relevance of psychological factors in patients with functional chest pain. First, the findings from acute experimental stress in functional heartburn reveal the importance of psychological symptoms and psychiatric comorbidity in the reporting esophageal symptoms [24, 36]. Second, acute stress induces spastic motor abnormalities including elevation of distal esophageal contraction amplitudes, findings that may reflect a correlated increment in sensitivity to esophageal stimuli [120–122]. This has not been tested directly. Third, a longitudinal study of subjects undergoing alcohol withdrawal demonstrated marked manometric changes occurring in parallel with changes in measures of stress [123]. High contraction wave amplitudes during early alcohol withdrawal were normalized 30 days following alcohol abstinence, indicating a longitudinal correlation of esophageal physiological measures with psychological status.

Psychological factors also influence behavior and global measures in chest pain patients. High rates of psychiatric comorbidity influence well-being, functioning, and quality of life. Psychological characteristics are accompanied by perceived vulnerability to serious heart disease. Latinga et al. found that chest pain patients without cardiac disease had higher levels of neuroticism and psychiatric morbidity before and after cardiac catheterization than patients with coronary heart disease [124]. This has prognostic significance since the chest pain patients with greater psychological distress displayed less improvement in pain, more frequent pain episodes, greater social maladjustment, and more anxiety symptoms at one year follow-up than patients with relatively low initial levels of psychological distress.

Collectively the available data reveal the following in functional chest pain patients: high rates of psychiatric comorbidity, importance of psychological factors in predicting the symptomatic state, potential mechanisms by which psychophysiological interactions can occur, and the influence of comorbidity on global measures and outcome in subjects without alternative explanations for pain. Although subjects with or without acid provoked symptoms are rarely segregated in the available reports, it is likely that the above findings apply substantially to the subset meeting criteria for functional chest pain.

— Treatment

Symptomatic management is recommended [125] since chest pain persists for most patients despite reassurance and exclusion of structural or progressive processes. Patients who are given an explanation for their pain, especially in the context of esophageal disorders have significantly reduced health resource use and improved work functioning [126–129]. However, reassurance solely about the non-cardiac nature of the pain rarely results in definitive relief of concern. In long-term follow-up studies, pain has a continued association with impaired functional status and health-care seeking [130–132]. Spontaneous recovery is rare [132].

The basic treatment approach resembles that for other painful FGIDs (Figure 4) [133]. Peripherally acting treatments are oriented toward reducing esophageal pain triggers and blocking up-regulated sensorimotor activity at the esophageal level. Centrally acting therapies are oriented either toward factors involved in altered signal processing and resultant heightened autonomic reactivity or the psychological/cognitive interface with these mechanisms. But before embarking on functional treatment strategies, management begins with exclusion of cardiac, extra-esophageal, and esophageal disorders that reasonably could be producing the symptoms. To satisfy criteria for functional chest pain, this includes exclusion of GERD [134].

Once the exclusionary evaluation is completed, therapeutic options for functional chest pain become limited. Results from four randomized controlled trials of calcium channel blockers do not demonstrate efficacy in symptom management [102, 135–137]. Calcium channel blockers and other smooth muscle relaxants primarily affect motor activity, which are physiological features no longer considered of primary importance in symptom production. Some data suggest that sensory stretch receptors are in series with esophageal intramural smooth muscle fibers, thereby explaining anecdotal benefits of these medications [138].

More consistent and established effects have been demonstrated for centrally acting treatments. The most encouraging outcomes have come from psychopharmacologic drugs and behavioral interventions. The treatment effect of antidepressants, the best studied agents, is independent of depression or anxiety modula-

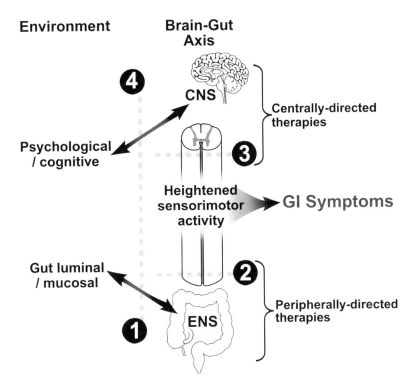

Environment

Brain-Gut Axis

4

CNS

Centrally-directed therapies

Psychological / cognitive

3

Heightened sensorimotor activity ➤ GI Symptoms

Gut luminal / mucosal

2

1 **ENS**

Peripherally-directed therapies

Figure 4. Treatment targets for managing functional chest pain. Up-regulated sensorimotor activity is susceptible to initiating, provoking, or perpetuating stimuli at both central (psychological/cognitive) and peripheral (gut luminal/mucosal) levels. The dashed lines (1–4) represent common treatment targets that may have varying utility from patient to patient. CNS = central nervous system; ENS = enteric nervous system; GI = gastrointestinal. (Adapted from [133])

tion, although the actual mechanism of action remains unknown [139, 140]. Other potential benefits include direct effects on pain, improvement in sleep pattern, reversal of autonomic dysregulation, anti-somatization effect, or blockade of stress effect on cortical activation [140]. Clouse and associates found that low doses of the antidepressant trazodone (100–150 mg daily) produced global improvement and reduced distress from esophageal symptoms over six weeks in patients with chest pain and nonspecific spastic esophageal motility disorders [117]. Symptom improvement was not related to changes in manometric parameters. Similarly, Cannon et al. found imipramine (50 mg at bedtime for two months) to be superior to clonidine or placebo in the treatment of unexplained chest pain [141]. The response to imipramine was not predicted by baseline psychologic or physiologic abnormalities, including esophageal manometry or balloon distension studies, and was not dependent on their change at outcome. These antidepressant doses are lower than those used in treating psychiatric disorders, further supporting an unconventional mechanism as being responsible for patient improvement.

The outcomes from these two antidepressant trials are similar to results found when antidepressants, particularly tricyclic agents, are used for other painful functional gastrointestinal disorders [142]. Treatment with tricyclic antidepressants successfully managed more than 75% of patients with functional chest pain, and remissions were sustained in the vast majority of initial responders [143]. An 8-week controlled trial of sertraline (a selective serotonin re-uptake inhibitor) also demonstrated a favorable effect on daily chest pain in an intention-to-treat analysis, suggesting a potential role of contemporary antidepressants in the management strategy [144]. Unlike the tricyclic agents, contemporary antidepressants may function primarily by treating the interface between psychological disturbance and up-regulated sensorimotor activity, as suggested in Figure 4. They may be best for patients with active anxiety or depression symptoms, although this remains conjectural [145]. At a minimum, these medications are capable of treating uncomfortable emotional symptoms that may interfere with global improvement or coping abilities. Pain modulation with antidepressants, whether tricyclic or contemporary agents, is becoming a more common recommendation in treatment algorithms [146–148].

Behavioral therapy is also effective in patients with functional chest pain. Hegel and colleagues [149] reported outcome of three chest pain patients with anxiety disorders who were treated with relaxation training and controlled diaphragmatic breathing exercises, practicing the techniques during increasingly complex activities. Two had substantial reductions in frequency and intensity of chest pain, a response that was maintained for 12 months after treatment ceased. Klimes and colleagues performed a controlled study of behavioral treatment in 31 patients with chest pain [150]. The intervention consisted of education, controlled breathing, training in relaxation and diversion of attention from pain, and practice of newly learned skills in the home environment. Active intervention, compared with a waiting-list control, produced significant improvement in chest pain episodes, functional capacity, and psychological distress that was maintained for 46 months after treatment. Some reported benefit could be attributed to methodological factors in the design of this investigation.

The value of psychological management was confirmed in an 8-week treatment trial of 60 patients with continuing chest pain despite negative cardiologic evaluations [151]. Besides reducing chest pain episodes, the combination of cognitive and behavioral treatments improved anxiety and depression scores, disability ratings, and exercise tolerance—effects maintained at 6-month follow-up. Cognitive behavioral therapy (CBT) alone was superior to usual care in another study of unexplained chest pain, with 48% of the subjects remaining pain-free at 12 months compared to 13% in the control group [152]. This is not surprising considering the general efficacy of this form of psychotherapy in unexplained somatic symptoms and syndromes [153]. Interest in a medical psychological intervention is reported by the majority of patients who are asked, and limitation of activities rather than intensity or frequency of pain is the strongest predictor of this interest [132]. A stepped approach depending on measures of disability has been recommended [154].

Botulinum toxin injection into the lower esophageal sphincter has been offered in open-label, uncontrolled fashion for patients with functional chest pain [94]. Seventy-two percent of subjects responded with at least 50% reduction in chest pain in one large series [155]. Most subjects had a spastic motor disorder. Early response was rated as excellent by most, repeated injections were required, and placebo response cannot be excluded [94]. Prolonged response in open-label use was more likely in female subjects, and adverse events were insignificant. A favorable open-label response also was seen when botulinum toxin was injected at multiple esophageal levels in 9 patients with diffuse esophageal spasm [156].

Other treatments have been limited to anecdotal experience, uncontrolled use, or speculation. Theophylline potentially can alter adenosine-mediated nociception and reduce pain sensitivity to balloon distention in 75% of hypersensitive chest pain patients in one study [157]. Seven of eight subjects subsequently reported sustained improvement in pain after oral theophylline [157]. Sildenafil and other agents that increase esophageal nitric oxide can improve manometric features of spastic disorders, but effects on symptoms are not yet established [158, 159]. Transcutaneous electrical nerve stimulation (TENS) is used for cardiac pain in severe angina. In a placebo-controlled study, TENS reduced sensitivity to intraesophageal balloon distention with unexplained chest pain and was suggested as a potential treatment [104].

Surgical intervention is ill advised. Lack of objective evidence of reflux disease, poor response to medical antireflux therapy, and lack of reflux-symptom association for atypical symptoms predict poor outcome from antireflux surgery [160, 161]. Early responses of chest pain associated with significant hypermotility to long esophagomyotomy can be favorable, but the long-term results for pain management are not good [162].

In summary, careful exclusion of cardiac disease and GERD is required before embarking on treatment of functional chest pain, using therapeutic trials for GERD if an invasive investigation is not performed. Treatment of functional chest pain then proceeds with reassurance and may include trials of smooth muscle relaxants or anticholinergic agents, recognizing the limited utility of these approaches. Patients with persistent symptoms or disability are best managed with antidepressants or psychological/behavioral interventions. A variety of other treatments have been examined in anecdotal fashion, but none is advised for widespread application. Surgery is not advised.

— Definition

The disorder is characterized by a sensation of abnormal bolus transit through the esophageal body. Thorough exclusion of structural lesions, GERD and histopathology-based esophageal motor disorders is required to establish the diagnosis.

— Epidemiology

Little information is available to ascertain reliably the prevalence of functional dysphagia. In a survey of the general population for functional disorders, between 7% and 8% of respondents reported dysphagia that was unexplained by the exclusionary criteria [50]. Forty-one percent of these had seen a physician for the complaint. More recently, in a validation study of the Rome II criteria in an Asian population, 0.6% of 1012 patients with functional gastrointestinal disease complained of frequent dysphagia [163]. Up to 80% of patients suffering from dysphagia can be classified into the non-functional dysphagia subset of patients [164]. Thus, by survey methods, functional dysphagia is the least prevalent of the functional esophageal disorders [50]. The prevalence is likely to be even lower than surveys estimate given that some of these individuals likely would be re-classified if subjected to intensive testing.

A3. Diagnostic Criteria* for Functional Dysphagia

Must include *all* of the following:
1. **Sense of solid and/or liquid foods sticking, lodging, or passing abnormally through the esophagus**
2. **Absence of evidence that gastroesophageal reflux is the cause of the symptom**
3. **Absence of histopathology-based esophageal motility disorders**

*Criteria fulfilled for the last 3 months with symptom onset at least 6 months prior to diagnosis

— Justification for Change in Criteria

Dysphagia is not easily linked to reflux events. Nevertheless, the modification of the threshold used for the second criterion (see introduction) would attribute the symptom to GERD rather than a functional diagnosis if the link were established, even in absence of other objective GERD indicators.

— Clinical Evaluation

The diagnosis of functional dysphagia is established only after a fastidious exclusion of structural disorders that might cause dysphagia. Structural lesions are excluded by endoscopy (with biopsy) and a barium esophagram (with videofluoroscopy, if possible). These investigations also help identify reflux esophagitis and, in the case of fluoroscopy, screen for motility disorders. Barium-impregnated bolus challenge during fluoroscopy (e.g., tablets, food) can help identify mucosal rings or strictures that may be overlooked with standard radiographic studies [165]. In the event of an apparently normal endoscopy, a structural cause for dysphagia cannot be ruled out with certainty until esophageal mucosal biopsies have been undertaken. Indeed, esophageal biopsies can be helpful in diagnosing eosinophilic esophagitis (particularly in young males) which can cause solid bolus dysphagia although when a mucosal ring(s) is present. If no structural lesions (or esophagitis) are found in the course of endoscopy and barium swallow, these evaluations should be followed by manometry. In one study, food ingestion during manometry increased the diagnostic yield—88% of dysphagia patients reported complaints during manometry supplemented with food ingestion while none complained of dysphagia during conventional manometry [166]. However these data need confirmation before the tests are recommended for routine practice. Ambulatory pH monitoring generally is reserved for patients in whom dysphagia is associated with heartburn or regurgitation. In instances in which the balance of data is still equivocal, a brief therapeutic trial with a high-dose PPI regimen may help identify patients in whom subtle reflux disease is the ultimate cause of dysphagia.

A variety of nonspecific spastic esophageal motility abnormalities are found in 34% to 70% of patients with dysphagia who have no other explanation for this symptom [83]. These include peristaltic disturbances (intermittent simultaneous contractions, segmental aperistalsis), contraction wave abnormalities (increased wave durations and/or amplitude, multipeak waves), and hypertension or poor relaxation of the LES. The great variation encountered in published reports of these findings is likely related to differences in manometric technique and interpretations as well as an underappreciation of the role of reflux disease. In general, these motor abnormalities do not have a recognized pathologic cause, and their presence does not preclude the diagnosis of functional dysphagia. Although the manometric criteria for the diagnosis of diffuse esophageal spasm are well defined, the distinction between this entity and nonspecific motility disorders may be difficult in some cases [101, 167].

— Physiological Features

Several mechanisms may be responsible for functional dysphagia, and the intermittent complaints in some patients limit their clarification. Concurrent manometry and fluoroscopy have shown that simultaneous contraction sequences characterizing diffuse esophageal spasm (propagation velocity > 8 cm/sec) are invariably accompanied by poor barium clearance that may be perceived as dysphagia [168]. Simultaneous contraction sequences are found in few patients during stationary manometric evaluation for dysphagia, but are more frequently detected during ambulatory pressure monitoring. Intraesophageal balloon distention can induce simultaneous contractions in 70% of subjects with presumed functional dysphagia, but not in asymptomatic control subjects [169].

In contrast, peristaltic dysfunction caused by failed contraction sequences or low-amplitude contractions (i.e., < 30–35 mm Hg) may also cause symptoms. Concurrent manometric and fluoroscopic studies demonstrate that the efficacy of esophageal emptying is inversely related to peristaltic amplitude, such that emptying becomes progressively impaired with peristaltic amplitudes less than 40 mmHg [170]. Recently, this finding was confirmed using multichannel intraluminal impedance (with a cutoff for peristaltic amplitude of 35 mmHg) to assess esophageal emptying [171]. Hypotensive or failed peristalsis is possibly responsible for nonobstructive dysphagia accompanying GERD [172, 173]. Failed contraction sequences or markedly reduced peristaltic activity also can be produced by feeding patients during manometry, and the induced motor abnormality correlates well with sensation of dysphagia [174]. Considering the frequency with which this type of abnormality could be induced in patients with otherwise unexplained dysphagia, peristaltic failure may be an important physiological explanation in many patients with intermittent functional dysphagia [172].

Abnormal intraesophageal sensory perception may be a third physiological factor in the report of dysphagia. A feeling of "food sticking" as well as pain is induced in some normal subjects with intraesophageal balloon distension in the distal esophagus [170]. Likewise, dysphagia is reported during acidification of the distal esophagus in some patients with reflux esophagitis [173]. Because dysphagia can be produced by various intraluminal stimuli, an error in visceral perception could exist in patients with functional dysphagia as it is in patients with functional chest pain [85].

Deschner et al. demonstrate peristaltic dysfunction related to intraesophageal balloon distension that could be interpreted as increased sensitivity to the distension stimulus [169]. The concordance of provoked dysphagia and peristaltic dysfunction was high but imperfect (87%), and peristaltic dysfunction might be an epiphenomenon. Other data indicate that abnormal pain sensitivity to balloon distension is significantly associated with dysphagia in patients with functional esophageal symptoms [175]. Taken together, the observations in functional dysphagia suggest that both abnormal motility and abnormal visceral sensitivity contribute to symptoms.

— Psychological Features

Little information on the role of psychological factors in functional dysphagia is available for review. Acute stress experiments suggest that central factors can precipitate motor abnormalities potentially responsible for dysphagia. Barium transit is impaired in asymptomatic and symptomatic subjects during recollection of unpleasant topics or stressful, unpleasant interviews [176, 177]. Noxious auditory stimuli or difficult cognitive tasks alter manometric recordings by increasing contraction wave amplitude and occasionally induce simultaneous contraction sequences [121]. However, extrapolating acute stress experiments to chronic symptoms in a functional esophageal disorder is entirely conjectural. Reported associations of psychiatric and psychological factors with motility abnormalities in patients with functional chest pain may also be relevant to functional dysphagia [178]. Anxiety, depression, and somatization disorders are significantly more common in the subset of patients with dysphagia and nonspecific motility disorders compared with patients having other explanations for the symptom [10].

— Treatment

The management of patients with functional dysphagia generally involves reassurance, avoidance of precipitating factors, careful chewing of food, and modification of psychological abnormalities where possible. Functional dysphagia may regress over time, and an overzealous treatment approach is unwarranted in patients with mild symptoms. Patients with more severe symptoms warrant a comprehensive medical evaluation and pharmacologic trials. A trial of antireflux therapy (usually 2–4 weeks of a PPI) should be considered in all patients, but terminated if ineffective and reflux or esophagitis has not been demonstrated [179]. Other medications commonly used are similar to those given to patients with functional chest pain of presumed esophageal origin, including smooth-muscle relaxants, anticholinergics, and anxiolytics/antidepressants. None has proven efficacy for treatment of functional dysphagia, but can be tried nevertheless. The mechanisms by which these medications might influence the pathophysiology are unclear. Smooth muscle relaxants conceivably could improve symptoms if nonspecific spastic motor abnormalities (including poor LES relaxation) were interfering with transit. Some conflicting evidence is available regarding the effects of tricyclic antidepressants on visceral hypersensitivity [180, 181].

Mechanical interventions can be considered in some patients. Dilation (e.g., 54F Maloney or Savary dilator) has been used effectively for patients presenting with intermittent food dysphagia, as a subtle stricture or ring can be overlooked [182, 183]. This technique has been used in some patients with dysphagia associated with nonspecific spastic motor disorders [184]. Similar to the treatment of achalasia, patients with incomplete LES relaxation and associated nonspecific motility disorders may respond to pneumatic dilation or botulinum toxin injection. These procedures should be reserved for patients with a documented delay of distal esophageal emptying as defined by barium esophagram or scintigraphic studies [185].

A4. Globus

— Definition

The symptom of globus is defined as a sense of a lump or retained food bolus or tightness in the throat. A range of other foreign body-like descriptors are volunteered by patients including a sense of retained particulate matter, mucus accumulation or a restrictive or choking sensation. It is usually perceived in the midline between the thyroid cartilage and the manubriosternal notch. However, in 20% of cases it is perceived in the paramedian position [186]. There are additional qualifiers for which there seems to be broad agreement. The symptom is non-painful, frequently improves with eating, and is frequently episodic [186–189]. Conversely, there are a number of features that most would agree are incompatible with the diagnosis, including constant or intermittent pain or weight loss [188, 190], dysphagia or odynophagia [187, 191]. Weight loss should alert one to the possibility of a neoplastic process—laryngo-pharyngeal malignancy rarely presents with globus [189, 192, 193]. The qualifier "functional" requires that, along with the other diagnostic criteria, there is no identifiable structural or motor disturbance in the anatomical vicinity, pharynx or esophagus. Reflux disease can cause varying symptoms in the neck and throat and some cases of globus may be associated with reflux disease. However, both globus and GERD are extremely common and there is no high-level evidence of a causative link between reflux and globus (see below).

— Epidemiology

Globus is extremely common, being reported in 7–46% of apparently healthy individuals, with a peak incidence in middle age and low incidence in individuals under 20 [11, 50, 186, 188, 194]. Overall, the symptom accounts for around 4% of ENT referrals [195]. In healthy individuals who are not seeking health care for symptoms of globus, there is equal prevalence between men and women [188, 190, 196]. Women are more likely to seek health care for globus [186].

A4. Diagnostic Criteria* for Globus

Must include *all* of the following:
1. **Persistent or intermittent, nonpainful sensation of a lump or foreign body in the throat**
2. **Occurrence of the sensation between meals**
3. **Absence of dysphagia or odynophagia**
4. **Absence of evidence that gastroesophageal reflux is the cause of the symptom**
5. **Absence of histopathology-based esophageal motility disorders**

*Criteria fulfilled for the last 3 months with symptom onset at least 6 months prior to diagnosis

— Justification for Change in Criteria

By factor analysis, globus is distinct from pain [187]. Pain often is indicative of ulcerative or malignant pathology [192, 193]. As for other functional esophageal disorders, demonstration that the symptom is directly related to reflux events would indicate a diagnosis of GERD, even in the absence of other objective GERD evidence.

— Clinical Evaluation

Since the pathophysiology of globus is unclear and as there is no current biological marker for the condition, the diagnosis is made on clinical history. This history must ensure that the patient does not have true dysphagia. Most clinicians feel that this distinction can be made reliably, a belief that has been supported by systematic analysis of symptoms. Deary et al. [187] published a self-report globus symptom scale, the Glasgow Edinburgh Throat Scale, derived from 105 consecutive patients completing a 10-item questionnaire. Factor analysis of the responses on this questionnaire showed that globus symptoms could be segregated from dysphagia or pain. Physical examination of the neck followed by nasolaryngoscopic examination of the pharynx and larynx are advised. Only a small number of patients are referred to specialists. The latter usually will be done routinely when the patient is seen by an otolaryngologist. The risk of cancer is extremely low in globus, and it remains unproven whether nasolaryngoscopy should be done routinely. A series of 120 globus patients undergoing laryngoscopic examination under general anesthesia showed hypopharyngeal cancer in two, but both of these had additional symptoms including dysphagia and hoarseness [192]. Timon et al. [193] reported a tongue base tumor in 1 of 83 prospective cases referred to an ENT clinic. Furthermore, long term follow-up studies (up to 7 yrs) do not report the late appearance of upper respiratory or digestive tract malignancies in patients with simple globus sensation [189].

Beyond nasolaryngoscopy currently there is no uniform policy on investigation or treatment. In a survey of ENT surgeons in the UK only 14% did not perform any investigations (apart from nasolaryngoscopy) on patients with globus [197]. The most common investigation among the majority of the ENT surgeons was rigid esophagoscopy (61%) followed by barium swallow (56%). The argument for reflux notwithstanding (see below), there is little evidence to support esophagoscopy in the evaluation of simple globus sensation. Barium swallow, while detecting incidental findings in some, adds little diagnostic value in globus [198]. In contrast, there are grounds for a therapeutic trial of a PPI when uninvestigated patients present with the globus symptom, particularly when typical reflux symptoms coexist.

Although clear guidelines are lacking, it seems reasonable to perform nasolaryngoscopy for this isolated symptom. However, if additional alarm symptoms are present, such as dysphagia, odynophagia, pain, weight loss, or hoarseness, more extensive evaluation is necessary.

— Physiological Features

Unfortunately, there has been relatively little new information published on this aspect of globus in the last 10 years. This may reflect the benign nature of the condition and the low priority attached to it by funding agencies. Hiatal hernia, cervical osteophytes, cricopharyngeal bar, cervical web, peptic ulcer and gallstones have been reported in association with globus, but the prevalence of such findings varies dramatically among such studies [190, 199, 200]. A well-designed prospective analysis of 77 consecutive cases found normal radiological examinations in 53% and hiatal hernias in only 13% [201]. Hiatal hernia is unlikely to have etiological significance, as the reported prevalence of hiatal hernia in uncontrolled studies of globus patients (30–50%) [190, 200] is comparable to that estimated in the general population [202, 203]. The cricopharyngeal bar, found in up to 17% of individuals undergoing contrast radiography [204, 205], is not more prevalent in globus [190]. In summary, there is no solid evidence to attribute globus to any anatomical abnormality.

A range of *mechanisms* have been proposed that might link gastroesophageal reflux with globus including: (a) referred sensation from the esophagus to the neck (perhaps via hypersensitive vagal afferent pathways), (b) reflexive contraction of the upper esophageal sphincter (UES) in response to esophageal acidification, (c) esophago-pharyngeal regurgitation, and (d) reflexive cough or habitual throat clearing in response to esophageal acidification. Other postulated mechanisms for the symptom are pharyngeal, cricopharyngeal, or esophageal motor dysfunction.

Cricopharyngeal hypertonicity was initially suspected as a cause of globus when an early study, using a posteriorly oriented perfused catheter and pull-through technique, found higher resting upper esophageal sphincter (UES) pressures compared to controls [206]. However, UES pressure is labile and responsive to both emotional stress and local physical stimulation. Hence this finding may reflect an abnormal response to the mechanical stimulation induced by the pull-through itself or the associated discomfort [207]. Accordingly, subsequent studies, either using a stationary sleeve sensor [196, 208] or non-perfused manometric catheters and a station pull-through technique to measure UES tone [196, 209], found no difference in resting UES pressure in globus compared with controls. Although the symptom of globus anecdotally is precipitated by deep emotion, and although the UES normally contracts in response to emotional stress, such stress-induced augmentation in UES tone in globus patients is normal [208]. Additionally, UES pressure augmentation in response to esophageal balloon distention was found to be comparable to that of controls [210]. Importantly, that study found that esophageal balloon distention reproduced globus sensation in 80% of patients and at significantly lower balloon volumes than were required to produce discomfort in controls. Hence, perception of esophageal distention is heightened in this population.

Based on video radiographic and most manometric assessments, the pharyngeal swallow mechanism is normal in globus [199, 211]. This is not surprising as these patients do not have dysphagia, and symptoms generally improve during the meal. The urge to swallow, and hence the swallow frequency, increases between meals. It is uncertain whether this habitual dry swallowing, presumably to "dislodge" the apparent bolus, is a result of the foreign body sensation or whether it contributes to the sensation by periodically causing air entrapment in the proximal esophagus [212].

Given the observed esophageal hypersensitivity to distension in this group, it might be argued that esophageal motor or sensory dysfunction may better account for globus than pharyngo-cricopharyngeal dysfunction. A tertiary referral center, which carefully examined physiological and psychometric variables in globus patients, reported approximately 25% of those presenting with the symptoms to have manometrically proven achalasia [211, 213]. However, 21 of 24 of such patients had one or more of the typical symptoms of achalasia when questioned after the diagnosis was made. This is not a consistent finding among other studies. Other motor disorders, including diffuse esophageal spasm and non-specific motor disorders have been reported in a small proportion of patients [214–217] although the prevalence among such studies varies widely [196]. One controlled study found no difference in the prevalence of these motility abnormalities (25%) between patients and controls [216]. On the basis of current evidence, it is possible that esophageal dysmotility might have globus as one of its manifestations, but there is certainly no esophageal motor pattern that characterizes globus, and the majority of globus sufferers do not have significant esophageal dysmotility.

Relationship Between Globus and Gastroesophageal Reflux Disease

Gastroesophageal reflux is the most favored etiology for the globus symptom, although strong evidence for a causative link between these conditions is lacking. Because the population prevalence of both reflux (15–39%) and globus (see above) is high, the reportedly high association between the two conditions is only weak evidence for a causative link [10, 11, 188, 203, 217–219]. By chance, the two entities will coexist. For example, a Scandinavian population survey, found that 20% of respondents had heartburn and 20% had globus, while half of those with heartburn reported globus [219]. In contrast, a population survey in Olmstead country found the odds ratio of someone with reflux symptoms experiencing globus was 1.9 (95% CI, 1.0–3.6) when compared with subjects not having reflux symptoms [11]. Replication of the increased odds ratio by additional studies is needed.

Pooling data from studies utilizing ambulatory pH monitoring shows that increased esophageal acid exposure is present in approximately a third of patients with globus [199, 215, 216, 220–224]. Two key issues, however, are whether GERD is over-represented in globus compared with appropriate controls and whether esophageal acidification causes the symptom. There are only two adequately controlled studies that addressed these issues, and they had conflicting results [199,

216]. Wilson et al. [199] found that the ambulatory esophageal acid profile did not differ between those with globus and appropriate control subjects, nor was there any temporal relationship identified between the globus sensation and actual reflux events. Hill et al. [216] found abnormal pH profiles in a significantly higher proportion (31%) of globus patients compared with 5% of controls in a Chinese population. Despite the inherent difficulty in attributing temporal association between a symptom which may be present continuously for hours (globus) and discrete transient events (reflux), Curran et al. [222] found that 61% of 21 patients with globus had a positive symptom index on ambulatory pH testing. Therefore, a closer examination of ambulatory pH monitoring in globus may help explain fluctuations in the severity of symptoms during the test.

In examining potential temporal relationships between globus and reflux events, the disappearance of symptoms with treatment is the best indirect evidence available. Timon et al. [193] found that neither the presence of heartburn, independent evidence of reflux, nor medical antireflux therapy had any significant impact on the likelihood of symptom resolution. There is no good evidence supporting the efficacy of acid suppressive therapy in globus (see below).

In conclusion, there appears to be a reasonably strong, although quite variable, association between globus and reflux. However, a large proportion of globus patients do not have reflux, and there currently is no significant evidence supporting a causative relationship between reflux and globus. Therefore, while a subset of globus is likely attributable to GERD, proof of this assertion is still required.

— Psychological Features

A number of studies have demonstrated higher levels of anxiety and depression and greater introversion and neuroticism in affected patients when compared with healthy controls [208, 225–228]. However, psychoneurosis has not been linked causally to the symptom and may simply reflect health care seeking behavior or self-referral bias, as less than 10% of sufferers seek medical advice for it. For example, using the DSM III-R criteria, a psychiatric diagnosis can be attached to 25–60% of these patients [211–215], but these studies revealed no more anxiety and depression than was found in patients in a general medical outpatient clinic [193, 211]. Up to 96% of sufferers report symptoms exacerbated by strong emotion [188].

Life stress events might precipitate globus. Deary et al. [227] found that significantly more globus patients had life stress events within 2 months of symptom onset compared with controls. This phenomenon was confirmed by a subsequent controlled study of life events—globus patients reported significantly more severe life events than control subjects over the preceding year and fewer close confiding relationships than controls [229]. Personality traits that might influence responses to life events have been assessed in globus patients. Low extraversion levels were found in women but largely normal personality traits were found in men [230].

In summary, no psychometric or personality profile is specific for globus. Life stress might be a cofactor in genesis of, or exacerbation of the symptom. A proportion of the psychiatric diagnoses evident in clinic presenters may reflect health care seeking behavior.

— Treatment

Given the benign nature of the condition, the likelihood of long-term persistence of symptoms, and the absence of high-level efficacy data for pharmacotherapy, the mainstay of treatment rests with explanation and reassurance. There are grounds for a trial of a PPI in patients presenting with uninvestigated globus sensation in reaching the diagnosis of globus, particularly when typical reflux symptoms coexist. However, prior warning of the likelihood of persistence of globus sensation would seem prudent, as symptoms persist in up to 75% at 3 years following diagnosis [193].

Anti-reflux therapy is not likely to produce a symptomatic response. Only one randomized controlled therapeutic trial of acid suppressive therapy for globus has been published since 1990, and no benefit was reported for cimetidine over placebo [231]. In a small, controlled but non-randomized study, the response to omeprazole 20mg daily (in those with coexistent heartburn) was equivalent to that of reassurance alone (25% in patients and controls) [216]. In the remaining prospective uncontrolled studies of medical antireflux therapy (three evaluating PPIs and three evaluating H_2 receptor antagonists), the response rates ranged from 25%–77% (mean response rate 57%) [193, 222, 224, 232, 233]. An uncontrolled trial of cisapride showed marginal symptomatic benefit after 14 weeks [234]. There are no controlled trials of antidepressants, but there is some anecdotal evidence for their efficacy [235].

Recommendations for Future Research

The need for further investigation of the functional esophageal disorders remains extremely high. Areas for future research in these disorders are identified in four categories:

1. *Criteria examination and validation.* Studies enhancing the sensitivity and specificity of the diagnostic criteria for each functional esophageal disorder would be welcomed. The diagnosis of functional esophageal disorders relies entirely on the presence of typical symptoms and the exclusion of organic and structured diseases, including GERD and motor disorders with known histopathological basis. Methods of improving the accuracy of symptom-based criteria alone should be sought.

2. *Fundamental mechanisms of symptom production.* The mechanisms responsible for symptoms remain poorly understood. Better detection and classification of the different esophageal stimuli (e.g., acid, weakly acidic and non-acid reflux episodes; motor events) that cause esophageal symptoms is expected from newly available technologies such as multichannel intraluminal impedance monitoring, high-frequency ultrasound probes, and high-resolution manometry. The development of neuro-imaging techniques (e.g., functional MRI) should result in a better understanding of the cerebral processing mechanisms that are activated by different visceral signals such as esophageal acidification and distention. The contributions of motor and sensory dysfunction to esophageal symptoms should be studied and the influence of cognitive and emotional factors should be further explored. The independent contribution of psychological factors, including personality, should be studied in well-designed fashion. Explanations for site specificity should be sought, and initiating and perpetuating processes should be investigated.

3. *Treatment approaches.* Randomized trials of short- and long-acting treatments affecting the esophageal environment (e.g., high-dose antisecretory therapy or drugs reducing transient LES relaxations) are encouraged. The relative utility of such intraluminal modification over approaches affecting perception and reporting of symptoms remains understudied. Although short-term benefits of psychopharmacological treatments in some functional esophageal disorders are determined, long-term outcome is unreported and treatment mechanisms have been poorly delineated. Outcomes from psychological and behavioral interventions remain unknown in most functional esophageal disorders, yet these approaches may be very effective considering the nature of the disorders and associated psychological features.

4. *Health economics.* Important indicators of morbidity from functional esophageal disorders are measures of health care resource use and social dysfunction. Although indirect costs are difficult to measure, attention should be paid not only to absenteeism (i.e., time off work) but also to loss in work productivity [236], which seems to be a better indicator of the economic burden in several functional digestive disorders. Treatment interventions should include short-term and long-term measures of quality of life and functional outcome. The cost-utility value of PPI

tests and of testing over empirical treatment for most functional esophageal disorders remains inappropriately explored or understudied.

Studying the functional esophageal disorders is difficult and these recommendations encourage future research. However, because of the interaction of many factors involved in the pathogenesis of symptoms, studies of multidimensional design that are capable of multivariate analysis are most likely to provide important results.

References

1. Drossman DA, Richter JE, Talley NJ, et al. (eds). The Functional Gastrointestinal Disorders; Diagnosis, Pathophysiology, and treatment: Boston: Little, Brown and Company, 1994.
2. Trimble KC, Douglas S, Pryde A, Heading, RC. Clinical characteristics and natural history of symptomatic but not excess gastroesophageal reflux. Dig Dis Sci 1995; 40:1098–104.
3. Sacher-Huvelin S, Gournay J, Amouretti M, et al. Natural history and quality of life of patients with acid hypersensitive esophagus syndrome. Comparison with classical gastro-esophageal reflux disease. Gastroenterol Clin Biol 2000;24:911–6.
4. Shi G, Bruley des Varannes S, Scarpignato C, et al. Reflux related symptoms in patients with normal oesophageal exposure to acid. Gut 1995;37:457–64.
5. Martinez SD, Malagon IB, Garewal HS, et al. Non-erosive reflux disease (NERD)— acid reflux and symptom patterns. Aliment Pharmacol Ther 2003;17: 537–45.
6. Bruley des Varannes S. The proton-pump inhibitor test: Pros and Cons. Eur J Gastroenterol Hepatol 2004;16(9):847–52.
7. Numans ME, Lau J, de Wit J, Bonis PA. Short-term treatment with proton-pump inhibitors as a test for gastroesophageal reflux disease: a meta-analysis of diagnostic test characteristics. Ann Intern Med 2004;140:518–27.
8. Kahrilas PJ, Quigley EM. Clinical esophageal pH recording: a technical review for practice guideline development. Gastroenterology 1996;110:1982–96.
9. Sifrim D. Acid, weakly acidic and non-acid gastroesophageal reflux: differences, prevalence and clinical relevance. Eur J Gastroenterol Hepatol 2004;16:823–30.
10. Richter JE, Baldi F, Clouse R, et al. Functional esophageal disorders. In: Drossman, DA, et al, (eds). The Functional Gastrointestinal Disorders: Diagnosis, Pathophysiology, and Treatment. Boston: Little, Brown and Company 1994, p 5–70.
11. Locke GR, Talley NJ, Fett SL, et al. Prevalence and clinical spectrum of gastroesophageal reflux: a population-based study in Olmsted Country, Minnesota. Gastroenterology 1997;112:1448–56.
12. Jones RH, Hungin APS, Phillips J, Mills JG. Gastro-oesophageal reflux disease in primary care in Europe: clinical presentation and endoscopic findings. Eur J Gen Pract 1995;1:149–54.
13. Watson RGP, Tham TCK, Johnston BT, McDougall NI. Double blind cross-over pla-

cebo controlled study of omeprazole in the treatment of patients with reflux symptoms and physiological levels of acid reflux—the "sensitive esophagus". Gut 1997; 40:587–90.

14. Khajanchee YS, Hong D, Hansen PD, Swanström LL. Outcomes of antireflux surgery in patients with normal preoperative 24-hour pH test results. Am J Surg 2004; 187:599–603.

15. Thibault R, Sacher-Huvelin S, Gournay J, et al. Antireflux surgery for non erosive reflux disease: a comparative study with reflux esophagitis. Gut 2004;53 (suppl VI) A10.

16. Numans ME, Dewit JN. Reflux symptoms in general practice: diagnostic evaluation of the Carlson-Dent gastro-oesophageal reflux disease questionnaire. Aliment Pharmacol Ther 2003;17:1049–55.

17. Small PK, Loudon MA, Waldron B, et al. Importance of reflux symptoms in functional dyspepsia. Gut 1995;36:189–92.

18. Dent J, Armstrong D, Delanye B, Moayyedi P, Talley NJ, Vakil N. Symptom evaluation in reflux disease: workshop, background, process, terminology, recommendations, and discussion outputs. Gut 2004;53 (Suppl IV): iv1–iv24.

19. Dent J, Brun J, Fendrick M, et al. And the Genval Workshop Group. An evidence-based appraisal of reflux disease management—The Genval Workshop Report. Gut 1999;44 (suppl 2):S1–S16.

20. French-Belgian Consensus Conference on Adult Gastro-Oesophageal Reflux Disease "Diagnosis and Treatment". Eur J Gastroenterol Hepatol 2000;12:129–37.

21. Fletcher J, Wirz A, Henry E, McColl KE. Studies of acid exposure immediately above the gastro-oesophageal squamocolumnar junction: evidence of short segment reflux. Gut 2004;53:168–73.

22. Weusten BLAM, Roelofs JMM, Akkermans LMA, et al. The symptom-association probability: an improved method for symptom analysis of 24-hour esophageal pH data. Gastroenterology 1994;107:1741–5.

23. Van Herwaarden MA, Smout AJPM. Diagnosis of reflux disease. Baillieres Best Pract Res Clin Gastroenterol 2000;14(5):759–74.

24. Carlsson R, Holloway RH. Endoscopy-negative reflux disease. Baillieres Best. Pract Res Clin Gastroenterol 2000;14(5):827–37.

25. Galmiche JP, Bruley des Varannes S. Endoscopy-negative reflux disease. Current Gastroenterology Reports 2001;3:206–14.

26. Fass R. Epidemiology and pathophysiology of symptomatic gastroesophageal reflux disease. Am J Gastroenterol 2003;98:S2–S7.

27. Sifrim D, Holloway R, Silny J, et al. Acid, nonacid, and gas reflux in patients with gastroesophageal reflux disease during ambulatory 24-hour pH-impedance recordings. Gastroenterology 2001;120:1588–98.

28. Vela MF, Camacho-Lobato L, Srinivasan R, et al. Simultaneous intraesophageal impedance and pH measurement of acid and nonacid gastroesophageal reflux: effect of omeprazole. Gastroenterology 2001;120:1599–606.

29. Rodriguez-Stanley S, Robinson M, Earnest DL, et al. Esophageal hypersensitivity may be a major cause of heartburn. Am J Gastroenterol 1999;94:628–31.

30. Fass R, Tougas G. Functional heartburn: the stimulus, the pain, and the brain. Gut 2002;51:885–92.

31. Meyer JH, Lembo A, Elashoff JD, et al. Duodenal fat intensifies the perception of heartburn. Gut 2001;49:624–8.

32. Kern MK, Birn RM, Jaradeh S, et al. Identification and characterization of cerebral cortical response to esophageal mucosal acid exposure and distention. Gastroenterology 1998;115:1353–62.

33. Gregory LJ, Yagüez L, Williiams SC, et al. Cognitive modulation of the cerebral processing of human oesophageal sensation using functional magnetic resonance imaging. Gut 2003;52:1671–7.

34. Hu WHC, Wong WM, Lam CLK, et al. Anxiety but not depression determines health care-seeking behaviour in Chinese patients with dyspepsia and irritable bowel syndrome: a population-based study. Aliment Pharmacol Ther 2002;16:2081–8.

35. Fass R, Malagon I, Naliboff BD, et al. Effect of psychologically induced stress on symptom perception & autonomic nervous system response of patients (pts.) with erosive esophagitis (EE) and non-erosive reflux disease (NERD). Gastroenterology 2000;118:A637.

36. Bradley LA, Richter JE, Pulliam TJ, et al. The relationship between stress and symptoms of gastroesophageal reflux: The influence of psychological factors. Am J Gastroenterol 1993;88:11–9.

37. McDonald-Haile J, Bradley LA, Bailey MA, et al. Relaxation training reduces symptom reports and acid exposure in patients with gastroesophageal reflux disease. Gastroenterology 1994;107:61–9.

38. Tew S, Jamieson GG, Pilowsky I, Myers J. The illness behavior of patients with gastroesophageal reflux disease with and without endoscopic esophagitis. Dis Esophagus 1997;10:9–15.

39. Johnston BT, Lewis SA, Love AH. Stress, personality and social support in gastro-esophageal reflux disease. J Psychosom Res 1995;39:221–6.

40. Johnston BT, Lewis SA, Collins JS, et al. Acid perception in gastro-oesophageal reflux disease is dependent on psychosocial factors. Scand J Gastroenterol 1995;30:1–5.

41. DeVault KR, Castell DO. Updated guidelines for the diagnosis and treatment of gastroesophageal reflux disease. The Practice Parameters Committee of the American College of Gastroenterology. Am J Gastroenterol 1999;94:1434–42.

42. Lind T, Havelund T, Carlsson R, et al. Heartburn without oesophagitis: Efficacy of omeprazole therapy and features determining therapeutic response. Scand J Gastroenterol 1997;32:974–9.

43. Vaezi MF, Richter JE. Duodenogastroesophageal reflux and methods to monitor nonacidic reflux. Am J Med 2001;111(suppl 8A):160S-168S.

44. Koek GH, Sifrim D, Lerut T, et al. Effect of the GABA(B) agonist baclofen in patients with symptoms and duodeno-gastro-oesophageal reflux refractory to proton pump inhibitors. Gut 2003;52:1397–402.

45. Lidums I, Lehmann A, Checklin H, et al. Control of transient lower esophageal sphincter relaxations and reflux by the GABA(B) agonist baclofen in normal subjects. Gastroenterology 2000;118:7–13.

46. Zhang Q, Lehmann A, Rigda R, et al. Control of transient lower oesophageal sphincter relaxations and reflux by the GABA(B) agonist baclofen in patients with gastro-oesophageal reflux disease. Gut 2002;50:19–24.

47. Ciccaglione AF, Marzio L. Effect of acute and chronic administration of the $GABA_B$ agonist baclofen on 24 hour pH metry and symptoms in control subjects and in patients with gastro-oesophageal reflux disease. Gut 2003;52:464–70.

48. Kemp HG, Vokonas PS, Cohn PF, et al. The anginal syndrome associated with nor-

mal coronary arteriograms. Report of a six year experience. Am J Med 1973;54:735–42.

49. Richter JE, Bradley LA, Castell DO. Esophageal chest pain: current controversies in pathogenesis, diagnosis and treatment. Ann Intern Med 1989;110:66–78.

50. Drossman DA, Li Z, Andruzzi E, Temple RD, et al. U.S. householders survey of functional gastrointestinal disorders. Prevalence, sociodemography and health impact. Dig Dis Sci 1993;38:1569–80.

51. Kemp HG, Kronmal RA, Vlietstra RE, et al. Seven year survival of patients with normal or near normal coronary arteriograms. A CASS registry study. J Am College Cardiol 1986;7:479–83.

52. Pasternak RC, Thibault GE, Savoia M, et al. Chest pain with angiographically insignificant coronary arterial obstruction: clinical presentation and long-term follow-up. Am J Med 1980;68:813–7.

53. Wiekgosz AT, Gletcher RH, McCants CB, et al. Unimproved chest pain in patients with minimal or no coronary disease: a behaviorial problem. Am Heart J 1984;108:67–72.

54. Bruschke AVG, Proudfit WL, Sones FM. Clinical course of patients with normal, and slightly or moderately abnormal coronary angiogram. A follow-up study on 500 patients. Circulation 1973;47:936–45.

55. Proudfit WL, Bruschke AVG, Sones FM. Clinical course of patients with normal or slightly or moderately abnormal coronary arteriograms: 10 year follow-up of 521 patients. Circulation 1980;62:712–7.

56. Nevens F, Janssens J, Piessens J, et al. Prospective study on prevalence of esophageal chest pain in patients referred on an elective basis to a cardiac unit for suspected myocardial ischemia. Dig Dis Sci 1991;36:229–35.

57. Klingler, D, Green-Weir, R, Nerenz, D, Havstad, S, Rosman, HS, Cetner, L, et al. Perceptions of chest pain differ by race. Am Heart J 2002;144:51–9.

58. Lux G, Van Els J, The GS, et al. Ambulatory esophageal pressure, pH and ECG recording in patients with normal and pathological coronary angiography and intermittent chest pain. Neurogastroenterol Motil 1995;7:23–30.

59. Cannon RO, Epstein JE. "Microvascular angina" as a cause of chest pain with angiographically normal coronary arteries. Am J Cardiol 1988;61:1338–43.

60. Cannon RO, Quyyumi AA, Schenke WH. Abnormal cardiac sensitivity in patients with chest pain and normal coronary arteries. J Am College Cardiol 1990;16:1359–66.

61. Frobert O, Funch-Jensen P, Jacobsen NO, al. Upper endoscopy in patients with angina and normal coronary angiograms. Endoscopy 1995;27:365–70.

62. Pandak WM, Arezo S, Everett S, et al. Short course of omeprazole: a better first diagnostic approach to noncardiac chest pain than endoscopy, manometry, or 24-hour esophageal pH monitoring. J Clin Gastroenterol 2002;35:307–14.

63. Ho, KY, Ng WL, Kang JY, Yeoh KG. Gastroesophageal reflux disease is a common cause of noncardiac chest pain in a country with a low prevalence of reflux esophagitis. Dig Dis Sci 1998;43:1991–7.

64. Richter JE, Hewson EG, Sinclair JW, Dalton CB. Acid perfusion test and 24-hour esophageal pH monitoring with symptom index. Comparison of tests for esophageal sensitivity. Dig Dis Sci 1991;36:565–71.

65. Paterson WG, Abdollah H, Beck IT, Da Costa LR. Ambulatory esophageal manometry, pH-metry and Holter monitoring in patients with atypical chest pain. Dig Dis Sci 1992;38:795–802.

66. Hewson EG, Dalton CB, Richter JE. Comparison of esophageal manometry, provocative testing, and ambulatory monitoring in patients with unexplained chest pain. Dig Dis Sci 1990;35:302–9.

67. Wiener GJ, Richter JE, Copper JB, Wu WC, Castell DO. The symptom index: a clinically important parameter of ambulatory 24-hour esophageal pH monitoring. Am J Gastroenterol 1988;83:358–61.

68. Trimble KD, Pryde A, Heading RC. Lowered oesophageal sensory thresholds in patients with symptomatic but not excess gastro-oesophageal reflux: evidence for a spectrum of visceral sensitivity in GORD. Gut 1995;37:7–12.

69. Janssens J, Vantrappen G, Ghillebert G. 24-hour recording of esophageal pressure and pH in patients with non-cardiac chest pain. Gastroenterology 1986;90:1978–84.

70. de Caestecker JS, Blackwell J, Brown J, Heading RC. The oesophagus as a cause of recurrent chest pain: which patients should be investigated and which tests should be used? Lancet 1985;2:1143–6.

71. Lacima G, Grande L, Pera M, Francino A, Ros E. Utility of ambulatory 24-hour esophageal pH and motility monitoring in noncardiac chest pain: report of 90 patients and review of the literature. Dig Dis Sci 2003;48:952–61;

72. Breumelhof R, Nadorp JHSM, Akkermans LMA, Smout AJPM. Analysis of 24-hour esophageal pressure and pH data in unselected patients with noncardiac chest pain. Gastroenterology 1990;99:1257–64.

73. Soffer EE, Scalabrini P, Wingate DL. Spontaneous noncardiac chest pain: value of ambulatory esophageal pH and motility monitoring. Dig Dis Sci 1989;34:1651–5.

74. Ghillebert G, Janssens J, Vantrappen G, et al. Ambulatory 24 hour intraoesophageal pH and pressure recording v provocation tests in the diagnosis of chest pain of oesophageal origin. Gut 1990;31:738–44.

75. Lam HG, Dekker W, Kan G, et al, AJ Acute noncardiac chest pain in a coronary care unit. Evaluation by 24-hour pressure and pH recording of the esophagus. Gastroenterology 1992;102:453–60.

76. Voskuil JH, Cramer MJ, Breumelhof, et al. Prevalence of esophageal disorders in patients with chest pain newly referred to the cardiologist. Chest 1996;189:1210–4.

77. DeMeester TR, O'Sullivan GC, Bermudez G, et al. Esophageal function in patients with angina-type chest pain and normal coronary angiogram. Ann Surg 1982;196:488–98.

78. Schofield PM, Bennett DH, Whorwell PJ, et al. Exertional gastro-esophageal reflux: a mechanism for symptoms in patients with angina pectoris and normal coronary angiograms. Br. Med J 1987;294:1459–61.

79. Fass R, Fennerty MB, Ofman JJ, et al. The clinical and economic value of a short course of omeprazole in patients with noncardiac chest pain. Gastroenterology 1998;115:42–9.

80. Ofman JJ, Gralnek IM, Udani Y, et al. The cost-effectiveness of the omeprazole test in patients with noncardiac chest pain. Am J Med 1999;107:219–27.

81. Borzecki AM, Pedrosa MC, Prashker MJ. Should noncardiac chest pain be treated empirically? A cost-effectiveness analysis. Arch Intern Med 2000;160:844–52.

82. Fass R, Fennerty MB, Johnson C, et al. Correlation of ambulatory 24-hour esophageal pH monitoring results with symptom improvement in patients with noncardiac chest pain due to gastroesophageal reflux disease. J Clin Gastroenterol 1999;28:36–9.

83. Kahrilas PJ, Clouse RE, Hogan WJ. American Gastroenterological Association technical review on the clinical use of esophageal manometry. Gastroenterology 1994; 107:1865–84.

84. Galmiche JP, Scarpignato C. Oesophageal sensitivity to acid in patients with noncardiac chest pain: is the oesophagus hypersensitive ? Eur J Gastroenterol Hepatol 1995;7:1152–9.

85. Richter JE, Barish CF, Castell DO. Abnormal sensory perception in patients with esophageal chest pain. Gastroenterology 1986;91:845–52.

86. Barish CF, Castell DO, Richter, JE. Graded esophageal balloon distension. A new provocative test for noncardiac chest pain. Dig Dis Sci 1986;31:1292–8.

87. Rao SSC, Gregersen H, Hayek B, et al. J Unexplained chest pain: the hypersensitive, hyperactive, and poorly compliant esophagus. Ann Intern Med 1996;124:950–8.

88. Hu WHC, Martin CJ, Talley NJ. Intraesophageal acid perfusion sensitizes the esophagus to mechanical distension: a barostat study. Am J Gastroenterol 2000;95: 2189–94.

89. Sarkar S, Aziz Q, Woolf CJ, et al. Contribution of central sensitisation to the development of non-cardiac chest pain. Lancet 2000;356:1154–9.

90. Fass R, Naliboff B, Higa L, et al. Differential effect of long-term esophageal acid exposure on mechanosensitivity and chemosensitivity in humans. Gastroenterology 1998; 115:1363–73.

91. Howard PJ, Pryde A, Heading RC. Oesophageal manometry during eating in the investigation of patients with chest pain or dysphagia. Gut 1989.30:1179–86.

92. Kahrilas PJ, Dodds WJ, Hogan WJ. Dysfunction of the belch reflex. A cause of incapitating chest pain. Gastroenterology 1987;93:818–22.

93. Snedegar CT, Haroian LR, Clouse RE. High-resolution manometry (HRM) reveals bolus entrapment in the proximal esophagus with double swallows in patients with spastic motor disorders. Gastroenterology 2004;126 (suppl 2):A-635.

94. Clouse RE, Richter JE, Heading RC, et al. In: Drossman DA, Corazziari E, Talley NJ, Thompson WG, Whitehead WE. Rome II. The Functional Gastrointestinal Disorders. Diagnosis, Pathophysiology and Treatment: A Multinational Consensus (2nd edition). McClean, Virginia, Degnon Associates, 2000: 247–98.

95. Bradley LA, Scarinci IC, Richter JE. Pain threshold levels and coping strategies among patients who have chest pain and normal coronary arteries. Med Clin North Am 1991;75:1189–202.

96. Bradley LA, Richter JE, Scarinci IC, et al. Psychosocial and psychophysical assessments of patients with unexplained chest pain. Am J Med 1992;92 (suppl 5A):65–73.

97. Whitehead WE, Palsson OS. Is rectal pain sensitivity a biological marker for irritable bowel syndrome: psychological influences on pain perception. Gastroenterology 1998;115:1263–71.

98. Hollerbach S, Bulat R, May A, et al. Abnormal cerebral processing of oesophageal stimuli in patients with noncardiac chest pain (NCCP). Neurogastroenterol Motil 2000;12:555–65.

99. Fallen EL, Kamath MV, Tougas G, Upton A. Afferent vagal modulation. Clinical studies of visceral sensory input. Auton Neurosci 2001;90:35–40.

100. Tougas G, Spaziani R, Hollerbach S, et al. Cardiac autonomic function and oesophageal acid sensitivity in patients with non-cardiac chest pain. Gut 2001;49:706–12.

101. Clouse RE. Spastic disorders of the esophagus. Gastroenterologist 1997;5:112–27.

102. Richter JE, Dalton CB, Bradley LA, Castell DO. Oral nifedipine in the treatment of non-cardiac chest pain patients with the nutcracker esophagus. Gastroenterology 1987;93:21–8.

103. Balaban DH, Yamamoto Y, Liu J, Pehlivanov N, Wisniewski R, DeSilvey D, Mittal RK. Sustained esophageal contraction: a marker of esophageal chest pain identified by intraluminal ultrasonography. Gastroenterology 1999;116:29–37.

104. Borjesson, M, Pilhall, M, Eliasson, T, Norssel, H, Mannheimer, C, Rolny, P. Esophageal visceral pain sensitivity: effects of TENS and correlation with manometric findings. Dig Dis Sci 1998;43:1621–8.

105. Mujica VR, Mudipalli RS, Rao SS. Pathophysiology of chest pain in patients with nutcracker esophagus. Am J Gastroenterol 2001;96:1371–7.

106. Rao SSC, Hayek B, Summers RW. Functional chest pain of esophageal origin: hyperalgesia or motor dysfunction. Am J Gastroenterol 2001;96:2584–9.

107. Zhang X, Tack J, Janssens J, Sifrim DA. Neural regulation of tone in the oesophageal body: in vivo barostat assessment of volume-pressure relationships in the feline oesophagus. Neurogastroenterol. Motility 2004;16:13–21.

108. Eslick GD, Jones MP, Talley NJ. Non-cardiac chest pain: prevalence, risk factors, impact and consulting-a population-based study. Aliment Pharmacol Ther 2003; 17:1115–24.

109. Clouse RE, Lustman PJ Psychiatric illness and contraction abnormalities of the esophagus. N Engl J Med 1983309:1337–42.

110. Richter JE, Obrecht WF, Bradley LA, et al. Psychological comparison of patients with nutcracker esophagus and irritable bowel syndrome. Dig Dis Sci 1986;31:131–8.

111. Bass C, Wade C. Chest pain with normal coronary arteries: a comparative study of psychiatric and social morbidity. Psychol Med 198414:51–61.

112. Alexander PJ, Prabhu SG, Krishnamoorthy ES, Halkatti PC. Mental disorders in patients with noncardiac chest pain. Acta Psychiatr Scand 1994;89:291–3.

113. Aikens JE, Zvolensky MJ, Eifert GH. Differential fear of cardiopulmonary sensations in emergency room noncardiac chest pain patients. J Behav Med 2001;24:155–67.

114. Maunder RG. Panic disorder associated with gastrointestinal disease: review and hypotheses. J Psychosom Res 1998;44:91–105.

115. Fleet RP, Dupuis G, Marchand A, et al. Panic disorder in emergency department chest pain patients: prevalence, comorbidy, suicidal ideation, and physician recognition. Am J Med 1996;101:371–80.

116. Stollman NH, Bierman PS, Ribeiro A, et al. CO_2 provocation of panic: symptomatic and manometric evaluation in patients with noncardiac chest pain. Am J Gastroenterol 1997;92:839–42.

117. Clouse RE, Lustman PJ, Eckert TC, et al. Low-dose trazodone for symptomatic patients with esophageal contraction abnormalities: double-blind, placebo-controlled trial. Gastroenterology 1987;92:1027–36.

118. Ringel Y, Drossman DA, Dyson T, et al. Characterization of physiological and psychological factors in functional esophageal disorders. Gastroenterology 2004;126 (suppl 2):A-28.

119. Song CW, Lee SJ, Jeen YT, et al. Inconsistent association of esophageal symptoms, psychometric abnormalities and dysmotility. Am J Gastroenterol 2001;96:2312–6.

120. Rubin J, Nagler R, Sprio HM, Pilot ML. Measuring the effect of emotions on esophageal motility. Psychosom. Med 1962;24:170–6.

121. Stacher G, Schmierer C, Landgraf M. Tertiary esophageal contractions evoked by acoustic stimuli. Gastroenterology 1979;44:49–54.
122. Anderson KO, Dalton CB, Bradley LA, Richter JE. Stressinduces alteration of esophageal pressures in healthy volunteers and non-cardiac chest pain patients. Dig Dis Sci 1989;34: 83–91.
123. Keshavarzian A, Iber FL, Ferguson Y. Esophageal manometry and radionuclide emptying in chronic alcoholics. Gastroenterology 1987;92:651–7.
124. Lantinga LJ, Sprafkin RP, McCroskery JH, et al. One-year psychosocial follow-up of patients with chest pain and angiographically normal coronary arteries. Am J Cardiol 1988;62:209–13.
125. Clouse RE. Therapy of functional gastrointestinal syndromes. J Funct Syndr 2001; 1:61–8
126. Ward BW, Wu WC, Richter JE, et al. Long-term follow-up of symptomatic status of patients with non-cardiac chest pain: is diagnosis of esophageal etiology helpful? AmJGastroenterol 1987;82:215–8.
127. Ockene IS, Shay MJ, Alpart JA, et al. Unexplained chest pain in patients with normal coronary arteriograms. A follow-up study of functional status. N Engl J Med 1980;303:1249–52.
128. Schofield PM. Follow-up study of morbidity in patients with angina pectoris and normal coronary angiograms and the value of investigation for esophageal dysfunction. Angiology 1990;41:286–96.
129. Swift GL, Alban-Davies N, McKirdy H, et al. A long term clinical review of patients with esophageal pain. Q J Med 1994;29:937–44.
130. Tew R, Guthrie EA, Creed FH, et al. A long-term follow-up study of patients with ischaemic heart disease versus patients with nonspecific chest pain. J Psychosom Res 1995;39:977–85.
131. Roll M, Kollind M, Theorell T. Five-year follow-up of young adults visiting an emergency unit because of atypical chest pain. J Intern Med 1992;231:59–65.
132. Peski-Oosterbaan AS, Spinhoven P, van der Does AJ, Bruschke AV. Noncardiac chest pain: interest in a medical psychological treatment. J Psychosom Res 1998;45: 471–6.
133. Clouse RE. Central nervous system approaches for treating functional disorders: how, when, and why? J Pediatr Gastroenterol Nutr 2004;39(3):S763–5.
134. Xia HH, Lai KC, Lam SK, et al. Symptomatic response to lansoprazole predicts abnormal acid reflux in endoscopy-negative patients with non-cardiac chest pain. Aliment Pharmacol Ther 2003;17:369–77.
135. Davies HA, Lewis MJ, Rhodes J, Henderson AH. Trial of nifedipine for prevention of esophageal spasm. Digestion 1987;36:81–3.
136. Cattau EL, Castell DO, Johnson DA, et al. Diltiazem therapy of symptoms associated with nutcracker esophagus. Am J Gastroenterol 1991;86(3):272–6.
137. Frachtman RL, Botoman VA, Pope CE. A double-blind crossover trial of diltiazem shows no benefit in patients with dysphagia and/or chest pain of esophageal origin. Gastroenterology 1986;90:140.
138. de Caestecker JS, Pryde A, Heading RC. Site and mechanism of pain perception with esophageal balloon distension and intravenous edrophonium in patients with esophageal chest pain. Gut 1992;33:580–6.
139. Clouse RE. Antidepressants for functional gastrointestinal syndromes. Dig Dis Sci 1994;39:2352–63.

140. Clouse RE, Lustman PJ. Antidepressants for irritable bowel syndrome. In: Camilleri M, Spiller RC (eds.). Irritable Bowel Syndrome: Diagnosis and Treatment. London: WB Saunders, 2002;161–71.

141. Cannon RO, Quyyumi A, Mincemoyer R, et al. Imipramine in patients with chest pain despite normal coronary angiograms. N Engl J Med 1994;330:1411–7.

142. Jackson JL, O'Malley PG, Tomkins G, et al. Treatment of functional gastrointestinal disorders with antidepressant medications: a meta-analysis. Am J Med 2000; 108:65–72.

143. Prakash C, Clouse RE. Long-term outcome from tricyclic antidepressant treatment of functional chest pain. Dig Dis Sci 1999;44:2373–9.

144. Varia I, Logue E, O'connor C, et al. Randomized trial of sertraline in patients with unexplained chest pain of noncardiac origin. Am Heart J 2002;140:367–72.

145. Clouse RE. Antidepressants for irritable bowel syndrome. Gut 2003;52:598–9.

146. Eslick GD, Fass R. Noncardiac chest pain: evaluation and treatment. Gastroenterol Clin North Am 200332:531–52.

147. Botoman VA. Noncardiac chest pain. J ClinGastroenterol 2002;34: 6–14.

148. Shrestha S, Pasricha PJ Update on noncardiac chest pain. Dig Dis 2000;18:138–146.

149. Hegel MT, Abel GG, Etscheidt M, Cohen-Cole S, Wilmer, CI. Behavioral treatment of angina-like chest pain in patients with hyperventilation syndrome. J Behav Ther Exp Psychiatry 1989;20:31–9.

150. Klimes I, Mayou RA, Pearce MJ, Coles L, Fagg JP. Psychological treatment of atypical non-cardiac chest pain: a controlled evaluation. Psychol Med 1990;20:605–11.

151. Potts SG, Lewin R, Fox KAA, Johnstone EC. Group psychological treatment for chest pain with normal coronary arteries. Q J Med 1999;92:81–6.

152. Peski-Oosterbaan AS, Spinhoven P, van Rood Y et al. Cognitive-behavioral therapy for noncardiac chest pain: a randomized trial. Am J Med 1999;106: 424–9.

153. Looper KJ, Kirmayer LJ Behavioral medicine approaches to somatoform disorders. J Consult Clin Psychol 2002;70:810–27.

154. Mayou RA, Bass CM, Bryant BM. Management of non-cardiac chest pain: from research to clinical practice. Heart 1999;81:387–92.

155. Miller LS, Pullela SV, Parkman HP, et al. Treatment of chest pain in patients with noncardiac, nonreflux, nonachalasia spastic esophageal motor disorders using botulinum toxin injection into the gastroesophageal junction. Am J Gastroenterol 2002;97:1640–46.

156. Storr M, Allescher HD, Rosch T et al. Treatment of symptomatic diffuse esophageal spasm by endoscopic injections of botulinum toxin: a prospective study with long term follow-up. Gastrointest Endosc 2001;54:754–9.

157. Rao SS, Mudipalli RS, Mujica V, et al. An open-label trial of theophylline for functional chest pain. Dig Dis Sci 2002;47:2763–8.

158. Eherer, AJ, Schwetz, I, Hammer, HF, et al. Effect of sildenafil on oesophageal motor function in healthy subjects and patients with oesophageal motor disorders. Gut 2002;50:758–64.

159. Lee JI, Park H, Kim JH, et al.The effect of sildenafil on oesophageal motor function in healthy subjects and patients with nutcracker oesophagus. Neurogastroenterol Motil 2003;15:617.

160. Floch NR. Surgical therapy for atypical symptoms of GERD: patient selection and preoperative evaluation. J ClinGastroenterol 2000;30:S45–S47.

161. Campos GM, Peters JH, DeMeester TR, et al. Multivariate analysis of factors pre-

dicting outcome after laparoscopic Nissen fundoplication. J Gastrointest Surg 1999; 3:292–300.

162. Ellis FH Jr. Long esophagomyotomy for diffuse esophageal spasm and related disorders: an historical overview. Dis Esophagus 1998;11:210–4.

163. Kwan AC, Bao TN, Chakkaphak S, et al. Functional gastrointestinal disorders, validation of Rome II criteria for functional gastrointestinal disorders by factor analysis of symptoms in Asian patient sample. J Gastroenterol Hepatol 2003;18:796–802.

164. Lind CD. Dysphagia: evaluation and treatment. Gastroenterol Clin North Am 2003; 32:553–75.

165. Davies HA, Evans KT, Butler F et al. Diagnostic value of "bread-barium" swallow in patients with esophageal symptoms. Dig Dis Sci 1983;28:1094–100.

166. Cordier L, Bohn B, Bonaz B, et al. Evaluation of esophageal motility disorders triggered by ingestion of solids in the case of non-obstructive dysphagia. Gastroenterol Clin Biol 1999;23:200–6.

167. Richter JE, Castell O. Diffuse esophageal spasm: a reappraisal. Ann Intern Med 1984;100:242–5.

168. Hewson EG, Ott DJ, Dalton CB, et al. Manometry and radiology. Complementary studies in the assessment of esophageal motility disorders. Gastroenterology 1990;98:626–32.

169. Deschner WK, Maher KA, Cattau E, Benjamin SB. Manometric responses to balloon distention in patients with nonobstructive dysphagia. Gastroenterology 1989; 97:1181–5.

170. Kahrilas PJ, Dodds WJ, Hogan WJ The effect of peristaltic dysfunction on esopha geal volume clearance. Gastroenterology 1988;94:73–80.

171. Tutuian R, Castell DO. Clarification of the esophageal function defect in patients with manometric ineffective esophageal motility. Clin Gastroenterol Hepatol 2004; 2:230–6.

172. Jacob P, Kahrilas PJ, Vanagunas A. Peristaltic dysfunction associated with nonobstructive dysphagia in reflux disease. Dig Dis Sci 1990;35:939–42.

173. Triadafilopoulos G. Nonobstructive dysphagia in reflux esophagitis. Am J Gastroenterol 1989;84:614–8.

174. Howard PJ, Maher L, Pryde A, et al. Esophageal motor patterns during episodes of dysphagia for solids. J Gastrointest Motil 1991;3:123–30.

175. Clouse RE, McCord GS, Lustman PJ, Edmundowicz SA. Clinical correlates of abnormal sensitivity to intraesophageal balloon distention. Dig Dis Sci 1991;36:1040–5.

176. Faulkner WB, Rudenbaugh FH, O'Neill, Jr. Influence of the emotions on esophageal function: comparison of esophagoscopic and roentgenologic findings. Radiology 1942;37:443–7.

177. Wolf S, Almy RP. Experimental observations on cardiospasm in man. Gastroenterology 1949;13:401–2.

178. Clouse RE, Carney RM. The psychological profile of non-cardiac chest pain patients. Eur J Gastroenterol Hepatol 1995;7:1160–5.

179. Vakil NB, Traxler B, Levine D. Dysphagia in patients with erosive esophagitis: prevalence, severity, and response to proton pump inhibitor treatment. Clin Gastroenterol Hepatol 2004;2: 665–8.

180. Gorelick AB, Koshy SS, Hooper FG, et al. Differential effects of amitriptyline on perception of somatic and visceral stimulation in healthy humans. Am J Physiol 1998;275:G460–66.

181. Peghini PI, Katz PO, Castell DO. Imipramine decreases oesophageal pain perception in human male volunteers. Gut 1998;42:807–13.

182. Marshall JB. Dysphagia. Diagnostic pitfalls and how to avoid them. Postgrad Med 1989;85:243–60.

183. Clouse RE. Apporach to the patient with dysphagia orodynophagia. In: Yamada, T, Alpers, DH, Kaplowitz, N, Laine, L, Owynag, C, Poweln, DW (eds). Textbook of Gastroenterology (4th edition). Philadelphia: Lippincott Williams and Wilkins, 2003, p. 678–691.

184. Winters C, Artnak EJ, Benjamin SB, et al. Esophageal bougienage in symptomatic patients with nutcracker esophagus. JAMA 1984;252:363–6.

185. Ebert EC, Ouyang A, Wright SH, et al. Pneumatic dilatation in patients with symptomatic diffuse esophageal spasm and lower esophageal sphincter dysfunction. Dig Dis Sci 1983;28:481–5.

186. Batch AJG. Globus pharyngeus (part I). J Laryngol Otol 1988;102:152–8.

187. Deary IJ, Wilson JA, Harris MB, MacDougall G. Globus pharyngis: development of a symptom assessment scale. J Psychosom Res 1995;39:203–13.

188. Thompson W, Heaton K. Heartburn and globus on apparently healthy people. Can Med Assoc J 1982;126:46–8.

189. Rowley H, O'Dwyer TP, Jones AS, Timon CI. The natural history of globus pharyngeus. Laryngoscope 1995;105:1118–21.

190. Malcomson K. Radiological findings in globus hystericus. Br J Radiol 1966;39: 583–6.

191. Ravich WJ, Wilson RS, Jones B, Donner MW. Psychogenic Dysphagia and Globus: Reevaluation of 23 Patients. Dysphagia 1989;4:35–8

192. Wilson JA, Murray JM, Haacke NP. Rigid endoscopy in ENT practice: appraisal of the diagnostic yield in a district general hospital. J Laryngol Otol 1987;101:286–92.

193. Timon C, O'Dwyer T, Cagney D, Walsh M. Globus pharyngeus: long-term follow-up and prognostic factors. Ann Otol Rhinol Laryngol 1991;100:351–4.

194. Ruth M, Mansson I, Sandberg N. The prevalence of symptoms suggestive of esophageal disorders. Scand J Gastroenterol 1991;26:73–81.

195. Moloy P, Charter R. The globus symptom. Incidence, therapeutic response, and age and sex relationships. Arch Otolaryngol 1982;108:740–4.

196. Wilson J, Pryde A, Piris J, et al. Pharyngoesophageal dysmotility in globus sensation. Arch Otolaryngol Head Neck Surg 1989;115:1086–90.

197. Webb CJ, Makura ZG, Fenton JE, et al. Globus pharyngeus: a postal questionnaire survey of UK ENT consultants. Clin Otolaryngol 2000;25:566–9.

198. Back GW, Leong P, Kumar R, Corbridge R. Value of barium swallow in investigation of globus pharyngeus. J Laryngol Otol 2000;114:951–4.

199. Wilson J, Heading R, Maran A, et al.Globus sensation is not due to gastro-oesophageal reflux. Clin Otolaryngol 1987;12:271–5.

200. Delahunty J, Ardran G. Globus hystericus—a manifestation of reflux oesophagitis? J Laryngol Otol 1970;84:1049–54.

201. Mair IW, Schroder KE, Modalsli B, Maurer HJ Aetiological aspects of the globus symptom. J Laryngol Otol 1975;88:1033–40.

202. Dyer WH, Pridie RB. Incidence of hiatus hernia in asymptomatic subjects. Gut 1968;9:696–9.

203. Wienbeck M, Barnert J Epidemiology of reflux disease and reflux esophagitis. Scand J Gastroenterol 1989;156:7–13.

204. Clements JL, Cox GW, Torres WE, Weens HS. Cervical esophageal webs: a roentgenanatomic correlation. Observations on the pharyngoesophagus. Am J Roentgenol Radium Ther Nucl Med 1974;121(2): 221–31.

205. Curtis DJ, Cruess DF, Berg T. The cricopharyngeal muscle: a videorecording review. Am J Roentgenol 1984;142 :497–500.

206. Watson W, Sullivan S. Hypertonicity of the cricopharyngeal sphincter: a cause of globus sensation. Lancet 1974;2:1417–9.

207. Cook IJ, Dent J, Shannon S, Collins SM. Measurement of upper esophageal sphincter pressure. Effect of acute emotional stress. Gastroenterology 1987;93:26–32.

208. Cook IJ, Dent J, Collins SM. Upper esophageal sphincter tone and reactivity to stress in patients with a history of globus sensation. Dig Dis Sci 1989;34:672–6.

209. Linsell J, Anggiansah A, Owen W. Manometric findings in patients with the globus sensation. Gut 1987;28:A1378.

210. Cook I, Shaker R, Dodds W, Hogan W, Arndorfer R. Role of mechanical and chemical stimulation of the esophagus in globus sensation. Gastroenterology 1989;96: A99.

211. Moser G, Wenzel-Abatzi TA, Stelzeneder M, et al. Globus sensation: pharyngoesophageal function, psychometric and psychiatric findings, and follow-up in 88 patients. Arch Intern Med 1998;158:1365–73.

212. Gray L. The relationship of the 'inferior constrictor swallow' and 'globus hystericus' or the hypopharyngeal syndrome. J Laryngol Otol 1983;97:607–18.

213. Moser G, Vacariu-Granser G, Schneider C, et al. High incidence of esophageal motor disorder in consecutive patients with globus sensation. Gastroenterology 1991;101:1512–21.

214. Leelamanit V, Geater A, Sinkitjaroenchai W. A study of 111 cases of globus hystericus. J Med Assoc Thai 1996;79:460–7.

215. Farkkila MA, Ertama L, Katila H, et al. Globus pharyngis, commonly associated with esophageal motility disorders. Am J Gastroenterol 1994;89:503–8.

216. Hill J, Stuart RC, Fung HK, et al. Gastroesophageal reflux, motility disorders, and psychological profiles in the etiology of globus pharyngis. Laryngoscope 1997;107: 1373–7.

217. Andersen LIB, Madsen PV, Dalgaard P, Jensen G. Validity of clinical symptoms in benign esophageal disease, assessed by questionnaire. Acta Med Scand 1897;221: 171–7.

218. Ollyo JB, Monnier P, Fontolliet C, Savary M. The natural history, prevalence and incidence of reflux oesophagitis. Gullet 1993;3:1–10.

219. Lindgren S, Janzon L. Prevalence of swallowing complaints and clinical findings among 50–79–year-old men and women in an urban population. Dysphagia 1991; 6:187–92.

220. Ott DJ, Ledbetter MS, Koufman JA, Chen MY. Globus pharyngeus: radiographic evaluation and 24-hour pH monitoring of the pharynx and esophagus in 22 patients. Radiology 1894;191:95–7.

221. Corso MJ, Pursnani KG, Mohiuddin MA, et al. Globus sensation is associated with hypertensive upper esophageal sphincter but not with gastroesophageal reflux. Dig Dis Sci 1998;43:1513–7.

222. Curran AJ, Barry MK, Callanan V, Gormley PK. A prospective study of acid reflux and globus pharyngeus using a modified symptom index. Clin Otolaryngol 1995; 20:552–4.

223. Woo P, Noordzij P, Ross JA. Association of esophageal reflux and globus symptom: comparison of laryngoscopy and 24-hour pH manometry. Otolaryngology—Head & Neck Surgery 1996;115:502–7.

224. Chevalier JM, Brossard E, Monnier P. Globus sensation and gastroesophageal reflux. Eur Arch Otorhinolaryngol 2003;260:273–6.

225. Puhakka H, Lehtinen V, Aalto T. Globus hystericus—a psychosomatic disease? J Laryngol Otol 1976;90:1021–6.

226. Pratt LW, Tobin WH, Gallagher RA. Globus hystericus—office evaluation by psychological testing with the MMPI. Laryngoscope 1976;86:1540–51.

227. Deary IJ, Smart A, Wilson JA. Depression and "hassles" in globus pharyngis. Br J Psychiatry 1992;161:115–7.

228. Deary IJ, Wilson JA, Kelly SW. Globus pharyngis, personality, and psychological distress in the general population. Psychosomatics 1995;36:570–7.

229. Harris MB, Deary IJ, Wilson JA. Life events and difficulties in relation to the onset of globus pharyngis. J Psychosom Res 1996;40:603–15.

230. Deary IJ, Wilson JA, Mitchell L, Marschall T. Covert psychiatric disturbance in patients with globus pharyngis. Br J Med Psychol 1989;62: 381–9.

231. Kibblewhite DJ, Morrison MD. A double-blind controlled study of the efficacy of cimetidine in the treatment of the cervical symptoms of gastroesophageal reflux. J Otolaryngol 1990;19:103–9.

232. Koufman JA. The otolaryngologic manifestations of gastroesophageal reflux disease (GERD): A clinical investigation of 225 patients using ambulatory 24-hour pH monitoring and an experimental investigation of the role acid and pepsin in the development of laryngeal injury. Laryngoscope 1991;101:1–78.

233. Tokashiki R, Yamaguchi H, Nakamura K, Suzuki M. Globus sensation caused by gastroesophageal reflux disease. Auris Nasus Larynx 2002;29:347–51.

234. Leelamanit V, Geater A, Ovartlarnporn T. Cisapride in the treatment of globus hystericus. Adv Otorhinolaryngol 1997;51:112–24.

235. Brown SR, Schwartz JM, Summergrad P, Jenike MA. Globus hystericus syndrome responsive to antidepressants. Am J Psychiatry 1986;143:917–8.

236. Dean BB, Crawley JA, Schmitt CM, Wong J, Ofman JJ The burden of illness of gastro-oesophageal reflux disease: impact on work productivity. Aliment Pharmacol Ther 2003;17:1309–17.

Chapter 8

Functional Gastroduodenal Disorders

Jan Tack, Chair

Nicholas J. Talley, Co-Chair

Michael Camilleri

Gerald Holtmann

Pinjin Hu

Juan-R. Malagelada

Vincenzo Stanghellini

Introduction

A numerically important group of patients with functional gastrointestinal disorders have chronic symptoms that, somewhat arbitrarily, are attributed to the gastroduodenal region. This includes patients who experience

- symptoms in the epigastrium, which is the region between the umbilicus and lower end of the sternum and marked by the midclavicular lines, in the absence of peptic ulceration or other organic upper gastrointestinal diseases,
- excess belching, or
- recurrent unexplained nausea or vomiting.

Based on the consensus opinion of an international panel of clinical investigators who reviewed the available evidence, a classification of the functional gastroduodenal disorders into functional dyspepsia (category B1, comprising postprandial distress syndrome or PDS and epigastric pain syndrome or EPS), belching disorders (category B2, comprising aerophagia and unspecified belching), functional nausea and vomiting disorders (category B3, comprising chronic idiopathic nausea or CIN, functional vomiting, and cyclic vomiting syndrome or CVS), and the rumination syndrome (category B4) is recommended (Table 1).

B1. Functional Dyspepsia

— Definition of Dyspepsia

Many different sets of symptoms have been used synonymously with the term dyspepsia, often resulting in confusion. Most patients do not recognize the term dyspepsia, and historically, physicians have interpreted the meaning of dyspepsia very variably [1–3]. Some authorities have restricted dyspepsia to refer to meal-related symptoms [4–6] but this is inadequate since conditions such as peptic ulcer disease, which is considered to be a classical organic cause of epigastric pain, do not cause symptoms that are confined to the pre- or post-prandial period [7–10].

The Rome I and II committees defined dyspepsia as pain or discomfort centered in the upper abdomen, and excluded reflux symptoms. However, it has remained unsettled whether discomfort is a mild variant of pain or a separate symptom complex [11]. In the Rome I and II definitions, pain was considered a subjective unpleasant sensation of tissue damage or extreme bothersomeness,

Table 1. Functional Gastrointestinal Disorders

A. Functional Esophageal Disorders

A1. Functional heartburn
A2. Functional chest pain of
presumed esophageal origin

A3. Functional dysphagia
A4. Globus

B. Functional Gastroduodenal Disorders

B1. Functional dyspepsia
B1a. Postprandial distress syndrome (PDS)
B1b. Epigastric pain syndrome (EPS)
B2. Belching disorders
B2a. Aerophagia
B2b. Unspecified excessive belching

B3. Nausea and vomiting disorders
B3a. Chronic idiopathic nausea (CIN)
B3b. Functional vomiting
B3c. Cyclic vomiting syndrome (CVS)
B4. Rumination syndrome in adults

C. Functional Bowel Disorders

C1. Irritable bowel syndrome (IBS)
C2. Functional bloating
C3. Functional constipation

C4. Functional diarrhea
C5. Unspecified functional bowel disorder

D. Functional Abdominal Pain Syndrome (FAPS)

E. Functional Gallbladder and Sphincter of Oddi (SO) Disorders

E1. Functional gallbladder disorder
E2. Functional biliary SO disorder
E3. Functional pancreatic SO disorder

F. Functional Anorectal Disorders

F1. Functional fecal incontinence
F2. Functional anorectal pain
F2a. Chronic proctalgia
F2a1. Levator ani syndrome
F2a2. Unspecified functional
anorectal pain

F2b. Proctalgia fugax
F3. Functional defecation disorders
F3a. Dyssynergic defecation
F3b. Inadequate defecatory propulsion

G. Functional Disorders: Neonates and Toddlers

G1. Infant regurgitation
G2. Infant rumination syndrome
G3. Cyclic vomiting syndrome
G4. Infant colic

G5. Functional diarrhea
G6. Infant dyschezia
G7. Functional constipation

H. Functional Disorders: Children and Adolescents

H1. Vomiting and aerophagia
H1a. Adolescent rumination syndrome
H1b. Cyclic vomiting syndrome
H1c. Aerophagia
H2. Abdominal pain-related FGIDs
H2a. Functional dyspepsia
H2b. Irritable bowel syndrome
H2c. Abdominal migraine

H2d. Childhood functional abdominal pain
H2d1. Childhood functional abdominal pain syndrome
H3. Constipation and incontinence
H3a. Functional constipation
H3b. Nonretentive fecal incontinence

Table 2. Dyspeptic Symptoms and Their Definition

Symptom	Definition
Epigastric pain	Epigastric refers to the region between the umbilicus and lower end of the sternum and marked by the midclavicular lines. Pain refers to a subjective, unpleasant sensation; some patients may feel that tissue damage is occurring. Epigastric pain may or may not have a burning quality. Other symptoms may be extremely bothersome without being interpreted by the patient as pain.
Postprandial fullness	An unpleasant sensation like the prolonged persistence of food in the stomach
Early satiation	A feeling that the stomach is overfilled soon after starting to eat, out of proportion to the size of the meal being eaten, so that the meal cannot be finished. Previously, the term "early satiety" was used, but satiation is the correct term for the disappearance of the sensation of appetite during food ingestion.
Bloating in the upper abdomen	An unpleasant sensation of tightness located in the epigastrium; it should be distinguished from visible abdominal distension
Epigastric burning	Epigastric refers to the region between the umbilicus and lower end of the sternum and marked by the midclavicular lines. Burning refers to an unpleasant subjective sensation of heat.
Nausea	Queasiness or sick sensation; a feeling of the need to vomit
Vomiting	Forceful oral expulsion of gastric contents associated with contraction of the abdominal and chest wall muscles. Vomiting is usually preceded by and associated with retching, repetitive contractions of the abdominal wall without expulsion of gastric contents.
Belching	Venting of air from the stomach or the esophagus

while discomfort meant one or more specific symptoms with a subjective, negative feeling that the patient does not interpret as pain [11]. Whether or not some symptoms such as upper abdominal fullness, early satiation, bloating, belching, nausea, retching, or vomiting are labeled as pain by the patient may depend on cultural factors, linguistic factors, and possibly education level [12]. There is also disagreement in the literature whether pain represents a more extreme intensity of any discomfort or whether it is an entirely different sensation. It has not been established whether visceral pain is mediated by separate pathways, or by more intense stimulation of pathways that mediate discomfort at lower stimulus intensities [13].

Hence, the Rome III committee recommended the following pragmatic definition: Dyspepsia refers to a symptom or set of symptoms that are considered by most physicians to originate from the gastroduodenal region. The specific symptoms (postprandial fullness, early satiation, and epigastric pain or epigastric burning) and their interpretation are summarized in Table 2. Patients with one or more of these symptoms are referred to as patients with dyspepsia.

Functional dyspepsia is the umbrella term that refers to unexplained dyspepsia i.e., no structural explanation on standard investigations. Functional dyspepsia is defined as the presence of one or more dyspepsia symptoms that are considered to originate from the gastroduodenal region, in the absence of any organic, systemic, or metabolic disease that is likely to explain the symptoms. These symptoms are listed in Table 2. However, particularly for experimental purposes, the term functional dyspepsia should preferably be replaced by more distinctively defined disorders, for which there is now increasing evidence in the literature. These are the new diagnostic categories of (1) meal-induced dyspeptic symptoms (PDS), and (2) epigastric pain (EPS).

Heartburn has been defined by the esophageal committee. (See Chapter 7.) A burning sensation confined to the epigastrium is not considered heartburn unless it also radiates retrosternally. In the past, heartburn (as well as acid regurgitation) has often been included as sufficient on its own to define dyspepsia [2]. The Rome II committee concluded, based primarily on expert opinions, that patients with typical heartburn as a dominant complaint almost invariably have gastroesophageal reflux disease (GERD), and should be distinguished from patients with dyspepsia [11]. The current committee concurs with this recommendation. There is evidence that heartburn has moderate specificity for GERD and the positive predictive value for heartburn is high in countries where GERD is a common disease [10, 14]. Heartburn is not considered a symptom that primarily arises from the gastroduodenum; hence this is excluded from the definition of dyspepsia even though heartburn commonly co-occurs with gastroduodenal symptoms. Similarly, retrosternal pain suggestive of esophageal disease or of a type embraced by the terms functional or noncardiac chest pain should also be excluded from dyspepsia.

Uninvestigated versus Investigated Dyspepsia

Especially when considering epidemiological data, it is important to distinguish the subjects with dyspeptic symptoms that have not been investigated from patients with a diagnostic label after investigation, with or without an identified causal abnormality.

Organic versus Idiopathic Dyspepsia

From an etiological viewpoint, patients with dyspeptic symptoms can be subdivided into two main categories:

1. Those with an identified organic or metabolic cause for the symptoms where, if the disease improves or is eliminated, symptoms also improve or resolve (e.g., chronic peptic ulcer disease, GERD with or without esophagitis, a subset of *H. pylori* gastritis, malignancy, pancreatico-biliary disease, medication use), or

2. Those with no identifiable explanation for the symptoms. In some of these patients, an identifiable pathophysiological or microbiologic abnormality of uncertain clinical relevance (e.g., *H. pylori* gastritis where symptoms persist despite eradication therapy eliminating the infection) may be present that is not thought to explain the symptoms.

Previously, those patients who have no definite structural or biochemical explanation for their symptoms were considered to have nonulcer dyspepsia, essential dyspepsia, idiopathic dyspepsia, or functional dyspepsia. The term nonulcer dyspepsia remains in popular usage but is not recommended here because some patients with functional dyspepsia will have symptoms typical of ulcer disease while others will have symptoms not at all like an ulcer, and peptic ulcer is not the only disease of exclusion in patients with dyspepsia.

Symptom patterns alone are unable to adequately discriminate organic from idiopathic dyspeptic symptoms [10, 15]. Patients need to be investigated to rule out relevant organic disease and there should be no evidence of structural or metabolic abnormalities that definitely explain the symptoms. There is agreement that symptoms should run a chronic course before a patient is labeled as having functional dyspepsia symptoms.

Heterogeneity of Dyspeptic Symptoms in Functional Dyspepsia: Identifying the Predominant Symptom and Subgroups

It seems likely that functional dyspepsia includes different types of patients with distinct underlying pathophysiologies who require different management approaches. However, it has been particularly difficult to identify these subgroups reliably. The approach has been to try to identify types or groups of symptoms that would reliably identify patients with different underlying pathophysiologies who would respond to therapy directed towards the underlying pathophysiology [16]. Several attempts have been undertaken to classify patients according to their symptom profile. Subclasses based on symptom clusters have been proposed [6, 17, 18]. In clinical practice, however, this classification showed great overlap between subclasses, limiting its value [19, 20]. More recent attempts to distinguish subgroups of patients with dyspeptic symptoms were based on identifying the predominant symptom, on the association of symptoms with pathophysiology, and on factor analyses of the symptom pattern.

Identifying the *predominant symptom* was shown to distinguish two subgroups with different demographic and symptomatic properties, and have some relationship to putative pathophysiological mechanisms such as delayed gastric emptying and the presence of *H. pylori* [20]. The predominant symptom also seemed to identify the group of patients who were most likely to respond to proton pump inhibitor therapy [16], but this was most obvious in a group with predominant heartburn, a subgroup who actually is no longer considered to belong to functional dyspepsia [11]. Thus, the Rome II committee proposed a subdivision according to the predominant symptom being pain vs. discomfort. However, the subdivision has been criticized because of the difficulty in distinguishing pain from discomfort, the lack of a widely accepted definition of predominant, the significant overlap between the symptom subgroups, the number of patients who do not fit into one of the subgroups, and the lack of stability over short time periods [10, 19, 21–23]. Moreover, a more detailed analysis has revealed that the predominant symptom does not reliably identify pathophysiological subsets [24].

There are inevitable limitations in the use of *symptom patterns* to identify relevant subgroups of patients with symptoms of functional dyspepsia in daily clinical practice. It is well known that the distinguishing features of visceral symptoms are not very precise. A symptom-based approach is also hampered by cultural and linguistic differences in different places of the world, which will inevitably affect and bias responses to symptom questionnaires. Finally, it is possible that the dyspepsia symptom pattern per se is not stable over time, given the already considerable fluctuation over time of dyspepsia as a syndrome [19].

A different approach was based on attempts to identify *pathophysiology-based subgroups* in functional dyspepsia. Thus, associations were demonstrated between delayed gastric emptying and symptoms of fullness, nausea, and vomiting [25–27], between impaired fundic accommodation and early satiety and weight loss [28], and between visceral hypersensitivity and epigastric pain and belching [29]. A practical implication of these findings could be that specific treatment with prokinetics, fundic relaxants, or visceral analgesics, respectively, may be selected based on symptomatology. However, these pathophysiological abnormalities do not identify distinct groups of patients, since there is overlap between different abnormalities within the dyspeptic symptom population [24]. Moreover, the association of these pathophysiological mechanisms with symptoms has not been confirmed in some studies [30–32]. Furthermore, some symptoms (e.g., weight loss) occurred in association with more than one mechanism, and given the diversity and number of additional nondyspeptic symptoms that patients with functional dyspepsia may report [33], an approach based on the presence or severity of multiple different individual symptoms seems impractical.

— Epidemiology

The prevalence of uninvestigated dyspeptic symptoms in the general population is now well documented. If predominant heartburn is not included in dyspepsia, then approximately 20% to 30% of people in the community each year report chronic or recurrent dyspeptic symptoms [18, 19, 34–36] and this percentage is reasonably consistent around the world [37–39]. Although these data represent uninvestigated dyspepsia, an organic cause is found in only a minority of dyspeptic subjects who are investigated and hence it is reasonable to assume that the majority would have functional dyspepsia [40–43].

The prevalence of dyspeptic symptoms is lower in the elderly and slightly higher in men than in women overall. In recent decades the prevalence rates of *Helicobacter pylori* has clearly decreased. As a result, the incidence of *H. pylori*-related structural diseases in the upper gut has probably decreased. Thus, the relative proportion of functional gastrointestinal disorders may have increased but this is speculative. To date, the available data do not provide evidence that the prevalence of dyspeptic symptoms has changed in recent decades [39].

The incidence of dyspeptic symptoms is substantially lower than the prevalence estimates. Based on prospective studies of subjects who report dyspeptic symptoms for the first time, the incidence is approximately 1% per year [19, 44]. Those who appear to develop symptoms are balanced by a similar number of people who lose their symptoms over time, which accounts for the prevalence being stable from year to year.

The majority of patients with functional dyspepsia symptoms continue to be symptomatic over the long term despite periods of remission [45]. Approximately one third of patients lose their symptoms spontaneously [19, 44]. In patients with functional dyspepsia, the risk of developing peptic ulcer disease appears to be no different from that of the background asymptomatic population [21, 45–47].

Approximately one in two subjects, it is estimated, seek health care for their dyspeptic symptoms at some time in their life [18, 38, 48]. Pain severity and anxiety (including fear of serious disease) appear to be factors associated with consulting behavior [37, 38, 48, 49].

The committee proposed to define functional dyspepsia at two levels while further research on more specific definitions is ongoing. A general, umbrella definition of functional dyspepsia to be used mainly for clinical purposes is provided under category B1. However, particularly for pathophysiological and therapeutic research purposes, newly defined entities of (1) meal-induced dyspeptic symptoms (PDS, defined under category B1a), and (2) epigastric pain (EPS, defined under category B1b), should be used.

B1. Diagnostic Criteria* for Functional Dyspepsia

Must include:
1. One or more of the following:
   a. Bothersome postprandial fullness
   b. Early satiation
   c. Epigastric pain
   d. Epigastric burning
AND
2. No evidence of structural disease (including at upper endoscopy) that is likely to explain the symptoms

*Criteria fulfilled for the last 3 months with symptom onset at least 6 months prior to diagnosis

B1a. Diagnostic Criteria* for Postprandial Distress Syndrome

Must include *one or both* of the following:
1. Bothersome postprandial fullness, occurring after ordinary-sized meals, at least several times per week
2. Early satiation that prevents finishing a regular meal, at least several times per week

*Criteria fulfilled for the last 3 months with symptom onset at least 6 months prior to diagnosis

Supportive Criteria
1. Upper abdominal bloating or postprandial nausea or excessive belching can be present
2. Epigastric pain syndrome may coexist

BIb. Diagnostic Criteria* for Epigastric Pain Syndrome

Must include *all* of the following:
1. **Pain or burning localized to the epigastrium of at least moderate severity, at least once per week**
2. **The pain is intermittent**
3. **Not generalized or localized to other abdominal or chest regions**
4. **Not relieved by defecation or passage of flatus**
5. **Not fulfilling criteria for gallbladder or sphincter of Oddi disorders**

*Criteria fulfilled for the last 3 months with symptom onset at least 6 months prior to diagnosis

Supportive Criteria
1. The pain may be of a burning quality, but without a retrosternal component
2. The pain is commonly induced or relieved by ingestion of a meal, but may occur while fasting
3. Postprandial distress syndrome may coexist

— Justification for Changes to Criteria

The rationale for the proposed new classification was based on the inadequacy of prior approaches such as the predominant symptom, the results of factor analyses in tertiary care and in the general population, clinical experience, and new observations in the peer-reviewed literature.

Previously, all patients without definite structural or biochemical explanation for dyspeptic symptoms were considered to have functional dyspepsia. It is clear that there is a lack of uniform interpretation and acceptance of the term "functional dyspepsia" at different levels of practice, in different countries and with regulatory authorities. Investigators in several large studies included heartburn and even acid regurgitation as "typical symptoms of dyspepsia" [50–54].

There is also increasing evidence for the existence of different entities within the "dyspepsia symptom complex." There is no single symptom that is present in all patients with functional dyspepsia, and there is considerable variation in the symptom pattern between patients [33]. Factor analysis studies in the general population and in investigated patients [55–62] have failed to support the existence of functional dyspepsia as a homogeneous condition. Pathophysiological studies have provided evidence for heterogeneity of putative underlying pathophysiological mechanisms and the association of symptoms with mechanisms is better for certain symptoms than for the overall dyspepsia symptom complex [24–33]. Moreover, there is evidence for different response to therapy for different subgroups in therapeutic studies in functional dyspepsia [50, 53, 54, 63].

Proposed Nomenclature and Classification

In clinical practice, therapy is usually directed towards individual symptoms (e.g., symptomatic treatment of nausea), rather than the full symptom complex. In many clinical trials, different therapeutic response for different subgroups seems to be expected, as strategies are used to enrich the patient population for certain symptom profiles [50, 64–66]. Based on these limitations, the committee proposed the development of a new nomenclature and a classification that was more evidence-based. Although the notion "functional dyspepsia" is not discarded, the committee proposes to include more distinctively defined disorders, for which there is now increasing evidence in the literature.

Factor analysis studies in the general population and in patients with functional dyspepsia all found that dyspeptic symptoms comprise three or four different symptom groupings [55–62]. Factor analysis in tertiary care patients did not support the existence of functional dyspepsia as a homogeneous condition, but found a model based on four different factors to be valid: (1) nausea, vomiting, satiety; (2) weight loss, bloating; (3) fullness, pain; and (4) burning, and belching [56]. Each of these factors was correlated with a putative pathophysiological abnormality and two of the factors were associated with psychosocial abnormalities, a dimension that so far had not been taken into account in defining the heterogeneity of dyspeptic patients. A population study in the same cultural and linguistic environment reported that the same factors are found in dyspepsia in the general population. Studies in the general population are generally supportive of the applicability of similar symptom groupings (Table 3).

By definition, certain symptoms such as early satiation or postprandial fullness are related to the ingestion of a meal. All factor analysis studies identified a separate factor of meal-related symptoms. Systematic studies revealed that symptoms are induced or worsened by meal ingestion in the majority of patients with dyspeptic symptoms, but there are patients in whom symptoms are not related to ingestion of a meal [61, 67–69]. The committee agreed that a distinction between meal-induced symptoms and meal-unrelated symptoms might be pathophysiologically and clinically relevant.

Although there is some heterogeneity between studies, consistent symptom groupings include an epigastric pain factor, a factor of meal-induced symptoms including postprandial fullness or early satiation, and a nausea factor (with or without vomiting) [55–62] (Table 3). In some studies, belching also appears as a separate symptom group [56, 62]. The epigastric pain factor is reminiscent of

Table 3. Factor Analysis Studies of Dyspeptic Symptoms in the General Population and in Tertiary Care Functional Dyspepsia Patients

Study	Setting	Symptom groupings
Westbrook 2002 [55]	Dyspepsia questionnaire in random population sample (n=2300)	*Three dyspeptic symptom factors:* an epigastric pain factor, an early satiety/fullness factor, and a nausea factor. In addition, a heartburn/regurgitation factor.
Fischler 2003 [56]	Dyspepsia questionnaire in 438 tertiary care patients with idiopathic dyspeptic symptoms	*Four dyspeptic symptom factors:* an epigastric pain factor, a fullness/bloating factor, a nausea/vomiting/satiation factor and a belching factor.
Tack 2003 [57]	Dyspepsia questionnaire in 636 tertiary care patients with idiopathic dyspeptic symptoms	*Three dyspeptic symptom factors:* an epigastric pain/burning/belching factor, a fullness/bloating/satiation factor, and a nausea/vomiting/satiation factor.
Jones 2003 [58]	Dyspepsia questionnaire in random population sample (n=888)	*Three dyspeptic symptom factors:* an epigastric pain factor, a fullness/satiation factor, and a nausea/vomiting factor.
Kwan 2003 [59]	Rome II questionnaire in 1012 functional gastrointestinal patients	*Three dyspeptic symptom factors:* an epigastric pain/discomfort factor, a fullness/satiation/bloating factor, and a nausea/vomiting factor.
Whitehead 2003 [60]	Rome II questionnaire in 1041 functional gastrointestinal patients	*Four dyspeptic symptom factors:* two epigastric pain factors, a nausea/vomiting/satiation factor, and an upper abdominal bloating factor.
Camilleri 2005 [61]	Telephone survey in random population U.S. sample (n=21 128)	*Three dyspeptic symptom factors:* an epigastric pain/bloating/fullness factor, an early satiety/loss of appetite/fullness factor and a nausea factor. In addition, a heartburn/regurgitation factor.
Piessevaux 2005 [62]	Face-to-face interview of general population sample (n = 2025)	*Four dyspeptic symptom factors:* an epigastric pain factor, a fullness/satiation factor, a nausea factor, and a belching factor.

430

ulcer-like dyspepsia, and the factor of meal-induced symptoms is reminiscent of dysmotility-like dyspepsia, as defined by the Rome II criteria [11]. However, this approach was based on the predominant symptom approach, which varies strongly from week to week [22, 23], and regarded both as subgroups of a single homogeneous diagnostic and clinically useful category. In the Rome II criteria, nausea was considered a symptom of dysmotility-like dyspepsia [11], but the committee decided to revise this on the basis of factor analysis data, on clinical experience that persistent nausea is often of central or psychological origin, and on responsiveness of this symptom to symptomatic therapy.

Overlap with GERD and IBS

Heartburn, considered an esophageal symptom, and dyspepsia are extremely common, and some overlap between both is likely. The Rome II definition proposed to exclude patients with predominant heartburn from the dyspepsia spectrum [11], but recent studies have demonstrated that the predominant symptom approach does not reliably identify all patients with GERD [54, 70, 71]. Although GERD may be accompanied by some dyspeptic symptoms that may respond to proton pump inhibitor (PPI) therapy [54], data have been published suggesting that PPIs are less effective in the absence of heartburn [53, 71]. The committee, therefore, recommends that the presence of frequent and typical reflux symptoms should lead to a provisional diagnosis of GERD [72]. In clinical practice and for clinical trials, recognition of frequent heartburn in dyspepsia may be improved by a simple descriptive questionnaire [70, 71]. In general, overlap of GERD or functional heartburn with PDS or EPS is probably frequent and needs to be carefully considered in both clinical practice and experimental trials.

Overlap between dyspeptic symptoms and irritable bowel syndrome (IBS) is also commonly observed, and overlap between IBS on one hand and PDS or EPS on the other hand is likely to occur [73]. Conditions identified as potential explanations for dyspepsia in patients with no evidence of ulcer disease, reflux esophagitis, or cancer at upper endoscopy are shown in Figure 1. The presence of IBS does not exclude the diagnosis of any of these functional gastroduodenal disorders, as coexisting IBS was found to have a minor impact on symptom pattern and putative pathophysiological mechanisms [74].

— Clinical Evaluation

The evaluation and management of the patient with uninvestigated dyspeptic symptoms should not be confused with the approach to the patient whose dyspepsia has been investigated.

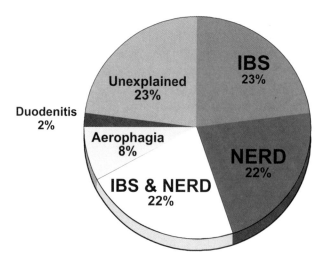

Figure I. Conditions identified as potential explanations for dyspepsia in patients with no evidence of ulcer disease, reflux esophagitis, or cancer at upper endoscopy and cholelithiasis excluded by radiology. NERD = nonerosive reflux disease; IBS = irritable bowel syndrome. From ref. 73.

Patients with Uninvestigated Dyspeptic Symptoms

Evidence-based analysis [75] suggests the following five-point management strategy for primary care physicians first seeing patients with dyspepsia:

1. Gather clinical evidence that symptoms probably arise in the upper gastrointestinal tract.
2. Investigate alarm features, which are less common in general practice, but that have a low positive predictive value for organic disease when present [72, 76].
3. Exclude ingestion of aspirin and nonaspirin nonsteroidal anti-inflammatory drugs (NSAIDS) since they increase the risk of dyspepsia by up to 36% (if not excluded, either withdraw the drug or add PPI) [77].
4. In the presence of typical reflux symptoms a provisional diagnosis of GERD should be made (erosive esophagitis has been found in as many as 43% of unselected dyspeptic patients subsequently endoscoped) [75]. Physicians may initially prescribe PPIs empirically in patients who also have heartburn, but should take into account that these drugs may be less effective in functional dyspepsia without heartburn. Long-term administration of PPIs may be needed since short-course PPI therapy in uninvestigated dyspepsia is followed by recurrence of symptoms in most patients, even in those who responded during acid inhibition [78–80].
5. The indications for upper gastrointestinal endoscopy, the role of *H. pylori* testing, and empirical treatment in the management of uninvestigated dyspepsia are no longer controversial. Guidelines have proposed prompt endos-

copy in patients with alarm symptoms or patients over a threshold age (45 to 55 years, depending on health care access and incidence of malignant disease). Noninvasive testing of *H. pylori* infection ("test and treat" *H. pylori* strategies), followed by eradication has been established to be a cost-effective approach that decreases the number of endoscopies [81–83]. Test and treat is usually recommended, as this strategy will cure most underlying peptic ulcer disease and prevent future gastroduodenal disease, although many infected patients with functional dyspepsia will not gain symptomatic benefit [43, 84–89]. The yield of this approach is therefore highest in places with a high prevalence of *H. pylori* and peptic ulcer disease [90]. Other evidence indicates that prompt endoscopy first may be more cost-effective in older patients where organic disease is more likely [91], that *H. pylori* testing followed by endoscopy in *H. pylori* positive patients is not cost-effective [92], and that many patients with negative *H. pylori* tests should have a trial of PPI therapy prior to endoscopy because of its low yield [93]. Test and treat becomes less attractive in areas of a low prevalence that makes false positive testing more likely [90].

Patients with Functional Dyspepsia

The available data in the literature are based on functional dyspepsia patients as a group; no data are available on diagnostic approaches to the categories EPS or PDS as defined by the Rome III committee.

The current best first test for excluding structural causes of dyspepsia is upper gastrointestinal endoscopy. Thus, for a patient to be considered as suffering from functional dyspepsia an endoscopy has to be performed first. Upper endoscopy would be best performed during a symptomatic period off all acid-suppressant therapy. It is recommended that biopsies be routinely obtained at the time of endoscopy to detect *H. pylori* infection. In view of the association of *H. pylori* with peptic ulcer disease and dyspepsia, eradication is recommended in all positive cases whether or not ulcer disease is detected, although this will often not improve dyspeptic symptoms [43, 81–88, 90]. A barium meal study is less sensitive and specific than upper endoscopy and hence is not generally recommended. Ultrasonography is not recommended as a routine clinical test, as the yield is low in the absence of symptoms or clinical features or biochemical tests suggestive of biliary tract or pancreatic disease [94]. Barium x-ray study of the small bowel is only useful in case of suspected mechanical obstruction.

A gastric emptying study (e.g., scintigraphy, ^{13}C-octanoic acid, or ultrasonography) is not currently recommended as a routine clinical test because the results uncommonly alter management. Indeed, recent studies have shown that less than 25% of patients with functional dyspepsia have delayed gastric emptying, even when considering exclusively the subgroup of dysmotility-like dyspepsia [27, 32] as shown in Figure 4A and B. *H. pylori* eradication appears to have no impact on gastric emptying [95]. There is some question as to whether electrogastrography (EGG) may provide a reliable indicator of gastric emptying [96–98]. Some clinicophysiological correlations have been demonstrated between symptoms and abnormalities of gastric function including gastric accommodation, gastric sensitivity to distention, and duodenal chemo- and mechanosensitivity (see section below). However, none of these tests can be advocated in routine clinical practice.

— Physiological Features

The literature shows that different definitions of functional dyspepsia have been used in different studies, and these definitions do not conform to the specific subcategories of dyspepsia proposed by the Rome III committee. Hence, prospective studies are needed in order to characterize the pathophysiology of the new categories. The following summary applies to the umbrella disorder of functional dyspepsia, which typically includes patients who were at least endoscopy-negative.

Dyspepsia shares pathophysiological disturbances with other disorders of gastrointestinal function, such as dysmotility and hypersensitivity. This may also account for the overlap in the syndromes, which has been demonstrated in epidemiological [19] as well as laboratory-based studies [99]. However, clearly other "players" participate in the development of the syndrome. In addition, it needs to be noted that some of the presumably "underlying" pathophysiologies are simply markers of disease and may not be directly linked to the manifestation of symptoms. Clinical experience and scholarly reviews have emphasized the importance of the environment, diet, and ingestion of food [6, 100, 101].

The role of *H. pylori*, salmonella, and other acute infections [102, 103] in the development of functional dyspepsia is still incompletely understood, although increasing evidence suggests that such environmental factors may play a role and mediate the induction of symptoms by altering physiology of the upper gut. For example, Figure 2 shows the increased incidence of postinfectious dyspepsia and IBS following acute *Salmonella* gastroenteritis. This section of the chapter summarizes the principle concepts on the pathophysiology of functional dyspepsia.

Diet and Environmental Factors

Little is known about the effect of diet and environmental factors on the etiology of dyspepsia. Two studies from Ireland provide conflicting information about the influence of food, nutrient intake, and feeding patterns in functional

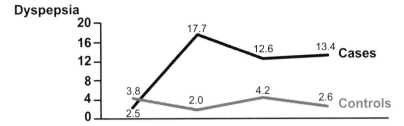

Figure 2. Incidence of post-infectious dyspepsia following *Salmonella* gastroenteritis. Cases postgastroenteritis were significantly more likely to have the new onset of dyspepsia than controls. From Mearin F, et al. Dyspepsia and irritable bowel syndrome after a Salmonella gastroenteritis outbreak: one-year follow-up cohort study. Gastroenterology 2005;129:98–104 with permission from Elsevier.

dyspepsia [104, 105]. Dyspeptic symptoms in functional dyspepsia are commonly exacerbated by meals rich in fat [106], but it is unclear whether this affects a subgroup of dyspeptic patients, or all patients [33]. Moreover, an aggravating effect of lipids is not unique to dyspepsia, and has been reported in other functional disorders as well [107, 108].

In 653 outpatients presenting for endoscopy with dyspepsia, neither smoking, alcohol, nor NSAIDs were identified as risk factors for functional dyspepsia [109]. However, as previously mentioned, patients with functional dyspepsia are more likely to develop symptoms when treated with NSAIDs [110].

Gastric Acid Secretion

Basal gastric acid secretion is within normal limits in patients with functional dyspepsia [111] but acid-related symptoms (perhaps through gastric or duodenal hypersensitivity—see below) may arise in a subgroup of patients. Proton pump inhibitors appear to be effective in this subset of patients, though it has been generally difficult to separate these patients from those with a significant GERD component.

Bombesin (gastrin-releasing peptide, GRP)-stimulated acid secretion was higher in *H. pylori*-positive functional dyspepsia patients than in the *H. pylori*-positive healthy volunteers or *H. pylori*-negative healthy volunteers. The *H. pylori*-positive functional dyspepsia patients, however, had lower acid output than duodenal ulcer controls. These findings are consistent with approximately 50% of functional dyspepsia patients having a similar disturbance of GRP-stimulated acid secretion to duodenal ulcer patients [112].

Though the pathogenic role of a mechanism cannot be clearly evaluated from therapeutic studies, it is useful to note that, in general, suppression of acid secretion is associated with limited efficacy in the treatment of functional dyspepsia in single studies or in large meta-analyses. The number needed to treat is nine [75, 113].

Helicobacter Pylori and Chronic Gastritis

The role of *H. pylori* infection in functional dyspepsia has been controversial [114–117]. However, recent meta-analyses suggest a small but consistent benefit from *H. pylori* eradication in infected patients [87].

An etiological role of the infection may be supported by small studies that have demonstrated disturbances of motor or sensory function of the upper gut in *H. pylori*-infected individuals [118–120]. However, the data are equivocal and not supported by larger studies [28, 29, 103, 121].

It is interesting nevertheless that patients with erosive prepyloric changes have been noted to have dyspepsia [122] and that when these patients are infected with *H. pylori* they appear to respond well to eradication of *H. pylori* [123]. These observations may help explain why in some trials eradication has been effective in approximately 20% of patients with dyspeptic symptoms [124]. Overall, the number needed to treat (NNT) of approximately 17 determined from meta-analyses of clinical trials suggests that only a small proportion of patients have dyspeptic symptoms that are convincingly attributable to *H. pylori* infection [75] (see p. 446).

Duodenitis

A few quantitative morphometric studies have shown that duodenitis associated with increased inflammatory infiltration is associated with dyspeptic symptoms even in the absence of erosions or ulcers [40, 125]. Whether this is a primary etiological entity for dyspeptic symptoms or is simply associated either with acid hypersecretion [111] or *H. pylori* infection [123] is unclear.

Gastrointestinal Dysmotility

There are several lines of evidence that suggest that gastrointestinal motility is abnormal in a proportion of patients with functional dyspepsia [126]. One study (Figure 3) showed that gastric emptying was slower in patients with functional dyspepsia compared to healthy controls [127]. However, the relationship between delayed gastric emptying and dyspepsia symptoms needs further study, since while symptoms may be related to the prevalence of delayed gastric emptying, they may not correlate with the rate of gastric emptying [27, 32] (Figure 4A and B). The contribution of motor abnormalities to symptom generation is incompletely established. Impaired (typically delayed) gastric emptying of solids is the most widely studied motility disorder in dyspepsia, both in patients and in non-consulting dyspeptics [126, 127]. The delay in gastric emptying appears to be more common in women and among patients with fullness, nausea, and vomiting [25–27]. Other disturbances of upper gut motility are postprandial antral hypomotility [128–130] and

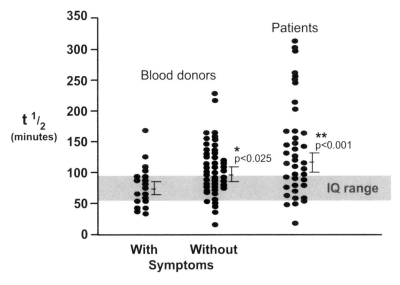

Figure 3. Prevalence of gastric emptying in the community: blood donors without and with dyspepsia, and patients with documented functional dyspepsia. Gastric emptying was significantly slower in healthy blood donors with symptoms versus those without, and was slower in patients with functional dyspepsia compared with healthy asymptomatic blood donors. IQ = interquartile. From Haag S, et al. Symptom patterns in functional dyspepsia and irritable bowel syndrome: relationship to disturbances in gastric emptying and response to disturbances in gastric emptying and response to a nutrient challenge in consulters and non-consulters. Gut. 2004;53:1445–51 with permission from BMJ Publishing Group.

reduced frequency of interdigestive migrating motor complexes [131, 132]. There are preliminary data to suggest that the duodenal motor responses to acid and nutrient infusions are impaired in functional dyspepsia [133].

More recently, intriguing data suggest that the stomach may have an excess of phasic contractions of the fundus after a meal in dyspeptic patients. Experimental data suggest that these contractions may actually induce an increase in tension in the fundus and hence activate tension receptors inducing pain or discomfort [134, 135]. Disturbances in antro-fundic coordination have also been reported, though the relationship with symptoms is unclear [136]. This is consistent with disturbances in the intra-gastric distribution of a meal in the early postprandial period [137–139] in some, but not in all studies [140].

As with discussion of other mechanisms, review of the results of treatment may provide some insights on the clinical relevance of the pathophysiology. Thus a detailed meta-analysis of prokinetics for dyspeptic disorders shows a favorable NNT (4), though it is important to note that the funnel plot suggested there was publication bias, which may influence the NNT estimate [141].

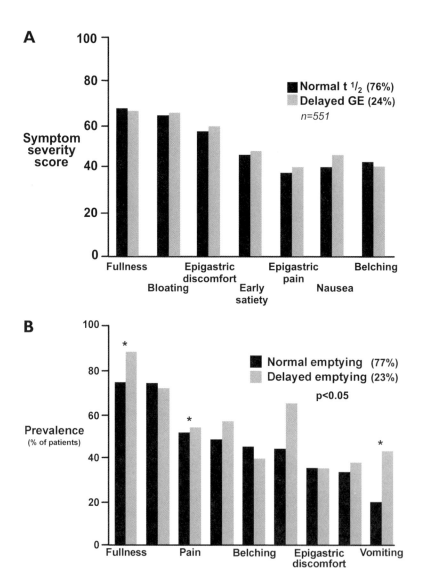

Figure 4. Relationship between symptoms and delayed gastric emptying in functional dyspepsia is controversial. (A) Several large randomized multicenter clinical trials, mainly from the US, found no association between symptoms and emptying rate. This example is taken from ref. 32. (B) Several large single-center studies from Europe found associations between delayed gastric emptying and the prevalence and severity of symptoms like postprandial fullness, nausea, and vomiting. From Sarnelli G, et al. Symptoms associated with impaired gastric emptying of solids and liquids in functional dyspepsia. Am J Gastro 2003;98:783–8, with permission from Blackwell Publishing.

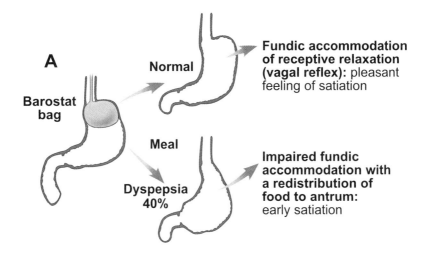

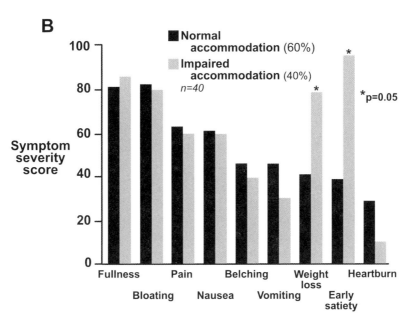

Figure 5. Role of impaired fundic accommodation in functional dyspepsia. (A) Gastric accommodation to a meal in health and in functional dyspepsia. Impaired fundic accommodation occurs in approximately 40% of patients with functional dyspepsia. (B) Some studies have identified an association between impaired fundic accommodation and early satiation as well as weight loss. From Tack et al. Gastroenterology 1998;115:1346–52, with permission.

Gastric Accommodation

Several studies show that the accommodation or volume response of the stomach after a meal is reduced in approximately 40% of patients with functional dyspepsia (Figure 5A and 5B), whether this is measured by the volume response to a non-compliant system linked to an infinitely compliant balloon [142], or a barostat of low compliance linked to an infinitely compliant balloon [28, 56, 140] or transabdominal ultrasonography [143, 144], or single-photon emission computed tomography (SPECT) imaging [145, 146].

Gastric Myoelectric Activity

Several studies in adults and children have documented the presence of gastric dysrhythmias especially in the postprandial period in patients with functional dyspepsia [147–150]. Although there are data that associate the symptoms with dysrhythmia in functional dyspepsia [151], attribution of the dysrhythmia as a causative factor is not yet convincing given the fact that therapies cannot be aimed at selectively correcting the dysrhythmia without affecting other pathophysiological disturbances. At present, it is reasonable to assume that some of the underlying motor abnormalities result from disorders of underlying myoelectrical activity.

Gastric Hypersensitivity

Evidence of gastric hypersensitivity or the irritable stomach in functional dyspepsia is well documented in the literature [152–157]. Figure 6A and 6B show that gastric barostat balloon distension is associated with greater abdominal discomfort and lower sensory thresholds in patients with functional dyspepsia compared with controls [152–155]. However, it is clear that not all patients will demonstrate evidence of hypersensitivity or hyperalgesia in response to distension [29, 158]. The symptoms associated with gastric hypersensitivity in dyspepsia have been described [29] and corroboration from other centers is eagerly awaited to determine whether symptoms could be used as surrogates of physiological studies.

The physiological and clinical relevance of reported reflex hyporeactivity is unclear [159]. Caldarella et al. have also recently reported antrofundic hyporeactivity in dyspepsia and also showed that there was no difference in the hyporeactivity of ulcer-like vs. dysmotility-like dyspepsia [136]. The brain centers involved in sensation of gastric stimuli like distension have been documented in health [160, 161] and full reports of the brain centers involved in functional dyspepsia are awaited.

In some patients, the sensitivity can be elicited with intraluminal contents, such as gastric acid or duodenal content [162]. The interaction of sensitivity and

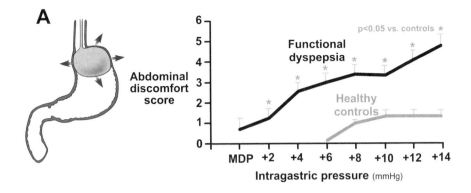

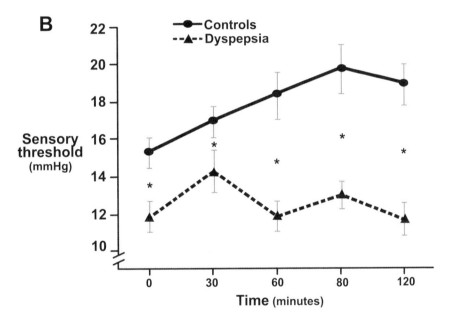

Figure 6. Visceral hypersensitivity in functional dyspepsia. (A) Reduced visceral pain thresholds have been identified in functional dyspepsia compared with healthy controls using a gastric barostat balloon distention protocol. From Mearin F, et al. The origin of symptoms on the brain-gut axis in functional dyspepsia. Gastroenterology. 1991;101:999–1006 with permission from Elsevier. (B) Repeated distention of the stomach with the barostat balloon increases sensory thresholds in controls (that is, reduces visceral hypersensitivity) but does not change visceral sensory thresholds in patients with functional dyspepsia. From Holtmann G, et al. Differences in gastric mechanosensory function after repeated ramp distensions in non-consulters with dyspepsia and healthy controls. Gut. 2000;47:332–6 with permission from BMJ Publishing Group.

intraluminal content in eliciting dyspeptic symptoms is important given the observation that symptoms due to aspirin may be related to hypersensitivity to distension [110].

The hypothesis that gastric hypersensitivity is key to the control of functional dyspepsia will be given considerable credence if a visceral analgesic is proven efficacious in clinical trials in relieving dyspepsia, but convincing data are still lacking.

Duodenal / Intestinal Sensitivity

Intestinal sensitivity has been observed in response to balloon distension, or in response to intraluminal content. For example, there is evidence of increased sensitivity to mechanical distension of a barostat balloon [163], or increased sensitivity (shown by enhanced orad contraction) in response to latex balloon distension [129].

Duodenal sensitivity was documented by directly infusing acid into the duodenum and measuring sensation in response to gastric mechanical stimuli in health [164–166] and in dyspepsia [167]. A subset of dyspeptic patients has spontaneously increased duodenal acid exposure, and this is associated with higher symptom intensity [167]. It is intriguing that there are also specific chemicals that elicit this hypersensitivity [133], and that inhibition of gastric acid secretion can restore the sensitivity of the duodenum towards normal [168].

Autonomic Dysfunction

In a minority of studies, patients with functional dyspepsia have evidence of decreased vagal tone [126, 169, 170]. When prospectively assessed, it was also shown that a minority of patients seen in two tertiary referral centers had evidence of vagal dysfunction [140, 163]. In a different study, patients were classified as falling into two groups: a sympathetic-predominant group and a parasympathetic-predominant group [171]. In another study, patients with functional dyspepsia had pancreatic polypeptide levels in response to an insulin hypoglycemic stimulus fall between patients with vagotomy and controls, suggesting vagal efferent dysfunction [163] (Figure 7). In general, the findings on parasympathetic and sympathetic activity have been contradictory in the limited literature available to date [172].

Hormonal Changes

There are insufficient data regarding the gastrointestinal hormones and their perturbations in dyspepsia [129]. Moreover, the changes in gut hormone levels may reflect the timing of arrival of nutrients in segments of the gut from which the hormones are secreted.

It has been reported that basal cholecystokinin (CCK) levels were higher in *H.*

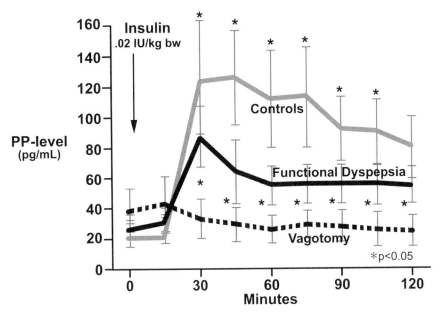

Figure 7. Evidence of vagal dysfunction in patients with functional dyspepsia. In response to an insulin hypoglycemic stimulus, pancreatic polypeptide (PP) levels rise in controls. In patients with a vagotomy, there is no rise in pancreatic polypeptide levels. In functional dyspepsia, the response of pancreatic polypeptide falls between patients with a vagotomy and controls, indicating vagal efferent dysfunction. From Holtmann G, et al. Altered vagal and intestinal mechanosensory function in chronic unexplained dyspepsia. Gut. 1998;42:501–6 with permission from BMJ Publishing Group.

pylori-negative patients than *H. pylori*-positive patients and controls [173]; conversely, there were conflicting results in gastrin levels reported by the same group, being the same in one study [173] and higher in *H. pylori*-positive patients in the second study [174]. Differences in gastric acid secretory status and degree of antral gastritis or atrophy may account in part for these differences. The clinical and physiological significance of the reported changes in gastrin and CCK levels is unclear. Furthermore, G-protein polymorphisms might be involved since there may be an association between $GN\beta_3$ and functional dyspepsia [175]. This could either cause altered responses after receptor stimulation or even directly influence the release of other hormones via augmented or diminished inhibitory influences.

Other authors evaluated a variety of patients with bloating-associated dyspepsia (which is closer to IBS according to current definitions) and concluded that circulating levels of these hormones are not related to symptoms [176].

A provocative report suggested that mucosal somatostatin levels were significantly higher in the ulcer-like disorder group than in the peptic ulcer, motility-like disorder, or control groups [177]. However, it is unclear whether this merely reflects differences in *H. pylori* colonization in the different groups [178]. In another inno-

vative study, but with low numbers of subjects studied, sensitivity to gastric distention was correlated with higher mucosal levels of calcitonin gene related-peptide
(CGRP) and substance P in *H. pylori*-positive dyspeptic patients [179].

Summary

The predominant pathophysiological factors involved in functional dyspepsia are gastric motor and sensory disorders; the underlying cause is unclear.
Gastric acid secretion and *H. pylori* infection probably play a role in a subgroup of
patients. There are many inconsistencies between studies.

— Psychological Features

There is evidence of an association of dyspepsia with psychopathological
factors and comorbidity with psychiatric disorders, especially anxiety disorders
[33, 38, 49, 180, 181]. It is still unclear whether these psychopathological factors
determine health care-seeking behavior, whether they play a key role in the pathophysiology of the dyspepsia symptom complex, or whether they reflect a common
predisposition for functional and psychological disorders. Abnormalities of several psychosocial dimensions were found to be associated with epigastric pain and
with hypersensitivity to gastric distention in functional dyspepsia [56].

— Treatment

General Measures

The available data in the literature are based on studies in functional
dyspepsia patients as a group; no data are available on treatment approaches to
the categories EPS or PDS as defined by the Rome III committee. Evaluation of
pharmacotherapy in functional dyspepsia is further confounded by high placebo
response rates that range from 20% to 60% [182].

Reassurance and explanation represent the first management step. Coffee may
aggravate symptoms in some cases [183] and should be avoided if considered a factor. Stopping smoking and ceasing consumption of alcohol may be helpful, but
there is no convincing evidence of efficacy [109]. The avoidance of aspirin and
other NSAIDs is commonly recommended; although not of established value, this
seems sensible advice as these drugs may cause symptoms that are confused with
functional dyspepsia [109]. If the patient has a coexistent anxiety disorder or depression, appropriate treatment should be considered.

Diet

Anecdotal reports suggest that avoiding offending foods may lessen post-prandial symptoms; spicy and fatty foods are common offenders. It is often recommended that patients take six small low-fat meals per day to decrease the intensity of the symptoms of early satiety, postprandial fullness or bloating, or nausea. This recommendation seems plausible but its impact on symptoms has not been formally investigated. When the neuromuscular function of the stomach is abnormal, the normal work of mixing and emptying ingested food can be seriously impaired. Dietary recommendations in this situation aim at maintaining adequate hydration and varying the gastric workload.

Medications

1. Antacids

While patients with dyspepsia often take antacids, this is not supported by randomized controlled trials in functional dyspepsia [184, 185]. However, this may reflect selection bias since subjects who would have responded to over-the-counter medications are unlikely to present for clinical trials.

Sucralfate has been tested in functional dyspepsia, with one positive [186] and one negative study [187]. Misoprostol is of uncertain efficacy; in one controlled trial reported, patients with erosive prepyloric changes and dyspepsia had a worsening of symptoms [188]. Bismuth is of uncertain efficacy but a trend towards improvement has been observed [189, 190].

2. H$_2$ Blockers

A Cochrane meta-analysis of 11 randomized placebo-controlled trials evaluating the efficacy of H$_2$-receptor antagonists in functional dyspepsia reported a significant benefit over placebo with a relative risk reduction of 22% (95% confidence interval, or CI, 7–35%) [141]. The estimated number needed to treat was eight. H$_2$ blockers thus appear to have a modest efficacy in functional dyspepsia. However, these trials were relatively small and heterogeneous, and often misclassified reflux disease as functional dyspepsia, which may account for much of the benefit.

3. Proton Pump Inhibitors

A Cochrane meta-analysis of seven placebo-controlled, randomized trials in functional dyspepsia reported that this class of agents was superior to placebo [141]. The number needed to treat was calculated to be nine in an updated review [75]. A subanalysis of six of the trials showed no difference in efficacy between half-dose and full-dose PPIs. Double-dose PPI therapy was also not superior to single-dose therapy in functional dyspepsia. How much of this benefit is explained by unrecognized GERD remains unknown. The benefit of symptom subgrouping in functional dyspepsia using previous Rome definitions is less clear. The BOND and OPERA studies when combined showed that ulcer-like dyspepsia but not dysmotility-like dyspepsia or predominant nausea responded to a PPI versus placebo [50]. On the other hand, a negative trial from Hong Kong failed to support any value of symptom subgrouping in terms of response to PPI [191].

4. Eradication of *H. pylori* Infection

A Cochrane meta-analysis reported a 9% pooled relative-risk reduction compared to placebo at 12 months of followup [84]. The number needed to treat was calculated to be 17 in an updated review [75]. Another meta-analysis reported no significant benefit of *H. pylori* eradication [192], but this appears to be primarily explained by a more limited inclusion of the available clinical trials [88]. As *H. pylori* eradication can induce sustained remission in a small minority of patients, this approach can be considered once the benefit and risks have been carefully discussed with the patient.

5. Prokinetics

Metoclopramide
Metoclopramide has multiple mechanisms of action, including dopamine D_2 receptor antagonism and serotonin (5-HT$_3$) antagonism. Metoclopramide appears to be efficacious in functional dyspepsia but has been poorly studied [193, 194], and the side-effect profile limits it use. Most of the studies with metoclopramide have been equivalence trials and therefore have not included placebo. Metoclopramide can prolong the Q-T interval, indicating it has arrhythmogenic properties. Side effects include drowsiness, anxiety, depression, and extra pyramidal symptoms; in the elderly in particular, irreversible tardive dyskinesia can occur.

Domperidone
Domperidone is a substituted benzamide and peripheral dopamine D_2 antagonist [195]. Unlike metoclopramide, domperidone does not cross the blood-brain barrier. Domperidone binds D_2 receptors in the circumventricular organs in the fourth ventricle, and especially in the area postrema and at gastric D_2 receptors. Because domperidone does not readily cross the blood-brain barrier, central nervous system symptoms are rare.

Davis et al. showed that domperidone improved symptoms in patients with functional dyspepsia and idiopathic gastroparesis, but did not increase the rate of gastric emptying, suggesting that domperidone improves symptoms by other mechanisms [196]. A few other trials suggest that domperidone is superior to placebo in reducing symptoms [197, 198]. Pooled estimates from a meta-analysis have indicated that domperidone was superior to placebo on global investigator- and patient-rated assessments of dyspeptic symptoms [197]. However, these studies had substantial heterogeneity.

Domperidone increases plasma prolactin levels, which is associated with breast tenderness and galactorrhea in less than 5% of patients.

Cisapride

Cisapride is a 5-HT_4 agonist that releases acetylcholine from cholinergic motor neurons; it is also a 5-HT_3 antagonist. Two meta-analyses showed significant benefits of cisapride compared with placebo on a number of symptoms including epigastric pain, early satiety, abdominal distention, and nausea [141, 197]. Publication bias may also account in part for the positive results in the literature [75, 141]. However, cisapride has been withdrawn from most markets in the world because of rare fatal arrhythmias.

Tegaserod

This drug is a partial 5-HT_4 agonist. Tegaserod may increase preprandial and postprandial gastric volumes, suggesting that it may be useful in functional dyspepsia where fundic dysaccommodation contributes to the symptoms [199]. A preliminary 12-week phase-two trial showed no significant benefit of tegaserod over placebo in all functional dyspepsia patients, but potential benefit for specific symptoms in female patients [66]; further work is in progress with this agent.

Motilin Agonists

Erythromycin is a macrolide antibiotic; administered by mouth or intravenously, erythromycin increases the gastric emptying rate in patients with diabetic and idiopathic gastroparesis [200, 201]. The erythromycin molecule acts at motilin receptor sites on nerve and smooth muscle to produce strong antral contractions. Macrolide compounds also increase small-bowel contractions and may produce abdominal cramps and diarrhea. A third of patients who were given erythromycin for gastroparesis were not able to tolerate the drug because of these side effects [193]. Synthetic motilin-like molecules that increase gastric emptying and possess no antibacterial activity are being developed, but so far do not appear to be of value in functional dyspepsia. For example, ABT 229 was of no significant benefit in functional dyspepsia over placebo, possibly because the drug impairs fundic relaxation [64].

6. Antidepressants

Antidepressants modulate central processing of visceral stimuli as well as potentially altering gut sensations. For this reason, this class of agents may be of value in functional dyspepsia [202, 203]. In one trial of seven patients, amitriptyline in low doses improved symptoms but not visceral hypersensitivity or sleep [202]. While antidepressants may be of value in other functional bowel disorders, their value in functional dyspepsia is not established. Selective serotonin reuptake inhibitors (SSRIs) have been studied in terms of their effects on gastric function but the results have been mixed [204, 205]. No studies of the clinical efficacy of SSRIs have been conducted in functional dyspepsia patients.

7. Other Drug Treatments

Itopride
Itopride is a novel prokinetic agent that acts both as a dopamine D_2 receptor antagonist and as an acetylcholinesterase inhibitor. A recent phase II study confirmed that itopride was significantly better than placebo for improvement of symptoms in patients with functional dyspepsia [206].

Antispasmodics
The antispasmodic drug dicyclomine was no better than placebo in reducing global symptoms in dyspeptic patients in two small crossover studies [207, 208]. Likewise, a double-blind trial with a 4-week crossover protocol showed that trimebutine was no better than placebo in 24 dyspeptic patients [209]. Newer, more selective M3 antispasmodics have been developed but have not been tested in functional dyspepsia.

Herbal Preparations
Various studies reported improvement of symptoms during treatment with an herbal preparation containing various plant extracts, including plant extract from bitter candy tuft, matricaria flower, peppermint leaves, caraway, licorice root, lemon balm [210]. The data support the assumption that these specific preparations are effective. The question, however, remains which component or components are responsible for the clinical efficacy. Furthermore, the stability and the concentration of the active components might be an issue that impairs the widespread use.

8. Potential Future Treatment Approaches

Visceral Analgesics
A number of different drugs may modulate gastric and duodenal sensation and hence improve the symptoms of functional dyspepsia. Kappa opioid agonists are currently under development. Fedotozine was a kappa opioid agonist that increased gastric distention pain thresholds [211–213]. In a multicenter, randomized placebo-controlled study of 271 patients, fedotozine led to significant reductions of global individual symptom scores compared with placebo, although the differences observed were very small and the outcome measures reported in the study were based primarily on post- versus pretreatment differences in symptom scores [213]. Fedotozine is no longer under development, but asimadoline is another promising kappa opioid agonist in testing.

Asimadoline significantly delayed the onset of satiety and reduced postprandial fullness in healthy volunteers [214]; its efficacy in functional dyspepsia is under testing. Alvimopan is a peripheral mu receptor antagonist that may increase gastric emptying and appears to be effective in postoperative ileus [215]. Whether this drug will have any benefit in functional dyspepsia is unknown.

N-methyl-D-aspartate (NMDA) receptor antagonists represent another group of potential visceral analgesics. However, the NMDA antagonist dextromethorphan did not reduce gastric perception scores compared with placebo and in fact was linked to increased reports of nausea, bloating, and satiation following gastric wall distention in one study [216].

The tachykinin system is considered to have an important role in transmission of afferent and efferent stimuli [217, 218]. The neurokinin (NK)$_1$ antagonist aprepitant is currently available for the treatment of chemotherapy-induced nausea and vomiting but has not been tested in functional dyspepsia [219, 220]. The NK$_3$ antagonists talnetant and osanetant have also not been tested in functional dyspepsia [221], but may have potential therapeutic value.

Capsaicin has analgesic properties related to its binding to the vanilloid receptor (VR)$_1$ [222]. In a double-blind placebo-controlled study, red pepper, which contains capsaicin, reduced overall symptom scores as well as epigastric pain and fullness in functional dyspepsia compared with placebo, although the benefit was small [223].

Fundus-Relaxing Drugs

If the hypothesis that impaired fundic relaxation is a major mechanism in induction of dyspeptic symptoms, then drugs that relax the fundus may have therapeutic benefit.

A number of agents appear to potentially be useful. These include the 5-HT$_1$ agonists, such as sumatriptan and buspirone (which also slow gastric emptying) [224, 225]. Tegaserod appears to relax the gastric fundus as does cisapride, presumably via 5-HT$_4$ agonist actions [199]. On the other hand, the 5-HT$_3$ antagonists (e.g., alosetron) do not alter gastric accommodation [226] but may improve dyspepsia [65]. Certain SSRIs can relax the gastric fundus, presumably by release of serotonin and hence stimulation of 5-HT$_1$ or 5-HT$_4$ receptors [204, 205]. Nitric oxide donor agents can also relax the gastric fundus [227] although nitroglycerin failed to relieve dyspeptic symptoms in one study [228]. On the other hand, the CCK antagonist dexloxiglumide has been shown to significantly reduce gastric accommodation and compliance [229]. It has been suggested that fundus-relaxing drugs such as nitrates were less effective in reducing sensitivity to gastric distention compared to alpha-2 agonists with antinociceptive properties such as clonidine [230], but these studies were conducted in healthy subjects with normal gastric accommodation. Further work is needed to establish the therapeutic place of fundic relaxing drugs in functional dyspepsia, but this is a promising area.

CCK Antagonists

Symptoms induced by duodenal infusion of lipids can be reduced by the CCK_1 receptor antagonist dexloxiglumide [229, 231]. The exact mechanism of action here is uncertain and randomized controlled trials with this class of agents in functional dyspepsia are awaited with interest. Dexloxiglumide significantly accelerated gastric emptying in patients with constipation-predominant irritable bowel syndrome [232].

Psychotherapy and Hypnotherapy

In one trial, psychotherapy was superior to supportive therapy in reducing patient-rated dyspepsia at the end of the 12-week intervention, although there was no difference at one year of followup [233]. In a study of hypnotherapy in functional dyspepsia, excellent results were reported in terms of improvement in patient-rated symptoms and quality of life as well as subsequent use of medications after therapy was ceased [234]. More studies are required to confirm these initial results, but hypnotherapy appears particularly promising.

9. Novel Approaches

Gastric Electrical Stimulation

Gastric stimulation, while not accelerating gastric emptying, significantly reduced symptoms in patients with gastroparesis, suggesting there may be some effect on afferent function [235, 236]. In patients with very resistant symptoms, this may be worth considering.

Acupuncture, Acupressure, and Acustimulation

Acupuncture stimulates a specific site during insertion and rotation of the acupuncture needle. In acupressure treatment, pressure with the fingers or a device is applied to the specific acupuncture point. Acupuncture and acupressure appear to decrease nausea and vomiting related to cancer chemotherapy [237]. Dundee et al. showed that acupuncture and acustimulation were significantly better in reducing these symptoms postoperatively compared with placebo stimulation [238]. Acustimulation and acupressure may also decrease the nausea that is part of motion sickness induced by illusory self-motion [239, 240]. Acupressure and acupuncture have not been systematically evaluated in patients with functional dyspepsia, but preliminary results have not been encouraging [241].

B2. Belching Disorders

Air swallowing during eating and drinking is a normal physiological event. In a study in volunteers, each swallow of a 10-mL liquid bolus was accompanied by ingestion of 8 to 32 mL of air [242]. Transient relaxation of the lower esophageal sphincter (LES), triggered by distention of the proximal stomach, is the mechanism that allows the ingested air to be vented from the stomach [243–245]. Hence, belching is common and this symptom can only be considered a disorder when it becomes troublesome [17].

— Epidemiology

The epidemiology of troublesome belching in the general population remains to be carefully defined but clinical impression suggests it is rare. A survey of consecutive new patients with a diagnosis of functional bowel disorder in an Asian specialized care center reported that only 1% of these met the Rome II criteria for aerophagia [59], while a prevalence of 6% was reported in a series evaluated in a Western referral center [246].

B2. Diagnostic Criteria* for Belching Disorders

B2a. Aerophagia
Must include *all* of the following:
1. **Troublesome repetitive belching at least several times a week**
2. **Air swallowing that is objectively observed or measured**

*Criteria fulfilled for the last 3 months with symptom onset at least 6 months prior to diagnosis

B2b. Unspecified Excessive Belching
Must include *all* of the following:
1. **Troublesome repetitive belching at least several times a week**
2. **No evidence that excessive air swallowing underlies the symptom**

*Criteria fulfilled for the last 3 months with symptom onset at least 6 months prior to diagnosis

— Justification for Changes to the Criteria

In the previous classification of gastroduodenal disorders, all excessive belching was considered to reflect aerophagia. Aerophagia is an unusual disorder in which patients are believed to have excessive belching due to air swallowing. The committee confirmed that aerophagia couldn't be diagnosed without observing the occurrence of excessive air swallowing or ingestion, which may or may not be obvious at the office assessment. The committee decided to expand the category based on consensus that excessive belching can be a presenting symptom and may be assessed with intraluminal impedance measurement of air transport in the esophagus [244], which confirms that different mechanisms of excessive belching occur [247]. In aerophagia, belching activity follows a distinct pattern, characterized by rapid antegrade and retrograde flow of air in the esophagus that usually does not reach the stomach. This phenomenon of "supragastric belching," clearly distinct from "gastric" belching, is not accompanied by transient relaxation of the LES and is only observed in aerophagia [247]. Patients with functional dyspepsia were more likely to have abdominal pain, nausea, vomiting, weight loss, and early satiety than patients with aerophagia [248] (Figure 8).

— Clinical Evaluation

A positive diagnosis is based on a careful history and observation of air swallowing [248]. In addition to belching, excess rectal flatus may occur with excessive air ingestion [249]. In typical cases, no investigation is required. Rumination can usually be distinguished by the history and observation. It is important to screen for psychiatric disease, including depression and anxiety. Excessive belching may also accompany or contribute to GERD. In difficult cases, pH monitoring or empirical acid-suppressive therapy may be considered to recognize GERD as an underlying cause [250]. Although not formally tested, it is likely that esophageal intraluminal impedance monitoring may be useful to explore the nature of troublesome belching that is not clinically clear-cut.

— Physiological Features

Air swallowing is normal; an approximate mean of 18 mL is swallowed with each bolus of a liquid meal [242]. By consequence, postprandial belching as a venting mechanism is also normal, with 3 to 4 belches per hour occurring with a normal diet. Belching is usually an unconscious act, and the motility patterns of belching are quite similar to those found in gastro-esophageal reflux [245, 251].

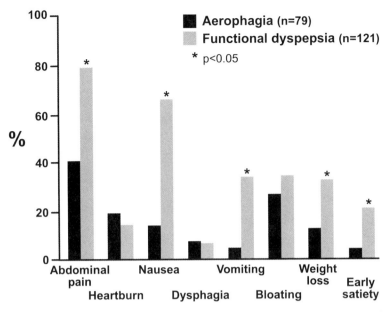

Figure 8. Prevalence of symptoms in patients with aerophagia compared with patients with functional dyspepsia. Patients with functional dyspepsia were more likely to have abdominal pain, nausea, vomiting, weight loss, and early satiety. From Chitkara et al. Aerophagia in adults: a comparison with functional dyspepsia. Published in Aliment Pharmacol Ther 2005;22:855–58 with permission from Blackwell Publishing.

With gastric belching, certain key reflex events need to occur: The lower esophageal sphincter has to relax in response to distension of the stomach from gas that has been swallowed, and this has to be followed by relaxation of the upper esophageal sphincter, which can occur when a large volume of gas abruptly distends the esophagus.

In patients with belching disorders, the belching must be repetitive and troublesome. There should be no evidence of structural or metabolic abnormalities to explain the symptoms. Repetitive belching alone is common and may be due to causes other than aerophagia; observation of air swallowing and belching is unequivocal evidence of aerophagia. The patient with aerophagia ingests air into the esophagus by expanding the chest and lowering the diaphragm against a closed glottis. The air is then released, often with a loud noise. The maneuver may relieve abdominal discomfort or even be pleasurable. While usually unconscious, presumably the habit is learned. Data on habitual air swallowers are lacking but excess gas is probably not present in patients with aerophagia, based on inert gas washout studies [249] and on x-ray evaluation of the intragastric air bubble [247].

The intraluminal impedance recording technique allows detection of the passage of air through the esophagus, either in aboral or oral direction [244]. A recent study using this technique in aerophagia patients revealed swallowing of air that enters the esophagus very rapidly and is expulsed almost immediately in the oral direction [247]. Use of impedance in the investigation of belching cannot be recommended for clinical practice at this point, but the field is rapidly evolving.

Belching is often an associated symptom in GERD. A tertiary care study reported that up to 70% of GERD patients were reporting belching and a close temporal association between acid reflux events detected on pH monitoring and belching was reported [250]. Belching is also reported in dyspepsia, where it does not respond to acid-suppressive therapy [50]. It has been suggested that disturbed upper gastrointestinal tract motility may account for the symptoms, but this has not been carefully studied [251]. In functional dyspepsia, belching is associated with hypersensitivity to gastric distension, which supports the concept that belching is induced to relieve upper abdominal discomfort [29, 56].

— Psychological Features

Changes in emotional state can lead to increases in spontaneous swallowing in health [252]. Psychological factors have been presumed to be of importance in aerophagia, but there is no objective evidence of excess major psychopathology in aerophagia [253]. In functional dyspepsia, no psychopathology was associated with symptoms of belching [56]. However, this does not rule out a role for psychiatric disease in some patients.

— Treatment

General Measures

Explanation of the symptoms and reassurance are important. It is probably useful to demonstrate chest expansion and air ingestion as the patient belches. The habit, if not firmly established, can be sometimes unlearned by behavioral techniques. Treatment of associated psychiatric disease or employment of stress reduction techniques, when present, may theoretically be of benefit.

Diet

Dietary modification (avoiding sucking hard candies or chewing gum, eating slowly and encouraging small swallows at mealtime, and avoiding carbonated beverages) is often recommended but has not been rigorously tested and is usually disappointing in practice.

Medications

Studies investigating drug therapy specifically in aerophagia are lacking. Information of efficacy of drug therapy in aerophagia can be derived from a number of studies conducted in functional disorders in a broader sense. While tranquillizers [254] may occasionally be useful in severe cases, drug therapy is not generally recommended. Simethicone and activated charcoal preparations are usually ineffective [255]. An uncontrolled study suggested that belching improved after botulinum toxin injection in idiopathic gastroparesis [256].

Other Treatments

Sustained improvement has been reported with hypnotherapy in a case report [257]. The value of other psychological interventions is unknown. In GERD, coexisting aerophagia is associated with a less favorable outcome of anti-reflux surgery [258].

B3. Nausea and Vomiting Disorders

— Definitions

Nausea is a subjective symptom and can be defined as an unpleasant sensation of the imminent need to vomit typically experienced in the epigastrium or throat. Nausea is a common symptom and the differential diagnosis is wide. Possible dimensions of nausea have been identified; queasiness and epigastric discomfort, systemic symptoms including sweating and light-headedness, and emotional symptoms including fatigue and depression [259].

Vomiting refers to the forceful oral expulsion of gastric or intestinal content associated with contraction of the abdominal and chest wall muscles. Vomiting must be distinguished from regurgitation and rumination. Regurgitation refers to food being brought back into the mouth without any abdominal or chest muscle contraction, while rumination is the voluntary repeated regurgitation of food.

— Epidemiology

Nausea is a common symptom but is less prevalent than epigastric pain or meal-related symptoms in the community. In one study, 8% of otherwise normal subjects reported nausea [260].

Unexplained (functional) vomiting, which refers to chronic vomiting at least once a week, is believed to be rare. It should be distinguished from occasional vomiting that can occur in patients with documented functional dyspepsia. Population-based data suggest that vomiting once a month or more occurs in about 2% of women and 3% of men [18]. However, how many of these subjects have functional or cyclical vomiting has not been ascertained [261]. In cases of functional or cyclic vomiting, no structural or biochemical cause for the vomiting can be identified. A prevalence of 5% was reported among selected patients fully investigated in a tertiary referral center [246]. The term psychogenic vomiting has been used synonymously with functional vomiting but has no standard definition in the literature [262–265]. Hence, the committee recommends the term psychogenic vomiting be abandoned in favor of functional vomiting.

Cyclic vomiting syndrome is characterized by episodes of vomiting with a stereotypical onset and duration; there are varying intervals of absence of vomiting in between episodes. No structural or biochemical cause can be identified. In children with cyclic vomiting, approximately 80% of cases have a strong family history of migraine headaches [266–270]. Adults are reported to develop cyclical vomiting in middle age but it is rare; the condition may affect over 1% of school-age children [268]. In 70 adult patients accrued over a 10-year period in a referral center, cyclical vomiting occurred at a mean age of 35 with a range of 14 to 73 years, although diagnosis was delayed until a mean age of 41 years; it affected both men and women [271]. Only one in four adults had a history of migraine headaches [258, 269]. The vomiting may be linked to the menstrual cycle or precipitated by pregnancy. Adult patients have a mean of four cycles per year of vomiting compared with a mean of 12 cycles per year in children [271]. In a study of 17 adult patients, the average duration was 6 days but ranged from 1 to 21 days; the symptom-free intervals had a mean of 3 months, but ranged between 0.5 to 6 months [271]. Episodes may only be related to the onset of menses in some cases.

Many drugs can induce nausea or vomiting. Chronic cannabis use has been recognized as a possible cause of recurrent vomiting [272]. Cessation of cannabis use led to cessation of the vomiting illness in patients who exhibited cyclical vomiting episodes [272].

B3. Diagnostic Criteria* for Nausea and Vomiting Disorders

B3a. Chronic Idiopathic Nausea
Must include *all* of the following:
1. Bothersome nausea occurring at least several times per week
2. Not usually associated with vomiting
3. Absence of abnormalities at upper endoscopy or metabolic disease that explains the nausea

*Criteria fulfilled for the last 3 months with symptom onset at least 6 months prior to diagnosis

B3b. Functional Vomiting
Must include *all* of the following:
1. On average one or more episodes of vomiting per week
2. Absence of criteria for an eating disorder, rumination, or major psychiatric disease according to **DSM-IV**
3. Absence of self-induced vomiting and chronic cannabinoid use and absence of abnormalities in the central nervous system or metabolic diseases to explain the recurrent vomiting

*Criteria fulfilled for the last 3 months with symptom onset at least 6 months prior to diagnosis

B3c. Cyclic Vomiting Syndrome
Must include *all* of the following:
1. Stereotypical episodes of vomiting regarding onset (*acute*) and duration (*less than one week*)
2. Three or more discrete episodes in the prior year
3. Absence of nausea and vomiting between episodes

Supportive Criterion
History or family history of migraine headaches

— Rationale for Changes in Diagnostic Criteria

After review of the available literature, a new category, chronic idiopathic nausea (CIN) was added. In the Rome II criteria, nausea was considered a symptom of dysmotility-like dyspepsia [11], but the committee decided to revise this on the basis of factor analysis data, on clinical experience that persistent nausea is often of central or psychological origin, and on the lack of responsiveness of this symptom to empiric therapy for dyspepsia.

The committee slightly modified the previous definition of functional vomiting based on the setting of threshold frequencies and on the recognition of cannabinoid use as a mechanism. A new category, cyclical vomiting in adults, was added based on expert opinion and a better appreciation that those with stereotypical attacks of cyclical vomiting differ from those with functional vomiting.

Differential Diagnosis

The differential diagnosis of recurrent vomiting is extensive (Table 4) [275]. Rumination and eating disorders need to be excluded.

Rumination

This may occur in normal adults as well as mentally impaired children [273, 274]. Typically there is effortless regurgitation of undigested food within minutes of starting or completing a meal. It often occurs daily and with each meal ingested. The food does not taste bitter or sour but like it has just been eaten. There is no associated nausea or retching. Weight is usually maintained although there may be weight loss. The patient may reswallow the food or spit it out depending on the social circumstances. The history is diagnostic. Gastric emptying may be delayed and esophageal pH testing may show reflux [273]. Characteristic rumination waves (i.e., synchronous pressure increases in stomach and esophagus creating a common channel) are seen in 40% with gastroduodenal manometry testing [273].

Eating Disorders

Patients with bulimia may have self-induced vomiting associated with binge episodes and generally a distorted body image. Careful clinical evaluation is essential to avoid overlooking an eating disorder causing recurrent vomiting.

Cannabinoid Hyperemesis

Patients should be asked for habitual and chronic use of marijuana. Urine drug screens may help to recognize this cause in noncooperative patients [272].

Table 4. Differential Diagnosis of Nausea and Vomiting

Disorders of the gut and peritoneum
Mechanical obstruction
 Gastric outlet obstruction
 Small bowel obstruction
Functional gastrointestinal disorders
 Gastroparesis
 Chronic intestinal pseudo-
  obstruction
 Functional dyspepsia
 Irritable bowel syndrome
 Roux-en-Y syndrome
Organic gastrointestinal disorders
 Pancreatic adenocarcinoma
 Inflammatory intraperitoneal disease
 Peptic ulcer disease
 Cholecystitis
 Pancreatitis
 Hepatitis
 Crohn's disease
 Mesenteric ischemia
 Retroperitoneal fibrosis
 Mucosal metastases

Medications and toxic etiologies
Cancer chemotherapy
 Severe-cisplatinum, dacarbazine,
  nitrogen mustard
 Moderate-etoposide, methotrexate,
  cytarabine
 Mild-fluorouracil, vinblastine,
  tamoxifen
Analgesics
 Aspirin
 Nonsteroidal anti-inflammatory
  drugs
 Auranofin
 Antigout drugs
Cardiovascular medications
 Digoxin
 Antiarrhythmics
 Antihypertensives
 ß-blockers
 Calcium channel antagonists
 Diuretics
Hormonal preparations/therapies
 Oral antidiabetics
 Oral contraceptives
Antibiotics/antivirals
 Erythromycin

Tetracycline
Sulphonamides
Antituberculous drugs
Acyclovir
Gastrointestinal medications
 Sulfasalazine
 Azathioprine
 Nicotine
CNS active medications
 Narcotics
 Antiparkinsonian drugs
 Anticonvulsants
Antiasthmatic
 Theophylline
Miscellaneous
 Ethanol abuse
 Jamaican vomiting sickness
 Hypervitaminosis

Infectious causes
Gastrointestinal
 Viral gastroenteritis
 Bacterial gastroenteritis
Nongastrointestinal
 Otitis media

Endocrine/metabolic disorders
Pregnancy
Diabetic ketoacidosis
Hyperthyroidism
Uremia
Addison's disease
Hyperparathyroidism
Hypoparathyroidism
Acute intermittent porphyria

Postoperative nausea and vomiting

CNS disorders
Migraine
Increased intracranial pressure
 Malignancy
 Hemorrhage
 Infarction
 Abscess
 Meningitis
 Congenital malformation
 Hydrocephalus
 Pseudotumor cerebri

Table 4 continued. Differential Diagnosis of Nausea and Vomiting

Seizure disorders	**Anxiety disorders**
Demyelinating disorders	Depression
Labyrinthine disorders	Pain
Motion sickness	Anorexia nervosa
Labyrinthitis	Bulimia nervosa
Tumors	
Menieres disease	**Miscellaneous causes**
Iatrogenic disease	Cardiac disease
Fluorescein angiography	Myocardial infarction
	Congestive heart failure
	Radiofrequency ablation
Psychiatric disorders	Starvation
Emotional response	
Psychogenic vomiting	

Adapted from Quigley et al. Gastroenterology 2001;120:263–86.

Diagnostic Tests

It is particularly important to exclude gastroparesis, intestinal obstruction, and intestinal pseudo-obstruction as well metabolic and central nervous system disease in adult patients presenting with recurrent unexplained vomiting [275–276]. An upper endoscopy and a small-bowel x-ray or computed tomography (CT) enterography are performed to exclude gastroduodenal disease and small-bowel obstruction. Biochemical testing is also essential to exclude electrolyte abnormalities, hypercalcemia, hypothyroidism, and Addison's disease. If these tests are normal, then it is reasonable to consider gastric emptying evaluation, although this may not significantly alter management based on current evidence. In typical cases where gastric emptying results are normal or equivocal, but severe symptoms persist, it is useful to ensure that enteric neuropathy is not being missed by undertaking gastroduodenal manometry. In this setting, a completely normal antroduodenal manometry is of most value. The use of electrogastography is not widely accepted, although gastric dysrhythmias may be recorded in some patients with unexplained nausea and vomiting with normal gastric emptying [98]. It is unknown how commonly gastric emptying disturbances and EGG abnormalities occur in patients with a clinical diagnosis of functional vomiting or cyclical vomiting [98]. Vomiting can be an atypical presentation of GERD and if endoscopy is negative, esophageal pH testing should be considered [276].

Certain mitochondrial disorders associated with intermittent vomiting episodes may rarely be confused with cyclical vomiting such as medium-chain acyl co-enzyme A dehydrogenase deficiency or mitochondrial encephalopathy, lactic acidosis, and stroke-like syndrome (MELAS) [269]. Food allergy such as sensitivity to cow's milk, soy, or egg white protein as well as food intolerance to chocolate, cheese, or monosodium glutamate may cause vomiting which can also be confused with the cyclical vomiting syndrome [270].

— Physiological Features

The mechanisms of explaining functional and cyclic vomiting remain unknown. There could be central, peripheral, or combined abnormalities in these patients.

— Psychological Features

Major depression has been linked to habitual postprandial and irregular vomiting, while conversion disorder may explain some cases of continuous vomiting [277]. There is no information on the psychological profile of patients with functional vomiting where major psychiatric diseases have been excluded and there is no evidence for structural or metabolic explanation for the symptoms. In cyclical vomiting in adults, psychiatric disease appears to be uncommon, with the largest adult series suggesting only 20% having anxiety or another psychiatric disorder [261].

— Treatment

Antinausea Drugs

The treatment of chronic idiopathic nausea is not defined. The 5-HT$_3$ antagonist drugs have been remarkably successful in controlling nausea and vomiting specifically related to cancer chemotherapy agents and in postoperative care. The exact mechanism of beneficial action of the 5-HT$_3$ antagonists is not known, although blockade of 5-HT$_3$ receptors in the area postrema, and/or vagal afferent fibers in the stomach and duodenum have been reported. Modest symptom improvement in functional dyspepsia has been shown with ondansetron and alosetron over placebo [65]; more potent agents are yet to be tested.

Prochlorperazine is an antinauseant drug with nonspecific actions in the central nervous system. The side effects can be formidable and range from hypotension to spastic torticollis and dystonia.

Diphenhydrinate and cyclizine are anti-motion-sickness drugs. These H$_1$ antagonists have not been studied for efficacy in controlling nausea due to gastrointestinal disorders. Diphenhydrinate and cyclizine, however, decrease gastric dysrhythmias and motion sickness symptoms, suggesting that a portion of the drug action is at a peripheral site, namely the stomach [275]. Promethazine is used to treat mild, nonspecific nausea. These drugs frequently induce unacceptable drowsiness. Tricyclic antidepressant therapy is useful by anecdotal accounts [275].

Functional Vomiting

In functional vomiting, management of nutritional status and psychosocial support is important. The role of dietary and pharmacological therapy, both frequently used, has not been specifically tested. There is also no evidence that medications are particularly useful in this group, although anecdotal reports suggest that tricyclic antidepressants are helpful even at low doses [275]. Anti-emetic drugs are often of little value. One case has documented the value of cognitive and social skills training [278]. Self-monitoring with suppression of urge to vomit has been reported to be of value [279]. Data otherwise are lacking on the value of behavioral or psychotherapy, but these approaches may be worth trying.

Cyclic Vomiting Syndrome

Patients may require hospital admission and supportive care during severe bouts. Empiric treatments of antimigraine medications have been used with anecdotal reports of success, and a trial of antimigraine medications is worth considering, especially when there is a family history of migraine headaches. Even if there is no such history, the medications sometimes appear to be of value. The serotonin-1 agonists (triptans) can be given as a subcutaneous injection, as a nasal spray, or orally, depending on the drug. All of the triptans appear to be effective for the treatment of acute migraine. They are contraindicated because of the risk of vascular disease in ischemic heart disease, ischemic stroke, and uncontrolled hypertension. Beta blockers seem to be useful in some patients with cyclic vomiting [281]. A tricyclic antidepressant (e.g., amitriptyline, doxepin, or nortriptyline at a median dose of 50 mg) or an SSRI (e.g., fluoxetine) may help [261]. Other drugs that have been tried empirically include cyproheptadine, ketorolac, prochlorperazine, metoclopramide, ondansetron, naloxone, carnitine, and erythromycin [266, 280]. In menstrual-related cyclic vomiting, low-dose estrogen oral contraceptive treatment may help. The Cyclic Vomiting Syndrome Association (CVSA) was established in the U.S. in 1993 and provides patient support.

B4. Rumination Syndrome

— Definition

Rumination is a well-known phenomenon [281] that occurs in animals such as sheep, cattle, and goats, with compartmentalized stomachs consisting of multiple chambers [282, 283]. In these animals, food residue in the proximal two chambers of the stomach moves by retrograde peristalsis into the mouth in a coordinated manner associated with relaxation of the lower esophageal sphincter. The animals then rechew and reswallow the regurgitated food. This process aids in the digestion and absorption of food by reducing particle size and enhancing acid exposure [284].

In humans, rumination syndrome is a condition characterized by the repetitive, effortless regurgitation of recently ingested food into the mouth followed by rechewing and reswallowing or expulsion [285]. Although initially described in infants [286–289] and the developmentally disabled [290–292], it is now widely recognized that rumination syndrome occurs in males and females of all ages and cognitive abilities [273, 274, 291–295]. In general, rumination is more common in females than males [273, 274, 295].

Rumination syndrome is an underappreciated condition in adults who are often misdiagnosed as having vomiting secondary to gastroparesis or gastroesophageal reflux. Difficulties in arriving at the correct diagnosis may be caused by the lack of awareness of the condition among physicians. It must be considered in the differential diagnosis of a patient with regurgitation, vomiting (especially postprandial), and weight loss.

— Epidemiology

The epidemiology of rumination syndrome in the adult general population remains to be carefully defined but clinical impression suggests it is rare.

B4. Diagnostic Criteria* for Rumination Syndrome

Must include *both* of the following:
1. Persistent or recurrent regurgitation of recently ingested food into the mouth with subsequent spitting or remastication and swallowing
2. Regurgitation is not preceded by retching

***Criteria fulfilled for the last 3 months with symptom onset at least 6 months prior to diagnosis**

Supportive Criteria
1. Regurgitation events are usually not preceded by nausea
2. Cessation of the process when the regurgitated material becomes acidic
3. Regurgitant contains recognizable food with a pleasant taste

Rumination is well described in infants with the typical age of onset between 3 and 6 months and is fully described in the chapter on disorders of gastrointestinal function in infants (Chapter 13). The committee based adult diagnostic criteria on the pediatric criteria.

— Rationale for Changes to Criteria

The committee changed the criteria based on the recognition that rumination syndrome occurs in males and females of all ages and cognitive abilities.

— Clinical Evaluation

Rumination syndrome is an underappreciated condition in adults who are often misdiagnosed as having vomiting secondary to gastroparesis or gastroesophageal reflux or anorexia or bulimia nervosa. Typical clinical features include:

1. Repetitive regurgitation of gastric contents starting within minutes of the start of a meal; this is to be contrasted with the typical history of vomiting in the later postprandial period in patients with gastroparesis.

2. Episodes often last 1 to 2 hours.
3. The regurgitant consists of partially recognizable food, which often has a pleasant taste according to the patients.
4. The regurgitation is effortless or preceded by a sensation of belching immediately prior to the regurgitation or arrival of food in the pharynx.
5. There is usually lack of retching or nausea preceding the regurgitation.

Patients make a conscious decision regarding the regurgitant once it is present in the oropharynx. The choice may depend on the social situation at the time. Rumination is typically a "meal in, meal out, day in, day out" behavior

Clinical experience suggests that many individuals with rumination have additional symptoms including nausea, heartburn, abdominal discomfort, diarrhea, and/or constipation. Weight loss can also be a prominent feature of rumination syndrome, particularly in the adolescent population [273, 274, 285, 286, 295, 296]. Patients often report that the regurgitant may be sour or bitter tasting and the behavior does not stop when the regurgitant becomes "acidic." Patients with additional symptoms may require further medical evaluation before rumination syndrome can be confidently confirmed as a singular diagnosis. Weight loss can also be a prominent feature of rumination syndrome, particularly in the adolescent population [273, 274, 295, 296]. Considering the female predominance of the condition and the frequent occurrence of weight loss, patients are often misdiagnosed as having bulimia and/or anorexia nervosa [298, 299]. Although weight loss is a concerning symptom, particularly in children and adolescents, we do not believe that weight loss alone is an indication for more exhaustive diagnostic testing in the presence of classical clinical features of rumination syndrome.

Many patients have evidence of "pathological gastroesophageal reflux" because the 24-hour pH study will show >4% of the time with intraesophageal pH below 4 [273]. However, careful study shows that this is typically in the first hour postmeal, associated with rapid oscillations in pH caused by regurgitation and reswallowing of food and most often there is no nocturnal acidification of the esophagus. The other clue is that despite repetitive changes in pH, the total time that the esophageal pH is < 4 may be paradoxically low, since food buffers the gastric acid and the pH of gastric contents may be > 4 during the postprandial period when repetitive regurgitation occurs. Many patients have evidence of macroscopic or microscopic damage to the lower esophagus due to the regurgitant [273].

— Physiological Features

Pathophysiological mechanisms involved in rumination syndrome remain somewhat unclear, though all observations suggest there is an adaptation of the belch reflex [273]. Thus one hypothesis proposes simultaneous relaxation of the lower esophageal sphincter during episodes of increased intra-abdominal pressure [300]. A second hypothesis is a learned, voluntary relaxation of the diaphragmatic crura that allows the normal postprandial increase in intragastric pressure to overcome the resistance to retrograde flow provided by the lower esophageal sphincter.

— Psychological Features

Thumshirn et al. [301] demonstrated that patients of normal intelligence with rumination syndrome required significantly lower fundic pressures to induce LES relaxation and had increased gastric sensitivity to balloon distention compared to healthy controls. The data suggest that the pressure of food within the fundus may result in reflex inhibition of lower esophageal pressure leading to the induction of a modified belch reflex. Smout et al. showed that the behavior was akin to the self-induction of a transient LES relaxation [302]. In some cases, stressful life events can be identified around the time of symptom onset [273]. However, in most cases rumination occurs in the absence of such identifiable predisposing factors.

An association between rumination and bulimia nervosa has been described. In one study 20% of bulimics were found to ruminate [299] and in another study, 17% of female ruminators had a history of bulimia [274]. An important difference between ruminators who are bulimic and those who are not is that the bulimics tend to expel rather than reswallow food and may self-induce vomiting by digital stimulation of the hypopharynx. It has been speculated that in this group of patients, rumination may be a learned behavior as a measure to control their weight and purge themselves without frank vomiting. Treatment of rumination in bulimics has been reported to be less successful because of the incentive of weight control. Treatment that resulted in control of overeating was more successful than treatments that directly targeted rumination. Rumination in such patients can be considered a variant of an eating disorder.

— Treatment

PPIs are frequently used to suppress the symptom of heartburn and protect the esophageal mucosa while therapy is instituted. The mainstay of treatment for rumination syndrome involves behavioral modification. The preferred behavioral treatment for rumination syndrome in this patient population consists of habit reversal using special breathing techniques to compete with the urge to regurgitate [303–305]. Habit reversal techniques are used in such a way that the target behavior (rumination) is eliminated by the consistent use of an incompatible or competing behavior. The rumination behavior is eliminated because rumination and the competing response cannot be performed at the same time. Consistent practice of diaphragmatic breathing during rumination effectively eliminates rumination activity after proper training in both habit reversal and diaphragmatic breathing.

Recommendations for Future Research

1. Rome III Definitions for Gastroduodenal Disorders

The relationship of the newly defined disorders (PDS, EPS, CIN, CVS) to each other, to pathophysiological mechanisms, and response to therapy needs to be assessed. The epidemiology of these disorders will also need to be studied carefully.

2. Mechanisms of Symptom Production

The goal should be that the field moves from appraisal of symptoms and empirical trials of therapy to therapy based on identified mechanisms. This requires more extensive understanding of the physiological mechanisms causing symptoms, or simply acknowledging that symptoms are multidetermined and may be caused by a variety of different physiological disturbances. The latter will lead to a focus on eliciting the pathophysiology. For this to be a practical goal, the diagnostic tests need to be enhanced and brought to the clinical arena.

3. Diagnostic Issues

Given the diverse etiologies described above, there is a great need for validated noninvasive diagnostic methods to help the clinician evaluate the etiology of symptoms and to target the appropriate treatment.

To date, these methods have been adequately assessed for face validity, reproducibility, and applicability in primary/secondary as well as tertiary care. To date, the methods have often involved radiation exposure; noninvasive imaging and stable isotope measurements are needed that measure accommodation and gastric emptying

The pros and cons of nutrient drink tests need to be thoroughly understood;

recent data propose that the nutrient drink test be used as a surrogate for measuring accommodation or visceral hypersensitivity. This approach is deserving of further study since it is a very practical and feasible test for the clinical practice.

Mail-in tests need to be developed for these common conditions seen in primary and secondary care.

4. Therapeutic Issues

No treatment without diagnosis: the field has to move from appraisal of symptoms and empirical therapy trials to therapy based on identified mechanism. Validated endpoints need to be used as biomarkers to test the validity of novel approaches to treatment in pharmacodynamic studies. Initially, studies may be proposed in healthy volunteers to characterize the mechanism of action of medications and to limit the dose range that would need to be tested in patients.

As a next step, pharmacodynamic studies in patients should be performed with new medications before embarking on costly and potentially dangerous phase IIb clinical trials before the true potential of a medication is tested in humans.

Medications affecting the different pathophysiological mechanisms require further development: prokinetics, gastric relaxants, and antinociceptive agents are some examples. However, this traditional approach has failed in recent years since some of the physiological abnormalities found only poorly correlated with symptoms and thus may simply reflect markers for an underlying abnormality.

The peripheral and central effects of SSRIs, tricyclic antidepressants, and selective noradrenaline reuptake inhibitors in health and dyspepsia require thorough characterization before a recommendation to use these medications indiscriminately in practice.

Ultimately, combination therapies need to be tested to either enhance correction of underlying single pathophysiology or to correct more than one pathophysiology.

Appropriate pharmacoeconomic studies are also needed to test the true value of available and future therapies.

References

1. Kingham JGC, Fairclough PD, Dawson AM. What is indigestion? J R Soc Med 1983; 76:183–186.
2. Colin-Jones DG, Bloom B, Bodemar G, Crean G, Freston J, Gugler R, Malagelada J, Nyren O, Petersen H, Piper D. Management of dyspepsia: Report of a working party. Lancet 1988;1:576–579.
3. Talley NJ, Phillips SF. Non-ulcer dyspepsia: potential causes and pathophysiology. Ann Intern Med 1988;108:865–879.

4. Thompson WG. Nonulcer dyspepsia. Can Med Assoc J 1984;130:565–569.
5. Malagelada J-R, Stanghellini V. Manometric evaluation of functional upper gut symptoms. Gastroenterology 1985;88:1223–1231.
6. Barbara L, Camilleri M, Corinaldesi R, Crean GP, Heading RC Johnson AG, Malagelada JR, Stanghellini V, Wienbeck M. Definition and investigation of dyspepsia: Consensus of an International Ad Hoc working party. Dig Dis Sci 1989;34:1272–1276.
7. Earlam R. A computerized questionnaire analysis of duodenal ulcer symptoms. Gastroenterology 1976;71:314–317.
8. Crean GP, Holden RJ, Knill-Jones RP, Beattie AD, James WB, Marjoribanks FM, Spiegelhalter DJ. A database on dyspepsia. Gut 1994;35:191–202.
9. Talley NJ, McNeil D, Piper DW. Discriminant value of dyspeptic symptoms: A study of the clinical presentation of 221 patients with dyspepsia of unknown cause, peptic ulceration and cholelithiasis. Gut 1987;28:40–46.
10. Talley NJ, Weaver AL, Tesmer DL, Zinsmeister AR. Lack of discriminant value of dyspepsia subgroups in patients referred for upper endoscopy. Gastroenterology 1993;105:1378–1386.
11. Talley NJ, Stanghellini V, Heading RC, Koch KL, Malagelada JR, Tytgat GNJ. Functional gastroduodenal disorders. Gut 1999;45(suppl. II):37–42.
12. Stanghellini V. Review Article: pain versus discomfort—is differentiation clinically useful? Aliment Pharmacol Ther 2001 Feb;15(2):145–9.
13. Mayer EA, Raybould HE. Role of visceral afferent mechanisms in functional bowel disorders. Gastroenterology 1990;99(6):1688–704.
14. Klauser AG, Schindlbeck NE, Muller-Lissner SA. Symptoms in gastro-esophageal reflux disease. Lancet 1990;335:205–208.
15. Bytzer P, Hansen JM, Schaffalitzky de Muckadell OB, Malchow-Moller A. Predicting endoscopic diagnosis in dyspeptic patients. The value of predictive score models. Scand J Gastroenterol 1997;32:118–25.
16. Talley NJ. Functional dyspepsia: Should treatment be targeted on disturbed physiology? Aliment Pharmacol Ther 1995;9:107–115.
17. Drossman DA, Thompson GW, Talley NJ, Funch-Jensen P, Janssens J, Whitehead WE. Identification of subgroups of functional gastrointestinal disorders. Gastroenterol Int 1990;3:159–172.
18. Talley NJ, Zinsmeister AR, Schleck CD, et al. Dyspepsia and dyspepsia subgroups: a population based study. Gastroenterology 1992;102:1259-1268.
19. Agreus L, Svardsudd K, Nyren O, et al. Irritable bowel syndrome and dyspepsia in the general population: overlap and lack of stability over time. Gastroenterology 1995;109:671–80.
20. Stanghellini V, Tosetti C, PaternicoÁ A, et al. Predominant symptoms identify different subgroups in functional dyspepsia. Am J Gastroenterol 1999;94:2080–5.
21. Hsu PI, Lai KH, Lo GH, Tseng HH, Lo CC, Chen HC, Tsai WL, Jou HS, Peng NJ, Chien CH, Chen JL, Hsu PN. Risk factors for ulcer development in patients with non-ulcer dyspepsia: a prospective two year follow up study of 209 patients. Gut 2002;51:15–20.
22. Laheij RJ, De Koning RW, Horrevorts AM, Rongen RJ, Rossum LG, Witteman EM, Hermsen JT, Jansen JB. Predominant symptom behavior in patients with persistent dyspepsia during treatment. J Clin Gastroenterol 2004;38:490–5.
23. Talley NJ, Locke GR, Lahr BD, Zinsmeister AR, Cohard-Radice M, D'Elis TV, Tack

J, Earnest DL. Predictors of placebo response in functional dyspepsia. Aliment Pharmacol Ther. 2006;23:923–936.

24. Karamanolis G, Caenepeel P, Arts J, Tack J. Association of the predominant symptom with clinical characteristics and pathophysiological mechanisms in functional dyspepsia. Gastroenterology 2006;130:296–303.

25. Stanghellini V, Tosetti C, Paternico A, et al. Risk indicators of delayed gastric emptying of solids in patients with functional dyspepsia. Gastroenterology 1996;110:1036–1042.

26. Perri F, Clemente R, Festa V, Annese V, Quitadamo M, Rutgeerts P, Andriulli A. Patterns of symptoms in functional dyspepsia: Role of Helicobacter pylori infection and delayed gastric emptying. Am J Gastroenterol 1998;93:2082–2088.

27. Sarnelli G, Caenepeel P, Geypens B, Janssens J, Tack J. Symptoms associated with impaired gastric emptying of solids and liquids in functional dyspepsia. Am J Gastroenterol 2003;98:783–8.

28. Tack J, Piessevaux H, Coulie B, Caenepeel P, Janssens J. Role of impaired gastric accommodation to a meal in functional dyspepsia. Gastroenterology 1998;115:1346–52.

29. Tack J, Caenepeel P, Fischler B, Piessevaux H, Janssens J. Symptoms associated with hypersensitivity to gastric distention in functional dyspepsia. Gastroenterology 2001;121:526–35.

30. Boeckxstaens GE, Hirsch DP, Kuiken SD, Heisterkamp SH, Tytgat GN. The proximal stomach and postprandial symptoms in functional dyspeptics. Am J Gastroenterol 2002;97:40–8.

31. Rhee PL, Kim YH, Son HJ, Kim JJ, Koh KC, Paik SW, hee, JC, Choi KW. Evaluation of individual symptoms acannot predict presence of gastric hypersensitivity in functional dyspepsia. Dig Dis Sci 2000;45:1680–4.

32. Talley NJ, Verlinden M, Jones M. Can symptoms discriminate among those with delayed or normal gastric emptying in dysmotility-like dyspepsia? Am J Gastroenterol 2001;96:1422–8.

33. Tack J, Bisschops R, Sarnelli G. Pathophysiology and treatment of functional dyspepsia. Gastroenterology 2004;127(4):1239–55.

34. Jones RH, Lydeard SE, Hobbs FDR, et al. Dyspepsia in England and Scotland. Gut 1990;31:401–405.

35. Drossman DA, Li Z, Andruzzi E, et al. U.S. householder survey of functional gastrointestinal disorders: Prevalence, sociodemography and health impact. Dig Dis Sci 1993;38:1569–1580.

36. Locke GR III, Talley NJ, Fett S, et al. Prevalence and clinical spectrum of gastroesophageal reflux in the community. Gastroenterology 1997;112:1448–1456.

37. Hu WH, Wong WM, Lam CL, et al. Anxiety but not depression determines health care-se behaviour in Chinese patients with dyspepsia and irritable bowel syndrome: a population-based study. Aliment Pharmacol Ther 2002;16(12):2081–2088.

38. Talley NJ, Boyce P, Jones M. Dyspepsia and health care seeking in a community: How important are psychological factors? Dig Dis Sci 1998;43:1016–1022.

39. Gschossmann JM, Haag S, Holtmann G. Epidemiological trends of functional gastrointestinal disorders. Dig Dis 2001;19:189–194.

40. Jonsson K-A, Gotthard R, Bodemar G, et al. The clinical relevance of endoscopic and histologic inflammation of gastroduodenal mucosa in dyspepsia of unknown origin. Scand J Gastroenterol 1989;24:385–395.

41. Johnsen R, Bernersen B, Straume B, et al. Prevalence of endoscopic and histological findings in subjects with and without dyspepsia. BMJ 1991;302:749–752.

42. Klauser AG, Voderholzer WA, Knesewitsch PA, et al. What is behind dyspepsia? Dig Dis Sci 1993;38:147–154.

43. Talley NJ, Silverstein M, Agreus L, et al. AGA Technical Review-Evaluation of dyspepsia. Gastroenterology 1998;114:582–595.

44. Talley NJ, Weaver AL, Zinsmeister AR, et al. Onset and disappearance of gastrointestinal symptoms and functional gastrointestinal disorders. Am J Epidemiol 1992; 136:165–177.

45. Talley NJ, McNeil D, Hayden A, et al. Prognosis of chronic unexplained dyspepsia. A prospective study of potential predictor variables in patients with endoscopically diagnosed nonulcer dyspepsia. Gastroenterology 1987;92:1060–1066.

46. Lindell GH, Celebioglu F, Graffner HO. Non-ulcer dyspepsia in the long-term perspective. Eur J Gastroenterol Hepatol 1995;7:829–833.

47. Heikkinen M, Farkkila M. What is the long-term outcome of the different subgroups of functional dyspepsia? Aliment Pharmacol Ther 2003;18:223–229.

48. Jones R, Lydeard S. Factors affecting the decision to consult with dyspepsia: comparison of consulters and non-consulters. J Roy Coll Gen Pract 1989;39:495–498.

49. Koloski NA Talley NJ, Boyce PM. Predictors of health care seeking for irritable bowel syndrome and nonulcer dyspepsia: a critical review of the literature on symptom and psychosocial factors. Am J Gastroenterol 2001;96(5):1340–1349.

50. Talley NJ, Meineche-Schmidt V, Pare P, Duckworth M, Raisanen P, Pap A, Kordecki H, Schmid V. Efficacy of omeprazole in functional dyspepsia: double-blind, randomized, placebo-controlled trials (the Bond and Opera studies). Aliment Pharmacol Ther 1998;12:1055–65.

51. Armstrong D, Kazim F, Gervais M, Pyzyk M. Early relief of upper gastrointestinal dyspeptic symptoms: a survey of empirical therapy with pantoprazole in Canadian clinical practice. Can J Gastroenterol 2002;16(7):439–50.

52. Chiba N, Van Zanten SJ, Sinclair P, Ferguson RA, Escobedo S, Grace E. Treating Helicobacter pylori infection in primary care patients with uninvestigated dyspepsia: the Canadian adult dyspepsia empiric treatment-Helicobacter pylori positive (CADET-Hp) randomised controlled trial. BMJ 2002;324(7344):1012–6.

53. Moayyedi P, Delaney BC, Vakil N, Forman D, Talley NJ. The efficacy of proton pump inhibitors in nonulcer dyspepsia: a systematic review and economic analysis. Gastroenterology 2004;127:1329–37. Review.

54. Peura DA, Kovacs TO, Metz DC, Siepman N, Pilmer BL, Talley NJ. Lansoprazole in the treatment of functional dyspepsia: two double-blind, randomized, placebo-controlled trials. Am J Med 2004;116:740–8.

55. Westbrook JI, Talley NJ. Empiric clustering of dyspepsia into symptom subgroups: a population-based study. Scand J Gastroenterol 2002;37:917–23.

56. Fischler B, Vandenberghe J, Persoons P, De Gucht V, Broekaert D, Luyckx K, Tack J. Evidence-based subtypes in functional dyspepsia with confirmatory factor analysis: Psychosocial and physiopathological correlates. Gastroenterology 2003; 124: 903–10.

57. Tack J, Talley NJ, Coulie B, Dubois D, Jones M. Association of weight loss with gastrointestinal symptoms in tertiary-referred functional dyspepsia patients. Gastroenterology 2003;124:A396.

58. Jones M, Talley N, Coulie B, Dubois J, and Tack J. Clustering of weight loss with symptoms of functional dyspepsia: a population-based study. Gastroenterology 2003; 124:A390.

59. Kwan AC, Bao TN, Chakkaphak S, Chang FY, Ke MY, Law NM, Leelakusolvong S, Luo JY, Manan C, Park HJ, Piyaniran W, Qureshi A, Long T, Xu GM, Xu L, Yuen H. Validation of Rome II criteria for functional gastrointestinal disorders by factor analysis of symptoms in Asian patient sample. J Gastroenterol Hepatol 2003;18:796–802.

60. Whitehead WE, Bassotti G, Palsson O, Taub E, Cook III EC, Drossman DA. Factor analyisis of bowel symptoms in US and Italian populations. Dig Liv Dis 2003;35:774–83.

61. Camilleri M, Dubois D, Coulie B, Jones M, Stewart WF, Sonnenberg A, Stanghellini V, Tack J, Talley NJ, Kahrilas P, Whitehead W, and Revicki D. Results from the US upper gastrointestinal study: prevalence, socio-economic impact and functional gastrointestinal disorder subgroups identified by factor and cluster analysis. Clin Gastroent Hep 2005;3:543–52.

62. Piessevaux H, De Winter B, Tack J, et al. Heterogeneity of dyspepsia in the general population in Belgium. Gastroenterology 2004;126(Suppl 2):A440–441.

63. Meineche-Schmidt V, Christensen E. Which dyspepsia patients will benefit from omeprazole treatment? Am J Gastroent 2000;95:2777–83.

64. Talley NJ, Verlinden M, Snape W, et al. Failure of a motilin receptor agonist (ABT-229) to relieve the symptoms of functional dyspepsia in patients with and without delayed gastric emptying: a randomized double-blind placebo-controlled trial. Aliment Pharmacol Ther 2000;14:1653–61.

65. Talley NJ, Van Zanten SV, Saez LR, Dukes G, Perschy T, Heath M, Kleoudis C, Mangel AW. A dose-ranging, placebo-controlled, randomized trial of alosetron in patients with functional dyspepsia. Alimentary Pharmacology & Therapeutics. 15(4):525–37, 2001b.

66. Tack J, Delia T, Ligozio G, et al. A phase II placebo controlled randomized trial with tegaserod (T) in functional dyspepsia (FD) patients with normal gastric emptying (NGE) Gastroenterology 2002;122(Suppl 1):154.

67. Castillo EJ, Camilleri M, Locke GR, Burton DD, Stephens DA, Geno DM, Zinsmeister AR. A community-based, controlled study of the epidemiology and pathophysiology of dyspepsia. Clin Gastroenterol Hepatol 2004;2:985–96.

68. Arts J, Caenepeel P, Verbeke K, and Tack J. Influence of erythromycin on gastric emptying and meal related symptoms in functional dyspepsia with delayed gastric emptying. Gut 2005;54:455–60.

69. Tack J, Bisschops R, Caenepeel P, et al. Comparison of functional dyspepsia patients with or without meal-related symptoms. Gastroenterology 2004;126(Suppl 2):A375.

70. Tack J, Caenepeel P, Arts J, et al. Prevalence of acid-reflux in functional dyspepsia and its association with symptom profile. Gut 2005;54:1370–6.

71. Carlsson R, Dent J, Bolling-Sternevald E, et al. The usefulness of a structured questionnaire in the assessment of symptomatic gastroesophageal reflux disease. Scand J Gastroenterol 1998;33:1023–9.

72. Thomson AB, Barkun AN, Armnstrong D, Chiba N, White RJ, Daniels S, Escobedo S, Chakraborty B, Sinclair P, Van Zanten SJ. The prevalence of clinically significant endoscopic findings in primary care patients with uninvestigated dyspepsia: the Canadian Adult Dyspepsia Empiric Treatment—Prompt Endoscopy (CADET-PE) study. Aliment Pharmacol Ther 2003;17(12):1481–1491.

73. Talley NJ, Piper DW. The association between non-ulcer dyspepsia and other gastrointestinal disorders. Scand J Gastroenterol 1985;20:896–900.

74. Corsetti M, Caenepeel P, Fischler B, Janssens J, Tack J. Impact of coexisting irritable bowel syndrome on symptoms and pathophysiological mechanisms in functional dyspepsia. Am J Gastroenterol 2004;99:1152–9.

75. Talley NJ, Vakil NB, Moayyedi P. American Gastroenterological Association Technical Review on the evaluation of dyspepsia.

76. Hammer J, Eslick GD, Howell SC, Altiparmak E, Talley NJ. Diagnostic yield of alarm features in irritable bowel syndrome and functional dyspepsia. Gut 2004 May;53(5):666–72.

77. Straus WL, Ofman JJ, MacLean C, Morton S, Berger ML, Roth EA, Shekelle P. Do NSAIDs cause dyspepsia? A meta-analysis evaluating alternative dyspepsia definitions. Am J Gastroenterol 2002;97(8):1951–1958.

78. Koelz HR, Arnold R, Stolte M, Fischer M, Blum AL; FROSCH Study Group. Treatment of Helicobacter pylori in functional dyspepsia resistant to conventional management: a double blind randomised trial with a six month follow up. Gut 2003; 52(1):40–46.

79. Manes G, Menchise A, de Nucci C, Balzano A. Empirical prescribing for dispepsia: randomised controlled trial of test and treta versus omeprazole treatment. BMJ 2003;326(7399);1118.

80. Rabeneck L, Souchek J, Wristers K, Menke T, Ambriz E, Huang I, Wray N. A double blind, randomised, placebo-controlled trial of proton pump inhibitor therapy in patients with uninvestigated dyspepsia. Am J Gastroenterol 2002;97(12):3045–3051.

81. Arents NL, Thijs JC, van Zwet AA, Oudkerk Pool M, Gotz JM, van de Werf GT, Reenders K, Sluiter WJ, Kleibeuker JH. Approach to treatment of dyspepsia in primary care: a randomised trial comparing "test-and-treat" with prompt endoscopy. Arch Intern Med 2003;163(13):1606–1612.

82. Lassen AT, Pedersen FM, Bytzer P, Schaffalitzky de Muckadell OB. Helicobacter pylori test-and-eradicate versus prompt endoscopy for management of dyspeptic patients: a randomised trial. Lancet 2000;356(9228):455–460.

83. McColl KE, Murray LS, Gillen D, Walker A, Wirz A, Fletcher J, Mowat C, Henry E, Kelman A, Dickson A. Randomised trial of endoscopy with testing for Helicobacter pylori compared with non-invasive H pylori testing alone in the management of dyspepsia. BMJ 2002;324(7344):99–1002.

84. Moayyedi P, Soo S, Deeks J, Delaney B, Harris A, Innes M, Oakes R, Wilson S, Roalfe A, Bennett C, Forman D. Eradication of Helicobacter pylori for non-ulcer dyspepsia. Cochrane Database Sys Rev 2003;(1):CD002096.

85. Moayyedi P, Feltbower R, Brown J, Mason S, Mason J, Nathan J, Richards ID, Dowell AC, Axon AT. Effect of population screening and treatment for Helicobacter pylori on dyspepsia and quality of life in the community: a randomised controlled trial. Leeds HELP Study Group. Lancet 2000;355(9216):1665–1669.

86. Malfertheiner P, Megraud F, O'Morain C, Hungin AP, Jones R, Axon A, Graham DY, Tytgat G; European Helicobacter Pylori Study Group (EHPSG). Current concepts in the management of Helicobacter pylori infection—the Maastricht 2–2000 Consensus Report. Aliment Pharmacol Ther. 2002 Feb;16(2):167–80.

87. Moayyedi P, Deeks J, Talley NJ, Delaney B, Forman D. An update of the Cochrane systematic review of *Helicobacter pylori* eradication therapy in nonulcer dyspepsia: resolving the discrepancy between systematic reviews. Am J Gastroenterol 2003c; 98:2621–6.

88. Laheij RJ, van Rossum LG, Verbeek AL, Jansen JB. Helicobacter pylori infection treatment of nonulcer dispepsia an analysis of meta-analyses. J Clin Gastroenterol 2003;36(4):315–320.

89. Talley NJ. Dyspepsia: management guidelines for the millennium. Gut 2002 May; 50 Suppl 4:iv72–8.

90. Madisch A, Hotz J, Grabowski G, Guth A, Malfertheiner P, Plein K, Schneider B. Efficacy of Helicobacter pylori eradication in uninvestigated chronic dyspeptic staff members of a large factory: a prospective long-term, follow-up, workplace outcome study. Eur J Gastroenterol Hepatol 2002;14(1):61–69.

91. Delaney BC, Wilson S, Roalfe A, Roberts L, Redman V, Wearn A, Briggs A, Hobbs FD. Cost effectiveness of initial endoscopy for dyspepsia in patients over age 50 years: a randomised controlled trial in primary care. Lancet 2000;356(9246):1965–1969.

92. Delaney BC, Wilson S, Roalfe A, Roberts L, Redman V, Wearn A, Hobbs FD. Randomised controlled trial of Helicobacter pylori testing an endoscopy for dyspepsia in primary care. BMJ 2001;322(7291):898–901.

93. Perri F, Ricciardi R, Merla A. Piepoli A, Gasperi V, Quitadamo M, Andriulli A. Appropriateness of urea breath test: a prospective observation study based on Maastricht 2000 guidelines. Aliment Pharmacol Ther 2002;16(8):1443–1447.

94. Berger MY, van der Velden JJ, Lijmer JG, de Kort H, Prins A, Bohnen AM. Abdominal symptoms: do they predict gallstones? A systematic review. Scan J Gastroenterol 2000;35(1):70–76.

95. Koskenpato J, Korppi-Tommola T, Kairemo K, Farkkila M. Long-term follow-up study of gastric emptying and Helicobacter pylori eradication among patients with functional dyspepsia. Dig Dis Sci 2000;45(9):1763–1768.

96. Van der Voort IR, Osmanoglou E, Seybold M, Heymann-Monnikes I, Tebbe J, Wiedenmann B, Klapp BF, Monnikes H. Electrogastrography as a diagnostic tool for delayed gastric emptying in functional dyspepsia and irritable bowel syndrome. Neurogastroenterol Motil 2003;15(5):467–473.

97. Lin X, Chen JZ. Abnormal gastric slow waves in patients with functional dyspepsia assessed by multichannel electrogastrography. American Journal of Physiology—Gastrointestinal & Liver Physiology. 280(6):G1370–5, 2001.

98. Parkman HP, Hasler WL, Barnett JL, Eaker EY. Electrogastrography: a document prepared by the gastric section of the American Motility Society Clinical GI Motility Testing Task Force. Neurogastroenterol Motil 2003;15:89–102.

99. Zighelboim J, Talley NJ, Phillips SF, Harmsen WS, Zinsmeister AR. Visceral perception in irritable bowel syndrome. Rectal and gastric responses to distension and serotonin type 3 antagonism. Digestive Diseases & Sciences 1995;40(4):819–27.

100. Camilleri M, Thompson DG, Malagelada JR. Functional dyspepsia. Symptoms and underlying mechanism. Journal of Clinical Gastroenterology 1986;8(4):424–9.

101. Camilleri M. Nonulcer dyspepsia: a look into the future. Mayo Clinic Proceedings 1996;71(6):614–22.

102. Tack J, Demedts I, Dehondt G, Caenepeel P, Fischler B, Zandecki M, Janssens J. Clinical and pathophysiological characteristics of acute-onset functional dyspepsia. Gastroenterology 2002;122:1738–47.

103. Mearin F, Perez-Oliveras M, Perello A, Vinyet J, Ibanez A, Coderch J, Perona M. Dyspepsia and irritable bowel syndrome after a Salmonella gastroenteritis outbreak: one-year follow-up cohort study. Gastroenterology 2005;129(1):98–104.

104. Cuperus P, Keeling PW, Gibney MJ. Eating patterns in functional dyspepsia: a case control study. European Journal of Clinical Nutrition 1996;50(8):520–3.

105. Mullan A, Kavanagh P, O'Mahony P, Joy T, Gleeson F, Gibney MJ. Food and nu-

trient intakes and eating patterns in functional and organic dyspepsia. European Journal of Clinical Nutrition 1994;48(2):97–105.

106. Houghton LA, Mangnall YF, Dwivedi A, et al. Sensitivity to nutrients in patients with non ulcer dyspepsia. Eur J Gastroenterol Hepatol 1993;5:109–13.)

107. Caldarella MP, Milano A, Laterza F, Sacco F, Balatsinou C, Lapenna D, Pierdomenico SD, Cuccurullo F, Neri M. Visceral sensitivity and symptoms in patients with constipation- or diarrhea-predominant irritable bowel syndrome (IBS): effect of a low-fat intraduodenal infusion. Am J Gastroenterol 2005 Feb;100(2):383–9.

108. Simren M, Simms L, D'Souza D, Abrahamsson H, Bjornsson ES. Lipid-induced colonic hypersensitivity in irritable bowel syndrome: the role of 5-HT3 receptors. Aliment Pharmacol Ther 2003 Jan;17(2):279–87.

109. Talley NJ, Weaver AL, Zinsmeister AR. Smoking, alcohol, and nonsteroidal anti-inflammatory drugs in outpatients with functional dyspepsia and among dyspepsia subgroups. American Journal of Gastroenterology 1994;89(4):524–8.

110. Holtmann G, Gschossmann J, Buenger L, Gerken G, Talley NJ. Do changes in visceral sensory function determine the development of dyspepsia during treatment with aspirin? Gastroenterology 2002;123(5):1451–8.

111. Collen MJ, Loebenberg MJ. Basal gastric acid secretion in nonulcer dyspepsia with or without duodenitis. Digestive Diseases & Sciences 1989;34(2):246–50.

112. El-Omar E, Penman I, Ardill JE, McColl KE. A substantial proportion of non-ulcer dyspepsia patients have the same abnormality of acid secretion as duodenal ulcer patients. Gut 1995;36(4):534–8.

113. Delaney BC, Moayyedi P, Forman D. Initial management strategies for dyspepsia. Cochrane Database Syst Rev 2003;(2):CD001961.

114. Holtmann G, Gschossmann J, Holtmann M, Talley NJ. H. pylori and functional dyspepsia: increased serum antibodies as an independent risk factor? Digestive Diseases & Sciences 2001;46(7):1550–7.

115. Blum AL, Talley NJ, O'Morain C, van Zanten SV, Labenz J, Stolte M, Louw JA, Stubberod A, Theodors A, Sundin M, Bolling-Sternevald E, Junghard O. Lack of effect of treating Helicobacter pylori infection in patients with nonulcer dyspepsia. Omeprazole plus Clarithromycin and Amoxicillin Effect One Year after Treatment (OCAY) Study Group. N Engl J Med 1998;339(26):1875–81.

116. Talley NJ, Janssens J, Lauritsen K, Racz I, Bolling-Sternevald E. Eradication of Helicobacter pylori in functional dyspepsia: randomised double blind placebo controlled trial with 12 months' follow up. The Optimal Regimen Cures Helicobacter Induced Dyspepsia (ORCHID) Study Group BMJ 1999;318(7187):833–7.

117. Talley NJ, Vakil N, Ballard ED II, Fennerty MB. Absence of benefit of eradicating Helicobacter pylori in patients with nonulcer dyspepsia. N Engl J Med 1999; 341:1106–11.

118. Holtmann G, Talley NJ, Goebell H. Association between H. pylori, duodenal mechanosensory thresholds, and small intestinal motility in chronic unexplained dyspepsia. Digestive Diseases & Sciences 1996;41(7):1285–91.

119. Saslow SB, Thumshirn M, Camilleri M, Locke GR 3rd, Thomforde GM, Burton DD, Hanson RB. Influence of H. pylori infection on gastric motor and sensory function in asymptomatic volunteers. Digestive Diseases & Sciences 1998;43(2):258–64.

120. Mearin F, de Ribot X, Balboa A, Salas A, Varas MJ, Cucala M, Bartolome R, Armengol JR, Malagelada JR. Does Helicobacter pylori infection increase gastric sensitivity in functional dyspepsia? Gut 1995;37(1):47–51.

121. Sarnelli G, Cuomo R, Janssens J, Tack J. Symptom patterns and pathophysiological mechanisms in dyspeptic patients with and without Helicobacter pylori. Dig Dis Sci 2003;48(12):2229–36.

122. Nesland A, Berstad A. Erosive prepyloric changes in persons with and without dyspepsia. Scandinavian Journal of Gastroenterology 1985;20(2):222–8.

123. Olafsson S, Hatlebakk JG, Berstad A. Patients with endoscopic gastritis and/or duodenitis improve markedly following eradication of Helicobacter pylori, although less so than patients with ulcers. Scandinavian Journal of Gastroenterology 2002; 37(12):1386–94, .

124. McColl K, Murray L, El-Omar E, et al. Symptomatic benefit from eradicating Helicobacter pylori infection in patients with nonulcer dyspepsia. N Engl J Med 1998;339:1869–74.

125. Collins JS, Hamilton PW, Watt PC, Sloan JM, Love AH. Quantitative histological study of mucosal inflammatory cell densities in endoscopic duodenal biopsy specimens from dyspeptic patients using computer linked image analysis. Gut 1990;31(8):858–61.

126. Quartero AO, de Wit NJ, Lodder AC, Numans ME, Smout AJ, Hoes AW. Disturbed solid-phase gastric emptying in functional dyspepsia: a meta-analysis. Digestive Diseases & Sciences 1998;43(9):2028–33.

127. Haag S, Talley NJ, Holtmann G. Symptom patterns in functional dyspepsia and irritable bowel syndrome: relationship to disturbances in gastric emptying and response to a nutrient challenge in consulters and non-consulters. Gut 2004 Oct; 53(10):1445–51.

128. Ahluwalia NK, Thompson DG, Mamtora H, Hindle J. Evaluation of gastric antral motor performance in patients with dysmotility-like dyspepsia using real-time high-resolution ultrasound. Neurogastroenterology & Motility 1996;8(4):333–8.

129. Greydanus MP, Vassallo M, Camilleri M, Nelson DK, Hanson R, Thomforde JM. Neurohormonal factors in functional dyspepsia: insights on pathophysiological mechanisms. Gastroenterology 1991;100:1311–1318.

130. Camilleri M, Malagelada JR, Kao PC, Zinsmeister AR. Gastric and autonomic responses to stress in functional dyspepsia. Digestive Diseases & Sciences 1986b; 31(11):1169–77.

131. Bortolotti M, Cucchiara S, Sarti P, Brunelli F, Del Campo L, Barbara L. Interdigestive gastroduodenal motility in patients with ulcer-like dyspepsia: effect of ranitidine. Hepato-Gastroenterology 1992;39(1):31–3.

132. Wilmer A, Van Cutsem E, Andrioli A, Tack J, Coremans G, Janssens J. Ambulatory gastrojejunal manometry in severe motility-like dyspepsia: lack of correlation between dysmotility, symptoms, and gastric emptying. Gut 1998;42(2):235–42.

133. Schwartz MP, Samsom M, Smout AJ. Chemospecific alterations in duodenal perception and motor responses in functional dyspepsia. Am J Gastroenterol 2001; 96:2596–602.

134. Simren M, Vos R, Janssens J, Tack J. Unsuppressed postprandial phasic contractility in the proximal stomach in functional dyspepsia: relevance to symptoms. American Journal of Gastroenterology 2003;98(10):2169–75.

135. Di Stefano M, Vos R, Lee KJ, Janssens J, Tack J. Neostigmine-induced postprandial phasic contractility in the proximal stomach and dyspeptic symptoms in healthy subjects. Submitted for publication, 2005.

136. Caldarella MP, Azpiroz F, Malagelada JR. Antro-fundic dysfunctions in functional dyspepsia. Gastroenterology 2003;124(5):1220–9.

137. Scott AM, Kellow JE, Shuter B, Cowan H, Corbett AM, Riley JW, Lunzer MR, Eckstein RP, Hoschl R, Lam SK, et al. Intragastric distribution and gastric emptying of solids and liquids in functional dyspepsia. Lack of influence of symptom subgroups and H. pylori-associated gastritis. Digestive Diseases & Sciences 1993;38(12):2247–54.

138. Piessevaux H, Tack J, Walrand S, Pauwels S, Geubel A. Intragastric distribution of a standardized meal in health and functional dyspepsia: correlation with specific symptoms. Neurogastroenterol Motil 2003; 15(5): 447–455.

139. Troncon LE, Bennett RJ, Ahluwalia NK, Thompson DG. Abnormal intragastric distribution of food during gastric emptying in functional dyspepsia patients. Gut 1994;35(3):327–32.

140. Thumshirn M, Camilleri M, Saslow SB, Williams DE, Burton DD, Hanson RB. Gastric accommodation in non-ulcer dyspepsia and the roles of Helicobacter pylori infection and vagal function. Gut 1999;44(1):55–64.

141. Moayyedi P, Soo S, Deeks J, Delaney B, Innes M, Forman D. Pharmacological interventions for non-ulcer dyspepsia. Cochrane Upper Gastrointestinal and Pancreatic Diseases Group Cochrane Database of Systematic Reviews 2004;4:CD0003840.

142. Ahluwalia NK, Thompson DG, Barlow J, Troncon LE, Hollis S. Relaxation responses of the human proximal stomach to distension during fasting and after food. American Journal of Physiology 1994;267(2 Pt 1):G166–72.

143. Berstad A, Hausken T, Gilja OH, Hveem K, Undeland KA, Wilhelmsen I, Haug TT. Gastric accommodation in functional dyspepsia. Scand J Gastroenterol 1997;32:193–197.

144. Gilja OH, Hausken T, Wilhelmsen I, Berstad A. Impaired accommodation of proximal stomach to a meal in functional dyspepsia. Dig Dis Sci 1996;41:689–696.

145. Kim DY, Delgado-Aros S, Camilleri M, Samsom M, Murray JA, O'Connor MK, Brinkmann BH, Stephens DA, Lighvani SS, Burton DD. Noninvasive measurement of gastric accommodation in patients with idiopathic nonulcer dyspepsia. Am J Gastroenterol 2001;96(11):3099–3105.

146. Bredenoord AJ, Chial HJ, Camilleri M, Mullan BP, Murray JA. Gastric accommodation and emptying in evaluation of patients with upper gastrointestinal symptoms. Clinical Gastroenterology and Hepatology 2003;1:264–272.

147. Jebbink HJ, Van Berge-Henegouwen GP, Bruijs PP, Akkermans LM, Smout AJ. Gastric myoelectrical activity and gastrointestinal motility in patients with functional dyspepsia. Eur J Clin Invest 1995;25(6):429–37.

148. Pfaffenbach B, Adamek RJ, Bartholomaus C, Wegener M. Gastric dysrhythmias and delayed gastric emptying in patients with functional dyspepsia. Digestive Diseases & Sciences 1997;42(10):2094–9.

149. Lin X, Levanon D, Chen JD. Impaired postprandial gastric slow waves in patients with functional dyspepsia. Digestive Diseases & Sciences 1998;43(8):1678–84.

150. Lin Z, Eaker EY, Sarosiek I, McCallum RW. Gastric myoelectrical activity and gastric emptying in patients with functional dyspepsia. American Journal of Gastroenterology 1999;94(9):2384–9.

151. Koch KL, Hong SP, Xu L. Reproducibility of gastric myoelectrical activity and the water load test in patients with dysmotility-like dyspepsia symptoms and in control subjects. Journal of Clinical Gastroenterology 2000;31(2):125–9.

152. Mearin F, Cucala M, Azpiroz F, Malagelada J-R. The origin of symptoms on the brain-gut axis in functional dyspepsia. Gastroenterology 1991;101:999–1006.

153. Bradette M, Paré P, Douville P, Morin A. Visceral perception in health and functional dyspepsia: crossover study of gastric distension with placebo and domperidone. Dig Dis Sci 1991;36:52–58.

154. Lémann M, Dederding JP, Flourié B, Franchisseur C, Rambaud JC, Jian R. Abnormal perception of visceral pain in response to gastric distension in chronic idiopathic dyspepsia. The irritable stomach syndrome. Dig Dis Sci 1991;36:1249–1254.

155. Holtmann G, Gschossmann J, Neufang-Huber J, Gerken G, Talley NJ. Differences in gastric mechanosensory function after repeated ramp distensions in nonconsulters with dyspepsia and healthy controls. Gut 2000;47(3):332–6.

156. Salet GA, Samsom M, Roelofs JM, van Berge Henegouwen GP, Smout AJ, Akkermans LM. Responses to gastric distension in functional dyspepsia. Gut 1998;15:823–9.

157. Troncon LE, Thompson DG, Ahluwalia NK, Barlow J, Heggie L. Relations between upper abdominal symptoms and gastric distension abnormalities in dysmotility like functional dyspepsia and after vagotomy. Gut 1995;37(1):17–22.

158. Klatt S, Pieramico O, Guenthner C, Glasbrenner B, Beckh K, Adler G. Gastric hypersensitivity in nonulcer dyspepsia. An inconsistent finding. Dig Dis Sci 1997;42:720–723.

159. Coffin B, Azpiroz F, Guarner F, Malagelada JR. Selective gastric hypersensitivity and reflex hyporeactivity in functional dyspepsia. Gastroenterology 1994;107:1345–1351.

160. Ladabaum U, Minoshima S, Hasler WL, Cross D, Chey WD, Owyang C. Gastric distention correlates with activation of multiple cortical and subcortical regions. Gastroenterology 2001;120(2):369–76.

161. Vandenberghe J, Dupont P, Fischler B, Bormans G, Persoons P, Janssens J, Tack J. Regional brain activation during proximal stomach distention in man: a positron emission tomography study. Gastroenterology 2005;128(3):564–73.

162. George AA, Tsuchiyose M, Dooley CP. Sensitivity of the gastric mucosa to acid and duodenal contents in patients with nonulcer dyspepsia. Gastroenterology 1991;15:3–6.

163. Holtmann G, Goebell H, Jockenhoevel F, Talley NJ. Altered vagal and intestinal mechanosensory function in chronic unexplained dyspepsia. Gut 1998;15:501–6.

164. Simren M, Vos R, Janssens J, Tack J. Acid infusion enhances duodenal mechanosensitivity in healthy subjects. Am J Physiol Gastrointest Liver Physiol 2003c;285(2):G309–15.

165. Lee KJ, Vos R, Janssens J, Tack J. Influence of duodenal acidification on the sensorimotor function of the proximal stomach in humans. Am J Physiol Gastrointest Liver Physiol 2004 Feb;286(2):G278–84.

166. Samsom M, Verhagen MAMT, van Berge Henegouwen GP, Smout AJPM. Abnormal clearance of exogenous acid and increased acid sensitivity of the proximal duodenum in patients with functional dyspepsia. Gastroenterology 1999;15: 515–20.

167. Lee KJ, Demarchi B, Demedts I, Sifrim D, Raeymaekers P, Tack J. A pilot study on duodenal acid exposure and its relationship to symptoms in functional dyspepsia with prominent nausea. Am J Gastroenterol 2004;99(9):1765–73.

168. Schwartz MP, Samsom M, Van Berge Henegouwen GP, Smout AJ. Effect of inhibition of gastric acid secretion on antropyloroduodenal motor activity and duodenal

acid hypersensitivity in functional dyspepsia. Alimentary Pharmacology & Therapeutics 2001b;15(12):1921–8.

169. Hausken T, Svebak S, Wilhelmsen I, Haug TT, Olafsen K, Pettersson E, Hveem K, Berstad A. Low vagal tone and antral dysmotility in patients with functional dyspepsia. Psychosom Med 1993;55:12–22.

170. Haug TT, Svebak S, Hausken T, Wilhelmsen I, Berstad A, Ursin H. Low vagal activity as mediating mechanism for the relationship between personality factors and gastric symptoms in functional dyspepsia. Psychosom Med 1994;56:81–186.

171. Muth ER, Koch KL, Stern RM. Significance of autonomic nervous system activity in functional dyspepsia. Digestive Diseases & Sciences 2000;45(5):854–63.

172. Tougas G. The autonomic nervous system in functional bowel disorders. Gut 2000; 47 Suppl 4:iv78–80; discussion iv87.

173. Chiloiro M, Russo F, Riezzo G, Leoci C, Clemente C, Messa C, Di Leo A. Effect of Helicobacter pylori infection on gastric emptying and gastrointestinal hormones in dyspeptic and healthy subjects. Dig Dis Sci 2001;46(1):46–53.

174. Riezzo G, Chiloiro M, Russo F, Clemente C, Di Matteo G, Guerra V, Di Leo A. Gastric electrical activity and gastrointestinal hormones in dyspeptic patients. Digestion 2001;63(1):20–9.

175. Holtmann G, Siffert W, Haag S, Mueller N, Langkafel M, Senf W, Zotz R, Talley NJ. G-protein beta 3 subunit 825 CC genotype is associated with unexplained (functional) dyspepsia. Gastroenterology 2004;126(4):971–9.

176. Watson RG. Shaw C. Buchanan KD. Love AH. Circulating gastrointestinal hormones in patients with flatulent dyspepsia, with and without gallbladder disease. Digestion 1986;35(4):211–6.

177. Kaneko H, Mitsuma T, Fujii S, Uchida K, Kotera H, Furusawa A, Morise K. Immunoreactive-somatostatin concentrations of the human stomach and mood state in patients with functional dyspepsia: a preliminary case-control study. Journal of Gastroenterology & Hepatology 1993;8(4):322–7.

178. Moss SF, Legon S, Bishop AE, Polak JM, Calam J. Effect of Helicobacter pylori on gastric somatostatin in duodenal ulcer disease. Lancet 1992;340:930–2.

179. Monnikes H, Van der Voort I, Wollenberg B, Heymann-Monnikes I, Tebbe JJ, Alt Z, Arnold R, Klapp BF, Wiedenmann B, McGregor GP. Gastric perception thresholds are low and sensory neuropeptide levels high in H. pylori positive functional dyspepsia. Digestion 2005;71(2):111–23.

180. Wilhelmsen I, Haug TT, Ursin H, Berstad A. Discriminant analysis of factors distinguishing patients with functional dyspepsia from patients with duodenal ulcer. Significance of somatization. Dig Dis Sci 1995;40:1105–11.

181. Cheng C. Seeking Medical Consultation: Perceptual and Behavioral Characteristics Distinguishing Consulters and Nonconsulters With Functional Dyspepsia. Psychosom Med 2000;62:844–852.

182. Veldhuyzen van Zanten SJO, Cleary C, Talley NJ, et al. Drug treatment of functional dyspepsia: a systematic analysis of trial methodology with recommendations for the design of future trials: report of an international working party. Am J Gastroenterol 1996;91:660–73.

183. Elta GH, Behler EM, Colturi TJ. Comparison of coffee intake and coffee-induced symptoms in patients with duodenal ulcer, nonulcer dyspepsia and normal controls. Am J Gastroenterol 1990;85:1339–42.

184. Gotthard R, Bodemar G, Brodin U, et al. Treatment with cimetidine, antacid or

placebo in patients with dyspepsia of unknown origin. Scand J Gastroenterol 1988; 23:7–18.

185. Nyren O, Adami H-O, Bates S, et al. Absence of therapeutic benefit from antacids or cimetidine in non-ulcer dyspepsia. New Engl J Med 1986;314:339–43.

186. Kairaluoma MI, Hentilae R, Alavaikko M, et al. Sucralfate versus placebo in treatment of non-ulcer dyspepsia. Am J Med 1987;83(Suppl 3B):51–55.

187. Gudjonsson H, Oddsson E, Bjornsson S, et al. Efficacy of sucralfate in treatment of non-ulcer dyspepsia: a double-blind placebo-controlled study. Scand J Gastroenterol 1993;28:969–72.

188. Hausken T, Stene-Larsen G, Lange O, et al. Misoprostol treatment exacerbates abdominal discomfort in patients with non-ulcer dyspepsia and erosive prepyloric changes: a double-blind placebo-controlled multicentre study. Scand J Gastroenterol 1990;25:1028–1033.

189. Rokkas T, Pursey C, Uzoechina E, et al. Non-ulcer dyspepsia and short term De-Nol therapy: a placebo controlled trial with particular reference to the role of *Campylobacter pylori*. Gut 1988;29:1386–91.

190. Kang JY, Tay HH, Wee A, et al. Effect of colloidal bismuth subcitrate on symptoms and gastric histology in non-ulcer dyspepsia: a double-blind placebo controlled study. Gut 1990;31:476–80.

191. Wong WM, Wong BC, Hung WK, Yee YK, Yip AW, Szeto ML, Fung FM, Tong TS, Lai KC, Hu WH, Yuen MF, Lam SK. Double blind, randomised, placebo controlled study of four weeks of lansoprazole for the treatment of functional dyspepsia in Chinese patients. Gut 2002;51:502–6.

192. Laine L, Schoenfeld P, Fennerty MB. Therapy for *Helicobacter pylori* in patients with nonulcer dyspepsia. Ann Intern Med 2001;134:361–9.

193. Johnson AG. Controlled trial of metoclopramide in the treatment of flatulent dyspepsia. Brit Med J 1971;2:25–26.

194. Perkel MS, Moore C, Hersh T, et al. Metoclopramide therapy in patients with delayed gastric emptying: a randomized, double-blind study. Dig Dis Sci 1979;24:662–66.

195. Brogden RN, Carmine AA, Heel RC, et al. Domperidone: a review of its pharmacological activity, pharmacokinetics and therapeutic efficacy in the symptomatic treatment of chronic dyspepsia and as an antiemetic. Drugs 1982;24:360–400.

196. Davis RH, Clench MH, Mathias JR. Effects of domperidone in patients with chronic unexplained upper gastrointestinal symptoms: a double-blind, placebo-controlled study. Dig Dis Sci 1988;33:1505–11.

197. Veldhuyzen van Zanten SJ, Jones MJ, Verlinden M, Talley NJ. Efficacy of cisapride and domperidone in functional (nonulcer) dyspepsia: a meta-analysis. Am J Gastroenterol 2001;96:689–96.

198. Koch KL, Stern RM, Stewart WR, Vasey MW. Gastric emptying and gastric myoelectrical activity in patients with diabetic gastroparesis: effect of long-term domperidone treatment. Am J Gastroenterol 1989 Sep;84(9):1069–75.

199. Tack J, Vos R, Janssens J, et al. Influence of tegaserod on proximal gastric tone and on the perception of gastric distension. Aliment Pharmacol Ther 2003;18:1031–7.

200. Janssens J, Peeters TI, Vantrappen G, et al. Improvement of gastric emptying in diabetic gastroparesis by erythromycin: preliminary studies. New Engl J Med 1990; 322:1028–31.

201. Richards RD, Davenport K, McCallum RW. The treatment of idiopathic and dia-

betic gastroparesis with acute intravenous and chronic oral erythromycin. Am J Gastroenterol 1993;88:203–206.

202. Mertz H, Fass R, Kodner A, et al. Effect of amitriptyline on symptoms, sleep, and visceral perception in patients with functional dyspepsia. Am J Gastroenterol 1998; 93:160–65.

203. Tanum L, Malt UF. A new pharmacologic treatment of functional gastrointestinal disorder: a double-blind placebo-controlled study with mianserin. Scand J Gastroenterol 1996;31:318–25.

204. Ladabaum U, Glidden D. Effect of the selective serotonin reuptake inhibitor sertraline on gastric sensitivity and compliance in healthy humans. Neurogastroenterol Motil 2002;14:395–402.

205. Tack J, Broekaert D, Coulie B, et al. Influence of the selective serotonin reuptake inhibitor paroxetine on gastric sensorimotor function in man. Aliment Pharmacol Ther 2003;17:603–8.

206. Holtmann G, Talley NJ, Liebregts T, Adam B, Parow C. A placebo-controlled trial of itopride in functional dyspepsia. N Eng J Med 2006;354(8):832–40.

207. Kagan G, Huddlestone L, Wolstencroft P. Comparison of dicyclomine with antacid and without antacid in dyspepsia. J Internat Med Res 1984;12:174–78.

208. Walters JM, Crean P, McCarthy CF. Trimebutine, a new antispasmodic in the treatment of dyspepsia. Irish Med J 1980;73:380–81.

209. Melzer J, Rosch W, Reichling J, Brignoli R, Saller R. Meta-analysis: phytotherapy of functional dyspepsia with the herbal drug preparation STW 5 (Iberogast). Aliment Pharmacol Ther 2004 Dec;20[11–12]:1279–87.

210. Bensoussan A, Talley NJ, Hing M, Menzies R, Guo A, Ngu M. Treatment of irritable bowel syndrome with Chinese herbal medicine: a randomized controlled trial. JAMA 1998 Nov 11;280(18):1585–9.

211. Coffin B, Bouhassira D, Chollet R, et al. Effect of the kappa agonist fedotozine on perception of gastric distension in healthy humans. Aliment Pharmacol Ther 1996; 10:919–25.

212. Fraitag B, Homerin M, Hecketsweiler P. Double-blind dose-response multicenter comparison of fedotozine and placebo in treatment of nonulcer dyspepsia. Dig Dis Sci 1994;39:1072–77.

213. Read NW, Abitbol JL, Bardhan KD, et al. Efficacy and safety of the peripheral kappa agonist fedotozine versus placebo in the treatment of functional dyspepsia. Gut 1997;41:664–68.

214. Delgado-Aros S, Chial HJ, Camilleri M, et al. Effects of a kappa-opioid agonist, asimadoline, on satiation and GI motor and sensory functions in humans. Am J Physiol—Gastrointest Liver Physiol 2003;284:G558–66.

215. Kurz A, Sessler DI. Opioid-induced bowel dysfunction: pathophysiology and potential new therapies. Drugs 2003;63:649–71.

216. Kuiken SD, Lei A, Tytgat GN, et al. Effect of the low-affinity, noncompetitive N-methyl-d-aspartate receptor antagonist dextromethorphan on visceral perception in healthy volunteers. Aliment Pharmacol Ther 2002;16:1955–62.

217. Holzer P, Holzer-Petsche U. Tachykinins in the gut. Part I. Expression, release and motor function. Pharmacol Ther 1997;73:173–217.

218. Holzer P, Holzer-Petsche U. Tachykinins in the gut. Part II. Roles in neural excitation, secretion and inflammation. Pharmacol Ther 1997;73:219–63.

219. Poli-Bigelli S, Rodrigues-Pereira J, Carides AD, et al. Addition of the neurokinin 1

receptor antagonist aprepitant to standard antiemetic therapy improves control of chemotherapy-induced nausea and vomiting. Results from a randomized, double-blind, placebo-controlled trial in Latin America. Cancer 2003;97:3090–8.

220. Chawla SP, Grunberg SM, Gralla RJ, et al. Establishing the dose of the oral NK1 antagonist aprepitant for the prevention of chemotherapy-induced nausea and vomiting. Cancer 2003;97:2290–300.

221. Fioramonti J, Gaultier E, Toulouse M, et al. Intestinal anti-nociceptive behaviour of NK3 receptor antagonism in conscious rats: evidence to support a peripheral mechanism of action. Neurogastroenterol Mot 2003;15:363–9.

222. Szallasi A, Nilsson S, Farkas-Szallasi T, et al. Vanilloid (capsaicin) receptors in the rat: distribution in the brain, regional differences in the spinal cord, axonal transport to the periphery, and depletion by systemic vanilloid treatment. Brain Res 1995; 703:175–83.

223. Bortolotti M, Coccia G, Grossi G, et al. The treatment of functional dyspepsia with red pepper. Aliment Pharmacol Ther 2002;16:1075–82.

224. Coulie B, Tack J, Sifrim D, et al. Role of nitric oxide in fasting gastric fundus tone and in 5-HT$_1$ receptor-mediated relaxation of gastric fundus. Am J Physiol 1999;276 (2Pt1):G373–7.

225. Tack J, Coulie B, Wilmer A, Andrioli A, Janssens J. Influence of sumatriptan on gastric fundus tone and on the perception of gastric distension in man. Gut 2000; 46:468–73.

226. Kuo B, Camilleri M, Burton D, et al. Effects of 5-HT(3) antagonism on postprandial gastric volume and symptoms in humans. Aliment Pharmacol Ther 2002;16: 225–33.

227. Kuiken SD, Vergeer M, Heisterkamp SH, et al. Role of nitric oxide in gastric motor and sensory functions in healthy subjects. Gut 2002b;51:212–8.

228. Hausken T, Berstad A. Effect of glyceryl trinitrate on antral motility and symptoms in patients with functional dyspepsia. Scand J Gastroenterol. 1994;29:23–8.

229. Lal S, McLaughlin J, Barlow J, et al. Cholecystokinin pathways modulate sensations induced by gastric distension in man. Am J Physiol Gastrointest Liver Physiol 2004 Jul;287(1):G72–9.

230. Thumshirn M, Camilleri M, Choi MG, Zinsmeister AR. Modulation of gastric sensory and motor functions by nitrergic and alpha2-adrenergic agents in humans. Gastroenterology 1999;116:573–85.

231. Feinle C, Meier O, Otto B, D'Amato M, Fried M. Role of duodenal lipid and cholecystokinin A receptors in the pathophysiology of functional dyspepsia. Gut 2001; 48:347–55.

232. Cremonini F, Camilleri M, McKinzie S, Burton D, Thomforde D, Zinsmeister A. Effect of a CCK1 antagonist, dexloxiglumide, on gastrointestinal and colonic transit in female patients with irritable bowel syndrome and predominant constipation Neurogastroenterology and Motility 2004 October; Volume 16 Issue 5: 647.

233. Hamilton J, Guthrie E, Creed F, Thompson D, Tomenson B, Bennett R, Moriarty K, Stephens W, Liston R. A randomized controlled trial of psychotherapy in patients with chronic functional dyspepsia. Gastroenterology 2000; 119:661–9.

234. Calvert EL, Houghton LA, Cooper P, et al. Long-term improvement in functional dyspepsia using hypnotherapy. Gastroenterology 2002;123:1778–85.

235. Jones MP, Maganti K. A systematic review of surgical therapy for gastroparesis. Am J Gastroenterol 2003;98:2122–9.

236. Lin Z, Forster J, Sarosiek I, McCallum RW. Treatment of gastroparesis with electrical stimulation. Dig Dis Sci 2003;48:837–48.

237. Dundee JW, Yang J, McMillan C. Non-invasive stimulation of the P6 (Neiguan) antiemetic acupuncture point in cancer chemotherapy. Royal Soc Med 1993;8:603–606.

238. Dundee JW, Ghaly RG, Bill KM, et al. Effect of stimulation of the P6 antiemetic point on postoperative nausea and vomiting. Brit J Anaesthesiol 1989;63:612–18.

239. Hu S, Stern RM, Kock KL. Electrical acustimulation relieves vection-induced motion sickness. Gastroenterology 1992;102:1854–58.

240. Hu S, Stritzel R, Chandler A, et al. P6 acupressure reduces symptoms of vection-induced motion sickness. Aviat Space Environ Med 1995;66:631–34.

241. Paterson C, Ewings P, Brazier JE, Britten N. Treating dyspepsia with acupuncture and homeopathy: reflections on a pilot study by researchers, practitioners and participants. Complement Ther Med 2003;11:78–84.

242. Pouderoux P, Ergun GA, Lin S, Kahrilas PJ. Esophageal bolus transit imaged by ultrafast computerized tomography. Gastroenterology 1996;110(5):1422–1428.

243. McNally EF, Kelly E, Ingelfinger F. Mechanism of belching: effects of gastric distention with air. Gastroenterology 1964;46:254–259.

244. Sifrim D, Silny J, Holloway RH, Janssens JJ. Patterns of gas and liquid reflux during transient lower oesophageal sphincter relaxation: a study using intraluminal electrical impedance. Gut 1999;44:47–54.

245. Wyman JB, Dent J, Heddle R, Dodds WJ, Toouli J, Downton J. Control of belching by the lower oesophageal sphincter. Gut 1990;31(6):639–646.

246. Tosetti C, Stanghellini V, Corinaldesi R. The Rome II Criteria for patients with functional gastroduodenal disorders. J Clin Gastroenterol 2003;37(1):92–3.

247. Bredenoord AJ, Weusten BL, Sifrim D, Timmer R, Smout AJ. Aerophagia, gastric, and supragastric belching: a study using intraluminal electrical impedance monitoring. Gut 2004;53(11):1561–5.

248. Chitkara DK, Bredenoord AJ, Rucker MJ, Talley NJ. Aerophagia in adults: a comparison with functional dyspepsia. Aliment Pharmacol Ther 2005 Nov 1;22(9):855–8.

249. Levitt MD, Bond JH. Flatulence. Annu Rev Med 1980;31:127–37.

250. Lin M, Triadafilopoulos G. Belching: dyspepsia or gastroesophageal reflux disease? Am J Gastroenterol 2003;98(10):2139–45.

251. Straathof JW, Ringers J, Lamers CB, Masclee AA. Provocation of transient lower esophageal sphincter relaxations by gastric distension with air. Am J Gastroenterol 2001;96(8):2317–2323.

252. Cuevas JL, Cook EW III, Richter JE, McCutcheon M, Taub E. Spontaneous swallowing rate and emotional state. Possible mechanism for stress-related gastrointestinal disorders. Dig Dis Sci 1995;40:282–86.

253. Talley NJ, Piper DW. Comparison of the clinical features and illness behaviour of patients presenting with dyspepsia of unknown cause (essential dyspepsia) and organic disease. Aust NZ J Med 1986;16:352-359.

254. Baume P, Tracey M, Dawson L. Efficacy of two minor tranquillizers in relieving symptoms of functional gastrointestinal distress. Aust NZ J Med 1975;5:503–6.

255. Friis H, Bode S, Rumessen JJ, Gudmand-Hoyer E. Effect of simethicone on lactulose-induced H_2 production and gastrointestinal symptoms. Digestion 1991;49:227–30.

256. Arts J, Van Gool S, Caenepeel P, Sifrim D, Janssens J, Tack J. Intra-pyloric Botulinum toxin injection improves gastric emptying of solids and symptoms in dyspeptic patients with delayed gastric emptying. Aliment Pharmacol Ther 2006; in press.

257. Spiegel SB. Uses of hypnosis in the treatment of uncontrollable belching: a case report. Am J Clin Hypnosis 1996;38:263–70.

258. Kamolz T, Bammer T, Granderath FA, Pointner R. Comorbidity of aerophagia in GERD patients: outcome of laparoscopic antireflux surgery. Scand J Gastroenterol 2002;37(2):138–43.

259. Muth ER, Stern RM, Thayer JF, Koch KL. Assessment of the multiple dimensions of nausea: The nausea profile (NP). J Psychosom Res 1996;40:511–520.

260. Delgado-Aros S, Locke GR 3rd, Camilleri M, Talley NJ, Fett S, Zinsmeister AR, Melton LJ 3rd. Obesity is associated with increased risk of gastrointestinal symptoms: a population-based study. Am J Gastroenterol 2004;99:1801–6.

261. Prakash C, Clouse RE. Cyclic vomiting syndrome in adults: clinical features and response to tricyclic antidepressants. Am J Gastroenterol 1999;94:2855–60.

262. Anonymous. Psychogenic vomiting: A disorder of gastrointestinal motility? Lancet 1992;339:279.

263. Morgan HG. Functional vomiting. J Psychosomat Res 1985;29:341–52.

264. Rosenthal RH, Webb WL, Wruble LD. Diagnosis and management of persistent psychogenic vomiting. Psychosomatics 1980;21:722–30.

265. Wruble LD, Rosenthal RH, Webb WL Jr. Psychogenic vomiting: a review. Am J Gastroenterol 1982;77:318–21.

266. Li BU, Isimman RM, Sanna SK. Consensus statement: second international symposium on CVS-the faculty of the second international scientific symposium on cyclic vomiting syndrome. Dig Dis Sci 1999a;44:9S.

267. Li BUK, Murray RD, Heitlinger LA, Robbins JL, Hayes JR. Is cyclic vomiting syndrome related to migraine? J Pediatr 1999b;134:567–72.

268. Fleisher DR, Matar M. The cyclic vomiting syndrome: a report of 71 cases and literature review. J Pediatr Gastroenterol Nutr 1993;17:361–9.

269. Boles RG, Chun M, Senadheera D, Wong LJ. Cyclic vomiting syndrome and mitochondrial DNA mutations. Lancet 1997;350:1299–1300.

270. Lucarelli S, Corrado G, Pelliccia A, D'Ambrini GD, Cavaliere M, Barbato M, Lendvai D, Frediani T. Cyclic vomiting syndrome and food allergy/intolerance in seven children: a possible association. Eur J Pediatr 2000;159:360–3.

271. Prakash C, Staiano A, Rothbaum RJ, Clouse RE. Similarities in cyclic vomiting syndrome across age groups. Am J Gastroenterol 2001;96:684–88.

272. Allen JH, de Moore GM, Heddle R, Twartz JC. Cannabinoid hyperemesis: cyclical hyperemesis in association with chronic cannabis abuse. Gut 2004;53(11):1566–70.

273. Chial HJ, Camilleri M, Williams DE, Litzinger K, Perrault J. Rumination syndrome in children and adolescents: diagnosis, treatment, and prognosis. Pediatrics 2003;111:158–62.

274. O'Brien MD, Bruce BK, Camilleri M. The rumination syndrome: clinical features rather than manometric diagnosis. Gastroenterology 1995;108:1024–29.

275. Quigley EMM, Hasler WL, Parkman HP. AGA technical review on nausea and vomiting. Gastroenterology 2001;120:263–86.

276. Brzana RJ, Koch KL. Gastroesophageal reflux disease presenting with intractable nausea. Ann Intern Med 1997;126:704–7.
277. Muraoka M, Mine K, Matsumoto K, Nakai Y, Nakagawa T. Psychogenic vomiting: the relation between patterns of vomiting and psychiatric diagnoses. Gut 1990; 31:526–8.
278. Olden KW. Rumination syndrome. Curr Treat Options Gastroenterol 2001;4: 351–8.
279. Stravynski A. Behavioral treatment of psychogenic vomiting in the context of social phobia. J Nerv Ment Dis 1983;171:448–51.
280. Dura JR. Successful treatment of chronic psychogenic vomiting by self-monitoring. Psychol Rep 1988;62:239–42.
281. Forbes D, Withers G. Prophylactic therapy in cyclic vomiting syndrome. J Pediatr Gastroenterol Nutr 1995;21 Suppl 1:S57–9.
282. Levine DF, Wingate DL, Pfeffer JM, et al. Habitual rumination: a benign disorder. Br Med J (Clin Res Ed) 1983;287:255–6.
283. Winship DH, Shoralski FF, Weber WN, et al. Esophagus in rumination. Am J Physiol 1964;207:1189–94.
284. Dougherty RW. Eructation in ruminants. Ann N Y Acad Sci 1968;150(1):22–6.
285. Malcolm A, Thumshirn MB, Camilleri M, et al. Rumination syndrome. Mayo Clin Proc 1997;72:646–52.
286. Whitehead WE, Drescher VM, Morrill-Corbin E, et al. Rumination syndrome in children treated by increased holding. J Pediatr Gastroenterol Nutr 1985;4:550–6.
287. Sheagren TG, Mangurten HH, Brea F, et al. Rumination—a new complication of neonatal intensive care. Pediatrics 1980;66:551–5.
288. Fleisher DR. Infant rumination syndrome: Report of a case and review of the literature. Am J Dis Child 1979;133:266–69.
289. Fleisher DR. Functional vomiting disorders in infancy: innocent vomiting, nervous vomiting, and infant rumination syndrome. J Pediatr 1994;125:S84–94.
290. Ball TS, Hendricksen H, Clayton J. A special feeding technique for chronic regurgitation. Am J Ment Defic 1974;78:486–93.
291. Rogers B, Stratton P, Victor J, et al. Chronic regurgitation among persons with mental retardation: A need for combined medical and interdisciplinary strategies. Am J Ment Retard 1992;96:522–27.
292. Fredericks DW, Carr JE, Williams WL. Overview of the treatment of rumination disorder for adults in a residential setting. J Behav Ther Exp Psychiatry 1998; 29(1):31–40.
293. Brown WR. Rumination in the adult. A study of two cases. Gastroenterology 1968; 54:933–9.
294. Soykan I, Chen J, Kendall BJ, et al. The rumination syndrome: clinical and manometric profile, therapy, and long-term outcome. Dig Dis Sci 1997;42:1866–72.
295. Khan S, Hyman PE, Cocjin J, et al. Rumination syndrome in adolescents. J Pediatr 2000;136:528–31.
296. Amarnath RP, Abell TL, Malagelada JR. The rumination syndrome in adults. A characteristic manometric pattern. Ann Intern Med 1986;105:513–8.
297. Eckern M, Stevens W, Mitchell J. The relationship between rumination and eating disorders. Int J Eat Disord 1999;26:414–9.
298. Larocca FE, Della-Fera MA. Rumination: its significance in adults with bulimia nervosa. Psychosomatics 1986;27:209–12.

299. Fairburn CG, Cooper PJ. Rumination in bulimia nervosa 1985;88:826–827.
300. Shay SS, Johnson LF, Wong RK, Curtis DJ, Rosenthal R, Lamott JR, Owensby LC. Rumination, heartburn, and daytime gastroesophageal reflux. A case study with mechanisms defined and successfully treated with biofeedback therapy.
301. Thumshirn M, Camilleri M, Hanson RB, et al. Gastric mechanosensory and lower esophageal sphincter function in rumination syndrome. Am J Physiol 1998;275: G314–21.
302. Smout AJ, Breumelhof R. Voluntary induction of transient lower esophageal sphincter relaxations in an adult patient with the rumination syndrome. Am J Gastroenterol 1990;85:1621–5.
303. Johnson WG, Corrigan SA, Crusco AH, et al. Behavioral assessment and treatment of postprandial regurgitation. J Clin Gastroenterol 1987;9:679–84.
304. Prather CM, Litzinger KL, Camilleri M, et al. An open trial of cognitive behavioral intervention in the treatment of rumination syndrome. Gastroenterology 1997;112: A808 (Abstract).
305. Wagaman JR, Williams DE, Camilleri M. Behavioral intervention for the treatment of rumination. J Pediatr Gastroenterol Nutr 1998;27:596–8.

Chapter 9

Functional Bowel Disorders

George F. Longstreth, Chair

W. Grant Thompson, Co-Chair

William D. Chey

Lesley A. Houghton

Fermin Mearin

Robin C. Spiller

Introduction

Functional bowel disorders are functional gastrointestinal disorders with symptoms attributable to the middle or lower gastrointestinal tract. These include the irritable bowel syndrome (IBS), functional bloating, functional constipation, functional diarrhea, and unspecified functional bowel disorder.

In 1984, an international working team began to define and establish diagnostic criteria for the diagnosis of IBS. Initially based on the study by Manning et al. [1], diagnostic symptom criteria have evolved through the Rome I, Rome II, and Rome III criteria [2]. Early diagnostic criteria for IBS, notably the Manning [1] and Kruis criteria [3], were derived from clinical data that differentiated patients with IBS from those with organic abdominal disease. In contrast, the Rome criteria, while largely drawn from the Manning and Kruis data, were intended to provide comprehensive clinical definitions of disorders of gastrointestinal function in order to better identify clinical syndromes and ensure homogeneity of clinical trial patients.

The present working team considered new evidence for over a year before meeting in Rome in December 2004. New data were considered judiciously, and the penultimate draft was circulated to six expert gastroenterologists throughout the world. We considered their comments in preparing the manuscript.

Subjects with a functional bowel disorder (FBD) (Table 1) may be divided into the following groups:

1. *Nonpatients.* Those who have never sought health care for the FBD.
2. *Patients.* Those who have sought health care for the FBD.
   a. *Incident Cases.* Those who have initially sought health care for the FBD over a specified period of time.
   b. *Prevalent Cases.* Those who have ever sought health care for the FBD.

To separate the chronic FBDs from transient gut symptoms, symptoms must have occurred for the first time at least 6 months prior to diagnosis and be present on at least 3 days a month during the last 3 months to demostrate current activity. Previous diagnostic criteria presumed the absence of a structural or biochemical disorder. However, research advances will likely confirm that FBDs may coexist with other gastrointestinal (GI) disorders. It is also assumed that IBS, functional bloating, functional constipation, and functional diarrhea may have multiple etiologies.

Table 1. Functional Gastrointestinal Disorders

A. Functional Esophageal Disorders

A1. Functional heartburn
A2. Functional chest pain of presumed esophageal origin
A3. Functional dysphagia
A4. Globus

B. Functional Gastroduodenal Disorders

B1. Functional dyspepsia
    B1a. Postprandial distress syndrome (PDS)
    B1b. Epigastric pain syndrome (EPS)
B2. Belching disorders
    B2a. Aerophagia
    B2b. Unspecified excessive belching
B3. Nausea and vomiting disorders
    B3a. Chronic idiopathic nausea (CIN)
    B3b. Functional vomiting
    B3c. Cyclic vomiting syndrome (CVS)
B4. Rumination syndrome in adults

C. Functional Bowel Disorders

C1. Irritable bowel syndrome (IBS)
C2. Functional bloating
C3. Functional constipation
C4. Functional diarrhea
C5. Unspecified functional bowel disorder

D. Functional Abdominal Pain Syndrome (FAPS)

E. Functional Gallbladder and Sphincter of Oddi (SO) Disorders

E1. Functional gallbladder disorder
E2. Functional biliary SO disorder
E3. Functional pancreatic SO disorder

F. Functional Anorectal Disorders

F1. Functional fecal incontinence
F2. Functional anorectal pain
    F2a. Chronic proctalgia
        F2a1. Levator ani syndrome
        F2a2. Unspecified functional anorectal pain
    F2b. Proctalgia fugax
F3. Functional defecation disorders
    F3a. Dyssynergic defecation
    F3b. Inadequate defecatory propulsion

G. Functional Disorders: Neonates and Toddlers

G1. Infant regurgitation
G2. Infant rumination syndrome
G3. Cyclic vomiting syndrome
G4. Infant colic
G5. Functional diarrhea
G6. Infant dyschezia
G7. Functional constipation

H. Functional Disorders: Children and Adolescents

H1. Vomiting and aerophagia
    H1a. Adolescent rumination syndrome
    H1b. Cyclic vomiting syndrome
    H1c. Aerophagia
H2. Abdominal pain-related FGIDs
    H2a. Functional dyspepsia
    H2b. Irritable bowel syndrome
    H2c. Abdominal migraine
    H2d. Childhood functional abdominal pain
        H2d1. Childhood functional abdominal pain syndrome
H3. Constipation and incontinence
    H3a. Functional constipation
    H3b. Nonretentive fecal incontinence

CI. Irritable Bowel Syndrome

— Definition

Irritable bowel syndrome is a functional bowel disorder in which abdominal pain or discomfort is associated with defecation or a change in bowel habit, and with features of disordered defecation.

— Epidemiology

About 10% to 20% of adults and adolescents have symptoms consistent with IBS, and the disorder affects all races throughout the world [4–9]. Some studies suggest that females may be more likely to consult a physician [4, 10, 11], while others do not [12, 13]. IBS symptoms come and go over time and often overlap with dyspeptic symptoms [14, 15]. The lifetime prevalence exceeds the point prevalence.

Direct medical expenses and indirect costs associated with IBS are considerable [4, 16–22]. In US managed-care populations, total direct costs incurred by subjects with IBS are about 50% higher than by individuals without IBS [18, 20]. Drug use is common and costs for outpatient visits, hospitalizations, and diagnostic tests are high [4, 17, 18, 20]. Work absenteeism is considerable [4], and reduced quality of life is common [23, 24]. Severity of IBS-associated pain/discomfort is related to medical costs [20] and quality of life impairment [24]. Some studies find that severity is related to functional status, phone calls to physicians, other behaviors, and psychological disturbance [25]. While psychosocial factors are believed to play a role in clinical outcomes such as health care-seeking in severely affected patients (see Chapter 6 on psychosocial aspects), little correlation between psychological factors and health care-seeking is reported in population surveys or patients with mild symptoms [26, 27]. IBS is associated with surgery independent of other variables such as age or comorbid conditions. For example, California Kaiser Permanente examinees with an IBS diagnosis report rates of cholecystectomy threefold higher, appendectomy and hysterectomy twofold higher and back surgery 50% higher than individuals without IBS [28].

C1. Diagnostic Criterion* for Irritable Bowel Syndrome

Recurrent abdominal pain or discomfort** at least 3 days/ month in the last 3 months associated with _two or more_ of the following:

1. **Improvement with defecation**
2. **Onset associated with a change in frequency of stool**
3. **Onset associated with a change in form (appearance) of stool**

*Criterion fulfilled for the last 3 months with symptom onset at least 6 months prior to diagnosis

**"Discomfort" means an uncomfortable sensation not described as pain.

In pathophysiology research and clinical trials, a pain/discomfort frequency of at least 2 days a week during screening evaluation is recommended for subject eligibility.

Supportive symptoms that are not part of the diagnostic criteria include abnormal stool frequency (a) fewer than three bowel movements per week, or (b) greater than three bowel movements per day; abnormal stool form (c) lumpy/hard stool, or (d) loose/watery stool; (e) defecation straining; (f) urgency, or also feeling of incomplete bowel movement, passing mucus, and bloating.

The Rome II working team suggested two systems for classifying patients into diarrhea-predominant (IBS-D) and constipation-predominant (IBS-C) subgroups based on the first six of these features.[1] Subclassification of IBS into these bowel patterns may be necessary for treatment trials and patient care. Both classification variations exclude patients with hard stools from IBS-D [29, 30], but one version can include patients with watery stools in IBS-C [30]. Straining, urgency, and incomplete evacuation occur across the spectrum of stool form [31, 32], and when subgroups are identified by cluster analysis [33] or symptoms [34], most subjects have a stool frequency within the normal range regardless of bowel pattern. On the other hand, stool form (from watery to hard) reflects intestinal transit time.

Therefore, assuming no use of antidiarrheals or laxatives, we propose the following system shown in Table 2. Researchers and practitioners should consider

---

[1] The Rome II classification based on the first six supportive symptoms noted above include _diarrhea-predominant:_ 1 or more of b, d, f, and none of a, c, e, or 2 or more of b, d, f, and 1 of a or e [c, hard/lumpy stool excluded]; and _constipation-predominant:_ 1 or more of a, c, e, and none of b, d, f, or 2 or more of a, c, e, and 1 of b, d, f.

Table 2. Subtyping IBS by Predominant Stool Pattern

To subtype patients according to bowel habit for research or clinical trials, the following subclassifications may be used (see Figure 1). The validity and stability of such subtypes over time is unknown and should be subjects of future research.

1. IBS with constipation (IBS-C)—hard or lumpy stools[a] at least 25% *and* loose (mushy) or watery stools[b] < 25% of bowel movements*

2. IBS with diarrhea (IBS-D)—loose (mushy) or watery stools[b] at least 25% *and* hard or lumpy stool[a] < 25% of bowel movements*

3. Mixed IBS (IBS-M)—hard or lumpy stools[a] at least 25% *and* loose (mushy) or watery stools[b] at least 25% of bowel movements*

4. Unsubtyped IBS—insufficient abnormality of stool consistency to meet criteria for IBS-C, D, or M*

---

* In the absence of antidiarrheal or laxative use

[a] Bristol Stool Form Scale 1–2 (Separate hard lumps like nuts [difficult to pass] or sausage shaped but lumpy)

[b] Bristol Stool Form Scale 6–7 (Fluffy pieces with ragged edges, a mushy stool or watery, no solid pieces, entirely liquid)

Figure 1. The Bristol Stool Form Scale with the standard description for each of the seven types.

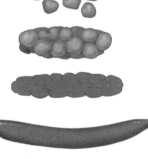
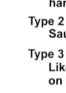
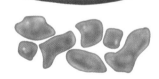
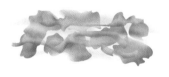

Type 1
  Separate hard lumps, like nuts, hard to pass

Type 2
  Sausage shaped, but lumpy

Type 3
  Like sausage, but with cracks on surface

Type 4
  Like sausage or snake, smooth and soft

Type 5
  Soft blobs with clear cut edges (passed early)

Type 6
  Fluffy pieces with ragged edges, a mushy stool

Entirely liquid

Type 7
  Watery, no solid pieces

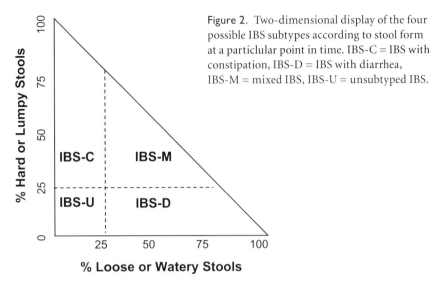

Figure 2. Two-dimensional display of the four possible IBS subtypes according to stool form at a particlular point in time. IBS-C = IBS with constipation, IBS-D = IBS with diarrhea, IBS-M = mixed IBS, IBS-U = unsubtyped IBS.

using the Bristol Stool Form Scale (Figure 1). We suggest the identification of constipation as Bristol types 1 and 2 and diarrhea as types 6 and 7.

Figure 2 describes the four possible bowel pattern subtypes at a particular point in time. Subjects with neither diarrhea nor constipation by these characteristics have unsubtyped IBS (IBS-U). Subjects not fitting the IBS-D or IBS-C subtypes have variably been termed mixed IBS (IBS-M) [35] or alternating IBS (IBS-A), or these terms have been used synonymously [34]. To reduce semantic confusion, the committee suggests that IBS-M be applied to individuals with both diarrhea and constipation for at least 25% of bowel movements at a given point in time and IBS-A refer to a change between IBS-D and IBS-C over time [35].

— Rationale for Changes in Diagnostic Criteria

The symptom criteria can be used for clinical practice, epidemiological surveys, pathophysiology research, and therapeutic trials. The required FBD symptom frequencies are arbitrary and may require modification, depending on how they are used. Since symptom frequency data on general populations are scanty, epidemiologists should investigate various frequencies to extend knowledge. In therapeutic trials, the higher the frequency threshold for subject enrollment, the larger the potential treatment effect and the smaller the number of subjects that may be needed to show a significant difference. However, such patients may be less likely to achieve satisfactory relief, and such studies are less generalizable. Therefore, enrollment symptom criteria are crucial. The Rome III recommended research threshold for pain/discomfort frequency is reported by a majority of IBS patients [36]. About three fourths of patients who rated their pain as at least moderate (not ignorable, but without effect on lifestyle) also had pain at least two days a week [37]. "Improved" with defecation replaces "relieved" because relief of pain or discomfort may be incomplete [32].

Subgrouping IBS patients according to bowel pattern is controversial. The Rome II subtyping schemes using multiple criteria were complex and difficult to use, so we simplified them by using only the most reliable criteria based on stool form, not bowel movement frequency [31–34, 38, 39]. There is particular support for the use of this method to classify IBS-M [40]. Although the committee recommends a change in subtyping from the multisymptom Rome II classification, to one based on stool form only, there are insufficient data to exclude either classification at this time. Further validation studies are needed.

We emphasize that bowel pattern subtypes are highly unstable. Prospective evaluation reveals (1) The point prevalences of IBS-D, IBS-C, and IBS-M are approximately equal (each about 1/3 of subjects) [34, 35]; (2) These patterns are retained over relatively short periods, as 29% evolve from IBS-C to IBS-D over one year [35]; and (3) IBS-C and IBS-M share similar characteristics, while IBS-D tends to be distinct [35]. Furthermore, the IBS-M subtype has been reported in about 50% of referred patients according to three sets of criteria [40], and IBS-M is the most prevalent group in primary care [36]. A majority of patients have rapidly fluctuating symptoms lasting from less than one hour to less than one week [36, 40]. Therefore, the rate of measured bowel pattern change is a function of the data collection frequency. There are insufficient data upon which to recommend a time period for defining IBS-A. In drug studies on patients subtyped by stool form, investigators may want to assess pharmacological effects on stool frequency, straining, urgency, and incomplete evacuation as well as stool form.

This great symptom instability underlies our preference for the terms IBS with diarrhea and IBS with constipation instead of diarrhea- and constipation-predominant IBS. As with any categorical system, many people whose features place them close to a subtype boundary will change pattern without a major change in pathophysiology. Subclassification may increase diagnostic precision in short-term clinical studies, but may have limited usefulness in patient care because bowel pattern varies so much. The heterogeneity and variable natural history of IBS significantly limit clinical trials of motility-active drugs and drug therapy in practice. In both research and practice, it may be desirable to base drug use on a stronger bowel pattern predominance than what is required by this system.

— Clinical Evaluation

The temporal relationship of pain, bowel habit and stool characteristics is the most prominent feature of IBS. Pain related to defecation is likely to be a bowel pain, while that associated with exercise, movement, urination or menstruation usually has a different cause. IBS should be suspected from the medical history taken at the initial clinical evaluation. "Alarm" symptoms or signs of anatomic disease include fever, rectal bleeding, weight loss, anemia and other alarm symptoms or signs that are not explained by a functional disorder. The presence of typical symptoms and absence of alarm features predict IBS accurately [3, 41, 42], but alarm features are of doubtful utility in predicting organic disease when patients are evaluated for IBS [43]. Nevertheless, the presence of alarm features does not exclude the possible coexistence of IBS with another GI disorder [44].

Many women with IBS consult a gynecologist for "chronic pelvic pain" [45]. In addition to gastrointestinal and gynecological symptom overlap, there is remarkable similarity between the psychosocial factors underlying IBS and the gynecologic patient's disorder [46]. The common occurrence of dyspareunia or other sexual dysfunction in women with IBS and worsening of IBS symptoms during menstruation [47, 48] may obscure the diagnosis, but the association of pain with defecation and bowel dysfunction point to an intestinal origin. Clearly, a specialist's point of view can influence the diagnosis and the approach to diagnosis and treatment [49]. Incorrect symptom attribution by clinicians leads to inappropriate hospitalization [50] and surgery, especially cholecystectomy, appendectomy, and hysterectomy [28]. Obtaining a history of bowel dysfunction from so-called "pelvic pain" patients may reduce hysterectomies [51].

Patient self-reports of "diarrhea" and "constipation" may be misleading. The stool may be solid even though defecation is frequent (pseudodiarrhea) [38]. Conversely, straining to defecate may occur with soft or watery stools. Some patients may feel they are constipated because they have unproductive calls to stool or feelings of incomplete evacuation that prompt them to strain after the stool is passed [52]. In a Spanish survey using Rome II criteria, most people with both diarrhea and constipation reported constipation, and concordance for IBS-D or IBS-C was better between the Rome II subclassification and individuals' opinions than between the Rome II subclassification and bowel movement frequency [34].

Obviously, a common disorder such as IBS may coexist with organic gastrointestinal disease [44, 53]. Specialists' patients often report other gastrointestinal, somatic, and psychological symptoms. These include heartburn and other upper gastrointestinal symptoms, fibromyalgia, headache, backache, genitourinary symptoms [54–56] and psychosocial dysfunction (see below). While these symptoms increase in number as the severity of IBS increases [57], they are not essential for the diagnosis. Although one group found that these "noncolonic" symptoms helped distinguish IBS from organic disease [58], other investigators did not [59]. Whitehead et al. proposed that multiple comorbid disorders are associated with psychological factors [60], and support for this hypothesis was provided by a Norwegian general practice survey [61].

While there are no proven discriminating physical signs of IBS, abdominal tenderness may be present. Focal abdominal wall tenderness detected by the Carnett test (examining for increased or unchanged focal abdominal tenderness during muscle contraction) identifies abdominal wall pain, which is a distinct disorder that many physicians overlook. It may occur with IBS, other chronic painful disorders, and depression [62].

Usually, only limited laboratory and structural evaluation is needed when IBS is suspected, with selective further testing based on the patient's age, duration and severity of symptoms, psychosocial factors, and family history of gastrointestinal disease [63–65]. Sigmoidoscopy, colonoscopy, or barium enema radiography may be indicated. Endoscopy can rule out inflammation, tumors, or melanosis coli, which indicates regular laxative use [66]. Some physicians think sigmoidoscopy can elicit hypersensitivity [67, 68]. Reproduction of the pain during sigmoidoscopy may help convince the patient of its source. Nevertheless, most primary care physicians do not perform sigmoidoscopy [69, 70]. Endoscopic colon examination is expensive [71], and a majority of cases are diagnosed without a colon imaging procedure [72] or any other tests [70]. Rectal biopsy is not normally indicated [73]. No standard battery of diagnostic tests can be recommended for patients who have typical symptoms and no alarm features [65, 74].

Unnecessary investigations may be costly or harmful, and they should be avoided [75]. A complete blood cell count, erythrocyte sedimentation rate, or C-reactive protein test are rarely abnormal from patients identified by symptom criteria [76]. Some investigators tested fecal calprotectin and intestinal permeability to differentiate IBS from organic diseases [77], but these are not in common use. Other tests may include a stool examination for occult blood, leukocytes, or ova and parasites (*Giardia*) where they are endemic. Notably, one third of people who report severe lactose intolerance absorb lactose normally, and lactose malabsorbers can consume eight ounces of milk a day with negligible symptoms [78]. Therefore, lactose absorption usually need not be tested unless the patient consumes more than this amount of milk. Documentation of lactase deficiency seldom leads to improvement of IBS symptoms [79]. Diverticulosis determined by barium enema does not change the diagnosis of IBS [80, 81], and incorrect diagnosis and treatment of "diverticulitis" should be avoided. Routine abdominal ultrasound examination is not helpful [82]. Often, no test is indicated.

Celiac sprue can be accompanied by IBS-type symptoms [83]. Fourteen of 300 Rome II-positive patients had histologic evidence of sprue [84]. Other patients had IBS symptoms and intestinal antibodies against gliadin and common foods. Stool frequency and intestinal immunoglobin A levels decreased significantly after gluten restriction in the subgroups of HLA-DQ2-positive and intestinal

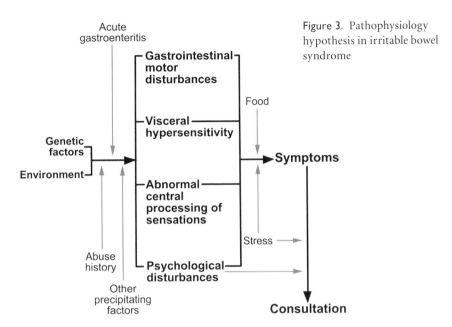

Figure 3. Pathophysiology hypothesis in irritable bowel syndrome

antibody-positive patients compared with those lacking these markers [85]. However, the available data do not support testing in all IBS patients but rather, selective testing based on clinical features and local prevalences [86–88].

Thus, careful history-taking is the most important diagnostic procedure, and lack of explanatory abnormalities on physical examination lends further support. A confident diagnosis that holds up over time [89] can usually be achieved through limited laboratory and structural evaluations that are individualized to each patient's needs [90]. There is no evidence that either liability to other diseases or life expectancy is altered by the IBS, but most patients remain symptomatic or experience relapses for many years following diagnosis. A change in the clinical picture may warrant additional investigation, but the simple symptom persistence does not justify suspicion of another diagnosis. Indeed, such persistence is to be expected, and further needless investigation only undermines the patient's confidence in the diagnosis and the physician.

— Physiological Features

No unique pathophysiological abnormality underlies IBS. Diverse pathophysiological mechanisms appear to generate some IBS symptoms. These include altered motility, visceral hyperalgesia, brain-gut disturbances, genetic and environmental factors, postinfectious sequels, and psychosocial disturbance. Historically, the disorder was often considered as purely psychosomatic in origin, but this was a gross oversimplification. In fact, the physiological and psychological hypotheses were antagonistic, and IBS is better understood using a model that emphasizes the importance of both biologic and psychosocial factors [91] (Figure 3).

Gastrointestinal Motor Disturbances

For many years, IBS was attributed to gut motor disturbances, since exaggerated motility induces diarrhea, decreased motility induces constipation, and intestinal "spasms" cause abdominal pain. Indeed, several motor disturbances occur in IBS patients, but none specifically explains the entire syndrome, likely because the motility pattern shifts with the changeable symptoms.

About 40 years ago, rectosigmoid motility was described as increased in constipation and decreased in diarrhea, suggesting a sphincteric action of the sigmoid colon, which controlled fecal transit [92, 93]. Later, a 3-cycle/min colonic myoelectric rhythm was found to be more prevalent in IBS patients than control subjects [94], but this finding was also present in psychoneurotic patients without IBS [95] and did not change once IBS symptoms improved [96]. Colonic transit is accelerated in IBS-D [97] and delayed in constipation [98], but no data confirm that these observations continue for a long time.

Digestive motility is normal during the basal state, but is exaggerated or altered in response to various stimuli, including food, fatty acids, bile salts, cholecystokinin, and physical and psychological stress [99]. Some small bowel motor patterns may be related to symptoms [100]. The frequency of retrograde pressure waves in phase II is correlated with symptom severity in diarrhea-predominant IBS [101]. In nonconstipated IBS patients, abdominal pain correlates with colonic high amplitude propagated pressure waves [102, 103]. Also, reduction of duodenal motility by colonic distension in controls but not IBS patients suggests an impaired intestinal reflex [104].

Among a subgroup of patients with IBS and delayed gastric emptying [105–107], gastric emptying of solids is slower in those with predominant constipation than in patients with predominant diarrhea [105]. Such gastric dysmotility in IBS patients is associated with concomitant dyspeptic symptoms [106]. Curiously, anger decreases antral motor activity in IBS patients and increases it in healthy controls [108]. None of these observations explain IBS's varied symptoms.

Visceral Hypersensitivity and Abnormal Central Processing of Sensations

IBS patients have lower pain thresholds to gut distention than healthy people. Recent insight into this pathophysiological phenomenon has challenged some previously accepted concepts. An earlier notion that visceral hypersensitivity was exclusive for mechanical stimuli is undermined by electrical stimulation studies that show lower discomfort thresholds in IBS patients than healthy controls [109, 110]. Moreover, early studies failed to show somatic hypersensitivity in IBS and led to the conclusion that pain intolerance was exclusive for visceral perception. New evidence indicates that IBS patients have both visceral and cutaneous hyperalgesia [109–112]. Somatic hyperalgesia seems to depend on the presence of painful nongastrointestinal comorbidity. For example, visceral stimulus was more unpleasant than a somatic stimulus for IBS patients without fibromyalgia, whereas both stimuli were equally unpleasant in the IBS patients with fibromyalgia [113]. However, diffuse hyperalgesia is not always found [114].

Some investigators find that intestinal wall tone and compliance are normal [109, 115, 116], but others have described a lower rectal compliance in both IBS-D and IBS-C [117] or noted increased rectal tone compared with healthy controls [118].

Investigation of visceral perception in humans usually employs barostat distention tests. Patients with IBS perceive the first sensation and pain at lower volumes or pressures than healthy controls [119]. Using 40-mmHg distention as the lower limit of normal, Bouin et al. obtained a sensitivity of 95% and a specificity of 72% in IBS [120]. The putative clinical-physiological correlation of visceral hypersensitivity is unconfirmed. Hypersensitivity has not been linked to the intensity of IBS symptoms [115], and there is disagreement on whether IBS-D and IBS-C differ [115, 121]. Pain thresholds are increased with effective amytriptyline therapy but not during effective psychological treatment [122].

Peripheral mechanisms, such as transient gut inflammation, may enhance visceral sensitivity. Intraluminal injection of the mucosal irritant glycerol in healthy volunteers decreases perception thresholds to rectal distension [123]. Barbara et al. correlated the severity and frequency of abdominal pain with activated mast cells near colonic mucosal nerve endings [124]. However, rectal perception is attenuated in ulcerative colitis patients with low-grade mucosal inflammation of the rectum [125]. Chronic mild inflammation activating antinociceptive mechanisms or central adaptation may prevent the experience of visceral hyperalgesia.

Techniques to map and quantify the activity of the brain, such as PET and functional magnetic resonance imaging (MRI), evaluate where and how visceral stimuli are centrally processed in healthy individuals and explore possibile differences in IBS. Preliminary studies suggest aberrant brain activation both during noxious rectal distention and in the anticipation of rectal pain in IBS patients [126]. The anterior cingulate cortex (ACC) (a limbic center that processes pain suffering), prefrontal cortex (PFC), insular cortex and thalamus seem to be crucial in pain perception [127, 128]. Using MRI, Bernstein et al. found a significantly higher activation of the anterior cingulate gyrus in the control group than in IBS patients and a greater deactivation of the left somatosensory cortex in IBS [129].

Another study demonstrated that patients with IBS have lateral activation of the right prefrontal cortex, reduced activation of the perigenual cortex, temporal lobe, and brain stem, but enhanced activation of rostral anterior cingulate and posterior cingulate cortices [130]. These differences in brain activation patterns may relate to study design. Often, anticipation of rectal distension produces as much activation as actual distension, so patterns of activation need very circumspect interpretation. IBS patients with and without a history of abuse have different brain responses to rectal distension [131]. Also, there are sex-related differences in cortical activity associated with visceral sensation [131, 132]. In a patient with elevated emotional distress and severe IBS, altered brain activation during rectal distension correlated with changes in IBS symptoms [133]. Finally, some studies point to increased afferent processing in ascending pathways rather than to selectively increased activity at higher cortical levels [133–135]. Cerebral evoked potential recordings after rectal stimulation support visceral afferent hypersensitivity as the underlying mechanism [136].

Postinfectious IBS

Overall, 7% to 30% of subjects suffering acute bacterial gastroenteritis develop IBS. Some IBS patients have increased inflammatory cells in the colonic and ileal mucosa, and human and animal studies indicate even minimal inflammation may perturb gastrointestinal reflexes and activate the visceral sensory system [137–140]. Moreover, rectal biopsy on patients with postinfectious IBS show increased chronic inflammatory cells (enteroendocrine cells and lymphocytes) 3 months after acute gastroenteritis [141, 142]. Biopsies from patients after recovery from infectious enteritis reveal increased expression of inflammatory mediators, such as interleukin 1beta, in patients with postinfectious IBS compared with those without IBS [139, 143]. Postinfectious IBS may depend on a genetic predisposition to produce lower amounts of the anti-inflammatory cytokine interleukin 10 [144].

Why some subjects develop IBS after enteric infections and others do not is unknown, but psychosocial difficulties as well as mucosal abnormalities seem equally important [141, 145]. Some studies report that the duration of initial diarrhea [146], hypochondriasis [147], and female sex [146] predict postinfectious IBS, though the latter ceases to be predictive if the effect of anxiety and depression are considered [141, 145]. In a large Spanish outbreak, no risk factors were identified [140]. Infection with *Campylobacter* or *Shigella* is more likely than *Salmonella* enteritis to provoke IBS; however, 10% of Spanish victims of a *Salmonella* outbreak had developed IBS at one year followup, and postinfectious dyspepsia was even more common [140]. Clinical manifestations of postinfectious IBS resemble those of spontaneous IBS except for more days with loose stools [138, 148, 149]. Gwee hypothesizes that exposure to various micororganisms in early life enhances immune tolerance and decreases the risk of subsequent IBS [8].

Bacterial Overgrowth

Some clinicians believe that small bowel bacterial overgrowth is a cause of IBS [150]. They diagnosed bacterial overgrowth by lactulose hydrogen breath testing in 78% of IBS patients and reported that antibiotic treatment eliminated IBS in 48% of patients [151]. However, methodological weaknesses undermined the credibility of this report [152]. Subsequently, it was reported that neomycin more often improved symptoms than placebo, and 75% of patients responded when the breath test normalized after neomycin therapy [153]. However, the short followup of the treated patients leaves the role of bacterial overgrowth unproven. Any benefit could be due to suppression of colonic gas-fermenting bacteria. Furthermore, other investigators did not identify an association of IBS with bacterial overgrowth [154].

Autonomic Function and Hormonal Control

Autonomic function of patients with IBS is abnormal. Mainly cholinergic excess is observed in those with predominant constipation and adrenergic excess in those with predominant diarrhea [155]. Acute psychological and physical stress alters rectal efferent autonomic innervation in controls and IBS patients, in whom the effect may be more prolonged [156]. Central autonomic dysregulation has been suggested [157]. Twenty four-hour electrogastrogram (EGG) recordings identify high- (HF) and low- (LF) frequency variations thought to reflect parasympathetic and sympathetic tone, respectively. However, the LF/HF ratio was similar in IBS patients and controls [158].

Gastrointestinal hormone release in response to jejunal perfusion of lipids is similar in IBS patients and healthy controls, but motilin levels are higher in IBS patients. Corticotrophin-releasing factor levels are lower in IBS-C versus IBS-D patients [159, 160]. IBS-D is associated with a significant postprandial increase in cortisol, which is not evident in controls or IBS-C patients [159]. The meaning of these observations is unclear.

Psychological Features

Psychological disturbance is associated with IBS, especially in patients who seek medical care [161, 162]. Regardless of care-seeking status, IBS is associated with more psychiatric distress [163–165], sleep disturbance [166], "affective vulnerability," and "overadjustment to the environment" [167]. Also, psychosocial factors affect outcome [27].

Community studies reveal that stressful life events, psychological distress, depression, and anxiety are associated with medical symptoms without identified pathology and with increased healthcare utilization and costs [168]. Sudden cultural change may increase the prevalence of IBS, as occurs when Israeli Bedouins move from rural to urban environments [169]. The most severe IBS patients have a poor sense of coherence and of quality of life [167], work absenteeism, frequent medical consultation, and psychosocial distress [164]. In China, anxiety but not depression independently determines healthcare utilization [170]. In traditional Chinese medicine, emotions are regarded as the main pathogenetic factors underlying diseases, especially functional gastrointestinal disorders, and Chinese patients more often report negative life events and demonstrate a negative coping style than healthy controls and peptic ulcer patients [170–172].

Common comorbid psychiatric diagnoses in IBS patients include panic disorder, generalized anxiety disorder, and post-traumatic stress disorder. Common comorbid mood disorders include major depression, dysthymic disorder, and somatoform disorders. Measurement methods could account for the observed differences in psychopathology between male and female patients [173–175]. The nature of the link between psychosocial factors and IBS is unclear [176–178], but Labus et al. developed a scale to measure gastrointestinal symptom-specific anxiety [179]. Sustained and acute life-threatening stressors affect the onset and modulation of GI symptoms [180].

Intestinal reactivity to emotional experiences is poorly understood. IBS patients selectively recall words describing GI sensations compared with neutral words and words describing respiratory sensations [181]. Moreover, exposure of IBS patients with phobic anxiety to words with emotional content causes increased brain responses and rectal activity compared to exposure of IBS patients without psychiatric comorbidity [134].

Abuse History

More than 40% of patients referred to gastroenterologists for functional gastrointestinal disorders, including IBS, are reported to have been physically and/or sexually abused [182–184]. A combination of childhood and adulthood abuse increases the risk of IBS threefold [185]. A positive abuse history seems associated with a tendency toward expressing psychological stress through physical symptoms [164, 186]. The underlying mechanism for greater pain-reporting and poorer health status is unclear, but self-blame and self-silencing may mediate the connection between emotional abuse and functional bowel symptoms [187]. One study found no relation of these factors with rectal pain sensitivity [188].

Some investigators challenge the hypothesis that abuse experiences lead to functional bowel disorders and emphasize instead a relationship of abuse with psychopathology [189, 190]. Other investigators find no associations between early abuse and psychiatric disorder, suggesting that individuals with psychological distress are a different group than those with an abuse history [191]. Nevertheless, both IBS and an abuse history can independently predispose patients to poor health status. The abuse effects on outcome are mediated by psychosocial factors. Therefore, it is important to identify psychological disturbance and an abuse history [192]. However, we do not know whether abuse and IBS are causally related.

Genetic and Environmental Factors

Clustering of IBS in families suggests genetic and/or environmental pathogenetic factors. Locke et al. [193] showed that subjects who have a family member with a history of abdominal pain or bowel dysfunction have a greater than twofold odds increase of self-reporting IBS, whereas those whose spouses have abdominal complaints are not more likely to report IBS. People with digestive symptoms may be aware of family members' similar symptoms or discuss them more, leading to a reporting bias. There is a concordance for functional bowel disorders in 33% of monozygotic twins compared with 13% of dizygotic twins, suggesting that genetics account for approximately 57% of the variance in reporting of functional bowel symptoms [194]. Similar conclusions apply to extraintestinal manifestations [195].

Genetic polymorphisms have been investigated in IBS. Serotonin, a key mediator of intestinal peristalsis, is eliminated from the neuronal gap by a high-affinity substance, serotonin transporter (SERT). SERT polymorphisms in patients with IBS suggest a role for SERT dysfunction in symptom pathogenesis, but ethnic, racial, and other factors require further research before the importance of this is known [196, 197].

Other Factors

Other causes of altered intestinal function have been proposed, including malabsorption of sugars [198] and/or bile acids [199]. Many IBS patients report food intolerance and think their symptoms, especially gas symptoms and pain, are related to meals, but data from dietary elimination and rechallenge studies are inconclusive. Foods rich in carbohydrates, as well as fatty food, coffee, alcohol, and hot spices are frequently reported to cause symptoms. Also, anxiety seems to predict food-related symptoms in IBS patients [200]. Many etiopathological mechanisms have been postulated to relate IBS symptoms to foods. The gut has an extensive immune system, but current understanding of food antigen processing in health and disease is limited [201]. More than 50% of IBS patients are sensitive to some food or inhalant with no typical clinical sign of food allergy. Often, patients are unable to identify offending foods [202]. Postprandial symptoms in female IBS-D patients may be related to increased postprandial platelet-depleted plasma 5-hydroxytryptamine concentrations [203]. Food seems an obvious source of symptom generation, but much more research is required to establish this.

Changes in digestive and psychological symptoms across the menstrual cycle in IBS are related to [47] or possibly due to the effect of menstrual events on rectal sensitivity [204]. Speculation that testosterone protects against IBS is undermined by similar testosterone levels in males with and without IBS. Paradoxically, patients' sensory thresholds correlated negatively with testosterone levels [205].

— Treatment

General Measures

Sensible management depends on a confident diagnosis. Patients often have little knowledge of their disorder [206], and an explanation of why symptoms occur should accompany suggestions for coping with them. Education about healthy lifestyle behaviors can be provided in individual [207] and class settings [208], and patients have greater expectation of benefit from advice about diet, lifestyle, and exercise than drugs [209]. Fear of cancer is a major concern for IBS patients in primary care, and one study suggests that patient reassurance is infrequent [210]. Explanation and reassurance may be the physician's most important therapeutic tools [211]. Repeated or inappropriate tests communicate physician insecurity and can lead to fear and uncertainty on the part of the patient and a cycle of ineffective management [75].

Patient and Physician Agendas

Many IBS patients feel frustrated, isolated, helpless, and worried [212]. These feelings may be more important to the patient than the physical symptoms, so it is important to identify them. Physicians may have attitudes that are not conducive to a therapeutic relationship [213–215]. Compared to other patients with chronic painful disorders, family practitioners may think IBS patients are difficult to satisfy, require a lot of physician time [216], and somatisize psychological distress [217]. Some university internists report that IBS is more difficult to diagnose but easier to treat in women than men [218]. Since the primary aim is to help patients cope, physicians should have and transmit realistic treatment expectations. They can be gratified with making a confident diagnosis and assisting, but not curing, patients [215].

Placebo Response

The "placebo effect" can assist patient improvement and should be understood and valued [219]. A therapeutic effect includes the physiological effects of drug or other therapy, the natural history of the disorder, and the placebo benefit [220]. The natural fluctuation in type and severity of symptoms is great [34, 35]. The placebo effect can be augmented through a physician's efforts to relieve anxiety, explain symptoms, avoid negative conditioned responses, maximize positive patient expectations and take proper advantage of authoritarian power and symbolism. The high placebo response rates that characterize clinical trials reflect the disorder's natural history and the power of the physician/patient interaction [221, 222]. It is clear that these phenomena occur with the test treatment as well. Thus, the wise physician ensures they are used to advantage with any treatment.

A Graded, Multicomponent Approach

Primary care physicians care for the majority of IBS patients [210] and are best positioned to know their histories, personalities, and families. Patients in primary care tend to attribute symptoms to stress [223], giving physicians an opportunity to explain and reassure. In contrast, patients in specialists' practices are more likely to have severe symptoms, depression, anxiety, panic or other psychosocial disorders, and to disagree that stress is important [210].

The type and severity of symptoms and the nature of associated psychosocial issues determine treatment [99, 224]. In addition to allaying fear of serious disease, it is important to uncover any unstated factors. The physician should assess the patient's quality of life and level of daily functioning, taking into account the patient's personality, recent life stress (e.g., divorce, bereavement, and job loss), anxiety, and depression. The patient's reaction to the symptoms may be more important than the symptoms themselves, and psychological factors may alter symptom perception. Most patients respond to psychological support. For example, Dutch patients with functional abdominal pain showed reduced anxiety, cancerphobia, somatic attribution, and catastrophizing cognitions after a series of clinic visits [225]. A strong physician-patient relationship influences health care utilization, as evidenced by the finding that notations in the medical record about psychosocial history, precipitating factors, and discussion of diagnosis and treatment were associated with fewer visits for IBS-related symptoms and fewer hospitalizations over the long term [226]. Canadian patients manifested reduced health care utilization and less pain after a multicomponent approach [227].

Unsatisfied patients may consult multiple physicians, undergo unjustified and hazardous investigation, take unproven medication and even have unneeded surgery [9]. One fifth of Australian subjects with IBS had sought alternative therapy, most often naturopathic care [228]. The physician in charge should maintain patient contact, try to prevent overtesting and harmful treatments, and provide the understanding that these patients require.

Diet

If lactose seems to provoke diarrhea and flatus, a trial of restriction may be advisable. However, the poor correlation between reported lactose intolerance and true lactose malabsorption [78], the failure of lactose restriction to improve symptoms [79, 229] and the potential exclusion of an important calcium source dictate caution in advising lengthy dairy product restriction. Artificial sweeteners, such as sorbitol or mannitol, found in some diet gums and confections, should be used sparingly. Occasionally, a trial of fructose restriction might be worthwhile [198]. Diets may have placebo effects. Exclusion of foods to which patients have immunoglobin G antibodies is reportedly more effective than placebo diets (number-needed-to-treat [NNT] value = 4) [230]. If replicated, this finding may promote the design of more effective food elimination diets than the current tedious elimination process. Nutritionally depleted diets should be avoided, and regular, unhurried meals encouraged.

Dietary fiber is a time-honored therapy that is inexpensive and safe, but the high placebo response, studies limited to specialists' patients, and methodological problems compromise interpretation of clinical trials. Global symptom improvement is marginal, and insoluble fiber (wheat and corn bran) may increase symptoms, including flatulence [231, 232].

Drugs

Dependable pharmacological relief of IBS symptoms remains elusive. Many drugs have been proposed for the treatment of IBS. However, the variety and interchange of symptoms, poor understanding of IBS pathophysiology, and complex central nervous system (CNS) and enteric nervous system (ENS) interactions and their many receptors make it unlikely that a single drug could correct IBS. A search for biomarkers and genetic polymorphisms that could identify patients most likely to respond to drugs is underway. Complicating the development and evaluation of new drugs are psychosocial and recruitment source effects on studied patients [233] and the need for numerous patients and multiple investigators [234]. Validated outcome measures should be employed [235, 236]. Naturally, variable symptom severity and bowel habit [34, 35] are particularly important.

Klein reported many methodological inadequacies in clinical trials before 1986: unstated, unclear, or irrelevant entry criteria; small patient samples; excessive dropouts; short study periods; and/or improper use of statistics or study design [237]. Trials have improved since then and reveal drugs to benefit some symptoms in selected patients [99, 238–241]. However, studies reporting placebo responses below about 40% are suspect. Furthermore, a publication bias favors positive trials.

Drugs should be directed toward the dominant symptom or symptoms (Table 3). Loperamide may prevent diarrhea when taken before a meal or an activity such as traveling that may cause diarrhea. Constipation should be treated initially with dietary fiber supplementation. If response is unsatisfactory, commercial fiber preparations may help. If they increase bloating, lactulose, sorbitol, or polyethylene glycol may be useful. Many physicians recommend one of the het-

Table 3. Possible Drugs for a Dominant Symptom in Irritable Bowel Syndrome[a]

Symptom	Drug	Dose
Diarrhea	Loperamide	2 to 4 mg when necessary, maximum 6 tablets daily
	Cholestyramine	4 g with meals
	Alosetron[b]	0.5 to 1 mg bid (for severe IBS, females)
Constipation	Psyllium	3.4 g bid with meals, then adjust
	Methylcellulose	2 g bid with meals, then adjust
	Calcium polycarbophil	1 g qd to qid
	Lactulose	10 to 20 g bid
	Sorbitol (70%)	15 mL bid
	Polyethylene glycol	17 g in 8 oz water qd
	Tegaserod[c]	6 mg bid
	Magnesium hydroxide	2 to 4 Tbsp qd
Abdominal pain	Smooth muscle relaxant[d]	qd to qid ac
	Tricyclic antidepressants	Start 25 to 50 mg hs, and then adjust
	Selective serotonin reuptake inhibitors	Begin low dose, increase as needed

[a] Local cost should be considered in drug choice.

[b] Available only in the U.S.

[c] Unavailable in the European Union.

[d] Selective antimuscarinic agents unavailable in the U.S.

erogeneous smooth-muscle relaxants (e.g., dicyclomine, cimetropium, pinaverium, otilonium and trimebutine) [240]. However, there is little credible evidence of their efficacy, and their availability varies in Australia, Canada, Europe, and the U.S. [242]. Pain sometimes responds to tricyclic antidepressant drugs in doses lower than those used to treat depression [243]. Desipramine and nortryptyline cause fewer side effects than imipramine and amitriptyline [244], but 28% of patients in one trial discontinued desipramine prematurely, mainly due to adverse effects [245]. The benefit of desipramine is unrelated to dose [246]. Paroxetine improves quality of life but not IBS-related pain [247, 248].

Serotonin has multiple peripheral actions on smooth muscle, secretion, peristalsis and extrinsic, neuronal sensory and vagal, spinal afferent activity. Alosetron, a selective 5-HT_3 receptor antagonist, decreases pain, urgency, and stool frequency in women with IBS-D. The margin of benefit between drug and placebo groups is about 15 %, and the NNT is 7 [249]. Cases of ischemic colitis [250] and obstipation with bowel perforation led to its withdrawal from the US market, but it was reintroduced under a restricted access program. One group reported that the incidence of ischemic colitis is 3.4 times higher in subjects with IBS than other people [251]. Tegaserod, a partial 5-HT_4 receptor agonist, decreases pain, and improves overall status, stool frequency and form, ease of evacuation and bloating in women with IBS-C [252–255]. An American College of Gastroenterology task force gave tegaserod a Grade A recommendation [256]. A Cochrane Review of studies through 2003 reported modest effects for this medication [257]. However, this conclusion should be interpreted with caution in the face of more recent, better-designed trials showing greater benefit.

Preliminary trials of probiotic therapy are encouraging. Notably, *Bifidobacterium infantis* reduced IBS symptoms in patients with various types of bowel habit disturbance and normalized the ratio of an anti-inflammatory to a proinflammatory cytokine in peripheral mononuclear blood cells [258]. However, more studies are needed before probiotics can be established as effective. Antibiotic therapy of small bowel overgrowth, as diagnosed by lactulose hydrogen breath testing, causes only transient benefit [153]. Furthermore, antibiotics can cause chronic functional symptoms [259] as well as *Claustridium difficile* infection, allergic reactions, and antimicrobial resistance. Furthermore, the role of bacterial overgrowth is disputed [154], so antibiotics cannot be recommended.

Psychological and Behavioral Treatment

Cognitive-behavioral therapy, standard psychotherapy, and hypnotherapy for selected patients may be beneficial. A single-blind trial of cognitive-behavioral therapy for 12 weeks yielded a 70% overall response rate compared with 37% from weekly educational sessions; depressed patients did not respond, and improvement was seen in global satisfaction and quality of life, not pain [245]. Combined, multicomponent behavioral therapy may be more effective than medical therapy alone [260]. Hypnotherapy normalizes rectal sensation [261], and it is the most thoroughly evaluated psychological treatment for IBS [262]. Twelve sessions benefit quality of life, anxiety, and depression in refractory patients, except males with IBS-D [263], and the benefits last at least 5 years [264]. Eight sessions of individual psychotherapy can improve the physical aspects of quality of life and reduce health care costs compared with usual care [247]. However, trials of psychological therapy cannot be double-blind, and treatment is time-consuming, costly, and often unavailable.

Non-Western Treatment

Medical concepts are different in non-Western societies. For example, in traditional Chinese medicine, various diseases are explained by disturbances in how the human body is seen to interact with the external universe. The complex etiological illness concepts include 6 climatic conditions, 7 emotions, 5 endogenous factors, excessive fatigue and leisure, and external injury. Therapeutic principles are also numerous and include herbal therapy to target the predominant symptom, agents that assist the main agent, agents that treat minor symptoms, and those that modulate the actions of other herbs. Therapy usually consists of at least four herbs [265]. Herbal mixtures can cause global improvement and reduce pain and other symptoms [266, 267]. However, the contents of the mixtures are varied and unknown to prescribers, and the active principle(s) are unknown. Moreover, some herbal mixtures are toxic [268].

C2. Functional Bloating

— Definition

Functional bloating is a recurrent sensation of abdominal distension that may or may not be associated with measurable distension but is not part of another functional bowel or gastroduodenal disorder.

The word "bloat" means to inflate or become inflated. Although subjective abdominal bloating is often viewed as synonymous with physical abdominal distension, a bloated feeling is not always associated with increased abdominal girth [48, 269–271]. This symptom is further confused by the frequent co-occurrence of borborygmi (audible bowel sounds), excessive flatulence, and frequent eructations [272, 273]. These symptoms can also occur with IBS, chronic constipation, dyspeptic symptoms, and premenstrual syndrome [1, 47, 204, 270, 274–279]. Translation of "bloating" into non-English languages may be difficult. For example, the Chinese term *furzhang* requires further description to clarify what the patient means. Thus, bloating can mean different things depending on the individual, the disorder with which it occurs, and the patient's language.

Abdominal distension was reported by Manning [1] as one of six factors that discriminated patients with IBS from those with organic disease. However, factor analyses show weak clustering of bloating with the three pain-related Manning IBS symptoms in males [280] and limited or no clustering in females [280, 281]. Some investigators find no clustering of bloating and/or distension with IBS but strong clustering with chronic constipation [276], while others find that bloating discriminates IBS patients from those with organic disease or food allergy [282]. Wiklund et al. [236] found that bloating, visible distension, and flatus cluster as a subgroup of IBS, while Ragnarsson and Bodemar [33] identified two subgroups, one with little and the other with considerable pain/bloating. Bloating with visible abdominal distension also clusters with epigastric pain [279, 283] and with visible distension, early satiety, and a sensation of food staying in the stomach [277]. Thus, bloating with or without distension occurs with various symptoms or alone.

— Epidemiology

Most of the epidemiology and physiological research on bloating has dealt with subjects who also have other functional gastrointestinal disease. Bloating affects 10% to 30% of individuals in the general population, women about twice as often as men [4, 277, 284–286], but without relation to age [4]. More female than male patients report distension [270]. In one survey, 16% of respondents reported recent bloating or distension [284]. Of these, 65% complained of moderate to severe bloating, 54% reported that it reduced their daily activities, 43% had taken medication for bloating and 16% had sought medical advice. More women [19%] than men [10%] were affected, but symptoms were unrelated to menstruation. Other studies report perimenstrual exacerbation of bloating in IBS patients [270, 278]. IBS patients may report bloating as their most frequent [41, 48], second most frequent [273, 287] or most bothersome symptom [41, 288]. Bloating seems more common in IBS with constipation than in IBS with diarrhea [41, 48, 270, 289], but the severity is similar [33, 290]. Seventy-five percent of IBS patients believe their bloating is associated with distension, especially with constipation [270].

C2. Diagnostic Criteria* for Functional Bloating

Must include *both* of the following:
1. **Recurrent feeling of bloating or visible distension at least 3 days/month in the last 3 months**
2. **Insufficient criteria for a diagnosis of functional dyspepsia, irritable bowel syndrome, or other functional GI disorder**

***Criteria fulfilled for the last 3 months with symptom onset at least 6 months prior to diagnosis**

— Rationale for the Change in Diagnostic Criteria

We deleted "abdominal" as a modifier of "bloating" because it is redundant. We also deleted "fullness," as the term implies postprandial satiety to some patients, yet bloating occurs throughout the day. Functional bloating overlaps with other functional disorders (e.g., functional constipation, IBS, and functional dyspepsia) and epidemiological surveys and factor analyses do not convincingly demonstrate a distinct bloating subgroup. Additional epidemiological research is needed.

— Clinical Evaluation

Sufferers typically report worsening as the day progresses, particularly after meals, and alleviation overnight [270, 274]. In tape-measure studies of abdominal girth to assess distension, diurnal worsening of bloating is accompanied by increased girth [291, 292]. However, patients and investigators can bias tape measurements. For example, patients can voluntarily protrude their abdomens, and investigators can inadvertently measure different positions on the abdomen or apply the tape with varying degrees of tightness. Furthermore, tape measures only allow intermittent, static determinations. These problems have been overcome with the development and validation of abdominal inductance plethysmography, which permits objective ambulatory measurement of abdominal girth throughout the day [293, 294]. This technique confirms that abdominal girth increases during the day in most patients with IBS and to a greater extent than in healthy volunteers [295]; however, not all patients exhibit abdominal distension beyond the normal reference range [269]. The symptom of bloating only correlates with increased abdominal girth in constipated patients [269, 295], suggesting different, constipation-related pathophysiological mechanisms.

— Physiological Features

Early theories such as hysterical bloating, excess lumber lordosis, depression of the diaphragm, and voluntary protrusion of the abdomen [296] have largely been dismissed [274, 292, 297]. Recent hypotheses include gas accumulation, food intolerance, fluid retention, abdominal muscle wall weakness and altered sensorimotor function.

Intestinal Gas

The normal intestine contains approximately 200 ml of gas [272], mainly nitrogen, oxygen, hydrogen, carbon dioxide, and methane [298]. Most of the nitrogen and oxygen comes from swallowed air, while hydrogen and methane result from colonic bacterial fermentation of carbohydrate and protein. Carbon dioxide is produced by fermentation and by the interaction of gastric acid and bicarbonate. Since it is rapidly reabsorbed and exhaled, it is unimportant in distension [299]. The average adult passes flatus 5 to 15 times per day, more after meals and less overnight [300, 301].

Studies using an argon washout technique showed no difference in endogenous gas production or composition between patients with gas-related complaints and controls [302]. However, using labeled sulphurhexafluoride (SF6), Barcelona investigators found that gas retention in IBS patients exceeded that in healthy volunteers [303, 304]. Computerized tomography discloses no excess gas in IBS patients, despite abdominal distension [305], while studies that measured gas production by calorimetry reveal increased hydrogen production but similar total gas production [306]. Two studies using computer-digitized radiology, however, suggest increased gas volume in IBS patients compared with healthy volunteers, with little or no symptom correlation [307, 308]. Thus, gas retention in bloating patients can vary, and those without retention might have a transit disturbance or visceral hypersensitivity.

Strategies to reduce bowel gas [309, 310] or modulate gut flora [153, 311–313] have not corroborated excess gas. *Lactobacillus planetarum* improves some gas-related symptoms but not bloating [311], while the probiotic VSL#3 may improve bloating but not flatulence [312]. Antibiotics do not improve bloating [153, 313], although rifaximin reduces flatus episodes and abdominal girth [313]. Compared with psyllium (a fermentable fiber) and methylcellulose (a nonfermentable fiber), only lactulose ingestion increased flatus and feelings of rectal gas in health volunteers, but all three substances increased bloating [314]. Therefore, some gas-related symptoms are associated with increased gas production, but bloating may not be.

Most healthy volunteers tolerate large gas infusions into the jejunum due to expeditious gas transit and evacuation [315], but patients with disorders of gut function exhibit gas retention, abdominal distension, and symptoms unrelated to voluntary gas retention [303, 304, 316]. Obstructive evacuation (self-restrained) and relaxation of the gut (via intravenous glucagons) lead to similar gas retention, but only subjects who voluntarily inhibit flatus have symptoms, suggesting functional obstruction to gas passage might underlie bloating and other abdominal symptoms [317].

Duodenal infusion of lipid mimicking the postprandial load induces retention of gas infused into the jejunum, increasing girth without perception, whereas gastric distension induces perception without gas retention or increased girth [318]. Compared with controls, slow duodenal lipid infusion increases intestinal gas retention, perception, and abdominal girth in bloated IBS patients, suggesting lipid-induced gas transit delay is upregulated in IBS [316]. Jejunal gas induces more bloating than an equivalent volume of gas in the rectum [319], and distension is directly related to the volume of retained gas [316, 318, 319]. Notably, about 10 times the amount of gas normally present in the gut must be infused to cause a 2-cm increase in girth [304, 320]. However, the average change in girth in IBS patients throughout the day may reach 12 cm [290, 321], discounting the attribution of distension entirely to gas retention.

Food Intolerance

Bloating is more common in IBS patients compared with patients who have lactose malabsorption, but is unrelated to increased gas production from carbohydrate fermentation [322]. Also, lactase-deficient IBS patients who restrict lactose intake have bloating similar to that of IBS patients without lactase deficiency [79]. Lactase supplementation for deficient IBS patients does not improve symptoms [323].

Body Fluid

Since the diurnal variation of bloating/distension is unaccompanied by changes in body weight, fluid retention is not a likely cause [292, 305].

Abdominal Muscle Strength

Patients with visible distension are more likely than controls to have recent weight gain and increased girth with bloating [292]. Rectal gas infusion produces paradoxical relaxation of the internal abdominal oblique muscle of patients with bloating, whereas healthy subjects react with increased muscle tone [324]. However, surface electrode electromyography without gas infusion reveals no differences in muscle activity between IBS patients reporting visible distension and healthy volunteers [325]. Likewise, abdominal inductance plethysmography reveals no relationship between bloating or distension and age, body mass index, or parity, which might be expected if abdominal muscles were weak [326].

Altered Sensorimotor Function

Altered visceral sensation may contribute to bloating: (1) IBS patients with bloating and distension have higher rectal sensory thresholds than those with bloating alone [271]; (2) duodenal lipid infusion lowers sensory thresholds in IBS patients [160] and increases gas retention, distension, and bloating more than in healthy volunteers [316]; and (3) bloating but not distension increases during menses [327] when IBS patients have increased rectal sensitivity [204].

Breath hydrogen tests show prolonged small bowel transit in IBS patients with predominant pain and distension [328]. Ileal emptying and clearance of ^{99m}Tc-bran is delayed in IBS patients with bloating compared with healthy volunteers [329]. However, scintigraphic studies show accelerated small bowel transit in IBS patients with moderate to severe bloating [330] and increased ileocecal transit in constipated IBS patients [331]. Bran ingestion increases pain and bloating. Bran speeds up small bowel transit in healthy controls but not IBS patients, suggesting that the symptom increase is attributable to the bulking effect of bran [330]. Small and large bowel motility does not vary with bloating in IBS patients [332]. Motility after intestinal gas infusion is also similar in IBS patients and controls [333]. Despite this, IBS patients exhibit poor gas clearance [303, 304, 316], exacerbation of gas retention after glucagon, and reversal by the prokinetic neostigmine [303, 327]. Jejunal gas infusion in healthy volunteers increases duodenal tone and causes symptoms [319, 320]. The available data support no unified concept of motility in the pathogenesis of abdominal pain and bloating.

— Psychological Features

In the late 1940s, Alvarez thought bloating was hysterical [296]. More recent population surveys correlate bloating with depression, insomnia, coping problems [334], panic disorder, and agoraphobia [334, 335]. In women with IBS, there is a temporal correlation between anxiety, depression, and bloating [31]. One third of IBS patients report that stress and anxiety exacerbate abdominal distension, and one quarter say that relaxation improves it [270].

However, anxiety and depression are similarly present in healthy controls and patients with bloating [297]. IBS patients with pain or bloating as their most bothersome symptom resemble each other in Symptom Check List (SCL)-90-R scores [288]. Factor analyses reveal no psychosocial associations with bloating in patients with dyspeptic symptoms [283]. Therefore, bloating is not convincingly related to psychopathology.

— Treatment

Although the functional bloating criteria require the absence of other disorders, most research has been done on patients who have IBS or another disorder; therefore, treatment of bloating is similar whether it is isolated or associated with another functional disorder. There is no evidence-based therapy. Indeed, treatments such as wheat bran for constipation, can sometimes worsen bloating, distension, and flatulence [231]. Worsening after ingesting dairy products, fresh fruits, or juices suggests lactose or fructose intolerance, which might warrant further investigation or a dietary exclusion trial [198]. However, even patients with proven lactase deficiency experience little or no bloating after drinking 240 mL milk [78]. Avoiding flatogenic foods and additives, exercising regularly, losing excess weight, and taking activated charcoal lack supporting evidence [336–338]. Surfactants, such as simethicone, have proven beneficial in some studies but not others [339, 340]. Antibiotics are unlikely to help [153], but trials of probiotics are encouraging [311, 312, 341]. Beano[TM], an over-the-counter oral solution that digests glucose linkages in complex carbohydrates, may reduce episodes of flatus without decreasing bloating and pain [342]. Pancreatic enzymes reduce bloating, gas, and fullness during and after high-calorie, high-fat meal ingestion [343]. The effect of hypnotherapy on bloating alone is unknown [262–264]. The 5-HT$_4$ receptor partial agonist, tegaserod, improves bloating (a secondary outcome measure) in some female IBS-C patients [252–254].

Bloating may be ameliorated if an associated syndrome, such as IBS or constipation, is improved. The routine withdrawal of milk, administration of pancreatic enzymes, or prescription of a drug cannot be routinely advised. Beano[TM], charcoal, and simethacone appear safe, but cannot be confidently recommended.

C3. Functional Constipation

— Definition

Functional constipation is a functional bowel disorder that presents as persistently difficult, infrequent, or seemingly incomplete defecation, and that does not meet IBS criteria.

Constipation can be defined by subjective or measurable definitions: (1) straining, hard stools or scybala, unproductive calls ["want to but can't"], infrequent stools, or incomplete evacuation [344]; (2) <3 bowel movements per week [345], daily stool weight <35 g/day) [346], or straining >25% of the time [345, 347, 348]; and (3) prolonged whole-gut or colonic transit [349, 350].

None of these definitions is ideal. Results of physiological tests are controversial [351, 352], and stool frequency correlates poorly with colonic transit [38, 353, 354]. However, transit can be estimated from stool form (Figure 1) [38]. In some patients, there is a poor correlation between physiological tests and symptoms [351].

Moreover, patient perception of constipation is variable. Young individuals define constipation as straining at stool [52%], hard stools [44%], defecation urge with inability to evacuate [34%], infrequent stools [32%], abdominal discomfort [20%], sense of incomplete evacuation [19%], and excessive time on the toilet [11%][344]. The elderly often perceive constipation as straining [355]. Obviously, simply asking patients if they are constipated is unsatisfactory.

A survey of 731 women in south Wales sought the prevalence of constipation by three means: patient complaint, Rome I criteria, and transit time using the Bristol Stool Form Scale [52]. Approximately 8% had constipation by each definition, but only 2% were constipated by all three definitions. Discussion of constipation will remain difficult so long as patients and doctors disagree so much about its nature and the physiological data conflict with patient reports.

— Epidemiology

Constipation occurs in up to 27% of the population depending on demographic factors, sampling, and definition [4, 286, 347, 356]. Only a minority complain to doctors. Constipation affects all ages and is most common in females and nonwhite persons. About 63 million people in North America meet Rome II criteria for functional constipation [357]. Nearly one third of children with severe constipation have constipation as adults [358]. Constipation increases with age [347, 348], but the stool frequency is unchanged [344, 359].

C3. Diagnostic Criteria* for Functional Constipation

1. Must include *two or more* of the following:
   a. **Straining during at least 25% of defecations**
   b. **Lumpy or hard stools in at least 25% of defecations**
   c. **Sensation of incomplete evacuation for at least 25% of defecations**
   d. **Sensation of anorectal obstruction/blockage for at least 25% of defecations**
   e. **Manual maneuvers to facilitate at least 25% of defecations (e.g., digital evacuation, support of the pelvic floor)**
   f. **Fewer than three defecations per week**
2. **Loose stools are rarely present without the use of laxatives**
3. **Insufficient criteria for irritable bowel syndrome**

*Criteria fulfilled for the last 3 months with symptom onset at least 6 months prior to diagnosis

— Rationale for Changes to Diagnostic Criteria

A required frequency of at least 25% instead of greater than 25% maintains consistency with other FBD criteria. Studies using Rome II criteria yield a lower prevalence than those using Rome I criteria [286], possibly because the Rome II criteria did not allow laxative-induced loose stools, which are accepted now.

— Clinical Evaluation

The history and physical examination provide the most diagnostic information and should guide subsequent evaluation. For patients who fulfill these criteria, investigations may exclude disorders that cause constipation and identify physiological subgroups that may require specific treatments.

Factors that are associated with or exacerbate constipation include: (1) poor general health and physical inactivity; (2) medication use (opiates, psychotropics, anticonvulsants, calcium channel blockers, anticholinergics, dopaminergics, and bile acid binders); (3) psychological status; (4) a history of sexual abuse; (5) low-fiber diet; and (6) medical disease (diabetes, hypothyroidism, porphyria, amyloidosis, pseudoobstruction, and hypercalcemia) [360–362]. The chronicity, severity, and nature of symptoms indicate the needed tests. For example, straining with soft stools and manual maneuvers to assist defecation suggest anorectal dysfunction [361, 362]. An estimate of transit time can be obtained from the Bristol Stool Form Scale as a surrogate measure of transit time [38] (Figure 1).

Physicians should perform perianal and digital rectal examination to detect fecal impaction, anal stricture, rectal prolapse or mass, and abnormal perineal descent with straining. Laboratory tests may include a blood count, serum calcium, and thyroid-stimulating hormone, although these are rarely abnormal. Colonoscopy in constipated patients identifies structural lesions, such as colon cancer, as frequently as in nonconstipated individuals [363]. Routine colonic imaging may be unnecessary for patients with new symptoms unless they have alarm features, such as bleeding, weight loss, recent onset, or family history of colon cancer. Some physicians recommend such tests for patients over 50. It is not justified to apply all tests listed in Table 4 to all patients. Testing should be individualized according to responsiveness to fiber supplementation and other clinical features.

If no cause is recognized, the next step is a therapeutic trial with fiber supplements. In general, patients who do not respond to proper fiber supplementation (see below) should undergo diagnostic evaluation to identify physiological subgroups.

Measurement of Colon Transit

Using radiopaque markers, measurement of whole-gut transit time (primarily colon transit) is inexpensive, simple, and safe. Several methods produce similar results [360–362]. A high-fiber diet during measurement controls for dietary fiber content. Retention of markers in the proximal colon suggests colonic dysfunction, and retention in the rectosigmoid area suggests obstructed defecation. A radioisotope technique involves less radiation than plain x-rays and may provide more information, helping to differentiate proximal colon emptying, pancolonic inertia and obstructed defecation [98].

Additional Studies

If the symptoms and marker studies suggest anorectal dysfunction, anorectal manometry and balloon expulsion testing may help. Anorectal manometry and balloon expulsion help identify disorders of defecation such as Hirschsprung's disease and pelvic floor dyssynergia [361, 362, 364, 365]. Defecography may detect anatomical etiologies, such as intussusception and rectocele with stool retention. Defecography also identifies the failure to decrease the anorectal angle with straining and abnormal pelvic floor descent, features that are typical of dyssynergic defecation [364]. Electromyography and pudendal nerve latency testing are adjuctive techniques. (See Chapter 12, "Functional Anorectal Disorders.")

— Physiological Features

At least two physiological abnormalities can produce functional constipation: slow colonic transit and anorectal dysfunction. In slow colonic transit, radiopaque markers are delayed in passing through the colon. Evidence suggests that patients with slow-transit constipation have impaired colonic motor activity [362], abnormal autonomic function [366] and reduced interstitial cells of Cajal [367], and colonic enteroglucagon- and serotonin-containing endocrine cells [368]. Some authors restrict the term slow-transit constipation to patients with very slow transit that responds poorly to all therapeutic measures [369, 370]. Very few patients with slow transit have a megacolon, which could be the cause or consequence of slow transit [371]. Its pathogenesis is unknown, and it can be suspected on plain abdominal x-rays and proved by barium enema. Anorectal dysfunction describes failure of the anal sphincter or pelvic floor to function normally during defecation. Although many constipated tertiary care patients have manometric dyssynergia, slow transit and dyssynergia may coexist, and many such patients with refractory symptoms have normal manometry and normal ability to expel a balloon [372–374].

Disorders of smooth muscle, the ENS, its neurotransmitters and receptors, or the CNS-ENS axis may cause severe constipation. Some patients have morphological changes within the myenteric and submucous plexus [375]. The widely held belief that such damage may be due to laxatives now seems unlikely. The "cathartic colon" is defined radiologically and is no longer recognized, perhaps because the causative laxatives have been withdrawn [376].

Fiber increases stool bulk and weight [377]. However, (1) there is little or no relationship between dietary fiber intake and whole gut transit time [373]; (2) the fiber intake of constipated patients resembles that of controls [378]; and (3) patients have lower stool weights and more delayed transit than controls, whether or not they take wheat bran [379]. Voluntary retention of stool is accompanied by delayed gastric emptying [380], and some severely constipated patients have slow gastric emptying and small bowel transit [381]. Nevertheless, an empirical trial of fiber supplementation is usually the best initial step.

Although long-distance travelers may become constipated [382], constipated patients have similar physical activity and drink similar amounts of fluids as controls [376]. Increased colonic water absorption is an unproven cause of constipation. The effect of acute or chronic physical exercise on colonic function is also controversial [376].

— Psychological Features

Constipation reporting, stool output, and gut dysmotility may be affected by personality, stress, and early toilet training [383, 384]. Patients with severe constipation and normal intestinal transit often have increased psychological distress [385].

Constipation behavior can be learned in early life. A child may learn to contract the sphincters to retain stool to avoid defecation [386]. Some data suggest that faulty toilet training produces anorectal disorders such as pelvic floor dyssynergia and encopresis [387]. Deliberate suppression of defecation leads to reduced stool frequency and weight and increased transit time [388]. Suppression of defecation is common, and in a quarter of subjects the urge may not return for several hours [389].

— Treatment

General Measures

Reassurance may help some patients who fear that failure to evacuate for 2 or 3 days is harmful. Other measures such as regular visits to the toilet, increased fluid intake, and physical exercise are recommended but unproven. Some physicians recommend assumption of the "squat position" on the toilet by raising the feet with a footstool. Sometimes, constipation is cured by discontinuing a constipating medication, treating depression or, less often, correcting an endo-

Table 4. Constipation: Diagnosis and Specific Treatment

Pathology	Diagnosis	Specific Treatment
Constipating drug (opiates, psychotropics, anticonvulsants, anticholinergics, dopaminergics, calcium channel blockers, bile acid binders, NSAIDs, calcium and iron supplements)	History	Stopping or switching to alternative medication
Endocrine disorder (diabetes mellitus, hypothyroidism, hyperparathyroidism, pheochromocytoma)	Clinical status, endocrine function test	Hormone replacement, operation, etc.
Neurologic diseases - Systemic (e.g., diabetic neuropathy, Parkinson's disease, Shy-Drager syndrome) - Traumatic (e.g., spinal cord lesion)	History, neurologic examination	Scheduled bowel training, facilitated by suppositories or enemas
Slow transit due to neuropathy of colonic nerve plexus	Transit time measurement, transmural colon biopsy	Colectomy (laxatives fail) if small bowel motility normal
Megacolon	X-ray	Colectomy (laxatives fail)
Pelvic floor dyssynergia (anismus)	No confirmatory test available, exclusion by proctologic examination, anorectal manometry, electromyography, defecography, balloon expulsion test	Behavioral training, biofeedback training
Short-segment Hirschsprung's disease	Lack of internal sphincter relaxation with rectal distention, aganglionic segment on deep rectal biopsy	Internal anal sphincter myomectomy
Megarectum	X-ray	Regular emptying with enemas and laxatives
Internal rectal prolapse, solitary rectal ulcer	Proctologic examination, defecography	Fiber supplementation, transabdominal rectopexy, perineal rectosigmoidectomy (Altemeier procedure), Delorme procedure
Rectocele with stool retention	Proctologic examination, defecography	Transanal repair

NSAIDs = nonsteroidal anti-inflammatory drugs

crine disease. Treatment should be guided by the severity of the symptoms and, if necessary, the results of physiological tests (Table 4).

Fiber Supplementation and Bulk Laxatives

Most patients with mild to moderate constipation respond to fiber therapy [373], which should be recommended before extensive evaluation. Its laxative action is complex and probably includes intestinal distension by the bulking effect of increased intraluminal water and bacteria [390]. Experiments with plastic models demonstrate that less effort is required to expel large stools than small ones [391]. The larger, softer stools induced by fiber ease defecation, suggesting that mechanical stimulus prompts defecation [392]. Fiber increases intestinal transit and stool frequency. Tactile stimulation of multimodal receptors in the intestinal mucosa may explain why coarse bran is more effective than fine bran [393]. The effect of dietary fiber on stool weight is dose-dependent and requires a week to reach a steady state [394, 395]. Patients may require more fiber than healthy controls to produce a similar increase in stool volume and transit [379]. Wheat bran, whole grain food products, soluble fiber bulk laxatives (e.g. psyllium products), methycellulose, or any combination are suitable [396–398].

Compliance with fiber supplementation is low, as many patients starting fiber complain of flatulence, distension, bloating, and poor taste [399]. Psyllium can cause gaseous symptoms by both increasing colonic gas production and retarding intestinal gas transit [400]. Rare allergic reactions, including anaphylaxis and asthma, have been reported with psyllium [401]. Patients with defecation disorders or slow transit may not respond [373].

Osmotic Laxatives

Although laxatives are commonly used, surprisingly few randomized, controlled trials have evaluated their efficacy [402].

Unabsorbed mono- and disaccharides: The osmotic properties of lactulose, lactitol, mannitol, and sorbitol increase intraluminal bulk and stimulate peristalsis [403–405]. They are rapidly metabolized by colon bacteria to short-chain fatty acids and may act as small-molecule, soluble dietary fiber [406]. Fifteen to 30 mL twice a day is effective in mild constipation, and there is moderately strong evidence for using lactulose [398]. Side effects include abdominal cramping and bloating [405]. Sorbitol is cheaper than lactulose and lactitol and may be as effective [404]. Glycerin suppositories act osmotically in the rectum.

Saline laxatives: Incompletely absorbed salts such as magnesium citrate, sodium and disodium phosphate, and magesium sulphate produce net osmotic flux of water into the small intestine and colon. Excessive use may lead to electrolyte imbalances, particularly in the elderly or among patients with renal impairment [401].

Other Water-Binding Compounds

Polyethylene glycol (PEG): An oral, isotonic solution of PEG was introduced to purge the colon for colonoscopy [407], and there is good evidence for its use in constipation [398]. Low doses are superior to placebo [408] and lactulose[409] in adults and children [410]. PEG is not absorbed and is safe, has a low sodium content, and does not cause net ion absorption or loss. Calcium polycarbophil has a similar mode of action [411].

Stimulant Laxatives

Stimulant laxatives include diphenylmethane derivatives, such as phenolphthalein (no longer included in US or Canadian preparations), bisacodyl, sodium picosulfate and conjugated anthraquinone derivatives, including cascara sagrada, aloin, and senna. They decrease absorption and stimulate motility and prostaglandin release [360–362]. Sodium picosulfate (bisacodyl conjugated with sulfate) and the anthraquinone derivatives are cleaved by bacteria in the colon, where the active (unconjugated) agent may stimulate enteric nerves. These over-the-counter agents are the most popular and the most likely to be abused [412, 413]. Melanosis coli, a brown mucosal discoloration, is a harmless, reversible consequence of prolonged anthraquinone intake that results from apoptosis of colonic epithelial cells and deposition of pigment in macrophages [414–416]. Melanosis typically disappears within 6 months of stopping the anthraquinone.

Enemas

Enema volume stimulates the rectum to defecate and may be necessary for constipation due to disordered defecation or megacolon [371]. Phosphate enemas have an intracolonic osmotic effect.

Prokinetic Agents

Serotonin is actived in gastrointestinal motility, secretion, and sensation [417]. 5-HT_4 receptor agonists stimulate the peristaltic reflex [418] and accelerate gastrointestinal transit [419, 420]. Tegaserod, a highly selective, partial 5-HT_4 receptor agonist, is superior to placebo for patients with chronic constipation; NNT values were reported from two large trials as 8 to 20, depending on the dose (6 mg bid or 2 mg bid) [421, 422].

The prostaglandin E_1 analog misoprostol (1200 µg/day) was effective in a 3-week study, but its long-term efficacy remains unproven. It stimulates uterine contractility, prohibiting its use by women who are pregnant or could become pregnant [423]. Other candidates include recombinant methionyl-human neurotrophin-3 [424] and colchicine [425]. The effectiveness of other agents such as macrolide antibiotics, bethanechol, domperidone, and metoclopramide is un-proven.

Surgery

Subtotal colectomy with ileorectal anastomosis is performed in rare, fully evaluated patients with severe colonic inertia and normal small-bowel motility and anorectal function. About 50% to 90% of these patients improve, but com-plications are common, including small-bowel obstruction in over one third, di-arrhea, incontinence, and recurrence of constipation. Although stool frequency often improves, other symptoms, including bloating and abdominal pain, may not [381, 426]. Therefore, colectomy should be performed only in disabled pa-tients with normal motility above the colon when all nonsurgical treatments have failed. Surgical treatment for anorectal dysfunction from paradoxical contraction of the puborectalis has been disappointing [427, 428].

C4. Functional Diarrhea

— Definition

Functional diarrhea is a continuous or recurrent syndrome character-ized by the passage of loose (mushy) or watery stools without abdominal pain or discomfort.

— Epidemiology

There are few studies where functional diarrhea was specifically diag-nosed as distinct from IBS-D, so it is impossible to provide a precise frequency. Using the Rome I criteria, the US Householder Survey found the prevalence of unspecified diarrhea to be 1.6%, compared to 9.4% for IBS and 3.0% for func-tional constipation [4]. In Olmsted County, Minnesota, 9.6% of residents have loose watery stools, females less often than males [429]. In the UK, 5.3% of males and 4.3% of females report mushy stools [353]. Similarly, 4.8% of people reported diarrhea in a US study [347], and 3.6% of university students reported diarrhea often [344]. In Asia, functional diarrhea occurred in 4.5% of people, compared with functional constipation in 3.9% and IBS in 2.3% [430]. These reports do not report how frequently the symptoms occur or how consistent they are. Most surveys have required diarrhea to be "often" (greater than 25% of the time).

C4. Diagnostic Criterion* for Functional Diarrhea

Loose (mushy) or watery stools without pain occurring in at least 75% of stools

***Criterion fulfilled for the last 3 months with symptom onset at least 6 months prior to diagnosis**

— ## Rationale for Changes in Diagnostic Criteria

When asked what they mean by "diarrhea," most people report loose or watery stools. Fewer individuals choose increased frequency and urgency [344]. Since rapid transit increases the percentage of water in stool, stool consistency correlates well with colon transit [38]. Despite wide variations in diet and stool weight, fecal water content remains remarkably constant in normal subjects at around 70%. Soft stools are 85% water, and watery stools 90% with greatly reduced stool viscosity [431]. Stool viscosity is the critical parameter because of its impact on rectal sensation and continence. Continence of watery stool is difficult and anal contact with fluid causes extreme urgency. However, urgency by itself is an unreliable indicator of diarrhea and may be reported by individuals with hard, pellet-like stools. Thus, stool form, not its frequency, defines diarrhea.

How often a symptom needs to occur to be significant depends on its troublesomeness. To a patient, infrequent fecal incontinence is a serious problem, while an occasional loose stool may not be. Fewer than 1% of respondents in a general population survey met the 75% threshold definition [432]; however, the completeness of evaluation cannot be readily determined in community surveys. Thus, retaining this requirement distinguishes these patients from those with IBS-D and ensures that it will remain a rare diagnosis after a full diagnostic evaluation.

— ## Clinical Evaluation

The combination of abdominal pain with intermittent diarrhea and constipation is highly suggestive of IBS, and small-volume, frequent defecation is likely functional. Diarrhea occurs with many gut disorders (Table 5), and is a common reason for consulting a physician. The evaluation should start with a careful history. Erratic bowel habit with episodes of constipation is highly sugges-

Table 5. Differential Diagnosis of Functional Diarrhea

Dietary-induced	Giardiasis
Drug-induced	Chronic pancreatic insufficiency
Lactose intolerance	Crohn's disease
Bile acid malabsorption	Microscopic colitis
Celiac disease	Small-bowel bacterial overgrowth

tive of IBS. Small-volume, frequent defecation is likely functional. A stool diary incorporating the Bristol Stool Form Score helps verify the bowel habit (Figure 1) and exclude pseudodiarrhea [433]. The diet should be assessed because stool volume and form can be markedly increased by ingestion of fiber or poorly absorbed carbohydrate, such as lactose by patients with hypolactasia, fructose and sorbitol or mannitol, which are common constituents of "sugar-free" preparations. Alcohol impairs sodium and water absorption from the small bowel [434], and excessive beer can cause increased ileal flow, accelerated colonic transit, and loose stools [435]. Alarm features, such as weight loss, nocturnal symptoms, tenesmus (painful urge to defecate), recent antibiotic use, hematochezia, high-volume diarrhea (>250mL/day), family history of colorectal neoplasia or celiac disease, and relevant abnormalities on physical examination should stimulate further investigations [436].

Physical examination should include examination for anemia, clubbing, and abdominal tenderness. An abdominal mass suggests Crohn's disease in the young and cancer in the elderly. Rectal examination and proctosigmoidoscopy are needed to exclude perianal Crohn's disease and colitis. Visualization of the stool may suggest further investigations. Simple screening blood and stool tests are recommended.

Evidence of malabsorption (malnutrition, weight loss, non-blood-loss anemia, electrolyte abnormalities) suggests celiac disease in Western countries and should provoke the appropriate antibody tests and/or duodenal biopsy. Where relevant, giardiasis and tropical sprue should be excluded. If there is no suggestion of malabsorption, colonoscopy and terminal ileoscopy may be needed to exclude microscopic colitis and Crohn's disease. If these procedures are negative and suspicion of an organic etiology persists, barium small-bowel radiography is indicated. Persistent, unexplained diarrhea may require tests for lactose intolerance when the patient's milk intake exceeds 240 mL/day and bile acid malabsorption, especially if diarrhea occurs at night or is of high volume [437].

Although single abnormalities of erythrocyte sedimentation rate, hemoglobin, and serum potassium and albumin yielded few diagnoses, more than one abnormality was found in 62% of patients with organic diarrhea but in only 3% of idiopathic cases [438]. In 20 of 21 patients with organic diarrhea, fat malabsorption, inflammatory bowel disease, or secretory diarrhea was identified with three simple tests (stool fat, rectal biopsy, and fecal water). Tolliver and colleagues found little benefit from performing simple blood tests and stool examination for parasites on patients who met Rome I criteria for IBS [76]. In 1452 IBS patients, the prevalence of lactose malabsorption [23%] was similar to the general US population rate, and there were low frequencies of thyroid dysfunction [6%], ova and parasite infestation [2%], and colonic inflammation [1%] [74]. There are no comparable data for functional diarrhea. Reportedly, about 3% of referred patients in northern England diagnosed to have IBS have unrecognized celiac disease [84]. One study identified lymphocytic colitis in 7 of 30 patients previously diagnosed to have IBS [439]. Lymphocytic colitis occurs in 5% of Swedish patients with non-bloody diarrhea and 10% of those over 70 years old [440].

Rare conditions may be encountered in referral practice. For example, bile acid malabsorption (BAM) may be associated with microscopic colitis [199], and the irritant effect of bile acids could cause diarrhea [441]. Clues are sudden-onset and nocturnal diarrhea, as all 23 patients with severe idiopathic acid salt malabsorption (bile acid retention <5% at 7 days) reported these features [442]. Another clue is increased stool weight, which averaged 285 g/day in another series [437]. Persistent BAM may follow acute *Salmonella* infection [443]. Watery diarrhea due to functioning endocrine tumors are rare but should be obvious from a high 24-hour stool output, which may be many liters. IBS patients rarely have a stool weight greater that 250 g per 24 hours [444, 445]. There are no stool volume data for functional diarrhea.

— Physiological Features

Few studies have specifically addressed the physiology of functional diarrhea as distinct from that found in IBS. Colonic transit is rapid in functional diarrhea, particularly after a meal, which is associated with reduced postprandial colonic motility [446, 447]. This paradox may result from the mixing rather than propulsive nature of most postprandial contractions [448].

Rectal sensitivity is increased in IBS, including postinfectious IBS [147], particularly when diarrhea alternates with constipation [117, 449]. While 7% of acute infectious gastroenteritis patients develop IBS, a further 18% of patients without Rome I criteria for IBS report continued abnormal bowel habit, mostly painless diarrhea. It seems likely that the mechanisms are similar. Increased sensitivity may be the effect rather than the cause of diarrhea, since inducing diarrhea with laxatives increases visceral hypersensitivity [450].

— Psychological Features

While anxiety often accompnaies IBS, few data apply specifically to functional diarrhea. Acute stress accelerates colonic transit in humans and animals [451], but the relevance of this finding to chronic stress is uncertain. However, patients with generalized anxiety have accelerated small-bowel and whole-gut transit [452, 453]. One study indicates anxiety tends to preceed IBS onset, particularly if diarrhea predominates [177]. In animals, corticotrophin-releasing factor mediates the acceleration of colonic transit [454, 455].

— Treatment

If a careful history and examination suggests functional diarrhea, the diagnosis should be explained to the patient at the first consultation. The Hospital Anxiety and Depression Scale is particularly useful to assess anxiety and depression [453, 456]. Explanation of normal gut physiology and how dietary factors, stress, and/or low-grade inflammation might accelerate colonic transit is helpful, as is the reassurance that the symptoms are unlikely to develop into other diseases.

Therapeutic diets have never been formally assessed, but wheat bran and vegetable and fruit fibers are laxative [457]. Therefore, some physicians advocate a low-residue diet. Whether patients with functional diarrhea malabsorb fructose and sorbitol more than do normal subjects is disputed, but IBS patients tend to develop symptoms when challenged with poorly absorbed sugars, and some claim benefit from excluding them [198]. Nonmedical practitioners often advise exclusion of wheat, lactose, and fructose. Provided a dietician supervises, this satisfies patients' desire to contribute to their own management. Enthusiasts claim that up to 50% of IBS patients respond to such diets, but the data are uncontrolled [458, 459]. Drinks containing caffeine or sorbitol or mannitol as noncalorie sweetener [460] should be limited.

Opiates are the principle drug treatments, loperamide being the best tolerated [461]. It controls diarrhea and reduces urgency and stool frequency in IBS-D [461–463]. The NNT value is 1.2. Loperamide is started at 2 mg twice daily and adjusted as necessary. This drug controls urgency because of its effects on anal tone and transit and may be used before leaving home to achieve control during social or work engagements.

The 5-HT$_3$ antagonist alosetron (available only in the US) is effective in some women with IBS-D; the NNT is about 7 [249]. Since it slows transit and reduces the gastrocolonic response in normal volunteers, it may help functional diarrhea patients, although there are no published, randomized, controlled trials. Its access is restricted owing to potential ischemic colitis and profound constipation. Cholestyramine is an ion-exchange resin that binds bile acids and renders them biologically inactive, reversing BAM. The drug is highly effective (NNT = 1) if the Se[75]HCAT bile acid test shows a retention of < 5% [437, 442]. If retention exceeds 10%, the benefit is no greater than that of a placebo. Some physicians prescribe a trial of cholestyramine, avoiding the Se[75]HCAT test. No published trials specifically address the use of psychotropic drugs in functional diarrhea, but some of them have mild constipating effects.

The prognosis of functional diarrhea is poorly documented. All patients in a tertiary referral center recovered after about 3 years [464], but such referred patients may not be typical of usual patients with functional diarrhea regarding outcome.

C5. Unspecified Functional Bowel Disorder

Individual symptoms discussed in the previous sections are very common in the population. These occasionally lead to medical consultation, yet are unaccompanied by other symptoms that satisfy criteria for a syndrome. Such symptoms are best classified as unspecified.

C5. Diagnostic Criterion* for Unspecified Functional Bowel Disorder

Bowel symptoms not attributable to an organic etiology that do not meet criteria for the previously defined categories

*Criterion fulfilled for the last 3 months with symptom onset at least 6 months prior to diagnosis

Future Research Directions

Development of the Rome criteria is a continuing process, and the criteria should be updated as data allow. We suggest the following topics for research:

1. Perform long-term, longitudinal studies on patients with disorders of bowel function to better determine the natural history, specifically regarding changing severity and interchange among disorders and the predominant symptom.
2. Direct more research to patients in primary care.
3. Compare the efficacy of new drugs with that of older ones (e.g., antidiarrheal agents, laxatives, and antidepressants) and placebos.
4. Study bloating with distension defined as a true increase in abdominal girth.
5. Further investigate the epidemiology of functional bloating.
6. Determine what the symptom terms (e.g., bloating and discomfort) mean to patients with different disorders and whether the meanings change across cultures and countries.
7. Use unobtrusive and ambulatory, objective measures of abdominal girth to investigate the pathophysiology of distension in functional disorders and its response to drugs.
8. Investigate pharmacological modulation of sensorimotor function and the gut microflora to identify mechanisms of bloating and/or distension.
9. Develop effective psychological treatments that can be provided by primary physicians.
10. Determine the features of colonic transit and stool water content in idiopathic diarrhea.
11. Investigate histological changes in mucosal biopsies from patients with idiopathic diarrhea; e.g., lymphocytic infiltration that does not meet criteria for lymphocytic colitis.
12. Investigate the main differences between functional diarrhea and IBS-D, including demographic features and symptom pattern and whether they require different treatments.
13. Perform repeated physiological evaluation, including visceral sensitivity and motility, on IBS patients during periods of changing bowel habit and symptom severity.

References

1. Manning AP, Thompson WG, Heaton KW, Morris AF. Towards positive diagnosis of the irritable bowel. Br Med J 1978;2:653–654.
2. Thompson WG. The Road to Rome. Gut 1999;45:80–81.
3. Kruis W, Thieme CH, Weinzierl M, Schussler P, Hall J, Paulus W. A diagnostic score for the irritable bowel syndrome. Its value in the exclusion of organic disease. Gastroenterology 1984;87:1–7.
4. Drossman DA, Li Z, Andruzzi E, Temple R, Talley NJ, Thompson WG, Whitehead WE, Janssens J, Funch-Jensen P, Corazziari E, Richter JE, Koch GG. U.S. householder survey of functional gastrointestinal disorders: prevalence, sociodemography and health impact. Dig Dis Sci 1993;38:1569–1580.
5. Thompson WG. A world view of IBS. In: Spiller R and Camilleri M, eds. The Irritable Bowel Syndrome. Diagnosis and treatment. 1 ed. WB Saunders, 2002:17–26.
6. Saito YA, Schoenfeld P, Locke GRI. The epidemiology of irritable bowel syndrome in North America: a systemic review. Am J Gastroenterol 2002;97:1910–1915.
7. Lau EM, Chan FK, Ziea ET, Chan CS, Wu JC, Sung JJ. Epidemiology of irritable bowel syndrome in Chinese. Dig Dis Sci 2002;47:2621–2624.
8. Gwee K-A. Irritable bowel syndrome in developing countries—a disorder of civilization or colonization? Neurogastroenterol Motil 2005;17:317–324.
9. Longstreth GF. Definition and classification of IBS: current consensus and controversies. Gastroenterol Clin North Am 2005;34:173–187.
10. Heaton KW, O'Donnell LJD, Braddon FEM, Mountford RA, Hughes AO, Cripps PJ. Symptoms of irritable bowel syndrome in a British urban community: consulters and nonconsulters. Gastroenterology 1992;102:1962–1967.
11. Thompson WG. Gastrointestinal symptoms in the irritable bowel compared with peptic ulcer and inflammatory bowel disease. Gut 1984;25:1089–1092.
12. Talley NJ, et al. Irritable bowel syndrome in a community: symptom subgroups, risk factors and health care utilization. Am J Epidemiol 1995;142:76–83.
13. Talley NJ, et al. Predictors of health care seeking for health care seeking: a population based study. Gut 1997;41:395–398.
14. Talley NJ, Weaver AL, Zinsmeister AR, Melton LJ. Onset and disappearance of gastrointestinal symptoms and functional gastrointestinal disorders. Am J Epidemiol 1992;136:165–177.
15. Agreus L, Svardsudd K, Talley NJ, Jones MP, Tibblin G. Natural history of gastro-esophageal reflux disease and functional abdominal disorders: a population-based study. Am J Gastroenterol 2001;96:2905–2914.
16. Everhart JE, Renault PF. Irritable bowel syndrome in office-based practice in the united states. Gastroenterology 1991;100:998–1005.
17. Talley NJ, Gabriel SE, Harmsen WS, Zinsmeister AR, Evans RW. Medical costs in community subjects with irritable bowel syndrome. Gastroenterology 1995;109:1736–1741.
18. Levy RL, Von Korff M, Whitehead WE, Stang P, Saunders K, Jhingran P, Barghout V, Feld AD. Costs of care for irritable bowel syndrome patients in a health maintenance organization. Am J Gastroenterol 2001;96:3120–3129.
19. Sandler RS, Everhart JE, Donowitz M, et al. The burden of selected digestive diseases in the United States. Gastroenterology 2002;122:1500–1511.

20. Longstreth GF, Wilson A, Knight K, et al. Irritable bowel syndrome,health care use, and costs: a U.S. managed care perspective. Am J Gastroenterol 2003;98:600–607.
21. Leong SA, Barghout V, Birnbaum HG, Thibeault CE, Ben Hamadi R, Frech F, Ofman JJ. The economic consequences of irritable bowel syndrome: a US employer perspective. Arch Intern Med 2003;163:929–935.
22. Inadomi JM, Fennerty MB, Bjorkman D. Systematic review: the economic impact of irritable bowel syndrome. Aliment Pharmacol Ther 2003;18:671–682.
23. Longstreth GF, Bolus R, Naliboff B, Chang L, Kulich KR, Carlsson J, Mayer EA, Naesdal J, Wiklund IK. Impact of irritable bowel syndrome on patients' lives: development and psychometric documentation of a disease-specific measure for use in clinical trials. Eur J Gastroenterol Hepatol 2005;17:411–420.
24. Wilson A, Longstreth G, Knight K, Wong J, Wade S, Chiou C, Barghout V, Frech F, Ofman J. Quality of life in managed care patients with irritable bowel syndrome. Manage Care Interface 2004;17:24–28.
25. Drossman DA, Whitehead WE, Toner BB, Diament NE, Hu YJB, Bangawala SI, Jia H, e. What determines severity among patients with painful functional bowel disorders. Am J Gastroenterol 2002;95:974–980.
26. Koloski NA, Talley NJ, Boyce PM. Epidemiology and health care seeking in the functional GI disorders: a population-based study. Am J Gastroenterol 2002;97:2290–2299.
27. Blewett A, Allison M, Calcraft B, Moore R, Jenkins P, Sullivan G. Psychiatric disorder and outcome in irritable bowel syndrome. Psychosomatics 1996;37:155–160.
28. Longstreth GF, Yao JF. Irritable bowel syndrome and surgery: a multivariable analysis. Gastroenterology 2004;126:1665–1673.
29. anon. Straining, sitting and squatting at stool. Lancet 1975;2:18.
30. Thompson WG, Longstreth GF, Drossman DA, Heaton KW, Irvine EJ, Muller-Lissner SA. Functional Bowel Disorders and D. Functional Abdominal Pain. In: Drossman DA, Corazziari E, Talley NJ, Thompson WG, and Whitehead WE, eds. The Functional Gastrointestinal Disorders. 2 ed. Washington: Degnon, 2000.
31. Heaton KW, Ghosh S, Braddon FEM. How bad are the symptoms and bowel dysfunction of patients with the irritable bowel syndrome? A prospective, controlled study with emphasis on stool form. Gut 1991;32:73–79.
32. Ragnarsson G, Bodemar G. Pain is temporally related to eating but not to defaecation in the irritable bowel syndrome [IBS]. Patients' description of diarrhea, constipation and symptom variation during a prospective 6-week study. Eur J Gastroenterol Hepatol 1998;10:415–421.
33. Ragnarsson G, Bodemar G. Division of the irritable bowel syndrome into subgroups on the basis of daily recorded symptoms in two outpatients samples. Scand J Gastroenterol 1999;34:993–1000.
34. Mearin F, Balboa A, Badia X, et al. Irritable bowel syndrome subtypes according to bowel habit: revisiting the alternating subtype. Eur J Gastroenterol Hepatol 2003; 15:165–172.
35. Drossman DA, Morris CB, Hu Y, Toner BB, Diamont N, Leserman J, Shetzline M, Dalton C, Bangdiwala SI. A prospective assessment of bowel habit in irritable bowel syndrome: defining an alternator. Gastroenterology 2005;128:580–589.
36. Guilera M, Balboa A, Mearin F. Bowel habit subtypes and temporal patterns in irritable bowel syndrome: systematic review. Am J Gastroenterol 2005;100:1174–1184.
37. Hahn BA, Kirchdoerfer LJ, Fullerton S, Mayer E. Patient-perceived severity of irri-

table bowel syndrome in relation to symptoms, health resource utilization and quality of life. Aliment Pharmacol Ther 1997;11:553–559.

38. O'Donnell LJD, Virjee J, Heaton KW. Detection of pseudodiarrhoea by simple clinical assessment of intestinal transit rate. Br Med J 1990;300:439–440.

39. Whitehead WE, Bassotti G, Palsson O, Taub E, Cook EC, III, Drossman DA. Factor analysis of bowel symptoms in US and Italian populations. Dig Liver Dis 2003;35:774–783.

40. Tillisch K, Labus JS, Naliboff BD, Bolus R, Shetzline M, Mayer EA, Chang L. Characterization of the alternating bowel habit subtype in patients with irritable bowel syndrome. Am J Gastroenterol 2005;100:896–904.

41. Schmulson M, Lee O-Y, Chang L, et al. Symptom differences in moderate to severe IBS patients based on predominant bowel habit. Am J Gastroenterol 1999;94:2929–2935.

42. Hammer J, Eslick GD, Howell SC, Altiparmak E, Talley NJ. Diagnostic yield of alarm features in irritable bowel syndrome and functional dyspepsia. Gut 2004;53:666–672.

43. Ganguli S, Fergani H, Profiti R, Longstreth G, Tougas G. Value of red flags in excluding organic disease in irritable bowel syndrome. Neurogastrodnetrol Motil 16[5], 666. 2004.

44. Isgar B, Harman M, Kaye MD, Whorwell PJ. Symptoms of irritable bowel syndrome in ulcerative colitis in remission. Gut 1984;24:190–192.

45. Williams RE, Hartmann KE, Sandler RS, Miller WC, Steege JF. Prevalence and characteristics of irritable bowel syndrome among women with chronic pelvic pain. Obstet Gynecol 2004;104:452–458.

46. Longstreth GF. Irritable bowel syndrome and chronic pelvic pain. Obstet Gynecol Surv 1994;49:505–507.

47. Heitkemper MM, Cain KC, Jarrett ME, et al. Symptoms accross the menstruel cycle in women with irritable bowel syndrome. Am J Gastroenterol 2003;98:420–430.

48. Lee O-Y, Mayer EA, Schmulson M, Chang L. Gender-related differences in IBS symptoms. Am J Gastroenterol 2001;96:2184–2193.

49. Wessely S, Mimnuan C, Sharpe M. Functional somatic syndromes: one or many? Lancet 1999;354:936–939.

50. Doshi M, Heaton KW. Irritable bowel syndrome in patients discharged from surgical wards with non-specific abdominal pain. Br J Surg 1994;81:1216–1218.

51. Gambone JC, et al. Nonsurgical management of chronic pelvic pain. a multidisciplinary approach. Clin Obstet Gynecol 1990;33:205–211.

52. Probert CSJ, Emmett PM, Cripps HA, Heaton KW. Evidence for the ambiguity of the word constipation: the role of irritable bowel syndrome. Gut 1994;35:1455–1458.

53. Barratt HS, Kalantzis C, Polymeros D, Forbes A. Functional symptoms in inflammatory bowel disease and their potential influence in misclassification of clinical status. Aliment Pharmacol Ther 2005;21:141–147.

54. Whorwell PJ, McCallum M, Creed FH, Roberts CT. Non-colonic features of irritable bowel syndrome. Gut 1986;27:37–40.

55. Whorwell PJ, Lupton EW, Eduran D, Wilson K. Bladder smooth muscle dysfunction in patients with irritable bowel syndrome. Gut 1986;27:1014–1017.

56. Francis CY. High prevalence of irritable bowel syndrome in patients attending a urological clinic. Dig Dis Sci 1997;42:404–407.

57. Longstreth GF, Wolde-Tsadik G. Irritable bowel-type symptoms in HMO examinees: prevalence, demographics and clinical correlates. Dig Dis Sci 1993;38:1581–1589.

58. Maxton DG, Morris J, Whorwell PJ. More accurate diagnosis of irritable bowel syndrome by use of "non-colonic" symptomatology. Gut 1991;32:784–786.

59. Talley NJ, et al. Multisystem complaints in patients with the irritable bowel syndrome and functional dyspepsia. Eur J Gastroenterol Hepatol 1991;3:71–77.

60. Whitehead WE, Paulsson O, Jones KR. Systematic review of the comorbidity or irritable bowel syndrome with other disorders: what are the causes and implications. Gastroenterology 2002;122:1140–1156.

61. Vandvik PO, Wilhelmsen I, Ihlebaek C, Farup PG. Comorbidity of irritable bowel syndrome in general practice: a striking feature with clinical implications. Aliment Pharmacol Ther 2004;20:1195–1203.

62. Costanza C, Longstreth G, Liu A. Chronic abdominal wall pain: clinical features, health care costs, and long-term outcome. Clin Gastroenterol Hepatol 2004;2:395–399.

63. Fass R, Longstreth GF, Pimentel M, et al. Evidence and consensus-based practice guidelines for the diagnosis of irritable bowel syndrome. Arch Intern Med 2001; 161:2081–2088.

64. Camilleri M. Management of the irritable bowel syndrome. Gastroenterology 2001; 120:652–668.

65. Cash B, Schoenfeld P, Chey WD. The utility of diagnostic tests in irritable bowel syndrome. Am J Gastroenterol 2002;97:2812–2819.

66. Thompson WG. Laxative Abuse. In: Tytgat GNJ and van Blankenstein M, eds. Current Topics in Gastroenterology and Hepatology. New YorK: Springer-Verlag, 1990: 236–245.

67. Cullingford GL, et al. Irritable bowel syndrome: can the patient's response to colonoscopy help with the diagnosis? Digestion 1992;52:209–213.

68. Kang JY, Gwee KA, Yap I. The colonic air insufflation test indicates a colonic cause of abdominal pain. An aid in the diagnosis of the irritable bowel syndrome. J Clin Gastro 1994;18:19–22.

69. Glaser SR. Utilization of sigmoidoscopy by family physicians in Canada. Can Med Assoc J 1994;150:367–371.

70. Thompson WG, Heaton KW, Smyth GT, Smyth C. Irritable bowel syndrome: the view from general practice. Eur J Gastroenterol Hepatol 1997;9:689–692.

71. Suleiman S, Sonnenberg A. Cost-effectiveness of endoscopy in irritable bowel syndrome. Arch Intern Med 2001;161:369–375.

72. Yawn BP, Locke GR, III, Lydick E, Wollan PC, Bertram SL, Kurland MJ. Diagnosis and care of irritable bowel syndrome in a community-based population. Am J Manag Care 2001;7:585–592.

73. MacIntosh DG, Thompson WG, Patel DG, Barr R, Guindi M. Is rectal biopsy necessary in irritable bowel syndrome? Am J Gastroenterol 1992;87:1407–1409.

74. Hamm LR, Sorrells SC, Harding JP, Northcutt AR, Heath AT, Kapke GF, Hunt CM, Mangel AW. Additional investigations fail to alter the diagnosis of irritable bowel syndrome in subjects fulfilling the Rome criteria. Am J Gastroenterol 1999;94:1279–1282.

75. Longstreth GF, Drossman DA. Severe irritable bowel and functional abdominal pain syndromes: managing the patient and health care costs. Clin Gastroenterol Hepatol 2005;3:397–400.

76. Tolliver BA, Herrera JL, DiPalma JA. Evaluation of patients who meet clinical criteria for irritable bowel syndrome. Am J Gastroenterol 1994;89:176–178.

77. Tibble JA, Sigthorrson G, Foster R, Forgacs I, Bjarnason I. Use of surrogate markers of inflammation and Rome criteria to distinguish organic from nonorganic intestinal disease. Gastroenterology 2002;123:450–460.

78. Suarez FL, Savaiano DA, Levitt MD. A comparison of symptoms after the consumption of milk or lactose-hydrolyzed milk by people with self-reported severe lactose intolerance. New Engl J Med 1995;333:1–4.

79. Tolliver BA, et al. Does lactose maldigestion really play a role in the irritable bowel syndrome? J Clin Gastroenterol 1996;23:15–17.

80. Thompson WG. Do colonic diverticula cause symptoms? Am J Gastroenterol 1986; 81:613–614.

81. Sim GPG, Scobie BA. Natural history of diverticulosis of the colon. NZ Med J 1982; 95:611–613.

82. Francis CY, Duffy JN, Whorwell PJ, Martin JF. Does routine abdominal ultrasound enhance diagnostic accuracy in irritable bowel syndrome? Am J Gastroenterol 1996; 91:1348–1350.

83. O'Leary C, Wieneke P, Buckley S, O'Regan P, Cronin CC, Quigley EMM, Shanahan F. Celiac disease and irritable bowel-type symptoms. Am J Gastroenterol 2002; 6:1463–1467.

84. Sanders D, Carter MJ, Hurlstone DP, Pearce A, Ward AM, McAlindon ME, Lobo AJ. Association of adult coeliac disease with irritable bowel syndrome: a case-controlled study in patients fulfilling Rome II criteria referred to secondary care. Lancet 2001;358:1504–1508.

85. Wahnshaffe U, Ulrich R, Riechen EO, Schulzke J-D. Celiac disease-like abnormalities in a subgroup of patients with irritable bowel syndrome. Gastroenterology 2001; 121:1329–1338.

86. Spiegel BM, Derosa VP, Gralnek IM, Wang V, Dulai GS. Testing for celiac sprue in irritable bowel syndrome with predominant diarrhea: A cost-effectiveness analysis. Gastroenterology 2004;126:1721–1732.

87. Drossman DA. Irritable bowel syndrome: how far do you go in the work-up. Gastroenterology 2001;1329:1512–1515.

88. Thompson WG. Irritable bowel syndrome and coeliac disease. Lancet 2002;359 [Letter]:1346–1347.

89. El Serag HB, Pilgrim P, Schoenfeld P. Systemic review: Natural history of irritable bowel syndrome. Aliment Pharmacol Ther 2004;19:861–870.

90. Longstreth GF. Clinical diagnosis of IBS. In: Camilleri M SR, ed. Irritable bowel syndrome. Diagnosis and treatment. London: WB Saunders, 2002:1–10.

91. Lea R, Whorwell PJ. New insights into the psychosocial aspects of irritable bowel syndrome. Curr Gastroenterol Rep 2003;5:343–350.

92. Connell AM. The motility of the pelvic colon. Part II Paradoxical motility in diarrhoea and constipation. Gut 1962;3:342–348.

93. Wangel DG, Deller DJ. Intestinal motility in man: III mechanisma of constipation and diarrhoea with particular reference to the irritable bowel. Gastroenterology 1965;48:69–84.

94. Snape WJ, Carlson GM, Matarazzo SA, Cohen S. Evidence that abnormal myoelectric activity produces colon motor dysfunction in the irritable bowel syndrome. Gastroenterol 1977;72:383–387.

95. Latimer P, Sarna S, Campbell D, Latimer M, Waterfall W, Daniel EE. Colonic motor and myoelectric activity: a comparative study of normal subjects, psychoneurotic patients and patients with the irritable bowel syndrome. Gastroenterol 1981;80: 893–901.

96. Madhu SV, Vij JC, Bhatnagar OP, Krishnamurthy N, Anand BS, Chuttani HK. Colonic myoelectric activity in irritable bowel syndrome before and after treatment. Indian J Gastroenterol 1993;7:31–33.

97. Vassallo M, Camilleri M, Phillips SF, Brown ML, Chapman NJ, Thomforde GM. Transit through the proximal colon influences stool weight in the irritable bowel syndrome. Gastroenterology 1992;102:102–108.

98. Stivland T, Camilleri M, Vassallo M, Proano M, Rath D, Brown M, Thomforde G, Pemberton J, Phillips S. Scintographic measurement of regional gut transit in idiopathic constipation. Gastroenterology 1991;101:107–115.

99. Drossman DA, Camilleri M, Mayer EA, Whitehead WE. AGA technical review on irritable bowel syndrome. Gastroenterology 2002;123:2108–2131.

100. Kellow JE, Phillips SF. Altered small bowel motility in irritable bowel syndrome is correlated with symptoms. Gastroenterology 1987;92:1885–1893.

101. Simren M, Castedal M, Svedlund J, Abrahamsson H, Bjornsson E. Abnormal propagation pattern of duodenal pressure waves in the irritable bowel syndrome [IBS]. Dig Dis Sci 2000;45:2151–2161.

102. Chey WY, Jin HO, Lee MH, Sun SW, Lee KY. Colonic motility abnormality in patients with irritable bowel syndrome exhibiting abdominal pain and diarrhea. Am J Gastroenterol 2001;96:1499–1506.

103. Clemens CH, Samsom M, Roelofs JM, Berge Henegouwen GP, Smout AJ. Association between pain episodes and high amplitude propagated pressure waves in patients with irritable bowel syndrome. Am J Gastroenterol 2003;98:1838–1843.

104. Fukudo S, Kanazawa M, Kano M, Sagami Y, Endo Y, Utsumi A, Nomura T, Hongo M. Exaggerated motility of the descending colon with repetitive distention of the sigmoid colon in patients with irritable bowel syndrome. J Gastroenterol 2002;37 Suppl 14:145–150.

105. Caballero-Plasencia AM, Valenzuela-Barranco M, Herrerias-Gutierrez JM, Esteban-Carretero JM. Altered gastric emptying in patients with irritable bowel syndrome. Eur J Nucl Med 1999;26:404–409.

106. Stanghellini V, Tosetti C, Barbara G, De Giorgio R, Cogliandro L, Cogliandro R, Corinaldesi R. Dyspeptic symptoms and gastric emptying in the irritable bowel syndrome. Am J Gastroenterol 2002;97:2738–2743.

107. van dV, I, Osmanoglou E, Seybold M, Heymann-Monnikes I, Tebbe J, Wiedenmann B, Klapp BF, Monnikes H. Electrogastrography as a diagnostic tool for delayed gastric emptying in functional dyspepsia and irritable bowel syndrome. Neurogastroenterol Motil 2003;15:467–473.

108. Welgan P, Meshkinpour H, Ma L. Role of anger in antral motor activity in irritable bowel syndrome. Dig Dis Sci 2000;45:248–251.

109. Drewes AM, Petersen P, Rossel P, Gao C, Hansen JB, Arendt-Nielsen L. Sensitivity and distensibility of the rectum and sigmoid colon in patients with irritable bowel syndrome. Scand J Gastroenterol 2001;36:827–832.

110. Rossel P, Drewes AM, Petersen P, Nielsen J, Arendt-Nielsen L. Pain produced by electric stimulation of the rectum in patients with irritable bowel syndrome: further evidence of visceral hyperalgesia. Scand J Gastroenterol 1999;34:1001–1006.

111. Bouin M, Meunier P, Riberdy-Poitras M, Poitras P. Pain hypersensitivity in patients with functional gastrointestinal disorders: a gastrointestinal-specific defect or a general systemic condition? Dig Dis Sci 2001;46:2542–2548.

112. Verne GN, Robinson ME, Price DD. Hypersensitivity to visceral and cutaneous pain in the irritable bowel syndrome. Pain 2001;93:7–14.

113. Chang L, Berman S, Mayer EA, Suyenobu B, Derbyshire S, Naliboff B, Vogt B, FitzGerald L, Mandelkern MA. Brain responses to visceral and somatic stimuli in patients with irritable bowel syndrome with and without fibromyalgia. Am J Gastroenterol 2003;98:1354–1361.

114. Rossel P, Pedersen P, Niddam D, Arendt-Nielsen L, Chen AC, Drewes AM. Cerebral response to electric stimulation of the colon and abdominal skin in healthy subjects and patients with irritable bowel syndrome. Scand J Gastroenterol 2001;36:1259–1266.

115. Delvaux M. Role of visceral sensitivity in the pathophysiology of irritable bowel syndrome. Gut 2002;51 Suppl 1:i67–i71.

116. Penning C, Steens J, van der Schaar PJ, Kuyvenhoven J, Delemarre JB, Lamers CB, Masclee AA. Motor and sensory function of the rectum in different subtypes of constipation. Scand J Gastroenterol 2001;36:32–38.

117. Steens J, van der Schaar PJ, Penning C, Brussee J, Masclee AA. Compliance, tone and sensitivity of the rectum in different subtypes of irritable bowel syndrome. Neurogastroenterol Motil 2002;14:241–247.

118. Blomhoff S, Spetalen S, Jacobsen MB, Vatn M, Malt UF. Rectal tone and brain information processing in irritable bowel syndrome. Dig Dis Sci 2000;45:1153–1159.

119. Mertz H, Naliboff B, Munakata J, Niazi N, Meyer EA. Altered rectal perception is a biological marker of patients with irritable bowel syndrome. Gastroenterology 1995;109:40–52.

120. Bouin M, Plourde V, Boivin M, et al. Rectal distension testing in patients with irritable bowel syndrome: sensitivity, specificity, and predictive values of pain sensory thresholds. Gastroenterology 2002;122:1771–1777.

121. Schmulson M, Chang L, Naliboff B, Lee OY, Mayer EA. Correlation of symptom criteria with perception thresholds during during rectosigmoid distension in irritable bowel syndrome. Am J Gastroenterol 2000;95:152–156.

122. Poitras P, Riberdy PM, Plourde V, Boivin M, Verrier P. Evolution of visceral sensitivity in patients with irritable bowel syndrome. Dig Dis Sci 2002;47:914–920.

123. Bouin M, Delvaux M, Blanc C, Lagier E, Delisle MB, Fioramonti J, Bueno L, Frexinos J. Intrarectal injection of glycerol induces hypersensitivity to rectal distension in healthy subjects without modifying rectal compliance. Eur J Gastroenterol Hepatol 2001;13:573–580.

124. Barbara G, Stanghellini V, De Giorgio R, Cremon C, Cottrell GS, Santini D, Pasquinelli G, Morselli-Labate AM, Grady EF, Bunnett NW, Collins SM, Corinaldesi R. Activated mast cells in proximity to colonic nerves correlate with abdominal pain in irritable bowel syndrome. Gastroenterology 2004;126:693–702.

125. Chang L, Munakata J, Mayer EA, Schmulson MJ, Johnson TD, Bernstein CN, Saba L, Naliboff B, Anton PA, Matin K. Perceptual responses in patients with inflammatory and functional bowel disease. Gut 2000;47:497–505.

126. Silverman DHS, Munakata JA, Ennes H, Mandelkern MA, HoH CK, Mayer EA. Regional cerebral activity in normal and pathological perception of visceral pain. Gastroenterology 1997;112:64–72.

127. Mertz H, Morgan V, Tanner G, et al. Regional cerebral activation in irritable bowel syndrome and control subjects with painful and nonpainful rectal distension. Gastroenterology 2000;118:842–848.

128. Yuan YZ, Tao RJ, Xu B, Sun J, Chen KM, Miao F, Zhang ZW, Xu JY. Functional brain imaging in irritable bowel syndrome with rectal balloon-distention by using fMRI. World J Gastroenterol 2003;9:1356–1360.

129. Bernstein CN, Frankenstein UN, Rawsthorne P, Pitz M, Summers R, McIntyre MC. Cortical mapping of visceral pain in patients with GI disorders using functional magnetic resonance imaging. Am J Gastroenterol 2002;97:319–327.

130. Naliboff BD, Derbyshire SW, Munakata J, Berman S, Mandelkern M, Chang L, Mayer EA. Cerebral activation in patients with irritable bowel syndrome and control subjects during rectosigmoid stimulation. Psychosom Med 2001;63:365–375.

131. Ringel Y, Drossman DA, Turkington TG, Bradshaw B, Hawk TC, Bangdiwala S, Coleman RE, Whitehead WE. Regional brain activation in response to rectal distension in patients with irritable bowel syndrome and the effect of a history of abuse. Dig Dis Sci 2003;48:1774–1781.

132. Berman S, Munakata J, Naliboff BD, Chang L, Mandelkern M, Silverman D, Kovalik E, Mayer EA. Gender differences in regional brain response to visceral pressure in IBS patients. Eur J Pain 2000;4:157–172.

133. Drossman DA, Ringel Y, Vogt BA, Leserman J, Lin W, Smith JK, Whitehead W. Alterations of brain activity associated with resolution of emotional distress and pain in a case of severe irritable bowel syndrome. Gastroenterology 2003;124:754–761.

134. Blomhoff S, Spetalen S, Jacobsen MB, Malt UF. Phobic anxiety changes the function of brain-gut axis in irritable bowel syndrome. Psychosom Med 2001;63:959–965.

135. Verne GN, Robinson ME, Vase L, Price DD. Reversal of visceral and cutaneous hyperalgesia by local rectal anesthesia in irritable bowel syndrome [IBS] patients. Pain 2003;105:223–230.

136. Chan YK, Herkes GK, Badcock C, Evans PR, Bennett E, Kellow JE. Alterations in cerebral potentials evoked by rectal distension in irritable bowel syndrome. Am J Gastroenterol 2001;95:2413–2417.

137. Barbara G, De Giorgio R, Stanghellini V, Cremon C, Corinaldesi R. A role for inflammation in irritable bowel syndrome? Gut 2002;51 Suppl 1:i41–i44.

138. Spiller RC. Infection, immune function, and functional gut disorders. Clin Gastroenterol Hepatol 2004;2:445–455.

139. Wang LH, Fang XC, Pan GZ. Bacillary dysentery as a causative factor of irritable bowel syndrome and its pathogenesis. Gut 2004;53:1096–1101.

140. Mearin F, Perez-Oliveras M, Perello A, Vinyet J, Ibanez A, Coderch J, Perona M. Dyspepsia and irritable bowel syndrome after a Salmonella gastroenteritis outbreak: one-year follow-up cohort study. Gastroenterology 2005;129:98–104.

141. Dunlop SP, Jenkins D, Neal KR, Spiller RC. Relative importance of enterochromaffin cell hyperplasia, anxiety, and depression in postinfectious IBS. Gastroenterology 2003;125:1651–1659.

142. Spiller RC, Jenkins D, Thornley JP, Hebden JM, Wright T, Skinner M, Neal KR. Increased rectal mucosal enteroendocrine cells, T lymphocytes, and increased gut permiability following acute *Campylobacter enteritis* and post dysenteric irritable bowel syndrome. Gut 2000;47:804–811.

143. Gwee KA, Collins SM, Read NW, Rajnakova A, Deng Y, Graham JC, McKendrick

MW, Moochhala SM. Increased rectal mucosal expression of interleukin 1beta in recently acquired post-infectious irritable bowel syndrome. Gut 2003;52:523–526.

144. Gonsalkorale WM, Perrey C, Pravica V, Whorwell PJ, Hutchinson IV. Interleukin 10 genotypes in irritable bowel syndrome: evidence for an inflammatory component? Gut 2003;52:91–93.

145. Dunlop SP, Jenkins D, Spiller RC. Distinctive clinical, psychological and histological features of postinfective irritable bowel syndrome. Am J Gastroenterol 2003;98:1578–1583.

146. Neal KR, Hebden J, Spiller R. Prevalance of gastrointestinal symptoms six months after bacterial gastroenteritis and risk factors for the development of the irritable bowel syndrome: a postal survey of patients. Br Med J 1997;314:779–782.

147. Gwee KA, Leong YL, Graham C, McKendrick MW, Collins SM, Walters SJ, Underwood JE, Read NW. The role of psychological and biological factors in postinfective gut dysfunction. Gut 1999;44:400–406.

148. Dunlop SP, Jenkins D, Spiller RC. Distinctive clinical, psychological, and histological features of postinfective irritable bowel syndrome. Am J Gastroenterol 2003;98:1578–1583.

149. Neal KR, Barker L, Spiller RC. Prognosis in post-infective irritable bowel syndrome: a six year follow up study. Gut 2002;51:410–413.

150. Lin HC. Small intestinal bacterial overgrowth: a framework for understanding irritable bowel syndrome. JAMA 2004;292:852–858.

151. Pimentel M, Chow EJ, Lin HC. Eradication of small intestinal bacterial overgrowth reduces symptoms of irritable bowel syndrome. Am J Gastroenterol 2000;95:3503–3506.

152. Hasler WL. Lactulose breath testing, bacterial overgrowth, and IBS: just a lot of hot air? Gastroenterology 2003;125:1898–1900.

153. Pimentel M, Chow PP, Lin HC. Normalization of lactulose breath testing correlates with symptom improvement in irritable bowel syndrome: a double-blind, randomized controlled study. Am J Gastroenterol 2003;98:412–419.

154. Walters B, Vanner SJ. Detection of bacterial overgrowth in IBS using the lactulose H2 breath test: comparison with 14C-D-xylose and healthy controls. Am J Gastroenterol 2005;100:1566–1570.

155. Aggarwal A, Cutts TF, Abell TL, Cardoso L, et al. Prominent symptoms in irritable bowel syndrome correlate with specific autonomic nervous system abnormalities. Gastroenterology 1994;106:945–950.

156. Murray CD, Flynn J, Ratcliffe L, Jacyna MR, Kamm MA, Emmanuel AV. Effect of acute physical and psychological stress on gut autonomic innervation in irritable bowel syndrome. Gastroenterology 2004;127:1695–1703.

157. Gupta V, Sheffield D, Verne GN. Evidence for autonomic dysregulation in the irritable bowel syndrome. Dig Dis Sci 2002;47:1716–1722.

158. Heitkemper M, Jarrett M, Cain KC, Burr R, Levy RL, Feld A, Hertig V. Autonomic nervous system function in women with irritable bowel syndrome. Dig Dis Sci 2001;46:1276–1284.

159. Elsenbruch S, Orr WC. Diarrhea- and constipation-predominant IBS patients differ in postprandial autonomic and cortisol responses. Am J Gastroenterol 2001;96:460–466.

160. Simren M, Abrahamsson H, Bjornsson ES. An exaggerated sensory component of the gastrocolonic response in patients with irritable bowel syndrome. Gut 2001;48:20–27.

161. Kettell J, Jones R, Lydeard S. Reasons for consultation in irritable bowel syndrome: symptoms and patient characteristics. Brit J Gen Pract 1992;42:459–461.

162. Drossman DA, McKee DC, Sandler RS, Mitchell CM, Cramer EM, Lowman BC, Burger AL. Psychosocial factors in the irritable bowel syndrome. A multivariate study of patients and nonpatients with irritable bowel syndrome. Gastroenterology 1988;95:701–708.

163. Drossman DA. Do psychosocial factors define symptom severity and patient status in irritable bowel syndrome? Am J Med 1999;107:41S-50S.

164. Herschbach P, Henrich G, von Rad M. Psychological factors in functional gastro-intestinal disorders: characteristics of the disorder or of the illness behaviour? Psychosom Med 1999;61:148–153.

165. Osterberg E, Blomquist L, Krakau I, Weinryb RM, Asberg M, Hultcrantz R. A population study on irritable bowel syndrome and mental health. Scand J Gastroenterol 2000;35:264–268.

166. Elsenbruch S, Thompson JJ, Harnish MJ, Exton MS, Orr WC. Behavioural and physiological sleep characteristics in women with irritable bowel syndrome. Am J Gastroenterol 2002;97:2307–2314.

167. Sperber AD, Carmel S, Atzmon Y, Weisberg I, Shalit Y, Neumann L, Fich A, Buskila D. The sense of coherence index and the irritable bowel syndrome. A cross-sectional comparison among irritable bowel syndrome patients with and without coexisting fibromyalgia, irritable bowel syndrome non-patients, and controls. Scand J Gastroenterol 1999;34:259–263.

168. Katon W, Sullivan M, Walker E. Medical symptoms without identified pathology: relationship to psychiatric disorders, childhood and adult trauma, and personality traits. Ann Intern Med 2001;134:917–925.

169. Sperber AD, Friger M, Shvartzman P, Abu-Rabia M, Abu-Rabis R, Abu-Rashid M, Albedour K, Alkranawi O, Eisenberg A, Kazanoviz A, Mazinger L, Fich A. Rates of functional bowel disorders among Israeli Bedouins in rural areas compared with those who moved to permanent towns. Clin Gastroenterol Hepatol 2005;3:342–348.

170. Hu WH, Wong WM, Lam CL, Lam KF, Hui WM, Lai KC, Xia HX, Lam SK, Wong BC. Anxiety but not depression determines health care-seeking behaviour in Chinese patients with dyspepsia and irritable bowel syndrome: a population-based study. Aliment Pharmacol Ther 2002;16:2081–2088.

171. He JWWHP. Coping characters of patients with irritable bowel syndrome. Chin J Dig 2004;23:527–529.

172. Wang G, He J, Hu P, Lin J. The illness behavior and its correlative factors in patients with irritable bowel syndrome. Chin J Behavior Med Sci 2003;12:265–267.

173. Fock KM, Chew CN, Tay LK, Peh LH, Chan S, Pang EP. Psychiatric illness, personality traits and the irritable bowel syndrome. Ann Acad Med Singapore 2001;30:611–614.

174. Trikas P, Vlachonikolis I, Fragkiadakis N, Vasilakis S, Manousos O, Paritsis N. Core mental state in irritable bowel syndrome. Psychosom Med 1999;61:781–788.

175. Blanchard EB, Keefer L, Galovski TE, Taylor AE, Turner SM. Gender differences in psychological distress among patients with irritable bowel syndrome. J Psychosom Res 2001;50:271–275.

176. Weinryb RM, Osterberg E, Blomquist L, Hultcrantz R, Krakau I, Asberg M. Psychological factors in irritable bowel syndrome: a population-based study of patients, non-patients and controls. Scand J Gastroenterol 2003;38:503–510.

177. Sykes MA, Blanchard EB, Lackner J, Keefer L, Krasner S. Psychopathology in ir-

ritable bowel syndrome: support for a psychophysiological model. J Behav Med 2003;26:361–372.

178. Drossman DA. Psychosocial factors and the disorders of GI function: what is the link? Am J Gastroenterol 2004;99:358–360.

179. Labus JS, Bolus R, Chang L, Wiklund I, Naesdal J, Mayer EA, Naliboff BD. The Visceral Sensitivity Index: development and validation of a gastrointestinal symptom-specific anxiety scale. Aliment Pharmacol Ther 2004;20:89–97.

180. Bennett EJ, Tennant CC, Piesse C, Badcock CA, Kellow JE. Level of chronic life stress predicts clinical outcome in irritable bowel syndrome. Gut 1998;43:256–261.

181. Gibbs-Gallagher N, Palsson OS, Levy RL, Meyer K, Drossman DA, Whitehead WE. Selective recall of gastrointestinal-sensation words: evidence for a cognitive-behavioral contribution to irritable bowel syndrome. Am J Gastroenterol 2001;96: 1133–1138.

182. Drossman DA, Leserman J, Nachman G, Li Z, Gluck H, Toomey TC, Mitchell CM. Sexual and physical abuse in women with functional or organic gastrointestinal disorders. Ann Intern Med 1990;113:828–833.

183. Leroi AM, Bernier C, Watier A, Hemond M, Goupil G, Black R, Denis P, Devroede G. Prevalence of sexual abuse among patients with functional disorders of the lower gastrointestinal tract. Int J Colorectal Dis 1995;10:200–206.

184. Talley NJ, Fett SL, Zinsmeister AR. Self-reported abuse and gastrointestinal disease in outpatients: association with irritable bowel-type symptoms. Am J Gastroenterol 1995;90:366–371.

185. Talley NJ, Fett SL, Zinsmeister AR, Melton LJ. Gastrointestinal tract symptoms and self-reported abuse: a population-based study. Gastroenterol 1994;107:1040–1049.

186. Leserman J, Drossman DA, Li Z, Toomey TC, Nachman G, Glogau L. Sexual and physical abuse history in gastroenterology practice. Psychosom Med 1996;58:4–15.

187. Ali A, Toner BB, Stuckless N, Gallop R, Diamant NE, Gould MI, Vidins EI. Emotional abuse, self-blame, and self-silencing in women with irritable bowel syndrome. Psychosom Med 2000;62:76–82.

188. Ringel Y, Whitehead WE, Toner BB, Diamant NE, Hu Y, Jia H, Bangdiwala SI, Drossman DA. Sexual and physical abuse are not associated with rectal hypersensitivity in patients with irritable bowel syndrome. Gut 2004;53:838–842.

189. Hobbis IC, Turpin G, Read NW. A re-examination of the relationship between abuse experience and functional bowel disorders. Scand J Gastroenterol 2002;37:423–430.

190. Talley NJ. Is the association between irritable bowel syndrome and abuse explained by neuroticism? Gut 1998;42:47–53.

191. Blanchard EB, Keefer L, Payne A, Turner SM, Galovski TE. Early abuse, psychiatric diagnoses and irritable bowel syndrome. Behav Res Ther 2002;40:289–298.

192. Drossman DA, Li Z, Leserman J, Toomey TC, Hu YJB. Health status by gastrointestinal diagnosis and abuse history. Gastroenterology 1996;110:999–1007.

193. Locke GR, III, Zinsmeister AR, Talley NJ, Fett SL, Melton LJ, III. Familial association in adults with functional gastrointestinal disorders. Mayo Clin Proc 2000; 75:907–912.

194. Morris-Yates A, Talley NJ, Boyce PM, Nandurkar S, Andrews G. Evidence of a genetic contribution to functional bowel disorder. Am J Gastroenterol 1998;93:1311–1317.

195. Svedberg P, Johansson S, Wallander MA, Hamelin B, Pedersen NL. Extra-intestinal manifestations associated with irritable bowel syndrome: a twin study. Aliment Pharmacol Ther 2002;16:975–983.

196. Camilleri M. Is there a SERT-ain association with IBS? Gut 2004;53:1396–1399.

197. Yeo A, Boyd P, Lumsden S, Saunders T, Handley A, Stubbins M, Knaggs A, Asquith S, Taylor I, Bahari B, Crocker N, Rallan R, Varsani S, Montgomery D, Alpers DH, Dukes GE, Purvis I, Hicks GA. Association between a functional polymorphism in the serotonin transporter gene and diarrhoea predominant irritable bowel syndrome in women. Gut 2004;53:1452–1458.

198. Skoog SM, Bharucha AE. Dietary fructose and gastrointestinal symptoms: a review. Am J Gastroenterol 2004;99:2046–2050.

199. Wildt S, Norby RS, Lysgard MJ, Rumessen JJ. Bile acid malabsorption in patients with chronic diarrhoea: clinical value of SeHCAT test. Scand J Gastroenterol 2003; 38:826–830.

200. Simren M, Mansson A, Langkilde AM, Svedlund J, Abrahamsson H, Bengtsson U, Bjornsson ES. Food-related gastrointestinal symptoms in the irritable bowel syndrome. Digestion 2001;63:108–115.

201. Zar S, Kumar D, Benson MJ. Food hypersensitivity and irritable bowel syndrome. Aliment Pharmacol Ther 2001;15:439–449.

202. Dainese R, Galliani EA, De Lazzari F, Di L, V, Naccarato R. Discrepancies between reported food intolerance and sensitization test findings in irritable bowel syndrome patients. Am J Gastroenterol 1999;94:1892–1897.

203. Houghton LA, Atkinson W, Whitaker RP, et al. Increased platelet depleted plasma 5-hydroxytryptamine concentration following meal ingestion in symptomatic female subjects with diarrhoea-predominant irritable bowel syndrome. Gut 2003;52:633–670.

204. Houghton LA, Lea R, Jackson N, Whorwell PJ. The menstrual cycle affects rectal sensitivity in patients with irritable bowel syndrome but not healthy volunteers. Gut 2002;50:471–474.

205. Houghton LA, Jackson NA, Whorwell PJ, Morris J. Do male sex hormones protect from irritable bowel syndrome? Am J Gastroenterol 2000;95:2296–2300.

206. O'Sullivan MA, Mahmud N, Kelleher DP, Lovett E, O'Morain C. Patient knowledge and educational needs in the Irritable bowel syndrome. Eur J Gastroenterol Hepatol 1999;12:39–43.

207. Heitkemper MM, Jarrett ME, Levy RL, Cain KC, Burr RL, Feld A, Barney P, Weisman P. Self-management for women with irritable bowel syndrome. Clin Gastroenterol Hepatol 2004;2:585–596.

208. Saito YA, Prather CM, Van Dyke CT, Fett S, Zinsmeister AR, Locke GR, III. Effects of multidisciplinary education on outcomes in patients with irritable bowel syndrome. Clin Gastroenterol Hepatol 2004;2:576–584.

209. Whitehead WE, Levy RL, Von Korff M, Feld AD, Palsson OS, Turner M, Drossman DA. The usual medical care for irritable bowel syndrome. Aliment Pharmacol Ther 2004;20:1305–1315.

210. Thompson WG, Heaton KW, Smyth T, Smyth C. Irritable bowel syndrome in general practice: prevalence, management and referral. Gut 2000;46:78–82.

211. Bijkerk CJ, de Wit NJ, Stalman WA, Knottnerus JA, Hoes AW, Muris JW. Irritable bowel syndrome in primary care: the patients' and doctors' views on symptoms, etiology and management. Can J Gastroenterol 2003;17:363–368.

212. Bertram S, Kurland M, Lydick E, Locke GR, III, Yawn BP. The patient's perspective of irritable bowel syndrome. J Fam Pract 2001;50:521–525.

213. Dixon-Woods M, Critchley S. Medical and lay views of irritable bowel syndrome. Fam Pract 2000;17:108–113.

214. Dalton CB, Drossman DA, Hathaway JM, Bangdiwala S. Perceptions of physicians and patients with organic and functional gastrointestinal diagnoses. Clin Gastroenterol Hepatol 2004;2:121–126.

215. Drossman DA. Challenges to the physician-patient relationship: feeling "drained". Gastroenterology 2001;121:1037–1038.

216. Longstreth GF, Burchette RJ. Family practitioners' attitudes and knowledge about irritable bowel syndrome: effect of a trial of physician education. Fam Pract 2003; 20:670–674.

217. Gladman LM, Gorard DA. General practitioner and hospital specialist attitudes to functional gastrointestinal disorders. Aliment Pharmacol Ther 2003;17:651–654.

218. Borum ML. Physician perception of IBS management in women and men. Dig Dis Sci 2002;47:236–237.

219. Thompson W. The placebo effect and health. New York: Prometheus, 2005.

220. Thompson WG. Placebos: a review of the placebo response. Am J Gastroenterol 2000;95:1637–1643.

221. Thompson WG. Tegaserod and IBS : a perfect match? Gut 2003;52:621–622.

222. Pitz M, Cheang M, Bernstein CN. Defining the predictors of the placebo response in irritable bowel syndrome. Clin Gastroenterol Hepatol 2005;3:237–247.

223. van der Horst HE, van Dulman AM, Schellevis FG, van Eijk JThM, Fennis JFM, Bleigenberg G. Do patients with irritable bowel syndrome in primary care really differ from outpatients with irritable bowel syndrome? Gut 1997;41:669–674.

224. Spiller R. Treatment of irritable bowel syndrome. Curr Treat Options Gastroenterol 2003;6:329–337.

225. van Dulman A, Fennis J, Mokkink H, Van Der Velden H, Bleijenberg G. Doctor dependent changes in complaint-related cognitions and anxiety during medical consultations in functional abdominal complaints. Psychol Med 1995;25:1011–1018.

226. Owens DM, Nelson DK, Talley NJ. The irritable bowel syndrome: long term prognosis and the patient-physician interaction. Ann Intern Med 1995;122:107–112.

227. Ilnyckyj A, Graff LA, Blanchard JF, Bernstein CN. Therapeutic value of a gastroenterology consultation in irritable bowel syndrome. Aliment Pharmacol Ther 2003;17:871–880.

228. Koloski NA, Talley NJ, Huskic SS, Boyce PM. Predictors of conventional and alternative health care seeking for irritable bowel syndrome and functional dyspepsia. Aliment Pharmacol Ther 2003;17:841–851.

229. Parker TJ, Woolner JT, Prevost AT, Tuffnell Q, Shorthouse M, Hunter JO. Irritable bowel syndrome: is the search for lactose intolerance justified? Eur J Gastroenterol Hepatol 2001;13:219–225.

230. Atkinson W, Sheldon TA, Shaath N, Whorwell PJ. Food elimination based on IgG antibodies in irritable bowel syndrome: a randomised controlled trial. Gut 2004; 53:1459–1464.

231. Bijkerk CJ, Muris JW, Knottnerus JA, Hoes AW, de Wit NJ. Systematic review: the role of different types of fibre in the treatment of irritable bowel syndrome. Aliment Pharmacol Ther 2004;19:245–251.

232. Snook J, Shepherd AH. Bran supplimentation in the treatment of the irritable bowel syndrome. Aliment Pharmacol Therap 1994;8:511–514.

233. Longstreth GF, Hawkey CJ, Meyer EA, et al. Characteristics of patients with irritable bowel syndrome from three practice surveys. Aliment Pharmacol Therap 2000;15:959–964.

234. Kamm MA. Review article: maintenance of remission in ulcerative colitis. Aliment Pharmacol Ther 2002;16 Suppl 4:21–24.

235. Bijkerk BJ, deWit NJ, Mutis JWM, et al. Outcome measures in irritable bowel syndrome: comparison of psychometric and methodologic characteristics. Am J Gastroenterol 2003;98:122–127.

236. Wiklund IK, Fullerton S, Hawkey CJ, Jones RH, Longstreth GF, Mayer EA, Peacock RA, Wilson IK, Naesdal J. An irritable bowel syndrome-specific symptom questionnaire: development and validation. Scand J Gastroenterol 2003;38:947–954.

237. Klein KB. Controlled treatment trials in the irritable bowel syndrome: a critique. Gastroenterology 1988;95:232–241.

238. Akehurst R, Kaltenhaler.E. Treatment of irritable bowel syndrome: a review of randomized controlled trials. Gut 2001;48:272–282.

239. Jones J, Boorman J, Cann P, et al. British society of gastroenterology guidelines for the management of the irritable bowel syndrome. Gut 2000;47:1–19.

240. Jailwala J, Imperiale TF, Kroenke K. Pharmacologic treatment of the irritable bowel syndrome: a systemic review of randomised, controlled trials. Ann Intern Med 2000;133:136–137.

241. Mertz HR. Irritable bowel syndrome. N Engl J Med 2003;349:2136–2146.

242. Thompson WG, Heaton KW. Irritable Bowel Syndrome. 2 ed. Abbington, Oxford: Health Press, 2003.

243. Clouse R, Lustman P. Antidepressants for IBS. In: Camilleri M SR, ed. Irritable bowel syndrome. Diagnosis and treatment. Edinburgh: WB Saunders, 2002:161–171.

244. Clouse RE. Managing functional bowel disease from the top down: lessons from a well-designed treatment trial. Gastroenterology 2003;125:249–252.

245. Drossman DA, Toner BB, Whitehead WE, Diamant NE, Dalton CB, Duncan S, Emmott S, Proffitt V, Akman D, Frusciante K, Le T, Meyer K, Morris CB, Blackman CJ, Hu Y, Jia H, Li JZ, Koch GG, Bungdiwala SI. Cognitive-behavioural therapy versus education and desipramine versus placebo for moderate to severe functional bowel disorders. Gastroenterology 2003;125:19–31.

246. Halpert A, Dalton CB, Diamant NE, Toner BB, Hu Y, Morris CB, Bangdiwala SI, Whitehead WE, Drossman DA. Clinical response to tricyclic antidepressants in functional bowel disorders is not related to dosage. Am J Gastroenterol 2005;100:664–671.

247. Creed F, Fernandes L, Guthrie E, Palmer S, Ratcliff J, Read N, Rigby C, Thompson D, Tomenson B. The cost-effectiveness of psychotherapy and paroxetine for severe irritable bowel syndrome. Gastroenterology 2003;124:303–317.

248. Tabas G, Beaves M, Wang J, Friday P, Mardini H, Arnold G. Paroxetine to treat irritable bowel syndrome not responding to high-fiber diet: a double-blind, placebo-controlled trial. Am J Gastroenterol 2004;99:914–920.

249. Cremonini F, Delgado-Aros S, Camilleri M. Efficacy of alosetron in irritable bowel syndrome: a meta-analysis of randomized controlled trials. Neurogastroenterol Motil 2003;15:79–86.

250. Friedel D, Thomas R, Fisher RS. Ischemic colitis during treatment with alosetron. Gastroenterology 2001;120:557–560.

251. Cole JA, Cook SF, Sands BE, Ajene AN, Miller DP, Walker AM. Occurrence of colon ischemia in relation to irritable bowel syndrome. Am J Gastroenterol 2004;99:486–491.

252. Kellow JE, Lee O-Y, Chang FY, et al. An Asia-Pacific, double-blind, placebo-controlled, randomised study to evaluate the efficacy, safety, and tolerability of tegaserod in patient with irritable bowel syndrome. Gut 2003;52:671–676.

253. Muller-Lissner SA, Fumagalli I, Bardhan KD, Pace F, Pecher E, Nault B, Ruegg P. Tegaserod, a 5-HT4 receptor agonist, relieves symptoms in irritable bowel syndrome patients with abdominal pain, bloating and constipation. Aliment Pharmacol Therap 1999;15:1655–1666.

254. Novick J, Miner P, Krause R, Glebas K, Bliesath H, Ligozio G, Ruegg P, Lefkowitch J. A randomized, double-blind, placebo-controlled trial of tegaserod in female patients suffering with irritable bowel syndrome with constipation. Aliment Pharmacol Therap 2002;16:1877–1888.

255. Tougas G, Snape WJ, Jr., Otten MH, Earnest DL, Langaker KE, Pruitt RE, Pecher E, Nault B, Rojavin MA. Long-term safety of tegaserod in patients with constipation-predominant irritable bowel syndrome. Aliment Pharmacol Ther 2002;16:1701–1708.

256. American College of Gastroenterology Functional Gastrointestinal Disorders Task Force. Evidence-based position statement on the management of irritable bowel syndrome in North America. Am J Gastroenterol 2002;97[Suppl]:S1–S5.

257. Evans B, Clark W, Moore D, Whorwell, P.J. Tegaserod for the treatment of irritable bowel syndrome. Cochrane Database Syst Rev 2004;1:CD003960.

258. O'Mahony L, McCarthy J, Kelly P, Hurley G, Luo F, Chen K, O'Sullivan GC, Kiely B, Collins JK, Shanahan F, Quigley EM. Lactobacillus and bifidobacterium in irritable bowel syndrome: symptom responses and relationship to cytokine profiles. Gastroenterology 2005;128:541–551.

259. Maxwell PR, Rink E, Kumar D, Mendall MA. Antibiotics increase functional abdominal symptoms. Am J Gastroenterol 2002;97:104–108.

260. Heymanne-Monnikes I, Arnold R, Florin I, Herda C, Melfsen S. The combination of medical treatment plus multicomponent behavioural therapy is superior to medical treatment alone in the therapy of irritable bowel syndrome. Am J Gastroenterol 2001;95:981–995.

261. Houghton LA, Calvert EL, Jackson NA, Cooper P, Whorwell PJ. Visceral sensation and emotion: a study using hypnosis. Gut 2002;51:701–704.

262. Palsson OS, Whitehead WE. The growing case for hypnosis as adjunctive therapy for functional gastrointestinal disorders. Gastroenterology 2002;123:2132–2135.

263. Gonsalkorale WM, Houghton LA, Whorwell, P.J. Hypnotherapy in irritable bowel syndrome:a large-scale audit of a clinical service with examination of factors influencing responsiveness. Am J Gastroenterol 2002;97:954–961.

264. Gonsalkorale WM, Miller V, Afzal A, Whorwell PJ. Long term benefits of hypnotherapy for irritable bowel syndrome. Gut 2003;52:1623–1629.

265. Wang W. J. Traditional Chinese medicine and functional gastrointestinal: basic and clinical study. Textbook of functional gastrointestinal disorders; from basic science to clinical medicine. 2004.

266. Bensoussan A, Talley NJ, Hing M, et al. Treatment of irritable bowel syndrome with Chinese herbal medicine: a randomized controlled trial. JAMA 2001;280:1585–1589.

267. Madisch A, Holtmann G, Plein K, Hotz J. Treatment of irritable bowel syndrome with herbal preparations: results of a double-blind, randomized, placebo-controlled, multi-centre trial. Aliment Pharmacol Ther 2004;19:271–279.

268. Ernst E. Serious adverse effects of unconventional therapies for children and adolescents: a systematic review of recent evidence. Eur J Pediatr 2003;162:72–80.

269. Houghton L, Whorwell P. Towards a better understanding of abdominal bloating and distension in functional gastrointestinal disorders. Neurogastroenterol Motil 2005;17:1–12.

270. Chang L, Lee OY, Naliboff B, Schmulson M, Mayer EA. Sensation of bloating and visible abdominal distension in patients with irritable bowel syndrome. Am J Gastroenterol 2001;96:3341–3347.

271. Lea R, Reilly B, Whorwell P, Houghton L. Abdominal bloating in the absence of physical distension is related to increased visceral sensitivity. Gastroenterology 126, 432. 2004.

272. Zar S, Benson MJ, Kumar D. Review article: bloating in functional bowel disorders. Aliment Pharmacol Ther 2002;16:1867–1876.

273. Hungin AP, Whorwell PJ, Tack J, Mearin F. The prevalence, patterns and impact of irritable bowel syndrome: an international survey of 40,000 subjects. Aliment Pharmacol Ther 2003;17:643–650.

274. Maxton DG, Whorwell PJ. Abdominal distension in irritable bowel syndrome: the patient's perception. Eur J Gastroenterol Hepatol 1992;4:241–243.

275. Talley NJ, Phillips SF, Melton LJ, Mulvihill C, Wiltgen C, Zinsmeister AR. Diagnostic value of the Manning criteria in irritable bowel syndrome. Gut 1990;31:77–81.

276. Talley NJ, Holtmann G, Agreus L, Jones M. Gastrointestinal symptoms and subjects cluster into distinct upper and lower groupings in the community: a four nations study. Am J Gastroenterol 2000;95:1439–1447.

277. Talley NJ, Boyce P, Jones M. Identification of distinct upper and lower gastrointestinal symptom groupings in an urban population. Gut 1998;42:690–695.

278. Heitkemper MM, Jarett M, Cain KC, Shaver J, Walker E, Lewis L. Daily gastrointestinal symptoms in women with and without a diagnosis of IBS. Dig Dis Sci 1995;40:1511–1519.

279. Kwan AC, Bao TN, Chakkaphak S, Chang FY, Ke MY, Law NM, Leelakusolvong S, Luo JY, Manan C, Park HJ, Piyaniran W, Qureshi A, Long T, Xu GM, Xu L, Yuen H. Validation of Rome II criteria for functional gastrointestinal disorders by factor analysis of symptoms in Asian patient sample. J Gastroenterol Hepatol 2003;18:796–802.

280. Taub E, Cuevas JL, Cook EW, Crowell MD, Whitehead WE. Irritable bowel syndrome defined by factor analysis. Dig Dis Sci 1995;40:2647–2655.

281. Whitehead WE, Crowell MD, Bosmajian L, Zonderman A, Costa PTJr, Benjamin C, Robinson JC, Heller BR, Schuster MM. Existence of irritable bowel syndrome supported by factor analysis of symptoms in two community samples. Gastroenterology 1990;98:336–340.

282. Neri M, Laterza F, Howell S, Di Gioacchino M, Festi D, Ballone E, Cuccurullo F, Talley NJ. Symptoms discriminate irritable bowel syndrome from organic gastrointestinal diseases and food allergy. Eur J Gastroenterol Hepatol 2000;12:981–988.

283. Fischler B, Tack J, De G, V, Shkedy ZI, Persoons P, Broekaert D, Molenberghs G, Janssens J. Heterogeneity of symptom pattern, psychosocial factors, and pathophysiological mechanisms in severe functional dyspepsia. Gastroenterology 2003; 124:903–910.

284. Sandler RS, Stewart WF, Liberman JN, Ricci JA, Zorich NL. Abdominal pain,

bloating, and diarrhea in the United States: prevalence and impact. Dig Dis Sci 2000;45:1166–1171.

285. Kay L, Jorgensen T, Jensen KH. The epidemiology of irritable bowel syndrome in a random population: prevalence, incidence, natural history and risk factors. J Intern Med 1994;236:23–30.

286. Thompson WG, Irvine EJ, Pare P, Ferrazzi S, Rance L. Functional gastrointestinal disorders in Canada: first population-based survey using the Rome II criteria with suggestions for improving the questionnaire. Dig Dis Sci 2002;47:225–235.

287. Maxton DG, Morris JA, Whorwell PJ. Ranking of symptoms by patients with the irritable bowel syndrome. Br Med J 1989;299:1138.

288. Lembo T, Naliboff B, Munakata J, Fullerton S, Saba L, Tung S, Schmulson M, Mayer EA. Symptoms and visceral perception in patients with pain-dominant irritable bowel syndrome. Am J Gastroenterol 1999;94:1320–1326.

289. Talley NJ, Dennis EH, Schettler-Duncan VA, et al. Overlapping upper and lower gastrointestinal symptoms in irritable bowel syndrome patients with constipation or diarrhoea. Am J Gastroenterol 2003;98:2454–2459.

290. Lea R, Houghton L, Whorwell P, Reilly B. Relationship of abdominal bloating to physical distension on irritable bowel syndrome [IBS]: effect of bowel habit. Neurogastroenterol Motil 2003;15:587.

291. Maxton DG, Martin DF, Whorwell PJ, Godfrey M. Abdominal distension in female patients with irritable bowel syndrome: exploration of possible mechanisms. Gut 1991;32:662–664.

292. Sullivan SN. Prospective study of unexplained visible abdominal bloating. New Zealand Med J 1994;107:428–430.

293. Lewis MJ, Reilly B, Houghton LA, Whorwell PJ. Ambulatory abdominal inductance plethysmography: towards objective assessment of abdominal distension in irritable bowel syndrome. Gut 2001;48:216–220.

294. Reilly BP, Bolton MP, Lewis MJ, Houghton LA, Whorwell PJ. A device for 24 hour ambulatory monitoring of abdominal girth using inductive plethysmography. Physiol Meas 2002;23:661–670.

295. Lea R, Whorwell P, Houghton L. Abdominal distension in irritable bowel syndrome [IBS]: diurnal variation and its relationship to abdominal bloating. Gut 32 [Suppl VI], A32. 2003.

296. Alvarez WC. Hysterical type of non gaseous abdominal bloating. Arch Intern Med 1949;84:217–245.

297. Song JY, Merskey H, Sullivan SN, Noh S. Anxiety and depression in patients with bdominal bloating. Can J Psychiatry 1993;38:475–479.

298. Levitt MD. Volume and composition of human intestinal gas determined by means of an intestinal washout technic. N Engl J Med 1971;284:1394–1398.

299. Malagelada JR. Sensation and gas dynamics in functional gastrointestinal disorders. Gut 2002;51 Suppl 1:i72–i75.

300. Furne JK, Levitt MD. Factors influencing frequency of flatus emission by healthy subjects. Dig Dis Sci 1996;41:1631–1635.

301. Tomlin J, Lowis C, Read NW. Investigation of normal flatus production in normal volunteers. Gut 1991;32:665–669.

302. Lasser RB, Levitt MD. The role of intestinal gas in functional abdominal pain. New Engl J Med 1975;293:524–526.

303. Caldarella MP, Serra J, Azpiroz F, Malagalada J-R. Prokinetic effects in patients with intestinal gas retention. Gastroenterology 2002;122:1748–1755.

304. Serra J, Azpiroz F, Malagalada J-R. Impaired transit and tolerance of intestinal gas in irritable bowel syndrome. Gut 2001;48:14–19.

305. Maxton DG, Martin DF, Whorwell PJ, Godfrey M. Abdominal distension in female patients with irritable bowel syndrome: exploration of possible mechanisms. Gut 1991;32:662–664.

306. King TS, Elis M, Hunter JO. Abnormal colonic fermentation in irritable bowel syndrome. Lancet 1998;352:1187–1189.

307. Chami TN, Schuster MM, Bohlman M, Pulliam TJ, Kamal N, Whitehead WE. A simple radiologic method to estimate the quantity of bowel gas. Am J Gastroenterol 1991;86:599–602.

308. Koide A, Yamaguche T, Okada T, et al. Quantitative analysis of bowel gas using plain abdominal radiograph in patients with irritable bowel syndrome. Am J Gastroenterol 2000;95:1735–1741.

309. Fardy J, Sullivan SN. Gastrointestinal gas. CMAJ 1988;139:1137–1142.

310. Jain NK, Patel VP, Pitchumoni CS. Efficacy of activated charcoal in reducing gastrointestinal gas: a double blind clinical trial. Am J Gastroenterol 1986;81:532–535.

311. Nobaek S, Johanssen M-L, Molin G, Ahrne S, Jeppsson B. Alteration of intestinal microflora is associated with reduction of abdominal bloating and pain in patients with irritable bowel syndrome. Am J Gastroenterol 2000;95:1231–1238.

312. Kim HJ, Camilleri M, McKinzie S, Lempke MB, Burton DD, Thomforde GM, Zinsmeister AR. A randomized controlled trial of a probiotic, VSL#3, on gut transit and symptoms in diarrhoea-predominant irritable bowel syndrome. Aliment Pharmacol Ther 2003;17:895–904.

313. Di Stefano M, Strocchi A, Malservisi S, Veneto G, Ferrieri A, Corazza GR. Nonabsorbable antibiotics for managing intestinal gas production and gas-related symptoms. Aliment Pharmacol Ther 2000;14:1001–1008.

314. Levitt MD, Furne J, Olsson S. The relation of passage of gas and colonic bloating to colonic gas production. Ann Intern Med 1996;124:422–424.

315. Serra J, Azpiroz F, Malagalada J-R. Intestinal gas dynamics and tolerance in humans. Gastroenterology 1998;115:542–550.

316. Serra J, Salvioli B, Azpiroz F, Malagalada J-R. Lipid-induced intestinal gas retention in irritable bowel syndrome. Gastroenterology 2002;123:700–706.

317. Serra J, Azpiroz F, Malagelada J-R. Mechanisms of intestinal gas retention in humans: impaired propulsion versus obstructed evacuation. Am J Physiol 2001;281: G138–G143.

318. Serra J, Azpiroz F, Malagelada JR. Gastric distension and duodenal lipid infusion modulate intestinal gas transit and tolerance in humans. Am J Gastroenterol 2002; 97:2225–2230.

319. Harder H, Serra J, Azpiroz F, Passos MC, Aguade S, Malagalada J-R. Intestinal gas distribution determines abdominal symptoms. Gut 2003;52:1708–1713.

320. Hernando-Harder AC, Serra J, Azpiroz F, Malagelada JR. Sites of symptomatic gas retention during intestinal lipid perfusion in healthy subjects. Gut 2004;53:661–665.

321. Distrutti E, Azpiroz F, Soldevilla A, Malagelada JR. Gastric wall tension determines perception of gastric distention. Gastroenterology 1999;116:1035–1042.

322. Haderstorfer B, Psycholgin D, Whitehead WE, Schuster MM. Intestinal gas production from bacterial fermentation of undigested carbohydrate in irritable bowel syndrome. Am J Gastroenterol 1989;84:375–378.

323. Lisker R, Solomons NW, Perez BR, Ramirez MM. Lactase and placebo in the management of the irritable bowel syndrome: a double-blind, cross-over study. Am J Gastroenterol 1989;84:756–762.

324. Tremolaterra F, Serra J, Azpiroz F, Villoria A, Malagelada J-R. Bloating and abdominal wall dystony. Gastroenterology 126, 431. 2004.

325. McManis PG, Newall D, Talley NJ. Abdominal wall muscle activity in irritable bowel syndrome with bloating. Am J Gastroenterol 2001;96:1139–1142.

326. Lea R, Reilly B, Whorwell P, Houghton L. Relationship of bloating to abdominal distension in irritable bowel syndrome: differences between bowel habit subgroups. American Journal of Gastroenterology. (In Press.)

327. Lea R, Reilly B, Whorwell P, Houghton L. Peri-menstrual bloating in patients with irritable bowel syndrome is not associated with abdominal distension and may be related to visceral hypersensitivity. Gastroenterology 126, M1611. 2004.

328. Cann PA, Read NW, Brown C, Hobson N, Holdsworth CD. Irritable bowel syndrome: relationship of disorders in the transit of a single solid meal to symptom patterns. Gut 1983;24:405–411.

329. Trotman IF, Price CC. Bloated irritable bowel syndrome defined by dynamic 99mtc bran scan. Lancet 1986;2:364–366.

330. Hebden JM, Blackshaw E, D'Amato M, Perkins AC, Spiller RC. Abnormalities in GI transit in bloated irritabel bowel syndrome: effect of bran on transit and symptoms. Am J Gastroenterol 2002;97:2314–2320.

331. Hutchinson R, Notghi A, Smith NB, Harding LK, Kumar D. Scintigraphic measurement of ileocaecal transit in irritable bowel syndrome and chronic idiopathic constipation. Gut 1995;36:585–589.

332. Lewis MJV, Houghton LA, Whorwell PJ. Changes in small and large bowel phasic activity do not explain the increased perception of distension in patients with IBS. Gut 49 [Suppl. III], 3088. 2001.

333. Galati JS, McKee DP, Quigley EMM. Response to intraluminal gas in irritable bowel syndrome. Motility versus perception. Dig Dis Sci 1995;40:1381–1387.

334. Johnsen R, Jacobsen BK, Forde OH. Association between symptoms of irritable colon and psychological and social conditions and lifestyle. Br Med J 1986;292:1633–1635.

335. Walker EA, Katon WJ, Jemelka RP, Roy-Bryne PP. Comorbidity of gastrointestinal complaints, depression, and anxiety in the Epidemiologic Catchment Area [ECA] Study. Am J Med 1992;92:26S-30S.

336. Rao SS. Belching, bloating and flatulence. How to help patients who ahve troublesome abdominal gas. Postgrad Med 1997;101:263–269.

337. Suarez FL, Furne J, Springfield J, Levitt MD. Failure of activated charcoal to reduce the release of gases produced by the colonic flora. Am J Gastroenterol 1999;94:208–212.

338. Sullivan SN. Functional abdominal bloating. J Clin Gastroenterol 1994;19:23–27.

339. Friis H, Bode S, Rumessen JJ, Gudmand-Hoyer E. Effect of simethicone on lactu-

lose-induced H2 production and gastrointestinal symptoms. Digestion 1991;49:227–230.

340. Holtmann G, Gschossmann J, Karaus M, Fischer T, Becker B, Mayr P, Gerken G. Randomised double-blind comparison of simethicone with cisapride in functional dyspepsia. Aliment Pharmacol Ther 1999;13:1459–1465.

341. O'Sullivan MA, O'Morain CA. Bacterial supplementation in the irritable bowel syndrome. A randomised double-blind placebo-controlled crossover study. Dig Liver Dis 2000;32:294–301.

342. Ganiats TG, Norcross WA, Halverson AL, Burford PA, Palinkas LA. Does Beano prevent gas? A double-blind, crossover study of oral alpha-galactosidase to treat dietary oligosaccharide intolerance. J Fam Pract 1994;39:441–445.

343. Suarez F, Levitt MD, Adshead J, Barkin JS. Pancreatic supplements reduce symptomatic response of healthy subjects to a high fat meal. Dig Dis Sci 1999;44:1317–1321.

344. Sandler RS, Drossman DA. Bowel habits in young adults not seeking health care. Dig Dis Sci 1987;32:841–845.

345. Drossman DA, Sandler RS, McKee DC, Lovitz AJ. Bowel patterns among subjects not seeking health care. Use of a questionnaire to identify a population with bowel dysfunction. Gastroenterology 1982;83:529–534.

346. Rendtorff RC, Kashgarian M. Stool patterns of healthy adult males. Dis Colon Rectum 1967;10:222–228.

347. Everhart JE, Go VL, Johannes RS, Fitzsimmons SC, Roth HP, White LR. A longitudinal survey of self-reported bowel habits in the United States. Dig Dis Sci 1989;34,8:1153–1162.

348. Thompson WG, Heaton KW. Functional bowel disorders in apparently healthy people. Gastroenterology 1980;79:283–288.

349. Evans RC, Kamm MA, Hinton JM, Lennard-Jones JE. The normal range and a simple diagram for recording whole gut transit time. Int J Color Dis 1992;7:15–17.

350. Metcalf AM, Phillips SF, Zinsmeister AR, MacCarty RL, Beart RW, Wolff BG. Simplified assessment of segmental colonic transit. Gastroenterology 1987;92:40–47.

351. Mertz H, Naliboff B, Mayer EA. Symptoms and physiology in severe chronic constipation. Am J Gastroenterol 1999;94:131–138.

352. Koch A, Voderholzer WA, Heinrich CA, Muller-Lissner SA. Symptoms in chronic constipation. Dis Colon Rectum 1997;40:902–906.

353. Heaton KW, Radvan J, Cripps H, Mountford RA, Braddon FEM, Hughes AO. Defecation frequency and timing, and stool form in the general population—a prospective study. Gut 1992;33:818–824.

354. Davies GJ, Crowder M, Reid B, Dickerson JWT. Bowel function measurements of individuals with different eating patterns. Gut 1986;27:164–169.

355. Harari D, Gurwitz JH, Avorn J, Bohn R, Minaker KL. How do older persons define constipation? Implications for therapeutic management. J Gen Intern Med 1997;12:63–66.

356. Pare P, Ferrazzi S, Thompson WG, Irvine EJ, Rance L. An epidemiological survey of constipation in Canada: definitions, rates, demographics and predictors of health care. Am J Gastroenterol 2001;96:3131–3137.

357. Higgins PD, Johanson Jf. Epidemiology of constipation in North America: a systematic review. Am J Gastroenterol 2004;99:750–759.

358. van Ginkel R, Reitsma JB, Buller HA, et al. Childhood constipation: longitudinal follow-up beyond puberty. Gastroenterology 2003;125:357–363.

359. Heaton KW, Cripps HA. Straining at stool and laxative taking in an English population. Dig Dis Sci 1993;38:1004–1008.

360. Lembo A, Camilleri M. Chronic constipation. N Engl J Med 2003;349:1360–1368.

361. Locke GR, III, Pemberton JH, Phillips SF. AGA technical review on constipation. American Gastroenterological Association. Gastroenterology 2000;119:1766–1778.

362. Rao SS. Constipation: evaluation and treatment. Gastroenterol Clin North Am 2003; 32:659–683.

363. Pepin C, Ladabaum U. The yield of lower endoscopy in patients with constipation: survey of a university hospital, a public county hospital, and a Veterans Administration medical center. Gastrointest Endosc 2002;56:325–332.

364. Minguez M, Herreros B, Sanchiz V, Hernandez V, Almela P, Anon R, Mora F, Benages A. Predictive value of the balloon expulsion test for excluding the diagnosis of pelvic floor dyssynergia in constipation. Gastroenterology 2004;126:57–62.

365. Diamant NE, Kamm MA, Wald A, Whitehead WE. AGA technical review on anorectal testing techniques. Gastroenterology 1999;116:735–760.

366. Emmanuel AV, Kamm MA. Laser Doppler flowmetry as a measure of extrinsic colonic innervation in functional bowel disease. Gut 2000;46:212–217.

367. He CL, Burgart L, Wang L, Pemberton J, Young-Fadok T, Szurszewski J, Farrugia G. Decreased interstitial cell of cajal volume in patients with slow-transit constipation. Gastroenterology 2000;118:14–21.

368. El Salhy M, Norrgard O, Spinnell S. Abnormal colonic endocrine cells in patients with chronic idiopathic slow-transit constipation. Scand J Gastroenterol 1999;34: 1007–1011.

369. Kamm MA, Lennard-Jones JE, Thompson DG, Sobnack R, Garvie NW, Granowska M. Dynamic scanning defines a colonic defect in severe idiopathic constipation. Gut 1988;29:1085–1092.

370. Preston DM, Lennard-Jones JE. Severe chronic constipation of young women: 'idiopathic slow transit constipation'. Gut 1986;27:41–48.

371. Gattuso JM, Kamm MA. Clinical features of idiopathic megarectum and idiopathic megacolon. Gut 1997;41:93–99.

372. Mertz H, Naliboff B, Mayer E. Physiology of refractory chronic constipation. Am J Gastroenterology 1999;94:609–615.

373. Voderholzer WA, Schatke W, Muhldorfer BE, Klauser AG, Bickner B, Muller-Lissner SA. Clinical response to dietary fiber treatment of chronic constipation. Am J Gastroenterol 1997;92:95–98.

374. Rao SS, Mudipalli RS, Stessman M, Zimmerman B. Investigation of the utility of colorectal function tests and Rome II criteria in dyssynergic defecation [Anismus]. Neurogastroenterol Motil 2004;16:589–596.

375. Krishnamurthy S, Schuffler MD, Rohrmann CA, Pope CE. Severe idiopathic constipation is associated with a distinctive abnormality of the colonic myenteric plexus. Gastroenterology 1985;88:26–34.

376. Muller-Lissner S, Kamm M, Scarpignato C, Wald A. Myths and misconceptions about chronic constipation. Am J Gastroenterol 2005;100:232–242.

377. Wyman JB, Heaton KW, Manning AP, Wicks AC. The effect on intestinal transit and the feces of raw and cooked bran in different doses. Am J Clin Nutr 1976;29:1474–1479.

378. Klauser AG, Peyeri C, Schindlbeck NE, Muller-Lissner SA. Nutrition and physical activity in chronic constipation. Eur J Gastroenterol Hepatol 1992;4:227–223.
379. Muller-Lissner SA. Effect of wheat bran on weight of stool and gastrointestinal transit time: A meta analysis. Br Med J 1988;296:615–617.
380. Tjeerdsma HC, Smout AJPM, Akkermans LMA. Voluntary suppression of defecation delays gastric emptying. Dig Dis Sci 1993;38:832–836.
381. Glia A, Akerlund JE, Lindberg G. Outcome of colectomy for slow-transit constipation in relation to presence of small-bowel dysmotility. Dis Colon Rectum 2004;47:96–102.
382. Mearin F, Sardi JA, Moreno-Osset E. Traveller's constipation. Am J Gastroenterol 2003;98:507–508.
383. Tucker DM, Sandstead HH, Logan GMJr, Klevay LM, Mahalko J, Johnson LK, Inman L, Inglett GE. Dietary fiber and personality factors as determinants of stool output. Gastroenterology 1981;81:879–883.
384. Almy TP, Hinkle LEJr, Berle B, Kern FJr. Alterations in colonic function in man under stress. III. Experimental production of sigmoid spasm in patients with spastic constipation. Gastroenterology 1949;12:437.
385. Wald A, Hinds JP, Caruana BJ. Psychological and physiological characteristics of patients with severe idiopathic constipation. Gastroenterology 1989;97:932–937.
386. Wald A, Chandra A, Chiponis D, Gabel S. Anorectal function and continence mechanisms in childhood encopresis. J Pediatr Gastroenterol Nutr 1986;5:346–351.
387. Bellman M. Studies on encopresis. Acta Paediatr Scand 1966;56:1–151.
388. Klauser AG, Voderholzer WA, Heinrich CA, Schindlbeck NE, Muller-Lissner SA. Behavioral modification of colonic function: can constipation be learned? Dig Dis Sci 1990;35:1271–1275.
389. Heaton KW, Wood N, Cripps HA, Philipp R. The call to stool and its relationship to constipation: a community study. Eur J Gastroenterol Hepatol 1993;6:145–149.
390. Cummings JH. The effect of dietary fibre on fecal weight and composition. In: Spiller GA, ed. Handbook of dietary fiber in human nutrition. 1 ed. Boca Raton: CRC Press, 1986:211–280.
391. Bannister JJ, Davison P, Timms JM, et al. Effect of stool size on defecation. Gut 1987;28:1246.
392. Tomlin J, Read NW. Laxative effects of indigestible plastic particles. BMJ 1988; 297:1175–1176.
393. Brodribb AJM, Groves C. Effect of bran particle size on stool weight. Gut 1978;19:60–63.
394. Jenkins DJA, Peterson RD, Thorne MJ, Ferguson PW. Wheat fibre and laxation: dose response and equilibration time. Am J Gastroenterol 1987;82:1259–1263.
395. Kumar A, Kumar N, Vij JC. Optimum dosage of isphagula husk in patients with irritable bowel syndrome: Correlation of symptom relief with whole gut transit time and stool weight. Gut 1987;28:150–155.
396. Marlett JA, Buk L, Patrow CJ, Bass P. Comparative laxation of psyllium with and without senna in an ambulatory constipated population. Am J Gastroenterol 1987;82:333–337.
397. Hamilton JW, Wagner J, Burdick DD, Bass P. Clinical evaluation of methylcellulose as a bulk laxative. Dig Dis Sci 1988;33:993–998.
398. Ramkumar D, Rao SS. Efficacy and safety of traditional medical therapies for chronic constipation: systematic review. Am J Gastroenterol 2005;100:936–971.

399. Edwards CA, Tomlin J, Read NW. Fibre and constipation. Br J Clin Pract 1988;42:26–32.

400. Gonlachanvit S, Coleski R, Owyang C, Hasler WL. Inhibitory actions of a high fibre diet on intestinal gut transit in healthy volunteers. Gut 2004;53:1577–1582.

401. Xing JH, Soffer EE. Adverse effects of laxatives. Dis Colon Rectum 2001;44:1201–1209.

402. Jones MP, Talley NJ, Nuyts G, Dubois D. Lack of objective evidence of efficacy of laxatives in chronic constipation. Dig Dis Sci 2002;47:2222–2230.

403. Bass P, Dennis S. The laxative effect of lactulose in normal and constipated subjects. J Clin Gastroenterol 1981;3:23–28.

404. Lederle FA, Busch DL, Mattox KM, West MJ, Aske DM. Cost-effective treatment of constipation in the elderly: a randomized double-blind comparison of sorbitol and lactulose. Am J Med 1990;89:597–601.

405. Passmore AP, Wilson-Davies K, Stoker C, Scott ME. Chronic constipation in long-stay elderly patients: A comparison of lactulose and a senna-fibre combination. Br Med J 1993;303:769–771.

406. Brown RL, Gibson JA, Sladen GE, Hicks B, Dawson AM. Effects of lactulose and other laxatives on ileal and colonic pH as measured by a radiotelemetry device. Gut 1974;15:999–1004.

407. Ernstoff JJ, Howard DA, Marshall JB, Jumshyd A, McCullough AJ. A randomized blinded clinical trial of a rapid colonic lavage solution [Golytely] compared with standard preparation for colonoscopy and barium enema. Gastroenterology 1983;84:1512–1516.

408. Chaussade S, Minic M. Comparison of efficacy and safety of two doses of two different polyethylene glycol-based laxatives in the treatment of constipation. Aliment Pharmacol Ther 2003;17:165–172.

409. Attar A, Lemann M, Ferguson A, Halphen M, Boutron MC, Flourie B, Alix E, Salmeron M, Guillemot F, Chaussade S, Menard AM, Moreau J, Naudin G, Barthet M. Comparison of a low dose polyethylene glycol electrolyte solution with lactulose for treatment of chronic constipation. Gut 1999;44:226–230.

410. Voskuijl W, de Lorijn F, Verwijs W, Hogeman P, Heijmans J, Makel W, Taminiau J, Benninga M. PEG 3350 [Transipeg] versus lactulose in the treatment of childhood functional constipation: a double blind, randomised, controlled, multicentre trial. Gut 2004;53:1590–1594.

411. Mamtami R, Cimino JA, Cooperman JM. Comparison of total costs of administering calcium polycarbophil in an institutional setting. Clinical Therapeutics 1990;12:22–24.

412. Read NW, Krejs GJ, Read MG, Santa Ana CA, Morawski SG, Fordtran JS. Chronic diarrhea of unknown origin. Gastroenterology 1980;78:264–271.

413. Bytzer P, Stockholm M, Andersen I, Klitgaard NA, Schaffalitzky de Muckadell OB. Prevalence of surreptitious laxative abuse in patients with diarrhoea of uncertain origin: a cost benefit analysis of a screening procedure. Gut 1989;30:1379–1384.

414. Balazs M. Melanosis coli. Ultrastructural study of 45 patients. Dis Colon Rectum 1986;28:839–844.

415. Ghadially FN, Parry EW. An electron microscope and histological study of melanosis coli. J Pathol Bacteriol 1966;92:312–317.

416. Speare GS. Melanosis coli: experimental observations on its production and elimination in twenty-three cases. Am J Surg 1951;82:631–637.

417. Gershon MD. Serotonin and its implication for the management of irritable bowel syndrome. Rev Gastroenterol Disord 2003;3 Suppl 2:S25–S34.

418. Grider JR, Foxx-Orenstein AE, Jin JG. 5-Hydroxytryptamine4 receptor agonists initiate the peristaltic reflex in human, rat, and guinea pig intestine. Gastroenterology 1998;115:370–380.

419. Bouras EP, Camilleri M, Burton DD, Thomforde G, McKinzie S, Zinsmeister AR. Prucalopride accelerates gastrointestinal and colonic transit in patients with constipation without a rectal evacuation disorder. Gastroenterology 2001;120:354–360.

420. Prather CM, Camilleri M, Zinsmeister AJ, McKinzie S, Thomforde G. Tegaserod accelerates orocecal transit in patients with constipation-dominant irritable bowel syndrome. Gastroenterology 2000;118:463–468.

421. Johanson Jf, Wald A, Tougas G, Chey WD, Novick JS, Lembo AJ, Fordham F, Guella M, Nault B. Effect of tegaserod in chronic constipation: a randomized, double-blind, controlled trial. Clin Gastroenterol Hepatol 2004;2:796–805.

422. Kamm M, Muller-Lissner S, Talley N, Tack J, Boeckxstaens G, Minushkin O, Kalinin A, Dzieniszewski J, Haeck P, Fordham F, Hugot-Cournez A, Nault B. Tegaserod for the treatment of chronic constipation: a randomized, double-blind, placebo-controlled multinational study. Am J Gastroenterol 2005;100:362–372.

423. Schiller LR. Review article: the therapy of constipation. Aliment Pharmacol Ther 2001;15:749–763.

424. Parkman HP, Rao SS, Reynolds JC, Schiller LR, Wald A, Miner PB, Lembo AJ, Gordon JM, Drossman DA, Waltzman L, Stambler N, Cedarbaum JM. Neurotrophin-3 improves functional constipation. Am J Gastroenterol 2003;98:1338–1347.

425. Snisky C, Verne G, Gordon J, Eaker E, Davis R. Double-blind, placebo-controlled, cross-over study evaluating the effectiveness of colchicine in the treatment of severe constipation. Gastroenterology 114, A839. 1998. Ref Type: Abstract.

426. Mollen RM, Kuijpers HC, Claassen AT. Colectomy for slow-transit constipation: preoperative functional evaluation is important but not a guarantee for a successful outcome. Dis Colon Rectum 2001;44:577–580.

427. Kamm MA, Hawley PR, Lennard-Jones JE. Lateral division of the puborectalis muscle in the management of severe constipation. Br J Surg 1988;75:661–663.

428. Keighley MR, Shouler P. Outlet syndrome: is there a surgical option? J R Soc Med 1984;77:559–563.

429. Talley NJ, Zinsmeister AR, Van Dyke C, Melton III LJ. Epidemiology of colonic symptoms and the irritable bowel syndrome. Gastroenterology 1991;101:927–934.

430. Ho KY, Kang JY, Seow A. Prevalence of gastrointestinal symptoms in a multiracial Asian population, with particular reference to reflux-type symptoms. Am J Gastroenterol 1998;93:1816–1822.

431. Wenzl HH, Fine KD, Schiller LR, Fordtran JS. Determinants of decreased fecal consistency in patients with diarrhea. Gastroenterology 1995;108:1729–1738.

432. Mearin F, Roset M, Badia X, Balboa A, Baro E, Ponce J, Diaz-Rubio M, Caldwell E, Cucala M, Fueyo A, Talley NJ. Splitting irritable bowel syndrome: from original Rome to Rome II criteria. Am J Gastroenterol 2004;99:122–130.

433. Heaton KW, O'Donnell LJD. An office guide to whole gut transit time: patient's recollection of their stool form. J Clin Gastroeterol 1994;19:28–30.

434. Bode C, Bode JC. Effect of alcohol consumption on the gut. Best Pract Res Clin Gastroenterol 2003;17:575–592.

435. Bouchoucha M, Nalpas B, Berger M, Cugnenc PH, Barbier JP. Recovery from dis-

turbed colonic transit time after alcohol withdrawal. Dis Colon Rectum 1991;34:111–114.

436. Vanner SJ, Depew WT, Patterson WG, et al. Predictive values of the Rome criteria for diagnosing irritable bowel syndrome. Am J Gastroenterol 1999;94:2912–2917.

437. Sinha L, Liston R, Testa HJ, Moriarty KJ. Idiopathic bile acid malabsorption: qualitative and quantitative clinical features and response to cholestyramine. Aliment Pharmacol Ther 1998;12:839–844.

438. Bertomeu A, Ros E, Barragan V, Sachje L, Navarro S. Chronic diarrhoea with normal stool and colonic examinations: organic or functional? J Clin Gastro 1991;13:531–536.

439. Tuncer C, Cindoruk M, Dursun A, Karakan T. Prevalence of microscopic colitis in patients with symptoms suggesting irritable bowel syndrome. Acta Gastroenterol Belg 2003;66:133–136.

440. Olesen M, Eriksson S, Bohr J, Jarnerot G, Tysk C. Microscopic colitis: a common diarrhoeal disease. An epidemiological study in Orebro, Sweden, 1993–1998. Gut 2004;53:346–350.

441. Rampton DS, Baithun SI. Is microscopic colitis due to bile-salt malabsorption? Dis Colon Rectum 1987;30:950–952.

442. Williams AJK, Merrick MV, Eastwood MA. Idiopathic bile salt malabsorption—a review of clinical presentation, diagnosis, and response to treatment. Gut 1991;32:1004–1006.

443. Niaz SK, Sandrasegaran K, Renny FH, Jones BJ. Postinfective diarrhoea and bile acid malabsorption. J R Coll Physicians Lond 1997;31:53–56.

444. Arffmann S, Andersen JR, Hegnhoj J, et al. The effect of coarse wheat bran in the irritable bowel syndrome. A double-blind, cross-over study. Scand J Gastroenterol 1985;20:295–298.

445. Cann PA, Read NW, Holdsworth CD. What is the benefit of coarse wheat bran in patients with irritable bowel syndrome? Gut 1984;25:168–173.

446. Bazzocchi G, Ellis J, Villanueva-Meyer J, Reddy SN, Mena I, Snape WJ. Effect of eating on colonic motility and transit in patients with functional diarrhea. Gastroenterology 1991;101:1298–1306.

447. Jian R, Najean Y, Bernier JJ. Measurement of intestinal progression of a meal and its residues in normal subjects and patients with functional diarhea by a dual isotope technique. Gut 1984;25:728–731.

448. Steed KP, Bohemen EK, Lamont GM, Evans DF, Wilson CG, Spiller RC. Proximal colonic response and gastrointestinal transit after high and low fat meals. Dig Dis Sci 1993;38:1793–1800.

449. Rey E, Diaz-Rubio M. Prevalence of rectal hypersensitivity in patients with irritable bowel syndrome and its clinical subgroups. Rev Esp Enferm Dig 2002;94:247–258.

450. Houghton LA, Wych J, Whorwell PJ. Acute diarrhoea induces rectal sensitivity in women but not men. Gut 1995;37:270–273.

451. Cann PA, Read NW, Cammack J, Childs H, Holden S, Kashman R, Longmore J, Nix S, Simms N, Swallow K, Weller J. Psychological stress and the passage of a standard meal through the stomach and small intestine in man. Gut 1983;24:236–240.

452. Chaudhary HR. Study of intestinal transit time in patient with anxiety and depression. J Assoc Physicians India 1989;37:156–157.

453. Gorard DA, Gamberone JE, Libby GW, Farthing MJG. Intestinal transit in anxiety and depression. Gut 1996;39:551–555.

454. Griebel G. Is there a future for neuropeptide receptor ligands in the treatment of anxiety disorders? Pharmacol Ther 1999;82:1–61.

455. Monnikes H, Schmidt BG, Tache Y. Psychological stress-induced accelerated colonic transit in rats involves hypothalamic corticotropin-releasing factor. Gastroenterology 1993;104:716–723.

456. Zigmond AS, Snaith RP. The hospital anxiety and depression scale. Acta Psychiatr Scand 1983;67:361–370.

457. Cummings JH, Branch W, Jenkins DJ, Southgate DA, Houston H, James WP. Colonic response to dietary fibre from carrot, cabbage, apple, bran. Lancet 1978; 1:5–9.

458. Nanda R, James R, Smith H, Dudley CRK, Jewell DP. Food intolerance and the irritable bowel syndrome. Gut 1989;30:1099–1104.

459. Parker T, Naylor S, Riordan A, Hunter J. Management of patients with food intolerance in irritable bowel syndrome: the development and use of an exclusion diet. Journal of Human Nutrition & Dietetics 1995;8:159–166.

460. Symons P, Jones MP, Kellow JE. Symptom provocation in irritable bowel syndrome. Effects of differing doses of fructose-sorbitol. Scand J Gastroenterol 1992;27:940–944.

461. Palmer KR, Corbett CL, Holdsworth CD. Double blind cross-over study comparing loperamide, codeine and diphenoxylate in chronic diarrhea. Gastroenterology 1980;79:1272–1275.

462. Cann PA, Read NW, Holdsworth CD, Barends D. Role of loperamide and placebo in management of irritable bowel syndrome. Dig Dis Sci 1984;29:239–247.

463. Lavo B, Stenstam M, Nielsen A-L. Loperamide in treatment of IBS: a double-blind placebo-controlled study. In: Read NW, ed. Irritable bowel syndrome: pathogenesis and treatment. 1 ed. Sweden: Janssen Pharma AB, 1986:77–80.

464. Afzalpurkar RG, Schiller LR, Little KH, Santangelo WC, Fortran JS. The self-limited nature of chronic idiopathic diarrhoea. New Engl J Med 1992;327:1849–1852.

Chapter 10

Functional Abdominal Pain Syndrome

Ray E. Clouse, Chair

Emeran A. Mayer, Co-Chair

Qasim Aziz

Douglas A. Drossman

Dan L. Dumitrascu

Hubert Mönnikes

Bruce D. Naliboff

D. Functional Abdominal Pain Syndrome

Functional abdominal pain syndrome (FAPS) describes continuous, nearly continuous, or frequently recurrent pain localized to the abdomen but poorly related to gut function. Like other functional gastrointestinal disorders (FGIDs), FAPS cannot be explained by a structural or metabolic disorder using currently available diagnostic methods. This disorder appears highly related to alterations in endogenous pain modulation systems, including dysfunction of descending pain modulation and cortical pain modulation circuits. There is only one recognized diagnosis in this category of functional gastrointestinal disorders (Table 1). Previous editions of the Rome criteria included the diagnosis of unspecified functional abdominal pain [1]. Because of the poor specificity of the criteria and its limited utility, the diagnosis of unspecified functional abdominal pain has been removed from this version.

— Definition

FAPS, also called "chronic idiopathic abdominal pain" and "chronic functional abdominal pain," describes pain attributed to the abdomen that is poorly related to gut function, is associated with some loss of daily activities, and has been present for at least 6 months. The pain is constant, nearly constant, or at least frequently recurring. FAPS is distinguished from other painful FGIDs, such as irritable bowel syndrome (IBS) and functional dyspepsia, primarily by the poor relationship of pain with food intake or defecation and from chronic pelvic pain by its abdominal location—although there will be some overlap in subject groups with FAPS and these other conditions. This disorder commonly is associated with a tendency to experience and report other unpleasant somatic symptoms. Psychological comorbidities, such as depression and anxiety, are more likely when pain is persistent over a long period of time, is associated with chronic pain behaviors, and/or dominates the patient's life [1]. FAPS would qualify as a somatoform pain disorder and satisfy a pain criterion toward the diagnosis of somatization disorder in psychiatric nosology [2].

— Epidemiology

The epidemiology of FAPS is incompletely known because of limited available data and methodological difficulties in establishing a diagnosis, especially one that is distinct from IBS. FAPS appears to be an uncommon condition with descriptions often restricted to case reports [3]. Although many studies have

Table 1. Functional Gastrointestinal Disorders

A. Functional Esophageal Disorders

A1. Functional heartburn
A2. Functional chest pain of presumed esophageal origin
A3. Functional dysphagia
A4. Globus

B. Functional Gastroduodenal Disorders

B1. Functional dyspepsia
  B1a. Postprandial distress syndrome (PDS)
  B1b. Epigastric pain syndrome (EPS)
B2. Belching disorders
  B2a. Aerophagia
  B2b. Unspecified excessive belching
B3. Nausea and vomiting disorders
  B3a. Chronic idiopathic nausea (CIN)
  B3b. Functional vomiting
  B3c. Cyclic vomiting syndrome (CVS)
B4. Rumination syndrome in adults

C. Functional Bowel Disorders

C1. Irritable bowel syndrome (IBS)
C2. Functional bloating
C3. Functional constipation
C4. Functional diarrhea
C5. Unspecified functional bowel disorder

D. Functional Abdominal Pain Syndrome (FAPS)

E. Functional Gallbladder and Sphincter of Oddi (SO) Disorders

E1. Functional gallbladder disorder
E2. Functional biliary SO disorder
E3. Functional pancreatic SO disorder

F. Functional Anorectal Disorders

F1. Functional fecal incontinence
F2. Functional anorectal pain
  F2a. Chronic proctalgia
    F2a1. Levator ani syndrome
    F2a2. Unspecified functional anorectal pain
  F2b. Proctalgia fugax
F3. Functional defecation disorders
  F3a. Dyssynergic defecation
  F3b. Inadequate defecatory propulsion

G. Functional Disorders: Neonates and Toddlers

G1. Infant regurgitation
G2. Infant rumination syndrome
G3. Cyclic vomiting syndrome
G4. Infant colic
G5. Functional diarrhea
G6. Infant dyschezia
G7. Functional constipation

H. Functional Disorders: Children and Adolescents

H1. Vomiting and aerophagia
  H1a. Adolescent rumination syndrome
  H1b. Cyclic vomiting syndrome
  H1c. Aerophagia
H2. Abdominal pain-related FGIDs
  H2a. Functional dyspepsia
  H2b. Irritable bowel syndrome
  H2c. Abdominal migraine
  H2d. Childhood functional abdominal pain
    H2d1. Childhood functional abdominal pain syndrome
H3. Constipation and incontinence
  H3a. Functional constipation
  H3b. Nonretentive fecal incontinence

detailed the epidemiology of abdominal pain in general and of IBS in particular, few studies focus exclusively on FAPS. Abdominal pain frequently is produced by or attributed to nondigestive organs, such as those in the urinary or gynecological systems, and disorders in these locations must be excluded before the diagnosis of FAPS can be established. Likewise, chronic abdominal wall pain can be confused with FAPS [4, 5]. The lack of additional symptoms to add security to a symptom-based diagnosis of FAPS combined with the extensive differential diagnosis and difficulties in verifying adequate exclusionary work-up have interfered with establishing the epidemiology of this disorder.

Other methodological problems impair accurate identification of FAPS in the general population. Collecting data by postal or telephone survey is a valuable method but can be biased by patients' tendencies toward overestimation of symptoms. Variations in survey tools and health care-seeking behaviors [6] also may bias the collected data. Likewise, the term FAPS as used today was coined relatively recently [7], making collation of data from retrospective literature reviews difficult. Singular symptoms like bloating or abdominal pain often were labeled as colitis [8], limiting historical data on FAPS. Despite these limitations, some recent data are available regarding the prevalence of the disorder.

FAPS is considered less common than other FGIDs, such as functional heartburn, functional dyspepsia or IBS. The best available prevalence data were supplied by a US householders survey [9]. In this self-report investigation, the prevalence of chronic abdominal pain was 2.2%. Only half of the patients reporting chronic abdominal pain had visited a physician for the symptom. The national estimate for the US was 1.7% (95% confidence interval 1.3–2.2%) [9]. Because of the self-report method used, the true prevalence likely is lower. In a large Canadian survey [10], the prevalence of FAPS was 0.5%. Unspecified functional abdominal pain, a subthreshold form of FAPS, or a preliminary diagnosis described in previous versions of the Rome criteria, was found at a rate of 2.1%. This figure is not significantly different from the prevalence rate extracted from the US householders survey [9], wherein the diagnosis of unspecified functional abdominal pain was not segregated from the total group diagnosed with chronic abdominal pain. Results from other countries vary with methods used but generally suggest similarly low rates of FAPS when patients also meeting criteria for IBS are removed from consideration [11–13].

In the US householders survey, the diagnosis of FAPS was more common in women (F:M=1.5) [9]. In the Canadian study [10], FAPS was reported at similar rates by men and women, but unspecified functional abdominal pain was twice as common in women as men. Associations of FAPS with phases of the menstrual cycle, as have been described in IBS [14], have not been reported. Available data indicate that prevalence of FAPS reaches a peak in the fourth decade of life (35–44 years in the US householders survey) and decreases in later age [9, 15].

Patients with FAPS have high health care resource use and impose a significant economic burden. In the US householders survey, respondents with FAPS visited a medical doctor an average of 1.52 times in the previous year for abdominal pain and 5.66 times for nondigestive symptoms [9]. In the same survey, patients with FAPS visited a physician four times more frequently than people without abdominal complaints. In the Australian study, 75.9% of the subjects with FAPS had consulted a physician, and about half of them saw physicians 1 to 3 times a year [11]. Maxton and Whorwell showed that these patients required 5.7 consultant visits, completed 6.4 endoscopic or imaging investigations, and underwent 2.7 surgical interventions (primarily hysterectomy and exploratory laparotomy) over a follow-up period of 7 years [16]. In the US, FAPS patients missed work an average of 11.8 days in the previous year, three times more than subjects without abdominal symptoms, and felt too sick to go to work at the moment of the survey in 11.2% of cases, about three times more frequently than respondents without FGIDs [9]. The amount of work absenteeism likely correlates with perceived pain intensity in FAPS as it does in IBS, although this has not been studied specifically [17]. Some of the epidemiological findings in FAPS may be influenced by the presence of IBS patients in the study populations, but investigators attempted to exclude these patients from consideration.

Familial clustering of FAPS has not been investigated. Family data may be influenced by or reflect psychiatric comorbidity that commonly is present in patients with FAPS [3, 11, 18, 19]. In psychiatric classification, FAPS would qualify as a somatoform pain disorder and satisfy a pain criterion toward the diagnosis of somatization disorder [2]. As such, familial aggregation would be expected [20]. Among the somatoform disorders as identified by the International Classification of Disease (ICD)-10, functional pain disorder (including pain centered at any segment of the body) has a prevalence of up to 12% in the general population, 5% to 7% in general practice, and up to 30% in specialized pain ambulatory centers in Germany [21, 22].

D. Diagnostic Criteria* for Functional Abdominal Pain Syndrome

Must include *all* of the following:
1. **Continuous or nearly continuous abdominal pain**
2. **No or only occasional relationship of pain with physiological events (e.g., eating, defecation, or menses)**
3. **Some loss of daily functioning**
4. **The pain is not feigned (e.g., malingering)**
5. **Insufficient symptoms to meet criteria for another functional gastrointestinal disorder that would explain the pain**

*Criteria fulfilled for the last 3 months with symptom onset at least 6 months prior to diagnosis

— Rationale for Changes from Previous Criteria

Studies determining the reliability of these criteria in identifying a homogeneous population are lacking, and subjects with various different explanations for pain (particularly chronic pain attributed to pelvic viscera) may be represented [23]. Lack of or very limited relationship of pain in FAPS with physiological events such as altered bowel function separates this diagnosis from the functional bowel disorders. Qualifiers in the diagnostic criteria (e.g., "occasional," "some") remain subjectively defined. The requirements for some loss of daily functioning and for pain that is not feigned are derived from the diagnostic criteria for somatization disorder and undifferentiated somatoform disorder as stated in the Diagnostic and Statistical Manual of Mental Disorders, Fourth Edition (DSM-IV) [2]. These diagnoses encompass, from a psychiatric standpoint, physical symptoms that suggest a medical condition but are not fully explained by such a condition, cause clinically significant distress or impairment in functioning, and are not intentional. The time requirement for the diagnosis of FAPS was adjusted to match the criteria used across the FGIDs. For a description of and diagnostic criteria for functional abdominal pain in children, refer to Chapters 13 and 14.

— Clinical Evaluation

A host of disorders can produce chronic abdominal pain, and the clinician should be aware of the extended differential diagnosis [24]. Algorithms to manage FAPS are empirical, as objective scientific evidence to support a singular approach does not exist. It is suggested that evaluation consist of a clinical/psychosocial assessment, observation of symptom-reporting behaviors, a physical examination, and—in the absence of alarm features—conservative efforts to exclude other medical conditions in a cost-effective manner. Notably, for patients meeting diagnostic criteria for FAPS who exhibit a long-standing history of pain behaviors and certain psychosocial correlates, the clinical evaluation usually fails to disclose any other specific medical etiology to explain the illness [25]. However, the evaluation incidentally may identify other medical conditions of uncertain relation to the presentation (e.g., hepatic cysts in a patient with chronic right upper quadrant pain). Efforts then must be directed toward understanding the relative contributions of FAPS and the elicited findings or diagnoses to the pain reported. A number of clinical and behavioral features typify but are not specific for FAPS. Their presence may aid in the planning of diagnostic testing and are essential to designing the treatment approach.

Clinical/Psychosocial Assessment

By answering a few questions the physician effectively can appraise the clinical features of FAPS, identify the key psychosocial contributions to the disorder, and increase confidence in the diagnosis [25, 26]:

1. *What is the patient's life history of illness?* A long (more than 2-year) history of painful complaints and frequent health care visits for poorly documented diagnoses (e.g., "adhesions," "gastroenteritis") predicts a poorer prognosis [27]. Conversely, a brief symptom history, particularly in an individual who does not report other past illnesses, often requires a more directed search for other pain causes and has a better prognosis. A history of other chronic pain conditions (e.g., fibromyalgia, pelvic pain, headaches, and back pain) also should be sought.

2. *Why is the patient presenting now for medical care?* The long-term nature of this disorder (averaging 7 years in most case series) [16] makes it inefficient (and often unnecessary) to elicit a detailed history of all exacerbations, visits, and hospitalizations. However it is important to learn the circumstances relating to the first and other major presentations and the reason for the current visit. Visits may occur because of (a) increased concern about having a serious disease (e.g., a relative recently being diagnosed with cancer), (b) environmental stressors, (c) worsening of functional status, (d) a "hidden agenda" (e.g., seeking narcotics, litigation, acquiring disability status, or legitimization of illness to family or co-workers), (e) exacerbation of co-morbid psychiatric disturbance, or (f) any combination of these factors. At times the association of a particular stressor with illness exacerbation or a visit may be evident to the physician but not to the patient.

3. *Is there a history of traumatic life events?* Traumatic events can include childhood or adult emotional, sexual, or physical abuse, death or divorce within the family, or losses of personal impact including abortion, stillbirth, or hysterectomy. These events commonly occur in patients with FGIDs and independently predict a poorer clinical outcome [28]). Therefore, when a history of FAPS is being considered, the physician should explore these possibilities; the manner in which the history is elicited is detailed elsewhere [29]. If this history is obtained, the physician must appraise the patient's willingness to explore this issue further, usually with a mental health professional, to optimize proper treatment and the opportunity for clinical improvement [29].

4. *What is the patient's understanding of the illness?* When the patient's illness beliefs are consistent with the physician's understanding (e.g., a chronic "mind-body" disorder with psychosocial contributions to illness exacerbations), a mutual treatment plan easily is developed. However, when these

beliefs markedly differ or the patient's goals are unachievable (e.g., to "find the organic cause and obtain cure"), effective treatment requires addressing and negotiating these differences.

5. *What is the impact of the pain on activities and quality of life?* Diagnostic and treatment decisions are determined primarily by the patient's functioning and quality of life rather than by the severity of pain reported. Some important questions to ask include "How much is this affecting (the quality of) your life?" or "What would you do differently if you did not have this pain?"

6. *Is there an associated psychiatric diagnosis?* Up to 60% of patients with FAPS may have comorbid psychiatric diagnoses that specifically are treatable (e.g., Axis I depressive or anxiety disorders), or which are less treatable and which may interfere with the conduct of the care (e.g., Axis II personality disorders or substance abuse) [30]. However, by being aware of these possible diagnoses, the physician possibly can improve the care or in the least modify his or her treatment approach in a way that is more gratifying [31]. Psychiatric disorders may be diagnosed through psychological referral or with standardized symptom criteria (e.g., DSM-IV) [2].

7. *What is the role of family or culture?* Usually, family interactions around a patient's illness produce emotional support, and the focus is toward recovery. With dysfunctional family interactions, stresses are managed poorly, and the illness may in fact be adaptive as a means to divert family distress [32]. This is apparent when the spouse or parent indulges the patient, assumes undue responsibility in the management, or becomes the patient's spokesperson. During office visits it helps to spend separate time with the patient and then later see the family together, during which time communication occurs primarily with the patient. At times, the physician may suggest counseling to help the family develop better coping strategies around the illness. Cultural belief systems also will affect how the pain is reported and how the patient responds to treatment. For example, open recognition of psychological difficulties is stigmatized in Asian cultures, but physical symptoms are sanctioned socially [33], whereas communication of emotion is more acceptable socially in Italian and Jewish cultures [34]. Importantly, patients may not comply with treatments inconsistent with their cultural beliefs.

8. *What are the patient's psychosocial impairments and resources?* Maladaptive (e.g., emotion-based) coping styles are impairments commonly seen in FAPS and are associated with poorer health status, greater pain reports, and poorer clinical outcomes [35]. These include "catastrophizing" or perceived hopelessness and sense of poor control over the illness. Such factors are amenable particularly to psychological interventions such as cognitive-behavioral treatments [36]. Conversely, the availability of social networks

Table 2. Symptom-Related Behaviors Often Seen in Patients with FAPS

– *Expressing pain of varying intensity through verbal and nonverbal methods*; may diminish when the patient is engaged in distracting activities, but increase when discussing a psychologically distressing issue or during examination

– *Urgent reporting of intense symptoms* disproportionate to available clinical and laboratory data (e.g., always rating the pain as "10" on a scale from 1 to 10)

– *Minimizing or denying a role for psychosocial contributors*, or of evident anxiety or depression, or attributing them to the presence of the pain rather than to understandable life circumstances

– *Requesting diagnostic studies* or even exploratory surgery to validate the condition as "organic"

– *Focusing attention on complete relief of symptoms* rather than adaptation to a chronic disorder

– *Seeking health care* frequently

– *Taking limited personal responsibility for self-management*, while placing high expectations on the physician to achieve symptom relief

– *Making requests for narcotic analgesics* when other treatment options have been implemented

---

such as family, church, recreational clubs, and community organizations, as well as effective (problem-based) coping strategies help to buffer the adverse effects of stress and improve outcome [37].

Observations of Symptom Reporting and Behaviors

A variety of symptom features and behaviors have been observed in patients with FAPS. The pain may be described (a) in emotional terms, e.g., as "nauseating" or "like a knife stabbing" [27]; (b) as constant and not influenced by eating or defecation indicating little or no relationship to disturbances in gut activity; (c) as involving a large anatomic area rather than a precise location; (d) as one of several other painful symptoms; and (e) as a continuum of painful experiences beginning in childhood or recurring over time. While there are symptom-related behaviors that typify FAPS (Table 2), they are neither sensitive nor specific and have limited diagnostic value. These behaviors usually are considered maladaptive but modifiable by physicians or mental health professionals [25]. Requests for narcotic analgesics may result from beliefs that there are no other effective treatments, or that the drugs are a means of achieving a level of control over the condition.

FAPS can have a profound impact on the family. In turn, and for better or worse, the family's interaction with the patient can have major impact on the illness. On occasion, a spouse or parent may assume responsibility for reporting the patient's history, possibly interrupting the patient's commentary, or prioritizing the discussion. This may lead the patient either to engage in a competitive discussion or more passively withdraw. While the partner's behavior may reflect a degree of concern and desire to be involved, it may also reflect family dysfunction that can interfere with implementing an effective treatment strategy, unless the needs of all parties are considered and addressed. It is important that the physician allow sufficient time to the patient in such cases, and a large part of the visit should be conducted with the patient alone.

Physical Examination

The physical examination does not establish a diagnosis of FAPS, and only rarely does it identify other etiologies in chronic pain patients. Nevertheless, it is essential in a comprehensive office evaluation of chronic abdominal pain and has several important roles. First, there is no substitute for examining the patient to clarify pain location and radiation patterns. Additionally, in the previously uninvestigated patient, important physical findings can direct the diagnostic workup and may expeditiously lead to an underlying cause (e.g., abdominal wall pain). Clues favoring or disfavoring a diagnosis of FAPS are derived both from the abdominal evaluation and from other components of the physical examination. In the patient with previously unrevealing diagnostic studies, the physical examination is not only useful in focusing further testing, if required, but also provides a valuable opportunity for eliciting symptoms supporting a functional diagnosis and for understanding the emotional impact of pain for that patient.

Although a limited, focused physical examination is essential for all patients in the course of their evaluations, attention to particular diagnostic possibilities and appropriate extension of the examination is directed by the medical history. Historical features are important in differentiating somatoparietal from visceral pain, the former typically described with detailed characterization and localization of painful stimuli, the latter being more diffusely localized, vague, and typical of FAPS. The examination should evaluate carefully abdominal wall structures and neuropathic possibilities if somatoparietal features are suspected. Likewise, other features of the presentation, including associated symptoms and exacerbating or ameliorating factors, might suggest referred pain and alter the focus of the examination. Needless to say, the physical examination rarely stands alone in evaluating the patient with chronic abdominal pain, but when integrated with other available information, it can be an important contributor to the ultimate management plan.

Table 3. Features Detected During Physical Examination
that Support the Diagnosis of FAPS

Feature	Implication
No autonomic arousal	Tachycardia, hypertension, or diaphoresis are expected in acute pain and in presentations related to structural pain causes
Abdominal surgical scars [10]	Multiple scars related to surgical procedures with unclear indications suggest prolonged and severe pain and pain behaviors leading to unneeded procedures
"Closed-eyes sign" [11]	Wincing with closed eyes during abdominal examination in FAPS is unlike open eyes with fearful anticipation expressed by patients with acute pain or structural pain
"Stethoscope sign"	Palpation with the stethoscope reduces behavioral response to pain and affords more accurate appraisal of visceral sensory activity; pain reporting is reduced paradoxically during this maneuver in FAPS

General Observations

Evidence of fever or weight loss and other constitutional signs should be noted. "Alarm signs" of this type are considered sufficient to prompt a diagnostic investigation even when historical features otherwise suggest a functional diagnosis [38]. Patient behavior can be correlated with the degree of stated pain to pair a measure of disability with the level of symptom reporting. For example, reports of "severe, constant pain" can be compared with the patient's ability to move around the room or onto the examination table. The examination should be used to carefully identify pain location, as pain location is one of the most important pieces of information used in formulating the differential diagnosis and directing an investigative work-up [39]. Some general features that can be observed in FAPS during physical examination are listed in Table 3.

During the physical examination, efforts can be made to further clarify the nature of the pain and uncover additional symptoms. In one series, features supporting the diagnosis of IBS were extracted in fully 38% of patients during this component of the office encounter, leading to a diagnosis other than FAPS [40]. Poor eye contact and other emotional behaviors can help identify an unsuspected level of hostility, low self-esteem, mistrust, anxiety, or distress. These features help establish the patient's emotional attitude toward the problem or in communication with others (e.g., authority figures); thus, a supportive and nonjudgmental effort should be made to allow the patient to describe his or her feelings associated with the symptom. Understanding the emotional impact of the symptom, as well as simply performing a physical examination, are considered two of the essential steps toward providing effective reassurance—a therapeutic approach ultimately required in many cases of FAPS and other painful FGIDs [41, 42].

Abdominal Examination

The abdominal examination is an essential part of the initial assessment of a patient with chronic abdominal pain and can provide clues supporting the diagnosis of many organic diseases. Even when no structural explanation is detected, "laying on of the hands" may have therapeutic advantages [43]. Few of the components of the abdominal examination discussed below have been tested for sensitivity or specificity in patients presenting with chronic pain. Their usefulness derives largely from the fact that they enhance the likelihood of specific diagnoses and lead to the most appropriate next test.

A complete physical examination is defined as one that pursues all clues obtained from the medical history and other data available on presentation. During the examination it is necessary to look for extra-abdominal signs of abdominal disorders or for signs of diseases that can present with abdominal symptoms. The examination of the abdomen should be thorough in all patients and performed with the anatomy completely exposed. In most cases the examination should extend to the thorax, as evaluation of ribs, spine, and nervous system in that region may be necessary. Inspection, auscultation, percussion, and palpation all may provide information favoring diagnoses other than FAPS, but, of these, palpation is the most useful. During the inspection phase, the patient should be asked to select the location of greatest pain with one finger. Inability to do so provides evidence against a somatoparietal cause and may favor a functional diagnosis.

Palpation should begin at areas remote from the painful site. All regions should be examined, noting warmth, masses, guarding, tenderness, and organ abnormalities. Patient behavior during palpation and change in exam with distraction should be noted (Table 3). Guarding refers to contraction of abdominal wall muscles and can be either voluntary or involuntary. The latter is more suggestive of structural disease, but voluntary guarding does not exclude this possibility. If fullness or mass effect is detected, distinguishing intra-abdominal from abdominal wall disorders requires that the supine patient relax with the thighs partially flexed at the hips. Extending the thighs while raising the head to the chest will contract abdominal muscles. An intra-abdominal source is favored if the findings increase with abdominal wall relaxation (Fothergill's sign).

Other maneuvers are used to detect tenderness in retroperitoneal or pelvic regions not as approachable by anterior abdominal examination. The *obturator sign* is elicited by flexing the thigh and rotating it through its full range of motion; resultant hypogastric pain suggests inflammation in the lower pelvis. The *psoas sign* is detected by having the patient fully extend the thigh while lying on the side opposite the pain. Inflammation of the iliopsoas muscle group is suggested if pain is sensed in the low back or flank (not anteriorly near the iliac spine). *Rebound tenderness* is an overused and misunderstood maneuver, its purpose being to detect peritoneal inflammation. Involuntary abdominal rigidity from generalized inflammation interferes with this maneuver, but identifying focal peritonitis is more important in chronic pain evaluations. The maneuver begins with slow and deep palpation at a point remote from the area of pain. With rapid release of the pressure, pain is reproduced at its original site, suggesting focal peritoneal involvement. It is rarely useful to begin the maneuver with pressure over the most tender site; pain will typically worsen in a nonspecific fashion. Rebound tenderness is less specific than direct local tenderness for focal inflammatory processes, such as acute appendicitis, and pain sensitivity often is diffuse in FAPS and other painful FGIDs [44]. Consequently, rebound tenderness must be interpreted with caution. Palpation for organs should be routine. The aorta frequently is neglected during abdominal examination for pain, yet nearly one third of aneurysms can be detected by palpation [45].

Examination of the anterior abdominal wall should be included in any careful evaluation. Subcutaneous tissues can be lifted and palpated separately from the underlying muscle. Tenderness elicited when the patient is supine should be reassessed while the patient tenses abdominal muscles by raising the head and trunk or lower extremities off the examining table. If tenderness remains the same or increases with this maneuver, abdominal wall pain can be invoked (Carnett's test) [5]. Abdominal wall pain often is due to functional causes [46–48], but sensitivity of the test is low [47]. Focal abdominal wall tenderness also is seen with organic causes, such as spigelian hernias, panniculitis, nerve entrapment syndrome, neuromas, and rectus sheath hematomas. Neuropathic pain can be suspected from dermatomal distribution and allodynia (pain from a non-noxious stimulus, such as light touching or rubbing). Severe pain from neuropathic causes also can be present at a site that is either numb or insensate. Residual signs from previous herpetic lesions should be sought on affected dermatomal regions. The focused physical examination of a patient presenting with chronic abdominal pain should include a digital rectal examination and visual inspection of the perineum.

Focused Extra-abdominal Exam

Many systemic illnesses that originate in or involve gastrointestinal organs produce chronic abdominal pain. These same disorders may result in inflammation or infiltration of extra-abdominal organs, such as skin, eyes, lymph nodes, or joints. Some disorders involving single thoracic organs adjacent to the diaphragm (e.g., cardiac ischemia, lower lobe pulmonary processes) also can produce a chronic abdominal pain presentation. The skin and mouth should be examined carefully for ulcers, angiomata, bleeding or bruising, dryness, vesicles, erythema, or edema. Examination of the bones and joints, especially around the pelvic girdle and low back, can provide clues to a skeletal origin of pain that was incorrectly attributed to abdominal organs.

Some abdominal causes of chronic abdominal pain involve only those nerves innervating abdominal organs, and general neurological examination is not helpful (e.g., chronic idiopathic intestinal pseudo-obstruction, IBS, FAPS). However, a thorough neurological examination may detect conditions that involve somatic and autonomic nerves in more diffuse manner. Both motor weakness and somatic sensory involvement typically are found in acute porphyrias [49]. Autonomic dysfunction (e.g., postural hypotension) and peripheral neuropathy are found in diabetes mellitus and in some patients with malignancies, but attributing abdominal pain directly to the neuropathic condition must be done with caution. Thoracic disc herniation can present as chronic abdominal pain [50]. Abdominal pain also can accompany some overt neurological disorders, such as spinal cord injury, in which the deficit appears obvious, but the association with abdominal pain is appreciated less easily [51].

Exclusion of Other Disease

The physician should exclude pain etiologies other than FAPS in a cost-effective manner [26], and pursue abnormalities detected during a prudent screening evaluation. The concept of "alarm signs" or "red flags" has helped validate the positive predictive value of symptom-based criteria for IBS [52] and can be applied with FAPS. Abnormalities on physical examination or screening laboratory studies (e.g., anemia, high sedimentation rate, low serum albumin, or occult fecal blood) or evidence of significant weight loss should precipitate further investigation. In the absence of alarm features or screening abnormalities and in the presence of long-standing stable symptoms, the diagnosis of FAPS is highly probable if all criteria for this diagnosis have been met. In such cases, reassurance of the diagnosis and symptomatic treatment should be followed by reassessment in 3 to 6 weeks [53]. Variable effort is required to determine the relevance of nonspecific physical findings and laboratory, endoscopic, or imaging results, depending on the finding.

— Physiological Features

Human pain is a conscious experience with several interrelated dimensions: a sensory-afferent component, multiple modulatory components (emotional and cognitive factors), and a motivational component (behavioral responses). From a pathophysiological viewpoint it can be categorized into nociceptive pain (in response to an injury), inflammatory pain (in response to tissue inflammation), and neuropathic pain (generated by nervous-system alterations—central or peripheral, not necessarily in the presence of ongoing tissue injury or inflammation) [54]. Even though several clinical characteristics of FAPS are consistent with a neuropathic pain condition, with important alterations in modulatory and motivational pain dimensions, it is likely that patients with FAPS represent a heterogeneous group of disorders with variable combinations of these features. Since no definitive neurophysiological studies (functional brain imaging studies, nerve studies) have been reported in FAPS patients, the following discussion focuses on plausible mechanisms based on characteristic symptoms and neurophysiological concepts derived from preclinical and clinical studies in patient populations with various chronic pain conditions. (Also see Chapter 3.)

Evidence for Neuropathic Pain

The fact that symptoms are reported as constant and unrelated to such peripheral events as food intake or defecation suggests that phasic, physiological visceral afferent input from the gut plays an insignificant role in symptom generation. These observations, along with the common responsiveness of FAPS symptoms to low-dose tricyclic antidepressants, point toward neuropathic pain as a likely pathophysiological process. Both peripheral and central mechanisms of neuropathic pain have been reported [55]. Unfortunately, neither the characteristically enlarged pain referral areas nor the response to tricyclic antidepressants (which work on both peripheral and central neuropathic pain conditions) make it possible to differentiate between these possibilities. In a subgroup of patients, peripheral neuropathic pain conditions resulting from various types of nerve injury (related to ectopic activity in somatic or visceral afferent nerves) could provide ongoing afferent input to the spinal cord, keeping it in a constant state of central sensitization [55]. Such nerve injury could result from abdominal surgeries or injuries to pelvic nerves during pregnancy or delivery. However, once central sensitization is established, symptoms can persist in the absence of ongoing abnormal peripheral stimulation or worsen with minimal stimulation. An important role of genetic factors in the predisposition to develop peripheral neuropathic pain is suggested by animal models, indicating that preexisting factors separate from the degree of neural injury may influence these processes [56].

Evidence for Alterations in Descending Pain Modulation

The clinical observations that there is significant comorbidity of FAPS with psychiatric disorders (in particular anxiety, depression, and somatization), and that chronic abdominal pain is common in major depressive disorder, suggest a prominent role of altered brain modulation of pain (cognitive or emotional). This does not exclude the possibility that, as in other neuropathic pain condi-

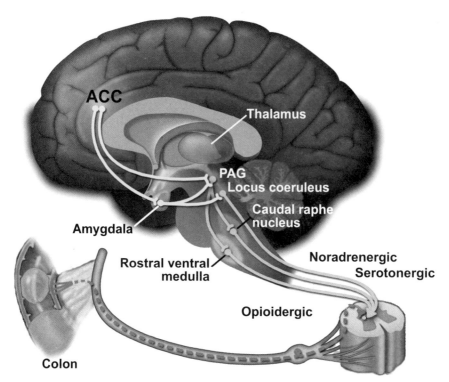

Figure 1. Descending inhibitory pathway for visceral pain. ACC = anterior cingulate cortex; PAG = periaqueductal gray (From Reference 26)

tions, peripheral factors play a role in initiating or perpetuating this chronic pain state; scientific evidence to support such a mechanism in FAPS, however, is not available. Brain mechanisms that are involved in the modulation of the pain experience include phasic pain modulation systems (both inhibitory and facilitatory) [57–59] that are engaged in response to noxious stimuli, and tonic modulation systems that are unrelated to acute noxious stimuli, but reflect the general homeostatic state of the organism [60]. The former includes preattentive and attentive hypervigilance as well as endogenous descending facilitatory and inhibitory pain modulation systems.

Descending pain modulation systems (i.e., opioidergic and noradrenergic pathways) originate in distinct brainstem regions and are activated automatically in a reflex-like fashion in response to a noxious stimulus (Figure 1). They modulate spinal cord (dorsal horn) excitability and thereby can determine how much of peripheral afferent input from the gut is allowed to ascend to the brain. Descending inhibitory systems can be diffuse (e.g., when activated by a specific noxious stimulus they can inhibit pain sensitivity throughout the body), and are designated as diffuse noxious inhibitory control (DNIC) [56]. Alternatively, these systems can be limited to attenuate the sensitivity to the noxious stimulus. It has been speculated that patients with chronic pain syndromes, including fibromyalgia and FAPS, may have a compromised ability to activate DNICs or exhibit an imbalance between facilitatory and inhibitory systems [61–62].

Tonic descending pain modulation systems originate from serotonergic nuclei in the brainstem and play a role in the central control of basal spinal cord excitability. They determine basal pain sensitivity even in the absence of a noxious stimulus. Activity of these systems is related to the general behavioral state of the organism, including mood and sleep-wake cycle, and to other homeostatic functions, such as thermoregulation and sexual function [60]. The involvement of decreased central serotonergic signaling in many psychiatric disorders—depression, in particular—suggests that the link between chronic pain conditions (including FAPS) and depression may be related to inadequate activity of these descending serotonergic pain modulation systems.

Corticolimbic and Corticopontine Pain Modulation Circuits

Cortical regions have well-documented connections to brain regions involved in pain modulation. Based on functional brain imaging studies, it has been suggested that different cortical regions have the ability to modulate the automatic spinal-bulbo-spinal pain modulation loops described above [63]. While lateral prefrontal cortical regions have been shown to exert primarily an inhibitory effect on pain perception, dorsomedial prefrontal cortical regions and subregions of the anterior cingulate cortex may be involved in cortical pain facilitation [64].

The belief systems and coping styles characteristically seen in FAPS patients (attention focused on symptoms, "catastrophizing," denial of psychosocial factors) are consistent with the possibility of altered influences of cortical networks (including prefrontal and parietal cortical regions) on pain modulation circuits [65]. The involvement of similar brain regions (anterior insular cortex, anterior cingulate cortex, medial prefrontal regions and amygdala) and circuits for both pain modulation [66] and emotional state [67] could be the basis for emotional characterizations of pain in FAPS. It also could explain the relationship of pain with symptom-related fears and anxiety.

Relationship of Pathological Stress and Trauma with FAPS

Clinical evidence suggests that there is a strong association of aversive early life events and certain types of psychosocial stressors, with increased pain reports among patients with FGIDs [68]. The relationship between early aversive life events and adult stress with visceral hypersensitivity also has been demonstrated in rodent models [69]. The combination of genetic factors, vulnerability factors, and adult stress may determine in part the effectiveness of endogenous pain modulation systems and thereby influence development of FAPS.

— Psychological Features

Relationship of Psychiatric Disorders and FAPS

Population- and patient-based studies have confirmed the significant association between chronic abdominal pain and affective disorders, especially anxiety and depression. For example, Bixo et al. [70] reported increased anxiety and depression in patients presenting to an obstetrics and gynecology clinic if the chief complaint was abdominal pain. Von Korff et al. [71], in a large random survey of enrollees attending a health maintenance organization, reported that abdominal pain and headache were associated significantly with mood disturbance; the level of family stress also was associated significantly with abdominal pain and facial pain. Halder et al. [72] in a one year prospective study found that psychological distress, fatigue, health anxiety, and illness behavior were predictors of future onset of abdominal pain rather than merely a consequence of symptoms.

Symptom-specific anxiety has been proposed recently as having a more direct influence on pain than general anxiety [73], and this construct also has been investigated in FGIDs including abdominal pain [74]. A measure of visceral-specific anxiety has been developed [75]. In addition to the presence of anxiety and depression, several other psychiatric diagnostic categories have been associated with FAPS. Abdominal pain patients seldom fit the criteria for a factitious disorder or malingering, but the syndrome does overlap with the psychiatric diagnosis of somatoform pain disorder (pain disorder associated with psychological factors) in the DSM-IV, wherein symptoms are localized to the abdomen [2]. Lack of the relationship between bowel activity and pain, differentiating IBS from FAPS, appears to indicate greater psychological dysfunction and contribution to the syndrome. When FAPS coexists with other structural or functional medical conditions, the patient may be classified as having "pain disorder associated with a general medical condition" [2]. The syndrome also may be seen with other somatoform disorders (e.g., somatization disorder, conversion disorder, hypochondriasis) [2]. In a study of somatization disorder identified in a primary care population, abdominal pain was present in 30% of subjects and was the third most frequent somatic symptom (following headache and back pain) [76].

Other Psychological Features and FAPS

Psychological disturbance and impaired quality of life are increased if abdominal pain is associated with presence of nonpainful somatic symptoms (e.g., faintness or dizziness, trouble getting your breath, feeling weak) [18]. Presence of widespread pain also is an important factor in predicting psychological disturbance. In a prospective study of the relationship between primary care visits over 25 years and current chronic pain problems, Howel et al. [18] reported that while all regional pain complaints were somewhat associated with prior mental health problems, the association was strongest for widespread pain. Interestingly, abdominal pain was most closely associated with prior history of intestinal complaints, showing some specificity of complaints over time.

As with most chronic pain conditions, there is little evidence for an association of abdominal pain with specific personality types. However, neuroticism or stress sensitivity has been linked to development of FGIDs and pain in subjects without other psychological disturbance [77] and may serve as markers of vulnerability from life events such as trauma [78]. Pain beliefs and coping strategies are important in chronic pain and somatoform disorders and are significant predictors of quality-of-life impairment and treatment response [79]. Patients may exhibit ineffective coping strategies (e.g., "catastrophizing") or have poor social or family support. These factors are associated with higher pain scores, more psychological distress, and poorer clinical outcomes [35, 80–82]. The main social support for the patient may be provided by the illness (e.g., increased attention from friends, family, and physicians). Despite these observations, patients with FAPS often deny or minimize a role for psychological factors [3]. Perhaps in childhood there was greater family attention to illness than to emotional distress [83, 84]. It has been shown recently that "catastrophizing" may be an important cognitive link to explain the relationship between depression and IBS symptoms [85].

Unresolved losses, including onset or exacerbation of symptoms after the death of a parent or spouse, personally meaningful surgery (e.g., hysterectomy, ostomy), or interference with the outcome of a pregnancy (abortion, stillbirth), are common in FAPS [86, 27]. Histories of sexual and physical abuse are prevalent [29, 87], but elevated rates are not specific for this diagnosis. These histories predict poorer health status [28], medical refractoriness, increased diagnostic and therapeutic procedures, and more frequent health care visits [29]. Such trauma may increase awareness of bodily sensations, although visceral pain thresholds are not reduced [88, 89].

In sum there is evidence that a bidirectional relationship exists between FAPS and psychological disturbance. The psychological disturbance associated with FAPS particularly is severe in the presence of comorbid pain complaints in other locations and/or nonpainful somatic symptoms. In many cases, FAPS may be part of a generalized disorder such as widespread pain or somatization disorder. A significant problem with the current literature is the lack of studies in which patients with FAPS as diagnosed by current criteria are separated clearly from those with other FGIDs or other somatic pain syndromes (e.g., fibromyalgia, referred visceral pain). This lack of differentiation interferes with the identification of unique biopsychosocial aspects of FAPS.

Table 4. Factors Contributing to an Effective Patient-Physician Relationship

Empathy
Education
Illness validation
Reassurance
Treatment negotiation
Establishment of reasonable limits in time and effort

— Management

In contrast to some other FGIDs, treatment recommendations for patients with FAPS are empirical and not based on results from well-designed clinical trials. The accepted basis for clinical management of FAPS relies on establishing an effective patient-physician relationship, following a general treatment approach (including setting treatment goals and basing treatment on symptom severity and degree of disability), and offering more specific management that often encompasses a combination of treatment options, including pharmacological and/or psychological management [90–91].

Establishing an Effective Patient-Physician Relationship

Several factors contribute to an effective patient-physician relationship [25, 91, 92]. These are listed in Table 4 and are summarized in the following paragraphs.

Empathy is at the cornerstone of the patient-physician relationship. It involves acknowledging the reality and distress associated with pain by understanding the patient's illness experience while maintaining an objective and observant position [93]. An empathetic approach improves patient satisfaction and adherence to treatment, reduces adversarial patient behaviors, and can improve clinical outcome [94]. Additional factors are less established by the scientific literature but have become accepted in clinical practice [33]. *Education* is provided by (a) eliciting the patient's understanding of FAPS and its causes, (b) addressing unrealistic patient concerns, (c) explaining the nature of the symptoms in a manner that is consistent with the patient's belief system, and (d) insuring the patient's understanding of what was discussed. One approach is to explain that FAPS is a true disorder relating to abnormal sensation and/or dysregulation of pain control pathways, and that it can be modified effectively by medications or psychological treatments which re-establish control over the condition.

Validation of the illness occurs by acknowledging the patient's experience, emotional responses, and beliefs. Examples include "I can understand how difficult it has been for you" or "This has really affected your life." Physicians must avoid unwittingly making personal judgments or closing the communication through quick reassurances or solutions. Patients usually see their condition as serious and, for various reasons, may not consider it caused by stress. Ineffective statements including "Don't worry, it's nothing serious" or "Your problem is due to stress," frequently are perceived by patients as dismissive or judgmental and are to be avoided.

Reassurance must be provided within a proper context. After the diagnostic evaluation, the physician should elicit and respond to the patient's worries and concerns clearly and objectively. Some physician statements that appear reassuring, e.g., "There is nothing to worry about," can be viewed as dismissive, particularly when given before an adequate evaluation or if stated before the patient is afforded the opportunity to express personal concerns. A more effective statement could be "Based on the evaluation thus far, you have a diagnosis of FAPS, and the focus now should be on helping you gain better control over your symptoms." If the patient still requests additional tests, the physician may state, "Of course we will stay vigilant to any changes that may require reassessment, but for the present I am satisfied that your studies are complete." Although some patients may exhibit early dissatisfaction by focusing on another diagnosis with the perception of achieving more effective and rapid treatment, the physician should not overreact by overmedicating or performing unneeded diagnostic studies or treatments. Diagnostic decisions are based on objective data rather than the patient's insistence that "something be done" [95].

Treatment negotiation is the next step. Here the physician begins to engage in a participatory form of care, wherein the patient learns to contribute to and take responsibility for the treatment options to follow. The physician should ask about the patient's personal experience, understanding, and interests in various treatments, and then provide choices rather than directives. A patient will accept a recommendation if he or she understands the reasons behind it and believes it will help.

Finally, *reasonable limits* in time and effort need to be established. Depending on the nature and severity of the condition, some patients may require that the global care be shared with a mental health professional. Scheduling brief but regular appointments of fixed duration is the best response to patients' requests for more time. The key to success is maintaining an ongoing relationship, regardless of any ancillary care by others, while maintaining proper boundaries.

General Treatment Approach

Several general aspects of care should be considered before implementing specific forms of treatment.

Setting Treatment Goals

Because some patients may hold unrealistic expectations for "cure," the physician must place the prognosis into proper perspective. Much as in the treatment of chronic arthritis or chronic pancreatitis, the physician can explain that a realistic treatment goal would be symptom relief with improved daily function. With younger patients, by using analogies to frequent headaches or recurrent injuries, FAPS can be presented as a condition where the focus is more on symptom reduction and rehabilitation rather than cure. This reframing of treatment goals is enhanced and supported by demonstrating the need for ongoing care through regular visits. Visits can be set up every 1 to 2 months, and when a trusting relationship is established (often after only two or three visits) the frequency can be reduced to every 3 to 6 months as needed.

Helping the Patient Take Responsibility

Shared responsibility in the care plan can help the patient obtain a sense of control over the illness. One way to do this is to ask the patient to keep a diary of symptoms [96] for a few weeks, particularly identifying the circumstances of the pain episodes and their emotional and cognitive responses. This approach not only helps the patient achieve insight into aggravating factors but also helps characterize the patient's coping style. Such information also may assist the mental health professional in choosing a behavioral treatment strategy.

Basing Treatment on Symptom Severity and the Degree of Disability

Patients who have intermittent pain episodes of moderate severity and who can relate symptom exacerbations to psychological distress often respond to psychological treatments [97]. If the pain is continuous and severe or if the patient is reluctant to participate in a psychological intervention, antidepressants (e.g., tricyclic antidepressants) are indicated for their analgesic effects [36]. There is some evidence that the improvement that occurs with antidepressants may help the patient later accept and engage in a psychological intervention for psychiatric or chronic medical conditions [98, 99].

Referring to a Mental Health Professional

Patients may be reluctant to see a psychologist or psychiatrist because they lack knowledge of the benefits of referral, feel stigmatized for possibly having a psychiatric problem, or see referral as a rejection by the medical physician. Therefore psychological referral is best presented as a means to help the patient manage the pain and reduce the psychological distress encumbered by the symptoms. Medical care should continue concurrent with psychological treatment.

Employing a Multidisciplinary Pain Treatment Center

Multidisciplinary pain treatment centers provide comprehensive rehabilitation of patients with chronic pain. The approach theoretically is rational and can be an efficient method of treating disability from refractory chronic pain symptoms and assisting with narcotic withdrawal or management [100]. An additional occasional outcome is the discovery of previously overlooked disorders and application of specific therapy (e.g., trigger point injection, intercostal nerve block), particularly if the pain has somatoparietal characteristics [101].

Pharmacological Therapy

Pharmacological therapy can be employed in FAPS in conjunction with the general treatment approaches outlined previously. These treatments more likely will be effective if the physician uses them within the context of a well-developed patient-physician relationship and with sound understanding of a comprehensive treatment plan.

Antidepressants and Anxiolytics

Antidepressants, particularly tricyclic antidepressants (TCAs), are helpful in treating chronic pain and other painful FGIDs—both for direct pain management effects and antidepressant effects. Evidence for their value in FAPS derives from rare controlled trials and extrapolation from outcomes in other pain-based FGIDs [36, 102], although success in FAPS has not been uniform [103]. Antidepressants have broad value in unexplained somatic symptoms and syndromes, and trials with TCAs generally have been more successful than contemporary antidepressants, such as the selective serotonin reuptake inhibitors (SSRIs) [104, 105]. Newer agents with combined norepinephrine and serotonin reuptake activity (serotonin noradrenaline reuptake inhibitors, e.g., venlafaxine, duloxetine) have pain reducing effects and may prove useful [106]. Unfortunately, patients may have poor adherence to therapy due to side effects of antidepressants and due to feeling stigmatized by taking a "psychiatric" drug [36, 107]. An effective patient-physician relationship and proper patient education can overcome these problems.

Initial selection of antidepressants for FAPS patients can follow a similar algorithm as suggested for use in IBS patients with at least moderately severe symptoms (Figure 2). High levels of somatization can be detected by patient endorsement of many symptoms on a review-of-systems checklist or from features of somatization disorder in the medical history. Very low doses of TCAs may be used in patients with high levels of somatization due to intolerance to the medications. After initiation, dosage incrementation and augmentation with other agents or psychological/behavioral treatments typically is required. Further methods of

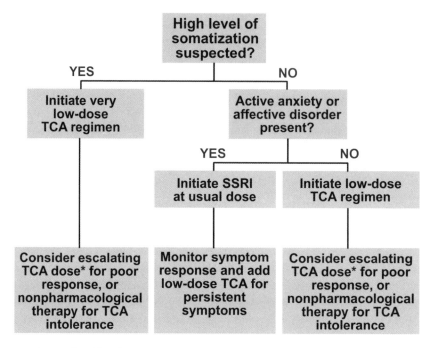

Figure 2. An algorithm for appropriate initiation of antidepressants in selected patients with functional abdominal pain syndrome (FAPS) that may be influenced by high levels of somatization.

*Monitoring for toxicity with tricyclic antidepressant (TCA) levels is required if the TCA is used in conjunction with medications that interfere with normal cytochrome p450 activity, such as selective serotonin reuptake inhibitors (SSRIs). (Modified from Clouse RE. Antidepressants for irritable bowel syndrome. Gut 2003;52:598–9.)

drug selection, introduction, and dose titration have been described in detail else-where [108]. (See Chapter 4.) Adherence to management can be increased by ex-plaining that antidepressants have analgesic properties. It is helpful to describe their use in other painful medical conditions like migraine, post-herpetic neu-ralgia and diabetic neuropathy. Patients should be informed of various aspects of antidepressant use in FAPS, including that (a) neurotransmitter changes in the brain induced by antidepressant treatment may reduce pain perception, (b) the doses used typically are lower than those used to manage psychiatric disorders, (c) the onset of effect may be delayed by several weeks, and (d) side effects may diminish with time.

Therapy with treatment combinations as used in psychiatric management may be helpful in some cases, but direct evidence for this approach in FAPS and other painful FGIDs is minimal [109]. Examples include combining a low-dose TCA with an SSRI, adding the anxiolytic buspirone to an antidepressant, or combin-ing an antidepressant with psychological treatment. The effects of antidepressants on comorbid depression symptoms also may reduce pain reporting [110]. Ben-zodiazepines are not recommended for chronic use because of dependency and abuse potential. These medications also may lower pain thresholds and exacerbate symptoms [111].

Analgesics

Most analgesics (e.g., aspirin and nonsteroidal anti-inflammatory drugs) offer little benefit, possibly because their actions primarily are peripheral in loca-tion. Both cyclooxygenase-1 (COX-1) and COX-2 are induced in the spinal cord after peripheral injury and reports support the efficacy of COX-2 inhibitors in neuropathic pain, but preliminary data have failed to demonstrate a benefit of COX-2 inhibition in a human model of acute esophageal central sensitization. Narcotic analgesics should be avoided because of the likelihood of addiction and possibility of narcotic bowel syndrome, wherein chronic use of narcotics leads to impaired motility and increased pain sensitivity [112]. New symptoms introduced by use of narcotic analgesics (e.g., constipation, nausea, vomiting) interfere with symptomatic improvement and complicate clinical presentation. In addition, chronic narcotic use may prevent implementation of more comprehensive treat-ment strategies by shifting the focus toward narcotic management.

The benefit or risks of brief, intermittent narcotic use for acute pain exacer-bations have not been tested formally in FAPS, although their use in this set-ting also is discouraged; if narcotics are required, guidelines for assessment of narcotic need and their subsequent use should be followed. When narcotics have been used chronically by a patient presenting with FAPS, withdrawal of the agents is recommended. This is accomplished over several days to weeks depend-ing on the degree of dependency and the specific medications, possibly while using a transient course of benzodiazepines for anxiety reduction and clonidine to reduce withdrawal effects and ongoing pain [113, 114]. Concurrently, a multi-component pharmacological and behavioral treatment plan for FAPS should be initiated [115].

Anticonvulsants

Anticonvulsants have been evaluated in chronic pain syndromes, such as chronic neuropathic pain, as alternatives to TCAs with fewer side effects. The most studied have been gabapentin, carbamazepine, and lamotrigine [116]. They have not been examined specifically in abdominal pain disorders or FAPS although a rationale exists [117], and evidence of efficacy in chronic pain management remains limited despite rather widespread use [118]. These agents are relatively safe and nonhabituating [119], also may interrupt the cycle between pain and depression [120], and might prove beneficial as adjunctive agents in some patients who are refractory to treatment, although direct evidence is lacking.

Other Medications

Other pharmacological treatments have been used, primarily in anecdotal fashion. Topically applied capsaicin has only moderate-to-poor efficacy in the treatment of chronic musculoskeletal or neuropathic pain syndromes, has not been used in FAPS, and would not be expected to have high utility, considering its peripheral mode of action [121]. Leuprolide acetate, a gonadotropin-releasing hormone analog provided in depot injection, may have a favorable effect in reducing pain in menstruating females with FAPS and painful functional bowel disorders [122]. The expected effects of this approach on reproductive hormone levels have limited enthusiasm for widespread evaluation. Management of coexistent sleep disorder is important, as insomnia can adversely affect pain perception. Breaking a circular, negative feedback process between chronic pain and sleep disorder is advantageous, and both pharmacological (sedative antidepressants, hypnotics, sedative antipsychotics) and nonpharmacological approaches (stimulus control, sleep restriction, progressive muscle relaxation) have been used [123].

— Psychological Therapy

No psychological treatment study specifically has targeted adult FAPS. However, studies in other painful FGIDs and pain conditions suggest psychological treatments would be beneficial. (See Chapter 6.) Based on outcomes from chronic pain centers [124, 125] and from treatment of patients with IBS [36, 126–128], several types of psychological intervention should be considered. Cognitive-behavioral therapy identifies maladaptive thoughts, perceptions, and behaviors, and is used to develop new ways for increasing symptom control [36, 129]. Dynamic or interpersonal psychotherapy seeks to reduce psychological distress and physical symptoms that are exacerbated by difficulties in interpersonal relationships [127, 130]. Hypnotherapy has been investigated primarily in IBS [131], wherein the focus is on "relaxation of the gut." Stress management attempts to counteract the physiological effects of stress or anxiety. Finally, referral to pain treatment centers for multidisciplinary treatment programs may be the most efficient method of treating disability from refractory chronic pain [132].

Behavioral therapies also have demonstrated benefits for patients with chronic somatic pain, including widespread pain of fibromyalgia. A recent controlled study also revealed the benefits of cognitive behavioral therapy in patients with primary hypochrondriasis [133]. Although the psychological treatments described above have been shown to improve mood, coping, quality of life, and health care costs, they have less demonstrable impact on specific visceral or somatic symptoms, suggesting that their best use may be in combination with symptomatic treatment [36]. For comparison, the combination of symptomatic medical treatment and multicomponent behavioral therapy is superior to medical treatment alone in managing IBS [134]. However, patients with FAPS may be reluctant to see a psychologist or psychiatrist because they fail to understand the benefits of referral, feel stigmatized for having a possible psychiatric problem, or see referral as a rejection by the physician. Psychological treatment may be most accepted if presented as a parallel intervention with ongoing medical care, a means for managing pain, and an attempt to reduce psychological distress from the symptoms. Considering the factors involved in the pathogenesis of FAPS, psychological therapy may be of benefit to many patients with this disorder. The timing of introduction varies depending on access, response to other approaches, and patient interest in the approach. Having a mental health professional closely associated with the medical practice setting may facilitate use of these interventions.

Other Interventions

Complementary therapies commonly are employed by patients with chronic pain disorders, including FAPS, although data supporting their use are limited. Spinal manipulation has no established role in chronic back pain—its most common application—and has no reported success in FAPS [135, 136]; the same presently is true for massage [137], particularly as a stand-alone therapy in back pain [138]. Whether generalized massage would have beneficial effects on FAPS through relaxation effects has not been studied. Data for acupuncture in chronic pain management remain limited, there are no trials in FAPS, and review of the existing literature cannot establish efficacy in chronic pain situations [139].

Few reports have described the use of transcutaneous electrical nerve stimulation (TENS) in patients with FAPS, and uncontrolled results are indeterminant [140]. Efficacy of TENS in chronic pain generally is lacking [141]. A variety of percutaneous neural blockade procedures have been developed for pain management [142], but these are directed at peripheral pain processes and not disorders such as FAPS. In patients with chronic abdominal pain, however, diagnostic blocks (controlled with saline injection) can be used to establish the presence of somatoparietal pain and diagnoses other than FAPS [143]. The saline control is essential in interpreting the outcome, and placebo response is high when trigger-point injections are used as therapeutic interventions [144]. Neurolytic celiac plexus blockade in benign disease has been restricted to chronic abdominal pain from suspected structural sources, such as chronic pancreatitis, with only modest success [125, 145].

Although uncontrolled studies suggest a significant diagnostic and therapeutic benefit of laparoscopic adhesiolysis in patients with chronic abdominal pain—tentatively attributed to adhesions from prior surgical procedures [146–148]—the outcome may be placebo-related, and unsuspected diagnoses are rare [149]. A blinded, randomized trial of 100 patients undergoing either laparoscopic adhesiolysis or diagnostic laparoscopy alone found no advantage to adhesiolysis [150]. This study also reported a significant improvement in chronic abdominal pain over 6 months whether laparoscopy alone or laparoscopic adhesiolysis were performed, suggesting spontaneous improvement in these patients over time.

— Topics for Future Research

FAPS remains an underinvestigated disorder with little evidence-based research appearing since the last edition of the Rome criteria. Evaluation of both diagnostic and treatment approaches for their effectiveness in clinical settings and studies of the long-term outcome of these approaches toward morbidity reduction are required. Specific areas of desired investigation include the following:

1. Further characterization of patients with FAPS to augment the diagnostic criteria and improve their specificity, especially with regard to overlap of this diagnosis with other FGIDs.
2. Better identification of the central neurophysiological processes involved in symptom production and effects of treatment on these processes.
3. Clearer definition of investigative and management algorithms depending on presenting characteristics or by identification of clinical subgroups.
4. Improved understanding of the relationship of somatization and somatization disorder to the presentation, management, and outcome of FAPS.
5. Assessment of physician role in management of FAPS patients and evaluation of patient-clinician interaction toward patient outcome.
6. Additional studies of antidepressants in patients with FAPS, with clarification of their optimal use.

7. Investigation of augmentative therapies, including combination pharmacological interventions and mixed pharmacological/nonpharmacological treatments.

8. Better identification of the roles of nonpharmacological treatments—including exercise and complementary/alternative therapies—in FAPS management.

References

1. Thompson WG, Longstreth G, Drossman DA, Heaton K, Irvine EJ, Muller-Lissner S. Functional bowel disorders and D. functional abdominal pain. In: Drossman DA, Corazziari E, Talley NJ, Thompson WG, and Whitehead WE, eds. Rome II: The Functional Gastrointestinal Disorders. Diagnosis, Pathohysiology and Treatment: A multinational Consensus. Mclean, VA: Degnon Associates, 2000:351–432.

2. American Psychiatric Association. Diagnostic and Statistical Manual of Mental Disorders—DSM-IV. Washington D.C.: American Psychiatric Association, 1994.

3. Drossman DA. Chronic functional abdominal pain. Am J Gastroenterol 1996;91:2270–2282.

4. Greenbaum DS, Greenbaum RB, Joseph JG, Natale JE. Chronic abdominal wall pain. Diagnostic validity and costs. Dig Dis Sci 1994;39:1935–1941.

5. Costanza CD, Longstreth GF, Liu AL. Chronic abdominal wall pain: clinical features, health care costs, and long-term outcome. Clin Gastroenterol Hepatol 2004;2:395–399.

6. Zuckerman MJ, Guerra LG, Drossman DA, Foland JA, Gregory GG. Health-care-seeking behaviors related to bowel complaints. Hispanics versus non-Hispanic whites. Dig Dis Sci 1996;41:77–82.

7. Thompson WG, the working team for functional bowel disorders. Functional bowel disorders and functional abdominal pain. In: Drossman DA, Richter JE, Talley NJ, Thompson WG, Corazziari E, Whitehead WE. The Functional Gastrointestinal Disorders: Diagnosis, Pathophysiology and Treatment. 1 ed. McLean, VA: Degnon Associates; 1994: 152–174.

8. Varay A. Précis de gastro-entérologie. Paris: Masson, 1966.

9. Drossman DA, Li Z, Andruzzi E, Temple RD, Talley NJ, Thompson WG, Whitehead WE, Janssens J, Funch-Jensen P, Corazziari E. U.S. householder survey of functional gastrointestinal disorders. Prevalence, sociodemography, and health impact. Dig Dis Sci 1993;38:1569–1580.

10. Thompson WG, Irvine EJ, Pare P, Ferrazzi S, Rance L. Functional gastrointestinal disorders in Canada: first population-based survey using Rome II criteria with suggestions for improving the questionnaire. Dig Dis Sci 2002;47:225–235.

11. Koloski NA, Talley NJ, Boyce PM. Epidemiology and health care seeking in the functional GI disorders: a population-based study. Am J Gastroenterol 2002;97:2290–2299.

12. Kwan AC, Bao TN, Chakkaphak S, Chang FY, Ke MY, Law NM, Leelakusolvong S,

Luo JY, Manan C, Park HJ, Piyaniran W, Qureshi A, Long T, Xu GM, Xu L, Yuen H. Validation of Rome II criteria for functional gastrointestinal disorders by factor analysis of symptoms in Asian patient sample. J Gastroenterol Hepatol 2003;18:796–802.

13. Thompson WG, Heaton KW, Smyth GT, Smyth C. Irritable bowel syndrome in general practice: prevalence, characteristics, and referral. Gut 2000;46:78–82.

14. Heitkemper MM, Jarrett M, Cain KC, Shaver J, Walker E, Lewis L. Daily gastrointestinal symptoms in women with and without a diagnosis of IBS. Dig Dis Sci 1995; 40:1511–1519.

15. Bharucha AE, Camilleri M. Functional abdominal pain in the elderly. Gastroenterol Clin North Am 2001;30:517–29.

16. Maxton DG, Whorwell PJ. Use of medical resource and attitudes to health care of patients with chronic abdominal pain. Br J Med Econ 1992;2:75–9.

17. Chiou CF, Wilson A, Longstreth G, Wade S, Wong J, Barghout V, Frech F, Offman J. The relationship between IBS abdominal pain/discomfort and indirect costs. Gastroenterology 2005;128:63–73.

18. Howell S, Poulton R, Caspi A, Talley NJ. Relationship between abdominal pain subgroups in the community and psychiatric diagnosis and personality. A birth cohort study. J Psychosom Res 2003;55:179–187.

19. Croft P, Lewis M, Hannaford P. Is all chronic pain the same? A 25-year follow-up study. Pain 2003;105:309–317.

20. Dumitrascu DL. Somatization: shall we believe the patient's complaints? In: Dumitrascu DL, ed. Psychosomatic Medicine. Recent progress and current trends. Med Univ Iuliu Hatieganu Cluj, 2003:109–118.

21. Egle UT, Nickel R. Somatoforme Schmerzstörungen. In: Kapfhammer HP and Gündel H, eds. Psychotherapie der Somatisierungstörungen. Thieme Stuttgart, 2001:235–250.

22. Nickel R, Egle UT, Schwab R. [Diagnostic subgroups and psychosocial characteristics in chronic non-malignant pain patients referred to an out-patient pain center]. Psychother Psychosom Med Psychol 2002;52:378–385.

23. Wong HY, Mayer EA. Gastrointestinal Pain. In: S McMahon and M Koltzenburg, eds. Wall and Melzack Textbook of Pain. 5 ed. Philadelphia: Elsevier, 2006.

24. Pasricha PJ. Approach to the patient with abdominal pain. In: Yamada T, Alpers DH, Kaplowitz N, Laine L, Owyang C, and Powell DW, eds. Textbook of Gastroenterology (4 [th edition]). Philadelphia: Lippincott Williams and Wilkins, 2003:781–801.

25. Drossman DA. Functional abdominal pain syndrome. Clin Gastroenterol Hepatol 2004;2:353–365.

26. Drossman DA. Diagnosing and treating patients with refractory functional gastrointestinal disorders. Ann Intern Med 1995;123:688–697.

27. Drossman DA. Patients with psychogenic abdominal pain: six years' observation in the medical setting. Am J Psychiatry 1982;139:1549–1557.

28. Drossman DA, Li Z, Leserman J, Toomey TC, Hu YJ. Health status by gastrointestinal diagnosis and abuse history. Gastroenterology 1996;110:999–1007.

29. Drossman DA, Talley NJ, Leserman J, Olden KW, Barreiro MA. Sexual and physical abuse and gastrointestinal illness. Review and recommendations. Ann Intern Med 1995;123:782–794.

30. Olden KW, Hom SS. The refractory functional GI patient: definition and implications for cost effective care. Gastroenterology 1998;114:G3343.

31. Drossman DA. Challenges in the physician-patient relationship: feeling "drained". Gastroenterology 2001;121:1037–1038.

32. Minuchin S, Rosman BL, Baker L. Psychosomatic Families: Anorexia Nervosa in Context. Cambridge: Harvard University Press, 1978.

33. Kleinman A, Eisenberg L, Good B. Culture, illness, and care: clinical lessons from anthropologic and cross-cultural research. Ann Intern Med 1978;88:251–258.

34. Zborowski M. Cultural components in responses to pain. Journal of Social Issues 1952;8:16–30.

35. Drossman DA, Whitehead WE, Toner BB, Diamant N, Hu YJ, Bangdiwala SI, Jia H. What determines severity among patients with painful functional bowel disorders? Am J Gastroenterol 2000;95:974–980.

36. Drossman DA, Toner BB, Whitehead WE, Diamant NE, Dalton CB, Duncan S, Emmott S, Proffitt V, Akman D, Frusciante K, Le T, Meyer K, Bradshaw B, Mikula K, Morris CB, Blackman CJ, Hu Y, Jia H, Li JZ, Koch GG, Bangdiwala SI. Cognitive-behavioral therapy versus education and desipramine versus placebo for moderate to severe functional bowel disorders. Gastroenterology 2003;125:19–31.

37. Berkman LF, Syme SL. Social networks, host resistance, and mortality: a nine-year follow-up study of Alameda County residents. Am J Epidemiol 1979;109:186–204.

38. Talley NJ, Silverstein MD, Agreus L, Nyren O, Sonnenberg A, Holtmann G. AGA technical review: evaluation of dyspepsia. American Gastroenterological Association. Gastroenterology 1998;114:582–595.

39. Bickston SJ, Clouse RE. Evaluation of the patient with abdominal pain. In: Bone RJ and Fitzgerald F, eds. Current Practice of Medicine. Philadelphia: Current Medicine, 1996.

40. Fielding JF. Detailed history and examination assist positive clinical diagnosis of the irritable bowel syndrome. J Clin Gastroenterol 1983;5:495–497.

41. Sapira JD. Reassurance therapy. What to say to symptomatic patients with benign diseases. Ann Intern Med 1972;77:603–604.

42. Clouse RE, Randall CW. Irritable bowel syndrome: Does making a confident diagnosis reassure an unhappy patient? In: Barkin JS and Rogers AI, eds. Difficult Decisions in Digestive Diseases [2nd Edition]. St. Louis: Mosby-Year Book, 1994:399–404.

43. Longstreth GF. Irritable bowel syndrome. Diagnosis in the managed care era. Dig Dis Sci 1997;42:1105–1111.

44. Dixon JM, Elton RA, Rainey JB, Macleod DA. Rectal examination in patients with pain in the right lower quadrant of the abdomen. BMJ 1991;302:386–388.

45. Chervu A, Clagett GP, Valentine RJ, Myers SI, Rossi PJ. Role of physical examination in detection of abdominal aortic aneurysms. Surgery 1995;117:454–457.

46. Thomson WH, Dawes RF, Carter SS. Abdominal wall tenderness: a useful sign in chronic abdominal pain. Br J Surg 1991;78:223–225.

47. Gray DW, Dixon JM, Seabrook G, Collin J. Is abdominal wall tenderness a useful sign in the diagnosis of non-specific abdominal pain? Ann R Coll Surg Engl 1988;70:233–234.

48. Alfven G. Preliminary findings on increased muscle tension and tenderness, and recurrent abdominal pain in children. A clinical study. Acta Paediatr 1993;82:400–403.

49. Meyer UA, Schuurmans MM, Lindberg RL. Acute porphyrias: pathogenesis of neurological manifestations. Semin Liver Dis 1998;18:43–52.

50. Whitcomb DC, Martin SP, Schoen RE, Jho HD. Chronic abdominal pain caused by thoracic disc herniation. Am J Gastroenterol 1995;90:835–837.

51. Stormer S, Gerner HJ, Gruninger W, Metzmacher K, Follinger S, Wienke C, Aldinger W, Walker N, Zimmermann M, Paeslack V. Chronic pain/dysaesthesiae in spinal cord injury patients: results of a multicentre study. Spinal Cord 1997;35:446–455.

52. Vanner SJ, Depew WT, Paterson WG, DaCosta LR, Groll AG, Simon JB, Djurfeldt M. Predictive value of the Rome criteria for diagnosing the irritable bowel syndrome. Am J Gastroenterol 1999;94:2912–2917.

53. Drossman DA, Camilleri M, Mayer EA, Whitehead WE. AGA technical review on irritable bowel syndrome. Gastroenterology 2002;123:2108–2131.

54. Scholz J, Woolf CJ. Can we conquer pain? Nat Neurosci 2002;5 Suppl:1062–1067.

55. Devor M. Neuropathic pain: what do we do with all these theories? Acta Anaesthesiol Scand 2001;45:1121–1127.

56. Lariviere WR, Wilson SG, Laughlin TM, Kokayeff A, West EE, Adhikari SM, Wan Y, Mogil JS. Heritability of nociception. III. Genetic relationships among commonly used assays of nociception and hypersensitivity. Pain 2002;97:75–86.

57. Fields HL, Basbaum AI. Central nervous system mechanisms of pain modulation. In: Wall PD and Melzack R, eds. Textbook of Pain. New York: Churchill Livingston, 1999:309–329.

58. Porreca F, Ossipov MH, Gebhart GF. Chronic pain and medullary descending facilitation. Trends Neurosci 2002;25:319–325.

59. Gebhart GF. Descending modulation of pain. Neurosci Biobehav Rev 2004;27:729–737.

60. Mason P. Contributions of the medullary raphe and ventromedial reticular region to pain modulation and other homeostatic functions. Annu Rev Neurosci 2001;24:737–777.

61. Le Bars D, Chitour D, Clot AM. The encoding of thermal stimuli by diffuse noxious inhibitory controls (DNIC). Brain Res 1981;230:394–399.

62. Edwards RR, Ness TJ, Weigent DA, Fillingim RB. Individual differences in diffuse noxious inhibitory controls (DNIC): association with clinical variables. Pain 2003; 106:427–437.

63. Petrovic P, Ingvar M. Imaging cognitive modulation of pain processing. Pain 2002; 95:1–5.

64. Lieberman MD, Jarcho JM, Berman S, Naliboff BD, Suyenobu BY, Mandelkern M, Mayer EA. The neural correlates of placebo effects: A disruption account. 2004.

65. Ringel Y, Drossman DA, Leserman J, Lin W, Liu H, Vogt B, Whitehead WE. Association of anterior cingulate cortex (ACG) activation with psychosocial distress and pain reports. Gastroenterology 2003;124:A97.

66. Chang L, Berman SM, Suyenobu B, Gordon WA, Mandelkern MA, Naliboff BD, Mayer EA. Differences in brain responses to rectal distension between patients with inflammatory and functional GI disorders. Gastroenterology 2004;126:A106.

67. Seminowicz DA, Mayberg HS, McIntosh AR, Goldapple K, Kennedy S, Segal Z, Rafi-Tari S. Limbic-frontal circuitry in major depression: a path modeling metanalysis. Neuroimage 2004;22:409–418.

68. Mayer EA, Derbyshire S, Naliboff BD. Cerebral activation in irritable bowel syndrome. Gastroenterology 2000;119:1418–1420.

69. Mayer EA, Collins SM. Evolving pathophysiologic models of functional gastrointestinal disorders. Gastroenterology 2002;122:2032–2048.

70. Bixo M, Sundstrom-Poromaa I, Bjorn I, astrom M. Patients with psychiatric disorders in gynecologic practice. Am J Obstet Gynecol 2001;185:396–402.

71. Von Korff M, Dworkin SF, Le Resche L, Kruger A. An epidemiologic comparison of pain complaints. Pain 1988;32:173–183.

72. Halder SL, McBeth J, Silman AJ, Thompson DG, Macfarlane GJ. Psychosocial risk factors for the onset of abdominal pain. Results from a large prospective population-based study. Int J Epidemiol 2002;31:1219–1225.

73. McCracken LM, Zayfert C, Gross RT. The Pain Anxiety Symptoms Scale: development and validation of a scale to measure fear of pain. Pain 1992;50:67–73.

74. Hazlett-Stevens H, Craske MG, Mayer EA, Chang L, Naliboff BD. Prevalence of irritable bowel syndrome among university students: the roles of worry, neuroticism, anxiety sensitivity and visceral anxiety. J Psychosom Res 2003;55:501–505.

75. Labus JS, Bolus R, Chang L, Wiklund I, Naesdal J, Mayer EA, Naliboff BD. The Visceral Sensitivity Index: development and validation of a gastrointestinal symptom-specific anxiety scale. Aliment Pharmacol Ther 2004;20:89–97.

76. El Rufaie OE, Al Sabosy MA, Bener A, Abuzeid MS. Somatized mental disorder among primary care Arab patients: I. Prevalence and clinical and sociodemographic characteristics. J Psychosom Res 1999;46:549–555.

77. Tanum L, Malt UF. Personality and physical symptoms in nonpsychiatric patients with functional gastrointestinal disorder. J Psychosom Res 2001;50:139–146.

78. Talley NJ, Boyce PM, Jones M. Is the association between irritable bowel syndrome and abuse explained by neuroticism? A population based study. Gut 1998;42:47–53.

79. Petrak F, Hardt J, Kappis B, Nickel R, Tiber EU. Determinants of health-related quality of life in patients with persistent somatoform pain disorder. Eur J Pain 2003;7:463–471.

80. Sarason IG, Sarason BR, Potter EH, III, Antoni MH. Life events, social support, and illness. Psychosom Med 1985;47:156–163.

81. Jamison RN, Virts KL. The influence of family support on chronic pain. Behav Res Ther 1990;28:283–287.

82. Scarinci IC, McDonald-Haile J, Bradley LA, Richter JE. Altered pain perception and psychosocial features among women with gastrointestinal disorders and history of abuse: a preliminary model. Am J Med 1994;97:108–118.

83. Psychosocial factors in the care of patients with gastrointestinal disorders. In: Drossman DA and Yamada T, eds. Textbook of Gastroenterology. Philadelphia: Lippincott Co., 1995:620–637.

84. Toner BB. Cognitive-behavioural treatment of functional somatic syndromes: integrating gender issues. Cognitive Behavioral Practice 1994;1:157–178.

85. Lackner JM, Gudleski GD, Blanchard EB. Beyond abuse: the association among parenting style, abdominal pain, and somatization in IBS patients. Behav Res Ther 2004;42:41–56.

86. Hislop IG. Childhood deprivation: an antecedent of the irritable bowel syndrome. Med J Aust 1979;1:372–374.

87. Wurtele SK, Kaplan GM, Keairnes M. Childhood sexual abuse among chronic pain patients. Clin J Pain 1990;6:110–113.

88. Mayer EA, Gebhart GF. Basic and clinical aspects of visceral hyperalgesia. Gastroenterology 1994;107:271–293.

89. Ringel Y, Whitehead WE, Toner BB, Diamant NE, Hu Y, Jia H, Bangdiwala SI, Drossman DA. Sexual and physical abuse are not associated with rectal hypersensitivity in patients with irritable bowel syndrome. Gut 2004;53:838–842.

90. Drossman DA. The Physician-Patient Relationship. In: Corazziari E, ed. Approach to the Patient with Chronic Gastrointestinal Disorders. Milan: Messaggi, 1999:133–139.

91. Drossman DA. Psychosocial factors in the care of patients with GI disorders. In: Yamada T, Alpers DH, Kaplowitz N, Laine L, Owyang C, and Powell DW, eds. Textbook of Gastroenterology (4th Edition). Philadelphia: Lippincott, WIlliams & Wilkins, 2003:620–637.

92. Chang L, Drossman DA. The psychosocial interview in the irritable bowel syndrome. Clinical Perspectives in Gastroenterology 2002;5:336–341.

93. Zinn W. The empathic physician. Arch Intern Med 1993;153:306–312.

94. Stewart M, Brown JB, Boon H, Galajda J, Meredith L, Sangster M. Evidence on patient-doctor communication. Cancer Prev Control 1999;3:25–30.

95. DeVaul RA, Faillace LA. Persistent pain and illness insistence. A medical profile of proneness to surgery. Am J Surg 1978;135:828–833.

96. Drossman DA. Diagnosing and treating patients with refractory functional gastrointestinal disorders. Ann Intern Med 1995;123:688–697.

97. Drossman DA, Creed FH, Olden KW, Svedlund J, Toner BB, Whitehead WE. Psychosocial aspects of the functional gastrointestinal disorders. In: Drossman DA, Corazziari E, Talley NJ, and Whitehead WE, eds. Rome II. The functional gastrointestinal disorders: Diagnosis, pathophysiology and treatment; A multinational consensus. 2nd ed. USA: Degnon and Associates, 2000:157–245.

98. Conte HR, Plutchik R, Wild KV, Karasu TB. Combined psychotherapy and pharmacotherapy for depression. A systematic analysis of the evidence. Arch Gen Psychiatry 1986;43:471–479.

99. Hunter MS, Ussher JM, Cariss M, Browne S, Jelley R, Katz M. Medical (fluoxetine) and psychological (cognitive-behavioural therapy) treatment for premenstrual dysphoric disorder: a study of treatment processes. J Psychosom Res 2002;53:811–817.

100. Barkin RL, Lubenow TR, Bruehl S, Husfeldt B, Ivankovich O, Barkin SJ. Management of chronic pain. Part I. Dis Mon 1996;42:389–454.

101. McGarrity TJ, Peters DJ, Thompson C, McGarrity SJ. Outcome of patients with chronic abdominal pain referred to chronic pain clinic. Am J Gastroenterol 2000; 95:1812–1816.

102. Jackson JL, O'Malley PG, Tomkins G, Balden E, Santoro J, Kroenke K. Treatment of functional gastrointestinal disorders with antidepressant medications: a meta-analysis. Am J Med 2000;108:65–72.

103. Loldrup D, Langemark M, Hansen HJ, Olesen J, Bech P. Clomipramine and mianserin in chronic idiopathic pain syndrome. A placebo controlled study. Psychopharmacology (Berl) 1989;99:1–7.

104. Fishbain DA, Cutler RB, Rosomoff HL, Rosomoff RS. Do antidepressants have an analgesic effect in psychogenic pain and somatoform pain disorder? A meta-analysis. Psychosom Med 1998;60:503–509.

105. O'Malley PG, Jackson JL, Santoro J, Tomkins G, Balden E, Kroenke K. Antidepressant therapy for unexplained symptoms and symptom syndromes. J Fam Pract 1999;48:980–990.

106. Briley M. Clinical experience with dual action antidepressants in different chronic pain syndromes. Hum Psychopharmacol 2004;19(Suppl 1):S21.

107. Clouse RE. Managing functional bowel disorders from the top down: lessons from a well-designed treatment trial. Gastroenterology 2003;125:249–253.

108. Clouse RE, Lustman PJ. Antidepressants for irritable bowel syndrome. In: Camilleri M and Spiller RC, eds. Irritable Bowel Syndrome: Diagnosis and Treatment. London: WB Saunders, 2002:161–171.

109. Nair D, Prakash C, Lustman PJ, Clouse RE. Added value of tricyclic antidepressants for functional gastrointestinal symptoms in patients on selective serotonin reuptake inhibitors (SSRIs). Am J Gastroenterol 2001;96 (Suppl.):S316.

110. Bradley RH, Barkin RL, Jerome J, DeYoung K, Dodge CW. Efficacy of venlafaxine for the long term treatment of chronic pain with associated major depressive disorder. Am J Ther 2003;10:318–323.

111. King SA, Strain JJ. Benzodiazepines and chronic pain. Pain 1990;41:3–4.

112. Sandgren JE, McPhee MS, Greenberger NJ. Narcotic bowel syndrome treated with clonidine. Resolution of abdominal pain and intestinal pseudo-obstruction. Ann Intern Med 1984;101:331–334.

113. Camilleri M, Kim DY, McKinzie S, Kim HJ, Thomforde GM, Burton DD, Low PA, Zinsmeister AR. A randomized, controlled exploratory study of clonidine in diarrhea-predominant irritable bowel syndrome. Clin Gastroenterol Hepatol 2003;1:111–121.

114. Malcolm A, Camilleri M, Kellow JE. Clonidine alters rectal motor and sensory function in irritable bowel syndrome. Gastroenterology 1999;116:A1035.

115. Drossman DA. A Biopsychosocial Understanding of Gastrointestinal Illness and Disease. In: Feldman M, Scharschmidt B, and Sleisenger MH, eds. Sleisenger and Fordtrans's Gastrointestinal Disease. Seventh Edition ed. Philadelphia: WB Saunders, 2002:2373–2385.

116. Guay DR. Adjunctive agents in the management of chronic pain. Pharmacotherapy 2001;21:1070–1081.

117. Bueno L, Fioramonti J, Garcia-Villar R. Pathobiology of visceral pain: molecular mechanisms and therapeutic implications. III. Visceral afferent pathways: a source of new therapeutic targets for abdominal pain. Am J Physiol Gastrointest Liver Physiol 2000;278:G670–G676.

118. Wiffen P, Collins S, McQuay H, Carroll D, Jadad A, Moore A. Anticonvulsant drugs for acute and chronic pain. Cochrane Database Syst Rev 2000;CD001133.

119. Hansen HC. Treatment of chronic pain with antiepileptic drugs: a new era. South Med J 1999;92:642–649.

120. Kudoh A, Ishihara H, Matsuki A. Effect of carbamazepine on pain scores of unipolar depressed patients with chronic pain: a trial of off-on-off-on design. Clin J Pain 1998;14:61–65.

121. Mason L, Moore RA, Derry S, Edwards JE, McQuay HJ. Systematic review of topical capsaicin for the treatment of chronic pain. BMJ 2004;328:991.

122. Mathias JR, Clench MH, Abell TL, Koch KL, Lehman G, Robinson M, Rothstein R, Snape WJ. Effect of leuprolide acetate in treatment of abdominal pain and nausea in premenopausal women with functional bowel disease: a double-blind, placebo-controlled, randomized study. Dig Dis Sci 1998;43:1347–1355.

123. Stiefel F, Stagno D. Management of insomnia in patients with chronic pain conditions. CNS Drugs 2004;18:285–296.

124. Peters JL, Large RG. A randomised control trial evaluating in- and outpatient pain management programmes. Pain 1990;41:283–293.

125. Hastings RH, McKay WR. Treatment of benign chronic abdominal pain with neurolytic celiac plexus block. Anesthesiology 1991;75:156–158.

126. Talal AH, Drossman DA. Psychosocial factors in inflammatory bowel disease. Gastroenterol Clin North Am 1995;24:699–716.

127. Creed F, Fernandes L, Guthrie E, Palmer S, Ratcliffe J, Read N, Rigby C, Thompson D, Tomenson B. The cost-effectiveness of psychotherapy and paroxetine for severe irritable bowel syndrome. Gastroenterology 2003;124:303–317.

128. Lackner JM, Mesmer C, Morley S, Dowzer C, Hamilton S. Psychological treatments for irritable bowel syndrome: A systematic review and meta-analysis. J Consult Psychol 2004;72:1100–13.

129. Keefe FJ, Dunsmore J, Burnett R. Behavioral and cognitive-behavioral approaches to chronic pain: recent advances and future directions. J Consult Clin Psychol 1992; 60:528–536.

130. Guthrie E, Creed F, Dawson D, Tomenson B. A randomised controlled trial of psychotherapy in patients with refractory irritable bowel syndrome. Br J Psychiatry 1993;163:315–321.

131. Whorwell PJ, Prior A, Colgan SM. Hypnotherapy in severe irritable bowel syndrome: further experience. Gut 1987;28:423–425.

132. Kames LD, Rapkin AJ, Naliboff BD, Afifi S, Ferrer-Brechner T. Effectiveness of an interdisciplinary pain management program for the treatment of chronic pelvic pain. Pain 1990;41:41–46.

133. Barsky AJ, Ahern DK. Cognitive Behavior Therapy for Hypochondriasis: A Randomized Controlled Trial. JAMA 2004;291:1464–1470.

134. Heymann-Monnikes I, Arnold R, Florin I, Herda C, Melfsen S, Monnikes H. The combination of medical treatment plus multicomponent behavioral therapy is superior to medical treatment alone in the therapy of irritable bowel syndrome. Am J Gastroenterol 2000;95:981–994.

135. Assendelft WJ, Morton SC, Yu EI, Suttorp MJ, Shekelle PG. Spinal manipulative therapy for low back pain. A meta-analysis of effectiveness relative to other therapies. Ann Intern Med 2003;138:871–881.

136. Assendelft WJ, Morton SC, Yu EI, Suttorp MJ, Shekelle PG. Spinal manipulative therapy for low back pain. Cochrane Database Syst Rev 2004;CD000447.

137. Ernst E. Manual therapies for pain control: chiropractic and massage. Clin J Pain 2004;20:8–12.

138. Furlan AD, Brosseau L, Welch V, Wong J. Massage for low back pain. Cochrane Database Syst Rev 2000;CD001929.

139. Lee TL. Acupuncture and chronic pain management. Ann Acad Med Singapore 2000;29:17–21.

140. Sylvester K, Kendall GP, Lennard-Jones JE. Treatment of functional abdominal pain by transcutaneous electrical nerve stimulation. Br Med J (Clin Res Ed) 1986;293:481–482.

141. McQuay HJ, Moore RA, Eccleston C, Morley S, Williams AC. Systematic review of outpatient services for chronic pain control. Health Technol Assess 1997;1:i-135.

142. Shah RV, Ericksen JJ, Lacerte M. Interventions in chronic pain management. 2. New frontiers: invasive nonsurgical interventions. Arch Phys Med Rehabil 2003;84: S39–S44.

143. Bogduk N. Diagnostic nerve blocks in chronic pain. Best Pract Res Clin Anaesthesiol 2002;16:565–578.

144. Garvey TA, Marks MR, Wiesel SW. A prospective, randomized, double-blind evaluation of trigger-point injection therapy for low-back pain. Spine 1989;14:962–964.

145. Gress F, Schmitt C, Sherman S, Ciaccia D, Ikenberry S, Lehman G. Endoscopic ultrasound-guided celiac plexus block for managing abdominal pain associated with chronic pancreatitis: a prospective single center experience. Am J Gastroenterol 2001;96:409–416.

146. Onders RP, Mittendorf EA. Utility of laparoscopy in chronic abdominal pain. Surgery 2003;134:549–552.

147. Mueller MD, Tschudi J, Herrmann U, Klaiber C. An evaluation of laparoscopic adhesiolysis in patients with chronic abdominal pain. Surg Endosc 1995;9:802–804.

148. Shayani V, Siegert C, Favia P. The role of laparoscopic adhesiolysis in the treatment of patients with chronic abdominal pain or recurrent bowel obstruction. JSLS 2002;6:111–114.

149. Di Lorenzo N, Coscarella G, Lirosi F, Faraci L, Rossi P, Pietrantuono M, Manzelli A, Russo F, Gaspari AL. [Impact of laparoscopic surgery in the treatment of chronic abdominal pain syndrome]. Chir Ital 2002;54:367–378.

150. Swank DJ, Swank-Bordewijk SC, Hop WC, Van Erp WF, Janssen IM, Bonjer HJ, Jeekel J. Laparoscopic adhesiolysis in patients with chronic abdominal pain: a blinded randomised controlled multi-centre trial. Lancet 2003;361:1247–1251.

Chapter 11

Functional Gallbladder and Sphincter of Oddi Disorders

Jose Behar, Chair

Enrico Corazziari, Co-Chair

Moises Guelrud

Walter J. Hogan

Stuart Sherman

James Toouli

Introduction

The integrated actions of the gallbladder (GB) and the sphincter of Oddi (SO) regulate bile flow from the liver through the biliary tract into the duodenum. The SO also plays a relevant role in regulating the flow of pancreatic secretions into the duodenum. Disorders of any of these components may lead to intermittent upper abdominal pain, transient elevations of liver and pancreatic enzymes, common bile duct dilatation, or episodes of pancreatitis. Functional GB disorder is characterized by motility abnormalities resulting in bile stasis caused by an initial metabolic disorder or, less commonly, by a primary motility alteration of the GB. Functional SO disorders encompass motility abnormalities of the biliary SO, the pancreatic SO or both (Table 1). The motility abnormalities of the GB and/or biliary SO produce similar patterns of biliary pain, whereas abnormalities of the pancreatic SO cause upper abdominal pain that is similar to that of pancreatitis. This chapter suggests that the diagnosis of these three entities, initially defined by functional abnormalities, should be made by eliciting specific symptoms and confirmed by objective tests. Disorders of the GB and SO share common diagnostic criteria that are summarized below. In addition to these criteria, criteria specific to either functional GB disorder, functional disorder of the biliary SO, or functional disorder of the pancreatic SO are discussed further on in the chapter.

Table 1. Functional Gastrointestinal Disorders

A. Functional Esophageal Disorders

A1. Functional heartburn	A3. Functional dysphagia
A2. Functional chest pain of presumed esophageal origin	A4. Globus

B. Functional Gastroduodenal Disorders

B1. Functional dyspepsia	B3. Nausea and vomiting disorders
B1a. Postprandial distress syndrome (PDS)	B3a. Chronic idiopathic nausea (CIN)
B1b. Epigastric pain syndrome (EPS)	B3b. Functional vomiting
B2. Belching disorders	B3c. Cyclic vomiting syndrome (CVS)
B2a. Aerophagia	B4. Rumination syndrome in adults
B2b. Unspecified excessive belching	

C. Functional Bowel Disorders

C1. Irritable bowel syndrome (IBS)	C4. Functional diarrhea
C2. Functional bloating	C5. Unspecified functional bowel disorder
C3. Functional constipation	

D. Functional Abdominal Pain Syndrome (FAPS)

E. Functional Gallbladder and Sphincter of Oddi (SO) Disorders

E1. Functional gallbladder disorder
E2. Functional biliary SO disorder
E3. Functional pancreatic SO disorder

F. Functional Anorectal Disorders

F1. Functional fecal incontinence	F2b. Proctalgia fugax
F2. Functional anorectal pain	F3. Functional defecation disorders
F2a. Chronic proctalgia	F3a. Dyssynergic defecation
F2a1. Levator ani syndrome	F3b. Inadequate defecatory propulsion
F2a2. Unspecified functional anorectal pain	

G. Functional Disorders: Neonates and Toddlers

G1. Infant regurgitation	G5. Functional diarrhea
G2. Infant rumination syndrome	G6. Infant dyschezia
G3. Cyclic vomiting syndrome	G7. Functional constipation
G4. Infant colic	

H. Functional Disorders: Children and Adolescents

H1. Vomiting and aerophagia	H2d. Childhood functional abdominal pain
H1a. Adolescent rumination syndrome	H2d1. Childhood functional abdominal pain syndrome
H1b. Cyclic vomiting syndrome	
H1c. Aerophagia	H3. Constipation and incontinence
H2. Abdominal pain-related FGIDs	H3a. Functional constipation
H2a. Functional dyspepsia	H3b. Nonretentive fecal incontinence
H2b. Irritable bowel syndrome	
H2c. Abdominal migraine	

E. Diagnostic Criteria for Functional Gallbladder and Sphincter of Oddi Disorders

Must include episodes of pain located in the epigastrium and/ or right upper quadrant and *all* of the following:
1. **Episodes lasting 30 minutes or longer**
2. **Recurrent symptoms occurring at different intervals (not daily)**
3. **The pain builds up to a steady level**
4. **The pain is moderate to severe enough to interrupt the patient's daily activities or lead to an emergency department visit**
5. **The pain is not relieved by bowel movements**
6. **The pain is not relieved by postural change**
7 **The pain is not relieved by antacids**
8. **Exclusion of other structural disease that would explain the symptoms**

Supportive Criteria
The pain may present with one or more of the following:
1. Associated nausea and vomiting
2. Radiates to the back and/or right subscapular region
3. Awakens from sleep in the middle of the night

E1. Functional Gallbladder Disorder

— Definition

Although several causes can affect GB function, we describe that it is characterized by a motility abnormality that manifests symptomatically with biliary-like pain as a consequence either of an initial metabolic disorder (supersaturated bile with cholesterol) [1] or of a primary motility alteration of the GB in the absence, at least initially, of any alteration of bile composition [2]. It is likely that the latter condition may cause altered bile recycling, bile stasis, and altered bile composition within the GB over a period of time. Both conditions may eventually lead over time to the development of organic abnormalities (e.g., gallstones and/or acute cholecystitis). The symptoms of both the primary functional and the metabolic causes appear to be indistinguishable from one another and therefore the definition of each one requires a careful diagnostic work-up.

— Epidemiology

The prevalence and incidence of GB dysfunction in the absence of lithogenic bile are not known. Large population based studies have reported that prevalence of biliary pain in US negative patients with GB in situ varies from 7.6% in men to 20.7% in women [3, 4].

E1. Diagnostic Criteria for Functional Gallbladder Disorder

Must include *all* of the following:
1. **Criteria for functional gallbladder and sphincter of Oddi disorder**
2. **Gallbladder is present**
3. **Normal liver enzymes, conjugated bilirubin, and amylase/lipase**

In some patients these symptoms may be superimposed on a background of low-grade chronic abdominal pain or nonspecific symptoms of functional etiology. Thus, the crucial step in the diagnosis of chronic functional (acalculous) GB disorder is a thorough history eliciting biliary pain as strictly defined above. Episodes of moderate to severe epigastric and right upper quadrant pain appear to be the most specific symptom attributed to GB disease. However, a thorough history may also elicit more chronic low-grade, poorly defined chronic abdominal pain or nonspecific symptoms of functional etiology suggestive of another functional gastrointestinal disorder.

The algorithm of the diagnostic work-up and management of functional GB disorders is shown in Figure 1. In general, the symptom of biliary pain that suggests the diagnosis of functional GB disorder should be confirmed by (a) absence of gallstones by ultrasound and if possible of micro-crystals in the bile (b) abnormal GB ejection fraction of less than 40% using a continuous intravenous cholecystokinin (CCK)-8 infusion over a 30 min period (c) positive therapeutic response to cholecystectomy with absence of the recurrent biliary pain for longer than 12 months.

— Rationale for Changes from Previous Criteria

The criteria proposed in this chapter modify the previously published criteria in Rome II by requiring both symptomatic and objective evidence in support of this functional disease entity and by emphasizing the need to elicit a history of

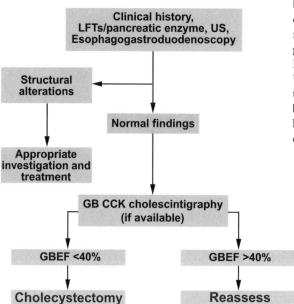

Figure 1. Algorithm of the diagnostic work-up and management of functional gallbladder disorders. LFTs = liver function tests; US = transabdominal ultrasonography; GB = gallbladder; CCK = cholecystokinin; GBEF = gallbladder ejection fraction.

moderate to severe biliary pain that is confirmed by an abnormal ejection fraction of less than 40%. This is recommended to reduce the false positivity rate.

— Clinical Evaluation

The symptoms arising from functional GB disorder are similar to those reported by patients with symptomatic GB disease due to gallstones or with lithogenic bile containing excess cholesterol. Our knowledge of the clinical manifestations originating from GB disease is mainly derived from the outcome of cholecystectomies performed in patients with symptomatic gallstone disease. The frequent association between symptoms and GB stones is not a sufficient indication that the GB is the origin of these symptoms, since more than 80% of patients with GB stones can be asymptomatic at the time of evaluation. In addition, "symptomatic" patients may also share some complaints that are similar to or may occur simultaneously with highly prevalent conditions such as gastroesophageal reflux disease (GERD), functional dyspepsia, peptic ulcer, and IBS.

Epigastric and right upper quadrant pain, dyspeptic symptoms such as upper abdominal discomfort, early satiety, bloating, belching, acid regurgitation, heartburn, and fatty food intolerance have been often attributed to GB stones. Preoperatively, "nonspecific" pain was still present after the cholecystectomy in 8%

to 27% of patients [3–6]. The more "specific" moderate to severe steady epigastric and right upper quadrant pain was still present in only 8% to 13% of the patients after cholecystectomy [5, 6]compared to 32% of colicky pain, 50% to 65% of flatulence, and 26% to 64% of abdominal distension. A multivariate logistic model indicates that the most frequently persistent symptoms after cholecystectomy are those belonging to the dyspeptic category including daily pain, bloating, flatulence, belching, and nausea whereas a previous episode of moderate to severe epigastric and right upper quadrant pain is the best predictor for a positive symptomatic outcome [7].

These findings are further supported by a multivariate analysis designed to identify signs and symptoms associated with GB stones in a population-based study [8]. It showed that the probability of having symptomatic gallstones increased progressively from 14.2% in the presence of only epigastric and right upper quadrant pain and progressively increased with the number of the following additional pain characteristics: radiation around the midback to the subscapular area, no relation with—or soon after—meals, unrelieved by bowel movements, forcing the patient to rest, and pain that was not associated with heartburn.

Screening Tests

Laboratory tests of liver biochemistries (LFTs) and pancreatic enzymes should be obtained in those patients with the above-mentioned symptomatology. These tests are normal in the presence of GB motility dysfunction. The findings of abnormal liver function tests, pancreatic enzyme levels, or both, indicate that diagnoses other than GB dysmotility should be considered. To rule out calculus biliary disease, which can produce similar symptoms, the following investigations have been used. However, some of them may not be available in some centers and some are obsolete.

Ultrasonography

Transabdominal ultrasonography (US) study of the entire upper abdomen is mandatory in patients with the above symptoms. In patients with functional GB disorders the ultrasound examination of the biliary tract and pancreas appear normal without evidence of gallstones or sludge. US usually detects stones within the GB equal to or greater than 3–5 mm in diameter but it has a low sensitivity to detect smaller stones [10]. Biliary sludge consists of cholesterol micro crystals, bilirubinate, and mucus but cannot be detected unless the crystals are greater than 3 mm. The ultrasound detection of stones or sludge within the common bile duct is more difficult. Because small echogenic precipitates are not always easily detected, microscopic analysis of bile may be necessary to exclude their presence [11].

Endoscopic ultrasonography is a technique more sensitive than traditional transabdominal ultrasonography in detecting microlithiasis (tiny stones < 3 mm) and sludge within the biliary tract [12, 13].

Endoscopy

In the presence of normal laboratory and ultrasonographic findings, an upper gastrointestinal endoscopy is usually indicated. The diagnosis of functional GB disorders is suspected in the absence of significant abnormalities in the esophagus, stomach, and duodenum.

Microscopic Bile Examination

To exclude microlithiasis as a cause for symptoms, a careful microscopic examination of GB bile could be performed [14–19]. The detection of microlithiasis and cholesterol microcrystal is best accomplished by a careful examination of GB bile obtained directly at the time of endoscopic retrograde cholangiopancreatography (ERCP) or by aspiration from the duodenum following cholecystokinin (CCK) stimulation using exogenous injection (e.g., CCK-8 5ng/kg IV over 10 min.) The resultant bile should appear deep, golden yellow to dark green-brown. Pale yellow bile from the common duct is not appropriate. Even in those patients with cholesterol gallstones or sludge, this hepatic bile is often free of cholesterol micro-crystals because it is insufficiently concentrated to nucleate. The collected bile should be immediately centrifuged and examined. Two types of deposits may be evident: cholesterol crystals and/or calcium bilirubinate granules. Cholesterol microcrystals are birefringent and rhomboid-shaped, best visualized by polarizing microscopy. If properly performed, the analysis of bile is highly accurate in the detection of cholesterol crystals and diagnosis of microlithiasis [14–19]. Bilirubinate granules are red-brown, and can be detected by simple light microscopy. These precipitants are significant only in freshly analyzed bile.

Tests of Gallbladder Motor Dysfunction

Assessment of Cystic Duct Patency

Cystic duct obstruction connotes organic disease. Filling of the GB with radionuclide at cholescintigraphy indicates patency of the cystic duct. Patency of the cystic duct can also be evaluated by ultrasound by measuring the reduction of GB volume after a test meal or other cholecystokinetic stimulus provided that it contracts after the stimulus.

Assessment of GB Emptying by Cholescintigraphy

Cholescintigraphy is performed following the administration of technetium 99m (Tc 99m)-labeled hepatobiliary iminodiacetic acid (HIDA) analogs. These compounds have a high affinity for hepatic uptake, are readily excreted into the biliary tract, and are concentrated in the GB. The test has low radiation exposure that is equivalent to that of a standard abdominal x-ray. A region of interest is drawn around the GB, as well as outside the GB to include the liver to determine background counts. Liver counts are subtracted to give the net GB counts. To minimize interference from hepatic bile activity one should wait 60 minutes after injecting the radionuclide to allow the liver to clear most of it.

The net activity-time curve for the GB is then derived from subsequent serial observations, after either CCK administration or the ingestion of a meal containing fat. GB emptying is usually expressed as the GB ejection fraction (GBEF), which is the percent reduction of net GB counts following the cholecystokinetic stimulus. A low GBEF has been considered evidence of impaired GB motor function that in the absence of lithiasis identifies patients with primary functional GB disorder.

The most widely used stimulus to contract the GB is the intravenous infusion of CCK analogs, especially CCK-8. In some countries CCK preparations have not been approved for human use. When CCK is used to stimulate GB contraction, it should be given by slow infusion instead of rapid bolus [21, 22]. Administration of CCK over a short period of 2 or 3 minutes produces variable GB evacuation activity. GB emptying following slow CCK infusion is reproducible in normal volunteers (Figure 2) [23]. A slow infusion of CCK-8 at 20 ng/kg over 30 minutes is most useful as a reproducible test for assessing GB emptying, resulting in a mean GBEF of 70% in normal individuals [24]. Fatty meals and variable bolus injections of CCK yield variable results [25].

Reduced emptying can arise from either depressed GB contraction or increased resistance such as an elevated tone in the SO due to a relatively uncommon paradoxical response of the SO to CCK stimulation. Furthermore, several additional conditions that do not necessarily present with biliary pain can be associated with reduced GB emptying (Table 2). Two systematic reviews have concluded that there is insufficient evidence to recommend the use of CCK-cholescintigraphy in selecting patients to undergo cholecystectomy [24, 25]. However, these reviews included papers that had not standardized their methodology, and, as indicated in the above-mentioned studies, they were based on bolus injections of CCK that are frequently associated with variable results. Furthermore the study of Amaral, et al. [26] indicates that the slow intravenous infusion of CCK-8 in vivo predicts human functional GB muscle disorders since it correlated well with contraction in dissociated muscle cells induced by CCK-8 (Table 3). These data revealed that there was a very good correlation between the reduction of GB volume and a defective muscle cell response to CCK-8.

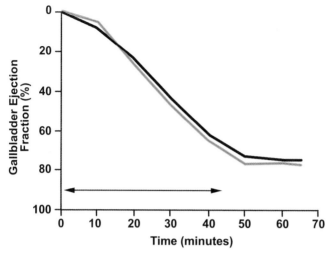

Figure 2. Comparison of the effect of a 45-minute infusion of cholecys-tokinin (CCK) on 20 normal volunteers on repeated testing. Mean GB ejection fractions (GBEFs) are indicated by the black line for the first test and by the gray line for the repeat test. The arrow indicates the du-ration of CCK infusion. The GBEF is highly reproducible. (Reproduced with permission from Yap L, et al. Acalculus biliary pain: cholecystec-tomy alleviates symptoms in patients with abnormal cholescintigraphy. Gastroenterology 1991;101:786).

Table 2. Causes of Impaired Gallbladder Emptying

1. Primary functional GB disorder

2. Cholesterol gallstones: prior to stone formation with microcrystals of cholesterol and after medical dissolution has occurred

3. Cholecystitis: acute or chronic, with or without stones

4. Metabolic disorders: obesity, diabetes, pregnancy, VIPoma, sickle hemoglobinopathy

5. Cirrhosis

6. Myotonia dystrophica

7. Denervation

8. Irritable bowel syndrome

9. Functional dyspepsia

10. Deficiency of cholecystokinin: celiac disease, fasting/total parenteral nutrition

11. Drugs: anticholinergic agents, calcium channel blockers, opioids, ursodeoxycholic acid

Table 3. Percent Decrease of Gallbladder Volume in Response to a 30-Min Continuous Intravenous Infusion of CCK-8

Groups	N	Δ GB volume (%)*	p value**
Control	8	57.8 ± 1.7	
Pigment stones (PS)	4	59.8 ± 2.0	NS
Cholesterol stones (ChS)	4	28.8 ± 3.9	< 0.0001
Chronic acalculous gallbladder disease (AGD)***	14	29.4 ± 2.0	< 0.0001

* Data are mean ± S.E.M.. ** Unpaired Student's t test. *** Described in this chapter as functional GB disease; CCK = cholecystokinin; NS = not significant.

Outcome is best predicted when patients are selected because of moderate to severe biliary pain described in the above-mentioned criteria supported by an abnormally low ejection fraction (<40%). The ejection fraction, however, may be abnormal in asymptomatic patients or patients with nonspecific upper gastrointestinal symptoms who may have an impaired GB contraction because of the presence of lithogenic bile with cholesterol that is frequently present in obese, overweight, and diabetic patients (Table 2). Thus, the ejection fraction is a useful clinical investigation to detect patients with functional GB disorders, but has a low prediction value in the selection of patients who will respond to cholecystectomy unless they are properly selected (e.g., patients with the symptomatic criteria suggested in this chapter). Further prospective randomized studies are needed to better understand the predictive value of CCK-cholescintigraphy in properly selected symptomatic patients to assess whether cholecystectomy is the appropriate treatment in patients with suspected functional symptomatic GB disorders.

Assessment of Volume Variations

Transabdominal Real-Time Ultrasonography
Unlike cholescintigraphy, this method measures GB volume and obtains serial measurements during fasting or following a meal stimulus. Simultaneous measurements with US and bolus cholescintigraphy have highlighted the differences of these two methods [27–29]. However, comparison between US and perfusion cholescintigraphy has shown that it is possible to derive a quantitative estimate of the bile emptied from (and stored in) the GB from frequent US GB volume measurements [30]. In addition, US allows for assessment of residual volume after emptying and the rate of refilling after GB contraction. US may be helpful when

radiation should be avoided. One deficiency in the technique is that it is operator-dependent and the results may not be reproducible between different centers. In conclusion, the diagnostic role, if any, of ultrasonographic assessment of GB emptying has not become the standard in functional GB disorders.

Pain Provocation Test

A stimulation test with CCK attempting to duplicate the pain has been historically used as a diagnostic investigation. This test has low sensitivity and specificity in selecting patients with functional GB disorders who respond to therapy [30]. This may relate to problems in the subjective assessment of pain and the use of bolus injections of CCK. The latter can induce intestinal contractions and therefore it can be falsely positive in patients with IBS.

— Physiological Factors

The biliary tract transports, stores, and regulates the continuous secretion of hepatic bile. Bile is transported by the intra- and extra-hepatic bile ducts and delivered into the duodenum to contribute to the digestion and absorption of fats. During the interdigestive phase the resistance of the SO, mainly due to its phasic contractions, increases intraductal pressures triggering a choledocho-cysto reflex that relaxes the GB [31, 32]. These pressure changes create a gradient between the common bile duct and the GB, diverting the bile flow through the cystic duct. However, about 25% of the hepatic bile enters the duodenum probably in between phasic contractions of the SO [33]. Moreover, during the interdigestive phase the cystic duct bile flow is complex [32, 33]. Although the net effect in this phase is storage of bile in the GB, double marker studies have shown that bile flow through the cystic duct is bidirectional. Bile may flow from the GB to the common bile duct because it contracts spontaneously. It also appears that during the interdigestive and digestive phases, bile is continuously mobilized by propulsive and nonpropulsive contractions. Some of the contractions are associated with emptying, whereas others are nonpropulsive and simply appear to stir bile contents [34]. These contractions become stronger and propulsive during phase III of the migrating motor complex (MMC) of the antrum, resulting in partial GB emptying. Thus, the bidirectional bile flow through the cystic duct can be best explained by the GB functioning as a bellows contracting and relaxing intermittently [35, 36]. The physiological significance of the nonpropulsive contractions is unclear, although they may stir the GB contents to avoid precipitation of relatively insoluble constituents such as cholesterol and bilirubin.

In the digestive phase, there is net bile emptying due to GB contraction and SO relaxation initiated by the sequential activation of cephalic, antral, and intestinal neurohormonal mechanisms [37, 38]. The cephalic phase is mediated by the vagus nerve and the antral phase through the activation of antral-cholecysto reflexes that result in the GB emptying of approximately 30% to 40% of its contents. Then, the intestinal phase is triggered by the entry of proteins and fats into the duodenum that stimulates CCK-containing cells of the upper small bowel. They release CCK that appears to act both as a paracrine peptide stimulating sensory vagal fibers and as a hormone released into the circulation [39]. Both mechanisms contract the GB muscle cells by stimulating postganglionic cholinergic neurons that releases acetylcholine. It is, however, unclear whether physiological serum concentrations of CCK can also contract the GB by direct action of its muscle cells. Although the net effect during this phase is GB emptying, double marker studies have also demonstrated that bile flows through the cystic duct in both directions.

The pathogenesis of most GB disorders appears to involve both metabolic and neurohormonal alterations that progressively lead to functional and then to specific organic disorders with the formation of gallstones and development of acute cholecystitis. These metabolic and neurohormonal abnormalities affect the motor function of the GB, probably by impairing the nonpropulsive and propulsive GB contractions involved in the stirring and emptying of bile. These motility disorders may occur as a result of a diverse group of disease states [40]. However, lithogenic bile with an excessive concentration of cholesterol is the most common condition that affects the GB motor function [1, 2]. GB muscle contraction and relaxation are affected by incorporation of increasing concentrations of cholesterol into the plasma membrane of the smooth muscle cells, probably as a result of increased cholesterol diffusion through the mucosa and lamina propia.

Pathological studies of gallbladders with cholesterol stones and cholesterolosis have shown the presence of macrophages in the lamina propia laden with cholesterol [41]. This increase in cholesterol in the plasma membrane of smooth muscle cells localizes in caveolae [42], membrane domains where free cholesterol is transported and where activated receptors translocate to couple with G proteins and stimulate pre-assembled signaling molecules [43, 44]. Increased cholesterol recruits higher concentrations of caveolin proteins that regulate negatively the function of G proteins and recycling of internalized receptors back to the bulk plasma membrane. This increased sequestration of receptors decreases the number of receptors in the bulk plasma membrane (plasma membrane without caveolae) able to respond to acetylcholine and CCK [45]. Removal of the excess cholesterol from the plasma membrane restores the function of these muscle cells [46, 47]. Thus conditions such as genetic disorders (Pima Indians), obesity, diabetes, and pregnancy may impair the GB motor function by inducing the liver to produce lithogenic bile with an excess of cholesterol. Supersaturated bile with cholesterol also is frequently complicated by acute cholecystitis because it appears that it creates a permissive environment. This inflammatory process causes additional impairment of the GB motor function through the generation of free radicals that initially damage transmembrane receptors.

The pathogenesis of acute cholecystitis is controversial. It has been suggested that this complication is due to obstruction of the cystic duct [48]. However, this hypothesis is based on anecdotic and circumstantial evidence, since gallstones are found in the cystic duct only in 14% of patients with acute cholecystitis [48] and this complication can develop in the absence of gallstones [49]. The hypothesis is based on the findings of HIDA scans showing absence of GB opacification. However, it is possible that the radioisotope fails to enter into a fully filled GB with bile because of the impaired contraction and relaxation or because the inflammatory process may also occlude the cystic duct. Cystic duct obstruction as the cause of acute cholecystitis is also not supported by experimental and therapeutic studies. Ligation of the cystic duct does not result in acute cholecystitis unless the bile is lithogenic and concentrated bile salts are introduced in the obstructed GB [50]. Moreover, treatment of ursodeoxycholic acid reduces the incidence of biliary pain and prevents the development of acute cholecystitis in patients with symptomatic gallstones and this therapeutic effect is independent of gallstone dissolution [51]. This trial is supported by experimental studies in guinea pigs that develop acute cholecystitis shortly after common bile duct ligation. This complication is averted in animals pretreated with ursodeoxycholic acids [52]. In addition, acute cholecystitis develops even in patients with lithogenic bile with excess cholesterol in the absence of gallstones, which has remained unexplained. It has also been shown that the abnormal bile that precedes this complication not only impairs the GB motor function but also affects the prostaglandin E_2-dependent cytoprotective functions [53, 54]. Thus, evidence is accumulating that lithogenic bile with cholesterol creates a permissive environment that facilitates the development of acute cholecystitis initiated by bile constituents, most likely hydrophobic bile acids.

In contrast, functional GB disorder can become symptomatic with biliary pain in the absence of lithogenic bile or gallstones and is frequently associated with poor GB contraction in response to a slow intravenous infusion of CCK-8 [55, 56]. Amaral, et al. [26] found a good correlation between recurrent episodes of biliary pain in patients with acalculous GBs and an abnormal reduction in GB volume of only 29 ± 2.0% induced by a slow intravenous infusion of CCK-8 (Table 3). The impaired GB contraction in vivo was associated with smooth muscle abnormalities. None of these patients had lithogenic bile with excess cholesterol as determined by the absence of cholesterol crystals and by the findings that the muscle defect responsible for the impaired GB contraction was quite different from the type of muscle dysfunction associated with lithogenic bile with excess cholesterol. In contrast to GBs with lithogenic with excess cholesterol, the binding of radio la-

Table 4. Proposed Progression of the Two Types of Acalculous Gallbladder (GB) Disease Characterized by Moderate to Severe Biliary Pain and Low Ejection Fraction [<40%]

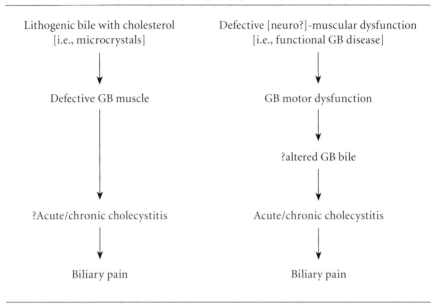

beled CCK-8 was normal [26]. These muscle cells responded poorly to agonists that act on membrane receptors, and activate G proteins and to second messengers, suggesting that the abnormality was present in the contractile apparatus.

— Treatment

Currently the treatment of this disorder is cholecystectomy once the diagnosis is made on the basis of recurrent episodes of moderate to severe biliary pain confirmed by an abnormal ejection fraction of less than 40%. There are no studies on the natural history of this functional disorders, on the pathogenesis of the biliary pain, or on whether these functional disorders lead to alteration of the gallbladder bile or to chronic or acute cholecystitis (Table 4). There are also no clinical studies or reports of treating this condition medically, including ursodeoxycholic acid. However, additional diagnostic studies should be done prior to cholecystectomy, including an evaluation of the SO if the ejection fraction is normal (higher than 40 %).

The diagnostic work-up reported in Figure 1 is recommended and is summarized in the following:

1. Symptoms consistent with a biliary tract etiology should be evaluated by US examination of the biliary tract, liver biochemistry, and pancreatic enzyme measurements. If the results are normal, upper gastrointestinal endoscopy is recommended.
2. If any of these investigations detect abnormalities, appropriate investigation and treatment should follow.
3. If no abnormal findings are detected, a dynamic cholescintigraphic gallbladder study with the administration of a CCK analog should be performed.
4. If gallbladder emptying is abnormal (less than 40%) and there are no other conditions associated with reduced GB emptying, the diagnosis of gallbladder dysfunction is likely; cholecystectomy is therefore the most appropriate treatment.

E2. Functional Biliary Sphincter of Oddi (SO) Disorder

— Definition

SO dysfunction is the term used to define motility abnormalities of the SO associated with pain, elevations of liver function tests or pancreatic enzymes, common bile duct dilatation, or episodes of pancreatitis [57].

The SO is situated strategically at the duodenal junction of the biliary and pancreatic ducts. Although functional disorders of the biliary SO may be present in patients with an intact GB, most of the clinical information concerning this entity refers to postcholecystectomy patients.

— Epidemiology

Symptoms suggesting SO dysfunction were noted in 1.5% of cholecystectomized patients in one survey of FGIDs [58]. This survey confirmed that SO dysfunction affects women more frequently than men and indicated a high association with work absenteeism, disability, and health care use [58]. SO dysfunction has been detected in less than 1% of cholecystectomized patients from a large consecutive series and in 14% of patients from a small selected group complaining of postcholecystectomy symptoms [59]. SO dysfunction was found in 12% of patients with symptomatic gallstones prior to cholecystectomy [60]. The frequency of SO manometric abnormalities differs in subgroups of patients categorized according to clinical history, laboratory results, and ERCP findings. In biliary type I, 65% to 95% of the patients have manometric evidence of biliary SO dysfunction, mainly due to what was thought to be structural alteration (stenosis). In biliary type II, 50% to 63% of the patients have manometric evidence of biliary SO dysfunction. In biliary type III, 12% to 59% of the patients have manometric evidence of biliary SO dysfunction [57].

Functional SO disorders can involve abnormalities in the biliary sphincter, pancreatic sphincter, or both. The true frequency would then depend on whether one or both sphincters were studied. One could be abnormal; the other normal. In a recent study, 360 patients were investigated by biliary and pancreatic manometry. Among the 214 patients labeled Type III, 31% had both sphincter pressures elevated, 11% had biliary alone, and 17% had the pancreatic alone. Overall, 59% of patients were found to have an abnormal basal sphincter pressure. In the same study, among the 123 patients categorized as biliary Type II, both sphincters were elevated in 32%, the biliary sphincter alone in 11%, and the pancreatic alone in 22%. Overall, 65% of Type II patients had an abnormal SO manometry [61].

E2. Diagnostic Criteria for Functional Biliary Sphincter of Oddi Disorder

Must include *all* of the following:
1. **Criteria for functional gallbladder and sphincter of Oddi disorder**
2. **Normal amylase/lipase**

Supportive Criterion
Elevated serum transaminases, alkaline phosphatase, or conjugated bilirubin temporally related to at least two pain episodes

In some patients these symptoms may be superimposed on a background of low-grade chronic abdominal pain or nonspecific symptoms of functional etiology. The diagnosis is supported by elevated serum transaminases, alkaline phosphatase, or conjugated bilirubin closely related to at least two pain episodes.

— Rationale for Changes from Previous Criteria

No recent studies have been performed to warrant a significant change in the criteria for the diagnosis of functional disorders of the biliary SO except to emphasize the importance of obtaining a history of biliary pain as defined in this chapter confirmed by laboratory and magnetic resonance cholangiopancreatography (MRCP studies), and, if necessary ERCP with SO manometry.

— Clinical Evaluation

Types of Clinical Presentation

Biliary SO dysfunction is characterized by motility abnormalities of the SO associated with biliary pain. These patients present with intermittent episodes of biliary-type pain sometimes accompanied by biochemical features of transient biliary tract obstruction such as elevated serum transaminases, alkaline phosphatase, or conjugated bilirubin. Although functional disorders of the biliary SO may be present in patients with an intact GB, most of the clinical information concerning this entity refers to postcholecystectomy patients.

SO dysfunction may also coexist with an intact biliary tract with the gallbladder in situ. As the symptoms of SO or GB dysfunction cannot be readily separated, the diagnosis of SO dysfunction is usually made following cholecystectomy or, less frequently, after proper investigations have excluded gallbladder abnormalities, including a normal gallbladder ejection fraction of higher than 40%.

Patients suspected of having biliary SO dysfunction are arbitrarily classified according to their clinical presentation, laboratory results, and ERCP findings [57]. The authors of this manuscript have revised this classification to make it more applicable to clinical practice as contrast drainage times—which used to be included—are almost never performed and noninvasive methods—instead of ERCP—are used to measure common bile duct diameter. Criteria for identifying Type I, II, and III patients are as follows:

- Type I patients present with moderate to severe biliary-type pain associated with transient increases in ALT, AST, alkaline phosphatase > 2 times normal values, or conjugated bilirubin documented on two or more occasions, and dilated common bile duct greater than 8 mm diameter at US.
- Type II patients present with biliary-type pain and only one or two of the previously mentioned criteria.
- Type III patients have only recurrent biliary-type pain and none of the above criteria.

The predictability of SO dysfunction based on these criteria varies between these groups, being highest in types I and II, but less so in type III. Conversely, the probability that the syndrome of functional abdominal pain (see Chapter 10 on functional abdominal pain) manifests itself as biliary pain is higher in type III patients and less likely in type I patients. It is therefore strongly suggested that other functional disorders be excluded before invasive procedures are carried out because they have significant morbidity.

The symptoms of biliary SO dysfunction must be differentiated from organic disease and other more common functional disorders: dyspepsia due to other causes and IBS where symptoms tend to occur daily for at least short intervals (a few days or weeks). The only method that can directly assess the motor function of the SO is manometry. This technique is not widely available and is invasive with potential and frequent complications. The incidence of complications relates to the degree of expertise associated with the performance of the procedure. Prolonged studies in inexpert hands not only result in suboptimal investigations, but also are associated with increased incidence in pancreatitis. In such circumstances, less invasive procedures should therefore be considered first and if a diagnosis cannot be made, the patient should be referred to an expert unit for further assessment.

Noninvasive Indirect Methods

Serum Biochemistries

A transient and significant elevation of liver enzymes in close temporal relationship to at least two episodes of biliary pain is suspect for SO dysfunction. Serum enzyme studies should be drawn during bouts of pain, if possible. The diagnostic sensitivity and specificity of abnormal liver biochemistry are relatively low [63]. However, the presence of abnormal liver tests in type II biliary SO dysfunction may predict a more favorable response to endoscopic sphincterotomy [63].

Pain Provocative Tests

These historic tests using morphine (± prostigmine) to detect SO dysfunction were greatly limited by their sensitivity and specificity [64]. They are no longer recommended. The clinical relevance of pain following intravenous administration of cholecystokinin (during ERCP manometry or during GB ejection fraction test) has not been critically evaluated but clinical experience suggests that there is no correlation with SO dysfunction.

Ultrasonographic Assessment of Duct Diameter

The normal duct diameter in the fasting state is 6 mm or less at ultrasound examination [65]. A dilated common bile duct may indicate the presence of increased resistance to bile flow at the level of the SO. However, the diagnostic usefulness is limited since 3% to 4% of asymptomatic patients have a dilated common bile duct after cholecystectomy [59].

Fatty Meal (Cholecystokinin) Stimulation Test

The fatty meal-induced bile flow caused by the endogenous release of CCK may be followed by dilation of the bile duct in the presence of a dysfunctional SO that causes obstruction to flow [66]. Typically the bile duct and pancreatic duct diameters are monitored by transabdominal ultrasound. The diagnostic yield has not been satisfactory when compared to the results of SO manometry [67]. It is likely that sensitivity and specificity of the test decreases markedly from group I to group III. However, the ultrasound with fatty meal is particularly advantageous in patients with a functioning GB. Although its diagnostic usefulness is limited, it can also be used to screen high-risk patients suspected of having partial bile duct obstruction. However, in the absence of appropriately designed outcome studies its diagnostic effectiveness remains to be ascertained.

Choledochoscintigraphy (HIDA Scan)

Dysfunction of the SO may become apparent when the radionuclide flow into the duodenum is delayed in subjects previously submitted to cholecystectomy. False positive results occur in the presence of a GB, liver diseases, ampullary tumors, and gallstones [68]. Several variables have been used to define a true positive (abnormal) study. A delayed duodenal arrival time, a prolonged hepatic hilum to duodenum transit time (choledochoscintigraphy) (Figure 3), and a high Johns Hopkins scintigraphic score are most widely used. The John Hopkins score had a 100% sensitivity and specificity although the number of patients included in this study was relatively small; fourteen normal postcholecystectomy patients with normal SO had a scintigraphy score of 0 to 4, whereas twelve patients with SO dysfunction by manometry had scores of 5 to 12 [69, 70]. Other studies have supported the correlation between hepatobiliary scintigraphy and SO manometry using the latter as the gold standard showing an overall sensitivity and specificity of 78% and 90% respectively [71]. Adding morphine provocation prior to the hepatobiliary scintigraphy appeared to increase sensitivity and specificity for SO dysfunction [72]. The level of sensitivity, however, has been reported to vary substantially according to the investigated variable and the employed method [69, 70]. Case studies have shown that choledochoscintigraphy may predict the outcome of SO sphincterotomy in SO dysfunction [73] but randomized studies are required to support this conclusion. Due to its high specificity hepatobiliary scintigraphy may be useful as a screening tool for suspected SO dysfunction in selecting patients to be submitted to SO manometry. Its role in selecting patients for treatment of the biliary SO, requires future studies on long-term therapeutic outcomes.

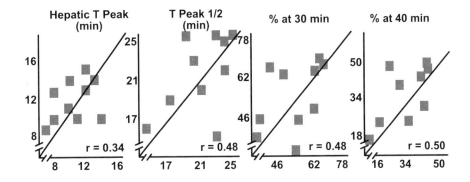

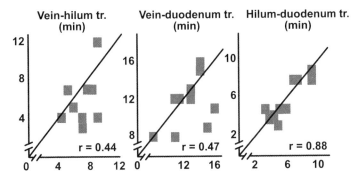

Figure 3. Correlation between values of the most commonly used cholescintigraphic variables derived from two duplicate studies performed at a 2-week interval in 10 asymptomatic cholecystectomized subjects. The solid line is the identity line. Note that only the value of the hepatic hilum-duodenum transit time shows a highly significant correlation between the duplicate studies. (Reproduced with permission from Cicala M, et al. Quantitative cholescintigraphy in the assessment of choledochoduodenal bile flow. Gastroenterology 1991;100:1106.)

Invasive Indirect Methods

Endoscopic Retrograde Cholangiopancreatography

ERCP alone is generally not recommended in the assessment of patients suspected of having SO dysfunction. Certain radiological features during ERCP such as a bile duct diameter exceeding 12 mm and delayed emptying of contrast media (>45 min) suggest SO dysfunction. However, the information obtained at ERCP to evaluate for SO dysfunction is indirect, uncontrolled, lacks sensitivity and specificity, and is influenced by a number of variables such as premedication, lack of standardization, and patient's posture.

When SO dysfunction is suspected, it is essential to rule out stones, tumors, or other obstructing lesions of the biliary tree that may mimic SO dysfunction.

Magnetic resonance cholangiopancreatography appears to be the most promising noninvasive method to obtain a cholangiogram. ERCP should be reserved when definitive therapy is planned or SO manometry is anticipated. ERCP with SO manometry and sphincterotomy should ideally be performed at specific referral centers and in controlled randomized clinical trials that will examine the impact of therapeutic maneuvers on clinical outcome [68].

Intraductal Ultrasound

Intraductal ultrasonography of the papilla of Vater demonstrates the sphincter as a thin hypoechoic circular structure. However, no correlation has been found between SO manometric findings of elevated basal pressures and the thickness of this hypoechoic layer [74].

Invasive Direct Methods: Manometry

SO manometry is done at the time of a diagnostic ERCP. Manometry allows direct measurements to be made in both the biliary and pancreatic segments of the sphincter. Recording periods are relatively short and may be influenced by drugs used for premedication, the presence of the endoscope within the duodenum, and insufflated air during the procedure. To avoid manometric artifacts, proper sedation is necessary. Drugs that interfere with SO motor function should be avoided. Current data demonstrates that benzodiazepines do not affect SO motor function. Meperidine, at a dose of less than 1 mg/kg also does not alter basal SO pressure but influences phasic activity [75]. Anticholinergic agents should be avoided as they inhibit SO motor activity. If necessary, glucagon 1.0 mg IV can be used because its effect on SO motor activity lasts less than 10 minutes. Propofol is being increasingly utilized for SO manometry [76]. However, further studies are required before its routine use can be advocated.

A three-lumen catheter with an outside diameter of 1.7 mm and distal side openings is the most widely used SO manometric catheter. Each lumen is continuously perfused by a minimally compliant pneumohydraulic capillary infusion system. Once the distal end of the manometric catheter is deeply inserted into the papilla of Vater, it is withdrawn through the SO by the station pull-through technique in 1 to 2 mm increments and then located, with the recording sensor stationed within the sphincter area to obtain a stable recording for at least 30 sec. Some authors indicate that a longer period of recording (3 to 4 min) at each station of the step-by-step pull-through reduces the risks of artifacts. During a pull-through maneuver (i.e., withdrawing a multilumen catheter across the SO), recordings of each port show, in orderly progression, an increase of the baseline pressure and then a relatively stable plateau, with phasic waves superimposed on it. The sphincter is identified as the zone of (1) elevated resting pressure between the duct (either pancreatic or choledochal) and (2) duodenal pressure with phasic waves

Table 5. Pressure Profile of Biliary and Pancreatic Sphincter of Oddi

	NORMAL*		ABNORMAL**
	CBD	*PD*	*CBD & PD*
Duct pressure (mm Hg)	7.4 ± 1.7	8.0 ± 1.6	
Basal pressure (mm Hg) (8–26)	16.2 ± 5.8	17.3 ± 5.8	>40
Phasic contractions			
Amplitude (mm Hg)	136.5 ± 25.9 (82–180)	127.5 ± 21.5 (90–160)	>350
Duration (sec)	4.7 + 0.9 (3–6)	4.8 ± 0.7 (4–6)	
Frequency (/min)	5.7 ± 1.4 (3–10)	5.8 ± 1.5 (3–10)	>7
Propagation sequence (%)			
Simultaneous	55 (10–100)	53 (10–90)	
Antegrade	34 (0–70)	35 (10–70)	
Retrograde	11 (0–40)	12 (0–40)	>50

* Values are means ± standard deviations; ranges are given in parentheses.

Source: Reproduced with permission from Guelrud M, et al. Sphincter of Oddi Manometry in healthy volunteers. Dig Dis Sci 1990;35:38. Published by Plenum

**Abnormal values for the common bile duct (CBD) and the pancreatic duct (PD) [75].

superimposed (Figure 4). The variables customarily assessed at SO manometry are basal pressure and amplitude, duration, frequency, and propagation pattern of the phasic waves. Normal reference values for the SO measured at the common bile duct and pancreatic (Wirsung) duct are reported in Table 5 [77].

Validation studies of SO manometry have shown that interobserver error can be significant in the absence of a standardized approach to the interpretation of manometric recordings [78]. Observer errors, however, become negligible when interpretation of the tracing follows an agreed standardized approach [79]. Repeated measurements of SO basal pressure are reproducible over days and even after a year [78, 79]. Nonetheless, in one study 42% of patients with suspected SO dysfunction with a normal SO manometric study who were reinvestigated, had an abnormal second study [80]. Phasic contractions vary in relation to the cyclical phases of the duodenal interdigestive motor complex [81] (Figure 5). Pancreatic enzyme elevation and episodes of pancreatitis can follow a manometric evaluation of the SO. Although such enzyme elevations occur in clinical situations in as

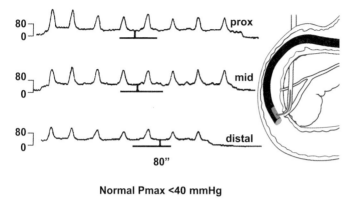

Figure 4. Perendoscopic manometry of the sphincter of Oddi (SO). On the right is shown the perendoscopic cannulation of the papilla of Vater, with the manometric catheter inserted in the choledochus. On the left, the manometric recording from the three sensors, proximal (prox), middle (mid), and distal (dist), positioned within the SO, shows phasic activity superimposed on the basal sphincter pressure, indicated by the solid line. P = pressure.

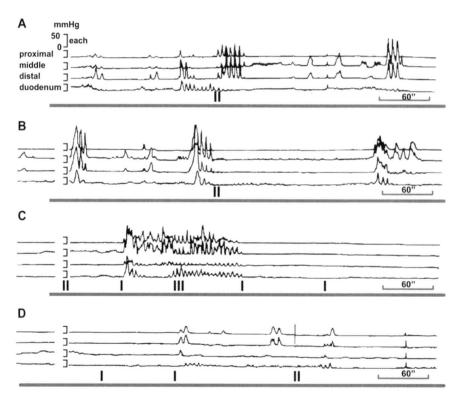

Figure 5. SO and duodenal phases of the interdigestive migrating motor complex in a prolonged manometric session (transductal and duodenal manometry). The 35-minute continuous recording shows phase II in a, b and d; phase III in c; and phase I in c and d. (Reproduced with permission from Torsoli A., et al. Frequencies and cyclical pattern of the human SO phasic activity. Gut 1986;27:363).

many as 61% of patients immediately after endoscopic manometry, overt pancreatitis may develop in as many as 24% of patients [82–85]. When perfused catheters are used, several maneuvers can be done to reduce the incidence of pancreatitis:

1. Gravity drainage of the pancreatic duct after manometry [86] may be helpful.
2. Continuous aspiration of the pancreatic duct with an aspiration catheter [83] can be used.
3. A back-perfused sleeve assembly, which has recently been developed, is associated with minimal complications and little artifact. It may prove to be the solution to current difficulties with SO manometry [87].
4. The use of a solid-state nonperfused manometry system appears to diminish the incidence of pancreatitis during SO manometry [88]. Further studies are required before their routine use for SO manometry can be recommended.

Basal sphincter pressure is routinely the only manometric criterion used to diagnose SO dysfunction (Table 5); other manometric alterations of the SO reported in patients with SO dysfunction include increased amplitude of phasic waves, paradoxical response to CCK analogs, increased frequency of phasic waves, and increased number of retrograde waves (Table 5). Moreover, more than one of these manometric findings may be found in postcholecystectomy patients with no apparent organic alterations. Thus, most experts accept only high basal sphincter pressures as an indicator of SO dysfunction.

Ideally, both the bile duct and pancreatic duct sphincters should be studied. In normal volunteers, pressures obtained from the bile duct and pancreatic duct are similar [77]. Abnormal SO function may be confined to one side of the sphincter [61, 89–90]. In patients with recurrent pancreatitis, the abnormal segment may be confined to the pancreatic duct. In contrast, patients with biliary symptoms may have the abnormality limited to the biliary sphincter. Elevated basal SO pressure indicates either stenosis or spasm of the sphincter. With sphincteric spasm, SO pressure decreases after administrating a smooth muscle relaxant [91].

Diagnostic Work-up in Patients with Suspected Biliary SO Dysfunction

The diagnostic work-up for suspected SO dysfunction as a cause of biliary-type pain is mostly considered in patients without a GB (Figure 6). It begins with liver biochemistries and pancreatic enzymes performed shortly after the episodes of pain and a careful elimination of potential structural causes for the symptoms and abnormal tests. This would include transabdominal ultrasound, abdominal CT scan, endoscopic ultrasound, magnetic resonance cholangiography

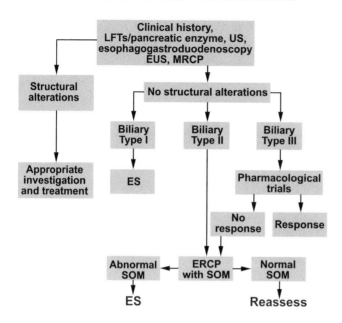

Figure 6. Algorithm of the history, diagnostic work-up, and treatment of patients suspected with functional biliary SO disorder with types I, II and III. ERCP = endoscopic retrograde cholangiopancreatography; ES = endoscopic sphincterotomy; EUS = endoscopic ultrasound; LFT = liver function test; MRCP = magnetic resonance cholangiopancreatography; SOM = sphincter of Oddi manometry; US = ultrasound.

and ERCP, depending upon circumstances of the patient and the resources available in the medical center. In patients with GB in situ the diagnostic work-up is similar to the diagnostic algorithm that is used to initially exclude the presence of a GB dysfunction without any structural abnormalities (i.e., without gallstones or cholesterol crystals). Therefore, biliary SO dysfunction is occasionally entertained in these patients with GB in situ if the biliary pain is not associated with structural abnormalities of the GB and have a normal ejection fraction >40% (Figure 1).

The diagnostic approach depends on the type of SO dysfunction. Biliary type I SO dysfunction may undergo endoscopic sphincterotomy without SO manometry. SO manometry is recommended in patients with suspected biliary type II and, if strongly suspected, in type III SO dysfunction. Invasive procedures should be avoided unless a proper clinical assessment has concluded that potential benefits exceed the risk of potential complications. Noninvasive investigations and therapeutic trials with proton pump inhibitors, spamolytic drugs, and psychotropic agents should be attempted before performing ERCP and SO manometry. ERCP with SO manometry is indicated if pain is disabling, noninvasive investigations have not detected structural alterations, and there is no favorable response to conservative therapy. As stated in the NIH State of the Science Conference, in ERCP perendoscopic SO manometry should ideally be performed at specific referral centers [92]. If SO stenosis or dyskinesia is detected at manometry, treatment is endoscopic sphincterotomy, since effective medical therapies have not demonstrated efficacy in SOD patients.

— Physiological Factors

The SO is situated strategically at the duodenal junction of the biliary and pancreatic ducts. The biliary SO exhibits basal pressures with superimposed phasic contractions of high amplitude with frequency of 4 to 6 per minute (Table 5). The high SO basal pressures prevent reflux of duodenal contents and appear to behave like resistors to the passage of bile into the duodenum, raising ductal pressures and diverting the bile flow to the cystic duct and GB. However 10% to 25% of bile drains directly into the duodenum. Cinefluorographic and manometric observations have shown that phasic contractions correspond to the closing movements of the SO. The closing movement appears as a ringlike contraction that takes place about half way down the sphincter and then extends upwards, obstructing the choledochus. At the same time the lower end of the sphincter empties into the duodenum. When phasic contractions end, the opening of the SO can be seen as a progressive filling from the proximal to the distal part of the sphincter segment, followed by flow of bile into the duodenum [93, 94]. Thus, both contraction and relaxation of the sphincter are accompanied by entry of bile into the duodenum, but the relative flow rate of choledochal bile differs markedly. The former actively squirts into the duodenum the tiny amount of bile retained in the ampulla, while the latter is followed by a flow of choledochal bile that varies in accordance with the duct duodenal pressure gradient. There are studies that suggest that the direct flow into the duodenum is facilitated by intermittent SO peristaltic contractions. However, the possibility that bile may flow through the sphincter in between phasic contractions, during the diastolic phase, has not been completely excluded. During phase III of the duodenal MMC, the phasic contractions of the SO are more frequent and of higher amplitude.

— Treatment

The therapeutic approach in patients with SO dysfunction is aimed at reducing the resistance caused by the SO to the flow of bile.

Medical Therapy

Several agents can affect the motility of the gallbladder and SO. Some agents have the potential because of their pharmacological actions but their therapeutic effectiveness has been limited. Pharmacological studies have shown that nitroglycerine decreases the biliary SO basal pressures [95] and the calcium channel blocker nifedipine at doses of 10 to 20 mg decreases SO pressure and reduces the amplitude, duration, and frequency of the phasic contractions in healthy volunteers and patients with biliary dyskinesia [96–99]. Two crossover clinical trials

Table 6. Clinical Outcome of Medical Treatment of Sphincter of Oddi (SO) Dysfunction

Treatment	Type SO dysfunction	N	Trial design	Follow-up period	Positive response
Nifedipine [97]	Biliary SO type II	28	crossover	12 weeks	21/28
Nifedipine [98]	Biliary SO type II	13	crossover	16 weeks	8/13

of relative short duration (12 or 16 weeks) showed symptomatic improvement over placebo (Table 6). Although medical therapy may be an attractive initial approach in patients with SO dysfunction, they all have several drawbacks. First, the side effects of calcium channel blockers and nitrates may be seen in up to one third of patients. Second, smooth muscle relaxants are unlikely to be of any benefit in patients with SO stenosis and the response is incomplete in patients with the other types of SO dysfunction. Third, there are no long-term studies (Table 6) on the outcome of medical therapy [97–99]. Botulinum toxin is a potent inhibitor of acetylcholine release from nerve endings. Botulinum injection into the sphincter has been shown to reduce the SO pressure and to improve bile flow [100]. This reduction in pressure may be accompanied by transient symptomatic improvement. Further studies are needed but botulinum toxin may serve as a diagnostic tool for SO dysfunction and as a predictor of outcome from subsequent sphincter ablation [101, 102].

Electroacupuncture has been shown to reduce the basal sphincter pressure of the SO in association with increased vasoactive intestinal polypeptide (VIP) levels or with increased plasma CCK levels [103, 104]. This therapeutic approach has not been investigated in the management of SO dysfunction.

Hydrostatic Balloon Dilatation

In an attempt to be less invasive and possibly preserve sphincter function, hydrostatic balloon dilation has been used to treat SO dysfunction [105]. Unfortunately because of the unacceptably high complication rates, i.e., primarily pancreatitis, this technique has little role in the management of SO dysfunction [106].

Endoscopic Therapy: Sphincterotomy

Division of the sphincter can be accomplished by endoscopic or trans-duodenal operative approach. Endoscopic sphincterotomy is the most widely used therapeutic procedure in patients with biliary-type SO dysfunction. Endoscopic sphincterotomy is less expensive, cosmetically more acceptable, and has a lower morbidity than open surgery. At present, surgical therapy is reserved for restenosis following endoscopic sphincterotomy and when endoscopic evaluation or therapy is not available or technically feasible.

Most studies reporting efficacy of endoscopic therapy in biliary SOD have been retrospective. Two randomized trials have been reported. In the first study 47 post-cholecystectomy type II biliary patients were randomized to biliary sphincterotomy or sham sphincterotomy [57, 107]. In the first study 47 post-cholecystectomy patients with type II biliary SO dysfunction were randomized to biliary sphincterotomy or sham sphincterotomy [57]. During a 4-year follow-up, the biliary pain was still improved after sphincterotomy in 95% of patients who were selected because of elevated basal sphincter pressures. In contrast, only 35% of patients improved after sham sphincterotomy. In a second study, post-cholecystectomy patients with biliary type pain (mostly type II) were prospectively randomized to sphincterotomy or sham treatment [107]. Eighty-five percent of patients with high SO basal pressures improved at 2 years following sphincterotomy, while only 38% of patients improved after a sham procedure. A third study compared endoscopic sphincterotomy and surgical biliary sphincteroplasty with pancreatic septoplasty for type II and III biliary patients with manometrically documented SO dysfunction [108]. During a 2.5-year follow-up period, 60% of patients undergoing endoscopic or surgical sphincter ablation improved with type II compared to 8% for type III SOD patients (p <0.01). Thus, because patients with type III lack objective evidence of SO dysfunction they should be approached with extreme caution before deciding to perform invasive diagnostic and therapeutic procedures [109]. Such procedures should be performed in patients with severe and disabling biliary pain who had structural abnormalities excluded and were unresponsive to trials of medical therapy (nifedipine, tricyclics, etc.).

Pancreatitis is the most common short-term complication of endoscopic sphincterotomy and its incidence is higher when this treatment is performed for functional SO disorders than for extraction of common bile duct stones [110]. This risk is even higher in patients without common bile duct dilatation or with hypertensive pancreatic sphincter. A multicenter study using multivariate analysis examined the risk factors for post-ERCP pancreatitis and identified SO dysfunction as an independent factor. It has been reported that SO dysfunction tripled the risk of post-ERCP pancreatitis to a frequency of 23%. Therefore the use of invasive diagnostic and therapeutic procedures in this functional condition are controversial, with some suggesting that in many cases the risk of complications exceeds the potential benefit [108]. A recent NIH consensus conference [92] concluded that "if ERCP is performed in these patients it must be coupled with diagnostic SO motility, possible dual sphincterotomy with placement of a

pancreatic stent" [111, 112]. Furthermore, a review on the evidence-based literature of patients with SO dysfunction type III concluded that about 60% might
benefit from sphincterotomy. These results clearly indicate that any enthusiasm
for sphincter ablation must be balanced against possible high complication rates
[113, 114]. Endoscopic techniques are being developed to reduce the incidence of
complications.

E3. Functional Pancreatic Sphincter of Oddi Disorder

— Definition

This entity is characterized by recurrent episodes of epigastric pain that
frequently radiates to the back, elevated pancreatic enzymes, and clearly defined
motility abnormalities of the pancreatic SO without being associated with any of
the well-known causes of pancreatitis (e.g., alcohol, gallstones, drugs, genetic abnormalities) and clearly defined motility abnormalities of the pancreatic SO [115,
116]. Patients report recurrent episodes of epigastric pain that frequently cannot
be distinguished from biliary pain, although it can radiate through to the back.
The pain episode is sometimes accompanied by elevated serum amylase and/or
lipase without classical abnormalities of pancreatitis. In the absence of the traditional causes of pancreatitis (gallstones, alcohol abuse, pancreas divisum, or any
of the other uncommon causes of pancreatitis), idiopathic recurrent pancreatitis
should be considered. In addition to idiopathic recurrent pancreatitis, the differential diagnosis of microlithiasis, in addition to SO dysfunction, needs to be
considered.

The association between the SO motility dysfunction and recurrent episodes of
pancreatitis has been reported in case studies [115, 116]. Manometric abnormalities of the pancreatic SO have been described in association with acute pancreatitis [117]. It has also been shown that total division of the SO in manometrically
identified patients with SO dysfunction results in abolition of the recurrent episodes of pancreatitis [115, 116]. However, randomized controlled studies are still
needed.

Many questions still remain with regards to the association between pancreatic SO dysfunction and episodes of acute pancreatitis. There is no evidence to explain the pathogenesis of the motility abnormality of the pancreatic SO in these
patients. While manometry provides an objective measure of identifying some of
the patients with SO dysfunction, even the most optimistic of investigators would
admit that manometry only identifies a percentage of these patients. Manome-

try per se is not without complication and most centers where it is practiced have evolved techniques to minimize these. Finally, the treatment of the pancreatic SO dysfunction can vary depending on the expertise available at the centers where patients are being treated. Both endoscopic and open surgical approaches have been described with variable results.

— Epidemiology

The majority of patients who present with SO dysfunction causing recurrent episodes of acute pancreatitis are female [115, 116]. This is similar to the incidence for biliary SO dysfunction. Patients with idiopathic recurrent pancreatitis have a median age in the forties and manometric evidence of pancreatic SO dysfunction varies from 39 to 72% [115, 116].

E3. Diagnostic Criteria for Functional Pancreatic Sphincter of Oddi Disorder

Must include *both* of the following:
1. **Criteria for functional gallbladder and sphincter of Oddi disorder**
2. **Elevated amylase/lipase**

— Clinical Evaluation

Episodes of pain occur at intervals of months rather than days and are associated with a significant rise in serum amylase and lipase [116]. Liver transaminases may also be elevated, dependent on the severity of the pancreatitis. In most instances, pancreatitis is not severe when standard severity scores are used to evaluate the patients. It is not uncommon for patients to associate episodes of pancreatitis with ingestion of opiate-containing substances such as codeine. An association with meals is not common. These episodes of pancreatitis usually needs in-hospital management to alleviate the pain and tend to resolve over 48 to 72 hours. Patients often describe lesser episodes of pain that do not require in-hospital management and that respond to oral analgesics.

The diagnostic work-up of patients presenting with pain episodes associated with elevated amylase/lipase requires a careful exclusion of potential structural abnormalities such as microlithiasis or pancreas divisum as the cause of pancreatitis and is summarized in Figure 7. As discussed below, this includes trans-abdominal US, computed tomography (CT) scan, endoscopic US, MRCP, and

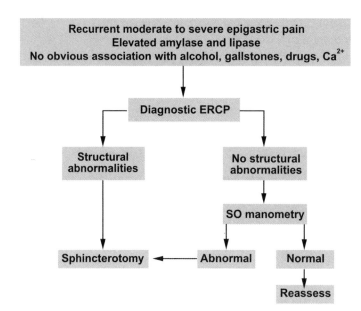

Figure 7. Algorithm of the diagnostic work-up and management of patients suspected with pancreatic sphincter of Oddi (SO) dysfunction. ERCP = endoscopic retrograde cholangiopancreatography.

ERCP, depending upon the patient's clinical picture and the resources available. The most practical diagnostic sequence in these patients suggested by the authors of this manuscript is as follows: that after all the traditional etiologies of pancreatitis have been excluded patients should undergo liver biochemistry and pancreatic enzymes followed by a US, endoscopic US and/or MRCP, and then ERCP with bile analysis and SO manometry as needed. Non-invasive procedures should be considered first [118].

Noninvasive Procedures

Ultrasonography

Ultrasonography of the upper abdomen does not normally reveal any abnormalities during an episode of acute pancreatitis. However, in the investigation of these patients, ultrasonography has been used to monitor the diameter of the pancreatic duct during secretin infusion. Following infusion of secretin (one unit per kilogram per minute), the pancreatic duct normally dilates as the secretin causes increased secretion of pancreatic juice. On cessation of the secretin infusion, the duct diameter returns to normal within 15 minutes. In contrast, it has been demonstrated that the pancreatic duct remains dilated in patients with SO dysfunction [119]. This investigation has been used to select patients to be treated with division of the pancreatic SO. However, the treatment outcomes have not fulfilled the expectation and therefore this investigation is not widely used.

Magnetic Resonance Cholangiopancreatography (MRCP)

MRCP has been used more recently to evaluate the pancreatic duct in patients presenting with recurrent episodes of pancreatitis. Secretin infusion has also been used to enhance the MR images of the pancreatic duct and these have detected abnormalities in the duct which were hitherto unidentified [120, 121]. However, the sensitivity and specificity of this investigation has not as yet been determined.

Endoscopic Ultrasonography

This diagnostic tool has also been used in patients who present with recurrent pancreatitis and this investigation has been important in identifying patients with microlithiasis as the cause of the recurrent episodes of pancreatitis [122]. The value of endoscopic ultrasonography is in its ability to select patients in whom a motility disorder of the sphincter may not be the primary cause of the episodes of pancreatitis.

Invasive Procedures

Manometry

Endoscopic manometry of the SO, which was first described over 30 years ago, remains as the objective investigation that selects patients with SO dysfunction associated with recurrent episodes of pancreatitis [89, 90]. The manometric technique has been well-described previously. Recording from the pancreatic SO in patients with recurrent pancreatitis is important because a normal biliary SO may exist in the presence of an abnormal pancreatic SO [89]. The most significant manometric abnormality is an elevated SO basal pressure in excess of 40 mmHg (Table 5). Patients with this manometric finding, and in the absence of other causes of pancreatitis, respond well to division of the sphincter.

Manometry of the SO has been in disrepute in certain centers due to the development of complications after the procedure [123, 124]. The major complication is that of pancreatitis [125], which may require hospital treatment for 48 to 72 hours. In order to minimize this complication, some units routinely use pancreatic duct stenting after the procedure [126]. Others use an aspiration manometry catheter in the belief that perfusion is the cause of the pancreatitis. Pharmacological agents have also been used during the procedure to minimize this complication [127]. While all of these techniques have been demonstrated to have effect, none have been universally adopted, as there are no major studies to demonstrate their efficacy. Most recently, a back-perfused sleeve manometric device has been developed [87]. Such a device accurately records SO pressures without perfusing into the pancreatic duct. Its efficacy and safety have not been determined as yet.

The morphine prostigmine provocation test (Nardi) test had been used in the past as an investigation to select patients for treatment [128]. This investigation is based on the knowledge that morphine produces SO contraction and prostigmine increases pancreatic flow. A positive test reproduces pain and is associated with abnormalities in liver enzymes and amylase. While this test reached popularity in the 1960s to 80s, it has not stood the test of time as an objective measure for selecting patients who respond to treatment of the SO.

More recently, injection of Botox into the SO has been used to select patients who will respond to division of the sphincter [129]. Botulinum toxin produces a chemical sphincterotomy that lasts for approximately 3 months. In a limited study, it has been shown to select patients who will respond well to division of the sphincter. Further randomized studies are required before this test can be recommended.

Drainage of the pancreatic duct by inserting a stent has also been used to select patients who may subsequently respond to sphincterotomy [120]. The results of this investigation are variable in different units and concern exists regarding the damage that a pancreatic stent may produce on the pancreatic duct.

When ERCP demonstrates no structural abnormality, SO manometry of both biliary and pancreatic sphincter is indicated [129, 130] (Figure 7). The investigation that has stood the test of time in selecting patients who will respond best to division of the sphincter is SO manometry. In a patient with the appropriate clinical presentation, a manometric finding of SO pressure in excess of 40 mmHg (Table 5) does predict a successful clinical outcome to treatment. In patients with idiopathic recurrent pancreatitis, it is important to record from both the biliary and the pancreatic duct sphincter since occasionally abnormalities in the pancreatic duct SO may be detected in the presence of a normal biliary SO manometry.

— Physiological Factors

(See previous comments on biliary SO physiology.) There is a paucity of firm data that provide a cause for pancreatic SO dysfunction. None of the hypotheses that have been proposed have been shown to be causally related. Long-term follow-ups of patients with recurrent episodes of pancreatitis have demonstrated that in time the features of chronic pancreatitis develop [111]. These include exocrine insufficiency and calcification of the gland. Consequently one may conclude that although the initial cause of pancreatitis differs pathogenetically, similarities appear to exist with other types of pancreatitis.

The passage of microlithiasis from the biliary system through the sphincter into the duodenum has been postulated to induce changes in the sphincter that may lead to motility dysfunction and hence pancreatitis. This is despite exclusion of microlithiasis in most of the series reported. However, it may still be an etiological cause, given that the majority of these patients have had gallstones in the past and prior to the development of recurrent pancreatitis.

In the last decade, there have been a number of studies that have looked at the genetic makeup of patients with idiopathic recurrent pancreatitis. These have resulted in mutations and polymorphisms that have been described. Mutations in three genes, PRSS1, CFTR, and SPINK1 have been associated with pancreatitis [131, 132]. These genetic mutations have been associated with early onset of pancreatitis. In addition, R122H or N29I mutations in cationic trypsinogen genes (PRSS1) responsible for classic autosomal dominant form of hereditary pancreatitis have been noted in patients with nonhereditary idiopathic recurrent pancreatitis. Although these mutations have been identified, their penetrance is low and indeed may only be sporadic in relationship to idiopathic recurrent pancreatitis. Their role in the pathogenesis of this disease has not been defined.

— Treatment

The best available treatment for SO dysfunction that produces recurrent pancreatitis is total division of the SO [129, 130]. The division ensures that both the biliary SO and the pancreatic sphincter are divided to allow free drainage of pancreatic juice and bile into the duodenum. Such treatment is recommended only in patients who have been shown by endoscopic manometry to have abnormal SO dysfunction as demonstrated by an elevated SO basal pressure in excess of 40 mmHg (Figure 7).

Traditionally, total division of the SO has been done by an open transduodenal approach to the SO [129]. The sphincter has been divided between sutures. It is noted at open surgery that for total division of the pancreatic sphincter, the incision normally extends beyond the outer wall of the duodenum. This is achieved via the surgical approach and the resultant perforation is dealt with by suturing of the edges. Long-term followup of patients who have undergone this procedure has demonstrated resolution of the episodes of pancreatitis. Restenosis of the sphincter has been reported in approximately 5% of patients, and this complication has been dealt with endoscopically by dilating the stricture and inserting a pancreatic stent.

More recently, division of the pancreatic duct sphincter for SO dysfunction has been done endoscopically [129, 130]. Similar to the surgical approach, these patients have undergone division of the biliary sphincter, and then subsequently the septum between the biliary and pancreatic duct has been divided using diathermy techniques. The stent is often left in the duct after the procedure and removed some weeks later [126]. The initial results of these procedures show an efficacy that is similar to that of the open surgical approach. However, at this time there are no long-term results and these are awaited. It is most important that the complication rate from an endoscopic approach is no greater than endoscopic division of the biliary sphincter. There are obvious advantages for the patients if adequate treatment can be achieved via this approach.

Botulinum toxin has been used to treat patients with SO dysfunction as previously discussed [133]. However, as a treatment option for SO dysfunction, botulinum is not efficacious, as its effects are limited by time. Consequently, it is best viewed as an investigational tool. Similarly with stenting of the pancreatic duct [109, 110]—this has not been demonstrated to have long-term positive outcome.

A number of pharmacological substances have been tried for the treatment of SO dysfunction without success. Calcium channel blockers have been shown to have a limited effect, but their side effects preclude their use long term [134].

Conclusion and Future Directions

Functional disorders of the GB and biliopancreatic SO cause significant clinical symptoms that are clearly associated with motility abnormalities of the GB and SO. However, several aspects of their pathophysiology and clinical symptomatology remain to be clarified.

Clinical studies can help clarify the following issues:

1. The natural history of functional GB disorders is clearly distinguished from that associated with lithogenic bile with excess cholesterol. Therefore, analysis of GB bile constituents and histological and biochemical parameters of inflammation in cholecystectomized specimens are needed.
2. The potential role of psychosocial conditions and genetic factors on the pathogenesis of functional biliary and pancreatic SO disorders should be studied.
3. The relation of these biliopancreatic disorders with other GI functional disorders—particularly with irritable bowel syndrome and nonulcer dyspepsia—needs to be better understood.
4. The relation to functional GB disorders—with or without lithogenic bile— with functional SO motility abnormalities should be studied.
5. The origin and pathogenesis of biliary pain in these functional conditions and whether they are associated with visceral hyperalgesia—particularly in the controversial biliary SO dysfunction type III—needs to be studied.

A number of noninvasive investigations have been developed that help to confirm the diagnosis of these conditions; however, further evaluations are needed to assess the specific roles of

1. Cholescintigraphy in the diagnosis and therapeutic outcome prediction of symptomatic functional disorders of the GB and SO
2. Magnetic resonance cholangiopancreatography (MRCP) in the visualization and dynamic assessment of the papillary region

Multicenter randomized clinical trials should be directed to the therapy of these conditions to assess

1. The medical treatment of functional disorders of the GB and SO (from bile acids [ursodeoxycholic acid], prokinetics, and relaxants to targeted analgesics) (Ursodeoxycholic acid may have a therapeutic potential since it has been recently shown that this hydrophilic acid not only decreases the excess of cholesterol from muscle cells in GBs with lithogenic bile but also normalizes the effects of oxidative stress, which may be applicable to the treatment of functional GB disorders.)
2. Improved modes of evaluation of outcome studies

References

1. Behar J, Lee KY, Thompson WR, et al. Gallbladder contraction in patients with cholesterol and pigment stones. Gastroenterology 1989;97:1479–1484.
2. Shaffer EA. Measurement of gallbladder emptying in response to cholecystokinin: the importance of GB emptying in the pathogenesis cholesterol gallstone disease and non-surgical of gallstones disease. J Lithotripsy Stone Dis 1991;3:369–80.
3. Rome Group for the epidemiology and prevention of cholelithiasis (GREPCO). The epidemiology of gallstone disease in Rome—Italy I. Prevance data in men. Hepatology 1988;8:904–6.
4. Gunn A and Kedolie N. Some clinical observations on patients with gallstones. Lancet 1972; 11:239–241.
5. Bates T, Ebbs SR, Harrison M. A'Hern RP. Influence of cholecystectomy on symptoms after laparoscopic cholecystectomy: a prospective study. Gut 1996;39:863–66.
6. Luman W, Adamy WA, Nixon SN, et al. Incidence of persistent symptoms after laparoscopic cholecystectomy: a prospective study. Gut 1996;39:863–66.
7. Ure BM, Troidl H, Spangenberger W, et al. Long-term results after laparoscopic cholecystectomy.Br J Surg 1995;82:267–70.
8. Weinert CR, Arnett D, Jacobs D, Kane RL. Relationship between persistence of abdominal symptoms and successful outcome after cholecystectomy. Arch Int Med 2000;160:989–995.
9. Festi D, Sottili S, Colecchia A, et al. Clinical manifestations of gallstones disease: Evidence from the multicenter Italian studies on cholelithiasis (MICOL). Hepatology 1999; 30:839–846.
10. Zeman RK, Garra BS. Gallbladder imaging. Gastrointerol. Clin. North Am 1991; 20: 27–56.

11. Wilkinson LS, Levin TS, Smith D, et al. Biliary sludge: can ultrasound reliably detect the presence of crystals in bile? Eur J Gastroenterol Hepatol 1996;8:999–1001.

12. Buscail L, Escourrou J, Delvaux M, et al. Microscopic examination of bile directly collected during endoscopic cannulation of the papilla: utility in suspected microlithiasis. Dig Dis Sci 1992;37:116–20.

13. Dill JE, Hill S, Callis J, et al. Combined endoscopic ultrasound and stimulated biliary drainage in cholecystitis and microlithiasis: diagnoses and outcomes. Endoscopy 1995;27:424–27.

14. Dahan P, Andant C, Levy P, et al. Prospective evaluation of endoscopic ultrasonography and microscopic examination of duodenal bile in the diagnosis of cholecystolithiasis in 45 patients with normal conventional ultrasonography. Gut 1996;38:277–81.

15. Lee SP, Maher K, Nicholls JF, et al. Origin and fate of biliary sludge. Gastroenterology 1988;94:170–176.

16. Juniper K, Burson EN. Biliary tract studies II. The significance of biliary crystals. Gastroenterology 1957;32:175–211.

17. Delchier JC, Beufredt P, Preaux AM, et al. The usefulness of microscopic bile examination in patients with suspected microlithiasis: a prospective evaluation. Hepatology 1986;6:118–22.

18. Gollish SH, Burnstein MJ, Ilson RG, et al. Nucleation of cholesterol monohydrate crystals from hepatic and gallbladder bile of patients. Gut 1983;24:831–44.

19. Sahlin S, Ahlberg J, Angelin B, et al. Occurrence of cholesterol monohydrate crystals in gallbladder and hepatic bile in man: influence of bile acid treatment. Eur J Clin Invest 1988;18:386–90.

20. Sarva RP, Shreiner DP, Van Thiel D, et al. GB function: methods of measuring filling and emptying. J Nucl Med 1985;26:140–44.

21. Shaffer EA. Measurement of gallbladder emptying in response to cholecystokinin: the importance of GB emptying in the pathogenesis of cholesterol gallstone disease and non-surgical therapy of gallstone disease. J Lithotripsy Stone Dis 1991;3:369–80.

22. Fullarton GM, Meek AC, Gray HW, et al. gallbladder emptying following cholecystokinin and fatty meal in normal subjects. Hepatogastroenterology 1980;37:(Supp II):45–48.

23. Yap L, Wycherley AG, Morphett AD, Toouli J. Acalculous biliary pain: cholecystectomy alleviates symptoms in patients with abnormal cholescintigraphy. Gastroenterology 1991;101:786–93.

24. Di Baise JK, Olejnikov D. Does gallbladder ejection fraction predict outcome after cholecystectomy for suspected chronic acalculus GB dysfunction? A systematic review. Am J Gastroenterol 2003;98:2605–11.

25. Delgado-Aros S, Cremonin F, Bredemoord AJ, Camilleri M. Systematic review and meta-analysis: does gallbladder ejection fraction on cholecystokinin cholescintigraphy predict outcome after cholecystectomy in suspected functional biliary pain? Ali Pharmacol Ther 2003;18:167–174.

26. Amaral J, Xiao ZL, Chen Q, et al. Gallbladder muscle dysfunction in patients with chronic acalculous disease. Gastroenterology 2001; 120: 506–511.

27. Jazrawi RP, Pazzi P, Petroni ML, et al. Postprandial GB motor function: refilling and turnover of bile in health and in cholelithiasis. Gastroenterology 1995;109:502–91.

28. Radberg G, Asztely M, Moonen M, et al. Contraction and evacuation of the gallbladder studied simultaneously by ultrasonography and 99mTc-labeled diethyliminodiacetic acid scintigraphy. Scand. J. Gastroenterol 1993;28:709–13.

29. Dunn FH,Christensen ED, Reynolds J, et al. Cholecystokinin cholecystography: controlled evaluation in the diagnosis and management of patients with possible acalculous GB disease. JAMA 1974;228:997–1003.

30. Pallotta N, Corazziari E, Scopinaro F, et al. Noninvasive estimate of bile flux through the gallbladder in humans. Am J Gastroenterol 1998;93:877–85.

31. Dahlstrand C, Edin R, Dahlstrom A. An in vivo model for the simultaneous study of motility of the GB, SO, and duodenal wall in the cat. Acta Physiol Scand 1985;123: 355–362.

32. Ryan JP. Motility of the GB and biliary tree. In : Physiology of the gastrointestinal tract. Ed. LR Johnson. Raven Press 1987: 695–722.

33. Dodds WJ, Hogan WJ and Geenen JE. Motility of the biliary system. The Gastrointestinal System. Chapter 28. Handbook of Physiology. Ed. JD Wood. Bethesda MD 1989.

34. Matsumoto T, Sarna SK, Condon RE, et al. Canine gallbladder cyclic motor activity. Am J Physiol. 1988 Oct;255(4 Pt 1):G409–16.

35. Itoh Z and Takahashi I. Periodic contractions of the canine GB during the interdigestive state. Am J Physiol 1981;240: G-183–G189.

36. Abiru H, Sarna SK, Condon RE. Contractile mechanisms of gallbladder filling and emptying in dogs.Gastroenterology. 1994;106(6):1652–61.

37. Hopman WPM, et al. Cephalic stimulation of gallbladder contraction in humans: role of cholecystokinin and the cholinergic systems. Digestion 1987; 38: 197–203.

38. Wiener I, Inoue K, Fagan CJ, et al. Release of cholecystokinin in man: correlation of blood levels with GB contraction. Ann Surg 1981;194: 321–327.

39. Li Y, Owyang C J, Pancreatic secretion evoked by cholecystokinin and non-cholecystokinin-dependent duodenal stimuli via vagal afferent fibres in the rat. Physiol. 1996 Aug 1;494 (Pt 3):773–82.

40. Strasberg SM. (1995). Acute calculus cholecystitis in *Gastroenterology* (Haubrich, W. S., Schaffner, F., and Berk, J. E., eds) Vol. 3, 5th Ed., pp.2635–2664, W.B. Saunders, Philadelphia; Vol. 3, 5th Ed., pp. 2665–2673, W.B. Saunders, Philadelphia.

41. Salmenkivi K. Cholesterolosis of the GB. A Clinical study. Acta Chirurgica Scandinavica. 1964;Suppl.324: 9–15.

42. Fielding CJ, Fielding PE. Cholesterol and caveolae: structural and functional relationships. Biocim Biophys Acta 2000;1529:210–22.

43. Okamoto T, Schlegel A, Scherer PE,et al. Caveolins, a family of scaffolding proteins for organizing "preassembled signalling complexes" at the plasma membrane. J Biol Chem 1998; 273:5419–5422.

44. Li S, Okamoto T, Chun M, et al. Evidence for a regulated interaction between heterotrimeric G proteins and caveolin. J Biol Chem 1995;270: 15693–15701.

45. Xiao ZL, Schmitz F, Biancani P, et al. Role of caveolin 3 proteins in the cholesterol induced impaired human gallbladder contraction in response to CCK-8. Gastroenterology april: abstract 2004.

46. Yu P, Chen Q, Biancani P, et al. Membrane cholesterol alters GB muscle contractility in prairie dogs. Am J Physiol Gastrointest Liver Physiol. 1996;271:G56–G61.

47. Lee S, Ko CW. Gallstones. Chapter 100, p.2177 in Textbook of Gastroenterology, Vol II, 4th Edition. Ed. Yamada T.

48. Mahmud S, Hamza Y, Nassar HM. The significance of cystic duct stones encountered during laparoscopic cholecystectomy. Surg.Endosc 2001; 15:460–62.

49. Strasberg SM. (1995) Acute acalculus cholecystitis in *Gastroenterology* Haubrich, W. S., Schaffner, F., and Berk, J. E., eds. Vol. 3, 5th Ed., pp.2665–2673, W.B. Saunders, Philadelphia; Vol. 3, 5th Ed., pp. 2665–2673, W.B. Saunders, Philadelphia.

50. Roslyn JJ, DenBesten L, Thompson JEJ, Silverman BF. Roles of lithogenic bile and cystic duct occlusion in the pathogenesis of acute cholecystitis. Am J Surg 1980;140: 126–130.

51. Tomida S, Abei M, Yamaguchi T, et al. Long-term ursodeoxycholic acid therapy is associated with reduced risk of biliary pain and acute cholecystitis in patients with gallbladder stones: a cohort analysis. Hepatology 1999; 30:6–13.

52. Zuo-Liang Xiao, Piero Biancani, Martin C. Carey, et al. Hydrophilic but not hydrophobic bile acids prevent gallbladder muscle dysfunction in acute cholecystitis. Hepatology 2003; 37: 1442–50.

53. Xiao ZL, Biancani P and Behar J. Role of PGE2 on GB muscle cytoprotection of guinea pigs. Am J Physiol Gastrointest Liver Physiol 2004;286: G82–8.

54. Xiao ZL, Amaral J, Biancani P, et al. Impaired cytoprotective function of muscle in human GBs with cholesterol stones. Am J Physiol Gastrointest. Liver Physiol. In press.

55. Barr RG, Agnes, JN, Schaub CR. Acalculus GB disease: US evaluation after slow-infusion of cholecystokinin stimulation in symptomatic and asymptomatic adults. Radiology 1997;2004:105–111.

56. Adam DB, Tarnasky PR, Hawes RH, et al. Outcome after laparoscopic cholecystectomy for chronic acalculus GB disease. Am Surg 1998; 64:1–5.

57. Geenen JE, Hogan WJ, Dodds WJ, et al. The efficacy of endoscopic sphincterotomy after cholecystectomy in patients with sphincter-of-Oddi dysfunction. N Engl J Med 1989;320:82–7.

58. Drossman DA, Li Z, Andruzzi E, et al. U.S. householder survey of functional gastrointestinal disorders. Prevalence, socio-demography, and health impact. Dig Dis Sci 1993;38:1569–80.

59. Bar-Meir S, Halpern Z, Bardan E, et al. Frequency of papillary dysfunction among cholecystectomized patients. Hepatology 1984;4:328–30.

60. Guelrud M MS, Mujica C: Sphincter of Oddi motor function in patients with symptomatic gallstones. Gastroenterology 1993;104:A361.

61. Eversman D, Fogel EL, Rusche M, et al. Frequency of abnormal pancreatic and biliary sphincter manometry compared with clinical suspicion of sphincter of Oddi dysfunction. Gastrointest Endosc 1999;50:637–41.

62. Steinberg WM: Sphincter of Oddi dysfunction: a clinical controversy. Gastroenterology 1988;95:1409–15.

63. Lin OS, Soetikno RM, Young HS: The utility of liver function test abnormalities concomitant with biliary symptoms in predicting a favorable response to endoscopic sphincterotomy in patients with presumed sphincter of Oddi dysfunction. Am J Gastroenterol 1998;93:1833–6.

64. Steinberg WM, Salvato RF, Toskes PP: The morphine-prostigmin provocative test—is it useful for making clinical decisions? Gastroenterology 1980;78:728–31.

65. Hunt DR, Scott AJ: Changes in bile duct diameter after cholecystectomy: a 5-year prospective study. Gastroenterology 1989;97:1485–8.

66. Simeone JF, Mueller PR, Ferrucci JT, Jr., et al. Sonography of the bile ducts after a fatty meal: an aid in detection of obstruction. Radiology 1982;143:211–5.
67. Cicala M PN, Corazziari E: Fatty meal ultrasonography is not reliable in the diagnosis of sphincter of Oddi dysfunction. Gastroenterology 1994;106:A337.
68. Corazziari E, Cicala M, Scopinaro F, et al. Scintigraphic assessment of SO dysfunction. Gut 2003;52:1655–6.
69. Sostre S, Kalloo AN, Spiegler EJ, et al. A noninvasive test of sphincter of Oddi dysfunction in postcholecystectomy patients: the scintigraphic score. J Nucl Med 1992; 33:1216–22.
70. Cicala M, Scopinaro F, Corazziari E, et al. Quantitative cholescintigraphy in the assessment of choledochoduodenal bile flow. Gastroenterology 1991;100:1106–13.
71. Corazziari E, Cicala M, Habib FI, et al. Hepatoduodenal bile transit in cholecystectomized subjects. Relationship with sphincter of Oddi function and diagnostic value. Dig Dis Sci 1994;39:1985–93.
72. Thomas PD, Turner JG, Dobbs BR, et al. Use of (99m)Tc-DISIDA biliary scanning with morphine provocation for the detection of elevated sphincter of Oddi basal pressure. Gut 2000;46:838–41.
73. Cicala M, Habib FI, Vavassori P, et al. Outcome of endoscopic sphincterotomy in post cholecystectomy patients with sphincter of Oddi dysfunction as predicted by manometry and quantitative choledochoscintigraphy. Gut 2002;50:665–8.
74. Wehrmann T, Stergiou N, Riphaus A, et al. Correlation between sphincter of Oddi manometry and intraductal ultrasound morphology in patients with suspected sphincter of Oddi dysfunction. Endoscopy 2001;33:773–7.
75. Sherman S, Gottlieb K, Uzer MF, et al. Effects of meperidine on the pancreatic and biliary sphincter. Gastrointest Endosc 1996;44:239–42.
76. Goff JS: Effect of propofol on human sphincter of Oddi. Dig Dis Sci 1995, 40: 2364–7.
77. Guelrud M, Mendoza S, Rossiter G, et al. Sphincter of Oddi manometry in healthy volunteers. Dig Dis Sci 1990;35:38–46.
78. Thune A, Scicchitano J, Roberts-Thomson I, et al. Reproducibility of endoscopic sphincter of Oddi manometry. Dig Dis Sci 1991;36:1401–5.
79. 79. Corazziari E, Torsoli A: Manometry of the sphincter of Oddi. Methodology and standardization. Z Gastroenterol Verh 1988;23:214–7.
80. Varadarajulu S, Hawes RH, Cotton PB: Determination of sphincter of Oddi dysfunction in patients with prior normal manometry. Gastrointest Endosc 2003;58:341–4.
81. Torsoli A, Corazziari E, Habib FI, et al. Frequencies and cyclical pattern of the human sphincter of Oddi phasic activity. Gut 1986;27:363–9.
82. Maldonado ME, Brady PG, Mamel JJ, et al. Incidence of pancreatitis in patients undergoing sphincter of Oddi manometry (SOM). Am J Gastroenterol 1999;94:387–90.
83. Sherman S, Troiano FP, Hawes RH, et al. Sphincter of Oddi manometry: decreased risk of clinical pancreatitis with use of a modified aspirating catheter. Gastrointest Endosc 1990;36:462–6.
84. Freeman ML, DiSario JA, Nelson DB, et al. Risk factors for post-ERCP pancreatitis: a prospective, multicenter study. Gastrointest Endosc 2001;54:425–34.
85. Rolny P, Anderberg B, Ihse I, et al. Pancreatitis after sphincter of Oddi manometry. Gut 1990;31:821–4.

86. Guelrud M: A technique for preventing pancreatitis during sphincter of Oddi manometry using the standard catheter. Gastrointest Endosc 1991;37:103–4.

87. Craig AG, Omari T, Lingenfelser T, et al. Development of a sleeve sensor for measurement of sphincter of Oddi motility. Endoscopy 2001;33:651–7.

88. Wehrmann T, Stergiou N, Schmitt T, et al. Reduced risk for pancreatitis after endoscopic microtransducer manometry of the sphincter of Oddi: a randomized comparison with the perfusion manometry technique. Endoscopy 2003;35:472–7.

89. Raddawi HM, Geenen JE, Hogan WJ, et al. Pressure measurements from biliary and pancreatic segments of sphincter of Oddi. Comparison between patients with functional abdominal pain, biliary, or pancreatic disease. Dig Dis Sci 1991;36:71–4.

90. Rolny P, Arleback A, Funch-Jensen P, et al. Clinical significance of manometric assessment of both pancreatic duct and bile duct sphincter in the same patient. Scand J Gastroenterol 1989;24:751–4.

91. Guelrud M: Papillary stenosis. Endoscopy 1988;20 Suppl 1:193–202.

92. NIH State of the Sciences Conference on ERCP Gastrointest Endosc 2002;56:803–809.

93. Torsoli A, Ramorino ML, Palagi L, et al Observations roentgencinématographiques et electromanométriques sur la motilité des voies biliaires. Sem Hop 1961;37:790–802.

94. Torsoli A, Corazziari E, Habib FI, Cicala M. Pressure relationships within the human bile tract. Normal and abnormal physiology. Scand J Gastroenterol 1990; 25(suppl 175):52–7.

95. Bar-Meir S, Halpern Z, Bardan E: Nitrate therapy in a patient with papillary dysfunction. Am J Gastroenterol 1983;78:94–5.

96. Guelrud M, Mendoza S, Rossiter G, et al. Effect of nifedipine on sphincter of Oddi motor activity: studies in healthy volunteers and patients with biliary dyskinesia. Gastroenterology 1988;95:1050–5.

97. Khuroo MS, Zargar SA, Yattoo GN: Efficacy of nifedipine therapy in patients with sphincter of Oddi dysfunction: a prospective, double-blind, randomized, placebo-controlled, cross over trial. Br J Clin Pharmacol 1992, 33:477–85.

98. Sand J, Norback I, Kostikenen M, et al. Nifedipine for suspected type II sphincter of Oddi dyskinesia. Eur J Gastroenterol Hepatol 1996;8:251–6.

99. Craig A, Toouli J: Sphincter of Oddi dysfunction: is there a role for medical therapy? Curr Gastroenterol Rep 2002;4:172–6.

100. Pasricha PJ, Miskovsky EP, Kalloo AN: Intrasphincteric injection of botulinum toxin for suspected sphincter of Oddi dysfunction. Gut 1994; 35:1319–21.

101. Sand J, Nordback I, Arvola P, et al. Effects of botulinum toxin A on the sphincter of Oddi: an in vivo and in vitro study. Gut 1998;42:507–10.

102. Wehrmann T, Seifert H, Seipp M, et al. Endoscopic injection of botulinum toxin for biliary sphincter of Oddi dysfunction. Endoscopy 1998;30:702–7.

103. Guelrud M, Rossiter A, Souney PF, et al. The effect of transcutaneous nerve stimulation on sphincter of Oddi pressure in patients with biliary dyskinesia. Am J Gastroenterol 1991;86:581–5.

104. Lee SK, Kim MH, Kim HJ, et al. Electroacupuncture may relax the sphincter of Oddi in humans. Gastrointest Endosc 2001;53:211–6.

105. Siegel JH, Guelrud M: Endoscopic cholangiopancreatoplasty: hydrostatic balloon dilation in the bile duct and pancreas. Gastrointest Endosc 1983;29:99–103.

106. Bader M GJ, Hogan WJ: Endoscopic balloon dilatation of the sphincter of Oddi

in patients with suspected biliary dyskinesia: results of a prospective randomized trial. Gastrointest Endosc 1986;32:A158.

107. Toouli J R-TI, Kellow J, et al. Prospective randomized trial of endoscopic sphincterotomy for treatment of sphincter of Oddi dysfunction. J Gastroenterol Hepatol 1996;11(suppl):A115.

108. Wehrmann T, Wiemer K, Lembcke B, et al. Do patients with SO dysfunction benefit from endoscopic sphincterotomy: a 5-year prospective trial. Eur J. Gastroenterol Hepatol 1996; 8: 251–6.

109. Lehman GA, Sherman S: Sphincter of Oddi dysfunction. Int J Pancreatol 1996;20: 11–25.

110. Freeman ML, Nelson DB, Sherman S, et al. Complications of endoscopic biliary sphincterotomy. N Engl J Med 1996;335:909–18.

111. Fogel EL, Eversman D, Jamidar P, et al. Sphincter of Oddi dysfunction: pancreatico-biliary sphincterotomy with pancreatic stent placement has a lower rate of pancreatitis than biliary sphincterotomy alone. Endoscopy 2002;34:280–5.

112. Tarnasky PR, Palesch YY, Cunningham JT, et al. Pancreatic stenting prevents pancreatitis after biliary sphincterotomy in patients with sphincter of Oddi dysfunction. Gastroenterology 1998;115:1518–24.

113. Petersen BT. An evidence-based review of sphincter of Oddi dysfunction: part 1 presentation with "objective" biliary findings. Gastrointest Endosc 2004; 59: 525–534.

114. Petersen BT. Sphincter of Oddi dysfunction, part 2: Evidence-based review of the presentations, with "objective" pancreatic findings (types I and II) and of presumptive type III. Gastrointest Endosc 2004;59:670–87.

115. Toouli J. The sphincter of Oddi and acute pancreatitis—revisited. HPB 2003;5: 142–5.

116. Toouli J, Roberts-Thomson IC, Dent J, Lee J. Sphincter of Oddi motility disorders in patients with idiopathic recurrent pancreatitis. Br J Surg 1985;72:859–63.

117. Eversman D, Sherman S, Bucksot L, et al. Frequency of abnormal biliary and pancreatic basal sphincter pressure at sphincter of Oddi manometry (SOM) in 593 patients. Gastrointest Endosc 1997; 45:131A.

118. Steinberg WM, Chari ST, Forsmark CE, Sherman S, REber HA, Bradley EL 3rd, DiMagno E. Controversies in clinical pancreatology : management of acute idiopathic recurrent pancreatitis. Pancreas. 2003;27(2):103–117.

119. Bolondi L, Gaiani S, Gullo L, Labo G. Secretin administration induces a dilatation of the main pancreatic duct. Dig Dis Sci 1948; 29:802–8.

120. Manfredi R, Lucidi V, Gui B, Brizi MG, Vecchioli A, Maresca G, Dall'Oglio L, Costamagna G, Marano P. Idiopathic chronic pancreatitis in children: MR cholangiopancreatography after secretin administration. Radiology 2002;224(3):675–82.

121. Mariani A, Curioni S, Zanello A, Passaretti S, Masci E, Rossi M, Del Maschio A, Testoni PA. Secretin MRCP and endoscopic pancreatic manometry in the evaluation of sphincter of Oddi function: a comparative pilot study in patients with idiopathic recurrent pancreatitis. Gastrointest Endosc 2003; 58:847–52.

122. Lee SP, Nicholls JF, Park HZ. Biliary sludge as a cause of acute pancreatitis. N Engl J Med 1992;326:589–93.

123. Coyle WJ, Pineau BC, Tarnasky PR, Knapple WL, Aabakken L, Hoffman BJ, Cunningham JT, Hawes RH, Cotton PB. Evaluation of unexplained acute and acute recurrent pancreatitis using endoscopic retrograde cholangiopancreatography,

sphincter of Oddi manometry and endoscopic ultrasound. Endoscopy 2002;34:617–23.

124. Elton E, Howell DA, Parsons WG, Qaseem T, Hanson BL. Endoscopic pancreatic sphincterotomy: indications, outcome and a safe stentless technique. Gastrointest Endosc 1998; 47:240–9.

125. Tarnasky P, Cunningham J, Cotton P, et al. Pancreatic sphincter hypertension increases the risk of post-ERCP pancreatitis. Endoscopy 1997;29:252–7.

126. Jacob L, Geenen JE, Catalano MF, Geenen DJ. Prevention of pancreatitis in patients with idiopathic recurrent pancreatitis: a prospective non-blinded randomized study using endoscopic stents. Endoscopy 2001; 33:559–62.

127. Di Francesco V, Mariani A, Angelini G, Masei E, Frulloni L, Talamini G, Passaretti S, Testoni P, Cavallini G. Effects of gabexate mesilate, a protease inhibitor, on human sphincter of Oddi motility. Dig Dis Sci 2002;47(4):741–5.

128. Roberts-Thomson I, Pannell PR, Toouli J. A relationship between morphine responses and sphincter of Oddi motility in undefined biliary pain after cholecystectomy. J Gastroenterology & Hepatology 1989;4:317–324.

129. Toouli J, Di Francesco V, Saccone G, Kollias J, Schloithe A, Shanks N. Division of the sphincter of Oddi for treatment of dysfunction associated with recurrent pancreatitis. Br J Surg 1996;83:1205–10.

130. Guelrud M, Plaz J, Mendoza S, Beker B, Rojas O, Rossiter. Endoscopic treatment of Type II pancreatic sphincter dysfunction. Gastrointest Endosc 1995;41:A398.

131. Etemad B, Whitcomb DC. Chronic pancreatitis: diagnosis, classification and new genetic developments. Gastroenterology 2001; 120:683–707.

132. Creighton J, Lyall R, Wilson DI, Curtis A, Charnley R. Mutations of the cationic trypsinogen gene in patients with chronic pancreatitis. Lancet 1999; 354:42–3.

133. Wehrmann T, Schmitt TH, Arndt A, Lembeke B, Caspary WF, Seifert H. Endoscopic injection of botulinum toxin in patients with recurrent cute pancreatitis due to pancreatic sphincter of Oddi dysfunction. Aliment Pharmacol Ther 2000; 14:1469–77.

134. Craig A, Toouli J Slow release nifedipine for patients with sphincter of Oddi dyskinesia: results of a pilot study Internal Med J 2002;32(3):119–23.

Chapter 12

Functional Anorectal Disorders

Arnold Wald, Chair

Adil E. Bharucha, Co-Chair

Paul Enck

Satish S. C. Rao

Introduction

Consistent with the other disorders encompassed in this textbook, the anorectal disorders are defined by specific symptoms and, in one instance (i.e., functional disorders of defecation), also by abnormal diagnostic tests. Our concepts of the pathophysiology of anorectal disorders continue to evolve with an increasing array of sophisticated tools that help to characterize anorectal structure and function [1]. These assessments may reveal disturbances of anorectal structure and/or function in patients who were hitherto considered to have an "idiopathic" or "functional" disorder. Likewise, the distinction between "organic" and "functional" anorectal disorders may be difficult to make in individual patients for the following reasons:

1. The causal relationship between structural abnormalities and anorectal function or bowel symptoms may be unclear, because such abnormalities are often observed in asymptomatic subjects. For example, up to one third of all women have small anal sphincter defects after vaginal delivery [2], and up to 80% of older asymptomatic women and 13% of older asymptomatic men have a rectocele [3]. Internal rectal intussusception is observed in up to 50% of healthy men and women [3].
2. Organic lesions are influenced by behavioral adaptations. For example, repeated straining to defecate may contribute to rectal prolapse or pudendal nerve injury.
3. The evaluation of the patient may reveal both structural and functional findings, any one of which could contribute to but not fully explain the symptoms. For example, diarrhea may lead to fecal incontinence in patients with previously asymptomatic sphincter weakness.

We also acknowledge that future research may reveal organic causes for some symptoms currently thought to be functional [e.g., in some patients, lactose malabsorption is a cause of abdominal symptoms formerly ascribed to irritable bowel syndrome (IBS)].

This report will be restricted to anorectal symptoms resulting from

1. abnormal functioning of normally innervated and structurally intact muscles, and/or
2. psychological or otherwise unexplained causes, and/or
3. minor abnormalities of muscle innervation with either minor or no structural abnormalities.

Consistent with the Rome II report, this report will not address anorectal symptoms secondary to a neurological or systemic disorder or a structural abnormality. Therefore, the following causes will be excluded:

1. abnormal innervation caused by lesion(s) within the brain (i.e., dementia), spinal cord, or sacral nerve roots, and those caused by mixed lesions (i.e., multiple sclerosis) or as part of a generalized peripheral or autonomic neuropathy (e.g., diabetes mellitus),
2. anal sphincter abnormalities associated with a multisystem disease, (e.g., scleroderma),
3. structural abnormalities believed to be the major or primary cause of fecal incontinence (FI).

Although the functional anorectal disorders have been defined primarily on the basis of symptoms [4], it is recognized that patients may not accurately recall bowel symptoms [5]. However, the reliability of symptom reports can be improved by prospectively obtained symptom diaries. In some instances (e.g., functional disorders of defecation), the clinical diagnosis must be substantiated by physiological testing. (See the section on functional defecation disorders, later in this chapter.)

The classification scheme for all functional gastrointestinal disorders is given in Table 1. In this report we will examine the prevalence of the functional anorectal disorders listed in section F of Table 1. We will summarize what is known about the pathophysiology of symptoms, and we will suggest recommendations for diagnostic evaluation and management. Readers are also referred to the working team report and practice guidelines on anorectal disorders published by the American Gastroenterological Association (AGA) [6], a consensus conference on fecal incontinence [7], and practice guidelines issued by the American College of Gastroenterology [8] for a more detailed review of this subject.

This report is based on an extensive review of the world literature by individuals with expertise in this area. The acknowledgement section lists expert reviewers whose advice was sought by the authors. The diagnostic criteria include a minimum duration of symptoms that were selected arbitrarily to avoid the inclusion of self-limited conditions.

FI. Functional Fecal Incontinence

— Definition

Fecal incontinence (FI) is defined as recurrent uncontrolled passage of fecal material for at least three months. Clear mucus secretion must be excluded by careful questioning. Patients with FI are also distressed by involuntary passage of flatus. However, involuntary passage of flatus alone should not be characterized as FI, in part because it is difficult to define when passage of flatus is abnormal

Table 1. Functional Gastrointestinal Disorders

A. Functional Esophageal Disorders

A1. Functional heartburn	A3. Functional dysphagia
A2. Functional chest pain of presumed esophageal origin	A4. Globus

B. Functional Gastroduodenal Disorders

B1. Functional dyspepsia	B3. Nausea and vomiting disorders
B1a. Postprandial distress syndrome (PDS)	B3a. Chronic idiopathic nausea (CIN)
B1b. Epigastric pain syndrome (EPS)	B3b. Functional vomiting
B2. Belching disorders	B3c. Cyclic vomiting syndrome (CVS)
B2a. Aerophagia	B4. Rumination syndrome in adults
B2b. Unspecified excessive belching	

C. Functional Bowel Disorders

C1. Irritable bowel syndrome (IBS)	C4. Functional diarrhea
C2. Functional bloating	C5. Unspecified functional bowel disorder
C3. Functional constipation	

D. Functional Abdominal Pain Syndrome (FAPS)

E. Functional Gallbladder and Sphincter of Oddi (SO) Disorders

E1. Functional gallbladder disorder
E2. Functional biliary SO disorder
E3. Functional pancreatic SO disorder

F. Functional Anorectal Disorders

F1. Functional fecal incontinence	F2b. Proctalgia fugax
F2. Functional anorectal pain	F3. Functional defecation disorders
F2a. Chronic proctalgia	F3a. Dyssynergic defecation
F2a1. Levator ani syndrome	F3b. Inadequate defecatory propulsion
F2a2. Unspecified functional anorectal pain	

G. Functional Disorders: Neonates and Toddlers

G1. Infant regurgitation	G5. Functional diarrhea
G2. Infant rumination syndrome	G6. Infant dyschezia
G3. Cyclic vomiting syndrome	G7. Functional constipation
G4. Infant colic	

H. Functional Disorders: Children and Adolescents

H1. Vomiting and aerophagia	H2d. Childhood functional abdominal pain
H1a. Adolescent rumination syndrome	H2d1. Childhood functional abdominal pain syndrome
H1b. Cyclic vomiting syndrome	
H1c. Aerophagia	
H2. Abdominal pain-related FGIDs	H3. Constipation and incontinence
H2a. Functional dyspepsia	H3a. Functional constipation
H2b. Irritable bowel syndrome	H3b. Nonretentive fecal incontinence
H2c. Abdominal migraine	

[7]. Table 2 lists conditions commonly associated with FI. This list includes organic disorders (e.g., central nervous system disease or inflammatory conditions) and so-called functional disorders. The spectrum of "functional" FI is broader compared to the Rome II criteria since limitations of diagnostic testing hinder a precise assessment of certain dysfunctions (e.g., pudendal neuropathy) or interpretation of the significance of certain findings (e.g., anal sphincter defects) to symptoms.

The age at which FI is considered inappropriate (the age of toilet training) varies among cultures, from less than 1 year in Switzerland [9] to 4 years in Sweden [10, 11]. In our opinion, incontinence should not be considered a medical problem earlier than age 4 years.

— Epidemiology

The epidemiology of FI in the general population and in selected groups has been characterized in several studies that have been summarized in a recent review [12]. The prevalence of FI in adults was 2.2% according to the Wisconsin Family Health Survey, which was based on a random telephone sampling of 2,570 households comprising 6,959 individuals [13]. Incontinence for solid stool was reported by 0.8%, incontinence for liquid stool by 1.2%, and incontinence for flatus by 1.3%. A postal survey of a stratified sample of 5,430 U.S. adults (i.e., the U.S. Householder Survey) reported a prevalence of 6.9% for frequent staining of underwear and 0.7% for frequent incontinence of at least 2 teaspoons of fecal matter (solid and liquid not distinguished) [14]. In a recent community survey of over 10,000 adults aged 40 years and older in the UK, 1.4% reported major FI and 0.7% major FI with bowel symptoms that had an impact on quality of life [15]. Fifteen percent of women and 11.2% of men aged 50 years and older in Olmsted County, MN reported FI in the past year [16]. Similar prevalence estimates have been reported in a study from Australia [17]. It is clear from the studies that FI is a common problem, although the data also underscore the effects of variation in survey methods, definitions of FI, and age distribution of populations surveyed on prevalence rates. For example, studies conducted by interviewing one member of the household (e.g., the Wisconsin Family Health Survey) may have underestimated the prevalence of incontinence because incontinent subjects are reluctant to disclose the symptom to others. These epidemiologic studies did not distinguish functional FI from FI due to structural or neurological causes.

The prevalence of FI in the community is comparable in men and women [15], and increases with age. The prevalence in nursing home residents is higher than in the general community and can be as high as 46% [18]. In the Wisconsin survey, age, gender, physical limitations, and general health were risk factors for FI [13]. Other identified risk factors for FI in the community include diarrhea and rectal urgency [17]. Among the elderly, cognitive and mobility impairment, diarrhea, and fecal retention are significant risk factors for functional FI [18–23]. The extent to which other risk factors (e.g., obstetric or iatrogenic anal sphincter trauma) contribute to FI in the community is unclear.

FI. Diagnostic Criteria* for Functional Fecal Incontinence

1. **Recurrent uncontrolled passage of fecal material in an individual with a developmental age of at least 4 years and *one or more* of the following:**
   a. **Abnormal functioning of normally innervated and structurally intact muscles**
   b. **Minor abnormalities of sphincter structure and/or innervation**
   c. **Normal or disordered bowel habits, (i.e., fecal retention or diarrhea)**
   d. **Psychological causes**

AND

2. **Exclusion of *all* of the following:**
   a. **Abnormal innervation caused by lesion(s) within the brain (e.g., dementia), spinal cord, or sacral nerve roots, or mixed lesions (e.g., multiple sclerosis), or as part of a generalized peripheral or autonomic neuropathy (e.g., owing to diabetes)**
   b. **Anal sphincter abnormalities associated with a multisystem disease (e.g., scleroderma)**
   c. **Structural or neurogenic abnormalities believed to be the major or primary cause of fecal incontinence**

* Criteria fulfilled for the last 3 months

— Rationale for Changes in Diagnostic Criteria

We recognize that increasingly sensitive diagnostic tools (e.g., anal ultrasonography, pelvic magnetic resonance imaging) may reveal disturbances of anorectal structure and/or function in patients with FI. The relationship of structural disturbances (e.g., small anal sphincter defects, excessive perineal descent) to symptoms is often unclear. Therefore, the presence of some structural abnormalities is not necessarily inconsistent with the diagnosis of functional FI.

It is now evident that measuring pudendal nerve terminal motor latencies (PNTML) are not accurate for identifying a pudendal neuropathy. Anal sphincter electromyography (EMG) is the only method that can indirectly assess pudendal neuropathy. The revised criteria recognize that many patients with anal sphincter weakness may exhibit evidence of denervation/re-innervation changes. However, the demonstration of such changes in the anal sphincters does not prove causality of FI, especially in the presence of coexistent small sphincter defects. Thus, such patients are included within the category of functional FI provided they do not have a generalized disease process that can cause pudendal neuropathy (e.g., diabetes with peripheral neuropathy).

— Clinical Evaluation

The diagnosis of FI is often made by history and physical examination. The important facts to be established are whether soiling is associated with altered bowel habits (e.g., constipation or diarrhea), whether dementia or behavioral problems lead to willful soiling or social indifference to continence, whether anal canal tone is normal, and whether the strength of voluntary contraction of the puborectalis and external anal sphincter are adequate. In addition, alternative causes of soiling must be excluded, including rectal prolapse, in which rectal mucosa extends out of the anus and secretes mucus onto the underclothes (this diagnosis requires physical exam), and impaired mobility or dexterity that makes it difficult to reach the toilet.

History

A comprehensive clinical assessment is useful to suggest the etiology and pathophysiology of FI, to evaluate the severity of incontinence, establish rapport with the patient, and guide diagnostic testing and treatment. The history should characterize the type and frequency of incontinence, bowel patterns, and the degree of awareness of the desire to defecate prior to incontinence, and elicit risk factors for anorectal injury. Staining, soiling, and seepage are terms that reflect the nature and severity of FI [15]. Soiling indicates leakage that is more extensive than staining of underwear and can be specified further (i.e., soiling of underwear, outer clothing, or furnishing/bedding). Seepage refers to leakage of small amounts of stool.

Pictorial stool scales and bowel diaries are extremely useful for accurately characterizing bowel habits, stool form, and consistency [24]. Patients with FI associated with fecal retention may report occasional passage of large, hard stools, but their incontinence more typically consists of the leakage of small amounts of liquid or pasty stool without awareness. Periods of more than three days between stools and the occurrence of hard or scybalous stools are suggestive of fecal retention, although defecation that is more frequent does not exclude significant fecal retention.

Symptoms also provide clues to the pathophysiology of FI. Incontinence for solid stool suggests more severe sphincter weakness than liquid stool alone. FI generally occurs during the day. Nocturnal incontinence is relatively uncommon and is most frequently encountered in conditions associated with altered gastrointestinal motility (e.g., diabetes, scleroderma). Patients with urge incontinence have an exaggerated sensation of the desire to defecate before leakage but cannot reach the toilet on time. Conversely, patients with passive incontinence have diminished awareness of the desire to defecate before the incontinent episode. Patients with urge incontinence have reduced squeeze pressures [25] and/or squeeze duration [26], whereas patients with passive incontinence have lower resting pressures [25]. Moreover, urge incontinence is also associated with reduced rectal capacity and increased perception of rectal balloon distention [27].

Risk factors to be elicited by a careful history include obstetric risk factors for pelvic trauma, (i.e., forceps delivery, episiotomy, and prolonged second stage of labor), medications that can cause or exacerbate incontinence, (e.g., laxatives, artificial stool softeners) and anorectal surgical procedures. Most "secondary" causes of FI (e.g., multiple sclerosis, diabetic neuropathy) are associated with other, (i.e., nonanorectal) manifestations of the underlying disease.

Scales for rating the severity of FI incorporate the nature and frequency of stool loss, number of pads used, severity of urgency, and the impact of FI on coping mechanisms and/or lifestyle-behavioral changes [28–32]. Quality of life not only includes items connected with coping, behavior, self-perception, and embarrassment, but also practical day-to-day limitations (e.g., the ability to socialize and leave the house) [33]. Patients are affected even by the possibility and unpredictability of incontinence episodes. The type and frequency of incontinent episodes alone may underestimate severity of FI in people who are housebound because of FI.

Physical Examination

A multisystem examination should be guided by the history and knowledge of underlying diseases. Figure 1 shows the anatomy of the anal canal and rectum, and summarizes the physiological mechanisms responsible for continence and defecation. A rectal examination should be conducted in the lateral position before enemas or laxatives are given. An absent anal "wink" reflex in response to gentle stroking of the perianal region or to perianal pinprick is sometimes observed in patients with a large fecal impaction, but persistence of this finding after disimpaction suggests nerve impairment. After inspection, anorectal digital palpation should be conducted when subjects are fully relaxed, while subjects con-

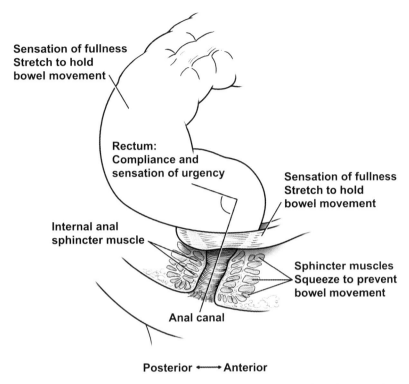

Sensation of fullness
Stretch to hold
bowel movement

Rectum:
Compliance and
sensation of urgency

Sensation of fullness
Stretch to hold
bowel movement

Internal anal
sphincter muscle

Sphincter muscles
Squeeze to prevent
bowel movement

Anal canal

Posterior ◄────► Anterior

Figure 1. Anatomy of the anal canal and rectum showing the physiologic mechanisms important to continence and defecation. (Reproduced with permission from Whitehead WE, Schuster MM. Gastrointestinal disorders: behavioral and physiological basis for treatment. Orlando, Florida: Academic Press, 1985.)

tract (i.e., squeeze) the anal sphincter and pelvic floor muscles, and while subjects try to expel the finger from the rectum, mimicking defecation. In patients with fecal retention, rectal palpation may disclose stool. Digital rectal examination is useful for assessing anal sphincter function. In one study, the positive predictive value of digital rectal examination for identifying low resting and squeeze pressures was 67% and 81%, respectively [34]. Inability to contract the external anal sphincter on command, or gaping of the external anal sphincter when the buttocks are parted or traction is applied to the anal canal, suggest significant structural injury to the anal sphincter(s) and/or neurological problem(s). In addition to the external anal sphincter, the puborectalis should also contract, lifting the palpating finger when subjects squeeze. Digital examination may also disclose dyssynergia (discussed later in this chapter). Dyssynergia is associated with contraction or failure to relax the puborectalis and/or anal sphincter muscle and reduced perineal descent when patients try to expel the examining finger.

After examination in the lateral position, patients should be examined in the seated position on a commode if the history and/or examination suggest a rectal prolapse, pouch of Douglas hernia, or excessive perineal descent, which may not be apparent in the lateral position.

In patients with FI or difficult defecation, the clinical assessment may identify significant disturbances in resting anal tone, the voluntary squeeze response, excessive perineal descent during straining, or fecal impaction. Digital palpation is a relatively insensitive technique for identifying anal sphincter defects compared to anal ultrasonography [2]. Thereafter, diagnostic testing is tailored to the patient's age, probable etiological factors, symptom severity, impact on quality of life, and lack of response to conservative medical management (e.g., loperamide or stool softeners).

Endoscopy

Endoscopic assessment of the rectosigmoid mucosa, with biopsies if necessary, should be considered in patients who have diarrhea or a recent change in bowel habit. A colonoscopy may be desirable in certain circumstances, (e.g., if the differential diagnosis includes colon cancer or age-appropriate colon cancer screening).

Manometric and Electromyographic Evaluation

The manometric evaluation assesses continence and defecatory mechanisms by determining the following:

1. resting anal pressure, which is predominantly (i.e. ~ 70%) attributable to internal sphincter function,
2. the amplitude and duration of voluntary external anal sphincter contraction,
3. the presence of an internal anal sphincter inhibitory reflex,
4. the threshold volume of rectal distention required to elicit the first sensation of distention, a sustained feeling of urgency to defecate, and the pain threshold or maximum tolerable volume, and
5. whether attempted defecation is accompanied by increased intra-abdominal pressure and relaxation of the pelvic floor muscles (normal), or by paradoxical contraction of the pelvic floor muscles, which may be abnormal. Though rectal compliance can also be evaluated by assessing the pressure-volume relationship during stepwise distention of a latex balloon, it is preferable to do so with a polyethylene balloon and a barostat.

Anal manometry is performed using a catheter assembly that includes a balloon positioned in the rectum, and water-perfused or solid-state pressure transducers located in the anal canal [35]. Electromyography (EMG) electrodes should not be used alone, but may provide helpful additional data if used in conjunction with pressure measurements. The methods for conducting and analyzing anorectal manometry are not standardized and are detailed elsewhere.

Water-perfused transducers are considerably cheaper and probably equivalent in other respects to solid-state manometry for measuring sphincter pressures. The station pull-through method is preferred to the rapid pull-through maneuver. Pressure measurements should take into consideration radial vector asymmetry in the anal canal, the length of the anal canal, and variations in patient effort. Lastly, both the pressure and duration of the squeeze response should be assessed. Because anal pressures and rectal sensory thresholds are influenced by age and sex, pressures and rectal sensory thresholds should be compared with normal values obtained in age- and sex-matched subjects by the same technique. With the advent of anal endosonography, vector manometry is not routinely used for identifying anal sphincter defects [36, 37].

Anal Endosonography

Anal endosonography (ultrasound, US) identifies anal sphincter thinning and defects [38] that are often clinically unrecognized [2] and may be amenable to surgical repair [39]. US may be performed with patients in the prone or left lateral positions. A rotating 7 MHz or 10 MHz transducer that provides a 360° view is inserted into the rectum and then slowly withdrawn to image the anal canal along its whole length. The possible advantages of 3-D imaging over available 2-D techniques are unknown [40].

US reveals the internal anal sphincter muscle as a dark homogeneous ring whereas the external anal sphincter has mixed echogenicity. US reliably identifies anatomic defects [41, 42] or thinning of the internal sphincter [43], whereas interpretation of external sphincter images is much more subjective, operator-dependent, confounded by normal anatomical variations of the external sphincter [38, 44], and subject to substantial interobserver variability [45, 46]. The external sphincter and perirectal fat are both echogenic and frequently indistinguishable, precluding accurate characterization of external sphincter thickness and identification of external sphincter atrophy. Moreover, the external sphincter is often asymmetric in the upper anal canal, particularly in women, impairing discrimination of normal variants from a sphincter defect [38, 47].

The accuracy of US identification of anal sphincter defects has been confirmed against EMG [41, 45] and histology in both in vivo and in vitro studies [42]. US may be used as a noninvasive test to identify anal sphincter abnormalities in FI.

Dynamic Proctography (Defecography)

During defecography, anorectal anatomy and pelvic floor motion are recorded on video at rest, and during coughing, squeezing, and straining to expel barium from the rectum. Pelvic floor motion is characterized by measuring the anorectal angle and position of the anorectal junction during these maneuvers. However, the methods for testing and interpretation are incompletely standardized [6] (e.g., for incontinent patients, a thick barium paste (Anatrast™, E-Z-EM, Westbury, NY) is probably preferable to liquid barium). Diagnostic utility is also hampered by the lack of appropriate age- and sex-matched subjects (e.g., since pelvic floor prolapse and rectoceles are relatively common in asymptomatic older women, findings should be compared to asymptomatic subjects, but only a handful of studies have characterized pelvic floor motion by evacuation defecography in asymptomatic subjects) [6].

Defecography is useful only for selected patients with FI, particularly prior to surgery, in order to identify or confirm rectal prolapse, excessive perineal descent, a significant rectocele, an enterocele, or internal rectal intussusception.

Pelvic Magnetic Resonance Imaging (MRI)

MRI is the only imaging modality that can visualize both anal sphincter anatomy and global pelvic floor motion (i.e., anterior, middle, and posterior compartments) in real time without radiation exposure [48]. In a small study of seven women with obstetric trauma, there was 100% concordance between MRI performed with an endoanal coil and surgical findings for presence, size, and location of anal sphincter tears [49]. Normal values for sphincter morphology by MRI differ from US, and also depend on whether images were acquired by an endoanal coil or phased-array imaging [50]. Interobserver variability may be slightly higher for endoanal MRI compared to US [46, 51]. Disagreement exists over whether MRI or US is the superior technique for the evaluation of the internal sphincter, although MRI performs the same or better than US for the assessment of the external sphincter [27, 51, 52].

Dynamic images are acquired every 1.4 to 2 seconds during rest, squeeze, defecation, and the Valsalva maneuver in the desired cross-sectional plane [53]. These acquisition rates overcome the limitations of relatively slow acquisition rates (i.e., 30 seconds per image) in breath-hold gradient imaging. The exam can be performed using conventional, closed-configuration MRI systems as there is little difference in the detection of clinically relevant findings between supine MRI and seated MRI using open-configuration magnets (with the exception of rectal intussusceptions) [54].

US is the first choice for anal sphincter imaging in FI, because it is widely available, reasonably accurate for identifying internal and external sphincter abnormalities, and cheaper than MRI. Endoanal MRI may be useful for identifying external sphincter atrophy [27], particularly prior to surgical repair of external sphincter defects. One study suggested that patients who underwent surgical repair of sphincter defects and had external sphincter atrophy did not fare as well as those patients who did not have atrophy [55]. Dynamic MRI provides a unique appreciation of global pelvic floor motion since, in addition to the anorectum, the bladder and genital organs are also visualized.

Neurophysiologic Tests

Neurophysiological tests can characterize disturbances in innervation of the external anal sphincter and pelvic floor muscles. These tests include pudendal nerve terminal motor latencies, concentric needle EMG recordings from single motor units in the external anal sphincter or puborectalis muscle, and surface recordings of EMG activity from the external anal sphincter from electrodes placed in the anal canal.

Pudendal Nerve Terminal Motor Latency (PNTML). PNTML is recorded by stimulating the pudendal nerve transrectally with a glove-mounted electrode and measuring the latency to onset of the anal sphincter EMG response, which is recorded from a second pair of electrodes at the base of the investigator's finger [56]. Prolonged conduction time is considered to be indicative of pudendal nerve damage, which may be caused by stretch from perineal descent or other trauma. Initial studies suggested that patients with a pudendal neuropathy would not fare as well as patients without a neuropathy after surgical repair of sphincter defects. More recently, the utility of measuring PNTML has been questioned since pudendal neuropathy is attributed to an axonopathy rather than demyelination. Since PNTML is dependent only on the fastest conducting fibers in the pudendal nerve, nerve latencies may be normal even if a few normally conducting fibers remain. There are several methodological limitations to PNTML. Test reproducibility is unknown, normative data are limited, and multiple factors (i.e., age, parturition, body-mass index) influencing nerve latencies are generally not taken into account. The "normal" ranges for nerve latencies are extremely stringent. Thus, latencies that would be regarded within normal limits for other peripheral nerve injuries are regarded as abnormal for the pudendal nerve. The sensitivity and specificity of the test is uncertain. In one study, approximately 50% of patients with prolonged PNTML had normal anal canal squeeze pressures [57]. Lastly, recent studies suggest the test does not predict improvement after surgical repair of anal sphincter defects [58]. An AGA technical review recommended that PNTML should not be used for evaluating patients with FI [6].

Alternative approaches for assessing the integrity of the motor pathways to the external anal sphincter involve spinal [59] or cortical stimulation with electrical or magneto-electrical stimulation techniques [60–62]. To date, these techniques have not been shown to correlate with clinical findings and are regarded as research tools only. Likewise, recording of cortical evoked potentials from electrical or mechanical stimulation of the rectum [63–65] to assess sensory innervation of the pelvic floor has not been shown to have clinical value in FI [65].

Concentric Needle EMG Recordings.   Concentric needle EMG is necessary when there is a clinical suspicion of a proximal neurogenic lesion such as one involving the sacral roots, conus, or cauda. EMG is sensitive for identifying denervation and can usually identify myogenic, neurogenic, or mixed injury affecting the external anal sphincter. In patients who do not have an underlying myopathy, myogenic injury indicates direct anal sphincter trauma. Neurogenic injury in the anal sphincter may be caused by damage anywhere along the lower motor neuron innervating the anal sphincter, including the nerve branches within the anal sphincter [66]. Neurogenic injury affecting the external anal sphincter and ischiocavernosus probably indicates a pudendal neuropathy. Needle EMG of the puborectalis muscle can be used to distinguish disorders that affect this muscle and the external sphincter muscle selectively, or in combination [67].

EMG recordings by an anal sponge or hard plug electrode correlate well with sphincter pressures, but cannot distinguish the causes of sphincter weakness specified above. Intraluminal electrodes are believed to be more accurate because they are closer to the external anal sphincter muscle and are less likely to pick up gluteal or other muscles [68]. Surface EMG is used as a biofeedback signal for pelvic floor retraining of the external anal sphincter in FI [69].

Surface Recordings of EMG Activity.   Surface EMG by means of multi-electrodes arrays has recently been developed to allow noninvasive recording of single motor-unit action potentials (MUAP) and their characteristics from large striated muscles [70]. This technique provides new insights into external sphincter innervation in healthy subjects [71].

— Physiological Features

Fecal continence is maintained by several mechanisms, including anatomical factors (i.e., the pelvic barrier, rectal curvatures, and transverse rectal folds), rectoanal sensation, and rectal compliance. In addition, disturbances of fecal delivery and/or consistency may be associated with FI [72].

Pelvic Barrier

Anal sphincter weakness is the most frequently identified disturbance in incontinent patients. Internal sphincter dysfunction may be characterized by exaggerated spontaneous relaxation of the internal anal sphincter (sampling reflex) [73, 74] or decreased resting pressure [73, 75]. Internal sphincter tone is primarily attributable to smooth muscle activity. Resting anal sphincter tone was not affected by spinal transection between vertebrae C_6 and L_1 [76, 77], whereas high spinal anesthesia reduced resting tone, suggesting extrinsic nerves may contribute to resting sphincter tone [78]. Decreased anal resting pressure may be associated with structural disturbances (i.e., defects and/or thinning) of the internal sphincter, as visualized by US. Internal sphincter thinning may be idiopathic or secondary to scleroderma. Farouk and colleagues [75] described electromechanical dissociation in patients with FI. Speakman and colleagues [79] documented reduced sensitivity of the internal anal sphincter to noradrenaline and alterations of α-adrenoceptors.

External anal sphincter weakness may result from one or more of the following factors: sphincter damage, neuropathy, myopathy, or reduced corticospinal input. In addition to the anal sphincters, the levator ani muscles also contribute to the pelvic barrier [67]. A recent study suggested that the reduced inward traction exerted by the puborectalis in patients with FI correlated more closely with symptoms than did squeeze pressures, and improved after biofeedback therapy [80]. Whereas the anal sphincters seal the anal canal, the levator ani maintain continence of solid stool by a flap-valve action [81]. Patients with excessive perineal descent have a more obtuse anorectal angle, impairing the flap valve that normally maintains continence when intra-abdominal pressure increases.

Although there are numerous studies of FI in women, few studies have evaluated the pathophysiology of FI in men [82–84]. FI may be associated with normal sphincteric function in men [83]. However, in the absence of iatrogenic injury (e.g., after perianal procedures), men generally have fecal soiling or leakage rather than gross incontinence. This may be associated with dyssynergic defecation [85], or high anal resting pressure that entraps small particles of feces during defecation and subsequently expels them, causing perianal soiling and discomfort [86], or isolated weakness of the internal anal sphincter.

Rectal Compliance and Rectoanal Sensation

Stool is often transferred into the rectum by colonic high-amplitude propagated contractions (HAPCs), which tend to occur after awakening or meals [87]. Rectal distention by stool is associated with several processes that serve to preserve continence, or if appropriate, proceed to defecation. Rectal distention induces reflex relaxation of the internal anal sphincter, and is perceived as a sensation of rectal fullness, as if the rectum were uncomfortably full of flatus or feces. If defecation is inconvenient, the urge to defecate prompts voluntary contraction of the external sphincter [88]; this sensation wanes together with the sense of urgency as the rectum accommodates to hold more stool.

Table 2. Common Causes of Fecal Incontinence

Anal sphincter weakness
  Traumatic—obstetric, surgical (e.g., hemorrhoidectomy, internal sphincterotomy)
  Nontraumatic—scleroderma, internal sphincter degeneration of unknown etiology

Neuropathy—peripheral (e.g., pudendal) or generalized (e.g., diabetes mellitus)

Disturbances of pelvic floor—rectal prolapse, descending perineum syndrome

Inflammatory conditions—radiation proctitis, Crohn's disease, ulcerative colitis

Central nervous system disorders—dementia, stroke, brain tumors, multiple sclerosis,
  spinal cord lesions

Diarrhea—irritable bowel syndrome, postcholecystectomy diarrhea

Other—fecal retention with overflow, behavioral disorders

The importance of rectal compliance and/or sensation for maintaining continence is emphasized by the finding that sphincter pressures alone do not always distinguish continent from incontinent subjects (see below). Reduced rectal sensation allows stool to enter the anal canal, and perhaps leak before the external sphincter contracts [73, 88, 89]. Decreased rectal sensitivity and increased rectal compliance may also contribute to fecal retention by decreasing the frequency and intensity of the urge (and hence the motivation) to defecate. Conversely, fecal retention may reduce rectal sensation, perhaps by altering rectal tone and viscoelastic properties, or by affecting afferent nerve pathways [90].

Enhanced rectal perception, perhaps a marker of concomitant IBS [73, 91] may be associated with reduced rectal compliance, and repetitive rectal contractions during rectal distention. Rectal capacity is also reduced in women with FI, and associated with the symptom of urgency [27]. Moreover, rectal hypersensitivity cannot be entirely explained by disturbances in rectal compliance. These observations confirm that FI is a heterogeneous disorder and that patients often suffer from more than one deficit (Table 2).

Anal sphincter relaxation may occur during, or be independent of, rectal distention, enabling the anal lining to periodically "sample" rectal contents and ascertain whether rectal contents are gas, liquid, or stool [92]. It is unclear if anal sampling normally contributes to maintaining fecal continence, because continence for saline is not affected when the anal canal is anesthetized by lidocaine [93]. However the anal sampling response occurred less frequently and anal sensation was reduced in incontinent patients, perhaps depriving them of sensory information [92].

Other Factors

In addition to anorectal dysfunctions, continence may also be affected by disturbances of stool consistency and/or delivery, impaired mental faculties, and mobility [94].

— Psychological Features

There is a paucity of data on psychological aspects of patients with FI. The results of two studies in adult patients with FI demonstrate high levels of psychological distress on the Symptom Checklist (SCL)-90R, and have impaired quality of life [15, 33]. Heymen and colleagues found normal Minnesota Multiphasic Personality Inventory (MMPI) profiles in fecally incontinent patients [95].

— Treatment

Management of FI must be tailored to clinical manifestations and includes treatment of underlying diseases as described below.

Bowel Habit Modification

Restoring normal bowel habits is often the cornerstone to effectively managing incontinence and accurate characterization of bowel habits is necessary to tailor therapy.

In addition to reducing diarrhea, loperamide given at an adequate dose, (i.e., 2 to 4 mg, 30 minutes before meals, up to 16 mg/day), slightly increased internal sphincter tone, thereby reducing incontinence [96]. In patients with constipation and diarrhea, effective loperamide dose titration to reduce diarrhea while avoiding constipation can be challenging. By taking loperamide before social occasions or when eating meals outside the home, incontinent patients may avoid having an accident and gain confidence in their ability to participate in social activities. In an open-label study of 18 patients treated with the tricyclic antidepressant (TCA) amitriptyline (20 mg daily), fecal continence improved significantly in 16 and normalized in 13 patients [97]. Diphenoxylate, which may be combined with atropine (Lomotil™), and the serotonin 5-hydroxytryptamine (5-HT$_3$) antagonist alosetron (Lotronex™) are alternative options for diarrhea [98, 99]. Patients with constipation, fecal impaction, and overflow incontinence often benefit from a regularized evacuation program that incorporates timed evacuation by digital stimulation and/or use of bisacodyl/glycerine suppositories, fiber supplementation, and oral laxatives [8, 100]. For example, a regimen consisting of a daily osmotic laxative (lactulose 10 ml twice daily) plus a weekly enema was curative in the majority of elderly patients with FI, including those with dementia [23].

Biofeedback Therapy

Biofeedback is based on the principle of operant conditioning [101]. Using a rectal balloon-anal manometry device, patients are taught to contract the external anal sphincter when they perceive balloon distention; perception may be reinforced by visual tracings of balloon volume and anal pressure, and the procedure is repeated with progressively smaller volumes. Many uncontrolled studies suggest continence improved in the majority of patients with FI [69]. Anal sphincter pressures improved modestly after biofeedback therapy in some studies. The improvement in anal pressures was small, and was not correlated to symptom improvement [102]. Perhaps these modest effects are attributable to inadequate biofeedback therapy, lack of reinforcement, and assessment of objective parameters at an early stage after biofeedback therapy [103]. In contrast, sensory assessments (i.e., preserved baseline sensation and improved sensory discrimination after biofeedback therapy) are more likely to be associated with improved continence after biofeedback therapy [104, 105].

A recent study randomized 171 incontinent patients to four treatment groups: standard medical/nursing care (i.e., advice only), advice plus verbal instruction on sphincter exercises, hospital-based computer-assisted sphincter pressure biofeedback, or hospital biofeedback plus use of a home EMG biofeedback device [106]. Based on intent-to-treat analysis, overall symptoms improved or resolved in ~ 50% and 5% patients, respectively. The improvement was sustained at one year after therapy. Symptoms and both resting and squeeze pressures improved to a similar degree in all four groups. These results underscore the importance of the patient-health care provider relationship in ensuring that patients understand their condition and benefit from practical advice regarding coping strategies (e.g., diet and skin care). Further controlled studies are necessary to define the effect of (1) pelvic floor retraining in patients who do not respond to advice only and (2) anorectal sensory retraining in incontinent patients.

Surgical Approaches

Surgical approaches are of unproven efficacy for functional FI and of uncertain long-term efficacy for incontinence associated with anal sphincteric defects. In short-term studies, up to 85% of patients with sphincter defects had improved continence after an overlapping anterior sphincteroplasty [107]. However, long-term results are disappointing; failure rates of ~ 50% are seen after 40 to 60 months [107–109]. A colostomy is the last resort for patients with severe incontinence. The impact of a colostomy on quality of life in FI has not been formally assessed [7].

Minimally Invasive Approaches

Sacral nerve stimulation involves implantation of an U.S. Food and Drug Administration (FDA)-approved device, and has been used in over 3000 patients with urinary incontinence in the United States. Observations from European studies suggest that sacral nerve stimulation augments squeeze pressure more than resting pressure and significantly improves continence [110–112]. Sacral stimulation may also modulate rectal sensation in incontinent patients [110]. Sacral stimulation is conducted as a staged procedure and patients whose symptoms respond to temporary stimulation over a 2-week period proceed to permanent subcutaneous implantation of the device. The procedure for device placement is technically straightforward, and device-related complications are less frequent or significant relative to more invasive artificial sphincter devices discussed above. A multicenter study assessing sacral nerve stimulation for FI is in progress in the United States.

F2. Functional Anorectal Pain

Two forms of functional anorectal pain have been described: chronic proctalgia and proctalgia fugax. They are distinguished on the basis of *duration* (hours of constant pain for chronic proctalgia vs. seconds to minutes for proctalgia fugax), *frequency* (constant or frequent pain for chronic proctalgia vs. infrequent pain in proctalgia fugax), and characteristic *quality of pain* (dull pain or urgency in chronic proctalgia vs. sharp pain in proctalgia fugax). Despite these differences there is significant overlap in the diagnoses [113] Factor analysis studies do not identify separate symptom clusters for the two disorders [114], giving rise to speculation that they are part of the same syndrome. However, indirect evidence suggests that there may be different physiological mechanisms for these two types of pain (striated muscle tension in chronic proctalgia and smooth muscle spasm in proctalgia fugax, see below). Consequently, the historical distinction between these two forms of anorectal pain has been preserved in this classification system.

F2a. Chronic Proctalgia

— Definition

Chronic proctalgia is also called levator ani syndrome, levator spasm, puborectalis syndrome, pyriformis syndrome, and pelvic tension myalgia. The pain is often described as a vague, dull ache or pressure sensation high in the rectum and is often worse with sitting than with standing or lying down. Physical examination may reveal overly contracted levator ani muscles and tenderness on palpation of the pelvic floor. For unknown reasons, tenderness is often asymmetric and may be noted on the left more often than on the right side [115].

— Epidemiology

The prevalence of rectoanal pain in a sample of the general population was 6.6% [14]. It is unclear what proportion of these people had symptoms suggestive of chronic proctalgia. Rectoanal pain was reported more frequently by women (7.4% of all women versus 5.7% of all men), and tended to decline after age 45 [14]. Though only 29% of people with rectoanal pain consulted a physician, the associated disability was significant; people with anorectal pain missed an average of 17.9 days from work or school in the previous year, and 11.5% reported that they were currently too sick to work or go to school [14]. In another study of over 300 patients with chronic proctalgia, ages ranged from 6 to 90 years with the majority aged 30 to 60 years [115]. There are no published data on the frequency with which chronic proctalgia is encountered in medical practice.

F2a. Diagnostic Criteria* for Chronic Proctalgia

Must include *all* of the following:
1. **Chronic or recurrent rectal pain or aching**
2. **Episodes last 20 minutes or longer**
3. **Exclusion of other causes of rectal pain such as ischemia, inflammatory bowel disease, cryptitis, intramuscular abscess, anal fissure, hemorrhoids, prostatitis, and coccygodynia.**

*Criteria fulfilled for the last 3 months with symptom onset at least 6 months prior to diagnosis

Chronic proctalgia may be further characterized into levator ani syndrome or unspecified anorectal pain based on digital rectal examination.

F2a1. Levator Ani Syndrome
Symptom criteria for chronic proctalgia and tenderness during posterior traction on the puborectalis

F2a2. Unspecified Functional Anorectal Pain
Symptom criteria for chronic proctalgia but no tenderness during posterior traction on the puborectalis

— Rationale for Changes in Diagnostic Classification System

In the previous classification, patients who had the symptom criteria specified above were characterized as "highly likely" or "possible" levator ani syndrome based on the presence or absence of tenderness during posterior traction on the puborectalis respectively. This distinction is emphasized by modifying the nomenclature in the current version. It is recognized that symptoms present for less than 3 months that are otherwise consistent with the diagnosis may warrant clinical diagnosis and treatment, but for research studies, symptoms should be present for at least 3 months.

— Clinical Evaluation

Diagnosis is based primarily on the presence of characteristic symptoms and physical examination findings (see definition above). During puborectalis palpation, tenderness may be predominantly left-sided, and massage of this muscle will generally elicit the characteristic discomfort. Evaluation often includes sigmoidoscopy and appropriate imaging studies such as ultrasonography, pelvic computed tomography (CT) or MRI to exclude alternative diseases.

— Physiological Features

The pathophysiology of unspecified functional anorectal pain is poorly understood. Levator ani syndrome is hypothesized to result from overly contracted pelvic floor muscles. Grimaud and colleagues [113] found elevated anal resting pressures in all patients (n=12) with levator ani syndrome. Moreover, anal canal pressures normalized in association with pain relief after biofeedback therapy. These observations suggest that elevated anal canal pressures or EMG levels may constitute a useful quantitative sign for the diagnosis of levator ani syndrome, but need confirmation in a controlled study with a larger number of patients.

— Psychological Features

Heymen, Wexner, and Gulledge [95] observed elevated hypochondriasis, depression, and hysteria scales on the MMPI in 11 patients with levator ani syndrome. This pattern is seen in chronic pain patients and often referred to as the "neurotic triad." Though clinical observations suggest that quality of life is significantly impaired in patients with this syndrome, there is limited evidence in this regard [116].

— Approach to Treatment

Treatments thought to be effective are those that are directed towards reducing tension in the striated pelvic floor muscles [113, 115, 117–119]. These include electrogalvanic stimulation [117, 119–121], biofeedback training [113, 119, 120, 122–124], muscle relaxants such as methocarbamol, diazepam, and cyclobenzaprine [115, 125], digital massage of the levator ani muscles [124, 126], and sitz baths [127]. A recent double-blind placebo-controlled study showed no efficacy of intrasphincteric injection of botulinum toxin A in levator ani syndrome [128].

Except as noted above, these therapeutic trials were uncontrolled, and patient selection criteria were variable. If the patient's distress or other circumstances require that treatment be undertaken, the only advice that can be offered at present is to do no harm, that is, to select a treatment such as biofeedback which has no significant adverse consequences. With the exception of internal sphincterotomy for chronic anal fissure refractory to conservative measures including pharmacological therapy, surgical procedures should be avoided because they do not correct the functional disorder and may lead to fecal incontinence.

— Definition

Proctalgia fugax is defined as sudden, severe pain in the anal area lasting several seconds to as long as 30 minutes, and then disappearing completely [129]. Only 10% of patients report a duration of more than 5 minutes. Pain is localized to the anus in 90% of cases [130]. Attacks are infrequent, typically occurring less than five times per year in 51% of patients [131].

The pain has been described as cramping, gnawing, aching, or stabbing and may range from uncomfortable to unbearable [132]. Thompson found that 49% of patients had to interrupt their normal activities during an attack [130]. The symptoms may awaken the patient from sleep.

— Epidemiology

The prevalence of proctalgia fugax has been difficult to determine because sufferers tend not to report episodes to their physician except in the most severe cases [129]. Estimates of the prevalence have ranged from 8% [14] to 18% [129], with only 17% to 20% reporting the symptoms to their physicians. There is no clear evidence for a gender difference in prevalence. Symptoms rarely begin before puberty, but cases have been reported in children as young as 7 years [130].

Although relatively few patients with proctalgia fugax consult physicians, there is a significant amount of disability associated with the disorder: According to the U.S. Householder Study [14], subjects with proctalgia fugax missed an average of 12.8 days from work or school in the past year, and 8.4% reported that they were currently too ill to work or attend school. It was not possible to determine whether the reported disability was the result of proctalgia fugax (unlikely) or was associated with other disorders in these patients.

F2b. Diagnostic Criteria* for Proctalgia Fugax

Must include *all* of the following:
1. **Recurrent episodes of pain localized to the anus or lower rectum**
2. **Episodes last from seconds to minutes**
3. **There is no anorectal pain between episodes**

*For research purposes criteria must be fulfilled for 3 months; however, clinical diagnosis and evaluation may be made prior to 3 months.

— Clinical Evaluation

Diagnosis is based on the presence of characteristic symptoms as described above and exclusion of anorectal and pelvic pathophysiology. Certain urogenital abnormalities may be mistaken for proctalgia fugax. Chronic benign prostatitis may also present with acute bouts of perianal pain.

— Physiological Features

The short duration and sporadic, infrequent nature of this disorder has made the identification of physiological mechanisms difficult. Several studies suggest that abnormal smooth muscle contractions may be responsible for the pain [133–135]. Three studies have reported families in which a hereditary form of proctalgia fugax was found to be associated with hypertrophy of the internal anal sphincter [136–138].

— Psychological Features

Karras and Angelo reported that attacks of proctalgia fugax are often precipitated by stressful life events or anxiety [139]. Pilling and colleagues [140], using the MMPI and structured psychiatric interviews, found that the majority of patients were perfectionistic, anxious, and/or hypochondriacal. However, there was no control group, and clinical inferences were not based on blind assessments.

— Approach to Treatment

Proctalgia fugax has been described as "harmless, unpleasant, and incurable" [141]. For the majority of patients, the episodes of pain are so brief that remedial treatment is impractical, and they are normally so infrequent that prevention is not feasible. Since the disorder is harmless, treatment will normally consist only of reassurance and explanation. However, a small group of patients have proctalgia fugax on a frequent basis and may require treatment. A randomized controlled trial showed that inhalation of salbutamol (a beta adrenergic agonist) was more effective than placebo for shortening the duration of episodes of proctalgia for patients in whom episodes lasted 20 minutes or longer [142]. Others have recommended an alpha agonist, clonidine [143], amylnitrite, or nitroglycerine.

The psychological findings in patients who consult for proctalgia include anxiety, depression, and a tendency towards hypochondriasis. When these symptoms are present, antidepressant or anxiolytic medications or behavioral therapies may be indicated. However, there are no studies on the outcome of such treatments for proctalgia fugax.

F3. Functional Defecation Disorders

— Definition

Functional constipation is commonly classified as slow colonic transit or outlet delay, although many patients have neither and some fulfill criteria for both. Functional defecation disorders are characterized by paradoxical contraction or inadequate relaxation of the pelvic floor muscles during attempted defecation (dyssynergic defecation) or inadequate propulsive forces during attempted defecation (inadequate defecatory propulsion). These disorders are frequently associated with symptoms such as excessive straining, feeling of incomplete evacuation, and digital facilitation of bowel movements [144].

Normal defecation is characterized by appropriate expulsion forces coordinated with relaxation of the puborectalis and the external anal sphincter. This can be demonstrated by simultaneously assessing intrarectal pressures and pelvic floor activity (by manometry, EMG, or imaging) [145–147]. In most healthy subjects, the pelvic floor muscles relax during defecation [148]. However, some chronically constipated patients either inappropriately contract [146] or inadequately relax the pelvic floor muscles, or alternatively do not generate adequate expulsion forces [149–151].

Beginning with Preston and Lennard-Jones [146], several investigators have described the association of paradoxical pelvic floor contraction with constipation [152, 153]. Dyssynergic defecation patterns have also been observed in asymptomatic controls [148, 154, 155]. A recent report suggested that dyssynergic patterns are reproducible in the laboratory in patients with difficult defecation [156]. Conversely, a previous report suggested that the laboratory findings of dyssynergic defecation were not well duplicated when using ambulatory monitors to record the response to straining at home [157]. This may be due, in part, to anxiety in which patients are unable to relax in the artificial and public laboratory setting.

Other terms have been used interchangeably to describe dyssynergic defecation. Preston and Lennard-Jones [146] coined the term "anismus," by analogy from "vaginismus," to describe this phenomenon. However, the term anismus implies a psychogenic etiology, which is unproven. The more general term "pelvic floor dyssynergia" is preferable to "anismus" or other terms that refer only to the puborectalis or to the external anal sphincter because the muscle dysfunction can affect either or both muscles. The pelvic floor is a complex structure that subserves three important functions, namely defecation, micturition, and sexual function. Though some patients with dyssynergic defecation also have obstructed micturition [158], many patients do not report sexual or urinary symptoms [144]. Therefore, we prefer the term dyssynergic defecation to pelvic floor dyssynergia.

Recent studies suggest that a functional defecation disorder may also be caused by inadequate propulsive forces. This pattern is characterized by a decreased or absent intrarectal pressure during attempted defecation. These patients may be clinically indistinguishable from patients with dyssynergic defecation [156, 159].

— Epidemiology

The prevalence of functional defecation disorders in the general population is unknown because the diagnosis requires laboratory testing. At tertiary referral centers, the prevalence of dyssynergic defecation among patients with chronic constipation has ranged widely, from 20% to 81% [147, 160–163]. The prevalence of dyssynergia may have been overestimated due to the high false-positive rates seen in some studies [157, 164]. In one tertiary care center, the prevalence of dyssynergia was three times higher in women than men but was similar in younger and older individuals [144].

Symptoms thought to be associated with functional defecation disorders include straining, feeling of incomplete evacuation after defecation, digital facilitation of defecation, and the sensation of trouble letting go when attempting to defecate. However, symptoms (e.g., digital disimpaction, anal pain) do not consistently distinguish patients with, from patients without, functional defecation disorders [156, 165–168]. Thus, the criteria for functional defecation disorders must rely on both symptoms of constipation and physiological testing.

F3. Diagnostic Criteria* for Functional Defecation Disorders

1. The patient must satisfy diagnostic criteria for functional constipation**
2. During repeated attempts to defecate must have *at least two* of the following:
   a. Evidence of impaired evacuation, based on balloon expulsion test or imaging
   b. Inappropriate contraction of the pelvic floor muscles (i.e., anal sphincter or puborectalis) or less than 20% relaxation of basal resting sphincter pressure by manometry, imaging, or EMG
   c. Inadequate propulsive forces assessed by manometry or imaging

* Criteria fulfilled for the last 3 months with symptom onset at least 6 months prior to diagnosis

** Diagnostic Criteria for Functional Constipation
1. Must include *two or more* of the following:
   a. Straining during at least 25% of defecations
   b. Lumpy or hard stools at least 25% of defecations
   c. Sensation of incomplete evacuation at least 25% of defecations
   d. Sensation of anorectal obstruction/blockage at least 25% of defecations
   e. Manual maneuvers to facilitate at least 25% of defecations (e.g., digital evacuation, support of the pelvic floor) and/or
   f. Fewer than three defecations per week
2. Loose stools are rarely present without the use of laxatives
3. Insufficient criteria for irritable bowel syndrome

F3a. Diagnostic Criterion for Dyssynergic Defecation

Inappropriate contraction of the pelvic floor or less than 20% relaxation of basal resting sphincter pressure with adequate propulsive forces during attempted defecation

F3b. Diagnostic Criterion for Inadequate Defecatory Propulsion

Inadequate propulsive forces with or without inappropriate contraction or less than 20% relaxation of the anal sphincter during attempted defecation

— Rationale For Changes In Diagnostic Criteria

The diagnostic criteria for functional defecation disorders still require symptoms of constipation and abnormal diagnostic tests and are similar to those of the previous Working Team Report. While retaining diagnostic criteria for dyssynergia (i.e., inappropriate contraction/inadequate relaxation of pelvic floor with adequate propulsive forces), the revised criteria acknowledge recent studies using manometry or imaging that suggest that inadequate propulsive forces may also cause functional defecation disorders [159, 169]. Four patterns of anal and rectal pressure changes during attempted defecation are recognized [156] (Figure 2). A normal pattern is characterized by increased intrarectal pressure associated with anal relaxation. Two patterns, types I and III, describe dyssynergic defecation. Type I pattern is characterized by increased intrarectal pressure ($\geq$ 45 mm Hg) and increased anal pressure reflecting contraction of the anal sphincter. Type III pattern is characterized by increased intrarectal pressure ($\geq$ 45 mm Hg) with absent or insufficient (< 20%) relaxation of the anal sphincter. The type II pattern reflects inadequate propulsion (intrarectal pressure < 45 mm Hg) with insufficient relaxation or contraction of the anal sphincter.

In a prospective study that assessed 100 patients presenting with difficult defecation, the prevalence of a normal pattern was 30%, type I pattern was 32%, type III pattern was 14% and type II pattern was 24% [156]. Similar findings were reported in another study [170]. When tested one month later, the abnormal patterns were reproduced in 51 of 53 patients [156]. Furthermore, the intrarectal pressure, anal residual pressure, and the defecation index were reproducible [156]. Another study compared rectal balloon expulsion with simultaneous imaging and measurement of intrarectal pressure to evacuation defecography in 74 constipated patients [171]. A combination of pelvic floor descent and evacuation time on defecography correctly predicted maximum intrarectal pressure in 74% of cases. No patient with both prolonged evacuation and reduced pelvic floor descent on defecography could void the balloon, as maximum intrarectal pressure was reduced in this group. Thus, a prolonged evacuation time on defecography, in combination with reduced pelvic floor descent, suggests that a functional disorder of defecation may be caused by inadequate propulsive forces.

— Clinical Evaluation, Investigations, and Diagnostic Utility of Tests

The recommended algorithm for the evaluation of chronic constipation and the indications for and extent of laboratory testing in constipation (e.g., for colon cancer) are addressed in Chapter 9 "Functional Bowel Disorders." This sec-

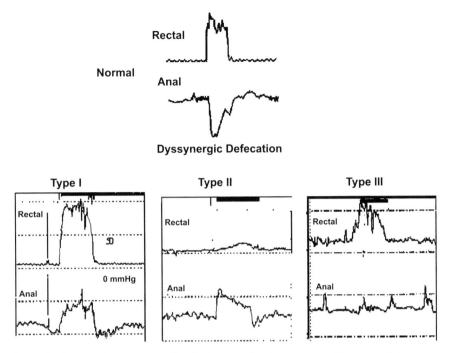

Figure 2. Rectoanal pressure profiles during simulated evacuation. Upper panel shows a normal pattern (i.e., increased rectal pressure associated with anal relaxation). Lower panel shows examples of dyssynergic defecation (types I and III) and inadequate propulsion (type II). (Reproduced with permission from WB Saunders; Gastroenterol Clin N Am 2003;32:659.)

tion will focus on the evaluation for functional disorders of defecation. In the absence of alarm symptoms (e.g., blood in the stools, a sudden change in bowel habits, weight loss) or a family history of colon cancer, anorectal testing is not recommended until patients have failed conservative treatment (e.g., education regarding normal bowel habits, increased dietary fiber and liquids, elimination of medications with constipating side-effects whenever possible). Patients who respond to conservative management require no further studies. If they do not respond, the next step in management is the use of osmotic or stimulant laxatives. Although efficacy of osmotic laxatives is better documented, there is sufficient experience to endorse both the safety and efficacy of stimulant laxatives [172]. Physiologic studies should be done if there is insufficient response to laxatives. These studies should include a colonic transit study and tests (i.e., balloon expulsion test, anorectal manometry and, if necessary, defecography) to aid in diagnosis of functional defecation disorders.

Balloon Expulsion Test

Rectal expulsion can be evaluated by asking patients to expel balloons filled with water or air from the rectum [145, 149, 166]. The time required to expel the balloon depends on the method used. Simultaneously, rectal and anal pressures and/or anal EMG may be monitored [149, 173]. Additional research is needed to standardize the method of conducting this test with respect to the following:

1. the position of the patient during straining (i.e., lateral recumbent versus sitting on a toilet chair);
2. the proportion of trials in which the patient fails to expel the balloon;
3. the length of time required to expel the balloon;
4. the intrarectal pressures produced by straining;
5. the minimum increase in anal pressure and/or EMG activity that defines a paradoxical contraction; and
6. the size and consistency of the balloon.

It is recommended that the patient sit on a commode chair behind a privacy screen and changes in rectal and anal pressures be recorded as the patient strains to defecate.

The balloon expulsion test is a useful screening test for a functional defecation disorder, but it does not define the mechanism of disordered defecation. Because the balloon may not mimic the patient's stool, patients with symptoms and with manometric and radiological evidence of a functional defecation disorder may have normal balloon expulsion. Hence, a normal balloon expulsion study does not always exclude a functional defecation disorder [156].

Manometric and EMG Assessment

A protocol for this assessment is given in category F1: functional fecal incontinence. The parts of the examination which are essential for diagnosis of functional defecation disorders are (1) measurement of intrarectal pressures during attempted defecation and (2) measurement of anal pressures and/or EMG activity during attempted defecation.

A recent international group of experts has recommended that patients be asked to attempt defecation on two separate occasions and that intrarectal pressures and anal residual pressures be examined to identify functional defecation disorders [35].

Defecography

Defecography is a dynamic radiological technique to evaluate the rectum and pelvic floor during attempted defecation. The technique for performing the test has been described and critically reviewed [3, 174]. Briefly, 150 to 300 ml of barium sulfate mixed with thickening agents to achieve the consistency of soft stool is injected into the rectum, and lateral radiographs (2 images/sec or higher) are taken during resting and straining to defecate. Preferably, video-fluoroscopy should be performed in addition. This test can detect structural abnormalities (rectocele, enterocele, intussusception, rectal prolapse, and megarectum) and assess functional parameters (anorectal angle at rest and during straining, perineal descent, anal diameter, indentation of the puborectalis, degree of rectal emptying).

The diagnostic value of defecography has been questioned on several grounds:

1. Some findings previously thought to be pathologic (e.g., rectoceles, intussusceptions) are common in asymptomatic control subjects [3, 175, 176];
2. Normal ranges for quantified measures are inadequately defined;
3. Some parameters such as the anorectal angle cannot be measured reliably because of variations in the shape of the rectum [175–180];
4. If liquid barium rather than paste is used, the consistency may not approximate stool consistency; and
5. Interobserver agreement is poor [177].

In a recent study of patients with difficult defecation, defecography did not provide clinically valuable information over and above that obtained from other physiological tests [156]. Magnetic resonance (MR) defecography provides an alternative approach to image anorectal motion and rectal evacuation in real time without radiation exposure. Whether MR defecography [48] will add a new dimension to the morphologic and functional assessment of these patients merits appraisal.

Radiopaque Marker Test of Whole Gut Transit Time

Colonic transit can provide useful physiologic information in constipated patients who fail to respond to conservative treatment. In part, this is because symptoms do not reliably identify different mechanisms of constipation. By itself, the test is not diagnostic of slow transit constipation because (1) slow transit constipation exists independent of or with functional defecation disorders and (2) defecation disorders can lead to proximal slowing of colonic markers.

There are several different methods to measure colonic transit time using commercially available radiopaque markers and obtaining abdominal radiographs on one or more days thereafter [181–183]. Information on the regional distribution of markers may prove useful in the diagnosis of functional defecation disorders when delayed transit occurs only in the sigmoid colon and rectum [184]. However, there may be a significant overlap between patients with functional defecation disorders and slow transit constipation [165, 185].

Other techniques for measuring whole gut transit time involve radioisotopes

[186, 187], or telemetric capsules [188]. These have no significant advantage over the relatively inexpensive and widely available marker technique for measurement of colonic transit time [189].

Utility of Anorectal Testing for Functional Defecation Disorders

The role of diagnostic testing was evaluated by assessing anorectal manometry, balloon expulsion test, defecography, and colonic transit in 100 consecutive patients with symptoms of difficult defecation [156]. In this group, anal manometry and balloon expulsion were normal in 30%. Among 70 patients with abnormal manometry, balloon expulsion was abnormal in 42 patients (60%) and indicative of a functional disorder of defecation. Among 28 patients with abnormal manometry and normal balloon expulsion, defecography was abnormal in seven patients (25%).

In another study of 130 patients with constipation, 24 patients had dyssynergic defecation, as defined by both manometry and defecography [166]. In contrast to other studies, the rectal balloon was distended with water until subjects reported a desire to defecate. Thereafter, subjects were asked to expel the balloon. Using this technique, the balloon expulsion had a sensitivity of 87% and specificity of 89% for dyssynergic defecation.

Based on these results, it appears that abnormal manometry and balloon expulsion testing are sufficient to diagnose a functional defecation disorder (Figure 3). On the other hand, further testing (e.g., defecography) may be required to confirm or exclude a functional defecation disorder in patients with abnormal manometry and normal balloon expulsion, or in patients with normal manometry and abnormal balloon expulsion.

— Physiological Factors

Functional defecation disorders are probably acquired behavioral disorders since at least two thirds of patients learn to relax the external anal sphincter and puborectalis muscles appropriately when provided with biofeedback training [190].

Many aspects concerning the physiologic mechanism for these disorders remain unresolved and complicate the interpretation of diagnostic tests, including the following:

1. Studies with needle EMG, defecography, and manometry suggest that the anal sphincter or puborectalis may not relax during defecation in a small proportion of asymptomatic subjects. It is unclear whether these observa-

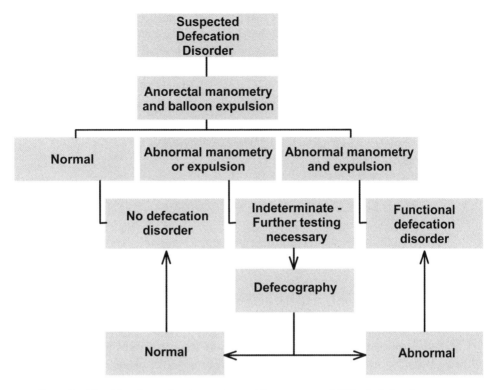

Figure 3. Algorithm for evaluating patients with symptoms of difficult defecation. Anorectal manometry and balloon expulsion are recommended.

tions reflect asymptomatic pelvic floor dysfunction or the inability to accurately characterize defecation in a laboratory setting.

2. Some investigators have [162] found a poor correlation between manometric evidence of dyssynergic defecation obtained with a balloon probe in the distal anal canal and the results of defecography; likewise others [189, 191] reported poor agreement between EMG evidence for dyssynergic defecation and defecography. One possible explanation is that these muscle groups can contract independently, since a balloon or surface EMG electrodes in the distal anal canal measure primarily from the external anal sphincter, whereas defecography also measures the puborectalis muscle (anorectal angle, puborectalis indentation). Lebel and Grandmaison [192] showed by needle EMG that dyssynergia can be limited to one of the two muscle groups. This is consistent with the observation that the puborectalis is innervated by both the sacral plexus and the pudendal nerves, whereas the

external anal sphincter is innervated only by the pudendal nerves [193]. However, one team of investigators [194] found agreement between defecography and anorectal manometry in 78% of patients if failure to relax on manometry was defined as less than a 20% decrease in anal canal pressure.

3. The voluntary inhibition of defecation [195] can be misdiagnosed as a functional defecation disorder. It is unknown how often false-positive diagnoses arise because of lack of privacy and the patient's fear of expelling stool during testing; many patients who test positive in the laboratory relax normally during straining at home [157].

— Psychological Factors

Functional defecation disorders are acquired disorders because they generally begin after the age of toilet training [156]. Conceptually, they are also regarded as behavioral disorders because they often improve with biofeedback training (see below). It has been speculated that pain associated with repeated attempts to defecate large, hard stools may lead to inadvertent anal sphincter contraction to minimize discomfort during defecation. This could result in a repetitive sequence of harder stools, difficult and painful defecation, stool retention, and worsening defecation. However, rectal discomfort did not occur more frequently in patients with functional defecation disorders than in normal or slow transit constipation [165]. Thus, avoidance behavior may account for only a small proportion of adult patients with functional defecation disorders.

Anxiety and/or psychological stress may also contribute to the development of dyssynergic defecation by increasing skeletal muscle tension. Heymen and colleagues [95] found elevated MMPI scales for hypochondriasis, depression, and hysteria in these patients. A recent study showed that patients (n=118) with a functional defecation disorder had significant impairment of their social life (74%), work life (69%), sexual life (56%), and interfamily relationships (35%) [144]. Other than studies published in abstract form [116], the impact of these disorders on psychological distress and quality of life has not been adequately characterized.

Uncontrolled studies have reported sexual abuse in 22% of women with functional defecation disorders, and 40% of women with functional lower gut disorders, including functional defecation disorders [144, 196]. It is speculated that after sexual abuse, a sensation of rectal fullness may trigger a memory of the original trauma and may lead to an involuntary contraction of the pelvic floor muscles. However, in the absence of appropriate controls, it is unclear if these observations are specific to patients with functional defecation disorders.

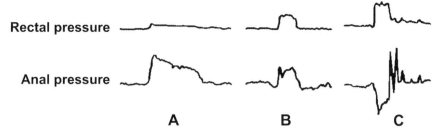

Rectal pressure

Anal pressure

A   B   C

Figure 4. Effect of biofeedback therapy on dyssynergia in one patient before and after treatment: Panel A shows baseline intrarectal and anal sphincter pressures. There is inadequate propulsion and paradoxical anal contraction. Panel B shows that after learning diaphragmatic breathing technique, the pushing effort has improved but patient still shows paradoxical contraction. Panel C shows coordinated relaxation, with an increase in intrarectal pressure and relaxation of the anal sphincter. (Adapted from Rao, Gastroenterol Clin N Am 2003;32:659).

— Approach to Treatment

Two types of pelvic floor training involving behavioral modification have been advocated: (1) biofeedback training in which EMG or pressure sensors in or adjacent to the anus are used to monitor and provide feedback to the patient on striated muscle activity [197–200] and (2) simulated defecation in which the patient practices evacuating an artificial stool surrogate [200, 201]. Simulated defecation has been combined with diaphragmatic muscle training by some investigators [200, 202].

Uncontrolled studies suggest an overall success rate of 67% after pelvic floor retraining for functional defecation disorders [200, 203, 204]. EMG biofeedback training was either more [198] or as effective as simulated defecation for functional defecation disorders. Effects of biofeedback therapy on dyssynergia in one typical patient are shown in Figure 4. Up to 60% of patients with dyssynergic defecation have impaired rectal sensation that often improves after sensory conditioning [200]. However the additional benefit of sensory conditioning is unknown.

Most studies have only reported changes in symptoms, not anorectal functions, after biofeedback therapy. Rao and colleagues reported improved coordination between rectal propulsive forces and anal relaxation, and the ability to expel an artificial stool that was maintained for at least 6 months after pelvic floor retraining [200]. Similarly, anorectal angles at rest and during expulsion were more obtuse and pelvic floor motion assessed by defecography improved after pelvic floor retraining [206].

Although results from uncontrolled studies are encouraging, controlled trials comparing biofeedback to either sham biofeedback or conventional treatment in adults are necessary. One study suggested that biofeedback was more effective than sham biofeedback but was no more effective than placebo when patient satisfaction was assessed [206]. A more recent study found that biofeedback was more effective than polyethylene glycol for treating dyssynergic defecation and that benefits last at least two years [207]. Also, there are no data identifying which components of treatment are most effective and data on long-term efficacy for dyssynergic defecation are limited. In one study using electrogalvanic stimulation for dyssynergic defecation in 30 patients, approximately 50% of patients showed symptomatic and objective improvement after one year, but the benefit was limited to patients with dyssynergia and normal colonic transit [208]. The mechanism(s) whereby electrogalvanic stimulation helps defecation is unclear. In a meta-analysis of 38 studies of biofeedback for dyssynergia, psychosocial symptoms were identified as an independent factor that influenced treatment outcome [209].

Directions for Future Research

1. Multicenter studies of the normal physiology of defecation and fecal continence in large groups of subjects stratified by age, gender, and (in women) by parity are needed. These would (a) help to define the normal ranges for diagnostic tests of FI and functional defecation disorders, and (b) help establish standardized technology for assessment of these conditions.

2. Studies are needed to define the role of rectal contraction and sensation in disordered defecation, to clarify the overlap between colonic motor dysfunction and functional defecation disorders, and to clarify the pathophysiology, natural history, and treatment outcomes of dyssynergic defecation versus inadequate defecation.

3. A randomized, blinded study of biofeedback treatment for dyssynergic and inadequate defecation should be carried out. This study could compare biofeedback to an equally credible (to patients) but nonphysiologic treatment to control for the sham response. Alternatively, a study incorporating the design of a recent study on biofeedback for FI [106] might involve randomization of patients into 1 of 4 treatment groups: (1) standard care including advice from experienced health care personnel; (2) standard care plus pelvic floor expulsion exercises taught verbally and by digital examination; (3) the above plus biofeedback involving coordinating exercise with visual feedback; (4) all of the above plus daily use of a home biofeedback device. These studies should enroll sufficient numbers of patients and should pro-

spectively obtain objective data. Outcomes should include standardized measures, patient assessments of adequacy of relief, a validated quality of life instrument, and a long-term assessment to determine durability of therapeutic success.

4. Studies are needed to clarify the clinical features, psychological characteristics, quality of life, and natural history of anorectal pain syndromes. A randomized, multicenter, blinded study comparing the effectiveness of electrogalvanic stimulation, biofeedback, and muscle relaxant drugs for the treatment of levator ani syndrome should be performed.

5. Studies are needed comparing sacral nerve stimulation to sham treatment in functional FI in order to clarify the effects of sacral nerve stimulation on anorectal functions and to identify patients who will respond to stimulation.

6. Studies are needed to assess the utility of biofeedback therapy in incontinent patients who do not respond to conservative approaches.

References

1. Bharucha AE. Fecal incontinence. Gastroenterology 2003;124:1672–1685.
2. Sultan AH, Kamm MA, Hudson CN, Thomas JM, Bartram CI. Anal-sphincter disruption during vaginal delivery. New Engl J Med 1993;329:1905–1911.
3. Shorvon PJ, McHugh S, Diamant NE, Somers S, Steveson GW. Defecography in normal volunteers: results and implications. Gut 1989;30:1737–1749.
4. Whitehead WE, Wald A, Diamant NE, Enck P, Pemberton JH, Rao SSC. Functional disorders of the anus and rectum. Gut 1999;45:II55–II59.
5. Ashraf W, Park F, Lof J, Quigley EM. An examination of the reliability of reported stool frequency in the diagnosis of idiopathic constipation. Gastroenterology 1996; 91:26–32.
6. Diamant NE, Kamm MA, Wald A, Whitehead WE. AGA technical review on anorectal testing techniques. Gastroenterology 1999;116:735–760.
7. Whitehead WE, Wald A, Norton NJ. Treatment options for fecal incontinence. Dis Colon Rectum 2001;44:131–144.
8. Rao SS. Diagnosis and management of fecal incontinence. American College of Gastroenterology Practice Parameters Committee. Am J Gastroenterol 2004;19:1585–1604.
9. Largo RH, Stutzle W. Longitudinal study of bowel and bladder control by day and at night in the first six years of life. I: Epidemiology and interrelations between bowel and bladder control. Dev Med Child Neurol 1977;19:598–606.
10. Bellman M. Studies on encopresis. Acta Paediatr Scand 1966;56:1–151.
11. Whiting JS, Child IL. Child training and personality. New Haven, Connecticut: Yale University Press, 1953.
12. Nelson RL. Epidemiology of fecal incontinence. Gastroenterology 2004;126:S3–S7.

13. Nelson R, Norton N, Cautley E, Furner S. Community-based prevalence of anal incontinence. JAMA 1995;274:559–561.

14. Drossman DA, Li Z, Andruzzi E, Temple R, Talley NJ, Thompson WG, Whitehead WE, Janssens J, Funch-Jensen P, Corazziari E, Richter JE, Koch GG. U.S. Householder Survey of Functional Gastrointestinal Disorders: Prevalence, Sociodemography and Health Impact. Dig Dis Sci 1993;38:1569–1580.

15. Perry S, Shaw C, McGrother C, Matthews RJ, Assassa RP, Dallosso H, Williams K, Brittain KR, Azam U, Clarke M, Jagger C, Mayne C, Castleden CM. Prevalence of faecal incontinence in adults aged 40 years or more living in the community. Gut 2002; 50:480–484.

16. Roberts RO, Jacobsen SJ, Reilly WT, Pemberton JH, Lieber MM, Talley NJ. Prevalence of combined fecal and urinary incontinence: a community-based study. J Am Geriatr Soc 1999;47:837–841.

17. Kalantar JS, Howell S, Talley NJ. Prevalence of faecal incontinence and associated risk factors; an underdiagnosed problem in the Australian community? Med J Aust 2002;176:54–57.

18. Nelson R, Furner S, Jesudason V. Fecal incontinence in Wisconsin nursing homes: prevalence and associations. Dis Colon Rectum 1998;41:1226–1229.

19. Read NW, Abouzekry L. Why do patients with faecal impaction have faecal incontinence? Gut 1986;27:283–287.

20. Read NW, Abouzekry L, Read MG, Howell P, Ottewell D, Donnelly TC. Anorectal function in elderly patients with fecal impaction. Gastroenterology 1985;89:959–966.

21. Drossman DA, Sandler RS, Broom CM, McKee DC. Urgency and fecal soiling in people with bowel dysfunction. Dig Dis Sci 1986;31:1221–1225.

22. Johanson JF, Irizarry F, Doughty A. Risk factors for fecal incontinence in a nursing home population. J Clin Gastroenterol 1997;24:156–160.

23. Tobin GW, Brocklehurst JC. Faecal incontinence in residential homes for the elderly: prevalence, aetiology and management. Age Ageing 1986;15:41–46.

24. Heaton KW, Parker D, Cripps H. Bowel function and irritable bowel syndrome symptoms after hysterectomy and cholecystectomy—A population-based study. Gut 1993;34:1108–1111.

25. Engel AF, Kamm MA, Bartram CI, Nicholls RJ. Relationship of symptoms in faecal incontinence to specific sphincter abnormalities. Int J Colorectal Dis 1995;10:152–155.

26. Chiarioni G, Scattolini C, Bonfante F, Vantini I. Liquid stool incontinence with severe urgency: anorectal function and effective biofeedback treatment. Gut 1993;34:1576–1580.

27. Bharucha AE, Fletcher JG, Harper CM, Hough D, Daube JR, Stevens C, Seide B, Riederer SJ, Zinsmeister AR. Relationship between symptoms and disordered continence mechanisms in women with idiopathic fecal incontinence. Gut 2005;54: 546–55.

28. Jorge JM, Wexner SD. Etiology and management of fecal incontinence. Dis Colon Rectum 1993;36:77–97.

29. Pescatori M, Anastasio G, Bottini C, Mentasti A. New grading and scoring for anal incontinence. Evaluation of 335 patients. Dis Colon Rectum 1992;35:482–487.

30. Rockwood TH, Church JM, Fleshman JW, Kane RL, Mavrantonis C, Thorson AG, Wexner SD, Bliss D, Lowry AC. Patient and surgeon ranking of the severity of symp-

toms associated with fecal incontinence: the fecal incontinence severity index. Dis Colon Rectum 1999;42:1525–1532.

31. Vaizey CJ, Carapeti E, Cahill JA, Kamm MA. Prospective comparison of faecal incontinence grading systems. Gut 1999;44:77–80.

32. Bharucha AE, Locke GR, III, Seide BM, Zinsmeister AR. A new questionnaire for constipation and faecal incontinence. Aliment Pharmacol Ther 2004;20:355–364.

33. Rockwood TH, Church JM, Fleshman JW, Kane RL, Mavrantonis C, Thorson AG, Wexner SD, Bliss D, Lowry AC. Fecal Incontinence Quality of Life Scale: quality of life instrument for patients with fecal incontinence. Dis Colon Rectum 2000;43:9–16.

34. Hill J, Corson RJ, Brandon H, Redford J, Faragher EB, Kiff ES. History and examination in the assessment of patients with idiopathic fecal incontinence. Dis Colon Rectum 1994;37:473–477.

35. Rao SS, Azpiroz F, Diamant N, Enck P, Tougas G, Wald A. Minimum standards of anorectal manometry. Neurogastroenterol Motil 2002;14:553–559.

36. Damon H, Henry L, Barth X, Mion F. Fecal incontinence in females with a past history of vaginal delivery: significance of anal sphincter defects detected by ultrasound. Dis Colon Rectum 2002;45:1445–1450.

37. Sentovich SM, Blatchford GJ, Rivela LJ, Lin K, Thorson AG, Christensen MA. Diagnosing anal sphincter injury with transanal ultrasound and manometry. Dis Colon Rectum 1997;40:1430–1434.

38. Bartram CI, Sultan AH. Anal endosonography in faecal incontinence. Gut 1995;37:4–6.

39. Nielsen MB, Hauge C, Pedersen JF, Christiansen J. Endosonographic evaluation of patients with anal incontinence: findings and influence on surgical management. Am J Roentgenol 1993;160:771–775.

40. Williams AB, Bartram CI, Halligan S, Spencer JA, Nicholls RJ, Kmiot WA. Anal sphincter damage after vaginal delivery using three-dimensional endosonography. Obstet Gynecol 2001;97:770–775.

41. Burnett SJ, Speakman CT, Kamm MA, Bartram CI. Confirmation of endosonographic detection of external anal sphincter defects by simultaneous electromyographic mapping. Br J Surg 1991;78:448–450.

42. Sultan AH, Kamm MA, Talbot IC, Nicholls RJ, Bartram CI. Anal endosonography for identifying external sphincter defects confirmed histologically. Br J Surg 1994;81:463–465.

43. Vaizey CJ, Kamm MA, Bartram CI. Primary degeneration of the internal anal sphincter as a cause of passive faecal incontinence. Lancet 1997;349:612–615.

44. Heyer T, Enck P, Gantke B, Schmitt A, Frieling T, Haussinger D. Anal endosonography: Are morphometric measurements of the anal sphincter reproducible? 108 ed. 1995:A613.

45. Enck P, Heyer T, Gantke B, Schmidt WU, Schafer R, Frieling T, Haussinger D. How reproducible are measures of the anal sphincter muscle diameter by endoanal ultrasound? Am J Gastroenterol 1997;92:293–296.

46. Gold DM, Halligan S, Kmiot WA, Bartram CI. Intraobserver and interobserver agreement in anal endosonography. Br J Surg 1999;86:371–375.

47. Hussain SM, Stoker J, Lameris JS. Anal sphincter complex: endoanal MR imaging of normal anatomy. Radiology 1995;197:671–677.

48. Fletcher JG, Busse RF, Riederer SJ, Hough D, Gluecker T, Harper CM, Bharucha AE.

Magnetic resonance imaging of anatomic and dynamic defects of the pelvic floor in defecatory disorders. Am J Gastroenterol 2003;98:399–411.

49. deSouza NM, Puni R, Zbar A, Gilderdale DJ, Coutts GA, Krausz T. MR imaging of the anal sphincter in multiparous women using an endoanal coil: correlation with in vitro anatomy and appearances in fecal incontinence. Am J Roentgenol 1996; 167:1465–1471.

50. Beets-Tan RG, Morren GL, Beets GL, Kessels AG, el Naggar K, Lemaire E, Baeten CG, van Engelshoven JM. Measurement of anal sphincter muscles: endoanal US, endoanal MR imaging, or phased-array MR imaging? A study with healthy volunteers. Radiology 2001;220:81–89.

51. Malouf AJ, Halligan S, Williams AB, Bartram CI, Dhillon S, Kamm MA. Prospective assessment of interobserver agreement for endoanal MRI in fecal incontinence. Abdom Imaging 2001;26:76–78.

52. Rociu E, Stoker J, Eijkemans MJ, Schouten WR, Lameris JS. Fecal incontinence: endoanal US versus endoanal MR imaging. Radiology 1999;212:453–458.

53. Busse RF, Riederer SJ, Fletcher JG, Bharucha AE, Brandt KR. Interactive fast spin-echo imaging. Magn Reson Med 2000;44:339–348.

54. Bertschinger KM, Hetzer FH, Roos JE, Treiber K, Marincek B, Hilfiker PR. Dynamic MR imaging of the pelvic floor performed with patient sitting in an open-magnet unit versus with patient supine in a closed-magnet unit. Radiology 2002;223:501–508.

55. Briel JW, Stoker J, Rociu E, Lameris JS, Hop WC, Schouten WR. External anal sphincter atrophy on endoanal magnetic resonance imaging adversely affects continence after sphincteroplasty. Br J Surg 1999;86:1322–1327.

56. Kiff ES, Swash M. Slowed conduction in the pudendal nerves in idiopathic (neurogenic) faecal incontinence. Br J Surg 1984;71:614–616.

57. Wexner SD, Marchetti F, Salanga VD, Corredor C, Jagelman DG. Neurophysiologic assessment of the anal sphincters. Dis Colon Rectum 1991;34:606–612.

58. Malouf AJ, Norton CS, Engel AF, Nicholls RJ, Kamm MA. Long-term results of overlapping anterior anal-sphincter repair for obstetric trauma. Lancet 2000;355:260–265.

59. Swash M. Anorectal incontinence: electrophysiological tests. Br J Surg 1985;72 Suppl: S14–S15.

60. Herdmann J, Bielefeldt K, Enck P. Quantification of motor pathways to the pelvic floor in humans. Am J Physiol 1991;260:G720–G723.

61. Enck P, Herdmann J, Bergermann K, Theisen U, Zacchi P, Luebke HJ. Up and down the spinal cord: afferent and efferent innervation of the human external and internal anal sphincter. J Gastrointest Mot 1992;4:271–277.

62. Loening-Baucke V, Read NW, Yamada T, Barker AT. Evaluation of the motor and sensory components of the pudendal nerve. Electroencephalogr Clin Neurophysiol 1994;93:35–41.

63. Frieling T, Enck P, Wienbeck M. Cerebral Responses Evoked by Electrical Stimulation of Rectosigmoid in Normal Subjects. Dig Dis Sci 1994;34(2):202–205.

64. Loening-Baucke V, Anderson RH, Yamada T, Zhu YX. Study of the afferent pathways from the rectum with a new distention control device. Neurology 1995;45:1510–1516.

65. Speakman CT, Kamm MA, Swash M. Rectal sensory evoked potentials: an assessment of their clinical value. Int J Colorectal Dis 1993;8:23–28.

66. Nyam DC, Pemberton JH. Long-term results of lateral internal sphincterotomy for

chronic anal fissure with particular reference to incidence of fecal incontinence. Dis Colon Rectum 1999;42:1306–1310.

67. Bartolo DC, Jarratt JA, Read MG, Donnelly TC, Read NW. The role of partial denervation of the puborectalis in idiopathic faecal incontinence. Br J Surg 1983;70:664–667.

68. Sorensen M, Tetzschner T, Rasmussen OO, Christiansen J. Relation between electromyography and anal manometry of the external anal sphincter. Gut 1991;32:1031–1034.

69. Heymen S, Jones KR, Ringel Y, Scarlett Y, Whitehead WE. Biofeedback treatment of fecal incontinence: a critical review. Dis Colon Rectum 2001;44:728–736.

70. Merletti R, Bottin A, Cescon C, Farina D, Gazzoni M, Martina S, Mesin L, Pozzo M, Rainoldi A, Enck P. Multichannel surface EMG for the non-invasive assessment of the anal sphincter muscle. Digestion 2004;69:112–122.

71. Merletti R, Bottin A, Cescon C, Farina D, Gazzoni M, Martina S, Mesin L, Pozzo M, Rainoldi A, Enck P. Multichannel surface EMG for the non-invasive assessment of the anal sphincter muscle. Digestion 69(2):112–22, 2004.

72. Rao SS. Pathophysiology of adult fecal incontinence. Gastroenterology 2004;126:S14–S22.

73. Sun WM, Donnelly TC, Read NW. Utility of a combined test of anorectal manometry, electromyography, and sensation in determining the mechanism of 'idiopathic' faecal incontinence. Gut 1992;33:807–813.

74. Kumar D, Waldron DL, Williams JS. Home assessment of anorectal motility and external sphincter EMG in idiopathic fecal incontinence. Br J Surg 1989;76:635–636.

75. Farouk R, Duthie GS, MacGregor AB, Bartolo DC. Evidence of electromechanical dissociation of the internal anal sphincter in idiopathic fecal incontinence. Dis Colon Rectum 1994;37:595–601.

76. Denny-Brown D, Robertson E. An investigation of the nervous control of defaecation. Brain 1935;58:256–310.

77. Frenckner B. Function of the anal sphincter in spinal man. Gut 1975;16:638–644.

78. Frenckner B, Ihre T. Influence of autonomic nerves on the internal anal sphincter in man. Gut 1976;17:306–312.

79. Speakman CT, Hoyle CH, Kamm MM, Henry MM, Nicholls RJ, Burnstock G. Abnormalities of innervation of internal anal sphincter in fecal incontinence. Dig Dis Sci 1993;38:1961–1969.

80. Fernandez-Fraga X, Azpiroz F, Malagelada JR. Significance of pelvic floor muscles in anal incontinence. Gastroenterology 2002;123:1441–1450.

81. Phillips SF, Edwards DA. Some aspects of anal continence and defaecation. Gut 1965;6:396–406.

82. Chen H, Humphreys MS, Kettlewell MG, Bulkley GB, Mortensen N, George BD. Anal ultrasound predicts the response to nonoperative treatment of fecal incontinence in men. Ann Surg 1999;229:739–743.

83. Mitrani C, Chun A, Desautels S, Wald A. Anorectal manometric characteristics in men and women with idiopathic fecal incontinence. J Clin Gastroenterol 1998;26:175–178.

84. Chun AB, Rose S, Mitrani C, Silvestre AJ, Wald A. Anal sphincter structure and function in homosexual males engaging in anoreceptive intercourse. Am J Gastroenterol 1997;92:465–468.

85. Rao SS, Ozturk R, Stessman M. Investigation of the pathophysiology of fecal seepage. Am J Gastroenterol 2004;99:2204–9.

86. Parellada CM, Miller AS, Williamson ME, Johnston D. Paradoxical high anal resting pressures in men with idiopathic fecal seepage. Dis Colon Rectum 1998;41:593–597.

87. Bassotti G, Crowell MD, Whitehead WE. Contractile activity of the human colon: Lessons from 24 hour studies. Gut 1993;34:129–133.

88. Sun WM, Read NW, Miner PB. Relation between rectal sensation and anal function in normal subjects and patients with faecal incontinence. Gut 1990;31:1056–1061.

89. Buser WD, Miner PB, Jr. Delayed rectal sensation with fecal incontinence. Successful treatment using anorectal manometry. Gastroenterology 1986;91:1186–1191.

90. Miller R, Bartolo DC, Roe A, Cervero F, Mortensen NJ. Anal sensation and the continence mechanism. Dis Colon Rectum 1988;31:433–438.

91. Whitehead WE, Palsson OS. Is rectal pain sensitivity a biological marker for irritable bowel syndrome: psychological influences on pain perception. Gastroenterology 1998;115:1263–1271.

92. Miller R, Bartolo DC, Cervero F, Mortensen NJ. Anorectal sampling: a comparison of normal and incontinent patients. Br J Surg 1988;75:44–47.

93. Read MG, Read NW. Role of anorectal sensation in preserving continence. Gut 1982; 23:345–347.

94. Devroede G. Functions of the anorectum: defecation and continence. In: Phillips SF, Pemberton JH, and Shorter R, eds. The Large Intestine: Physiology and Disease. New York: Raven Press, 2004:115.

95. Heymen S, Wexner SD, Gulledge AD. MMPI assessment of patients with functional bowel disorders. Dis Colon Rectum 1993;36:593–596.

96. Read M, Read NW, Barber DC, Duthie HL. Effects of loperamide on anal sphincter function in patients complaining of chronic diarrhea with fecal incontinence and urgency. Digestive Diseases and Sciences 1982;27:807–814.

97. Santoro GA, Eitan BZ, Pryde A, Bartolo DC. Open study of low-dose amitriptyline in the treatment of patients with idiopathic fecal incontinence. Am J Gastroenterol 2000;43:1676–1681.

98. Palmer KR, Corbett CL, Holdsworth CD. Double-blind cross-over study comparing loperamide, codeine and diphenoxylate in the treatment of chronic diarrhea. Gastroenterology 1980;79:1272–1275.

99. Cremonini F, Delgado-Aros S, Camilleri M. Efficacy of alosetron in irritable bowel syndrome: a meta-analysis of randomized controlled trials. Neurogastroenterol Motil 2003;15:79–86.

100. Locke GR, III, Pemberton JH, Phillips SF. AGA Technical Review on Constipation. Gastroenterology 2000;119:1766–1778.

101. Engel BT, Nikoomanesh P, Schuster MM. Operant conditioning of rectosphincteric responses in the treatment of fecal incontinence. N Engl J Med 1974;290:646–649.

102. Bharucha AE. Outcome measures for fecal incontinence: anorectal structure and function. Gastroenterology 2004;126:S90–S98.

103. Rao SS, Welcher KD, Happel J. Can biofeedback therapy improve anorectal function in fecal incontinence? Am J Gastroenterol 1996;91:2360–2366.

104. Miner PB, Donnelly TC, Read NW. Investigation of mode of action of biofeedback in treatment of fecal incontinence. Dig Dis Sci 1990;35:1291–1298.

105. Wald A, Tunuguntla AK. Anorectal sensorimotor dysfunction in fecal incontinence and diabetes mellitus. New Engl J Med 1984;310:1282–1287.

106. Norton C, Chelvanayagam S, Wilson-Barnett J, Redfern S, Kamm MA. Ran-

domized controlled trial of biofeedback for fecal incontinence. Gastroenterology 2003;125:1320–1329.

107. Cheung O, Wald A. Review article: the management of pelvic floor disorders. Aliment Pharmacol Ther 2004;19:481–495.

108. Halverson AL, Hull TL. Long-term outcome of overlapping anal sphincter repair. Dis Colon Rectum 2002;45:345–348.

109. Karoui S, Leroi AM, Koning E, Menard JF, Michot F, Denis P. Results of sphincteroplasty in 86 patients with anal incontinence. Dis Colon Rectum 2000;43:813–820.

110. Vaizey CJ, Kamm MA, Turner IC, Nicholls RJ, Woloszko J. Effects of short term sacral nerve stimulation on anal and rectal function in patients with anal incontinence. Gut 1999;44:407–412.

111. Ganio E, Ratto C, Masin A, Luc AR, Doglietto GB, Dodi G, Ripetti V, Arullani A, Frascio M, BertiRiboli E, Landolfi V, DelGenio A, Altomare DF, Memeo V, Bertapelle P, Carone R, Spinelli M, Zanollo A, Spreafico L, Giardiello G, de Seta F. Neuromodulation for fecal incontinence: outcome in 16 patients with definitive implant. The initial Italian Sacral Neurostimulation Group (GINS) experience. Dis Colon Rectum 2001;44:965–970.

112. Rosen HR, Urbarz C, Holzer B, Novi G, Schiessel R. Sacral nerve stimulation as a treatment for fecal incontinence. Gastroenterology 2001;121:536–541.

113. Grimaud JC, Bouvier M, Naudy B, Guien C, Salducci J. Manometric and radiologic investigations and biofeedback treatment of chronic idiopathic anal pain. Dis Colon Rectum 1991;34:690–695.

114. Palsson OS, Taub E, Cook E, III, Burnett CK, McCommons JJ, Whitehead WE. Validation of Rome Criteria for functional gastrointestinal disorders by factor analysis. Gastroenterology 1996;91:2000.

115. Grant SR, Salvati EP, Rubin RJ. Levator Syndrome: An analysis of 316 cases. Dis Colon Rectum 1975;18:161–163.

116. Burnett C, Palsson OS, Whitehead WE, Drossman DA. Psychological distress and impaired quality of life in patients with functional anorectal disorders. Gastroenterology 1998;114:A729.

117. Sohn N, Weinstein MA, Robbins RD. The levator syndrome and its treatment with high-voltage electrogalvanic stimulation. Am J Surg 1982;144:580–582.

118. Oliver GC, Rubin RJ, Salvati EP, Eisenstat TE. Electrogalvanic stimulation in the treatment of levator syndrome. Dis Colon Rectum 1985;28:662–663.

119. Nicosia JF, Abcarian H. Levator syndrome. A treatment that works. Dis Colon Rectum 1985;28:406–408.

120. Billingham RP, Isler JT, Friend WG, Hostetler J. Treatment of levator syndrome using high-voltage electrogalvanic stimulation. Dis Colon Rectum 1987;30:584–587.

121. Ware Jr JE. SF-36 health survey: Manual and interpretation guide. Boston: The Health Institute, New England Medical Center, 1993.

122. Ger GC, Wexner SD, Jorge MN, Lee E, Amaranath LA, Heymen S, Nogueras JJ, Jagelman DG. Evaluation and treatment of chronic intractable rectal pain—a frustrating endeavor. Dis Colon Rectum 1993;36:139–145.

123. Gilliland R, Heymen JS, Altomare DF, Vickers D, Wexner SD. Biofeedback for intractable rectal pain: outcome and predictors of success. Dis Colon Rectum 1997; 40:190–196.

124. Heah SM, Ho YH, Tan M, Leong AF. Biofeedback is effective treatment for levator ani syndrome. Dis Colon Rectum 1997;40:187–189.

125. Schuster MM. Rectal pain. In: Bayless T, ed. Current Therapy in Gastroenterology and Liver Disease. 1 ed. Ontario: B. C. Decker, 1990:378–379.
126. Thiele GH. Tonic spasm of the levator ani, coccygeus and piriformis muscle: Relationship to coccygodynia and pain in the region of the hip and down the leg. Trans Am Proctol Soc 1936;37:145–155.
127. Dodi G, Bogoni F, Infantino A, Pianon P, Mortellaro LM, Lise M. Hot or cold in anal pain? A study of the changes in internal anal sphincter pressure profiles. Dis Colon Rectum 1986;29:248–251.
128. Rao SC, McLeod M, Beaty J, Stessman M. Effects of botox on levator ani syndrome: a double blind, placebo controlled cross-over study. Gastroenterology 2004;99:S114–5.
129. Thompson WG, Heaton KW. Proctalgia Fugax. Roy Coll of Phys (London) 1980; 14:247–248.
130. Thompson WG. The irritable bowel. Gut 1984;25:305–320.
131. Thompson WG. Proctalgia Fugax in Patients with the Irritable Bowel, Peptic Ulcer, or Inflammatory Bowel Disease. Gastroenterology 1984;79:450–452.
132. Perry WH. Proctagia fugax: a clinical enigma. Southern Medical Journal 1988;81: 621–623.
133. Eckardt VF, Dodt O, Kanzler G, Bernhard G. Anorectal function and morphology in patients wiht sporadic proctalgia fugax. Dis Colon Rectum 2004;39:755–762.
134. Harvey RF. Colonic motility in proctalgia fugax. Lancet 1979;2:713–714.
135. Rao SS, Hatfield RA. Paroxysmal anal hyperkinesis: a characteristic feature of proctalgia fugax. Gut 1996;39:609–612.
136. Kamm MA, Hoyle CH, Burleigh DE, Law PJ, Swash M, Martin JE, Nicholls RJ, Northover JM. Hereditary internal anal sphincter myopathy causing proctalgia fugax and constipation. A newly identified condition. Gastroenterology 1991;100:805–810.
137. Celik AF, Katsinelos P, Read NW, Khan MI, Donnelly TC. Hereditary proctalgia fugax and constipation: report of a second family. Gut 1995;36:581–584.
138. Guy RJ, Kamm MA, Martin JE. Internal anal sphincter myopathy causing proctalgia fugax and constipation: further clinical and radiological characterization in a patient. Eur J Gastroenterol Hepatol 1997;9:221–224.
139. Karras JD, Angelo G. Proctalgia fugax. Clinical observations and a new diagnostic aid. Dis Colon Rectum 1963;6:130–134.
140. Pilling LF, Swenson WM, Hill JR. The psychologic aspects of proctalgia fugax. Dis Colon Rectum 1965;8:372–376.
141. Douthwaite AH. Proctalgia fugax. Br Med J 1962;5298:164–165.
142. Eckardt VF, Dodt O, Kanzler G, Bernhard G. Treatment of proctalgia fugax with salbutamol inhalation. Am J Gastroenterol 1996;91:686–689.
143. Swain R. Oral clonidine for proctalgia fugax. Gut 1987;28:1039–1040.
144. Rao SS, Tuteja AK, Vellema T, Kempf J, Stessman M. Dyssynergic defecation: demographics, symptoms, stool patterns, and quality of life. J Clin Gastroenterol 2004; 38:680–685.
145. Pezim ME, Pemberton JH, Levin KE, Litchy WJ, Phillips SF. Parameters of anorectal and colonic motility in health and in severe constipation. Dis Colon Rectum 1993;36:484–491.
146. Preston DM, Lennard-Jones JE. Anismus in chronic constipation. Dig Dis Sci 1985; 30 (5):413–418.
147. Lestar B, Pennickx FM, Kerremans RP. Defecometry: A new method for determining the parameters of rectal evacuation. Dis Colon Rectum 1989;32:197–201.

148. Rao SS, Hatfield R, Soffer E, Rao S, Beaty J, Conklin JL. Manometric tests of ano-rectal function in healthy adults. Am J Gastroenterol 1999;94:773–783.

149. Rao SS, Welcher KD, Leistikow JS. Obstructive defecation: a failure of rectoanal coordination. Am J Gastroenterol 1998;93:1042–1050.

150. Kuijpers HC, Bleijenberg G. The spastic pelvic floor syndrome: a cause of constipa-tion. Dis Colon Rectum 1985;28:66–672.

151. Kuijpers HC, Bleijenberg G, de Morree H. The spastic pelvic floor syndrome. Large bowel outlet obstruction caused by pelvic floor dysfunction: a radiological study. Int J Colorectal Dis 1986;1:44–48.

152. Rao SS. Dyssynergic defecation. Gastroenterol Clin North Am 2001;30:97–114.

153. Roberts JP, Womack NR, Hallan RI, Thorpe AC, Williams NS. Evidence from dy-namic integrated proctography to redefine anismus. Br J Surg 1992;79:1213–1215.

154. Jones PN, Lubowski DZ, Swash M, Henry MM. Is paradoxical contraction of pu-borectalis muscle of functional importance? Dis Colon Rectum 1987;30:667–670.

155. Voderholzer WA, Schatke W, Muhldorfer BE, Klauser AG, Birkner B, Muller-Lissner SA. Clinical response to dietary fiber treatment of chronic constipation. Am J Gastroenterol 1997;92:95–98.

156. Rao SSC, Mudipalli RS, Stessman M, Zimmerman B. Investigation of the utility of colorectal function tests and Rome II criteria in dyssynergic defecation (Anismus). Neurogastroenterol Motil 2004;16:1–8.

157. Duthie GS, Bartolo DC. Anismus: the cause of constipation? Results of investiga-tion and treatment. World J Surg 1992;16:831–835.

158. Thorpe AC, Williams NS, Badenoch DF, Blandy JP, Grahn MF. Simultaneous dy-namic electromyographic proctography and cystometrography. Br J Surg 1993;80: 115–120.

159. Rao SSC, Welcher KD, Leistikow BS. Obstructive defecation: A failure of rectoanal coordination. Amer J Gastroenterol 1998;93:1042–1050.

160. Surrenti E, Rath DM, Pemberton JH, Camilleri M. Audit of constipation in a ter-tiary referral gastroenterology practice. Am J Gastroenterol 1995;90:1471–1475.

161. Kuijpers HC. Application of the colorectal laboratory in diagnosis and treatment of functional constipation. Dis Colon Rectum 1990;33:35–39.

162. Wald A, Caruana BJ, Friemanis MG, Bauman DH, Hinds JP. Contributions of evac-uation proctography and anorectal manometry to evaluation of adults with consti-pation and defecatory difficulty. Dig Dis Sci 1990;35:481–487.

163. Rao SS, Patel RS. How useful are manometric tests of anorectal function in the management of defecation disorders? Am J Gastroenterol 1997;92:469–75.

164. Schouten WR. Anismus: Fact or Ficton. Dis Colon Rectum 1997;40:1033–1041.

165. Grotz RL, Pemberton JH, Talley NJ, Rath DM, Zinsmeister AR. Discriminant value of psychological distress, symptom profiles, and segmental colonic dysfunction in outpatients with severe idiopathic constipation. Gut 1994;35:798–802.

166. Minguez M, Herreros B, Sanchiz V, Hernandez V, Almela P, Anon R, Mora F, Bena-ges A. Predictive value of the balloon expulsion test for excluding the diagnosis of pelvic floor dyssynergia in constipation. Gastroenterology 2004;126:57–62.

167. Glia A, Lindberg G, Nilsson LH, Mihocsa L, Akerlund JE. Clinical value of symptom assessment in patients with constipation. Dis Colon Rectum 1999;42:1401–1408.

168. Koch A, Voderholzer WA, Klauser AG, Muller-Lissner S. Symptoms in chronic con-stipation. Dis Colon Rectum 1997;40:902–906.

169. Halligan S, Thomas J, Bartram C. Intrarectal pressures and balloon expulsion re-lated to evacuation proctography. Gut 37(1):100–4, 1995.

170. Jung SH, Myung SJ, Jung HY, et.al. Manometric classification of pelvic floor dyssynergia and its clinical significance in constipated patients. 122 ed. 2002:446–447.
171. Halligan S, Thomas J, Bartram C. Intrarectal pressures and balloon expulsion related to evacuation proctography. Gut 1995;37:100–4.
172. Muller-Lissner SA, Kamm MA, Scarpignato C, Wald A. Myths and misconceptions about chronic constipation. Am J Gastroenterol 2005;100:323–42.
173. Barnes PR, Lennard-Jones JE. Balloon expulsion from the rectum in constipation of different types. Gut 1985;26:1049–1052.
174. Ekberg O, Mahiew PHG, Bartram CI, Piloni V. Defecography: dynamic radiological imaging and proctology. Gastroenterology International 1990;3:93–99.
175. Goei R. Anorectal function in patients with defecation disorders and asymptomatic subjects: evaluation with defecography. Radiology 1990;174:121–123.
176. Halligan S, Bartram CI, Park HJ, Kamm MA. Proctographic features of anismus. Radiology 1995;197:679–682.
177. Muller-Lissner S, Bartolo DC, Christiansen J, Ekberg O, Goei R, Hopfner W, Infantino A, Kuijpers HC, Selvaggi F, Wald A. Interobserver agreement in defecography—an international study. Gastroenterol 1998;36:273–279.
178. Pennickx FM, Debruyne C, Lestar B, Kerremans R. Observer variation in the radiological measurement of the anorectal angle. Int J Colorectal Dis 1990;5:94–97.
179. Ferrante SL, Perry RE, Schreiman JS, Cheng SC, Frick MP. The reproducibility of measuring the anorectal angle in defecography. Dis Colon Rectum 1991;34:51–55.
180. Freimanis MG, Wald A, Caruana B, Bauman DH. Evacuation proctography in normal volunteers. Investigative Radiology 1991;26:581–585.
181. Hinton JM, Lennard-Jones JE, Young AC. A new method for studying gut transit times using radioopaque markers. Gut 1969;10:842–847.
182. Arhan P, Devroede G, Jehannin B, Lanza M, Faverdin C, Dornic C, Persoz B, Tetreault L, Perey B, Pellerin D. Segmental colonic transit time. Dis Colon Rectum 1981; 24:625–629.
183. Metcalf AM, Phillips SF, Zinsmeister AR, MacCarty RL, Beart RW, Wolff BG. Simplified assessment of segmental colonic transit. Gastroenterology 1987;92:40–47.
184. Dailianas A, Skandalis N, Rimkis MN, Koutsomanis D, Kardasi M, Archimandritis A. Pelvic floor study in patients with obstructie defecation: influence of biofeedback. J Clin Gastroenterol 2000;30:176–180.
185. Karlbom U, Pahlman L, Nilsson S, Graf W. Relationships between defecographic findings, rectal emptying, and colonic transit time in constipated patients. Gut 1995; 36:907–912.
186. Proano M, Camilleri M, Phillips SF, Brown ML, Thomforde GM. Transit of solids through the human colon: regional quantification in the unprepared bowel. Am J Physiol 1990;258:856–862.
187. Stivland T, Camilleri M, Vassallo M, Proano M, Rath D, Brown M. Scintigraphic measurement of regional gut transit in idiopathic constipation. Gastroenterology 1991; 101:107–115.
188. Waller SL. Differential measurement of small and large bowel transit times in constipation and diarrhoea: A new approach. Gut 1975;16:372–378.
189. van der Sijp JR, Kamm MA, Nightingale JM, Britton KE, Mather SJ, Morris GP, Akkermans LM, Lennard-Jones JE. Radioisotope determination of regional colonic transit in severe constipation: comparison with radio opaque markers. Gut 1993;34:402–408.

190. Whitehead WE, Devroede G, Habib FI, Meunier P, Wald A. Functional Disorders of the Anorectum. Gastroenterology International 1992;5:92–108.

191. Miller R, Duthie GS, Bartolo DC, Roe AM, Locke-Edmunds J, Mortensen NJ. Anismus in patients with normal and slow transit constipation. Br J Surg 1991;78:690–692.

192. Lebel ML, Grandmaison F. Etude electromyographique dynamique du plancher pelvien dans la constipation: importance de la EMG la aiguille. Can J Neurol Sci 1988;15:212.

193. Percy JP, Neill ME, Swash M, Parks AG. Electrophysiological study of motor nerve supply of pelvic floor. Lancet 1981;1:16–17.

194. Badiali D, Habib FI, Corazziari E, Viscardi A, Primerano L, Anzini F, Torsoli A. Manometric and defaecographic patterns of straining. J Gastrointest Mot 1991;3:171.

195. Enck P, Bielefeldt K, Legler T, Krasemann TFM, Erckenbrecht JF. Kann man Verstopfung lernen? Eine experimentelle Untersuchung bei gesunden Probanden. Zeitschrift fur Gastroenterol 1991;1:31.

196. Leroi AM, Berkelmans I, Denis P, Hemond M, Devroede G. Anismus as a marker of sexual abuse. Dig Dis Sci 1995;40:1411–1416.

197. Kawimbe BM, Papachrysostomou M, Binnie NR, Clare N, Smith AN. Outlet obstruction constipation (anismus) managed by biofeedback. Gut 1991;32:1175–1179.

198. Bleijenberg G, Kuijpers HC. Biofeedback treatment of constipation: a comparison of two methods. Am J Gastroenterol 1994;89:1021–1026.

199. Cox DJ, Sutphen J, Borowitz S, Dickens MN, Singles J, Whitehead WE. Simple electromyographic biofeedback treatment for chronic pediatric constipation/encopresis: preliminary report. Biofeedback & Self Regulation 1994;19:41–50.

200. Rao SS, Welcher KD, Pelsang RE. Effects of biofeedback therapy on anorectal function in obstructive defecation. Dig Dis Sci 1997;42:2197–2205.

201. Bleijenberg G, Kuijpers HC. Treatment of spastic pelvic floor syndrome with biofeedback. Dis Colon Rectum 1987;30:108–111.

202. Koutsomanis D, Lennard-Jones JE, Roy AJ, Kamm MA. Controlled randomised trial of visual biofeedback versus muscle training without a visual display for intractable constipation. Gut 1995;37:95–99.

203. Whitehead WE. Functional anorectal disorders. Semin Gastro Dis 1996;7:230–236.

204. Enck P. Biofeedback training in disordered defecation. A critical review. Dig Dis Sci 1993;38:1953–1960.

205. Glia A, Gylin M, Gullberg K, Lindberg G. Biofeedback retraining in patients with functional constipation and paradoxical puborectalis contraction: comparison of anal manometry and sphincter electromyography for feedback. Dis Colon Rectum 1997;40:889–895.

206. Papachrysostomou M, Smith AN. Effects of biofeedback on obstructive defecation—reconditioning of the defecation reflex? Gut 1994;35:252–256.

207. Chiarioni G, Whitehead WE, Pezza V, Morelli A, Bassotti G. Biofeedback is superior to laxatives for normal transit constipation due to pelvic floor dyssynergia. Gastroenterology 2006;130:657–664.

208. Chiarioni G, Chistolini F, Menegotti M, Salandini L, Vantini I, Morelli A, Bassotti G. One-year follow-up study on the effects of electrogalvanic stimulation in chronic idiopathic constipation with pelvic floor dyssynergia. Dis Colon Rectum 2004;47:346–353.

209. Heymen S. Psychological and cognitive variables affecting treatment outcomes for urinary and fecal incontinence. Gastroenterology 2004;126:S146–S151.

Chapter 13

Childhood Functional Gastrointestinal Disorders: Neonate/Toddler

Peter J. Milla, Chair

Paul E. Hyman, Co-Chair

Marc A. Benninga

Geoffrey Davidson

David Fleisher

Jan Taminiau

Introduction

Infant and toddler functional gastrointestinal disorders (FGIDs) include a variable combination of often age-dependent, chronic, or recurrent symptoms not explained by structural or biochemical abnormalities. Functional symptoms during childhood sometimes accompany normal development (e.g., infant regurgitation), or they may arise from maladaptive behavioral responses to internal or external stimuli (e.g., retention of feces in the rectum often results from painful defecation). The clinical expression of an FGID depends on an individual's stage of development particularly with regard to autonomic, affective, and intellectual development. Infant regurgitation is a problem for a few months during the first year. Functional diarrhea affects infants and toddlers. Many difficult-to-manage cases of functional constipation resolve once a child enters puberty, as thinking about the problem matures and motivation increases. Irritable bowel syndrome (IBS) and functional dyspepsia are diagnosed only after the child becomes a reliable reporter for pain, typically in the early school years (Table 1).

The decision to seek medical care for a symptom arises from a parent's or caretaker's concern for the child. The caretaker's threshold for concern varies with their own experiences and expectations, coping style, and perception of their child's illness. For this reason, the office visit is not only about the child's symptom, but also about the family's conscious and unconscious fears. The clinician must not only make a diagnosis, but also recognize the impact of the symptom on the family's emotional tone and ability to function. Therefore, any intervention plan must attend to both the child and the family. Effective management depends upon securing a therapeutic alliance with the parents.

Through the first years of life children cannot accurately report symptoms such as nausea or pain. The infant and preschool child cannot discriminate between emotional and physical distress. Therefore, the clinician depends upon the reports and interpretations of the parents, who know their child best, and the observations of the clinician, who is trained to differentiate between health and illness.

Disability from a functional symptom is related to maladaptive coping with the symptom. Childhood functional gastrointestinal disorders are not dangerous when the symptoms and parental concerns are addressed and contained. Conversely, failed diagnosis and inappropriate treatments of functional symptoms may be the cause of needless physical and emotional suffering. In severe cases, well-meaning clinicians inadvertently cocreate unnecessarily complex and costly solutions to functional symptoms, prolonging emotional stress and promoting disability.

Table 1. Functional Gastrointestinal Disorders

A. Functional Esophageal Disorders

A1. Functional heartburn
A2. Functional chest pain of presumed esophageal origin
A3. Functional dysphagia
A4. Globus

B. Functional Gastroduodenal Disorders

B1. Functional dyspepsia
    B1a. Postprandial distress syndrome (PDS)
    B1b. Epigastric pain syndrome (EPS)
B2. Belching disorders
    B2a. Aerophagia
    B2b. Unspecified excessive belching

B3. Nausea and vomiting disorders
    B3a. Chronic idiopathic nausea (CIN)
    B3b. Functional vomiting
    B3c. Cyclic vomiting syndrome (CVS)
B4. Rumination syndrome in adults

C. Functional Bowel Disorders

C1. Irritable bowel syndrome (IBS)
C2. Functional bloating
C3. Functional constipation
C4. Functional diarrhea
C5. Unspecified functional bowel disorder

D. Functional Abdominal Pain Syndrome (FAPS)

E. Functional Gallbladder and Sphincter of Oddi (SO) Disorders

E1. Functional gallbladder disorder
E2. Functional biliary SO disorder
E3. Functional pancreatic SO disorder

F. Functional Anorectal Disorders

F1. Functional fecal incontinence
F2. Functional anorectal pain
    F2a. Chronic proctalgia
        F2a1. Levator ani syndrome
        F2a2. Unspecified functional anorectal pain
    F2b. Proctalgia fugax
F3. Functional defecation disorders
    F3a. Dyssynergic defecation
    F3b. Inadequate defecatory propulsion

G. Functional Disorders: Neonates and Toddlers

G1. Infant regurgitation
G2. Infant rumination syndrome
G3. Cyclic vomiting syndrome
G4. Infant colic
G5. Functional diarrhea
G6. Infant dyschezia
G7. Functional constipation

H. Functional Disorders: Children and Adolescents

H1. Vomiting and aerophagia
    H1a. Adolescent rumination syndrome
    H1b. Cyclic vomiting syndrome
    H1c. Aerophagia
H2. Abdominal pain-related FGIDs
    H2a. Functional dyspepsia
    H2b. Irritable bowel syndrome
    H2c. Abdominal migraine
H2d. Childhood functional abdominal pain
    H2d1. Childhood functional abdominal pain syndrome
H3. Constipation and incontinence
    H3a. Functional constipation
    H3b. Nonretentive fecal incontinence

GI. Infant Regurgitation

— Introduction

Regurgitation of stomach contents into the esophagus, mouth, and/or nose is common in infants and is developmentally a normal physiological event. Unfortunately, distinguishing this benign event from the pathological problem of gastroesophageal reflux can be problematic and may lead to unnecessary doctor visits, investigations, and therapy. This will often lead to the infant being mislabeled with gastroesophageal reflux disease (GERD), and once this occurs it is often very difficult to reverse.

The aim of this guideline is to argue for treating uncomplicated regurgitation in otherwise healthy infants as a developmental issue rather than a disease.

— Definition

Regurgitation is the involuntary return of previously swallowed food or secretions into or out of the esophagus, mouth, and/or nose. Regurgitation is distinguished from vomiting, which is defined by a central nervous reflex involving both autonomic and skeletal muscles in which gastric contents are forcefully expelled through the mouth because of coordinated movements of the small bowel, stomach, esophagus, and diaphragm. Regurgitation is also different from rumination in which previously swallowed food is voluntarily returned to the pharynx and mouth, chewed and swallowed again. Regurgitation, vomiting, and rumination are examples of gastroesophageal reflux. Gastroesophageal reflux refers to retrograde movement of gastric contents out of the stomach. When gastroesophageal reflux causes or contributes to tissue damage or inflammation (e.g., esophagitis, obstructive apnea, reactive airway disease, pulmonary aspiration, feeding and swallowing difficulties, or failure to thrive), it is called gastroesophageal reflux disease (GERD).

— Epidemiology

Daily regurgitation is common in the first year, is more common in neonates than in older infants and children, and is found with higher rates in premature neonates [1]. Regurgitation occurs more than once a day in 67% of healthy four-month-old infants. Unfortunately many parents believe this is abnormal; 24% of parents report regurgitation symptoms by the time their infants are sixth months old [2]. Daily regurgitation decreases with age to 5% of infants ten-to-twelve months old. Occasional regurgitation may persist until the third year in a few healthy children. Most of these infants have no symptoms other than regurgitation.

G1. Diagnostic Criteria for Infant Regurgitation

Must include *both* of the following in otherwise healthy infants 3 weeks to 12 months of age:
1. **Regurgitation two or more times per day for 3 or more weeks**
2. **No retching, hematemesis, aspiration, apnea, failure to thrive, feeding or swallowing difficulties, or abnormal posturing**

— Rationale for Changes in Diagnostic Criteria

There have been no changes from the Rome II criteria. The forcefulness of the regurgitation or its outflow through the mouth or nares does not carry any diagnostic relevance. The duration of three weeks was chosen because infants come to medical attention more quickly and symptoms cause more parental anxiety than in older children and adults.

— Clinical Evaluation

History and physical examination may provide evidence of disease outside the gastrointestinal tract including a large number of metabolic infectious and neurological conditions associated with vomiting. Prematurity, developmental delay, and congenital abnormalities of the oropharynx, chest, lungs, central nervous system, heart, or gastrointestinal tract are considered risk factors for GERD [3].

Physical signs that may indicate a systemic condition associated with chronic regurgitation include eczema (milk allergy) [4] and an abnormal neurological examination. Evidence of failure to thrive, hematemesis, occult blood in the stool, anemia or food refusal (particularly tolerance of only smooth purees at an inappropriate age), and swallowing difficulties should prompt an evaluation for GERD.

Assessment to exclude an upper gastrointestinal anatomical abnormality such as malrotation or a gastric outlet obstruction should be done if regurgitation persists past the first year of life, and if it has not been done previously as part of an evaluation for GERD.

— Physiological Features

Infant regurgitation is usually a transient problem, possibly due in part to postnatal maturation of upper gastrointestinal motility. In premature infants, large volume or high osmolality feeds delay gastric emptying by inducing postprandial duodenal hypomotility. A full gastric fundus in turn predisposes to transient lower esophageal sphincter (LES) relaxations, which in turn leads to regurgitation [5]. In children, there is no evidence to support a delay in gastric emptying as a contributing factor to GERD [5, 6]. As the postprandial duodenal motility changes to a more mature pattern over the first weeks and months of life, meal volume has less effect on the rate of emptying and the duodenal motility increases with larger more complex meals [7]. As the infant develops and esophageal volume increases, visible regurgitation reduces markedly although it may still be noted by frequent swallowing, particularly after meals. As suggested by Orenstein [3], regurgitation in an otherwise healthy infant may simply serve as a pop-off valve to cope with the high fluid volume they receive compared to adults.

Esophageal volume is another contributor to regurgitation. The volume of the esophagus is a few milliliters in the newborn infant—about 1/20th of the adult esophageal volume. Because of this, reflux material is likely to travel much further up the esophagus of the infant than in an adult.

— Psychological Features

Parent anxiety or maternal postnatal depression, infant temperament, and environmental stresses may interact to cause an aberrant parent-child interaction [8]. Infants may regurgitate as one symptom of emotional distress. Feeding problems such as early satiety, food refusal, and excessive crying may occur and lead to failure to thrive [9, 10].

— Treatment

A natural history of infant regurgitation is one of spontaneous improvement [2]. Therefore, treatment goals are to provide effective reassurance and symptom relief while avoiding complications.

Effective reassurance includes (a) an empathetic, satisfactory response to the stated and unstated fears of the parents (i.e., What is wrong with my baby? Is it dangerous? Will it go away? What can we do about it?) and (b) a promise of continuing availability and reassessment.

Symptom relief includes adjustment in infant care and medication. Prone positioning is no longer recommended [10], but the left-sided and prone position have been shown to reduce regurgitation and may help in reducing regurgitation frequency [11]. An analysis of randomized controlled trials has failed to support or refute the efficacy of thickening agents in infant formula [12], although efficacy is suggested by several recent studies [13, 14]. The most convincing is the study by Wenzl et al. [14] using intraluminal impedance to measure flow of the refluxate. While frequent smaller volume feedings are recommended, there is little direct evidence to support the efficacy of this approach.

Improving the parental-child interaction is often aided by relieving the parent's fears about the condition of the infant, identifying sources of physical and emotional distress, and making plans to eliminate them. Stress relief may be aided by periods of respite for the parents and an assurance of clinician availability for follow up. Because of the anxiety generated by these symptoms in infants, feed, play, or sleep patterns are often abandoned, and re-establishing a routine for infant and caretaker is often helpful. Infants who are breast fed tend to regurgitate less for a variety of reasons, including stress reduction in mother and infant and faster gastric emptying. At the present time no medical interventions improve esophageal and gastric motility and reduce symptoms [15, 16].

G2. Infant Rumination Syndrome

— Definition

Rumination is the voluntary, habitual regurgitation of stomach contents into the mouth for the purpose of self-stimulation. Nonruminative gastroesophageal reflux may play a role in its development [16].

Rumination has three clinical presentations (1) infant rumination syndrome [18], (2) rumination in neurologically impaired children and adults, and (3) rumination in healthy older children and adults. The latter two presentations are discussed in Chapter 14.

— Epidemiology

Infant rumination syndrome is rare. It seems to have been more prevalent earlier in this century, as indicated by Kanner's report of seven cases per thousand admissions to an acute care pediatric hospital [19]. It is five times more prevalent in male than female infants [20].

G2. Diagnostic Criteria for Infant Rumination Syndrome

Must include *all* of the following for at least 3 months:
1. **Repetitive contractions of the abdominal muscles, diaphragm, and tongue**
2. **Regurgitation of gastric content into the mouth, which is either expectorated or rechewed and reswallowed**
3. **Three or more of the following:**
   a. **Onset between 3 and 8 months**
   b. **Does not respond to management for gastroesophageal reflux disease, or to anticholinergic drugs, hand restraints, formula changes, and gavage or gastrostomy feedings**
   c. **Unaccompanied by signs of nausea or distress**
   d. **Does not occur during sleep and when the infant is interacting with individuals in the environment**

— Rational for Change in Diagnostic Criteria

There have been no changes from the Rome II criteria.

— Clinical Evaluation

Observing the ruminative act is essential for diagnosis. However, such observations require time, patience, and stealth because rumination may cease as soon as the infant notices the observer.

No readily available diagnostic test identifies rumination as the etiology of vomiting or regurgitation (antroduodenal manometry identifies rumination in adults and children evaluated at special centers). In the past, the diagnosis of infant rumination depended on the resolution of symptoms with empathetic and responsive nurturing [21, 22].

Diagnostic efforts should be directed toward the parents as well as the infant because infant rumination syndrome results from malfunction in the infant caregiver relationship [23]. Interviews with each parent and the infant and parents together are important.

— Physiologic Features

Reversal of the abdominal-thoracic pressure gradient coupled with relaxation of the LES mechanism is probably similar in infants and adults who ruminate. (See Chapter 7.) One feature that makes infant rumination much more dangerous than adult rumination is the infant's inability to retain enough regurgitated nutrients for nutritional sufficiency. This causes potentially lethal malnutrition, a complication that seldom if ever occurs in older ruminators [18].

— Psychological Features

The emotional and sensory deprivation that prompts rumination may occur in sick infants living in environments that prevent normal handling (e.g., neonatal intensive care units) [24]. It may also occur in otherwise healthy infants whose mothers are emotionally unconnected. Maternal behavior may appear to be neglectful or slavishly attentive, but in every case, there is no enjoyment in holding the baby or sensitivity to the infant's needs for comfort and satisfaction [18, 25–30]. The aberrant nurturing relationship is one aspect of more pervasive difficulties the parents have with interpersonal relationships. There is often a history of traumatic emotional deprivation during childhood, and of marital dysfunction [17, 20–25].

The pathogenesis of infant rumination syndrome can be understood in light of developmental phenomena that emerge at about three months of age [18]. The infant develops a sense of self. The infant learns that the infant and mother are physically separate and have different affective experiences. The awareness of separateness from the need-gratifying maternal figure is the condition that makes possible feelings of helplessness in the infant.

Fortunately, two means of coping also develop at about three months. The infant (1) becomes able to evoke a social response from caregivers and (2) gains the ability to entertain and self-satisfy by producing interesting noises and activities. If the infant's efforts fail to elicit sufficient tension-relieving responses from caregivers, he/she may resort to more self-stimulation. The concept of rumination as self-stimulating behavior provides both a theoretical basis for its pathogenesis and an effective approach to its management [18, 26].

— Management

Loss of previously swallowed food may cause progressive inanition and death [16, 17, 26, 28, 30–32].

Behavioral therapy that employs aversive techniques and positive reinforcement is useful in eliminating rumination in highly motivated adults or children with neurological impairment [33]. The use of such measures in infants [34] may be harmful if therapeutic goals are limited to symptom suppression without addressing the infant's unmet needs for nurturing and the mother's inability to engage her baby in a mutually satisfying relationship. The most humane, developmentally appropriate, and comprehensive management aims at reversing the baby's weight loss by eliminating its need for ruminative behavior. This can be achieved by providing a temporary substitute care giver to hold, comfort, and feed the infant. The nurturing person should be sufficiently sensitive and observant to know when the infant withdraws into the self-absorbed state that fosters rumination and promptly respond by engaging the baby socially [18, 20–23]. Treatment also aims at helping the parents to address their feelings toward the infant and to improve their ability to recognize and respond to the infant's physical and emotional needs.

The weight loss and rumination rapidly respond to nurturing that is sensitive and interactive. It may be exacerbated by withdrawal of reciprocal care-giving, and by the noxious stress of the work-up that accompanies "diagnosis by exclusion." After rumination with failure-to-thrive subsides, it usually does not recur, even in families whose overall mental health remains poor [35].

G3. Cyclic Vomiting Syndrome

— Definition

Cyclic vomiting syndrome (CVS) consists of recurrent, stereotypic episodes of intense nausea and vomiting lasting hours to days that are separated by symptom-free intervals [36]. The frequency of episodes in a series of 71 patients ranged from 1 to 70 per year and averaged 12 per year [37]. Attacks may occur at fairly regular intervals or sporadically. Typically, episodes begin at the same time of day, most commonly during the night or in the morning. The duration of episodes tend to be the same in each patient over months or years [37]. Once vomiting begins, it reaches its highest intensity during the first hours. The frequency of vomiting tends to diminish thereafter, although nausea continues until the episode ends. Episodes usually end as rapidly as they begin and are marked by prompt recovery of well-being, provided the patient has not incurred major deficits of fluids and electrolytes.

Signs and symptoms that may accompany cyclic vomiting include pallor, weakness, increased salivation, abdominal pain, intolerance to noise, light and/or odors, headache, loose stools, fever, tachycardia, hypertension, skin blotching, and leukocytosis [38].

Eighty percent of patients can identify circumstances or events that trigger some or most of their attacks. The most common triggers are heightened emotional states, which may be either noxious (e.g., anxiety) or pleasant excitement (e.g., birthdays or vacations), infections (e.g., upper respiratory infection), asthma, or physical exhaustion [37, 39, 1].

— Epidemiology

CVS affects equal numbers of boys and girls and less commonly adults [40, 2, 3], occurs from infancy to midlife, and is most common in the toddler age range between 2 and 7 years [40]. Population-based studies have shown the prevalence of cyclic vomiting syndrome to be 2.3% in Western Australian children [44], and 1.9% in the school children from Aberdeen, Scotland [45]. The prevalence in adult life is uncertain with few data available at the present time. Migraine, increased susceptibility to motion sickness, and functional bowel disorders are more prevalent in patients with CVS as well as in their families.

G3. Diagnostic Criteria for Cyclic Vomiting Syndrome

Must include *both* of the following:
1. **Two or more periods of intense nausea and unremitting vomiting or retching lasting hours to days**
2. **Return to usual state of health lasting weeks to months**

— Rationale for Changes in Diagnostic Criteria

To encourage early diagnosis and treatment, the number of episodes required for diagnosis has been changed from three to two.

— Clinical Evaluation

Patients do not vomit between episodes, but two thirds of them have symptoms of IBS, and 11% have migraine headaches. Motion sickness is a problem for about 40% of those affected by CVS. Over half have family histories of IBS and nearly half have a family history of migraine headache.

The differential diagnosis of CVS includes diseases having similar presentations during at least part of their courses [36, 46]. Brain stem gliomas may infiltrate the vomiting centers and cranial nerves around the medulla, causing intermittent vomiting without obstruction of flow of cerebral spinal fluid or signs of increased intracranial pressure. Occult upper respiratory tract infection, particularly if associated with vestibulitis and obstructive uropathy, may cause symptoms indistinguishable from cyclic vomiting syndrome. Gastrointestinal disorders mimicking cyclic vomiting include peptic disease with pyloric outlet obstruction, enteropathy (especially if there is a marked duodenitis), recurrent pancreatitis, intermittent small bowel obstruction, chronic intestinal pseudo-obstruction, and the vomiting crises of familial dysautonomia. Endocrine and metabolic conditions to be considered include pheochromocytoma, adrenal insufficiency, diabetes mellitus, ornithine transcarbamylase deficiency, and other urea cycle defects, medium-chain acyl coenzyme A dehydrogenase deficiency, proprionic acidemia, isovaleric acidemia (the chronic intermittent form), and porphyria [36, 46].

— Physiological Features

CVS is a paroxysmal disorder related to the episodic and recurrent activation of the emetic reflex. Current understanding suggests that the reflex consists of a variety of afferent inputs from vagal afferents, higher cranial nuclei, the cortex and metabolites/toxins via the area postrema all accessing the chemotactic trigger zone in the floor of the fourth ventricle; if the intensity of afferent input exceeds the vomiting threshold interneurones activate the vagal motor nuclei resulting in the efferent output. This consists of a pre-ejection phase accompanied by autonomic activation (pallor, headache, nausea, drooling, etc.) followed by an ejection phase with repeated retching and vomiting. Cyclic vomiting episodes are accompanied by intense autonomic discharge and release of adrenocorticotrophic hormone (ACTH), vasopressin, norepinephrine, and prostaglandin F_2 in some or most patients.

— Psychological Features

A majority of parents in one study (with no control population) described their affected children as having one or more of the following personality traits: competitive, perfectionistic, high-achieving, strong-willed, moralistic, caring, and enthusiastic [36]. The natural course of CVS in any individual is unpredictable. Patients and parents feel oppressed and fearful because of the mysterious, uncertain nature of the illness. Depression and anxiety disorders complicate nearly a third of CVS patients [38].

— Treatment

There are four phases to CVS: interepisodic, pre-ejection, ejection, and recovery. Prevention becomes a goal in patients whose episodes are frequent, severe, and prolonged. Conditions that trigger episodes may be identified and treated. Prophylactic daily treatment with cyproheptadine, amitriptyline, phenobarbital, or propranolol may reduce the sensitivity of the chemotactic trigger zone. These measures succeed in reducing the frequency or eliminating episodes in many children [45–52].

The identification of the key role that corticotrophin releasing factor (CRF), 5-hydroxytryptamine$_3$ (5-HT$_3$) and neurokinin$_1$ (NK$_1$) [46, 47] receptors play in the emetic reflex has resulted in improvements in treating individual episodes. CRF has been implicated as an important factor in the midbrain response to stress and is responsible for the excessive cortisol release seen in CVS. 5-HT$_3$ and NK$_1$ are sensory receptors in the foregut and afferent receptors in the hind brain are involved in the afferent limb of the emetic reflex. Targeting these receptors is the logical way of controlling individual episodes of CVS [47]. Aborting episodes is possible in some children with a recognizable prodrome. Prior to the onset of nausea, oral medications such as ondansetron, erythromycin, and ibuprofen may be useful. Early in the episode it may be helpful to begin an oral acid-inhibiting drug agent to protect esophageal mucosa and dental enamel, and lorazepam for its anxiolytic, sedative, and anti-emetic effects. In some patients combinations of intravenous ondansetron, granisetron, diphenhydramine, and chlorpromazine are helpful. The addition of NK$_1$ antagonists such as aprepitant [47] to this therapeutic approach is logical and may be effective.

Patients whose episodes cannot be prevented or interrupted should be sedated starting early in the prodromal phase until the episodes end because sleep not only provides comfort for patients with intractable nausea but also reduces input from the cortex and activity of the chemotactic trigger zone. Symptoms may be interrupted by titrating intravenous lorazepam until the patient enters restful sleep. Intravenous fluids, electrolytes, and H$_2$-histamine receptor antagonists are administered until the episode is over. Complications arising during cyclic vomiting episodes include water and electrolyte deficits, hematemesis mostly due to prolapse gastropathy, peptic esophagitis and/or Mallory-Weiss tears, deficits in intracellular potassium and magnesium, hypertension, and inappropriate secretion of antidiuretic hormone.

CVS is a paroxysmal disorder involving interactions between the central nervous system and the gastrointestinal tract. CVS is differentiated from abdominal migraine, another paroxysmal disorder by the most distressing symptom. In CVS, vomiting is the most distressing symptom, but in abdominal migraine pain is the most distressing symptom [53].

G4. Infant Colic

— Definition

Infant colic has been described as a behavioral syndrome of early infancy involving frequent crying, long periods of crying, and hard-to-soothe behavior [54]. Infant colic is defined as crying during the first 3 months of life for 3 or more hours per day on 3 or more days per week in infants who do not suffer from other conditions that may cause crying [55, 56]. Crying bouts start and stop suddenly without obvious cause [56] and are more likely to occur late in the day [57, 58]. Colicky crying tends to resolve spontaneously by 3 to 4 months of age or, in the case of babies born prematurely, 3 to 4 months after term [59, 60]. Normal infants cry more during the early months of life than at any age thereafter [56]. On average, crying peaks at about 6 weeks and then steadily diminishes by 12 weeks [61, 62]. "Colicky" crying probably represents the upper end of the normal "crying curve" of healthy infants and is not the result of pain [63]. Colic "is something infants do, rather than a condition they have" [64]. There is no proof that the crying of infant colic is caused by pain in the abdomen or any other part of the infant's body [54]. Nevertheless, parents often assume that the cause of excessive crying is abdominal pain of gastrointestinal origin.

— Epidemiology

About 20% of infants are perceived by parents to be colicky by Wessel's criteria [55, 65]. However, the prevalence of infant colic is influenced by parents' perceptions of the intensity and duration of crying bouts [66], the method by which data on crying are collected, the psychosocial well-being of the parents [67], and culturally determined infant care practices. Barr found that among Kung San hunter-gathers of the Kalahari Desert, the frequency of crying onsets conformed to the Brazelton-Barr "crying curve," but the amount of crying was much less than in Western cultures. This may be due to the almost continuous contact taking place between parent and infant in the hunter-gatherer culture, resulting in consistent and prompt comforting responses provided to the infant [68].

G4. Diagnostic Criteria for Infant Colic

Must include *all* of the following in infants from birth to 4 months of age:

1. **Paroxysms of irritability, fussing, or crying that start and stop without obvious cause**
2. **Episodes lasting 3 or more hours/day and occurring at least 3 days/wk for at least 1 week**
3. **No failure to thrive**

— Rationale for Changes in Criteria

Rome II excluded infant colic from consideration as a functional gastrointestinal disorder. Nevertheless the abdominal pain attribution persists and pediatric gastroenterologists receive referrals of babies with refractory colic or infants who cry excessively due to unsuspected colic. The Working Team achieved consensus to include infant colic in the list of childhood functional gastrointestinal disorders as familiarity with the "colic syndrome" is necessary to avoid diagnostic and therapeutic misadventures.

— Clinical Evaluation

Many disorders cause irritability and crying that can mimic colic, including cow's milk protein intolerance, fructose intolerance, maternal drug ingestion during pregnancy causing withdrawal irritability in the infant, infantile migraine, GERD, and anomalous origin of the left coronary artery with meal-induced angina [54, 69, 70]. The colicky crying pattern results from organic disease in 10% or less of colicky babies [69]. Behaviors associated with colicky crying (e.g., prolonged crying, unsoothable crying, crying after feedings, facial expressions of pain, abdominal distension, increased gas, flushing, and legs over the abdomen) are not diagnostic clues indicative of pain or organic disease, but they do explain and justify parents' concerns [71, 72].

A presumptive diagnosis of colic can be made in any infant under four to five months of age whose crying has the temporal features of infant colic, who has no signs of CNS or intrinsic developmental difficulties, who is normal on physical examination and has normal growth patterns [54, 73]. It is reasonable to apply time-limited therapeutic trials appropriate for two possible etiologies of colic-like crying: elimination of cow's milk from the diet and elimination of reflux esophagitis. Switching to a protein-hydrolysate formula or deleting milk and milk products from the diet of a breast-feeding mother should result in sustained remission of colic-like behavior due to cow's milk sensitivity, particularly in atopic infants [74]. Relief should be apparent within 48 hours [75]. A similarly time-limited trial of gastric acid suppression may be useful as a test of the etiologic significance of reflux esophagitis. The satiated infant's response to nonanalgesic, nonnutritive soothing maneuvers, such as rhythmic rocking and patting two to three times per second in a quiet, nonalerting environment, may quiet the baby who may nevertheless resume crying as soon as it is put down [76, 77]. Repeated demonstration of a common maneuver that could not eliminate pain, but does quiet the colicky crying has great diagnostic and therapeutic value.

— Physiological Factors

Significant differences have been found in comparisons of colicky infants and infants who did not cry excessively, such as increased muscle tone [56], heart rate during feedings [56], ease of falling asleep and soundness of sleep [78], stool patterns, postprandial gallbladder contraction [79], and other features [74, 80–82]. However, none of these findings have been shown to be more than epiphenomena or have provided a basis for successful treatment in 90% or more of babies with colic syndrome. On the other hand, no differences between colicky and noncolicky infants were found with respect to gastrointestinal transit times [82], fecal alpha-1 antitrypsin [70], or intraluminal gas or flatulence [83, 84].

Current evidence suggests that colicky crying is behavior originating in the CNS rather than the gut. Colicky babies have been shown to have different temperament characteristics [85]. Another hypothesis for the genesis of colic is based on differences in infants' reactivity (i.e., the excitability and/or arousability of behavioral and physiologic responses to stimuli) and infants' inherent ability to self-regulate responses to stimuli and benefit from externally applied soothing procedures [86].

— Psychological Features

Understanding infant colic requires an appreciation of the subjective experience and development of the infant, the mother, their dyadic relationship, and the family and social milieu in which they exist [87].

At about 2 to 3 months of age, normal infants become more attentive, socially responsive, and aware of the distinction of "self" and "other." They become better able to soothe themselves, interact with, and give pleasure to their caregivers. This developmental shift occurs at about the age that colic subsides. These developmental advances are smoother if the infant's temperament is easy, the parents are caring, intuitive, and self-confident, and if the dyadic relationship between them proceeds with smooth reciprocity [87].

Parents usually have conscious and unconscious ambivalence toward their infant. If the infant isn't fussy or difficult to regulate, and if the circumstances of their lives are pleasant, positive feelings predominate and family life is happy. However, if the infant is colicky, resentful feelings may rise to the surface of the parents' awareness [88]. Recognition of angry feelings towards the infant triggers anxiety and guilt which may prompt the caregiver to intensify efforts at nurturing. If attempts at controlling crying are unsuccessful, guilty anxiety may develop into a vicious cycle causing profound physical and emotional exhaustion. This is made more likely when the parental relationship is unsupportive [89]. This stressful state impairs the caregiver's ability to sooth the infant and causes doubts regarding competence as a parent [89, 90]. The emergence of adversarial or alienated feelings towards the unsoothable infant lowers the threshold for abuse. Infant colic may then present as a clinical emergency. Even in noncritical cases, excessive crying may be associated with transient developmental delay in the infant and family dysfunction 1 to 3 years after the infant's birth [91].

— Treatment

Any measure that parents perceive as definitely helpful is worth continuing, provided it is harmless. If there is a question of milk intolerance [75] or reflux esophagitis [54, 72], a time-limited therapeutic trial of a hydrolysate formula or medication to suppress gastric acid secretion is warranted. Relief in such cases should become apparent within 48 hours [75]. However, in more than 90% of cases, management consists not of "curing the colic," but of helping the parents get through the challenging period in their baby's development [92].

There are at least 12 elements to consider in the clinic management of infant colic:

- Understand the history of the infant and the past and present conditions of family life that may impair coping.
- Acknowledge the importance of the problem and how disruptive it usually is to family life.
- Schedule the consultation during a time when the infant is likely to be fussy.
- A thorough, gentle physical examination impresses the parents that the physician is open-minded and looking for organic disease (the parents' chief concern).
- Gently dismantle the pain hypothesis in favor of the developmental hypothesis for colicky crying.
- Inform the parents that a colicky baby taxes even the most experienced, devoted parents.
- Affirm the infant's good health and that the symptoms will subside by 3 to 5 months of age.
- Offer suggestions for soothing maneuvers.
- Individualize advice.
- Relieve guilt and restore parents' confidence.
- Be available for support. The physician's promise to re-examine their baby enables worried parents to continue coping with their colicky infant without turning to unnecessary diagnostic procedures or false "cures."

— Definition

Functional diarrhea is defined by the daily painless recurrent passage of three or more large unformed stools for 4 or more weeks with onset in infancy or preschool years. There is no evidence for failure-to-thrive if the diet has adequate calories. Parents become aware of a problem when unformed stools containing easily identified pieces of undigested vegetables eaten just a few hours earlier run down or over the diaper. The child appears unperturbed by the loose stools, and the symptom resolves spontaneously by school age.

— Epidemiology

Functional diarrhea is the leading cause of chronic diarrhea in an otherwise well child from an industrialized country.

G5. Diagnostic Criteria for Functional Diarrhea

Must include *all* of the following:
1. **Daily painless, recurrent passage of three or more large, unformed stools**
2. **Symptoms that last more than 4 weeks**
3. **Onset of symptoms that begins between 6 and 36 months of age**
4. **Passage of stools that occurs during waking hours**
5. **There is no failure-to-thrive if caloric intake is adequate**

— Rationale for Changes in Diagnostic Criteria

There were no changes from the Rome II criteria.

— Clinical Evaluation

The evaluation of children with chronic diarrhea includes history concerning factors that may cause or exacerbate diarrhea, such as past enteric infections, laxatives, antibiotics, or diet. In toddlers with functional diarrhea, typical stools contain mucus and/or visible undigested food. Often stools become less solid with each bowel movement during the day. Problems in the diet that may cause diarrhea include overfeeding, excessive fruit juice consumption, excessive carbohydrate ingestion with low fat intake, and food allergy. Excessive sorbitol intake results in diarrhea.

The clinician examines the child, with special attention to height, weight, and signs of malnutrition, diaper rash, and fecal impaction (another cause for chronic loose stools). Laboratory screening tests include a complete blood count (increased eosinophils suggest allergy, microcytic anemia and thrombocytosis suggest iron deficiency), stool analysis for occult blood and leukocytes, reducing substances, fat globules, and stool collections for ova and parasites. Culture for enteric pathogens and for *Clostridium difficile* and its toxin may be necessary in selected cases. Although infectious gastroenteritis rarely causes chronic diarrhea, *Giardia lamblia, Dientamoeba fragilis,* and *Cryptosporidium* are agents implicated as causing diarrhea in toddlers attending day care centers. If there is growth deceleration, weight loss, and distended abdomen or a family history of celiac disease, then screening tests with IgA antitransglutaminase and IgA antiendomysial antibodies are important screening tests.

In children who fulfill the criteria for functional diarrhea, a malabsorption syndrome would be unexpected. Chronic diarrhea as the sole symptom in a thriving child makes cystic fibrosis and celiac disease unlikely. Mild celiac disease or cystic fibrosis with isolated pancreatic involvement are exceptions. If there is deceleration in growth or a family history for either of these two diseases exists, than a sweat test and blood tests (such as serum iron, ferritin, albumin, immunoglobulins, cholesterol, and fat-soluble vitamins) for malabsorption are indicated.

— Physiological Features

Both motility and mucosal factors have been proposed to explain functional diarrhea.

Mucosal Factors

Small-intestinal transport is not defective in children with functional diarrhea. Water and electrolyte secretion and glucose absorption are normal [93] and steatorrhea is absent.

In jejunal biopsies from children with functional diarrhea, activities of the mucosal enzymes Na-K ATPase and adenylate cyclase were elevated [94]. The increase in mucosal enzyme activity was associated with an increase in plasma prostaglandin E_2 and F concentrations [95]. Aspirin reduced plasma prostaglandin concentration and resolved the diarrhea [96]. Loperamide, an opiate agonist, has little effect on prostaglandins, but also reduced stool output. These results are intriguing in view of the normal jejunal secretion in children with functional diarrhea, and because of the action of prostaglandins on adenylate cyclase activation and intestinal secretion.

Intestinal Motility

The migrating motor complex (MMC)—the recurring sequence of three consecutive contraction patterns which cycles through the small bowel during fasting—is interrupted by a meal in healthy children and adults. A meal normally stimulates a pattern of frequent variable amplitude contractions, some of which mix the luminal contents and others that propagate. In functional diarrhea, food fails to interrupt the MMC [97]. As soon as phase 3 of the MMC begins in the stomach, a cluster of high amplitude gastric antral contractions sweep undigested gastric contents through a wide open pylorus, into and through the small bowel, with early arrival to the colon. The failure to induce a postprandial motility pattern results in a kind of colonic dumping accompanied by excess bile salts and incompletely digested food. Sodium and bile acid concentrations are elevated in the extractable water phase of stools from toddlers with functional diarrhea [98].

— Psychological Factors

The morbidity associated with functional diarrhea may be related to the caloric deprivation caused by the misuse of elimination diets [99]. The misuse of elimination diets can be related to an anxious parent's inability to accept the functional diarrhea diagnosis, or a clinician's attempt to assuage the parent's anxiety. Temperament may play a role in the etiology of functional diarrhea. Wender found that those with an active temperament had symptoms suggestive of functional diarrhea [100].

— Treatment

For the child, no treatment is necessary. For the parents, effective reassurance is of paramount importance. A daily diet and defecation diary helps to reassure parents that specific dietary items are not responsible for the symptom. Many families accept effective reassurance readily, and followup is unnecessary. For others, it helps to schedule regular visits for monitoring weight and responding to parents' questions. Diet modifications are occasionally effective (e.g., increasing dietary fiber helps to improve stool consistency). Although failure to induce a normal postprandial motor response seems to be the most likely mechanism for functional diarrhea, medications to slow motility are seldom necessary. If chronic diarrhea persists and is troublesome, a trial of amitriptyline or loperamide may improve the quality of life.

G6. Dyschezia and G7. Functional Constipation

The defecation frequency of healthy infants and children varies with age [101]. The normal range is broadest in healthy breast-fed infants, who may defecate as frequently as 12 times per day, or as infrequently as once in 3 or 4 weeks. Firm stools may occur from the first weeks of life in formula-fed infants. Although there is no identifiable enteric neuromuscular disorder, these infants may experience painful defecation, and so have a predisposition towards developing functional constipation (see below).

Complaints related to defecatory problems are responsible for 25% of outpatient visits to pediatric gastroenterologists [102].

G6. Infant Dyschezia

— Definition

Parents describe infants with dyschezia as straining for many minutes, screaming, crying, turning red or purple in the face with effort. The symptoms persist for 10 to 20 minutes, until there is passage of soft or liquid stool. Stools pass several times daily. The symptoms begin in the first months of life, and resolve spontaneously after a few weeks.

G6. Diagnostic Criteria for Infant Dyschezia

Must include *both of the following* in an infant less than 6 months of age:
1. At least 10 minutes of straining and crying before successful passage of soft stools
2. No other health problems

— Clinical Evaluation

The examiner performs a history (including diet), conducts a physical examination (including rectal examination) to exclude anorectal abnormalities, and charts the infant's growth.

— Physiological Features

Failure to coordinate increased intra-abdominal pressure with relaxation of the pelvic floor results in infant dyschezia. The infant's cries increase intra-abdominal pressure. Defecation requires increasing intra-abdominal pressure and simultaneously relaxing the pelvic floor. Coordination of these two independent events to effect successful defecation may occur by chance, but eventually defecation is learned.

— Psychological Features

The child's parents require effective reassurance to address their concerns that their child is in pain and that something is wrong with the infant.

— Treatment

Parents are reassured by a methodical physical examination completed in their presence. They are happy to accept the explanation that the child needs to learn to relax the pelvic floor at the same time as bearing down. To encourage the infant's defecation learning, the parents are advised to avoid rectal stimulation, which produces artificial sensory experiences which may be noxious, or that may condition the child to wait for stimulation before defecating. Laxatives are unnecessary.

G7. Functional Constipation

— Definition

Infants are considered to be constipated when they have either two bowel movements weekly or hard, painful bowel movements and at least one of the criteria listed below under diagnostic criteria.

There is a decline in stool frequency from an average of more than four stools daily in the first week of life to one or two each day at 4 years of age. The reduced number of stools with age occurs with a corresponding increase in stool volume. Approximately 97% of 1 to 4 year old children pass stool three times daily to once every other day [100, 103, 104].

— Epidemiology

Bowel frequency is influenced by diet, social habits, convenience, family cultural beliefs, relationships within the family, and daily time of activities. All these factors may vary in relation to psychological and physical development. A very early onset of constipation (before 6 months of age) and the presence of a family history of constipation could suggest a genetic tendency to develop functional constipation. In particular, a positive family history has been found in 28% to 50% of constipated children and a higher incidence has been reported in monozygotic than dizygotic twins [105–107].

Constipation represents the chief complaint in 3% of pediatric outpatient visits. Most problems with defecation are due to functional constipation. Approximately 40% of children with functional constipation develop symptoms during the first year of life [108, 109]. Sixteen percent of parents of 22-month-old children reported constipation [109].

G7. Diagnostic Criteria for Functional Constipation

Must include *one month of at least two* of the following in infants up to 4 years of age:
1. **Two or fewer defecations per week**
2. **At least one episode/week of incontinence after the acquisition of toileting skills**
3. **History of excessive stool retention**
4. **History of painful or hard bowel movements**
5. **Presence of a large fecal mass in the rectum**
6. **History of large diameter stools which may obstruct the toilet**

Accompanying symptoms may include irritability, decreased appetite and/or early satiety. The accompanying symptoms disappear immediately following passage of a large stool.

— Rationale for Change in Diagnostic Criteria

The change from 12 weeks to 1 month of symptoms is based both on clinical experience and data suggesting that the longer functional constipation goes unrecognized, the less successful is the treatment. In constipated young children (less than 4 years old) seen in a general pediatric practice, prognosis was more favorable when the referral had been made before the age of 2 years [110]. Recovery in children with fecal incontinence was associated with shorter duration of symptoms [111]. A recent long-term follow-up study of constipated children also found a trend toward a diminished number of successfully treated children in those with a longer period of symptoms before referral to a subspecialty clinic [112].

The previous diagnostic criteria for functional fecal retention (FFR) placed a high premium on *retentive posturing*, which was one of the two criteria that had to be present in order to make a diagnosis. We now prefer to assess the parents' impression of excessive stool retention—one of the six criteria supporting the diagnosis—but without the requirement to be present in all subjects. In some cases, parents may not have watched the child's retentive behavior or recognized it [113].

Fecal incontinence (involuntary passage of fecal material) may occur in infants and toddlers who accumulate a large rectal fecal mass. Loose stool that accumulates around the fecal mass may be involuntary extruded as the infant passes gas. Fecal incontinence may occur even if the infant or toddler has acquired toilet skills, because it is caused by the rectal fecal mass. Two studies that have looked at the applicability of the Rome II criteria for FFR both recommended that fecal incontinence should be added to the revised criteria [114, 115]. Incontinence may be useful as an objective marker for the severity of functional constipation and in monitoring effectiveness of treatment [114].

A *painful bowel movement* has been identified as an important cause for retentive behavior [115].

The presence of a *large fecal mass* either before evacuation (recognized during the physical examination) or after a huge bowel movement is a common feature in functional constipation, although is not a symptom. The painful evacuation of a fecal mass often leads a terrified child to try to avoid further bowel movements.

— Clinical Evaluation

Functional constipation is a clinical diagnosis that can be made on the basis of a typical history and physical examination. There are no well-designed studies that determine which aspects of a history are pertinent [116].

The differential diagnosis of constipation in infancy includes anatomic obstructions and Hirschsprung's disease. More than 99% of healthy infants pass their first stool within 48 hours of birth [117]. Ninety-four percent of children with Hirschsprung's disease fail to pass meconium within the first 24 hours of life [118]. A rectal biopsy should be done in an infant who does not pass meconium within 48 hours of birth and has accompanying symptoms (vomiting, food refusal, abdominal distension, fever, failure-to-thrive, blood in stool). Rectal biopsy is the best test to diagnose Hirschsprung's disease [119] and rectal biopsy with cholinesterase staining is the 'gold' standard [120]. If defecation problems begin after 3 months, Hirschsprung's disease is much less likely [121].

The history of painful defecation, passage of huge stools at infrequent intervals, and retentive posturing are diagnostic. Onset frequently occurs during one of three periods: (1) in infants with hard stools (often corresponding with the change from breast milk to commercial formula, or introduction of solids), (2) in toddlers learning toilet behavior, as they attempt to control bowel movements and find defecation painful, and (3) as school starts and children attempt to avoid defecation throughout the school day. All these events have in common the potential for making defecation an unpleasant experience resulting in fecal retention. Passing large stools may cause anal fissures, especially in the first 2 years. Blood in the stools alarms parents, but does not cause clinically important blood loss.

Affected children are often described as standing on their toes, holding onto furniture, stiffening their legs, and hiding in a corner. Fecal incontinence may be mistaken for diarrhea by some parents. Urinary infections are occasionally observed in these children [122].

A physical examination provides reassurance to the clinician and parents that there is no disease. The physical examination includes assessing the size of the rectal fecal mass, which is judged for height above the pelvic brim with bimanual palpation on either side of the rectus sheath. A rectal examination is performed after establishing rapport with patient and family. In functional constipation, the initial rectal examination occasionally causes the child to react with acute intense fear and negative behaviors. An irrational fear of the rectal examination typifies the child with functional constipation, and is rarely a problem in children with other complaints, including other defecatory disorders. When the history is typical for functional constipation, the perineum should be inspected but a digital rectal examination may be delayed, to facilitate the therapeutic alliance between the child and clinician, until after a treatment trial fails. In cases in which the clinician plans a consultation but no followup, a rectal examination is performed to evaluate the child for the rare obstructing mass.

Occult spinal dysraphism (e.g., lipoma of the cauda equina, tethered cord, anterior sacral meningocele) is a cause of retentive or nonretentive fecal soiling. Signs of spinal dysraphism include pelvic floor weakness (patulous anus, involuntary spurt of urine with the Crede maneuver, absence of reflex contraction of the external anal sphincter and pelvic floor with a voluntary cough, urinary incontinence), diminished tactile sensitivity in the sacral dermatomes, asymmetry of the buttocks, calves, or feet, hyperactive or absent Achilles tendon reflexes, abnormal plantar reflexes, pigmentary abnormalities, vascular nevi or sinuses in the lumbo-sacral region, scoliosis suggestive of vertebral malformation, or radiologic abnormalities of the lumbo-sacral spine [123].

Anorectal manometry, anal sphincter ultrasound, radiography, and blood tests are unnecessary for the routine evaluation of functional constipation.

— Physiological Features

All the child's symptoms are explained by voluntary efforts to avoid defecation. Pain results from colonic contractions pushing luminal contents against a closed anal sphincter. Incontinence occurs when stool seeps around the fecal mass, and leaks out when the child relaxes the pelvic floor or anal sphincter, either inadvertently (as in sleep), with fatigue, or with attempts to pass flatus.

Functional constipation is often the result of repeated attempts of voluntary withholding of feces by a child who tries to avoid unpleasant defecation because of fears associated with evacuation. In the first years of life, an acute episode of constipation due to a change in diet may lead to the passage of dry and hard stools, which may cause painful defecation. In toddlers the onset of constipation may coincide with toilet training when excessive parental pressure to maintain bowel control and/or inappropriate techniques such as the use of regular toilets that do not allow sufficient leverage may lead to stool withholding. The start of school may coincide with the child's decision to suppress the defecation. Other causes of painful and frightening evacuation are allergic or infectious colitis, perianal infections, or fissures. Occasionally, the fear may be linked to a specific event associated with anxiety or pain, such as an episode of perianal streptococcal disease [124], lichen sclerosus [125], sexual abuse [126], or even a horrifying television show or commercial [127].

When the child learns to ignore the defecatory urge in anticipation of painful defecation, a vicious cycle is created. Stools accumulate and chronically distend the rectum, dampening the sensory input normally elicited by the presence of feces. Over time, as water and electrolytes are reabsorbed, the fecal mass becomes too large and too firm to be extruded without great pain. Increasing fecal accumulation in the rectum causes decreased motility in the foregut leading to anorexia, abdominal distension, and abdominal pain. There may be two mechanisms linked to the decreased appetite noted in constipated children: gastric emptying is delayed by a full rectum and children may choose not to eat to avoid the colonic high amplitude propagating contraction usually induced by meals. When such contractions occur in the presence of a fecal mass and withholding, the child experiences abdominal pain. Over time, as the fecal mass becomes too large and pelvic floor muscles fatigue, the anal sphincter becomes less competent and any relaxation leads to fecal incontinence.

— Psychological Features

Development of bowel and bladder control is a maturational process that cannot be accelerated by early onset or high intensity of toilet training [129, 130]. The child's initiative is a reliable indicator that the child is developmentally capable of being clean and dry. Many children achieve partial voluntary bowel control at about 18 months, but the age of complete control varies. By 4 years 98% of normal children are toilet trained. Toilet training may be initiated inappropriately early. Initiation of intensive training before 27 months does not correlate with earlier completion of toilet training, suggesting little benefit in beginning intensive training before 27 months of age in most children [130, 73, 4]. Parents of children at risk for functional constipation seem to be inconsistent in their approach to toilet training, varying from excessive rigidity to permissiveness [131].

In most cases, the fear of painful defecation is the cause for fecal retention [132, 5, 75]. Indeed, constipated children display more anxiety related to toileting than well children or children with asthma. Although fear of painful defecation is the initial cause, parents may find themselves in a power struggle with their child concerning toilet learning.

When children provide an accurate report of their fears, the fears can be addressed with tact and sensitivity. Toddlers with functional constipation may attribute the pain associated with defecation to fantastic, living stuff coming out of them. This may be frightening, and create an emotional climate that does not favor toilet learning.

Parents worried about their child with functional constipation feel alone and frightened. They have fantasies that may include

1. They are the only one with this problem.
2. Their child's colon might burst, or leak toxic, rotten stuff into them.
3. Their child is incurable.
4. The problem will turn into cancer (e.g., Uncle Jack was constipated and he had cancer!).
5. Laxatives will damage the colon.

— Treatment

Even in infants, response to treatment improves with early intervention, preventing development of severe symptoms. The longer symptoms persist, the lesser the chance for treatment success [110]. Education for parents and child is the first step in treatment, beginning during the initial interview. The child and family appreciate a clinician who thoroughly assesses the history and physical examination, then explains the evolution of the problem, the absence of worrisome disease, and safe and effective management. The clinician addresses the myths and fears: the child has functional constipation, one of the most common problems in pediatrics. It goes away in time, and it is not dangerous. These statements assuage the child's and family's anxiety, and create an expectation for positive change. The parents then need to be helped to understand the child's point of view. For toddlers, toilet training will not proceed smoothly until the child's fear of painful defecation resolves. Parents who are anxious (*"We can not put him into day care until he's potty trained!"*) must understand that coercive toilet training tactics are likely to backfire into a struggle for control. The clinician, child, and parent then agree on a plan for evacuating the rectal fecal mass. Most experts favor a daily nonstimulant laxative such as polyethylene glycol, mineral oil, lactulose, or Milk of Magnesia, which slowly softens the mass until the child chooses to pass it, days or weeks later. In a biopsychosocial model, this developmentally sound, nonintrusive approach returns the control of the child's pelvic floor to the child. Many toddlers are frightened of any anal manipulation, and find enemas and any other anal intrusions scary.

The key to effective maintenance is assuring painless defecation until the child is comfortable and acquisition of toilet learning is complete. For the maintenance phase of treatment, the safe and effective stool softeners are continued for months to years. Stimulant laxatives may be helpful for episodes when the fecal mass returns, in order to "rescue" the child from entering another cycle of retention and fear. However, sodium docusate has no role in maintenance treatment of constipation in children. Although dietary fiber is important for a variety of reasons, fiber supplements are not adequate as a single agent for consistent stool softening. The goal of stool softening is to assure painless defecation for every stool until functional constipation resolves.

For preschool children, behavior modification utilizing rewards for successes in toilet learning is often helpful. A child may earn stars for a chart with each successful defecatory effort. Another behavior modification technique is to establish a daily routine for sitting on the commode. Sitting on the commode for 5 to 10 minutes after eating takes advantage of the gastrocolonic response, the increase in colonic motility following a meal. The child should be actively attempting to defecate during the sitting. Passivity is not useful, and sitting may be terminated if the child chooses not to try.

Functional constipation is as common in children and adolescents as it is in infants and toddlers. Aspects of this disorder in older children are covered in the next chapter, particularly with regard to biofeedback and physical therapies that are inappropriate for the treatment of functional constipation in infants and toddlers.

Conclusions and Recommendations for Future Research

Functional gastrointestinal disorders other than those mentioned in this chapter occur during childhood, but are defined adequately by the adult criteria. The list of adult functional bowel disorders also found in children and adolescents includes: functional chest pain, functional heartburn, functional dysphagia, and proctalgia fugax. We did not describe functional biliary disorders because documentation and experience with childhood gallbladder and sphincter of Oddi dysfunction are sketchy at this time.

Recommendations for future research include

1. Validating the diagnostic criteria for the childhood functional gastrointestinal disorders will be an important goal for the next decade. Epidemiologic community-based studies and studies of populations thought to be at risk (e.g., children of patients with functional gastrointestinal disorders, female child abuse victims) are needed to determine the applicability of the diagnostic criteria, which were arrived at by consensus rather than by data analysis.

2. Clinical trials measuring symptom change as the primary outcome measure will help us to learn which interventions improve outcomes in the childhood functional gastrointestinal disorders.

3. Definitions and diagnostic criteria for currently unrecognized childhood functional gastrointestinal disorders are needed.

4. A history of physical, sexual, and/or emotional abuse will be elicited from some children with functional bowel disorders. There is a need for education and training related to the evaluation and treatment of child abuse for all clinicians who care for children with functional gastrointestinal disorders.

5. The role of childhood functional gastrointestinal disorders in adult functional gastrointestinal disorders should be explored.

6. There is increasing evidence in adult practice of the role of inflammation in some FGIDs. There are virtually no such studies in childhood. The role of inflammation in childhood FGIDs requires systematic study.

References

1. Poets CF. Gastro esophageal reflux: A critical review of its role in preterm infants. Pediatrics 2004;113:e128–e132.
2. Nelson SP, Chen EH, Syniar GM et al. Prevalence of symptoms of gastro esophageal reflux during infancy. Arch Pediatr Adolesc Med 1997;15:569–72.
3. Orenstein S. Regurgitation and GERD. J Pediatr Gastroenterol Nutr 2001;32:516–518.
4. D'Netto MA, Herson VC, Hussain N et al. Allergic gastroenteropathy in preterm infants. J Pediatr 2000;137:480–486.
5. Ewer AK, Durbin GM, Morgan ME, Booth IW. Gastric emptying and gastro-oesophageal reflux in preterm infants. Arch Dis Child Foetal Neonatal Ed 1996;75: F117–F1211.
6. Omari T, Barnett CP, Benninga MA et al. Mechanisms of gastro oesophageal reflux in preterm and term infants with reflux disease. Gut 2002;51:475–479.
7. Baker JH, Berseth CL. Duodenal motor responses in preterm infants fed formula with varying concentrations and rates of infusion. Pediatr Res 1997;42:618–22.
8. Levy R. Mother-infant relations in the feeding situation. In. Lebenthal E, Editor. Textbook of Gastroenterology and Nutrition in Infancy. New York: Raven Press, 1981;633–44.
9. Fleisher DR. Functional vomiting disorders in infancy: innocent vomiting, nervous vomiting and infant rumination syndrome. J Pediatr 1994;125:584–594.
10. North American Society for Pediatric Gastroenterology and Nutrition. Pediatric Gastro oesophageal reflux practice guidelines. J Pediatr Gastroenterol Nutr 2001;32 (Suppl 2):S1–S31.
11. Ewer A, James ME, Tobin JM. Prone and left lateral position reduce gastro oesophageal reflux in preterm infants. Arch Dis Child Fetal Neonatal Ed 1999;81:2001–5.
12. Huang R-C, Forbes DA, Davies MW. Food thickener for new born infants with gastro oesophageal reflux (Cochrane Review). In: The Cochran Library, Issue 1, Chichester, UK: John Wiley & Sons, Ltd 2004.
13. Vanderhoof JA, Moran JR, Harris CL, Merkel KL, Orenstein SR. Efficacy of a pre-thickened infant formula: a multicentre, double-blind, randomized, placebo controlled parallel group trial in 104 infants with symptomatic gastroesophageal reflux. Clin Pediatr 2003;42:483–95.
14. Wenzl TG, Schneider S, Scheele F, Silmy J, Heimann G, Skopnik H. Effects of thickened feeding on gastroesophageal reflux in infants: a placebo-controlled crossover study using intra luminal impedance. Pediatrics 2003;111:e355–359.
15. Bourke B, Drumm B. Cochrane's epitaph for Cisapride in childhood gastro oesophageal reflux. Arch Dis Child 2002;86:1–2.
16. Moore DJ, Tao BS, Lines DR, Hirta C, Heddle ML, Davidson GP. Double-blind placebo-controlled trial of omeprazole in irritable infants with gastroesophageal reflux. J Pediatr 2003;143:219–23.
17. Cameron HC. Some forms of habitual vomiting in infancy. Brit Med J 1925;i:872–76.
18. Fleisher DR. Infant rumination syndrome: report of a case and review of the literature. Am J Dis Child. 1979 133(3):266–9.

19. Kanner L. Child Psychiatry. 4th Ed. Springfield, IL:Charles C. Thomas 1972;463–464.

20. Mayes SD, Humphrey FJ, Hanford HA, et al. Rumination disorder: differential diagnosis. J Am Acad Child Adolesc Psychiatry 1988;27(3):300–302.

21. Powell GF, Low JF, Speers MA. Behavior as a diagnostic aid in failure-to-thrive. J Devel Behav Pediatr 1987;8(1):18–24.

22. Singer L. Long-term hospitalization of nonorganic failure-to-thrive infants: patient characteristics and hospital course. J Devel Behav Pediatr 1987;8(1):25–31.

23. Hirschberg L. Clinical interviews with infants and their families. In: Zeanah C, Editor. Handbook of Infant Mental Health. New York:P Guilford Press, 1993;173–190.

24. Sheagren TG, Mangurten HH, Brea F, et al. Rumination: a new complication of neonatal intensive care. Pediatr 1980;66(4):551–555.

25. Sauvage D, Leddet I, Hameury L, et al. Infantile rumination: diagnosis and follow-up study of twenty cases. J Am Acad Child Psychiatry 1985;24(2):197–203.

26. Richmond JB, Eddy F, Green M. Rumination: a psychosomatic syndrome of infancy. Pediatr 1958;22:49–54.

27. Stein ML, Rausen AR, Blair A. Psychotherapy of an infant with rumination. JAMA 1959;171:2309–2312.

28. Gaddini R, Gaddini E. Rumination in infancy. In: Jessner L, Pavenstedt E, Editors. Dynamic Psychopathology in Childhood. New York:Grune & Stratton Inc., 1959;166–185.

29. Fullerton DT. Infantile rumination. Arch Gen Psychiatry 1963;9:593–600.

30. Menking M, Wagnitz JG, Burton JJ, et al. Rumination: a near-fatal psychiatric disease of infancy. New Engl J Med 1969;280:802–804.

31. Flanagan CH. Rumination in infancy. J Am Acad Child Psychiatry 1977;16:140–149.

32. Clark FH. Rumination. Arch Pediatr 1966;73:12–19.

33. Luckey R, Walson C, Music J. Aversive conditioning as a means of inhibiting vomiting and rumination. Am J Mental Deficiency 1968;73:139–142.

34. Lavigne J, Burns W, Cotter P. Rumination in infancy: recent behavioral approaches. Internat Eating Disorders 1981;1:70–82.

35. Sheinbein M. Treatment of the hospitalized infantile ruminator. Clin Pediatr 1975;14(8):719–724.

36. Li BUK, Guest Editor. Cyclic vomiting syndrome: proceedings of the international scientific symposium on CVS. J Pediatr Gastroenterol Nutr 1995;21 (suppl 1)S1–3.

37. Fleisher DR, Matar M. The cyclic vomiting syndrome: a report of 71 cases and a literature review. J Pediatr Gastroenterol Nutr 1993;17:361–369.

38. Fleisher DR. Cyclic vomiting syndrome: a paroxysmal disorder of brain-gut interaction. J Pediatr Gastroenterol Nutr 1997;25(suppl 1):s13–slS.

39. Withers GD, Silburn SR, Forbes DA. Precipitants and aetiology of cyclic vomiting syndrome. Acta Paediatr 1998;87:272–277.

40. Fleisher D. The cyclic vomiting syndrome described. The cyclic vomiting syndrome described. J Pediatr Gastroenterol Nutr. 1995;21 Suppl 1:S1–5. Review

41. Prakash C, Staiano A, Rothbaum RJ,ClouseRE. Similarities in cyclic vomiting syndrome across age groups. Am. J. Gastroenterol 2001;96:684–688.

42. Abell TL, Kim CH, Malagelada JR. Idiopathic cyclic nausea and vomiting—a disorder of gastrointestinal motility? Mayo Clin Proc 1988;63:1169–1175.

43. Prakash C, Clouse RE. Cyclic vomiting syndrome in adults: clinical features and response to tricyclic antidepressants. Am J Gastroenterol 1999;94:2855–2860.

44. Cullen KJ, MacDonald. The periodic syndrome: its nature and prevalence. Med I Australia 1963;2(5):167–172.

45. Abu-Arefeh I, Russell C. Cyclic vomiting in children: a population based study. J Pediatr Gastroenterol Nutr 1995;21(4):454–458.

46. Tache Y. Cyclic vomiting sydrome : the corticotrophin release factor hypothesis Dig Dis Sci 1999;44:795–868.

47. Andrews PL. Cyclic vomiting syndrome. Timing, targeting and treatment—a basic science perspective. Dig Dis Sci 1999;44:319–385.

48. Pasricha PJ, Schuster MM, Saudek CD, et al. Cyclic vomiting: association with multiple homeostatic abnormalities and response to ketorolac. Am J Gastroenterol. 1996; 91(10):2228–32.

49. Vanderhoof IA, Young R, Kaufman SS, et al. Treatment of cyclic vomiting in childhood with erythromycin. J Pediatr Gastroenterol Nutr 1995;21(suppl 1)S60–S62.

50. Forbes D, Withers C. Prophylactic therapy in cyclic vomiting syndrome. J Pediatr Gastroenterol Nutr 1995;21(suppl 1):s57–59.

51. Anderson I, Sugerman K, Lockhart JR, et al. Effective prophylactic therapy for cyclic vomiting syndrome in children using amitriplytine or cyproheptadine. Pediatr 1997;100:977–981.

52. Gokhale R, Huttenlocher PR, Brady L, et al. Use of barbituates in the treatment of cyclic vomiting during childhood. J Pediatr Gastroenterol Nutr 1997;25:64–67.

53. Welch KM. Scientific basis of migraine:speculationon the relationship to cyclic vomiting. Dig Dis Sci 1999;44:265–305.

54. Treem WR. Infant colic, a pediatric gastroenterologist's perspective. Pediatric Clinics of North America; 199441:1121–1138.

55. Wessel MA, Cobb IC, Jackson EB, et al. Paroxysmal fussing in infancy, sometimes called colic. Pediatr 1954;14(5):421–434.

56. Lester BM. Definition and Diagnosis of Colic. In: Sauls HS, Redfern DE, eds. Colic and Excessive Crying—Report of the 105th Ross Conference on Pediatric Research. Columbus, OH: Ross, 1997:18–29.

57. Paradise JL. Maternal and other factors in the etiology of infantile colic. J Am Med Assoc 1966;197:123–131.

58. St. James-Roberts I. Distinguishing Between Infant Fussing, Crying, and Colic: How Many Phenomena? In: Sauls HS, Redfern DE, eds. Colic and Excessive Crying— Report of the 105th Ross Conference on Pediatric Research. Columbus, OH: Ross, 1997:3–14.

59. Pierce P. Delayed onset of three months colic in premature infants. Am J Dis Child 1948;75:190–192.

60. Barr RG, Chen S, Hopkins B, Westra T. Crying patterns in pre-term infants. Dev Med Child Neurol 1996;38:345–355.

61. Brazelton TB. Crying in infancy. Pediatrics 1962;29:579–588.

62. Barr RG. The normal crying curve: what do we really know? Dev Med Child Neurol 1990;32:356–362.

63. Geertsma MA, Hyams JS. Colic—a pain syndrome of infancy? Pediatr Clin North Am 1987;36:905–919.

64. Barr RG. "Colic" is something infants do, rather than a condition they "have": a developmental approach to crying phenomena, patterns, pacification and (patho)genesis. In: Barr RG SJ-RI, Keefe, MR, ed. New Evidence on Unexplained Early Infant Cry-

ing: Its Origins, Nature and Management: Johnson & Johnson Pediatric Institute, 2001; 87–104.

65. St. James-Roberts I, Conroy S, Wilsher K. Clinical, developmental and social aspects of infant crying and colic. Early Dev Parenting 1995;4:107.

66. St. James-Roberts I, Halil T. Infant crying patterns in the first year: normal community and clinical findings. J Child Psychol Psychiatry. 1991 Sep;32(6):951–68.

67. Rautava P, Helenius H, Lehtonen L. Psychosocial predisposing factors for infantile colic. British Medical Journal 1993;307:600–604.

68. Barr RG, Konner M, Bakeman R, Adamson L. Crying in !Kung San infants: a test of the cultural specificity hypothesis. Dev Med Child Neurol 1991;33:601–610.

69. Gormally S. Clinical Clues to Organic Etiologies in Infants With Colic. In: Barr RG, St. James-Roberts I, Keefe MR, eds. New Evidence on Unexplained Early Infant Crying: Its Origins, Nature and Management: Johnson & Johnson Pediatric Institute, 2001;133–148.

70. Thomas DW, McGilligan K, Eisenberg LD, Liberman HM, Rissman EM. Infantile colic and type of milk feeding. Am J Dis Child 1987;141:451–453.

71. Barr RG. Infant Colic. In: E. HP, ed. Pediatric Functional Gastrointestinal Disorders. New York: Academy of Professional Information Services, Inc., 1999;2.1–2.23.

72. Dellert SF, Hyams JS, Treem WR, Geertsma MA. Feeding resistence and gastro-esophageal reflux in infancy. J Pediatric Gastroenterol Nutr1993;17:66–71.

73. Miller AR, Barr RG. Infantile colic—is it a gut issue? Pediatr Clin North Am 1991; 38:1407–1423.

74. Jakobsson I. Cow's milk protiens as a cause of infantile colic. In: Sauls HS, Redfern DE, eds. Report of the 105th Ross Conference on Pediatric Research. Columbus, OH: Ross, 1997;39–47.

75. Lothe L, Lindberg T, Jakobsson I. Cow's milk formula as a cause of infantile colic: a double blind study. Pediatrics 1982;70:7–10.

76. Dunn J. Distress and Comfort. Boston: Harvard University Press, 1977.

77. Brackbill Y. Continuous stimulation reduces arousal level: stability of the effect over time. Child Devel 1973;44:43–46.

78. Pinyerd BJ. Mother-Infant Interaction and Temperament When the Infant Has Colic. In: Sauls HS, Redfern DE, eds. Report of the 105th Ross Conference on Pediatric Research. Columbus, OH: Ross, 1997;101–112.

79. Lehtonen L, Korvenranta IT, Eerola E. Intestinal microflora in colicky and non-colicky infants: bacterial cultures and gas-liquid chromatography. J Pediatr Gastroenterol Nutr 1994;19:310–314.

80. Lothe L, Ivarsson SA, Lindberg T. Motilin and infantile colic. Acta Paediatr Scand 1990;79:410.

81. Lehtonen L, Svedstrom E, Korvenranta H. Gallbladder hypocontractility in infantile colic. Acta Paediatr Scand 1994;83:1174–1177.

82. Treem WR, Hyams JS, Blankenschen E, al. e. Evaluation of the effect of fiber-enriched formula on infant colic. Pediatrics 1991;119:695–701.

83. Illingworth RS. Three months colic. Arch Dis Child 1954;29:165.

84. Sferra TJ, Heitlinger LA. Gastrointestinal gas formation and infant colic. Pediatr Clin North Am 1996;43:489–510.

85. Carey WB. Clinical applications of infant temperament measures. J Pediatrics 1972; 81:823–828.

86. Barr RG, Gunnar M. Colic: the "transient responsivity" hypothesis. In: Barr RG, Hopkins B, Green JA, eds. Crying as a Sign, a Symptom, and a Signal. London: Mac Keith Press, 2000;41–66.

87. Brazelton TB. Joint regulation of neonate-parent behavior. In: Tronick EZ, ed. Social Interchange in Infancy. Baltimore: University Park Press, 1982;7–22.

88. Lyons-Ruth K, Zeanah CH. The Family Context of Infant Mental Health. In: Zeanah CH, ed. Handbook of Infant Mental Health. New York: Guilford Press, 1993; 14–37.

89. Murray L, Cooper P. The Impact of Irritable Infant Behavior on Maternal Mental State: A Longitudinal Study and a Treatment Trial. In: Barr RG, St. James-Roberts I, Keefe MR, eds. New Evidence on Unexplained Early Infant Crying: Johnson & Johnson Pediatric Institute, 2001;149–164.

90. Stifter CA, Bono MA. The effect of infant colic on maternal self-perceptions and mother-infant attachment. Child: Care, Health, and Development 1998;24:339–351.

91. Rautava P, Lehtonen L, Helenius H, et al. Infantile colic: child and family three years later. Pediatrics 1995;96:43–47.

92. Meyer E, Garcia C, LesterB,et al Family based intervention improves maternal psychological well being and feeding interaction of pre-term infants. Pediatrics 1994;93:241.

93. Milla PJ, Atherton DA, Leonard JV, et al. Disordered intestinal functions in glycogen storage disease. J Inher Metab Dis 1978;1:155–157.

94. Tripp JH, Muller DPR, Harries JT. Mucosal Na-K ATPase and adenylate cyclase activities in children with toddler diarrhea and postenteritis syndrome. Paediatr Res 1980;14:1382–1386.

95. Dodge JA, Hamdi IA, Burns GM, et al. Toddler's diarrhea and prostaglandins. Arch Dis Child 1981;56:705–707.

96. Hamdi I, Dodge JA. Toddler diarrhea: observations on the effects of aspirin and loperamide. J Pediatr Gastroenterol Nutr 1985;4:362–365.

97. Fenton TR, Harries JT, Milla PJ. Disordered small intestinal motility: a rational basis for toddler's diarrhea. Gut 1983;24:897–903.

98. Jonas A, Diver Haber A. Stool output and composition in the chronic nonspecific diarrhea syndrome. Arch Dis Child 1982;57:35–39.

99. Lloyd-Still JD. Chronic diarrhea of childhood and the misuse of elimination diets. J Pediatr 1979;95:10–13.

100. Wender EH. Chronic non-specific diarrhea: behavioral aspects. Postgrad Med 1977;62:83–88.

101. Weaver LT. Bowel habit from birth to old age. J Pediatr Gastroenterol Nutr 1988; 7:637–640.

102. Taitz LS, et al. Factors associated with outcome in management of defecation disorders. Arch Dis Child 1986;61:472–477.

103. Pettei MJ, Chronic constipation. Pediatr Ann 1987;16:796–811.

104. Weaver LT, Steiner A. The bowel habit of young children. Arch Dis Child 1984; 59:649–652.

105. Abrahamian FP, Lloyd-Still JD. Chronic constipation in childhood: a longitudinal study of 186 patients. J Pediatr Gastroenterol Nutr 1984;3:460–467.

106. Bakwin H, Davidson M. Constipation in twins. Am J Dis Child 1971;121:179–181.

107. Morris-Yates A, Talley NJ, Boyce PM, Nandurkar S, Andrews G. Evidence of a ge-

netic contribution to functional bowel disorder. Am J Gastroenterol 1998;93:1311–1317.

108. Davidson M, Kugler MM, Bauer CH. Diagnosis and management in children with severe and protracted constipation and obstipation. J Pediatr 1963;62:261–275.

109. Issenman RM, Hewson S, Pirhonen D, Taylor W, Tirosh A. Are chronic digestive complaints the result of abnormal dietary patterns? Diet and digestive complaints in children at 22 and 40 months of age. Am J Dis Child 1987;141:679–682.

110. Loening-Baucke V. Chronic constipation in children. Gastroenterology 1993;105:1557–1564.

111. Loening-Baucke V, Krishna R, Pashankar DS. Polyethylene glycol 3350 without electrolytes for the treatment of functional constipation in infants and toddlers. J Pediatr Gastroenterol Nutr 2004;39:536–539.

112. van Ginkel R, Reitsma JB, Buller HA, van Wijk MP, Taminiau JA, Benninga MA. Childhood constipation: longitudinal follow-up beyond puberty. Gastroenterology 2003;125:357–363.

113. Voskuijl WP, Heijmans J, Heijmans HS, Taminiau JA, Benninga MA. Use of Rome II criteria in childhood defecation disorders: applicability in clinical and research practice. J Pediatr 2004;145:213–217.

114. van der Plas RN, Benninga MA, Redekop WK, Taminiau JA, Buller HA. How accurate is the recall of bowel habits in children with defaecation disorders? Eur J Pediatr 1997;156:178–181.

115. Partin JC, Hamill SK, Fischel JE, Partin JS. Painful defecation and fecal soiling in children. Pediatrics 1992;89:1007–1009.

116. Baker SS, Liptak GS, Colletti RB, et al. Constipation in infants and children; evaluation and treatment, A medical position statement of the North American Society for Pediatric Gastroenterology and Nutrition. J Pediatr Gastroenterol Nutr 1999;29:613–626.

117. Clark DA. Times of first void and first stool in 500 newborns. Pediatrics 1977;60:457–459.

118. Swenson o, Sherman JO, Fisher JH. Diagnosis of congenital megacolon: an analysis of 501 patients. J Pediatr Surg 1973;8:587–594.

119. Lorijn F, Reitsma JB, Voskuijl WP, Aronson DC, Ten Kate FG, Smets AM, Taminiau JA, Benninga M. Diagnosis of Hirschsprung's disease:prospective, comparative study of common tests. J Pediatrics In press.

120. Lake BD,Puri P,Nixon HH, Claireaux AE Hirschsprung's disease an appraisal of histochemically demonstrated acetylcholiesterase activity in suction rectal biopsies, an aid to diagnosis. Arch Pathol Lab Med 1978;102:244–247.

121. Ghosh A, Griffiths DM. Rectal biopsy in the investigation of constipation. Arch Dis Child 1998;79:266–268.

122. Loening-Baucke V. Urinary incontinence and urinary tract infection and their resolution with treatment of chronic constipation of childhood. Pediatrics 1997;100:228–232.

123. Anderson FM. Occult spinal dysraphism. Pediatr 1975;55:826–835.

124. Spear M, Rothbaum R, Keating I, et al. Perianal streptococcal cellulitis. J Pediatr 1985;107:557–559.

125. Hurwitz S. Clinical Pediatric Dermatology. Philadelphia:WB Saunders, 1993;671–73.

126. Clayden CS. Anal appearances and child sexual abuse. Lancet 1987;1:620–621.

127. Pilapil VR. A horrifying television commercial that led to constipation. Pediatr 1990;85:592–593.
128. Tjeerdsma HC, Smout AJ, Akkermans LM. Voluntary suppression of defecation delays gastric emptying. Dig Dis Sci 1993;38:832–836.
129. Largo RH, Stutzle W. Longitudinal study of bowel and bladder control by day and night in the first 6 years of life. Epidemiology and interrelations between bowel and bladder control. Dev Med Child Neurol 1977;19:598–606.
130. Largo RH, Molinari L, Von Siebenthal K, Wolofensberger U, Does a profound change in toilet training affect development of bowel and bladder control Dev Med Child Neurol 1996;38:1106–1116.
131. Fishman L, Rappaport L, Cousineau D, Nurko S. Early constipation and toilet training in children with encopresis J Pediatr Gastroenterol Nutr 2002;34:385–388.
132. Borowitz SM, Cox DJ, Tam A, Ritterband LM, Sutphen JL, Penberthy JK. Precipitants of constipation during early childhood. J Am Board Fam Pract 2003;16: 213–218.

Chapter 14

Childhood Functional Gastrointestinal Disorders: Child/ Adolescent

Carlo Di Lorenzo, Chair

Andrée Rasquin, Co-Chair

David Forbes

Ernesto Guiraldes

Jeffrey S. Hyams

Annamaria Staiano

Lynn S. Walker

Introduction

Five years after the publication of the first symptom-based classification of pediatric functional gastrointestinal disorders (FGID) [1], this committee has been asked to update both the types of disorders that were initially described and the symptoms used to diagnose them. There are now sufficient data in the literature to make some of the changes evidence-based rather than based solely on expert opinion and consensus, as was the case in the first pediatric classification. Two pediatric committees have been created as part of the Rome III process and this committee has been charged with the task of discussing FGID occurring in children and adolescents (Table 1).

We defined childhood and adolescence as ranging from 4 to 18 years of age. Some of the pediatric FGIDs, such as cyclic vomiting and functional abdominal pain, overlap in age presentation with the neonatal-toddler committee and they were arbitrarily assigned to one of the two committees. Whenever possible, harmonization with terminology and diagnostic criteria used by the committees discussing similar entities in adults was sought. At times, the different duration of symptoms and dissimilar phenotypic presentation in children justified the use of different criteria in the pediatric group.

The committee elected to continue basing the pediatric classification of FGIDs on the main complaints reported by children or their parents rather than on targeted organs. Indeed, the criteria were designed to be used as diagnostic tools and the committee felt that this symptom-based classification would better serve the clinician. This was particularly true for abdominal pain-related FGIDs, where care providers can consider functional abdominal pain as a diagnostic option only after having eliminated the other abdominal pain-related FGIDs.

The committee members changed the required duration of symptoms from 3 to 2 months for all the disorders except for abdominal migraine and cyclic vomiting syndrome. This decision was based on the following considerations: (1) it is enough to establish chronicity; (2) although children presenting to tertiary care centers have symptoms of long duration, it was felt that primary care physicians should be able to make the diagnosis of FGIDs earlier than 3 months of symptom duration; (3) a duration of 2 months is more inclusive and facilitates clinical research of FGIDs in children, and (4) it was the consensus of the committee that 2 months better reflects clinical experience in children compared to adults.

Age-appropriate questionnaires have been created as part of the Rome III process and a threshold of "at least once per week" for inclusion of a diagnostic symptom has been chosen for all the disorders except the two cyclical ones: abdominal migraine and cyclic vomiting, and for nonretentive fecal incontinence, a condition in which monthly episodes of fecal incontinence are distressing enough to bring

Table 1. Functional Gastrointestinal Disorders

A. Functional Esophageal Disorders

A1. Functional heartburn	A3. Functional dysphagia
A2. Functional chest pain of presumed esophageal origin	A4. Globus

B. Functional Gastroduodenal Disorders

B1. Functional dyspepsia	B3. Nausea and vomiting disorders
B1a. Postprandial distress syndrome (PDS)	B3a. Chronic idiopathic nausea (CIN)
B1b. Epigastric pain syndrome (EPS)	B3b. Functional vomiting
B2. Belching disorders	B3c. Cyclic vomiting syndrome (CVS)
B2a. Aerophagia	B4. Rumination syndrome in adults
B2b. Unspecified excessive belching	

C. Functional Bowel Disorders

C1. Irritable bowel syndrome (IBS)	C4. Functional diarrhea
C2. Functional bloating	C5. Unspecified functional bowel disorder
C3. Functional constipation	

D. Functional Abdominal Pain Syndrome (FAPS)

E. Functional Gallbladder and Sphincter of Oddi (SO) Disorders

E1. Functional gallbladder disorder
E2. Functional biliary SO disorder
E3. Functional pancreatic SO disorder

F. Functional Anorectal Disorders

F1. Functional fecal incontinence	F2b. Proctalgia fugax
F2. Functional anorectal pain	F3. Functional defecation disorders
F2a. Chronic proctalgia	F3a. Dyssynergic defecation
F2a1. Levator ani syndrome	F3b. Inadequate defecatory propulsion
F2a2. Unspecified functional anorectal pain	

G. Functional Disorders: Neonates and Toddlers

G1. Infant regurgitation	G5. Functional diarrhea
G2. Infant rumination syndrome	G6. Infant dyschezia
G3. Cyclic vomiting syndrome	G7. Functional constipation
G4. Infant colic	

H. Functional Disorders: Children and Adolescents

H1. Vomiting and aerophagia	H2d. Childhood functional abdominal pain
H1a. Adolescent rumination syndrome	H2d1. Childhood functional abdominal pain syndrome
H1b. Cyclic vomiting syndrome	H3. Constipation and incontinence
H1c. Aerophagia	H3a. Functional constipation
H2. Abdominal pain-related FGIDs	H3b. Nonretentive fecal incontinence
H2a. Functional dyspepsia	
H2b. Irritable bowel syndrome	
H2c. Abdominal migraine	

the child to the medical provider's attention. The accompanying symptoms have to be present at least "sometimes" ($\geq$ 25% of the time) (see the section on pediatric questionnaires for more details).

The committee members acknowledge that, in some patients, both disorder and disease may coexist (e.g., irritable bowel syndrome (IBS) and Crohn's disease). They emphasize that when "absence of disease" is a criterion, a diagnosis of functional disorder can only be made if diseases that could account for the symptoms are absent or inactive.

HI. Vomiting and Aerophagia
HIa. Adolescent Rumination Syndrome

Rumination syndrome, characterized by regurgitation and reswallowing of food, has previously been acknowledged as a disorder of infants and of adults [1, 2, 3, 4], and has recently been recognized as a problem of older children and adolescents [5, 6]. The name rumination syndrome derives from similarities between this behavior, and that of the ruminant herbivores that regurgitate food from their stomach and "chew the cud." Some patient groups, such as adolescent girls, are at higher risk of rumination syndrome. The severity of this condition ranges from being mostly a benign disorder, amenable to behavioral therapies, to much more severe forms interfering with the ability to work or attend school [6]. It may be associated with weight loss and require treatment with naso-jejunal or gastro-jejunal feeding tubes [5].

— Definition

Rumination syndrome is characterized by the habitual regurgitation of recently ingested stomach contents into the mouth for remastication or expulsion. It is distinct from gastroesophageal reflux, chronic vomiting, gastroparesis, and intestinal pseudo-obstruction. It is more akin to a "tic" and it is has been described as an exaggerated "belch reflex."

— Epidemiology

The true frequency of rumination syndrome in adolescents is not known. Despite recent descriptions of this entity in the pediatric literature, rumination is still poorly recognized and often misdiagnosed. Symptom duration before diagnosis has been reported to average more than 2 years [6]. It can occur in any age group in childhood but is most frequent among infants and adolescents [7, 8]. In adolescence, girls are more likely to be affected than boys in a ratio of 2:1 [6], while among younger children, ruminators are more likely to be boys [8, 9]. In the largest published series concerning rumination in children and adolescents, the mean age of diagnosis was 15 years. Specific stressors were identified just before the onset of the symptoms in 10% of the subjects [6]. Two thirds of cases in this series had associated physical illnesses and one third concomitant psychological illness [6]. Rumination has been associated with intellectual handicap and emotional deprivation mostly in infants and young children [9, 10, 11]. Adolescents and young adults who ruminate have an increased risk of bulimia nervosa [3, 12]. It has been suggested that there may be overlap between a form fruste of eating disorders and rumination [5].

H1a. Diagnostic Criteria* for Adolescent Rumination Syndrome

Must include *all* of the following:
1. **Repeated painless regurgitation and rechewing or expulsion of food that**
   a. **begin soon after ingestion of a meal**
   b. **do not occur during sleep**
   c. **do not respond to standard treatment for gastroesophageal reflux**
2. **No retching**
3. **No evidence of an inflammatory, anatomic, metabolic or neoplastic process that explains the subject's symptoms**

* Criteria fulfilled at least once per week for at least two months prior to diagnosis

— Rationale for Change in Criteria

Universally acceptable diagnostic criteria for children and adolescents have not been previously established, although the American Psychiatric Association has published diagnostic criteria [13], and the Rome II document included criteria for rumination syndrome in infants [1] and in adults [14]. Recently, criteria for children and adolescents have been proposed [6]. The American Psychiatric Association in the Diagnostic and Statistical Manual of Mental Disorders IV (DSM IV) [13] uses a 4-week time period in its definition, investigators from the

Mayo Clinic have proposed a 6-week time period [6], and the Rome II definition for adult rumination syndrome utilizes a 12-week time period for the definition. None of these has been justified experimentally. Duration of 12 weeks may be unjustifiably restrictive and delay diagnosis or exclude patients with recent onset of symptoms from research studies. Two months is the proposed uniform duration of symptoms for pediatric functional disorders as part of the Rome III document. The Rome II definition for rumination in adults included also "absence of nausea and vomiting." The reporting of nausea has been noted in 17% and 33% of affected adolescents [5, 6]. As patients with rumination often expel food rather than reswallowing it, to exclude vomiting may be confusing and exclusion of vomiting has been eliminated from these revised criteria. In Rome II, one of the criteria was cessation of the symptom when the regurgitated material became acidic. The committee felt that it was difficult to demonstrate this feature in the pediatric population and elected to eliminate it, rather emphasizing the absence of heartburn by mentioning "*painless regurgitation.*" The "*absence of retching*" is now mentioned in order to emphasize that rumination is an effortless behavior and should be differentiated on clinical basis from vomiting. Clinical experience suggests that rumination behavior ceases during sleep, distinguishing this entity from pathologic gastroesophageal reflux, which often worsens when lying down.

— Clinical Evaluation

The classic history is the onset of effortless repetitive regurgitation of gastric contents within minutes of starting a meal. Although the regurgitated gastric contents may be reswallowed, they are frequently expelled, particularly in adolescents. Rumination persists a mean of 70 minutes after eating and rarely occurs at night [6]. Gastroesophageal reflux, achalasia, gastroparesis, bulimia nervosa, and functional or anatomical small-intestinal diseases must be considered as potential causes of recurrent regurgitation and vomiting. Weight loss is a common association of rumination syndrome, and may be significant. Other symptoms, particularly abdominal pain, heartburn, and dental damage are less frequently reported [3, 5, 6]. Evidence of fear of weight gain, disturbed body image, and low self-esteem should be sought in adolescents.

— Physiological Features

Both motor and sensory abnormalities have been reported in rumination syndrome. The characteristic manometric abnormality is a synchronous increase in pressure ("r" waves) across multiple parts of the upper gut. These pressure waves are thought to represent the effect of an increase in intragastric or intra-abdominal pressure generated by the voluntary contraction of the skeletal abdominal muscles. Fasting and postprandial motor patterns are essentially normal [2, 3, 5]. Mechano-sensory studies have demonstrated higher gastric sensitivity than in control subjects, with more frequent episodes of lower esophageal sphincter relaxation in response to gastric distension [15]. A subgroup of individuals also has impaired gastric accommodation in response to a meal. A mild degree of delayed gastric emptying of solids may be found in approximately 40% of adolescents with rumination [6], although scintigraphic studies must be interpreted with caution in individuals who continuously regurgitate during the test. These sensory and motor abnormalities lead to symptoms and regurgitation in response to food intake. The escape of gastric contents towards the mouth relieves the abdominal discomfort. Once this activity is perceived as pleasurable by the individuals, there may be a tendency to perpetuate it. It has also been proposed that rumination is a learned adaptation of the belch reflex, possibly acting through changes in pressure in the diaphragmatic crura [6].

— Psychological Features

Rumination syndrome has been recognized in both apparently normal individuals and in markedly disturbed individuals. It appears to serve the purposes of self-stimulation or as an aid to weight control. The proportion of patients with psychological disturbance has been quite variable, from very few up to one third of the studied populations [6, 7]. Detailed psychological analysis of these individuals and their families may provide additional evidence of disturbed family and interpersonal relationships. An association with eating disorders, particularly bulimia nervosa, has been reported by several investigators [3, 12]. Other psychiatric disturbances that have been recognized in association with rumination syndrome have been depression, anxiety disorder, obsessive-compulsive disorder, posttraumatic stress disorder, adjustment disorder, and attention deficit-hyperactivity disorder [6]. Disturbance of mother-child relationships, in particular the difficulty of the mother to nurture, is typically evident in younger children with rumination syndrome. (See Chapter 13 on infantile rumination.) This is frequently secondary to maternal psychiatric illness [8, 16]. Intellectually handicapped children and adolescents, including those with Prader-Willi syndrome, frequently ruminate [9, 11]. Self-stimulation is believed to be the motive in this group.

— Treatment

A broad range of treatments has been utilized in the management of rumination syndrome. In the absence of nutritional impairment, it needs to be remembered that rumination can occur over long periods of time, without harm [7]. In patients motivated to improve, behavioral therapy has been the main modality utilized, with benefit reported in 85% of subjects after a median followup of 10 months [6]. These programs have typically been built around relaxation techniques, which may be combined with diaphragmatic breathing. This is believed to inhibit both lower esophageal sphincter relaxation and the generation of increased intragastric pressure [17]. Other diversionary techniques, such as increased holding have also been employed [18]. Tricyclic antidepressants have been used with some success [5]. Special means of alimentation with postpyloric feedings, either through naso-jejunal or gastro-jejunal feeding catheters, are used when weight loss is significant. Antireflux surgery has been reported to be beneficial in a small group of adult patients [19]. However, a report of children with visceral pain-associated disability syndrome identified a subgroup with rumination in whom fundoplication was associated with worsening symptoms [20].

H1b. Cyclic Vomiting Syndrome

Although cyclic vomiting often presents in children and adolescents, this entity is discussed both in the neonatal/toddler chapter (Chapter 13) and the adult gastroduodenal chapter (Chapter 8). This committee did not believe there are enough distinguishing features in children to warrant different diagnostic criteria in this age group. The criteria discussed in the neonatal/toddler section (Chapter 13) should also be used for children and adolescents.

H1b. Diagnostic Criteria for Cyclic Vomiting Syndrome

Must include *both* of the following:
1. **Two or more periods of intense nausea and unremitting vomiting or retching lasting hours to days**
2. **Return to usual state of health lasting weeks to months**

H1c. Aerophagia

Aerophagia is a disorder that involves excessive air swallowing causing progressive abdominal distension. The symptoms in children are a nondistended abdomen in the morning; progressive abdominal distension during the day; visible, often audible, air swallowing; excessive burping; excessive flatus; and, sometimes, abdominal (usually colicky) pain [1, 21, 22, 23]. Abdominal distension is maximal in the evening and usually resolves during the night by absorption of gas and by flatulence.

— Epidemiology

There are no epidemiological studies addressing the prevalence of aerophagia in children. Among children presenting for the first time to a gastroenterology clinic and who received a diagnosis of FGID, aerophagia was diagnosed in 1.1% and 1.4% of children aged 4 to 9 years and 10 to 18 years respectively [24]. Aerophagia is a rarely observed behavior among healthy children and adults but involves 8.8% of the institutionalized mentally retarded population [21].

HIc. Diagnostic Criteria* for Aerophagia

Must include *at least two* of the following:
1. Air swallowing
2. Abdominal distention due to intraluminal air
3. Repetitive belching and/or increased flatus

***Criteria fulfilled at least once per week for at least 2 months prior to diagnosis**

— Rationale for Changes from Previous Criteria

Except for the change from 12 weeks to 2 months in the duration symptoms, these criteria have not been modified.

— Clinical Evaluation

Partly because it may mimic other entities, partly because the toddler and preschool child does not explain to the parents what is happening, and finally because the child's gulping of air goes unnoticed by parents, a diagnosis of aerophagia may not be appreciated early in its course [23]. Aerophagia may be confused with generalized motility disorders, such as chronic intestinal pseudo-obstruction and Hirschsprung's disease, because of the associated abdominal distention. Bacterial overgrowth and malabsorption (particularly celiac disease) are other causes of extensive gaseous abdominal distension and excessive flatus. Severe aerophagia may cause massive distention of the bowel, possibly leading to ileus or volvulus. This problem may be encountered more frequently in developmentally delayed children.

In infants, there may be a history of nursing from an empty bottle, or sucking on a pacifier. In older children, large amounts of air can be swallowed while drinking through a straw, while chewing gum, or from drinking excessive amounts of carbonated beverages. It may also be seen in association with respiratory disease such as asthma, which may be chronic, and overlooked by parents. A normal physical examination and growth history help to exclude disease. Breath hydrogen testing may be of use, with lactose to test for lactose malabsorption and with lactulose or glucose to test for bacterial overgrowth and transit time. It is important to ask about recent stressful life events in the family because anxiety is a frequent cause of excessive air swallowing.

— Physiological Features

Air is ingested with every swallow and gas is normally present throughout the lumen of the gut from the mouth to the anus and, under normal circumstances, swallowed air is the prevailing source of gastric gas, with a smaller contribution from gas refluxing through the pylorus [25, 26]. If air swallowing is excessive and repeated, air fills the gastrointestinal lumen resulting in excessive belching, abdominal distention, flatus, and pain, presumably a consequence of distention. There are no physiologic studies of aerophagia in children.

— Psychological Features

There are no studies of psychological features of children with aerophagia defined by Rome criteria.

— Treatment

In children, there are no controlled studies to guide therapy, which remains largely supportive but may include behavioral therapy and psychotherapy. Some commonly recommended agents (e.g., simethicone) do not have confirmed efficacy [26]. Treatment consists of effective reassurance and an explanation for the symptom for the parents and the child. Often, the clinician can help the child become aware of air swallows during the visit. Avoidance of gum chewing and carbonated beverages and refraining from talking during eating can all be helpful.

Behavioral modifications, relaxation and breathing techniques, and other psycho-therapeutic strategies may be helpful for the patient in some cases [27, 28]. In extreme cases, gastric decompression by nasogastric tube [23] or by the placement of a gastrostomy has alleviated the condition [22].

H2. Abdominal Pain-related FGIDs

In children with abdominal pain-related FGIDs the alarm features, signs, and symptoms listed in Table 1 are generally absent. The committee recognized the great variability in the severity and phenotypic presentation of children with ab-dominal pain-related FGIDs and therefore decided to split the previously inclusive category of functional abdominal pain (FAP) into two separate disorders, func-tional abdominal pain and functional abdominal pain syndrome (FAPS), so that studies done in this population may include more homogeneous patients.

Functional impairment, which is included in the FAP syndrome, can also be observed in other FGIDs such as abdominal migraine and functional dyspepsia or IBS. In abdominal migraine, it is now included in the definition, while in the other disorders it is not. Impairment of daily activity, though possibly present, has not traditionally been included in the definition of IBS and functional dys-pepsia in adults. Severity of symptoms is addressed in the questionnaire section developed as part of the Rome III process.

Clinical evaluation and treatment of children with abdominal pain-predomi-nant disorders have been recently reviewed in two documents of the American Academy of Pediatrics and the North American Society for Pediatric Gastroen-terology, Hepatology, and Nutrition and will only be very briefly addressed in this chapter [29, 30].

H2a. Functional Dyspepsia

Upper gastrointestinal discomfort is common in children and adolescents. In contrast to adult patients, the possibility of esophageal or stomach cancer is virtu-ally nil in children, and ulcer disease is much less common as well. Despite these reassuring facts, upper gastrointestinal pain, nausea, or vomiting cause significant morbidity in some pediatric patients, resulting in school absence. Upon investiga-tion, most cases prove to be functional in origin.

— Definition

Dyspepsia is defined by a persistent or recurrent pain or discomfort centered in the upper abdomen. Dyspepsia may occasionally arise from disease (gastroesophageal reflux, peptic ulcer, allergy, Crohn's disease), but is much more likely to be due to a disorder of upper gastrointestinal sensation and motility. In children and adolescents functional dyspepsia can have variable presentations, including predominantly pain or ulcerlike symptoms, presentation in which nausea, bloating, fullness, or early satiety predominate, or cases in which patients have both features [31]. The symptoms may arise following an intercurrent infectious illness or may develop in a more insidious way [32].

— Epidemiology

Criteria for defining dyspepsia have not been uniform among published reports. Hyams et al. [33] found that typical dyspeptic symptoms were reported by 5% to 10% of subjects in a community-based study of 507 adolescents in a suburban setting in the northeast United States. In a completely different setting in Novosibirsk, western Siberia, the prevalence of dyspepsia among adolescents was reported to be 27% in girls and 16% in boys [34]. Researchers in northern Italy investigated a school-based population for the presence of gastrointestinal tract symptoms and identified symptoms of ulcerlike dyspepsia in 3.5% and of dysmotilitylike dyspepsia in 3.7% of subjects [35]. In another study carried out in southern Italy [36], this time in a primary care setting, functional dyspepsia was described in 0.3% of the study population. Since the study population excluded children older than 12 years, the low prevalence of functional dyspepsia is most likely explained by the absence of adolescents in the sample. A recent study that applied a questionnaire to assess the symptoms defined by the pediatric Rome II criteria to parents of new patients with recurrent abdominal pain (RAP) referred to a university pediatric gastroenterology clinic in the United States [37], found that symptom criteria were met for functional dyspepsia in 16% of patients. Most patients met the criteria for either ulcerlike dyspepsia or unspecified dyspepsia. In another study performed in a pediatric gastroenterology unit, dyspepsia was diagnosed in 13.5% of 4- to 9-year-old children and in 10.2% of 10- to 18-year-old children who received a diagnosis of FGID [24].

H2a. Diagnostic Criteria* for Functional Dyspepsia

Must include *all* of the following:
1. **Persistent or recurrent pain or discomfort centered in the upper abdomen (above the umbilicus)**
2. **Not relieved by defecation or associated with the onset of a change in stool frequency or stool form (i.e., not irritable bowel syndrome)**
3. **No evidence of an inflammatory, anatomic, metabolic, or neoplastic process that explains the subject's symptoms**

***Criteria fulfilled at least once per week for at least 2 months prior to diagnosis**

There appear to be subjects with functional dyspepsia who have differing symptom presentations. In some, epigastric pain predominates. In others, upper abdominal discomfort characterized by nausea, satiety, bloating, or fullness predominates. In others, there may be a combination of both.

— Rationale for Change in Criteria

In the criteria proposed, we have changed the duration of symptoms from 12 weeks to 2 months. This change is not based on new data, but rather on clinical experience and in an effort to maintain uniform pediatric criteria. We have also eliminated the mandatory use of upper gastrointestinal endoscopy in order to make this diagnosis. In children, the likelihood of finding mucosal abnormalities responsible for dyspeptic symptoms is much lower than in adults. We have eliminated ulcerlike and dysmotilitylike subtypes since epidemiologic data suggest that young children do not fall into either category [24, 31, 37]. Finally, we decided that there should be no evidence of an inflammatory, anatomic, metabolic, or neoplastic process that explains the subject's symptoms. We recognize that there are children with FAP or FAPS who may have evidence of mild, chronic inflammatory changes on mucosal biopsies. In view of the evidence that an FGID may follow an acute inflammatory event [38], such changes should not impede a diagnosis of an FGID. We have used this terminology also for the other childhood FGIDs presenting with abdominal pain or discomfort.

Table 2. Alarm Symptoms, Signs, and Features in Children and
Adolescents with Noncyclic Abdominal Pain-Related
Functional Gastrointestinal Disorders.

- Persistent right-upper or right-lower quadrant pain
- Arthritis
- Pain that wakes the child from sleep
- Perirectal disease
- Dysphagia
- Involuntary weight loss
- Persistent vomiting
- Deceleration of linear growth
- Gastrointestinal blood loss
- Delayed puberty
- Nocturnal diarrhea
- Unexplained fever
- Family history of inflammatory bowel disease, celiac disease, or peptic ulcer disease

— Clinical Evaluation

There are no specific diagnostic tests for functional dyspepsia. The approach to the pediatric patient with dyspeptic symptoms starts with a detailed history (including dietary, psychological, and social factors), careful physical examination, and inspection of growth curves. Alarm signals (Table 2) should be identified and, if present, conditions other than functional dyspepsia should be suspected. Demographic factors such as family crowding, poor household living conditions, underprivileged socioeconomic condition, or a family history of *H. pylori* infection should raise suspicion for peptic disease associated with this microorganism [39, 40]. Persistent dyspeptic symptoms may follow a viral illness or an episode of diarrhea, even when the originating illness has abated. These individuals are presumed to be suffering from a postviral gastroparesis [32].

Children with dyspepsia can report occasional heartburn. Of note, heartburn as the predominant symptom suggests gastroesophageal reflux as the diagnosis and upper gastrointestinal endoscopy is warranted whenever symptoms are likely to represent foregut mucosal disease. Often this test is performed in children with persistent symptoms despite the use of acid-reducing medications or in those who have recurrent symptoms upon cessation of such medications. Abdominal ultrasonography does not appear to be helpful in children with dyspepsia except when pancreatic or biliary diseases are strongly suspected based on a typical history.

Measurements of serum amylase, lipase, and serum amino-transferases are important in assessing the latter conditions. The association of dyspeptic symptoms with a history of poor growth, diarrhea, or anemia should prompt the clinician to perform serological screening for celiac disease. It has been claimed—but not conclusively proven—that infection by *Giardia lamblia* may be a cause of dyspepsia [41]. Serologic tests for *H. pylori* in children with dyspepsia are not fully reliable in the pediatric population [42] and upper gastrointestinal endoscopy currently remains the standard technique for the diagnosis of *H. pylori*-associated peptic disease in these subjects. In the absence of peptic disease there is little evidence in the pediatric literature that *H. pylori* causes dyspeptic symptoms [42] and there are no specific characteristics of symptoms in dyspeptic *H. pylori*-infected children as compared with noninfected children [43].

— Physiological Features

There have been several physiological studies of dyspeptic children, though most have not used standardized clinical criteria to define their study population. Electrogastrography showed disordered gastric myoelectrical activity [44, 45, 46], and radionuclide imaging or ultrasound examination showed delayed gastric emptying [47, 48]. Antroduodenal manometry revealed disordered motility in some subjects [49]. Among 57 children with functional dyspepsia ingesting a standardized egg meal labeled with Technetium-99m sulfur colloid, 40% had slow small bowel transit [50]. Rapid gastric emptying and slow small bowel transit were associated with bloating in this population. Visceral hypersensitivity and impaired fundic accommodation have been shown to play a role in subgroups of dyspeptic adults [51].

— Psychological Features

There are no pediatric data on the psychological features of children with functional dyspepsia as defined by the Rome consensus criteria.

— Treatment

There are no adequately sized double-blind placebo-controlled studies of the treatment of children with functional dyspepsia, defined by the Rome pediatric criteria. Empiric therapy is often primarily directed toward the predominant symptoms of pain, nausea, bloating, fullness, or early satiety. Foods aggravating symptoms (e.g., caffeine-containing, spicy, and fatty foods) and nonsteroidal anti-inflammatory agents should be avoided. Psychological factors that may be contributing to the severity of the problem should be addressed. It is presumed that the placebo effect seen in drug trials in adults with functional dyspepsia is also present in children. Acid blockade with histamine receptor antagonists and proton pump inhibitors is offered for pain-predominant symptoms. One under-powered study suggested famotidine was superior to placebo for children with dyspepsia [52]. Acid reduction therapy may also be helpful when the relationship of symptoms to possible gastroesophageal reflux is not clear. Nausea, bloating, and early satiety are more difficult to treat and prokinetics such as cisapride (where available), metoclopramide, and domperidone can be offered. A recent study investigated 40 children and adolescents with dyspeptic symptoms and found a beneficial role for montelukast in the treatment of a subgroup of children with symptoms associated with duodenal eosinophilia [53].

— Addendum: Towards a More Evidence-Based Nomenclature and Classification

Functional dyspepsia is an entity that has been studied extensively in adult patients. (See Chapter 8, "Functional Gastrointestinal Disorders.") Despite the large body of literature on this entity, little improvement has been made in understanding its pathophysiology and in developing effective therapeutic interventions for its treatment. Several problems have contributed to this lack of progress. There is still disagreement on its definitions, with heartburn still being considered by some to be part of the spectrum of dyspeptic symptoms. Pathophysiological studies have uncovered different mechanisms associated with some dyspeptic symptoms but not with others. Patients with different phenotypic presentation respond differently to treatment, making it challenging to show efficacy with new drugs in the treatment of functional dyspepsia as currently defined. Factor analysis studies in adults have not supported the existence of functional dyspepsia as a homogeneous entity. Based on these and other observations, the adult committee on functional gastrointestinal disorders has suggested a new classification for dyspeptic disorder. Please see Chapter 8 for a more in-depth discussion of the adult literature leading to their recommendation.

The pediatric committee believes that there are no adequate data to suggest that this new nomenclature can be applied in children. It is also believed that the revised classification represents progress in the understanding of dyspepsia and supports the concept that such classification be used and validated in future pediatric studies.

H2b. Irritable Bowel Syndrome

Irritable bowel syndrome (IBS) comprises a group of functional bowel disorders in which abdominal discomfort or pain is associated with defecation or a change in bowel habit, and with features of disordered defecation.

— Epidemiology

Surveys of adult European and North American populations estimate the prevalence of IBS to range from 7% to 22% of adults, with a female predominance. Similar rates have been reported in non-European populations [54]. There is limited information available on the epidemiology of childhood IBS. Older studies reported prevalence rates for recurrent abdominal pain of 10% to 20% throughout childhood in both Western and non-Western populations [55, 56, 57, 58], but to date most studies have not adequately differentiated the recurrent abdominal pain disorders that include FAP, dyspepsia, abdominal migraine, or IBS, and the precision of the definition of FGIDs will affect the defined prevalence [54].

In a community-based study of 507 North American children, 6% of middle school (mean age 12.6 years) and 14% of high school students (mean age 15.6 years) fulfilled criteria for IBS adapted from Rome I criteria, with no significant differences in frequency of diagnosis for either gender (16% of girls and 11% of boys reporting abdominal pain) [33]. Limited data suggest that a socioeconomic gradient exists, with markers of increased affluence associated with increased risk of IBS [59].

In a tertiary pediatric gastroenterology service, Hyams et al. prospectively characterized the symptoms of 227 patients aged 5 to 18 years referred for recurrent abdominal pain [60]. Using Rome I adult criteria they found that 68% of the 171 patients without evidence of organic disease or physiological disturbance to account for their symptoms fulfilled the diagnostic criteria for IBS. In a separate retrospective review of 356 referred children with chronic abdominal pain, a quarter were found to meet modified Rome I diagnostic criteria for IBS [61]. By contrast, a recent population study [62] found IBS in only 0.2% of Italian children. Importantly, this population consisted of young children (mean age 52 months). It specifically excluded patients older than 12 years, and thus is unlikely to reflect childhood population prevalence.

Two studies have demonstrated that up to 50% of children and adolescents presenting to tertiary services with RAP fulfill Rome II pediatric criteria for IBS [24, 37]. Walker et al. assessed the presenting symptoms of 114 children presenting to a tertiary care children's medical center with abdominal pain [37]. Of the

107 children in whom there was no evidence of organic disease, 45% fulfilled the Rome II diagnostic criteria for IBS, while another 23% fulfilled the diagnostic criteria for functional dyspepsia, FAP, or abdominal migraine. In the study of Caplan et al., 315 consecutive new pediatric patients received a diagnosis of FGID by pediatric gastroenterologists [24]. Among 177 children aged 4 to 9 years, 22% had IBS according to the Rome II pediatric criteria and 35.5% of 138 children aged 10 to 18 years met the same criteria for IBS. This increase in incidence with age seems to confirm Hyams' previous findings in a community-based study, where the history was obtained totally from the children [33]. In the Caplan et al. study, diagnoses for the younger age group were derived from questionnaire data provided by parents, whereas diagnoses for the adolescent group were based on questionnaire data completed by the patients themselves [63].

In 2001, data on gastrointestinal motility and visceral sensitivity in pain-related FGIDs in children were published [64, 65]. These studies confirm findings from studies of adults and provide additional construct validity, as well as discriminant validity, for the pediatric Rome II criteria. Indeed, in the first study [64], children selected according to the pediatric Rome II criteria for IBS had different motility patterns and visceral sensitivity than healthy controls and children with FAP (also selected according to the pediatric Rome II criteria). The presence of visceral hypersensitivity was confirmed in the second study [65] in which children with IBS selected according to Rome II criteria had higher pain scores than children with non-IBS recurrent abdominal pain and controls. These two studies support the Rome II criteria for IBS in children by demonstrating that these criteria discriminate children whose pain is associated with visceral hypersensitivity from those whose pain is not associated with this physiological marker.

The relationship between childhood FAP and adult IBS is not clear. Walker et al. followed up a group of 76 patients 5 years after medical evaluation for RAP and found that 18% of female patients and none of the female control subjects fulfilled Rome I criteria for IBS [66]. Campo et al. reported that patients seen in a tertiary hospital clinic because of recurrent abdominal pain were not more likely than hospital controls to have IBS at followup 6 to 17 years later, although they were more likely to be disabled by symptoms [67]. This was similar to the findings of Hotopf who reported that children with persistent abdominal pain followed up as part of a large cohort were not more likely to express somatic symptoms as adults (mean age 43 years) [68].

H2b. Diagnostic Criteria* for Irritable Bowel Syndrome

Must include *both* of the following:
1. **Abdominal discomfort** or pain associated with *two or more* of the following at least 25% of the time:**
   a. **Improvement with defecation**
   b. **Onset associated with a change in frequency of stool**
   c. **Onset associated with a change in form (appearance) of stool**
2. **No evidence of an inflammatory, anatomic, metabolic, or neoplastic process that explains the subject's symptoms**

*Criteria fulfilled at least once per week for at least 2 months prior to diagnosis

**"Discomfort" means an uncomfortable sensation not described as pain.

— Rationale for Changes in Diagnostic Criteria

The only change has been the duration of symptoms, which has decreased from 12 weeks to 2 months in order to keep the criteria more uniform with the other pediatric Rome III criteria.

— Physiological Features

Two studies on adult twins have addressed the possibility of a genetic predisposition to the development of IBS [69, 70]. A genetic component in the pathogenesis of IBS is suggested by the fact that symptoms consistent with IBS are more common in monozygotic than dizygotic twins. However, for a dizygotic twin, having a parent with IBS doubles the risk for developing the same disorder. This raises the possibility that social learning is an even more important etiologic factor than genetics (see the section on psychological features).

In the literature pertaining to chronic abdominal pain in children, gastrointestinal motility disturbances [32, 71], hormonal changes [72], autonomic disorders [73], psychiatric disorders [74, 75], and family dynamics [76] have been proposed as factors contributing to chronic abdominal pain of functional origin. However, over the years no single abnormality has been found to explain the complexity of symptoms.

During the last decade, visceral hypersensitivity has been demonstrated in adults with IBS [77]. Recently, there have been two studies on the pathophysiology of IBS in children and adolescents. As mentioned above, subjects in these two studies were selected according to pediatric Rome II criteria for IBS and investigated for motility disorders and/or visceral hyperalgesia. Van Ginkel and his colleagues [64] found that IBS children had different rectal tone and rectal motor response after ingestion of a meal. All IBS children perceived pain earlier than controls or children with FAP, confirming the presence of visceral hypersensitivity associated with IBS. This last finding was confirmed by Di Lorenzo et al. [65] who showed that 10 children with IBS (again, selected according to pediatric Rome II criteria) had higher pain scores than 10 non-IBS children with recurrent abdominal pain and 15 healthy controls. Despite the small sample sizes in both studies, these data support the role of visceral hypersensitivity in IBS children.

Given that visceral hypersensitivity seems to exist in both children and adults with IBS, there is reason to believe that other findings concerning pathophysiology may also apply to both age groups (see the section on physiology for more details). Alterations in the brain-gut axis have been implicated in the development of the pain and disturbed motility associated with IBS. (See Chapter 3.) These neuronal changes can be very succinctly described as a hyper-excitable state, which can last long after the initial stimuli have disappeared [78]. (See Chapters 2 and 3 on basic science and physiology.) These stimuli, including infection, inflammation, allergy, and trauma, have been incriminated in the development of IBS after enteric infection or psychological stress [38]. The occurrence of IBS after an infectious episode of the gastrointestinal tract has been very well documented in the adult population [38, 79, 80]. Unfortunately, there are no data in the pediatric population on postinfectious IBS. However, it is the belief and experience of this committee that it also occurs in children and adolescents. Most pertinent to the pediatric population is the finding that in animals, the neonatal period appears to be a particularly sensitive period for the development of visceral hyperalgesia and altered motility. (See Chapter 5.) Indeed, early traumatic experiences and life events shape brain-gut connections and may have consequences during adult life [38, 81, 82, 83]. Early maternal separation and psychological stress predisposed pup rats to develop visceral hyperalgesia, reduced somatic analgesia, and increased colonic motility in response to stress during adult life. Early alterations in central circuits mediating autonomic and pain modulatory responses were also shown to develop in another rat model after colonic irritation. In contrast, the same colonic irritation performed in adult rats did not induce long-lasting consequences. Thus, the permanency of changes depended on the timing of the trigger (neonatal period or adulthood) in these animal models. Stress-induced exacerbation of IBS symptoms is a well-known and consistent finding in humans and anxiety specific to visceral sensation has been demonstrated [84]. Enhanced stress responsiveness acquired very early in life is a plausible underlying pathophysiological mechanism in a number of IBS patients. Along these lines is the recent report that gastric suction in the neonatal period may be a contributing factor to the development of functional gastrointestinal disorders later in life [85].

— Psychological Features

Existing research links IBS to internalizing behavior (anxiety, depression) in children and adolescents. In a study using the Rome II criteria, more than half (55%) of 29 pediatric patients with IBS, functional dyspepsia, or FAP showed significant internalizing problems, according to their parents' and their own reports [86]. Among adolescents, self-reported IBS symptoms were associated with depressive symptoms in a community sample [33] and a clinical sample [66]. In addition, more severe IBS symptoms reported by adolescents on the Bowel Disease Questionnaire, were related to significantly lower self-reported academic, social, and athletic competence [66, 87].

Regarding family environment, children with a parent who has IBS are significantly more likely than peers to have somatic complaints and have significantly more school absences and clinic visits than their peers [88]. These findings lend some support to the view that social learning contributes to the development of FGIDs and to their transmission across generations.

— Clinical Evaluation

With the advent of pediatric criteria for FGIDs, a positive diagnosis of IBS can now be made. IBS is no longer a diagnosis of exclusion [89]. Symptoms of abdominal pain that meet Rome II criteria for IBS, normal physical examination, normal growth curve, and the absence of alarm signals strongly suggest such a diagnosis. Alarm signs and symptoms are listed in Table 2. During the initial visit, considerable time should be devoted to the patient's history, family incidence of gastrointestinal disease or disorders, and infectious episodes or stressful events associated with the onset of symptoms. Inquiring about the psychosocial history of both the child and family helps establish a rapport and form a working alliance with the patient. The presence of anxiety, depression, and somatization symptoms should be particularly noted not only in the patient, but also in parents and siblings.

The physician should make a diagnosis based on the Rome criteria, confirm the child's experience of pain, and provide precise information about the disorder. This provides a new understanding of the disorder that will help parents accept a limited screening for organic disease. The predictive value of blood tests with or without alarm signs and symptoms has not yet been adequately tested in children [29, 30]. Recent data on adults suggest that screening for celiac disease in patients presenting with IBS symptoms may be cost-effective [90]. It is the responsibility of each clinician to elect when and if to use tests such as breath hydrogen analysis, ultrasound, and endoscopy [91].

— Treatment

There are no controlled studies of therapy in pediatric IBS using Rome criteria. Most studies of treatment relate to recurrent abdominal pain, and in general contain small numbers of subjects. Recent systematic reviews have outlined the inadequacy of these studies and of the scientific underpinning of therapeutic approaches [92, 93, 94, 95]. The Cochrane review concluded that "there is little evidence to suggest that recommended drugs are effective in the management of RAP. At present there seems little justification for the use of these drugs other than in clinical trials" [93]. It is noted that the evidence for a therapeutic effect is stronger in situations where a specific FGID is treated, rather than RAP [95]. Recommendations are based therefore largely on expert opinion, limited trials of therapy, and extrapolation from studies of adults, and from studies of therapies in children with recurrent abdominal pain. It is important to note that given the paucity of adequate trials, the lack of evidence for a therapeutic effect does not imply that there is no effect. This emphasizes the need for properly conducted scientific evaluation of therapies in pediatric populations.

Once there is a confident diagnosis of IBS, the first and most important part of the approach to treatment is to validate the symptoms that the child is experiencing and provide effective reassurance regarding the underlying well-being of the sufferer and the potential for symptom modification [96]. The presence and severity of the pain should be acknowledged. A review of the current understanding of IBS and the exacerbating effects of stress and anxiety helps the child and family to understand why the pain occurs. Psychosocial difficulties and triggering events for symptoms should be identified and management options explored. Usually, it is appropriate to initiate therapeutic interventions in a stepwise fashion, starting with the simplest and safest interventions, and progressing as necessary to the more complex and expensive therapeutic options. It is important that the clinician recognize that the consultation itself can be therapeutic [97, 98]. It may be useful to outline the specific goals of therapy, including the fact that resolution of symptoms may not be as possible as modifying severity and developing strategies for dealing with symptoms.

There is little evidence that dietary interventions alter intestinal motility or stool form. Despite this, supplementation with dietary fiber has been recommended on the basis of three studies in children [99, 100, 101]. A systematic review, however, found methodological issues with these studies and reports no support for the use of fiber in the management of childhood abdominal pain [94]. Dietary exclusion of lactose is not supported by the available evidence [94]. However, lactose intolerance may coexist and, if confirmed by a hydrogen breath test, a trial of lactose restriction is justified.

Drug therapy may be used as adjunctive therapy, especially for those individuals who are severely disabled by their symptoms. Anticholinergic medications are widely used but have not been demonstrated efficacious in placebo-controlled trials in adults [102], and there are no data from studies in children. Tricyclic antidepressants such as imipramine, desipramine, or amitriptyline in low doses improved symptoms in adults with diarrhea-predominant IBS in controlled, blinded studies [103, 104]. These drugs have been used extensively for chronic visceral pain, but there are only anecdotal reports concerning their use in children with chronic abdominal pain. Enteric-coated peppermint-oil capsules, believed to exert calcium channel blockade in smooth muscle, were shown in a randomized, placebo-controlled study to decrease the severity of abdominal pain, but not other symptoms in pediatric patients meeting the Manning criteria for adult IBS [105].

There is good support for the use of psychological therapies (e.g., hypnotherapy and cognitive behavioral therapy) in adults with IBS and children with abdominal pain[106] and limited data suggest that cognitive behavioral therapy, biofeedback, and self-hypnosis are beneficial in managing pediatric RAP [101, 107, 108]. Elucidation of the role of serotonin in the pathogenesis of IBS in adults has led to the development of serotonergic agents such as alosetron (a 5-hydroxytryptamine$_3$ (5-HT$_3$) receptor antagonist) and tegaserod (a 5-HT$_4$ receptor antagonist) [109]. No published data are available on their use in children.

H2c. Abdominal Migraine

Though controversy surrounded its very existence for many years, the syndrome of abdominal migraine first described in the 1920s [110, 111] is now recognized as a disorder affecting both children and adults [111, 112, 113, 114]. Much of the initial reluctance to accept abdominal migraine as a distinct disorder came from adult neurologists treating migraine who did not appreciate the protean nature of extracranial symptoms. The likelihood that episodic abdominal pain in the absence of headache may be the result of a migrainous phenomenon arises from four pieces of evidence: (1) the common coexistence of abdominal pain and migraine headaches; (2) the similar demographic and social factors, precipitating factors, and accompanying neurological, vasomotor, and gastrointestinal features in some children with episodic abdominal pain and those with migraine headaches; (3) the utility of antimigraine therapy in the treatment of children with abdominal migraine; and, (4) similar neurophysiological features in children with abdominal migraine and those with migraine headaches.

Confusion has also arisen from the lack of distinction between cyclic vomiting syndrome and abdominal migraine. Both syndromes have marked periodicity with asymptomatic periods in between. In the former, vomiting is the predominant symptom with or without abdominal pain, whereas in the latter abdominal pain dominates the clinical picture. Both disorders were likely included in the 1933 paper of Wyllie and Schlesinger who introduced the diagnosis of "periodic disorder of childhood" [115].

— Definition

Abdominal migraine is a paroxysmal disorder characterized by the acute onset of severe, noncolicky, periumbilical pain that generally lasts for several hours. Anorexia, nausea, vomiting, and pallor often accompany it. The affected individual is well between attacks. Attacks may occur at any time of the day or night, and they often awaken the patient from sleep or become manifest shortly after awakening. Associated features may include a history of migraine headaches in the proband or a family member, increased susceptibility to motion sickness, prodromal changes in mood and activity, or other accompaniments of migraine episodes (e.g., photophobia, headache, and phonophobia). Toward the end of an attack the individual often becomes lethargic and after a period of sleep the symptoms resolve. When these abdominal findings occur in an individual with a history of migraine headaches, and especially if the abdominal pain and headache occur simultaneously, the diagnosis of abdominal migraine is straightforward. In some children, there is no history of migraine headache in the proband or in the immediate family.

Many of the features of abdominal migraine are also present in children with cyclic vomiting syndrome. It has been suggested that abdominal migraine, cyclic vomiting syndrome, and migraine headache comprise a continuum of a single disorder, with affected individuals often progressing from one clinical picture to another [116].

— Epidemiology

It has been estimated that abdominal migraine affects 1% to 4% of children [113, 117]. It is more common in girls than in boys (3:2) with a mean age of onset at 7 years and a peak at 10 to 12 years. More recently, it has been noted to account for 5% of children presenting with chronic abdominal pain [37] and 2.2%

of new patients aged 10 to 18 years who received a diagnosis of FGID by pediatric gastroenterologists [24].

H2c. Diagnostic Criteria* for Abdominal Migraine

Must include *all* of the following:

1. **Paroxysmal episodes of intense, acute periumbilical pain that lasts for 1 hour or more**
2. **Intervening periods of usual health lasting weeks to months**
3. **The pain interferes with normal activities**
4. **The pain is associated with *two or more* of the following:**
   a. **Anorexia**
   b. **Nausea**
   c. **Vomiting**
   d. **Headache**
   e. **Photophobia**
   f. **Pallor**
5. **No evidence of an inflammatory, anatomic, metabolic, or neoplastic process considered that explains the subject's symptoms**

* Criteria fulfilled two or more times in the preceding 12 months

— Rationale for Changes in Criteria

The number of episodes required was changed from three to two. "Recurrent" implies two episodes, and a recent review by experts suggests that two episodes are sufficient for diagnosis [118]. The minimum duration of an episode was changed from 2 hours to 1 hour. The expert review suggested 1 hour was sufficient. Most episodes generally last several hours to days. Pain is now specified to be severe enough to affect activity. Indeed, a hallmark of this syndrome is that the pain is often incapacitating. The experts suggested adding this terminology to the definition [118]. Additional symptoms have been added to the definition. The gastrointestinal and vasomotor symptoms are an integral part of the syndrome. We removed the necessity for family history of migraine and aura. These features are indeed not necessary, and are internally somewhat redundant. The history of migraine in the proband and family is a supporting feature. The decision to change from "symptom-free interval between episodes" to "return to usual state of health" was made because some patients may have other chronic or recurrent symptoms unrelated to abdominal migraine.

— Clinical Evaluation

The clinical hallmark of abdominal migraine is the paroxysmal nature of symptoms and the absence of the characteristic severe abdominal pain between episodes. This pattern makes chronic inflammation from esophagitis, gastritis, duodenitis, ulcer, or inflammatory bowel disease unlikely. Therefore endoscopic evaluation is generally not useful. Rather, a search can be made for causes of intermittent severe pain such as obstructive uropathy, malrotation of the gut and its complications, intermittent bowel obstruction (e.g., intussusception), biliary tract disease, recurrent pancreatitis, familial Mediterranean fever, and metabolic disorders such as porphyria. Abdominal sonography can evaluate the hepatobiliary and renal systems, and contrast radiography can determine if a gastrointestinal anatomic abnormality is present. A favorable response to medications used for prophylaxis of migraine headaches supports the diagnosis of abdominal migraine.

— Physiological Features

Given the significant clinical overlap of abdominal migraine, cyclic vomiting syndrome, and migraine headache it has been thought that there may be similar underlying pathophysiological mechanisms. Similar abnormal visual evoked responses have been described in children with abdominal migraine, cyclic vomiting syndrome, and migraine headaches compared to controls [119, 120]. Abnormalities in the hypothalamic-pituitary-adrenal axis and autonomic dysfunction have been described in cyclic vomiting syndrome [116] but have not been well-characterized in individuals with abdominal migraine.

— Psychological Features

There are limited data detailing the psychological characteristics of these children, although there is an extensive literature relating to the psychological characteristics of migraine sufferers. In a case control study, Withers demonstrated higher scores on the Achenbach Child Behavior Checklist for internalizing behavior (e.g., anxiety and depression) in patients with cyclic vomiting syndrome in comparison with control subjects [121]. Older follow-up data on children with cyclic vomiting syndrome emphasize the risk of long-term chronic psychiatric morbidity in this group [122].

— Treatment

There are no well-designed trials of any therapy for abdominal migraine. In practice, therapy is directed toward avoidance of triggers, mitigation of symptoms once an episode starts, and prophylaxis. Potential triggers include stress (either good or bad), travel, prolonged fasting, altered sleep patterns, and exposure to flickering or glaring lights [123]. Avoidance of caffeine-containing foods (e.g., chocolate, colas), foods rich in nitrites, and foods rich in amines has been suggested [123]. Prophylactic drug therapy is undertaken when episodes are frequent. Pizotifen, an antihistaminic and serotonin antagonist, was shown effective in preventing recurrent abdominal migraine episodes in 70% of children in a small double blind-placebo-controlled trial [124]. Uncontrolled observations have suggested a prophylactic role for propranolol and cyproheptadine [125]. Anecdotal use of nasal sumatriptan has been reported to treat acute attacks [120].

H2d. Childhood Functional Abdominal Pain

Childhood functional abdominal pain (FAP) describes abdominal pain that occurs over a period of at least 2 months in children and adolescents with no evidence of an inflammatory, anatomic, metabolic, or neoplastic process considered likely to be an explanation for the subject's symptoms.

— Epidemiology

There have been no pediatric epidemiological studies of FAP based on the Rome criteria. Two studies have used Rome II criteria to distinguish FAP, IBS, dyspepsia, and abdominal migraine in pediatric patients with abdominal pain [24, 37]. Both studies were conducted in tertiary care centers and used the Questionnaire on Pediatric Gastrointestinal Disorders [24, 37]. The questionnaire has been partially validated in a recent study [63]. In the Walker study [37] the questionnaire was given to parents, while in the Caplan study [24] it was given to parents of children aged 4 to 9 years and to the children themselves aged 10 to 18 years. FAP was found to account for only a small percentage of the diagnoses in children with abdominal pain-related functional gastrointestinal disorders. Indeed, it represented only 7.5 % of the 4- to 18-year-old group in the Walker study, and in the Caplan study FAP was documented in only 3% of children aged 10 to 18 years.

Several factors contribute to the low prevalence of FAP in these studies. First, they were conducted with pediatric patients presenting for treatment in tertiary care settings and thus do not reflect FAP in children in the community. However, community-based surveys have also identified a low prevalence of FAP in adults. More specifically, the U.S. Householder Study of Functional Gastrointestinal Disorders identified FAP in only 1.7% (primarily women) of the sample [126]. Second, it should be stressed that this low prevalence is to be expected since the Rome II criteria required that children present with *continuous or nearly continuous pain* in order to be considered for a diagnosis of FAP. Furthermore, the Rome II criteria excluded children with pain centered in the upper abdomen and those whose pain was related to defecation, regardless of location. Finally, the Rome II criteria for FAP included impairment in daily activities as a measure of severity but no attempt was made to clearly specify the extent or frequency of activity interference required [37, 127].

In the absence of epidemiological studies on FAP in children, the Pediatric Working Team of Rome II chose to include FAP as defined in the adult population because they believed that this disorder also occurred in children and adolescents. They introduced a modification with respect to symptom duration. Symptoms needed to be present 3 months instead of 6 months. The team wanted to make clear that the term FAP was not meant to substitute for Apley's "recurrent abdominal pain of childhood" (RAP), a term that has been used historically to describe children who may or may not have an organic disease underlying the recurrent episodes of abdominal pain [55].

H2d. Diagnostic Criteria* for Childhood Functional Abdominal Pain

Must include *all* of the following:
1. **Episodic or continuous abdominal pain**
2. **Insufficient criteria for other FGIDs**
3. **No evidence of an inflammatory, anatomic, metabolic, or neoplastic process that explains the subject's symptoms**

***Criteria fulfilled at least once per week for at least 2 months prior to diagnosis**

H2d1. Diagnostic Criteria* for Childhood Functional Abdominal Pain Syndrome

Must satisfy criteria for childhood functional abdominal pain and have at least 25% of the time _one or more_ of the following:
1. Some loss of daily functioning
2. Additional somatic symptoms such as headache, limb pain, or difficulty sleeping

*Criteria fulfilled at least once per week for at least 2 months prior to diagnosis

— Rationale for Changes in Diagnostic Criteria

The committee is proposing several changes to the previous Rome II criteria that substantially simplify the diagnosis. It was felt that the previous criteria were unnecessarily restrictive and therefore responsible for the lower than expected incidence of childhood FAP [24, 37].

The duration of the symptoms has been reduced to _2 months_ as part of an effort of the pediatric committee to keep the criteria for the childhood functional GI disorders uniform. A duration of 2 months is sufficient to exclude most acute gastrointestinal illnesses in children. The requirement for _continuous or nearly continuous pain_ has been eliminated based on the clinical experience that children present with episodic or intermittent pain at least as frequently as they do with more continuous pain. The previous criteria mentioned that the pain had to have _no or only occasional relation with physiological events._ This criterion would exclude children who have some features of IBS or dyspepsia but do not meet criteria for those entities (for example children who only have one of the two bowel symptoms required for IBS). Children with FAP who have continuous abdominal pain will also sometimes have pain in association with physiological events. That _the pain is not feigned_ was a requirement of the Rome II criteria. This was a very challenging criterion to assess, because pain is a subjective experience reported by the individual child. We have elected to eliminate the requirement for _some loss of daily function_ in the criteria for FAP, because such a criterion confounded symptoms and function. It excluded motivated children who continued activity despite the pain and children whose parents insisted that they continue activities. However, we recognize that there is a subgroup of children in whom loss of daily functioning and/or accompanying somatic symptoms form an important component of their symptom complex. This group is now referred to as having _functional abdominal pain syndrome (FAPS)._ The current pediatric criteria for functional abdominal pain differ from the criteria in adults and further research may make these two sets of criteria converge. The committee decided (much like the adult group) to omit the category of "unspecified functional abdominal pain" because the new pediatric criteria are more inclusive.

— Clinical Evaluation

Children who meet the criteria for FAP do not have any symptoms demonstrably related to a specific gastric or intestinal anatomic or inflammatory abnormality. In these children, it is of the utmost importance to perform a careful physical examination. The growth chart is examined for involuntary weight loss or deceleration of linear growth. General appearance as well as behavior and pain during abdominal examination are noted. A child who is not easily distracted from pain during abdominal examination needs particular attention. The examiner focuses on the possible presence of masses, organomegaly, areas of tenderness, or guarding. Inspection of the perianal area should be part of the physical examination. The physician must decide to what extent investigative tests should be performed. A limited and reasonable screening includes a complete blood cell count, erythrocyte sedimentation rate or C-reactive protein measurement, urinalysis, and urine culture. A biochemical profile of kidney, liver, and pancreas functions may be performed at the discretion of the clinician. In certain cases, the history may justify requesting stool culture and examination for ova and parasites, and breath hydrogen testing for sugar malabsorption. Fecal calprotectin or lactoferrin determination may prove to be an attractive diagnostic tool to rule out the presence of mucosal inflammation [128, 129, 130]. In children who present with recurrent episodes of abdominal pain without suggestive alarms and symptoms, abdominal radiographs and ultrasound examination appear to be of little use [131]. In one study, ultrasound abnormalities were uncovered in less than 1% [132]. No data are presently available on the predictive value of blood tests in children using the previous Rome II criteria for FAP.

Abdominal wall pain caused by cutaneous nerve entrapment should be considered when severe pain can be elicited by light pinching of the skin in the affected area and the pain resolves completely after blockade of the cutaneous nerve in the abdominal wall [133].

— Physiological Features

The data on physiological mechanisms of FAP as defined by Rome II are very limited. Only one study has addressed this topic and the data consisted of negative findings [64]. In this study, patients were selected according to the Rome

II pediatric criteria for IBS and FAP. In contrast to eight children with IBS, eight children with FAP did not demonstrate visceral hypersensitivity in response to balloon distension of the rectum. This finding does not preclude the possibility that visceral hypersensitivity may exist more proximally in the gastrointestinal tract. In response to a water-load symptom provocation test, children with FAP (defined as abdominal pain of at least 3 months' duration without identifiable organic disease) reported significantly more gastrointestinal symptoms than healthy peers, a finding that could reflect either differences in sensory function or in symptom perception [134]. Much of our knowledge of the specific abdominal pain syndromes is extrapolated from children with RAP [55]. An increased prevalence of headache and limb pain has been found in children with RAP [135, 136]. In addition, some of these children were shown to have a lower pressure pain threshold [137]. It remains to be demonstrated whether these associated features are present in and restricted to children who meet the symptom-based Rome II criteria for FAP.

— Psychological Features

No studies have examined the psychological features of children with FAP as defined by the Rome criteria. To the extent that Apley's broad criteria for RAP include children who meet the more specific criteria for FAP, the frequent finding of anxiety and depression in children with RAP may also apply to children with FAP. Considerable evidence documents higher levels of anxiety and depression in patients with RAP compared to healthy community controls [74, 75, 138, 139, 140]. Furthermore, pediatric patients with RAP are at risk for anxiety and depression in adulthood [68, 141]. Several studies have reported higher levels of anxiety, depression, and somatization symptoms in parents of children with RAP compared to parents of well children [67, 140, 142]. There are also data to suggest that subjects with FAP who have additional somatic complaints more likely have significant psychosocial disturbances [143].

— Treatment

There are no studies on the management of children with abdominal pain that use the FAP criteria [29, 30]. The recommendation of a biopsychosocial approach to children with abdominal pain-related FGID is particularly relevant in the case of children with FAP. Indeed, as there are no specific treatment targets other than pain, it is very important to carefully investigate the possible contribution of psychosocial factors. Reassurance and a detailed explanation of possible mechanisms involving brain-gut interaction should be given to the child and parent. When consistent with the medical history, the possible roles of viral infection, psychosocial factors, or triggering events should be explained. Tricyclic antidepressants are sometimes useful but have not been empirically studied in children. In some children, pain can be severe enough to impair eating and school attendance. In one study, children who missed school or required tube feeding or parenteral alimentation for over 2 months were recruited to enter a rehabilitation program and treated for what the authors called "visceral pain-associated disability syndrome" [20]. The 40 patients met Rome II criteria for one or more functional disorders (15 FAP, 9 IBS, and 11 dyspepsia). Drug treatment and biopsychosocial management succeeded in helping 21 patients. Although no empirical research has been conducted on the behavioral treatment of FAP, two randomized controlled clinical trials have been conducted with children who met Apley's criteria for RAP [107, 144]. These cognitive-behavioral interventions had some success in reducing pain episodes in children with RAP and may be relevant more generally to children with FGIDs involving abdominal pain.

H3. Constipation and Incontinence
H3a. Functional Constipation

Most children with constipation do not have an organic disease responsible for their symptom. Instead, they suffer from functional constipation. Based on their different phenotypic presentation, the Rome II committee divided the non-organic forms of constipation into (1) infant dyschezia, (2) functional constipation, and (3) functional fecal retention (FFR). This subdivision was not evidence-based and engendered confusion, in view of the fact that most practitioners use the term "functional constipation" to describe *all* children in whom constipation does not have an organic etiology. There was also overlap between functional constipation and FFR, with patients likely transitioning from the first into the second condition. We now propose to merge the entities previously called "functional constipation" and "FFR" into one category named "*functional constipation.*"

Functional constipation is the most common cause of childhood constipation and fecal incontinence. It is most commonly caused by painful bowel movements with resultant voluntary withholding of feces by children who try to avoid an unpleasant defecation [145]. Withholding feces can lead to prolonged fecal stasis in the colon; consequently, the frequency of bowel movements per week decreases and there is an increase in size and hardness of the feces.

Fecal incontinence is the voluntary or involuntary passage of feces in the underwear or into socially inappropriate places in a child with a developmental age of at least 4 years [13, 146, 147]. It may be due to organic diseases or functional disorders and occurs in the majority of children with functional constipation. Based on characteristic clusters of symptoms, functional fecal incontinence should be classified as follows: (1) associated with fecal retention or (2) nonretentive fecal incontinence. The terms "encopresis" or "fecal soiling" have also been used extensively in the medical literature to describe the involuntary evacuation of stools. In different cultural environments, such as in the U.S. or in England, encopresis and soiling have different meanings. Thus, it was felt that the term *fecal incontinence* should be used whenever possible to avoid confusion or misunderstanding. Encopresis is a psychiatric term used in the Diagnostic and Statistic Manual (DSM). It has the disadvantage of being a medical term, and risks medicalizing a functional disorder that is often related to abnormal toilet learning. Soiling has a negative connotation (the child "being soiled") and is not easily accepted by some families.

— Epidemiology

Bowel frequency is influenced by diet, social habits, convenience, family cultural beliefs, relationships within the family, and daily time of activities. All these factors may vary in relation to psychological and physical development. A very early onset of constipation (before 6 months of age) and the presence of a family history of constipation could suggest a genetic tendency to develop functional constipation. In particular a positive family history has been found in 28% to 50% of constipated children and a higher incidence has been reported in monozygotic than dizygotic twins [70, 148, 149].

Estimates of constipation vary from 0.3% of the pediatric population to as high as 8% [150]. Approximately 3% to 5% of general pediatric outpatient visits and up to 25% of pediatric gastroenterology consultations reveal constipation as the chief complaint [151]. Using the Rome II criteria, functional constipation was diagnosed in 19.2% and 15.2% of children aged 4 to 9 years and 10 to 18 years respectively who received a diagnosis of FGID [24]. It has been reported that 34% of toddlers in the United Kingdom and 37% of Brazilian children younger than 12 years of age are considered constipated by their parents [152]. Peak incidence occurs at the time of toilet training, between 2 and 4 years of age [153]. In contrast to constipated adults, in children there seems to be a greater prevalence of constipation in boys [154]. Childhood constipation is distributed equally among social classes with no relationship to family size, ordinal position of the child in the family, or age of the parents. Obese children seem to be at higher risk for development of constipation and fecal soiling[155]. Most pediatric gastroenterologists estimate that 80% to 90% of defecation problems are due to functional constipation while nonretentive fecal incontinence, anatomic problems, and colonic neuromuscular disease account for the remaining defecation problems.

H3a. Diagnostic Criteria* for Functional Constipation

Must include *two or more* of the following in a child with a developmental age of at least 4 years with insufficient criteria for diagnosis of IBS:
1. **Two or fewer defecations in the toilet per week**
2. **At least one episode of fecal incontinence per week**
3. **History of retentive posturing or excessive volitional stool retention**
4. **History of painful or hard bowel movements**
5. **Presence of a large fecal mass in the rectum**
6. **History of large diameter stools which may obstruct the toilet**

*Criteria fulfilled at least once per week for at least 2 months prior to diagnosis

— Rationale for Change in Diagnostic Criteria

The change from 12 weeks to 2 months of symptoms is based both on clinical experience and data from the literature suggesting that the longer functional constipation goes unrecognized, the less successful is the treatment. Loening-Baucke studied the outcome in constipated young children (less than 4 years old) seen in a general pediatric practice and found that prognosis was more favorable when the referral had been made before the age of 2 years [150]. She also reported that recovery in encopretic children was associated with shorter duration of symptoms [145]. In addition, a recent long-term follow-up study of constipated children found a trend toward a diminished number of successfully treated children in those with a longer period of symptoms before referral to a subspecialty clinic [156].

In the previous diagnostic criteria for FFR *retentive posturing* was one of the two criteria that had to be present in order to make a diagnosis. It is now recommended that the history of retentive posturing or volitional stool retention be one of the six criteria for functional constipation, but without the requirement to be present in all subjects. Children who have been constipated for years may have had withholding behavior long before the visit to the physician. By the time they are evaluated the rectum has become dilated and has accommodated to the point that withholding is no longer necessary in order to delay the passage of stools. In other instances, the parents will deny withholding. Either they misinterpret the withholding for attempts to defecate, or they have not paid enough attention to the child's behavior to be able to describe it. It has been reported that 14% of parents of constipated children could not adequately answer questions regarding retentive posturing [157], and in a recent study, adolescents were not able to understand the concept of excessive withholding behavior [24]. In more than 20% of children older than 5 years presenting with incontinence due to constipation, parents do not report withholding behavior [145]. The term *excessive volitional stool retention* is used to describe older children who still withhold their stools without necessarily displaying retentive posturing.

Fecal incontinence (involuntary passage of fecal material in the underwear) is one of most common presentations of functional constipation and is found in up to 84% of children at presentation [157]. It causes a tremendous amount of distress for patients and their families. The two studies that have looked at the applicability of the Rome II criteria for FFR have both recommended fecal incontinence be incorporated in the revised criteria [145, 157]. Incontinence may be useful as an objective marker for the severity of functional constipation and in monitoring effectiveness of treatment [158]. A *painful bowel movement* has an important historical value in causing the retentive behavior [151].

The presence of a *large fecal mass* either before evacuation (recognized during the physical examination) or after having a bowel movement (obstructing the toilet or causing severe discomfort) is a critical feature of constipated children. The painful evacuation of such fecal mass often leads the terrified child to try to avoid further bowel movements. A large fecal mass in the rectum has been found in 98% of children fulfilling the previous Rome II criteria for FFR [145]. It is acknowledged that the mention of a "large" mass in the criteria introduces a subjective element that can be interpreted differently by different individuals. The mention of stools "clogging the toilet" represents an attempt to provide an objective measure of the size of the fecal mass.

— Clinical Evaluation

Functional constipation is a clinical diagnosis that can be made based on a typical history and physical examination. There are no well-designed studies that determine which aspects of a history are pertinent [159]. However, a careful history needs to elicit

- delayed passage of the initial bowel movement after birth
- the time of onset
- characteristics of the stools (frequency, consistency, caliber, volume)
- a history of a frightening defecation experience
- presence of associated symptoms (pain at defecation, abdominal pain, blood on the stool or the toilet paper, fecal incontinence)
- stool withholding behavior
- urinary problems
- neurological deficits

There are three periods when a child is particularly vulnerable to developing constipation: dietary transitions in infants (e.g., weaning from breast milk to formula or introduction of solid food), toilet training in toddlers, and start of school in children. All these events have the potential for making defecation an unpleasant experience resulting in fecal retention. Affected children are often described as standing on their toes, holding onto furniture, stiffening their legs, and hiding in a corner. Fecal incontinence may be mistaken for diarrhea by some parents. Urinary problems are occasionally observed in these children [160].

A thorough physical examination is recommended for the child who presents with constipation. The abdominal exam commonly identifies a fecal mass in the left lower quadrant and suprapubic region. External examination of the perineum and perianal area is essential. It is important to exclude signs of spinal dysraphism, such as the presence of sensory and motor deficits, a patulous anus, urinary incontinence, absent cremasteric reflex, pigmentary abnormalities, vascular nevi, and hair tufts in the sacrococcygeal area. Rectal examination is useful to assess muscle tone, stool consistency, amount of stool, presence of anatomic abnormalities, and size of rectal vault. Although controversy exists in regards to the necessity of a rectal examination during the initial and follow-up visits [161, 162], the medical position statement of the North American Society for Pediatric Gastroenterology and Nutrition recommends that the digital rectal examination should be performed at least once in a child presenting with constipation [159]. A moderate to large amount of stool found in the rectum has high sensitivity and positive predictive value (greater than 80%) for fecal retention as assessed by abdominal radiograph [163]. Consequently, an abdominal radiograph is not indicated to establish the presence of rectal impaction if the rectal examination reveals the presence of large amounts of stool. An x-ray can be useful in determining the presence of fecal retention in a child who is obese or who refuses a rectal examination. It should be noted that there seems to be a high interindividual variability among radiologists in assessing the presence of an "excessive" amount of stool in the colon [164].

Quantification of colonic transit time with radiopaque markers may be helpful in confirming the presence of constipation in cases lacking objective data [165]. However, when the history and the physical examination are typical of functional constipation no diagnostic testing is necessary. Anorectal manometry, suction rectal biopsies, barium enema, and colonic manometry may be indicated to diagnose organic causes of constipation.

— Physiological Features

Functional constipation often results from repeated attempts of voluntary withholding of feces to avoid unpleasant defecation because of fears associated with evacuation or because of social reasons. In the first years of life, an acute episode of constipation due to a change in diet may lead to the passage of dry and hard stools, which may cause painful defecation. In toddlers the onset of constipation may coincide with toilet training, when excessive parental pressure to maintain bowel control and/or use inappropriate techniques. The use of regular toilets that do not allow sufficient leverage (instead of a potty-chair) may lead to stool withholding. In children the start of school may coincide with a child's decision to suppress the defecatory urge in order to stay in class during school hours. Other causes of painful and frightening evacuation are allergic or infectious colitis, perianal infections, or fissures. Occasionally, the fear may be linked to a specific event associated with anxiety or pain, such as an episode of perianal streptococcal disease [166] or lichen sclerosus [167], sexual abuse [168], or even a horrifying television show or commercial [169]. Abnormal defecation dynamics or pelvic dyssynergia (the child contracts instead of relaxes the external anal sphincter and the pelvic floor), have been reported in 63% of children with chronic constipation [170].

When the child ignores the defecatory urge in anticipation of painful defecation, he or she creates a vicious cycle. Stools accumulate and chronically distend the rectum, dampening the sensory input normally elicited by the presence of feces. Over time, as water and electrolytes are reabsorbed, the fecal mass becomes too large and too firm to be extruded without great pain. Increasing fecal accumulation in the rectum causes decreased motility in the foregut leading to anorexia, abdominal distension, and abdominal pain [171]. There may be two mechanisms linked to the decreased appetite noted in constipated children: (1) gastric emptying is delayed by a full rectum and (2) a child may choose not to eat to avoid the onset of the colonic high amplitude propagating contraction usually induced by meal. When such contractions occur in the presence of a fecal mass, cramping abdominal pain ensues. As the fecal mass becomes too large and the pelvic floor muscle fatigues, the anal sphincter becomes less competent and any relaxation leads to fecal incontinence. Liquid stools arriving in the rectum encounter impacted stools and begin to seep around them. In most cases, the liquid stools are passed into the undergarment of the child.

— Psychological Features

When given a validated questionnaire, children presenting with constipation have lower quality-of-life scores than children presenting with gastroesophageal reflux or inflammatory bowel disease. The difference is particularly significant in the emotional and social domains [172]. Children with frequent incontinence exhibit poor self-esteem and social withdrawal [173]. All these characteristics are more likely to be secondary to the chronic struggle with defecation and bowel control rather than primary etiologic factors. In most cases, the fear of painful defecation is the cause for the fecal retention [174]. Indeed, constipated children display more anxiety related to toileting than well children or children with asthma [175]. Although fear of painful defecation is the initial cause, after several years affected children often evolve a coping style based on denial. School-aged children insist that they are unaware of the problem. They also frequently state that they are unaware that they are about to soil their underwear. This apparent nonchalance is part of the syndrome as the school-aged child attempts to avoid facing fears about defecation.

Parents may find themselves in a power struggle with their child concerning toilet learning. Toilet training may be initiated inappropriately early. It has been shown that initiation of intensive training before 27 months does not correlate with earlier completion of toilet training [176].

— Treatment

Education for both parents and child is the first step and probably the most important component of treatment, beginning during the initial interview. The child who is frightened and embarrassed appreciates a clinician with a direct approach. The clinician should address the myths and fears of children and parents. The child has functional constipation, which is the most common cause of childhood constipation and one of the most common problems in pediatrics. It is curable and it is not dangerous. Such statements decrease the child's and family's anxiety, and create an expectation for improvement. Next, parents need to be helped to understand the child's point of view. For toddlers, toilet training will not proceed smoothly until the child's fear of painful defecation resolves. Anxious parents must understand that coercive toilet training tactics are likely to backfire into a futile struggle for control. The clinician, child, and parent need to agree on a plan for evacuating the rectal fecal mass. Some experts favor daily oral agents, which slowly soften the mass until the child chooses to pass it, days or weeks later. There is evidence that a dose of 1 to 1.5 g/kg/day polyethylene glycol (PEG) 3350 for 3 days is effective in treating fecal impaction [177]. This developmentally sound, nonintrusive approach returns the control of the pelvic floor to the child. Many constipated toddlers are frightened of any anal manipulation, and find enemas particularly frightening. Other practitioners view the fecal mass as an obstruction, and favor enemas and stimulant laxatives to expedite its expulsion. They argue that early passage of the obstructing mass gives the child immediate relief and provides the confidence necessary for continuing toilet learning.

For maintenance, there are a variety of effective stool softeners [159]. A recent double-blinded, randomized, controlled study demonstrated that PEG 3350 provided a higher success rate with fewer side effects when compared with lactulose[178]. The authors recommended that PEG 3350 be the laxative of first choice in childhood constipation. Stimulant laxatives may be used to avoid buildup of a fecal mass and facilitate the expulsion of retained feces when stool softeners alone have failed. Although dietary fiber is important for a variety of reasons, fiber supplements are often not adequate as a single agent for consistent stool softening. The goal of stool softening is to assure painless defecation for every stool until the problem resolves. Despite the publication of guidelines for evaluation and treatment of constipated children [159], there is evidence that primary care physicians tend to undertreat childhood constipation [179].

Behavior modification utilizing rewards for successes in toilet learning is often helpful. A child may earn stars with each successful defecatory effort. Older children may ask for small amounts of money or special time with a parent, for example. Another behavior modification technique is to establish a daily routine for sitting on the commode. Sitting on the commode for 10 minutes after eating takes advantage of the gastrocolonic response, that is, the increase in colonic motility following a meal. Behavior modifications alone are successful in up to one third of encopretic children and lead to improvement in two thirds of them [180]. Several trials of biofeedback have concluded that, although this technique leads to normalization of defecation dynamics, it does not alter long-term outcome [181, 182].

Several long-term follow-up studies have shown that functional constipation, although a benign disorder, might be a long-lasting problem [156, 183, 184]. Approximately 60% of 418 Dutch children with functional constipation achieved a complete remission rate by 1 year. However, despite intensive initial medical and behavioral treatment, 30% to 50% of these children continued to have severe symptoms of constipation after 5 years of followup and constipation continued even beyond 18 years of age in approximately 20% [156, 183]. Furthermore, 50% of the Dutch children had a least one relapse within the first 5 years of initial treatment success. This underscores the need for frequent follow-up visits and prolonged medical treatment to prevent and monitor relapses. It should be acknowledged, however, that most of the children studied had presented with long-standing constipation to tertiary care centers.

H3b. Nonretentive Fecal Incontinence

The rationale for the use of the term "fecal incontinence" instead of soiling or encopresis was discussed in the previous section. It is believed that most cases of fecal incontinence are secondary to constipation. Levine [185] stated that virtually all children with encopresis retain stools. A more recent study, however, reported that one third of children referred for fecal incontinence showed no signs of constipation [186]. The latter patients were classified as functional nonretentive fecal soiling in the pediatric Rome II criteria.

— Definition

Nonretentive fecal incontinence represents the repeated, inappropriate passage of stool into a place other than the toilet, by a child older than 4 years [1, 146]. Fecal incontinence without fecal retention may occur in organic diseases such as colonic inflammation. Patients may be incontinent of stool because of damaged corticospinal pathways from any cause. This results in abnormal innervation of the rectum, with inability to maintain normal sphincter function. Progressive loss of function may also result from a spinal cord tumor or a tethered cord. Nonretentive fecal incontinence occurs after endorectal pull-through surgery, as high amplitude propagating ileal or colonic contractions push luminal contents directly through the anal sphincter because there is no rectosigmoid reservoir.

Functional nonretentive incontinence may be a manifestation of an emotional disturbance in a school-aged child and may represent impulsive action triggered by unconscious anger. Nonretentive incontinence has been reported in children with psychiatric morbidity, mental deficiency, learning disabilities, and behavioral problem. It can be a symptom of deep-rooted behavioral derangement. It has also been described as a sequel of sexual abuse in childhood.

— Epidemiology

Fecal incontinence is reported to be responsible for 3% of referrals to teaching hospitals. Its prevalence has been reported to be 4.1% in the 5-to-6 age group and 1.6% in the 11-to-12 age group in the Netherlands. Also it is noted to be more frequent among boys and children from families with lower socioeconomic status [187]. Interestingly, only 38% of the 5- to 6-year-olds and 27% of the 11- to 12-year-olds who had fecal incontinence had ever seen a physician for this problem. The prevalence of nonretentive fecal incontinence among these nonconsulters was not reported. Twenty-one percent of patients attending a subspecialty clinic fulfilled the Rome II criteria for functional nonretentive fecal incontinence [157].

H3b. Diagnostic Criteria* for Nonretentive Fecal Incontinence

Must include *all* of the following in a child with a developmental age at least 4 years:
1. **Defecation into places inappropriate to the social context at least once per month**
2. **No evidence of an inflammatory, anatomic, metabolic, or neoplastic process that explains the subject's symptoms**
3. **No evidence of fecal retention**

***Criteria fulfilled for at least 2 months prior to diagnosis**

— Rationale for Change in Diagnostic Criteria

The duration of symptoms to 2 months has been changed in agreement with the other Rome III pediatric criteria. The name of the condition has been modified from "soiling" to "incontinence" according to the rationale previously discussed.

— Clinical Evaluation

Most children with nonretentive fecal incontinence have bowel movements during waking hours and often pass stools in their undergarments. There are few complaints of associated constipation. The episodes of incontinence may be small in volume or consist of a large bowel movement. Pertinent items of information to be collected in the clinical history are [188]

- Stool pattern: size, consistency, interval
- History of constipation: age of onset
- History of fecal incontinence: age of onset, type, and amount of material
- Diet
- Abdominal pain
- Medications
- Urinary symptoms: enuresis, urinary tract infection
- Family history of defecatory disorders
- Family or personal stressors

Physical examination should emphasize the following features:

- Height and weight
- Abdominal examination: distention, mass (especially suprapubic)
- Rectal examination: sacral dimple, position of anus, anal fissures, sphincter tone, rectal vault size, presence or absence of stool in rectum, pelvic mass
- A thorough neurological examination

In children with nonretentive fecal incontinence, no fecal mass is found upon physical examination. Some clinicians believe it may be necessary to obtain an abdominal radiograph [163] before a diagnosis of occult fecal retention due to incomplete passage of stool is made.

— Physiological Features

Studies in patients with functional nonretentive fecal soiling have shown normal defecation frequencies, normal anorectal function on manometry, and normal colonic transit times. These suggest a different pathophysiological mechanism than that of patients with incontinence as a result of constipation. Identification of such children should be based on clinical symptoms—that is, normal defecation frequency and absence of abdominal or rectal palpable mass, normal marker studies, and normal anal manometric threshold of sensation. Benninga et al. [146] found that total and segmental colonic transit times were significantly prolonged in constipated children compared with children with nonretentive fecal incontinence. All manometric parameters were comparable between the two groups, except for a significantly higher threshold of sensation in children with functional constipation.

— Psychological Features

Incontinence along with several other behaviors (e.g., sloppiness, procrastination, lack of consideration for others) may occur in the child having a passive-aggressive relationship with his parents. Researchers from the Netherlands have recently shown [189] that children with functional nonretentive fecal incontinence have significantly more behavioral problems and more externalizing and internalizing problems than the local normative sample. Improvement of the fecal incontinence is associated with amelioration of the emotional disturbance [190].

— Treatment

Prospective, randomized, controlled trials of treatment options in children with nonretentive fecal incontinence are noticeably scarce and most current treatment protocols and guidelines have an intuitive or empirical basis [191]. Most treatment trials have not explicitly differentiated between the retentive form and the nonretentive form of incontinence. A recent review [192] showed no evidence to support the routine use of psychotherapy or anal sphincter biofeedback to treat pediatric fecal elimination dysfunctions. Nevertheless, there are benefits derived from a comprehensive medical-behavioral intervention. The same review indicated that paradoxical contraction of the external anal sphincter does not influence the treatment outcome of either biofeedback or medical-behavioral interventions. A multimodal treatment protocol in patients with functional nonretentive fecal incontinence comparing laxative treatment with and without biofeedback therapy showed poor clinical outcome in the two treatment groups at the end of the intervention period (39% and 19%, respectively) [190, 193]. One recent trial [193] concluded that laxatives seem to have no use in the treatment of children with functional nonretentive fecal incontinence in contrast to children with incontinence caused by constipation and that biofeedback training plays no or only a minor role in the treatment of these patients. Loperamide has been found to be helpful in one adolescent with nonretentive fecal incontinence [194].

One goal of treatment is to help the parents to acknowledge the absence of medical disease and to accept a referral to a mental health professional. The parents are often frustrated and angry at the child they view as exhibiting a willful oppositional behavior. Parents need guidance to understand that incontinence may be a symptom of emotional distress and represent a consequence of failed toilet training, rather than an intentional behavior. Education, a nonaccusatory approach, and regular toilet use with rewards are part of the therapeutic regimen [147]. Victims of sexual abuse should be referred for psychological services. These patients are more likely to have depression, anxiety disorders, behavioral problems, and post-traumatic stress disorder.

With regard to prognosis, it has been suggested that nonretentive incontinence may be a risk factor for persistent symptoms and that anorectal manometry findings are not useful to predict response to treatment [195, 196]. A recent long-term study showed that after 2 years of intensive medical and behavioral treatment, such as a strict toilet training program and biofeedback training, only 29% of the children were completely free of fecal incontinence. In contrast to children with constipation however, significantly fewer patients continued to have these problems beyond puberty [197].

Future Research

The committee identified several areas that are in need of research. Many of the recommendations listed by the Rome II committee remain valid [1]. Other future research topics in this area have recently been suggested by committees of several pediatric gastroenterology societies [198, 199].

1. Validation studies of the pediatric Rome criteria need to be developed. Such studies need to be performed in a wide range of clinical settings and patient populations using validated questionnaires. Specifically, the new proposed criteria for subgroups of dyspeptic disorders need to be studied in children.
2. Mechanistic studies will help us understand how clusters of symptoms may be related to different pathophysiological mechanisms, providing better targets for more tailored therapeutic interventions.
3. Large and well-designed studies need to be developed to assess the epidemiology and health care impacts of pediatric FGIDs.
4. The effect of early life events and intercurrent infections on the development of pediatric and adult FGIDs will need further investigation.
5. The interaction between the central nervous system, enteric nervous system, and immune system needs to be explored.
6. Studies are needed to explore the effects of different FGID treatments on quality of life.
7. Using standardized diagnostic criteria, multisite intervention studies of current and emerging pharmacological agents need to be completed.
8. Cohort studies need to address the natural history of pediatric FGIDs.

Acknowledgments

The members of the Rome III Pediatric Child/Adolescent committee thank the members of The Paris Consensus on Childhood Constipation Terminology (PACCT) group for their insightful suggestions regarding the definitions of pediatric disorders of defecations [200].

References

1. Rasquin-Weber A, Hyman PE, Cucchiara S, Fleisher DR, Hyams JS, Milla PJ, Staiano A. Childhood functional gastrointestinal disorders. Gut 1999;45 Suppl 2:II60–8.
2. Amnarath R, Abell T, Malagaleda J-R. The rumination syndrome in adults. Ann Int Med 1986;105:513–518.
3. O'Brien MD, Bruce BK, Camilleri M. The rumination syndrome: clinical features rather than manometric diagnosis. Gastroenterology 1995;108:1024–1029.
4. Fleisher DR. Functional vomiting disorders in infancy: innocent vomiting, nervous vomiting, and infant rumination syndrome. J Pediatr 1994;125:S84–S94.
5. Khan S, Hyman PE, Cocjin J, Di Lorenzo C. Rumination syndrome in adolescents. J Pediatr 2000;136:528–31.
6. Chial HJ, Camilleri M, Williams DE, Litzinger K, Perrault J. Rumination syndrome in children and adolescents: diagnosis, treatment, and prognosis. Pediatrics 2003; 111:158–162.
7. Levine DF, Wingate DL, Pfeffer JM, Butcher P. Habitual rumination: a benign disorder. Br Med J (Clin Res Ed) 1983;287:256–257.
8. Mayes S, Humphrey F, Handford H, Mitchell J. Rumination disorder: differential diagnosis. J Am Acad Child Adolesc Psychiatry 1988;27:300–302.
9. Sullivan PB. Gastrointestinal problems in the neurologically impaired child. Baillieres Clin Gastroenterol 1997;11:529–546.
10. Whitehead WE, Drescher VM, Morrill-Corbin E, Cataldo MF. Rumination syndrome in children treated by increased holding. J Pediatr Gastroenterol Nutr 1985; 4:550–556.
11. Alexander RC, Greenswag LR, Nowak AJ. Rumination and vomiting in Prader-Willi syndrome. Am J Med Genet 1987;24:889–895.
12. Eckern M, Stevens W, Mitchell J. The relationship between rumination and eating disorders. International Journal of Eating Disorders 1999;26:414–419.
13. American Psychiatric Association. Diagnostic and Statistical Manual of Mental Disorders. Fourth ed. Washington, DC 1994.
14. Clouse RE, Richter JE, Heading RC, Janssens J, Wilson JA. Functional esophageal disorders. Gut 1999;45(Suppl 2):II31–6.
15. Thumshirn M, Camilleri M., Hanson RB, Williams DE, Schei AJ, Kammer PP. Gastric mechanosensory and lower esophageal sphincter function in rumination syndrome. Am J Physiol Gastrointest Liver Physiol 1998;275(2 Pt 1):G314–321.
16. Fleisher DR. Infant rumination syndrome: report of a case and review of the literature. Am J Dis Child 1979;133:266–269.
17. Wagaman JR, Williams DE, Camilleri M. Behavioral intervention for the treatment of rumination. J Pediatr Gastroenterol Nutr 1998;27:596–598.
18. Sokel B, Devane S, Bentovim A, Milla P. Self hypnotherapeutic treatment of habitual reflex vomiting. Arch Dis Child 1990;65:626–627.
19. Oelschlager BK, Chan MM, Eubanks TR, Pope II CE, Pellegrini C. Effective treatment of rumination with Nissen fundoplication. J Gastrointest Surg 2002;6:638–644.
20. Hyman PE, Bursch B, Sood M, Schwankovsky L, Cocjin J, Zeltzer LK. Visceral pain-associated disability syndrome: a descriptive analysis. Journal of Pediatric Gastroenterology & Nutrition. 2002;35:663–8.

21. Loening-Baucke V. Aerophagia as cause of gaseous abdominal distention in a toddler. J Pediatr Gastroenterol Nutr 2000;31:204–207.
22. Lecine T, Michaud L, Gottrand F, al. e. Les enfants avaleurs d'air. Arch Pediatr 1998; 5:1224–1228.
23. Gauderer MW, Halpin Jr TC, Izant Jr. RJ. Pathologic childhood aerophagia: a recognizable clinical entity. J Pediatr Surg 1981;16:301–305.
24. Caplan A, Walker LS, Rasquin-Weber A. Validation of the pediatric Rome II criteria for functional gastrointestinal disorders using the questionnaire on pediatric gastrointestinal symptoms. J Pediatr Gastroenterol Nutr 2005 41:305–316.
25. Lasser RB, Bond JH, Levitt MD. The role of intestinal gas in functional abdominal pain. N Engl J Med 1976;293:524–526.
26. Sferra TJ, Heitlinger LA. Gastrointestinal gas formation and infantile colic. Pediatr Clin North Am 1996;43:489–510.
27. Barrett RP, McGonigle JJ, Ackles PK. ea. Behavioral treatment of chronic aerophagia. Am J Ment Def 1987;91:620–625.
28. Holburn CS, Dougher MJ. Behavioral attempts to eliminate air-swallowing in two profoundly mentally retarded clients. Am J Ment Def 1985;89:524–536.
29. Di Lorenzo C, Colletti RB, Lehmann HP, Boyle JT, Gerson WT, Hyams JS, Squires RH, Jr., Walker LS, Kanda PT. Chronic Abdominal Pain In Children: a Technical Report of the American Academy of Pediatrics and the North American Society for Pediatric Gastroenterology, Hepatology and Nutrition. J Pediatr Gastroenterol Nutr 2005;40:249–61.
30. Di Lorenzo C, Colletti RB, Lehmann HP, Boyle JT, Gerson WT, Hyams JS, Squires RH, Jr., Walker LS, Kanda PT. Chronic abdominal pain in children: a clinical report of the American Academy of Pediatrics and the North American Society for Pediatric Gastroenterology, Hepatology and Nutrition. J Pediatr Gastroenterol Nutr 2005;40:245–8.
31. Hyams JS, Davis P, Sylvester FA, Zeiter DK, Justinich CJ, Lerer T. Dyspepsia in children and adolescents: a prospective study. J Pediatr Gastroenterol Nutr 2000;30: 413–8.
32. Sigurdsson L, Flores A, Putnam PE, Hyman PE, Di Lorenzo C. Postviral gastroparesis: presentation, treatment, and outcome. Journal of Pediatrics. 1997;131:751–4.
33. Hyams JS, Burke G, Davis PM, Rzepski B, Andrulonis PA. Abdominal pain and irritable bowel syndrome in adolescents: a community-based study. J Pediatr 1996;129: 220–6.
34. Reshetnikov OV, Kurilovich SA, Denisova DV, Zav'ialova LG, Svetlova IO, Tereshonok IN, Krivenchuk NA, Eremeeva LI. [Prevalence and risk factors of the development of irritable bowel syndrome in adolescents: a population study]. Ter Arkh 2001;73:24–9.
35. De Giacomo C, Valdambrini V, Lizzoli F, Gissi A, Palestra M, Tinelli C, Zagari M, Bazzoli F. A population-based survey on gastrointestinal tract symptoms and Helicobacter pylori infection in children and adolescents. Helicobacter 2002;7:356–363.
36. Miele E, Simeone D, Marino A, Greco L, Auricchio R, Novek SJ, Staiano A. Functional gastrointestinal disorders in children: an Italian prospective survey. Pediatrics 2004;114:73–8.
37. Walker LS, Lipani TA, Greene JW, Caines K, Stutts J, Polk DB, Caplan A, Rasquin-Weber A. Recurrent Abdominal Pain: Symptom Subtypes Based on the Rome II Criteria for Pediatric Functional Gastrointestinal Disorders. J Pediatr Gastroenterol Nutr 2004;38:187–191.

38. Mayer EA, Collins SM. Evolving pathophysiologic models of functional gastrointestinal disorders. Gastroenterology 2002;122:2032–2048.

39. Graham DY, Malaty HM, Evans DG, Evans DJJ, Klein PD, Adam E. Epidemiology of Helicobacter pylori in an asymptomatic population in the United States. Effect of age, race, and socioeconomic status. Gastroenterology 1991;100:1495–1501.

40. Drumm B, Rowland M. The epidemiology of Helicobacter pylori: where to from here? J Pediatr Gastroenterol Nutr 2003;36:7–8.

41. Cotte-Roche C, Roche H, Chaussade S, Dupouy-Camet J, Tulliez M, Couturier D, Guerre J. [Role of giardiasis in non-ulcer dyspepsia]. Presse Med. 1991;25:936–938.

42. Gold BD, Colletti RB, Abbott M, Czinn SJ, Elitsur Y, Hassall E, Macarthur C, Snyder J, Sherman PM, The North American Society for Pediatric G, Nutrition. Helicobacter pylori infection in children: recommendations for diagnosis and treatment. J Pediatr Gastroenterol Nutr 2000;31:490–7.

43. Kalach N, Mention K, Guimber D, Michaud L, Spyckerelle C, Gottrand F. Helicobacter pylori infection is not associated with specific symptoms in nonulcer-dyspeptic children. Pediatrics 2005;115:17–21.

44. Cucchiara S, Riezzo G, Minella R, Pezzolla F, Giorgio I, Auricchio S. Electrogastrography in non-ulcer dyspepsia. Arch Dis Child 1992;67:613–617.

45. Chen JD, Lin X, Zhang M, al. e. Gastric myoelectrical activity in healthy children and children with functional dyspepsia. Dig Dis Sci 1998;43:2384–2391.

46. Cucchiara S, Minella R, Riezzo G, Vallone G, Vallone. P., Castellone F, Auricchio S. Reversal of gastric electrical dysrhythmias by cisapride in children with functional dyspepsia. Report of three cases. Dig Dis Sci 1992;37:1136–1140.

47. Riezzo G, Chiloiro M, Guerra V, Borrelli O, Salvia G, Cucchiara S. Comparison of gastric electrical activity and gastric emptying in healthy and dyspeptic children. Dig Dis Sci 2000;45:517–524.

48. Barbar M, Steffen R, Wyllie R, Goske M. Electrogastrography versus gastric emptying scintigraphy in children with symptoms suggestive of gastric motility disorders. J Pediatr Gastroenterol Nutr 2000;30:193–197.

49. Di Lorenzo C, Hyman PE, Flores AF, Kashyap P, Tomomasa T, Lo S, Snape WJ, Jr. Antroduodenal manometry in children and adults with severe non-ulcer dyspepsia.[erratum appears in Scand J Gastroenterol 1994 Dec;29(12):preceding 1057]. Scandinavian Journal of Gastroenterology. 1994;29:799–806.

50. Chitkara DK, Delgado-Aros S, Bredenoord AJ, Cremonini F, El-Youssef M, Freese D, Camilleri M. Functional dyspepsia, upper gastrointestinal symptoms, and transit in children. J Pediatr 2003;149:609–613.

51. Tack J, Caenepeel P, Fischler B, Piessevaux H, Janssens J. Symptoms associated with hypersensitivity to gastric distention in functional dyspepsia. Gastroenterology 2001;121:526–35.

52. See MC, Birnbaum AH, Schechter CB, Goldenberg MM, Benkov KJ. Double-blind, placebo-controlled trial of famotidine in children with abdominal pain and dyspepsia: global and quantitative assessment. Dig Dis Sci 2001;46:985–92.

53. Friesen CA, Kearns GL, Andre L, Neustrom M, Roberts CC, Abdel-Rahman SM. Clinical efficacy and pharmacokinetics of montelukast in dyspeptic children with duodenal eosinophilia. J Pediatr Gastroenterol Nutr 2004;38:343–51.

54. Thompson WG, Heaton KW, Smyth GT, C. S. Irritable bowel syndrome in general practice: prevalence, characteristics, and referral. Gut 2000;46:78–82.

55. Apley J, Naish N. Recurrent abdominal pain: a field survey of 1000 school children. Arch Dis Child 1958;33:165–70.

56. Boey C, Yap S, Goh KL. The prevalence of recurrent abdominal pain in 11- to 16-year-old Malaysian schoolchildren. J Paediatr Child Health 2000;36:114–6.

57. Cullen KJ, MacDonald WB. The periodic syndrome: its nature and prevalence. Med J Aust 1963;50:167–73.

58. Oster J. Recurrent abdominal pain, headache and limb pains in children and adolescents. Pediatrics 1972;50:429–36.

59. Mendall MA, Kumar D. Antibiotic use, childhood affluence and irritable bowel syndrome (IBS). Eur J Gastroenterol Hepatol 1998;10:59–62.

60. Hyams JS, Treem WR, Justinich CJ, Davis P, Shoup M, Burke G. Characterization of symptoms in children with recurrent abdominal pain: resemblance to irritable bowel syndrome [see comments]. J Pediatr Gastroenterol Nutr 1995;20:209–14.

61. Croffie JM, Fitzgerald JF, Chong SK. Recurrent abdominal pain in children—a retrospective study of outcome in a group referred to a pediatric gastroenterology practice. Clin Pediatr (Phila) 2000;39:267–74.

62. Miele E, Simeone D, Marino A, Greco L, Auricchio R, Novek SJ, Staiano A. Functional gastrointestinal disorders in children: an Italian prospective survey. Pediatrics 2004;114:73–78.

63. Caplan A, Walker LS, Rasquin A. Development and preliminary validation of the questionnaire on pediatric gastrointestinal symptoms to assess functional gastrointestinal disorders in children and adolescents. J Pediatr Gastroenterol Nutr 2005; 41:296–304.

64. Van Ginkel R, Voskuijl WP, Benninga MA, Taminiau JA, Boeckxstaens GE. Alterations in rectal sensitivity and motility in childhood irritable bowel syndrome. Gastroenterology 2001;120:31–8.

65. Di Lorenzo C, Youssef NN, Sigurdsson L, Scharff L, Griffiths J, Wald A. Visceral hyperalgesia in children with functional abdominal pain. J Pediatr 2001;139:838–43.

66. Walker LS, Guite JW, Duke M, Barnard JA, Greene JW. Recurrent abdominal pain: a potential precursor of irritable bowel syndrome in adolescents and young adults. J Pediatr 1998;132:1010–5.

67. Campo JV, Di Lorenzo C, Chiappetta L, Bridge J, Colborn DK, Gartner JC, Jr., Gaffney P, Kocoshis S, Brent D. Adult outcomes of pediatric recurrent abdominal pain: do they just grow out of it? Pediatrics 2001;108:E1.

68. Hotopf M, Carr S, Mayou R, Wadsworth M, Wessely S. Why do children have chronic abdominal pain, and what happens to them when they grow up? Population based cohort study [see comments]. BMJ 1998;316:1196–200.

69. Levy RL, Jones KR, Whitehead WE, Feld SI, Talley NJ, Corey LA. Irritable bowel syndrome in twins: heredity and social learning both contribute to etiology. Gastroenterology. 2001;121:799–804.

70. Morris-Yates A, Talley NJ, Boyce PM, Nandurkar S, Andrews G. Evidence of a genetic contribution to functional bowel disorder. Am J Gastroenterol 1998;93:1311–7.

71. Pineiro-Carrero VM, Andres JM, Davis RH, Mathias JR. Abnormal gastroduodenal motility in children and adolescents with recurrent functional abdominal pain. J Pediatr 1988;113:820–5.

72. Alfven G, Uvnas-Moberg K. Elevated cholecystokinin concentrations in plasma in children with recurrent abdominal pain. Acta Paediatr 1993;82:967–70.

73. Chelimsky G, Boyle JT, Tusing L, Chelimsky TC. Autonomic abnormalities in children with functional abdominal pain: coincidence or etiology? J Pediatr Gastroenterol Nutr 2001;33:47–53.

74. Dorn LD, Campo JC, Thato S, Dahl RE, Lewin D, Chandra R. DLC. Psychological co-

morbidity and stress reactivity in children and adolescents with recurrent abdominal pain and anxiety disorders. J Am Acad Child Adolesc Psychiatry 2003;42:66–75.

75. Walker LS, Garber J, Greene JW. Psychosocial correlates of recurrent childhood pain: a comparison of pediatric patients with recurrent abdominal pain, organic illness, and psychiatric disorders. J Abnorm Psychol 1993;102:248–58.

76. Walker LS, Claar RL, Garber J. Social consequences of children's pain: when do they encourage symptom maintenance? J Pediatr Psychol 2002;27:689–698.

77. Bouin M, Plourde V, Boivin M, Riberdy M, Lupien F, Laganiere M, Verrier P, Poitras P. Rectal distention testing in patients with irritable bowel syndrome: sensitivity, specificity, and predictive values of pain sensory thresholds. Gastroenterology 2002;122:1771–1777.

78. Milla PJ. Irritable bowel syndrome in childhood. Gastroenterology 2001;120:287–290.

79. Talley NJ, Spiller R. Irritable bowel syndrome: a little understood organic bowel disease? Lancet. 2002;360:555–64.

80. Gwee KA. Postinfectious Irritable Bowel Syndrome. 2001;4:287–291.

81. Drossman DA, Camilleri M, Mayer EA, Whitehead WE. AGA technical review on irritable bowel syndrome. Gastroenterology. 2002;123:2108–31.

82. Al Chaer ED, Kawasaki M, Pasricha PJ. A new model of chronic visceral hypersensitivity in adult rats induced by colon irritation during postnatal development. Gastroenterology 2000;119:1276–1285.

83. Coutinho SV, Plotsky PM, Sablad M, Miller JC, Zhou H, Bayati AI, McRoberts JA, Mayer EA. Neonatal maternal separation alters stress-induced responses to viscerosomatic nociceptive stimuli in rat. Am J Physiol Gastrointest Liver Physiol 2002;282: G307–G316.

84. Hazlett-Stevens H, Craske MG, Mayer EA, Chang L, Naliboff BD. Prevalence of irritable bowel syndrome among university students. The roles of worry, neuroticism, anxiety sensitivity and visceral anxiety. J Psychosom Res 2003;55:501–505.

85. Anand KJ, Runeson B, Jacobson B. Gastric suction at birth associated with long-term risk for functional intestinal disorders in later life. J Pediatr 2004;144:449–454.

86. Caplan A, Lambrette P, Joly L, Bouin M, Boivin M, Rasquin A. Intergenerational transmission of functional gastrointestinal disorders: children of IBS patients versus children with IBS, functional dyspepsia and functional abdominal pain. Gastroenterology 2003;124:A-533.

87. Claar RL, Walker LS, Smith CA. Functional disability in adolescents and young adults with symptoms of irritable bowel syndrome: the role of academic, social, and athletic competence. J Pediatr Psychol 1999;24:271–80.

88. Levy RL, Whitehead WE, Walker LS, Von Korff M, Feld AD, Garner M, Christie D. Increased Somatic Complaints and Health-Care Utilization in Children: Effects of Parent IBS Status and Parent Response to Gastrointestinal Symptoms. Am J Gastroenterol 2004;99:2442–51.

89. Hyams JS, Hyman PE. Recurrent abdominal pain and the biopsychosocial model of medical practice [see comments]. J Pediatr 1998;133:473–8.

90. Mein SM, Ladabaum U. Serological testing for coeliac disease in patients with symptoms of irritable bowel syndrome: a cost-effectiveness analysis. Aliment Pharmacol Ther 2004;19:1199–210.

91. Zeiter DK, Hyams JS. Recurrent abdominal pain in children. Pediatr Clin North Am 2002;49:53–71.

92. Eccleston C, Yorke L, Morley S, Williams AC, Mastroyannopoulou K. Psychological therapies for the management of chronic and recurrent pain in children and adolescents. Cochrane Database Syst Rev 2003:CD003968.

93. Huertas-Ceballos A, Macarthur C, Logan S. Pharmacological interventions for recurrent abdominal pain (RAP) in childhood. Cochrane Database Syst Rev 2002: CD003017.

94. Huertas-Ceballos A, Macarthur C, Logan S. Dietary interventions for recurrent abdominal pain (RAP) in childhood. Cochrane Database Syst Rev 2002: CD003019.

95. Weydert J, Ball T, Davis M. Systematic review of treatments for recurrent abdominal pain. Pediatrics 2003;111:e1–11.

96. Bursch B, Walco GA, Zeltzer L. Clinical assessment and management of chronic pain and pain-associated disability syndrome. J Dev Behav Pediatr 1998;19:45–53.

97. Owens DM, Nelson DK, Talley NJ. The irritable bowel syndrome: long-term prognosis and the physician-patient interaction.[comment]. Annals of Internal Medicine. 1995;122:107–12.

98. Ilnyckyj A, Graff LA, Blanchard JF, Bernstein CN. Therapeutic value of a gastroenterology consultation in irritable bowel syndrome. Aliment Pharmacol Ther 2003; 17:871–880.

99. Christensen MF. Recurrent abdominal pain and dietary fiber. Am J Dis Child 1986; 140:738–739.

100. Feldman W, McGrath P, Hodgson C, Ritter H, Shipman RT. The use of dietary fiber in the management of simple, childhood, idiopathic, recurrent, abdominal pain. Results in a prospective, double-blind, randomized, controlled trial. Am J Dis Child 1985;139:1216–8.

101. Humphreys PA, Gevirtz RN. Treatment of recurrent abdominal pain: components analysis of four treatment protocols. J Pediatr Gastroenterol Nutr 2000;31:47–51.

102. Talley NJ. Pharmacologic therapy for the irritable bowel syndrome. American Journal of Gastroenterology. 2003;98:750–8.

103. Greenbaum DS, Mayle JE, Vanegeren LE, Jerome JA, Mayor JW, Greenbaum RB, Matson RW, Stein GE, Dean HA, Halvorsen NA. Effects of desipramine on irritable bowel syndrome compared with atropine and placebo. Dig Dis Sci 1987;32: 257–266.

104. Drossman DA, Toner BB, Whitehead WE, Diamant NE, Dalton CB, Duncan S, Emmott S, Proffitt V, Akman D, Frusciante K, Le T, Meyer K, Bradshaw B, Mikula K, Morris CB, Blackman CJ, Hu Y, Jia H, Li JZ, Koch GG, Bangdiwala SI. Cognitive-behavioral therapy versus education and desipramine versus placebo for moderate to severe functional bowel disorders. Gastroenterology 2003;125:19–31.

105. Kline RM, Kline JJ, Di Palma J, Barbero GJ. Enteric-coated, pH-dependent peppermint oil capsules for the treatment of irritable bowel syndrome in children. J Pediatr 2001;138:125–8.

106. Blanchard EB, Scharff L. Psychosocial aspects of assessment and treatment of irritable bowel syndrome in adults and recurrent abdominal pain in children. J Consult Clin Psychol 2002;70:725–738.

107. Sanders MR, Shepherd RW, Cleghorn G, Woolford H. The treatment of recurrent abdominal pain in children: a controlled comparison of cognitive-behavioral family intervention and standard pediatric care. J Consult Clin Psychol 1994;62:306–14.

108. Youssef NN, Rosh JR, Loughran M, Schuckalo SG, Cotter AN, Verga BG, Mones RL. Treatment of functional abdominal pain in childhood with cognitive behavioral strategies. J Pediatr Gastroenterol Nutr 2004;39:192–6.

109. Camilleri M. Serotonergic modulation of visceral sensation: lower gut. Gut 2002;51 Suppl 1:i81–6.

110. Buchanan JA. The abdominal crises of migraine. J Nerv Ment Dis 1921;54:406–412.

111. Brams WA. Abdominal migraine. JAMA 1922;78:26–27.

112. Symon DN, Russell G. Abdominal migraine: a childhood syndrome defined. Cephalalgia 1986;6:223–8.

113. Mortimer MJ, Kay J, Jaron A. Clinical epidemiology of childhood abdominal migraine in an urban general practice. Dev Med Child Neurol 1993;35:243–8.

114. Long DE, Jones SC, Boyd N, al. e. Abdominal migraine: a cause of abdominal pain in adults. J Gastroenterol Hepatol 1992;7:210–213.

115. Wyllie WG, Schlesinger B. The periodic group of disorders in childhood. Br J Child Dis 1933;30:1–21.

116. Li BUK, Balint JP. Cyclic vomiting syndrome: evolution in our understanding of a brain-gut disorder. Adv Pediatr 2000;47:117–160.

117. Abu-Arafeh I, Russell G. Prevalence and clinical features of abdominal migraine compared with those of migraine headache. Arch Dis Child 1995;72:413–7.

118. Dignan F, Abu-Arafeh I, Russell G. The prognosis of childhood abdominal migraine. Arch Dis Child 2001;84:415–418.

119. Mortimer MJ, Good PA. The visual-evoked response as a diagnostic marker for childhood abdominal migraine. Headache 1990;30:642–645.

120. Good PA. Neurologic investigations of childhood abdominal migraine: a combined elecrophysiologic approach to diagnosis. J Pediatr Gastroenterol Nutr 1995;Suppl 1: S44–S48.

121. Withers G, Silburn ST, Forbes DA. Precipitants and etiology of cyclic vomiting syndrome. Acta Paediatr 1998;87:272–277.

122. Hammond J. The late sequelae of recurrent vomiting. Dev Med Child Neurol 1974; 16:15–22.

123. Russell G, Abu-Arafeh I, Symon DNK. Abdominal migraine. Evidence for existence and treatment options. Pediatr Drugs 2002;4:1–8.

124. Symon DN, Russell G. Double blind placebo controlled trial of pizotifen syrup in the treatment of abdominal migraine [see comments]. Arch Dis Child 1995;72:48–50.

125. Worawattanakul M, Rhoads JM, Lichtman SN, Ulshen MH. Abdominal migraine: prophylactic treatment and follow-up. J Pediatr Gastroenterol Nutr 1999;28:37–40.

126. Drossman DA, Li Z, Andruzzi E, Temple RD, Talley NJ, Thompson WG, Whitehead WE, Janssens J, Funch-Jensen P, Corazziari E, et al. U.S. householder survey of functional gastrointestinal disorders. Prevalence, sociodemography, and health impact. Dig Dis Sci 1993;38:1569–80.

127. von Baeyer CL, Walker LS. Children with recurrent abdominal pain: issues in the selection and description of research participants [see comments]. J Dev Behav Pediatr 1999;20:307–13.

128. Carroccio A, Iacono G, Cottone M, Di Prima L, Cartabellotta F, Cavataio F, Scalici C, Montalto G, Di Fede G, Rini G, Notarbartolo A, Averna M. Diagnostic accuracy of fecal calprotectin assay in distinguishing organic causes of chronic diarrhea from irritable bowel syndrome: a prospective study in adults and children. Clin Chem 2003;49:861–867.

129. Olafsdottir E, Aksnes L, Fluge G, Berstad A. Faecal calprotectin levels in infants with infantile colic, healthy infants, children with inflammatory bowel disease, chil-

dren with recurrent abdominal pain and healthy children. Acta Paediatr 2002;91: 45–50.

130. Kane SV, Sandborn WJ, Rufo PA, Zholudev A, Boone J, Lyerly D, Camilleri M, Hanauer SB. Fecal lactoferrin is a sensitive and specific marker in identifying intestinal inflammation. Am J Gastroenterol 2003;98:1309–14.

131. Shanon A, Martin DJ, Feldman W. Ultrasonographic studies in the management of recurrent abdominal pain. Pediatrics 1990;86:35–8.

132. Yip WC, Ho TF, Yip YY, Chan KY. Value of abdominal sonography in the assessment of children with abdominal pain. J Clin Ultrasound 1998;26:397–400.

133. Peleg R. Abdominal wall pain caused by cutaneous nerve entrapment in an adolescent girl taking oral contraceptive pills. J Adolesc Health 1999;24:45–7.

134. Walker LS, Williams SE, Smith CA, Garber J, Van Slyke DA, Lipani TA, Greene JW, Mertz H, Naliboff B. Validation of a symptom provocation test for laboratory studies of abdominal pain and discomfort in children and adolescents. J Pediatr Psychol 2005 (in press).

135. Perquin CW, Hazebroek-Kampschreur AA, Hunfeld JA, Bohnen AM, van Suijlekom-Smit LW, Passchier J, van der Wouden JC. Pain in children and adolescents: a common experience. Pain 2000;87:51–8.

136. Alfven G. One hundred cases of recurrent abdominal pain in children: diagnostic procedures and criteria for a psychosomatic diagnosis. Acta Paediatr 2003;92:43–49.

137. Duarte MA, Goulart EM, Penna FJ. Pressure pain threshold in children with recurrent abdominal pain. J Pediatr Gastroenterol Nutr 2000;31:280–5.

138. Garber J, Zeman J, Walker LS. Recurrent abdominal pain in children: psychiatric diagnoses and parental psychopathology. J Am Acad Child Adolesc Psychiatry 1990;29:648–56.

139. Wasserman A, Whitington P, Rivara F. Psychogenic basis for abdominal pain in children and adolescents. J Am Acad Child Adolesc Psychiatry. 1988;27:179–84.

140. Walker LS, Greene JW. Children with recurrent abdominal pain and their parents: more somatic complaints, anxiety, and depression than other patient families? J Pediatr Psychol 1989;14:231–43.

141. Hodges K, Kline JJ, Barbero G, Woodruff C. Anxiety in children with recurrent abdominal pain and their parents. Psychosomatics 1985;26:859, 862–6.

142. Hodges K, Kline JJ, Barbero G, Flanery R. Depressive symptoms in children with recurrent abdominal pain and in their families. J Pediatr 1985;107:622–6.

143. Little CA, Williams SE, Walker LS. Depression influences symptom presentation in pediatric patients with recurrent abdominal pain. J Pediatr Gastroenterol Nutr 2004;39:S372.

144. Sanders MR, Rebgetz M, Morrison M, Bor W, Gordon A, Dadds M, Shepherd R. Cognitive-behavioral treatment of recurrent nonspecific abdominal pain in children: an analysis of generalization, maintenance, and side effects. J Consult Clin Psychol 1989;57:294–300.

145. Loening-Baucke V. Functional fecal retention with encopresis in childhood. J Pediatr Gastroenterol Nutr 2004;38:79–84.

146. Benninga MA, Buller HA, Heymans HS, Tytgat GN, Taminiau JA. Is encopresis always the result of constipation? Arch Dis Child 1994;71:186–93.

147. Loening-Baucke V. Encopresis. Curr Opin Pediatr 2002;14:570–5.

148. Abrahamian FP, Lloyd-Still JD. Chronic constipation in childhood: a longitudinal study of 186 patients. J Pediatr Gastroenterol Nutr 1984;3:460–7.

149. Bakwin H, Davidson M. Constipation in twins. Am J Dis Child 1971;121:179–181.

150. Loening-Baucke V. Constipation in early childhood: patient characteristics, treatment, and longterm follow up. Gut 1993;34:1400–4.

151. Partin JC, Hamil SK, Fischel JE, Partin JS. Painful defecation and fecal soiling in children. Pediatrics 1992;89:1007–1009.

152. Loening-Baucke V. Constipation in children. N Engl J Med 1998;339:1155–6.

153. Loening-Baucke V. Chronic constipation in children. Gastroenterology 1993;105: 1557–64.

154. Di Lorenzo C. Pediatric anorectal disorders. Gastroenterol Clin North Am 2001; 30:269–87.

155. Fishman L, Lenders C, Fortunato C, Noonan C, Nurko S. Increased prevalence of constipation and fecal soiling in a population of obese children. J Pediatr 2004;145: 253–4.

156. van Ginkel R, Reitsma JB, Buller HA, van Wijk MP, Taminiau JA, Benninga MA. Childhood constipation: longitudinal follow-up beyond puberty. Gastroenterology. 2003;125:357–63.

157. Voskuijl WP, Heijmans J, Heijmans HAS, Taminiau AJM, Benninga MA. Use of Rome II criteria in childhood defecation disorders; applicability in clinical and research practice. J Pediatr 2004;145:213–217.

158. van der Plas RN, Benninga MA, Redekop WK, Taminiau JA, Buller HA. How accurate is the recall of bowel habits in children with defaecation disorders? Eur J Pediatr. 1997;156:178–81.

159. Baker SS, Liptak GS, Colletti RB, Croffie JM, Di Lorenzo C, Ector W, Nurko S. Constipation in infants and children: evaluation and treatment. J Pediatr Gastroenterol Nutr 1999;29:612–26.

160. Loening-Baucke V. Urinary incontinence and urinary tract infection and their resolution with treatment of chronic constipation of childhood. Pediatrics 1997;100: 228–32.

161. Beach RC. Management of childhood constipation. Lancet 1996;348:766–767.

162. Gold DM, Levine J, Weinstein TS, Kessler BH, Pettei MJ. Frequency of digital rectal examination in children with chronic constipation. Arch Pediatr Adolesc Med 1999;153:377–379.

163. Rockney RM, McQuade WH, Days AL. The plain abdominal roentgenogram in the management of encopresis. Arch Pediatr Adolesc Med 1995;149:623–7.

164. Leech SC, McHugh K, Sullivan PB. Evaluation of a method of assessing faecal loading on plain abdominal radiographs in children. Pediatr Radiol 1999;29:255–258.

165. Papadopoulou A, Clayden GS, Booth IW. The clinical value of solid marker transit studies in childhood constipation and soiling. Eur J Pediatr. 1994;153:560–564.

166. Spear M, Rothbaum R, Keating I, al. e. Perianal streptococcal cellulitis. J Pediatr 1985; 107:557–559.

167. Maronn ML, Esterly NB. Constipation as a feature of anogenital lichen sclerosus in children. Pediatrics 2005;115:e230–2.

168. Clayden CS. Anal appearances and child sexual abuse. Lancet 1987;1:620–21.

169. Pilapil VR. A horrifying television commercial that led to constipation. Pediatrics 1990;85:592–593.

170. Loening-Baucke V, Cruikshank B, Savage C. Defecation dynamics and behavior profiles in encopretic children. Pediatrics 1987;80:672–9.

171. Tjeerdsma HC, Smout AJ, Akkerman LM. Voluntary suppression of defecations delays gastric emptying time. Dig Dis Sci 1993;38:832.

172. Youssef NN, Langseder A, Schuckalo S, Irizarry R, Nussbaum E, Fehling BG, Mones RL, Rosh JR. Childhood constipation impairs quality of life. J Pediatr Gastroenterol Nutr 2003;37:327.

173. Landman GB, Rappaport L, Fenton T, Levine MD. Locus of control and self-esteem in children with encopresis. J Dev Behav Pediatr 1986;7:111–113.

174. Borowitz SM, Cox DJ, Tam A, Ritterband LM, Sutphen JL, Penberthy JK. Precipitants of constipation during early childhood. J Am Board Fam Pract 2003;16:213–218.

175. Ahmad T, Steffen R, Banez G, Mahajan L, Feinberg L, Worley S. Defecation anxiety in children with functional constipation. J Pediatr Gastroenterol Nutr 2003;37:328.

176. Blum N, J, Taubman B, Nemeth N. Relationship between age at initiation of toilet training and duration of training: a prospective study. Pediatrics 2003;111:810–814.

177. Youssef NN, Peters JM, Henderson W, Shultz-Peters S, Lockhart DK, Di Lorenzo C. Dose response of PEG 3350 for the treatment of childhood fecal impaction. J Pediatr 2002;141:410–414.

178. Voskuijl W, de Lorijn F, Verwijs W, Hogeman P, Heijmans J, Makel W, Taminiau J, Benninga M. PEG 3350 (Transipeg) versus lactulose in the treatment of childhood functional constipation: a double blind, randomised, controlled, multicentre trial. Gut 2004;53:1590–4.

179. Borowitz SM, Cox DJ, Kovatchev B, Ritterband LM, Sheen J, Sutphen J. Treatment of childhood constipation by primary care physicians: efficacy and predictors of outcome. Pediatrics 2005;115:873–7.

180. Nolan T, Debelle G, Oberklaid F, Coffey C. Randomised trial of laxatives in treatment of childhood encopresis. Lancet 1991;338:523–527.

181. van der Plas RN, Benninga MA, Buller HA, Bossuyt PM, Akkermans LM, Redekop WK, Taminiau JA. Biofeedback training in treatment of childhood constipation: a randomised controlled study. Lancet 1996;348:776–80.

182. Loening-Baucke V. Biofeedback training in children with functional constipation. A critical review. Dig Dis Sci 1996;41:65–71.

183. Staiano A, Andreotti MR, Greco L, Basile P, Auricchio S. Long-term follow-up of children with chronic idiopathic constipation. Dig Dis Sci 1994;39:561–4.

184. Procter E, Loader P. A 6-year follow-up study of chronic constipation and soiling in a specialist paediatric service. Child Care Health Dev 2003;29:103–9.

185. Levine MD. Encopresis: its potentiation, evaluation, and alleviation. Pediatr Clin North Am 1982;29:315–330.

186. Voskuijl WP, Heijmanws J, Taminau JA, Benninga MA. Functional defecation disorders in children (FGD'S): The pediatric Rome II criteria revised. J Pediatr Gastroenterol Nutr 2003;36:562.

187. van der Wal MF, Benninga MA, Hirasing RA. The prevalence of encopresis in a multicultural population. J Pediatr Gastroenterol Nutr 2005;40:345–8.

188. Kuhn BR, Marcus BA, Pitner SL. Treatment guidelines for primary nonretentive encopresis and stool toileting refusal. Am Fam Physician 1999;59:2171–2178, 2184–2186.

189. Benninga MA, Voskuijl WP, Akkerhuis GW, Taminiau JA, Buller HA. Colonic

transit times and behaviour profiles in children with defecation disorders. Arch Dis Child 2004;89:13–16.

190. van der Plas RN, Benninga MA, Redekop WK, Taminiau JA, Buller HA. Randomised trial of biofeedback training for encopresis. Arch Dis Child 1996;75:367–374.

191. McGrath ML, Mellon MW, Murphy L. Empirically supported treatments in pediatric psychology: constipation and encopresis. J Pediatr Psychol 2000;25:225–254.

192. Brooks RC, Copen RM, Cox DJ, Morris J, Borowitz S, Sutphen J. Review of the treatment literature for encopresis, functional constipation, and stool-toileting refusal. Ann Behav Med 2000;22:260–267.

193. van Ginkel R, Benninga MA, Blommaart PJ, van der Plas RN, Boeckxstaens GE, Buller HA, Taminiau JA. Lack of benefit of laxatives as adjunctive therapy for functional nonretentive fecal soiling in children. J Pediatr 2000;137:808–813.

194. Voskuijl WP, van Ginkel R, Taminiau JA, Boeckxstaens GE, Benninga MA. Loperamide suppositories in an adolescent with childhood-onset functional nonretentive fecal soiling. J Pediatr Gastroenterol Nutr 2003;37:198–200.

195. Rockney RM, McQuade WH, Days AL, Linn HE, Alario AJ. Encopresis treatment outcome: long-term follow-up of 45 cases. J Dev Behav Pediatr 1996;17:380–385.

196. Benninga MA, Taminiau JAJM. Diagnosis and treatment efficacy of functional non-retentive fecal soiling in childhood. J Pediatr Gastroenterol Nutr 2001;32:S42–S43.

197. Voskuijl W, Reitsma J, Van Ginkel R, Buller H, Taminiau J, Benninga M. Functional non-retentive fecal soiling in children: 12 years of lungitudinal follow-up. Gastroenterology 2005;128:A462.

198. Di Lorenzo C, Benninga MA, Forbes D, Morais MB, Morera C, Rudolph C, Staiano A, Sullivan PB, Tobin J. Functional gastrointestinal disorders, gastroesophageal reflux and neurogastroenterology: Working Group report of the second World Congress of Pediatric Gastroenterology, Hepatology, and Nutrition. J Pediatr Gastroenterol Nutr 2004;39 Suppl 2:S616–25.

199. Li BU, Altschuler SM, Berseth CL, Di Lorenzo C, Rudolph CD, Scott RB. Research agenda for pediatric gastroenterology, hepatology and nutrition: motility disorders and functional gastrointestinal disorders. Report of the North American Society for Pediatric Gastroenterology, Hepatology and Nutrition for the Children's Digestive Health and Nutrition Foundation. J Pediatr Gastroenterol Nutr 2002;35 Suppl 3:S263–7.

200. Benninga M, Candy DC, Catto-Smith AG, Clayden G, Loening-Baucke V, Di Lorenzo C, Nurko S, Staiano A. The Paris Consensus on Childhood Constipation Terminology (PACCT) Group. J Pediatr Gastroenterol Nutr 2005;40:273–5.

Chapter 15

Design of Treatment Trials for Functional Gastrointestinal Disorders

E. Jan Irvine, Chair

William E. Whitehead, Co-Chair

William D. Chey

Kei Matsueda

Michael Shaw

Nicholas J. Talley

Sander J.O. Veldhuyzen van Zanten

Introduction

For some functional gastrointestinal disorders (FGIDs) there is emerging evidence of treatment efficacy, while for others it remains uncertain whether truly efficacious treatments are yet available. Increasing attention has been paid to the methodological challenges in the design of treatment trials for FGIDs. The Rome diagnostic criteria and design recommendations are being increasingly incorporated in recent trials. However, several factors, such as symptom variability between subjects or groups and within subjects over time, contribute to problems with optimizing trial design. The lack of specific structural or (patho)physiological diagnostics for most FGIDs makes efficacy assessment for treatments difficult. Nevertheless, validated outcome measurement tools are accumulating. Establishing treatment efficacy also requires agreement among researchers and providers on the definition of a clinically meaningful change and what constitutes a treatment responder. Once efficacy is established in short duration studies, additional studies may be indicated to establish long-term efficacy, the utility of intermittent (on-demand) treatment, and treatment cost-effectiveness and cost-utility.

Goals of the Chapter

The committee's aims were to review the literature on trial design for the functional gastrointestinal disorders (FGIDs), to further develop guidelines [1–3] to assist researchers in conducting treatment trials for the FGIDs, provide standards to help explain the mechanisms of therapeutic success and enable regulatory agencies, researchers, and providers to better evaluate the quality of published studies. An additional goal was to enhance the homogeneity of future trials to permit pooling of results in meta-analyses.

Several reviews have examined the potential impact of study design problems on outcomes and interpretation of FGID trials [4–6]. Previous reports from the Rome I and II processes have addressed these issues for irritable bowel syndrome (IBS) and other FGIDs [2, 3]. Some recommendations from those reports are incorporated and expanded in this chapter. We have largely limited this review to design issues of clinical trials evaluating the efficacy of new treatments. Studies that address pathophysiology or mechanism of treatment effects are not included in this review because different and very diverse study designs are required for these purposes.

The report will follow the basic structure of a randomized clinical trial, that is, research question, study design, inclusion and exclusion criteria, treatment inter-

Table I. Goals of a Treatment Trial

To ascertain the ability of the intervention to
> Abolish symptoms or decrease severity
> Improve functional health status and quality of life
> Improve ability to cope with symptoms
> Decrease use of health care resources

vention, outcome measures and their validation, statistical issues, and interpretation of results. In each section, recommendations will be made with supporting evidence. Particular emphasis will be placed on examples of studies of IBS and functional dyspepsia (FD), as these disorders have been studied most extensively. Recommendations in this article are based largely on consensus of the literature, except where specifically indicated.

Identifying the Research Question and Hypothesis

A treatment trial may have several objectives. However, the goals of most intervention studies of FGIDs are to ascertain the impact of the intervention in one of the four categories listed in Table 1. Patients with IBS may wish a decrease in abdominal pain, physicians may want less frequent office visits or more satisfied patients, while third-party payers seek less health care resource use and employers want decreased sick leave or increased productivity. Finally, family members may hope for happier relatives who participate more fully in family life. While these are all legitimate and desirable definitions of success, it is unlikely that a single clinical trial can assess them all simultaneously or that one treatment will achieve improvement in all outcomes.

Investigators should select their most important research question(s) pertinent to the specific FGID, develop a hypothesis based on available evidence, and design a study that will most effectively answer the proposed research question.

Most treatment trials are designed to ask whether the study treatment is efficacious, (i.e., whether it reduces the severity or completely abolishes the symptoms prompting the health care visits). Consequently, the primary outcome measurement tools must include subjective reporting of the most important symptoms and/or a global assessment of overall disease severity. The secondary outcome measures are best determined by the particular disorder and research questions. For example, intestinal motility or gut transit time might be appropriate to assess in patients with constipation-variant IBS if the drug tested is expected to alter these parameters. This may then explain why patients' symptoms improve (or not) and whether improvement correlates with other outcome measures. No structural, pathophysiological, or functional abnormalities have been found to fully explain the origin and persistence of the FGID symptoms (see the chapter discussing pathophysiology). Therefore, pathophysiological parameters cannot yet be used as the primary outcome measure of a clinical trial.

Patient Population

A screening log, summarizing the most important clinical variables in patients entered or excluded and the reasons for exclusion, is strongly recommended. It is advisable to include a broad spectrum of patients to support the generalizability of the findings (applicability of results to patients not participating in the trial). This is particularly true for pharmaceutical research, where regulatory agencies may limit the licensed drug indication to patients similar to those in the trial population. However, this must be balanced against the risk of being overly inclusive. For example, if an investigational drug slows gut transit, constipated patients are likely to experience undesirable side effects and should be excluded [7–9]. Similarly, if an investigational drug accelerates transit, it may be inappropriate to include patients having frequent loose stools [10–12]. The putative mechanisms of new FGID treatments will vary greatly. Thus, no general recommendations can be given; investigators can select the study population based on pilot data, together with the likelihood that a positive or negative treatment effect is determined by patient characteristics.

A screening log, summarizing clinical variables in patients entered or excluded, is strongly recommended to support the generalizability of the results.

Explicit inclusion and exclusion criteria are mandatory for all studies. If researchers choose to target enrollment to a special population to maximize treatment efficacy or minimize side effects, the reasons for restriction must be carefully documented and patient selection methods should be clearly described. Examples of trials that targeted selected study populations expected to be more responsive and/or to experience fewer adverse effects of the treatment are alosetron [7, 9] and tegaserod [11, 13] phase III efficacy trials for IBS. These trials recruited patients with IBS with diarrhea or constipation, respectively, since phase II data suggested a greater potential treatment effect in these specific subgroups.

It is advisable to include as broad a spectrum of patients as possible, defined by the Rome-specific FGID criteria. Restricting the study population must be justified and inclusion and exclusion criteria must be specified.

The case definition for the particular FGID under study will also be part of the inclusion criteria. In clinical practice, many physicians avoid formal investigation for IBS and some other FGID patients in favor of a positive diagnosis, reassurance and—if indicated—life style modification. However, entry criteria for treatment trials must be more specific. The consensus view is that the minimum evaluation should include a complete blood count, imaging of the relevant part of the gastro-intestinal tract within the previous 5 years, and other investigations determined by symptoms and family history [14]. Emerging evidence suggests that screening IBS patients for gluten enteropathy in high risk patients may also be desirable [15]. Diagnostic testing should be consistent across all treatment arms, and the timing should be recorded, as delays for testing or reassurance after a normal test may lead to apparent spontaneous improvement [16].

The minimum screening for eligibility should be specified.

Most trials of FGIDs have been conducted in academic centers specifically interested in the FGIDs [3, 17]. Expert opinion [18] previously suggested that tertiary centers attract 'intractable' patients with more severe symptoms and /or psychosocial issues [5, 19]. Recent observations from community GI clinics show that IBS patients are neither more severe nor more intractable to medical management than those from primary care [20]. Nonetheless, two large FD trials did show significant differences in response rates between primary care and referred patients [21]. Thus, conducting some studies in primary care will ensure that results are germane to the 'average' patient. Researchers should strongly consider recruiting broadly and identifying when subjects are from primary, secondary, or tertiary care. The number of participating centers can also affect the trial generalizability, as patients from a study conducted in a single center are likely to be more homogeneous than those in a multicenter trial. Increasingly, trials are multicenter and multinational. Assessing patient homogeneity across centers can be undertaken easily if the distribution and demographic data are reported by center.

Patient characteristics should be documented sufficiently to test the comparability of patients among centers and allow comparisons with other populations.

Special recruitment strategies such as advertising have been accepted in some countries to accelerate recruitment. A recent IBS study observed that patients recruited by newspaper advertisement, in comparison to patients enrolled by gastroenterologists, were older, more highly educated, more often depressed but less anxious, and had less severe IBS symptoms; primary care patients were also anxious but had symptom severity that was intermediate between patients recruited by advertisement and patients recruited from gastroenterology clinics [22].

Recruitment strategies should be clearly identified to allow exploration of different patterns of treatment responses.

— Patient Characteristics

The FGIDs frequently overlap with each other and with other somatic and psychiatric disorders [23]. This raises multiple concerns for the trialist. First, the presence of comorbid disorders is associated with increased symptom severity, greater impact on quality of life, and greater psychological distress—all of which could modify the response to treatment. Second, when a patient meets symptom criteria for two or more FGIDs based in part on a shared symptom such as abdominal pain, the accuracy of the diagnosis may be questioned. Third, underlying motility or sensory disorders in different parts of the gastrointestinal tract may interact in ways that could affect the response to specific treatments; for example, comorbid pelvic floor dyssynergia (outlet obstruction) could affect the response to a prokinetic drug treatment for IBS or functional dyspepsia. The logical solution to this problem—excluding patients with overlapping diagnoses from the trial—is likely to be unacceptable because the overlap among disorders (e.g., IBS and FD) is so high that the exclusion of patients with overlap conditions would result in the recruitment of an atypical sample. The committee therefore recommends that in most situations, patients with overlapping conditions should be included in the trial and the presence and type of comorbid conditions should be documented.

Other important patient characteristics to measure include age, sex, race, disease severity, symptom duration, prior treatments for the condition, and the use of concurrent medications. Very few studies have reported the disease duration, prior treatments, or the use of nonstudy medications. Reporting all medications, including over the counter supplements or antidepressants, is recommended. Even those thought to be of limited importance (e.g., iron and calcium) may be relevant to the symptoms or proposed intervention.

Recently, gender differences in response to drug treatments for IBS have become evident in clinical trials of certain serotonergic drugs [24–26]. Depending on the hypothesis, investigators may choose to enroll only one sex. However, if both women and men are to be included, there should be sufficient numbers of both to allow meaningful subgroup analyses in phase III trials. As data accumulate describing the genetics of FGIDs and associated drug responsiveness [24], these parameters may become relevant to assess during clinical trials.

It is also advisable to assess for psychological distress or prior mental health problems, as these potential confounders could alter both baseline symptom severity and response to treatment [27]. Personality profiles are not specific for any FGID and, hence, psychological criteria are not part of the diagnostic criteria. Nevertheless, assessing psychological factors at baseline has been suggested, as they may alter the response to treatment [28–33]. Several validated instruments are available for this purpose and we refer readers to the report of the Working Party on Psychosocial Factors in FGIDs [31]. It may be important to collect other clinical information such as history of abdominal or pelvic surgeries, although further testing of this impact on outcome is needed [34].

Potential disease modifiers/confounders that might affect response to therapy should be assessed.

Clinical Trial Design

Clinical trials differ from clinical practice in several ways, including the application of strict inclusion and exclusion criteria, the use of a placebo, application of a standardized intervention, frequent follow-up visits with extensive data recording, and the use of study coordinators. Nonetheless, standard aspects of diagnosis and management, especially adequate explanation and reassurance about the disease, are part of standard care and should be provided to all patients in the trial. Novel interventions must show promise of a benefit over standard care.

Every trial should incorporate the principles of good clinical practice to ensure that the study results are relevant to real practice situations.

— Unique Challenges for the Design of Treatment Trials in FGIDs

Study designs for FGID treatment trials face several challenges: (1) a high placebo response rate that makes detecting treatment benefits difficult [5, 17], (2) symptoms that are of intermittent and fluctuating severity [35], (3) a potential need for multimodal therapy, given the limited efficacy of available treatments or

Table 2. Major Sources of Bias

Bias Type	Comments
1. Investigator bias	Conscious or unconscious bias, usually expressed through decisions about eligibility
2. Patient expectancy (placebo)	Especially a problem where endpoints are subjective
3. Ascertainment bias:	
a. Self-selection for treatment	Patients are more likely to respond positively to treatments they prefer and seek out
b. Changes in subject pool	Publicity or other factors may influence the subject pool over time
4. Nonspecific effects:	
a. Doctor-patient relationship	Especially important in psychological interventions
b. Regression to mean	Patients are usually enrolled when most symptomatic and inevitably "improve"
5. Publication bias	Authors are more likely to submit positive results and journals more likely to publish them

multiple etiological mechanisms affecting the disease process [18], (4) difficulty maintaining masking (blinding) of patients and investigators in trials of behavioral interventions [36], (5) contamination from over-the-counter treatments or medicines taken for other conditions, and (6) avoidance of significant harms [37, 38] in treating non-life-threatening conditions.

Bias, defined as 'systematic error' in estimating the treatment effect, may enter a clinical trial at any stage, from the design to publication of results [39, 40]. The major sources of bias addressed here are listed in Table 2. The roles of masking, randomization, and the use of a control group in minimizing bias in the study execution will be reviewed.

Masking

Double-masking (of both patients and research personnel) to the intervention is important to ensure the validity of the primary outcome measurement. "Triple-masking" is suggested and includes masking of monitors, data managers, statisticians, and others who interpret tests that are part of the outcome [41, 42].

In drug trials, investigators are encouraged to ask both the patient and the interventionist who interacts with the patient at the end of the trial whether they believe the active treatment was administered and to report these data. Interventions, such as psychotherapy, hypnotherapy, sphincterotomy, or drug trials in which the active drug causes predictable side effects or rapid symptom change, are difficult to mask from patients or investigators. Possible solutions to ensure a valid outcome assessment include using independent assessors, who are unaware of the intervention, or standardized interviewer-administered or self-administered questionnaires. This provides reassurance that the providers who performed the intervention do not influence the outcome assessment. Alternatively, using laboratory tests, (e.g., anal manometry in fecal incontinence) that are interpreted by individuals not interacting with the patients can ensure independent assessment.

It is mandatory to undertake the maximum masking possible, determined by the type of intervention and study design.

Randomization

Randomization is the process (equivalent to the flip of a coin) of assigning subjects to different treatment arms without bias. This allows the application of standard statistical methods. *Concealed allocation*, whereby investigators and research personnel cannot anticipate a patient's treatment assignment, can be accomplished either by (1) someone other than an investigator preparing a numbered series of sealed envelopes containing group assignments, with instructions that envelopes are to be opened only after a subject is deemed eligible and has provided written consent, or (2) use of a computer program to confirm patient eligibility prior to random allocation. Methods to ensure randomized concealed treatment allocation are well established [42, 43]. The most critical recommendations are that (1) the randomization code should be generated by a noninvestigator (preferably via a computer program), (2) randomization should be done within blocks of variable (permuted block randomization) or sufficient size to minimize unmasking due to side effects in previously exposed patients, (3) the list of patient treatment assignments should be available to the medical officer in charge of patient safety, and (4) a record should be kept of patients for whom the mask has been broken.

When reporting the trial, the randomization procedure should be explicitly described because it is a potential source of bias. Randomization protects against ascertainment bias (subject self-selection or changes in the subject pool over time), and assures a balance among treatment groups of potential effect modifiers or confounders [44]. Chalmers et al. [45] have shown that prognostic factors are unevenly distributed when treatment allocation is not concealed. Stratified randomization assures balance of the most important prognostic factors (e.g., sex and typical bowel habit for IBS) by using a separate randomization sequence for each stratum (e.g., male vs. female or constipation-predominant vs. diarrhea-predominant IBS) [46]. Stratification should be restricted to one or two factors. Readers are directed to the references for a more in-depth discussion of randomization [44, 47].

Investigators must include a detailed description of their randomization scheme in the report of the study.

— Selecting the Control Group

A control group is an absolute requirement to establish the efficacy of a new treatment. As treatments of proven efficacy accumulate, a comparison against active treatment can be considered. In some therapeutic areas (e.g., migraine headache) standard effective treatments are available, and clinical trials of new compounds can and should be compared to standard treatment [48]. However, comparisons between two active treatments require many more patients to establish efficacy and often fail to show a statistically significant difference between treatments [49, 50]. Consequently, inclusion of a placebo control group is recommended in studies that compare two active treatments to avoid an inconclusive trial in which the active treatments are similar.

Control Groups for Behavioral Trials

Creating a placebo control for behavioral therapy trials [36] is particularly challenging. The dilemma is to identify an inactive treatment that generates expectancy comparable to the behavioral intervention. Ingenious efforts include the use of low-level counseling plus a placebo tablet as control conditions for hypnosis [51], and use of a patient self-help group [52] or an educational intervention [53] in trials of cognitive behavioral therapy (CBT) for IBS. The use of untreated patients or those receiving standard medical care as controls is best avoided as it can lead to an overestimate of the potential treatment benefit since untreated waiting list patients or those who have failed standard medical care can experience a 'negative expectancy' [54]. Care should also be taken to ensure that the number of control visits is similar to the active treatment group. Recommendations to preserve the trial integrity include (a) administering a questionnaire to test the credibility of both active and control interventions after initial exposure to both (For example, the Credibility Scale developed by Borkovec and Nau [55] for psychotherapy research has been adapted for clinical trials of FGIDs [53].), or (b) using a process measure to determine whether the behavioral intervention is changing the anticipated physiological or psychological response in the active treatment group but not (or to a lesser degree) in the control group. An example is a trial of CBT in IBS patients undertaken by Blanchard and colleagues [52]. CBT was hypothesized to improve IBS symptoms by changing patients' self-defeating attitudes about their symptoms, while controls, participating in a support group, were anticipated to have no such benefit. Cognitions measured during and after the intervention using the Dysfunctional Attitudes Scale [56] demonstrated that the CBT group had significantly reduced dysfunctional attitudes compared to controls. Improved IBS symptoms could then be attributed to the CBT intervention and not to nonspecific effects or expectancy. Similar process measures were used by Drossman et al. [53] who compared CBT to an education control. A cognitive scale for functional bowel disorders has also been developed and validated [57]. These process measures are useful in discriminating nonspecific doctor-patient interactions that can alter outcome (e.g., reduced abdominal pain due to anxiety reduction) from the active treatment effects, or when masking of patients or investigators is difficult. In a study by Drossman et al., desipramine did not significantly improve well-being in patients with IBS in the intention-to-treat analysis but did show greater overall satisfaction and benefit of desipramine in the per-protocol analysis; the disparity between the two analyses likely arose because side effects caused a higher dropout rate in the group treated with desipramine [53].

A placebo control group is essential. In behavioral treatment trials, confirming that the control condition produces a similar expectation of benefit but does not act on the same physiological or psychological principle is recommended.

— Placebo Interventions

The definition of a placebo is an intervention that generates the expectation of benefit in the patient but is believed to lack any specific effect to change a particular disorder [58]. In FD and IBS trials, the 'placebo effect' is well established and reported placebo response rates range from 10% to 70% for FD [17] and 0% to 84% (median 47%) for IBS [5]. Although this seems to be of a rather substantial magnitude, placebo response rates in other gastrointestinal (GI) disorders are comparable (e.g., 18% remission (range 0% to 50%) in Crohn's disease [59] and 36% to 44% healing rates for peptic ulcer in H_2-receptor antagonist studies [60]).

This substantial placebo response rate makes it difficult to demonstrate superior efficacy of new treatments. An important feature of placebo treatment [58] is that a placebo administered by a physician appears to be more powerful than one given by other health professionals. Some treatments also demonstrate an 'order effect' in which an effective drug has a lesser benefit when given after a placebo. This is particularly germane if a "placebo run-in period" is implemented to exclude placebo responders or in crossover studies, where approximately half of patients will receive placebo first [58].

External factors may also contribute to changes in health status, including (1) a natural variation in symptoms (see below), (2) regression towards the mean, and (3) unidentified or unintended cointerventions. Regression to the mean refers to the likelihood that patients will present when symptoms are particularly severe and tend to improve with time, regardless of participation in a clinical trial [36, 61]. Important cointerventions for IBS or FD patients would be altering the diet or using over-the-counter remedies while initiating the new treatment. This could lead to a false interpretation that the intervention was effective (or ineffective). In addition, patients receive extra attention from researchers during clinical trials that could also lead to significant improvements in general well-being (Hawthorn effect) [39, 59, 62]. The magnitude of the placebo response may also be influenced by the wording of the question used to define treatment response or by the use of a compound question; a recently published meta-analysis suggests that the placebo response rate is larger when a responder is defined by a global improvement in IBS symptoms compared to defining a responder by reduction in abdominal pain (average placebo responses of 36% vs. 28%) [63].

The placebo response rate in treatment trials of FGIDs is substantial and largely unavoidable.

— Baseline Observation vs. Placebo Run-in

A placebo run-in period should be distinguished from a period of baseline measurement without treatment, which is useful to characterize patient eligibility since many patients have intermittent and fluctuating symptoms. It can also be used to test whether patients in the active and placebo groups are comparable prior to treatment and may permit a fuller evaluation of clinically important change in health status after treatment. Such baseline recordings can be made retrospectively. However, prospective evaluation is recommended to eliminate important recollection and reporting biases (discussed below in outcome assessment).

Several older studies employed a placebo run-in period where all patients received placebo for a specified period and their response was assessed using the study outcome measures [17]. Patients who significantly improved were excluded from further participation, theoretically to reduce the proportion of placebo responders and exclude patients with poor adherence. Although used in several trials of allergic rhinitis to remove placebo responders, and apparently acceptable to regulatory agencies, it may cause underestimation of the overall 'effect size' [64, 65]. Other potential disadvantages [66] include the inability to predict whether (1) the placebo response increases, plateaus, or diminishes after the run-in phase, (2) a differential dropout may occur in which patients removed have a different treatment response to those who continue in the trial, and (3) patients will be distressed if excluded, disrupting the doctor-patient relationship for future management.

The disadvantages of a placebo run-in appear to outweigh the benefits and it is best avoided. However, baseline observations are recommended.

— Choice of Study Design

The *double-masked randomized placebo-controlled trial* is the gold standard method to test for efficacy of new treatments. A *parallel-group* study design requires that patients be randomized to receive the assigned treatment for the entire trial. Variations of this basic design include different groups receiving different doses of the active treatment (dose-ranging), more than one control treatment, a baseline period of no treatment, and a washout period after treatment is completed.

Crossover designs have been popular in treatment trials of some FGIDs (33% of FD and 50% of IBS trials) [5, 17]. Subjects receive both treatments during distinct time periods, usually separated by a washout phase. Theoretically, a crossover design can increase sensitivity to detect an important change, due to less variability in measurements within rather than between subjects; thus, a smaller sample size can achieve the desired statistical power. However, patient dropout rates and missing data have a greater impact than in a parallel-group design, as subjects with missing data must be omitted from both study arms. The greatest disadvantages, however, are (1) the carry-over (period-by-treatment) effects that occur when the first treatment influences the response to the second treatment, and (2) the high likelihood of unmasking due to side effects [67–69]. It is mandatory that data analysis account for period and sequence effects and, if found, only the first treatment period should be used to determine efficacy [67], thereby rendering this design extremely inefficient. Although crossover designs are not recommended for treatment trials with subjective endpoints, they may be used in physiological studies where the endpoints are objectively measured.

The European Agency for the Evaluation of Medicinal Products (EMEA) may be willing to accept a crossover design for a phase III trial, but in Notes for Guidance in Clinical Trials, they highlight problems that could invalidate the results [70]. Their design guidelines are discussed below. For example, in the only completed trial that followed EMEA guidelines [71], 2,660 IBS patients were randomized to tegaserod 6 mg twice daily or placebo in a 4:1 ratio for an initial 4-week treatment period, and all responders were then withdrawn from drug but continued to monitor symptoms until a symptom recurrence occurred. Patients initially treated with tegaserod who were responders in the first treatment period and who experienced a recurrence (n=983) were then rerandomized to tegaserod or placebo in a 1:1 ratio for a second 4-week treatment period. Placebo responders and patients who did not experience symptom recurrence during the treatment-free period were dropped from the analysis of the second treatment period. The authors reported that the proportion of patients on active drug who met the responder criterion was significantly greater than the proportion of patients on placebo who met the responder criterion both in the initial treatment period and independently in the second treatment period. The results provided compelling evidence for efficacy on initial and on repeat administration. However, the design required 2 to 3 times the number of patients that would be required in a traditional parallel-group design. Period and sequence effects were not analyzed and, in particular, unmasking in the second treatment period was not assessed.

When comparing two efficacious compounds or two doses of an efficacious therapy, a crossover design can be used to test the influence of side effects on efficacy ratings. After both treatment periods, patients express and grade their preference for one treatment over another [48]. Multiple crossover trials (N of 1), described by the last working team report as acceptable for trials of treatments that have short durations, are not recommended for FGIDs because of difficulty in interpreting results, due to carry-over effects and lack of guidance in interpreting partial responses.

A *factorial design* is appropriate when evaluating combination treatments, which may be necessary in patients with severe FGID symptoms [72]. Illustrating the simplest factorial design to evaluate two treatments, A and B, subjects would be randomly assigned to one of four groups: no A and no B, A and no B, B and no A, or both A and B. Theoretically, a factorial design could reduce study costs by pooling comparator groups to examine the main effect (e.g., all subjects receiving treatment A can be compared to all subjects not receiving treatment A, independently of whether they receive treatment B). However, the added complexity of data analysis and interpretation frequently offset any savings, except when testing for treatment interactions. Importantly, the two treatments should have distinct mechanisms of action, to properly interpret the effects of combining treatments. Thus, a factorial design might test psychotherapy and a drug [73] but not two drugs in the same class or two doses of the same drug. Equally important, a control group is required for each intervention. For example, a trial testing CBT together with a drug such as a tricyclic antidepressant might use an educational control for CBT and a placebo tablet for the antidepressant. All patients would receive two treatments—a behavioral treatment (CBT or education) and a pill (antidepressant or inert tablet). Such trials are difficult to design and manage, and recently published trials in other conditions (as there are none for FGIDs) have shown significant compromises (e.g., high withdrawal rate and lack of placebo control group) [73, 74].

The *withdrawal trial* is an "enrichment design" in which all subjects receive the active treatment and at a predefined time point are classified as responders or nonresponders. The latter are then excluded and responders are randomly assigned to continue with treatment or placebo. The efficacy assessment is based only on the second part of the trial—the active treatment versus placebo. A major drawback of this design is that potential carry-over effects from active treatment can prevent an accurate estimate of the drug benefit. One study found no clinically important benefit from domperidone over placebo in diabetic gastroparesis due to a carry-over effect, but also due to investigator unmasking [75].

A variation of this design has been used in clinical trials for Crohn's disease to determine the contribution of maintenance azathioprine [76] and the efficacy of different induction and maintenance regimens for infliximab [77, 78]. The goal here was not to establish efficacy but to demonstrate that there was no inferiority of component treatments. Investigators should be mindful that withdrawal trials do not provide evidence of treatment superiority and statistical analyses are those for a noninferiority trial.

The EMEA guidelines [79] for testing drugs for short-term efficacy in IBS recommend the randomized withdrawal design as one option and indicate that two or more cycles of treatment, each demonstrating efficacy, are required. The EMEA provides the following two design examples: (1) an open-label 4-week treatment period followed by a randomized double-blind second treatment period for responders only (as above), and (2) an initial placebo-controlled, double-blind 4-week treatment period followed by a variable period off study drug, and rerandomization of all patients to drug versus placebo for a second 4-week treatment phase (effectively a crossover design). The EMEA guidelines do not address the statistical analysis of these study designs.

A trial that followed these EMEA guidelines [71] was described above under crossover designs. The treatment benefit in this study (difference between active drug and placebo response rates) increased from 10.6% during the initial 4-week treatment period to 17% during a second treatment period when patients who responded to active drug in the first period and then relapsed were rerandomized to active drug or placebo. These results suggest that this design probably overestimates the 'effect size' [80] by dropping nonresponders from the second treatment period and possibly by unmasking.

An additional EMEA recommendation [79] is that withdrawal or rebound effects should always be assessed in a blinded placebo-extension phase following the first treatment phase in which patients are exposed to the active drug. Recent phase III trials of tegaserod [11, 81, 82] and alosetron [9, 83] have included follow-up observations off treatment. After discontinuing active or placebo, both groups worsened but did not return to baseline. However, withdrawal effects were not examined in a masked fashion and no placebo was administered. No guidelines have been offered for the statistical analysis or interpretation of data collected during drug withdrawal, whether masked or not.

The parallel-group design remains the accepted standard for evaluation of efficacy for most treatments and is applicable to most experimental situations. The crossover design is best avoided.

Types of Trials

Superiority Trial

The strongest case supporting the efficacy of a new medication is to demonstrate clinical and statistical superiority to placebo or an active control treatment or by showing a dose-response relationship. The decision to use a placebo vs. an active control should be based on scientific and ethical considerations. Active controls must be proven effective at the dose used.

Equivalence or Noninferiority Trial

An equivalence study or noninferiority trial can be considered (1) when a known, effective treatment is available and it would be unethical to administer a placebo (e.g., cancer or inflammatory bowel disease, but not FGIDs), or (2) when a new treatment might be less costly, safer, or as good as standard therapy [50]. Such trials are usually more costly than superiority trials, as much larger sample sizes are required and there is a risk of obtaining uninterpretable results. Investigators must first estimate the expected difference between standard treatment and placebo, based on a meta-analysis or systematic review [49, 50, 84], and then define "equivalence margins" that are smaller than the expected difference. The trial will be judged to be positive only if the 95% confidence interval for the observed difference between the new and standard treatments falls within the equivalence margins. For a noninferiority trial, only the lower 95% confidence limit must fall within the margins.

Intermittent or On-demand Trials

Many patients with FGIDs experience episodic symptoms or "attacks" [35, 72, 85]. For IBS and FD, most drug trials have focused on administering new drugs continuously for symptom control and/or prevention [7, 8, 10, 12]. However, there is a growing interest in developing drugs for *intermittent* (short-course administration for a predetermined time period after symptom recurrence) *or on-demand treatment* (medication only taken during symptoms). On-demand studies are generally undertaken after a treatment has been found to be efficacious in short- or long-term trials. This approach has been successful in gastroesophageal reflux disease (GERD) [86, 87]. Guidelines developed for intermittent drug treatment of migraine [48] may provide a model for FGIDs, as they share two important characteristics: (a) symptom episodes are intermittent and last for hours to days, and (b) the pathophysiology is poorly understood, with symptom relief being the reference outcome. The guidelines for intermittent dosing in migraine [48] are summarized below:

The active drug or placebo for migraine should be tested on only one symptom episode per patient [48]. In early analgesic studies, the migraine drug was often administered during multiple pain episodes, assuming that repeated trials would provide a more reliable estimate of drug efficacy. However, this not only prolongs the trial, but the initial response may influence the patient's expectation and response to subsequent administrations, possibly increasing dropouts and biasing results. Potential gains in statistical power from repeated administrations may be offset by an increased dropout rate. The suggested primary outcome measure in migraine trials is the proportion of patients achieving a pain-free state within two hours of drug dosing. After two hours, migraine patients who are not pain-free or having "meaningful relief" are classed as treatment failures and offered alternative treatments. This is both reasonable and ethical since other treatments are available. Secondary outcomes, such as time to achieve a pain-free state or "meaningful relief," as defined by the patient, can also be adopted. Additionally, sustained response or absence of relapse within 48 hours is a valid outcome. Patients must first fulfill the responder criterion of meaningful relief within 2 hours, and one can then evaluate the proportion who achieved a sustained response or relapse within 48 hours. The time to symptom remission has also been used to assess outcome in trials of antidiarrheal agents for acute infectious diarrhea [88, 89].

Several trials of on-demand therapy for nonerosive GERD have demonstrated this strategy to be effective in controlling symptoms, improving quality of life, and to be cost-effective [86]. In these studies, the primary endpoints were the proportion of patients who discontinued the medication due to inadequate control [90] or who were unwilling to continue; secondary outcomes included time to control of heartburn and need for use of rescue medications [91–93]. A similar approach has been used in nausea and vomiting studies [94]. These studies suggest that when clearly beneficial short- and long-term therapies are accepted for the FGIDs, then on-demand trials can be considered.

Superiority trials (not equivalence or noninferiority trials) are recommended for FGIDs. If appropriate, on-demand trials or intermittent treatment trials should also be performed.

Duration of Treatment

Treatment duration should be based on natural history data describing the frequency and duration of episodes. Some FGIDs are characterized by frequent exacerbations and remissions. For IBS, this is highly variable [35] but for the majority of patients both flares and remissions appear to last less than one week [35,

95], and for dyspepsia there appears to be a high symptom turnover in the general population, with many individuals "losing" or "acquiring" symptoms [96, 97]. Prior recommendations for trials of 8 to 12 weeks were based on experience, together with considerations of cost and ability to retain patients. The EMEA guidelines [79] differentiate between trials to establish short-term efficacy, for which a treatment duration of 4 weeks would be acceptable, versus trials intended to establish long-term efficacy, for which a minimum of 6 months is recommended. This latter recommendation is supported by the observation of a rising placebo response in recent 12-week trials [98, 99]. While both types of trials require patients with active symptoms at randomization, long-term studies could include patients with intermittent symptoms. Further research on the natural history of individual FGIDs should be a high priority, to allow clearer recommendations based on real observations. Extended patient followup should be considered to determine the treatment durability and should also relate to the presumed treatment mechanism and periodicity of symptoms. Thus, for behavioral or surgical treatments that are expected to have long-lasting effects, a followup of a year would be appropriate, whereas for drugs that relieve symptoms, 2 to 6 weeks may be sufficient. Long-term studies of on-demand therapy have been undertaken in GERD and demonstrate low dropout rates (< 20%) when therapy effectively controlled heartburn [91, 92, 100]. Thus, a patient-centered approach to the treatment of GERD is feasible and can be considered for the FGIDs.

A minimum treatment duration of 4 to 12 weeks that reflects the symptom periodicity and anticipated treatment mechanism is recommended. If chronic use is anticipated, trials of at least 6 months should be undertaken to establish long-term efficacy. Followup after treatment discontinuation is recommended based on the expected durability of the intervention.

— Adherence to Treatment and Study Protocol

Standard methods to assess adherence include interviewing patients or counting unused medication [101–104]. A more definitive and more costly approach in drug trials is to measure blood levels of metabolites [53]. For studies of longer duration, adherence assessment may be more important than in short-duration studies in interpreting results. When measured by patient self-report (the usual method), it is important to reassure patients that missing medication doses (or missing homework assignments in behavioral trials) will not result in their exclusion from the trial. Nonetheless, the frequency of missed or late appointments and missing data from diaries or questionnaires should be reported.

Adherence to the protocol and to treatment should be measured.

Methods for Collecting Symptoms and Outcome Data

— Accuracy of Symptom Recall

An efficient method to assess symptoms is for patients to complete questionnaires before and at follow-up visits during treatment. However, concerns regarding the accuracy of retrospective questionnaires include (1) Are patient responses biased by symptoms experienced the day of completing the questionnaire rather than the typical symptoms over the reporting interval? (2) Does poor recall alter the accuracy of a retrospective report? and (3) Do patients feel pressured to give a more positive report if completing questionnaires in the presence of the investigator?

Jensen and colleagues [105] compared retrospective "usual" pain intensity ratings for the past two weeks to prospective averaged hourly ratings by the same subjects, using a paper diary. The correlations were relatively high (r=.80), suggesting acceptable accuracy. However, other studies have demonstrated that current pain intensity accounts for 15% to 30% of the variance in recalled pain [105–107]. Jensen et al. [105] also showed that the recall of "usual" and "lowest" pain intensities correlated more strongly with the averaged hourly pain ratings than did recall of "highest" pain intensity.

Means et al. [108] compared subjective recall of health-related events to the medical record, observing recall accuracy of 71% for events within the past month, 69% for events 2 to 3 months old, 39% for events 4 to 8 months old, and 26% for events 9 to12 months old. These results suggested acceptable accuracy for events within 3 months.

— Symptom Diaries

Diaries may be used either as the primary endpoint or to collect data for secondary endpoints. Some investigators believe daily diaries minimize recall bias at follow-up visits. Generally, fewer symptoms are recorded in a diary than in a questionnaire. Subjects may be instructed to rate symptoms at a fixed time of day (e.g., before going to sleep) or whenever symptoms occur. The former method is more commonly used, as the latter may require several entries each day or no entries for some days, making data analysis and interpretation more complex. Diaries also create potential methodological problems [109] as some patients miss entries, or complete them retrospectively (e.g., "parking lot compliance"), potentially invalidating the data. In one study [110], patients were asked to complete pain ratings at three specified times each day (within a 15-minute window) and the actual time of data entry was surreptitiously recorded and compared to the patient report: subject-reported compliance was 90%, compared to objectively measured compliance of only 11%. When the window was expanded to 90 minutes (specified time ± 45 minutes), actual compliance was 20%. On 32% of days, subjects did not even open the diaries. These same data collected using an electronic device increased compliance to 94% and satisfaction was similar for both methods [111]. Other studies, examining electronic "smart" medical devices revealed that diary entries were frequently completed immediately before a clinic visit [112, 113].

Harding and colleagues [114] carried out two studies in which subjects called once daily to enter ratings using a touch-tone telephone keypad. The reported compliance with data entry was 81% and 83% in the two cohorts, and 79% of patients were satisfied or very satisfied with the system. Only ten percent were dissatisfied or very dissatisfied. Techniques to remind subjects to record symptoms and prevent delayed completion include (1) using hand-held electronic devices with audio alarms to prompt patients and record the time of completion or Web-based recording [110], (2) collecting information by telephone at frequent (usually daily) intervals [114], and (3) requiring patients to mail in diaries at frequent intervals, allowing investigators to estimate the time of completion within 2 or 3 days and initiate reminder calls if needed.

Retrospective questionnaires are an acceptable method for assessing symptoms provided the recall interval is limited to 3 months. Patients should receive clear instructions on the use of a dairy, including the directive to leave it blank if they forget to record information. Electronic diaries are preferred over paper diaries. Methods to ensure adherence with completion should be implemented.

Outcome Measures

— General Considerations

The primary outcome variable provides the basis for judging the success or failure of an intervention and should thus be specified before the trial begins. The investigator should choose one, or at most two, primary outcome variables in advance, based on the primary outcome. Investigators must clearly define "success" and "failure" of the intervention before beginning the trial. If more than one primary outcome is selected, they must also specify whether results will be considered successful if only one parameter fulfills criteria for success or if both are required. Guidelines for choosing a primary outcome variable are discussed below.

The "minimal clinically important difference" in the primary outcome variable should be specified before the trial begins to ensure that results are interpretable.

The well-recognized distinction between "statistical significance" and "clinical significance" was first noted in large clinical trials of antihypertensive medications in which the experimental intervention lowered the systolic blood pressure by a mean of 2 mmHg more than placebo. Using the appropriate statistical test, this difference, although statistically significant (due to the large sample size) and unlikely to have occurred by chance, would not be clinically relevant. Although the minimal clinically important difference can be specified as an absolute difference between treatments for the primary outcome variable, the U.S. Food and Drug Administration (FDA) and EMEA have declared a preference that investigators provide rules, a priori, that allow classification of each participant as a treatment responder or nonresponder. The definition of a responder should reflect a clinically meaningful symptom improvement for each patient. For IBS and other FGIDs there is no consensus on what constitutes a clinically meaningful improvement. Some studies accept as little as a 10% reduction in a visual analog scale rating of symptom severity [115] or one step on a 7-step ordinal scale [71] as clinically meaningful, while other studies require a 50% reduction in an aggregate symptom severity index [52] or questionnaire [116]. However, the most commonly employed definition of clinically meaningful improvement in IBS has been a patient's report (yes or no) of "adequate relief of abdominal pain and discomfort" [7, 83, 117, 118] or "satisfactory relief of IBS symptoms" [11, 13]. These definitions are assumed to have face validity. However, empirical data are needed for each outcome measure to assess the clinical significance of different degrees of change from both the patient's perspective and the physician's perspective.

Most clinical trials also include a series of secondary outcome variables. These are chosen for several reasons: (1) to strengthen the results by showing concordance between changes in individual symptoms and the primary outcome measure, (2) to address the mechanism of the intervention, (3) to assess the safety or (4) cost-effectiveness of the investigational treatment, and (5) to identify variables that predict the patients who are most or least likely to benefit. Guidelines for choosing secondary outcome measures are discussed below.

One or at most two primary outcome measures should be specified in advance. Investigators should list criteria to classify each patient as a responder or nonresponder based on a clinically meaningful change in symptoms.

— Choosing a Primary Outcome Variable

In selecting a primary outcome, investigators should examine the trial objectives, the study population, and mechanism of action of the proposed treatment. Currently, there is no consensus regarding the pathophysiology of the FGIDs. Diagnosis is based on the presence of one or more symptoms, together with the absence of structural or biochemical abnormalities suggestive of an alternative diagnosis [119]. Symptoms of FGIDs also vary substantially among patients and change over time; furthermore, opinions differ among investigators and across cultures regarding which symptoms define a particular FGID and how specific symptoms should be described. Assessment of patients' response to treatment has been determined by physicians in some studies [2, 3], but physician assessments are likely to be less accurate and to have greater potential for inter- and intrarater variability than patient-reported assessments [120]. Therefore, for all these reasons, patient-reported measures are endorsed.

Only outcome measures that have been validated and shown to be psychometrically sound are recommended as primary outcome assessment tools. The validity of secondary outcome measures should also be assessed. Psychometric validation of an outcome measure (including a disease-specific quality-of-life instrument) requires that (1) it include symptoms relevant to and fully representative of the disorder (face validity), (2) it shows a predictable relationship with other measures (construct validity), (3) the assessment produces similar results when re-administered to patients whose health status has not changed (reliability), (4) it can detect clinically meaningful change in health status when a change has occurred (responsive), and (5) changes in the score can be related to clinical indicators that are meaningful to clinicians (criterion validity). Validation of a new outcome measure is best established in a separate study. We refer the reader to relevant references on this topic [121–123].

The frequency of data recording for each outcome should also be specified before the trial begins, as should the time frame for defining a patient as a responder or nonresponder. It is important to determine whether this judgment is based on the outcome assessment only at the end of the trial, during a prespecified proportion of weeks or months that responder criteria have been fulfilled, or for all time points assessed during the trial.

A patient-reported outcome assessment is recommended. Psychometric validation of each outcome measure is recommended before it is used in clinical trials.

Adequate or Satisfactory Relief as a Primary Outcome

Since the publication of the previous Rome Working Team Report on the Design of Treatment Trials for FGIDs [2, 31], several methodological standards have changed in response to recommendations by regulatory agencies. The Rome II report emphasized that the primary outcome measure should be an integrative, patient-based report of symptom change, comparing symptoms before the trial to those during the trial. An "adequate relief" measure that had been developed by investigators working with Glaxo Smith Kline [8] was described as an example. The use of comprehensive patient questionnaires was offered as an alternative primary outcome measure. Since 1998, several published trials evaluating investigational drugs have used "adequate relief" [7, 8] or "satisfactory relief" of IBS symptoms as their primary outcome measure [11, 13, 124]. Some published trials of psychological interventions [53, 125] have also used such measures, while others have used a validated symptom severity questionnaire [126], or have defined a responder as a patient reporting a 50% reduction in the primary IBS symptoms [127, 128].

Adequate relief was used as the primary outcome measure in the phase III clinical trials of alosetron [7, 8, 25]. Patients were asked the following question once weekly during 12 weeks of treatment: "In the past 7 days, have you had adequate relief of your IBS pain and discomfort?" Subjects could answer "yes" or "no," and a responder was defined as a subject who reported adequate relief for at least 2 of 4 weeks for each month. A patient could be a responder for any of months 1, 2, 3. In addition, participants in the alosetron trials kept a daily diary to record the occurrence and intensity of pain, discomfort, and altered bowel habits. A disease-specific quality-of-life instrument was given at week 12 or end of treatment. Mangel and colleagues [129] did a secondary analysis of the data from these trials to address the validity of the "adequate relief" measure based on a subset of patients examined during weeks 9 to 12. Responders, based on the adequate relief measure, differed significantly from nonresponders regarding number of pain-free days, pain severity ratings, days with urgency and decreased stool frequency, as well as on 6 of 8 scales of the Medical Outcomes Study Short-Form Health Survey (SF-36) quality-of-life instrument, and 8 of 9 scales of a disease-specific quality-of-life measure. Correlations among measurements and reliability assessment (test-retest and internal consistency) were not reported; however, the authors reported (personal communication) that patients rarely recorded a week without adequate relief after their first week of adequate relief.

A similar measure, satisfactory relief, was used in the most recent tegaserod trials [11, 13, 124]. Patients were asked, "Over the past week, do you consider that you have had satisfactory relief from your IBS symptoms?" (Implied symptoms were overall well-being, abdominal pain/discomfort and bowel function.) Patients were classified as responders if they reported satisfactory relief on at least 50% of weeks over a 1 to 3 month period. The validity of this dichotomous, satisfactory-relief measure was evaluated in a manner similar to the Mangel study of adequate relief [116, 130]: responders of satisfactory relief were shown to have greater reductions in pain intensity, pain frequency, abdominal distention, and dissatisfaction with bowel habits compared to nonresponders.

Early trials on the efficacy of tegaserod [10] employed a Subject's Global Assessment (SGA) of relief, which was a 5-step rating scale. At weekly intervals, subjects were asked the following question: "Please consider how you felt this past week in regard to your IBS, in particular your overall well-being, and symptoms of abdominal discomfort, pain, and altered bowel habit. Compared to the way you usually felt before entering the study, how would you rate your relief of symptoms during the past week?" Possible answers were "completely relieved," "considerably relieved," "somewhat relieved," "unchanged," or "worse." Muller-Lissner et al. [131] reported validation analysis of the data from two 12-week clinical trials of tegaserod, comparing the weekly SGA to a visual analog scale (VAS) of pain/discomfort, daily diary data for pain intensity, bloating, stool frequency and consistency, and disease-specific quality of life before and after 12 weeks. As in the tegaserod trials [10], responders were defined as patients who had symptoms "completely or considerably relieved" at least 50% of the time *or* who described themselves as at least "somewhat relieved" 100% of the time. The number of improved symptom parameters correlated well with responder status (r = 0.7). Reproducibility and responsiveness were partly evaluated, but more extensive reliability testing and a minimum clinically important change definition were not reported and are needed.

Bijkerk and colleagues [132], assembled six judges who rated five outcome measures and five disease-specific quality-of-life instruments using 12 predefined methodological and psychometric criteria. Adequate relief scored best of the symptom outcomes but the raters concluded that this measure had not been adequately assessed for internal consistency and did not fully assess the breadth of IBS symptoms (content validity). Adequate relief was also used as an outcome measure in a study of cilansetron [124].

The adequate relief definition of a responder has subsequently been used in several large trials, and data are available for several thousand patients. Furthermore, it has been used in pivotal trials to obtain registration approval from regulatory agencies. Although adequate relief is becoming the standard for efficacy trials in the FGIDs, investigators should be aware of some gaps in its validation, and the potential for similar drawbacks in examining satisfactory relief. Whitehead and colleagues [20] used the satisfactory relief measure from the tegaserod trials to assess response in health-maintenance-organization IBS patients who were given standard medical care for 6 months. Patients were classed as having mild, moderate, or severe IBS symptoms at enrollment and completed a validated symptom severity questionnaire [116] at entry and 6 months followup. Mild patients were the most likely, and severe patients the least likely, to report satisfactory relief after 6 months; but the mild patients showed the smallest mean decrease in symptom severity, and the severe patients showed the largest mean decrease in symptom severity. Thus, responses to the satisfactory relief question were linked to the baseline symptom severity and were discordant with the degree of symptom reduction (assessed by questionnaire). These findings suggest that satisfactory relief is confounded by initial symptom severity and may underestimate the "effect size" in patients with severe IBS symptoms. Similar effects may be found relating to baseline symptom severity with adequate relief, but this has not been tested.

An additional problem with multiple timepoint measurements is that patients can be classed as responders and nonresponders at different time points. More complex data analyses and statistical modeling should be undertaken to evaluate how best to classify patients as responders or nonresponders over time; this should be a research priority. All studies should report the proportion of patients responding at each time point and the proportion of patients who maintained response throughout the trial. The working team recommends that investigators consider other outcome measures, either as primary or as secondary outcome measures, such as a 50% decrease in symptoms [52, 127] or a reduction in symptoms below a clinically meaningful predefined threshold [133, 134]. However, like satisfactory relief and adequate relief, these require further validation.

Integrative Symptom Questionnaires

The Irritable Bowel Syndrome Symptom Severity Scale (IBS-SSS) [126] is the only IBS symptom severity scale that has been shown to be valid, reliable, and responsive to treatment effects. It has been used in hypnosis studies [135, 136] and a study assessing the effectiveness of standard medical care [20]. An alternative scale, the Functional Bowel Disease Severity Index [137], was shown to be valid and reliable to stratify patients by symptom severity [138], but was not designed to measure responsiveness. The Gastrointestinal Symptom Rating Scale for IBS (GSRS-IBS) [139] also assesses symptom severity for several FGIDs.

Blanchard and colleagues [127, 128] have consistently defined a treatment responder as a patient showing at least a 50% reduction in severity of the primary symptoms of IBS from baseline to the end of treatment. Psychometric properties of this scale have not been fully described, but it was responsive to change in IBS patients treated effectively with cognitive behavioral therapy [127, 128]. Whitehead and colleagues [20] later defined a responder to standard medical care as a patient with at least a 50% decrease in the total score of the IBS [126] symptom severity scale. This responder definition correlated significantly with graded symptom improvement and satisfactory relief, supporting its validity and responsiveness. Although reliability was not assessed, the IBS-SSS, on which the measure is based, has been shown to be reliable. Furthermore, this responder definition was not significantly influenced by the initial IBS severity, highlighting a potential advantage over "satisfactory relief" [140]. Defining a responder in an IBS therapeutic trial as a patient who reports a 50% reduction in symptoms was endorsed by a European panel of experts but will require further evaluation [6].

Several well validated outcome measures have been used in FD trials, including the Duration-Intensity-Behavior Scale (DIBS) score [141] (assesses duration, intensity, and behavioral symptoms due to dyspepsia), severity or absence of epigastric pain (using four-, five-, or seven-point Likert scales), the Glasgow Dyspepsia Severity Score (GDSS) [142], the sum score of baseline adjusted severity of dyspepsia symptoms (10 symptoms 4 point severity scale), the Leeds Dyspepsia Questionnaire [143], the Canadian Dyspepsia score [144], the Severity of Dyspepsia Assessment (SODA) [145], (pain intensity, non-pain symptoms and satisfaction with dyspepsia-related health), the Nepean Dyspepsia Index [146] and the Quality of Life in Reflux and Dyspepsia (QOLRAD) [139]. These use a single global outcome of a specific symptom, a global overall assessment of dyspepsia symptoms or several questions covering important dyspepsia and quality-of-life outcomes. For some FGIDs, such outcome measures are yet to be developed. Because Rome III has redefined dyspepsia as a cluster of three separate syndromes rather than a single entitiy, integrative outcome measures for FD may no longer be valid [147].

Pain

Pain or discomfort is a key feature of many FGIDs and is typically either the primary outcome variable or an important secondary outcome variable in clinical trials. Pain has three dimensions—intensity, duration, and frequency—that can be considered separately or integrated in a global assessment of pain. Pain can also be incorporated into a quality-of-life measure to assess the impact on normal daily activities or work. Different rating scales, whether ordinal (Likert) or visual analog scales (VAS), as discussed below, can be used, and both methods have been shown to be reproducible and sensitive to change [148]. If pain is chosen as the primary outcome, a meaningful clinical response should be defined beforehand, and the proportion of patients reaching this endpoint reported.

"Adequate relief" and "satisfactory relief" are the current standards for primary outcome assessment in treatment trials in IBS. They require additional validation. Alternative outcome measures such as integrative symptom questionnaires are also acceptable if appropriately validated.

Safety Issues and Absence of Harms

Recent attention has focused on the appropriate reporting of harms-related issues in randomized clinical trials [149]. An extension of the Consolidated Standards of Reporting Trials (CONSORT) statement [150] encouraged the use of the term "harms" rather than "safety," the term that has traditionally been used. In addition, if the collection of harms data is a key trial objective, this fact should be reflected in the title and abstract, as well as the body of the manuscript, reporting the study results. The methods section should clearly define how adverse events were measured.

Anticipated and unanticipated adverse events should be reported.

— Choosing Secondary Outcome Variables

Secondary outcome variables (including inclusion criteria) are meant to confirm the primary analysis by showing that individual symptoms also improve. Not all Rome symptom criteria for FGIDs are amenable to a severity assessment.

For example, the Rome criteria for IBS [85] require that the patient have abdominal pain satisfying at least two of three conditions: (1) the pain or discomfort is relieved by defecation, (2) onset is associated with a change in the frequency of stools, or (3) onset is associated with a change in the consistency of stools. These three criteria for IBS diagnosis would be difficult to assess in terms of severity. Secondary measures in an IBS trial should include the severity of pain or discomfort, stool consistency (using for example, the Bristol Stool Form [151]), and stool frequency [152].

Secondary outcome measures can also explain the mechanism of the intervention. These outcomes may be conceptualized as "process measures" that assess whether the intervention produces the anticipated physiological, psychological, or cognitive effects [53, 127, 128], or they may simply be exploratory analyses to test for changes in such variables as whole-gut transit time, gastric emptying, or psychological state.

"Credibility scales" in behavioral trials are another category of secondary outcome measures that can assess whether the control condition produces an expectation of benefit that is comparable to the investigational treatment [55]. "Predictor variables," such as psychological profile or manometry features, can be measured at baseline and examined for their ability to identify the patients who are most likely (or least likely) to benefit.

Health economic outcomes are now becoming an important class of secondary outcome variables. For example, recent trials of interpersonal psychotherapy [125] and hypnosis [51] have shown that these psychological interventions, although labor-intensive and costly, produce long-term savings. Analyses of health care outcomes could also provide a more rational way of pricing new drugs. The methodology to capture direct and indirect health care costs is complex [125] and may not be feasible to include in efficacy trials, but new questionnaire-based techniques show promise [153]. Moreover, simple outcomes such as the frequency of health visits or the number of prescriptions filled during a follow-up period are easily obtained [51].

Because multiple secondary outcome variables may be included in a trial, and for different purposes, the investigator should clearly identify the reasons for each secondary outcome and the plan for analysis before the trial begins. Sample size need not be based on the analysis of secondary outcome measures; however, it is advantageous to estimate the power of the planned comparisons of secondary variables to allow selection of the most meaningful secondary measures.

Secondary outcomes should be selected based on the study question, and should be validated measures that support or explain the results. Investigators should state the reasons for each secondary outcome and describe the plan for analysis before the trial begins. Integrating health economic outcomes is recommended when feasible.

Quality of Life (QOL) Assessment

FGIDs generally do not limit life expectancy, but do have a major impact on quality of life (QOL) [154, 155]. A measure of their impact on QOL would be a logical primary outcome measure, but concerns about their responsiveness to treatment have limited their use as primary outcome variables. One report focused on the health-related quality of life (HRQOL) data from two previously reported trials of alosetron and found a significantly greater improvement on active drug compared to placebo [156], challenging the belief that these measures are not responsive enough to be employed as primary outcome variables. It is strongly recommended that HRQOL measures be included routinely among secondary outcome variables to support (or qualify) any claim of efficacy.

QOL instruments can be divided into two categories: generic and disease-specific [121, 122]. Generic instruments assess QOL in large populations and across a wide spectrum of disorders. Examples of validated generic instruments include the Sickness Impact Profile [157], the Nottingham Health Profile [158], the Rand Corporation Instruments [159], the McMaster Health Index Questionnaire [160], the SF-36 [161], and the Psychological General Well-being Index (PGWB) [162]. A limitation of generic instruments is that they may not reflect the most important aspects of health status for any particular disorder, and thus may be less sensitive to detect important treatment effects. Their major advantage is to allow comparisons of the impact of FGIDs with other diseases and detect unexpected changes in health status or adverse effects after new treatments. Measuring generic QOL at baseline is recommended.

Disease-specific QOL instruments examine the impact of a specific disease on quality of life and include problems specific to the disease of interest (e.g., the fear of fecal incontinence in IBS). Theoretically, they can detect smaller changes in health status that are relevant for patients and that may be missed by the generic instruments. For FD, disease-specific QOL instruments include the QOLRAD and the Nepean Index. There are also published instruments for IBS that include the IBS-QOL [137], the IBS QOL [163] the Functional Digestive Disorders Quality of Life questionnaire (FDDQL) [164], Gastrointestinal Quality of Life Index (GIQLI) [165], and the IBS Questionnaire (IBSQ) [166]. Some have been more fully validated than others. It is wise to consider the use of both a generic and disease-specific QOL instrument. QOL assessment can also be applied in pharmaco-economic analyses when comparing costs to achieve a particular outcome (such as adequate relief), or costs per quality-adjusted life year gained. Readers are referred to the references for QOL instruments in specific FGIDs [123].

QOL assessments are important secondary outcomes. Investigators are encouraged to include both a baseline generic and a pre post disease-specific QOL instrument.

— Choice of Response Scales

A detailed discussion of measurement scales and their properties is beyond the scope of this report [2, 148, 167–175]. The most common scales assessing symptom severity are (1) categorical scales (ordinal or Likert scales), (2) visual analogue scales (VAS), and (3) numerical rating scales.

Likert Scales

A categorical scale has several response categories, each accompanied by a verbal descriptor (e.g. a seven-point scale ranging from 1= no problem to 7 = a severe problem). In constructing these scales, there are three methodological issues to consider: (1) the understandability of the verbal descriptors, (2) the number of categories employed, and (3) the appropriate statistical analysis for the data. The descriptors must be chosen carefully to ensure that they are interpreted and applied consistently: for example, do all subjects interpret "mild discomfort" as different from "minor discomfort" and do they all believe that "mild discomfort" represents a higher intensity of sensation than "minor discomfort"? The nature of the descriptors is especially important when scales must be translated for use by different cultures for a multinational trial.

The number of categories is frequently a compromise between sensitivity (more categories yield a more sensitive scale) and practicality (it is difficult to identify more than seven different verbal labels that are interpreted in the same way by all subjects). Consequently most scales use four to seven scale levels. However, in FGIDs, the extreme ends of the scale are often not used by patients, thereby potentially reducing a four-point scale to a two-point scale. An additional consideration is that an odd number of response options is preferred to allow subjects to select a middle or neutral value. Standardizing the number of levels has advantages, particularly when conducting meta-analyses. Therefore, five- to seven-point scales have been favored [169].

Parametric statistics (e.g., t tests or analysis of variance) are considered appropriate, in theory, only if scale divisions can be assumed to be of equal intervals (i.e., if the difference between a rating of 1 and 2 is equivalent to the magnitude of the difference between ratings of 3 and 4). Categorical scales have rarely been tested to verify that they are equal interval scales [176], and under these circumstances, nonparametric tests (e.g., Mann-Whitney U tests) are more appropriate. However, some investigators are prepared to assume that categorical scales with seven or more response options approximate equal interval scales closely enough to justify the use of (more powerful) parametric statistics [176].

Dichotomous or binary scales ("yes" vs. "no" scales) are a special case of categorical scales. An advantage of the binary adequate-relief and satisfactory-relief scales is a clear relationship to a clinically meaningful change for the patient. The disadvantage of binary response scales is a substantial decrease in sensitivity, specificity, and reliability due to the restricted number of response options. Adequate relief and satisfactory relief are examples of dichotomous scales that have been used in recent IBS trials and subjects have been required to respond to these scales at multiple visits. Studies should report the frequency and type of problems encountered in completing all scales during a trial.

Visual Analogue Scales (VAS)

A VAS is a horizontal line (usually 100 mm), with verbal anchors at each end (e.g., 0 = no pain and 100 = most severe pain imaginable, on which the patient must place a mark). The distance from the left-hand side to the subject's mark is measured and interpreted as the symptom severity. The use of VAS scales for pain has been extensively validated both for reliability and interval scaling [176], and parametric statistics are considered appropriate for analysis. However, concerns have been expressed about the complexity of VAS scales and their understandability in older or less educated subjects [177]. The FDA currently discourages the use of VAS scales in pivotal trials of investigational drugs.

Numerical Scales

Numerical scales are similar to VAS scales: the subject is asked to select a number representing the intensity of the symptom(s) between 0 and an arbitrary upper limit such as 20 or 100. "0" represents zero intensity and the upper limit represents the most intense symptom imaginable. The intermediate steps in the numerical scale are not assigned verbal labels. This type of scale is easily implemented, and may be more comprehensible for all subjects than a VAS. Studies show that numerical scales with more than nine categories have equal interval scaling properties and are equivalent to VAS scales [178].

Likert scales are acceptable primary or secondary outcome measures. VAS scales and numerical scales are acceptable as primary or secondary outcome measures and can be analyzed by parametric statistics. All newly developed scales should be independently validated prior to use.

Global Assessment Scales

A global assessment can be considered to be a patient-reported 'weighted average' of the overall impact of symptoms on their well-being. The response to this question implies a weighting of all aspects of the subject's well-being integrated in a single response. The global assessment used as outcome measures in clinical trials usually ask patients to consider specific FGID symptoms when they make these ratings.

There are two ways to measure change using a global outcome measure: (1) administer the same rating scale before and periodically during treatment to document the change by subtraction, or (2) use a separate global rating scale of change. Table 3 lists examples of both approaches. When a global rating scale of change is used, the patient is asked only if symptoms have changed compared to the beginning of the study and is not asked about their current severity. This can be either done on a single scale or by a combined scale (Table 3). For a combined scale, the patient is asked first if the symptoms have remained the same, improved, or deteriorated, and then to rate the degree of change on a seven-point scale (Table 3). Guyatt et al. have used a variation of this combined scale successfully as a 15-point scale (−7, 0, +7) of change in several asthma and heart failure studies [168, 175]. Whatever scale is chosen, it must be able to record both improvement and deterioration.

Another global change scale is the Clinical Global Impressions (CGI) [179]. The CGI was originally developed by the National Institutes of Health for use in schizophrenia studies. Ratings were made by clinicians on two scales that measured the disease and the intervention using seven-point Likert descriptors for (1) current severity of illness and (2) global improvement. The "severity of illness" scale ranges from "normal" (=1) to "among the most extremely ill" (=7) and the "global improvement" scale ranges from "very much improved" (=1) through "no change" (=4) to "very much worse" (=7). The severity of illness scale is administered at baseline and periodically during the trial. The global improvement scale is administered periodically during the study or, in short trials, only at the end of the treatment period. The advantage of combining these two scales is that the change scale can be standardized relative to the severity of illness at baseline, and there is a high correlation between the severity of illness and global improvement scales. These scales have high face validity and are simple, brief, and easy to understand across different languages and cultures. The Global Improvement Scale has undergone partial validation in IBS, using data from alosetron trials, and showed a good correlation (r = 0.8) between responder status and satisfaction with overall treatment [180].

Global rating scales of change in symptom intensity are acceptable and are commonly employed outcome measures in randomized controlled trials. Adequate relief and satisfactory relief are binary scale versions of global ratings scales of change in symptoms. It is recommended that global rating scales of change in symptoms be validated in the target disease entity, patient population, and language prior to initiating the trial.

Table 3. Examples of Scales to Measure Outcome

1. Seven-point Likert scale to measure epigastric discomfort, which can be administered before and after the intervention. Patients indicate how much discomfort they have in the epigastric region.
   - No discomfort at all
   - Minor discomfort
   - Mild discomfort
   - Moderate discomfort
   - Moderately severe discomfort
   - Severe discomfort
   - Very severe discomfort

2. Global rating of change. Patients indicate how much they have improved.
   - No improvement at all
   - Minor improvement
   - Mild improvement
   - Moderate improvement
   - Quite a bit of improvement
   - A lot of improvement
   - Great improvement

3. Seven-point scale to rate deterioration or improvement.
   - Markedly worse
   - Somewhat worse
   - A little bit worse
   - No change
   - A little better
   - Somewhat better
   - Markedly better

4. Combined scale to measure change. Patients first report if they have improved, remained the same, or deteriorated. If a change occurs, the degree of change is then scored on a seven-point Likert scale, providing a 15-point scale of change from −7 to 0 to +7. Only deterioration is shown here.
   1 Worse
   2 About the same
   3 Better

   1 Almost the same, hardly any worse at all
   2 A little worse
   3 Somewhat worse
   4 Moderately worse
   5 A good deal worse
   6 A great deal worse
   7 A very great deal worse

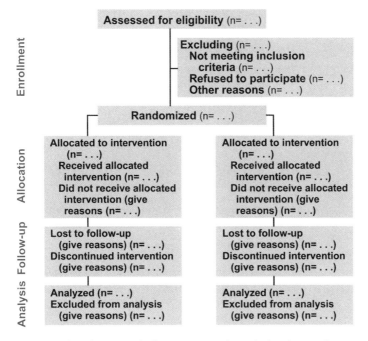

Figure I. Flow diagram of subject progress through the phases of a randomized trial

Analysis and Data Reporting

The original CONSORT statement, published in 1996, was developed to improve the quality of reporting of two-group, parallel, randomized, controlled trials [181, 182]. In response to investigator feedback and accumulating evidence, the CONSORT guidelines have recently been revised [150]. The latest iteration re-emphasized the importance of clearly and transparently reporting the reason the study was undertaken, and how it was carried out and analyzed. It includes a 22-item checklist (Table 4) and a flow diagram (Figure 1). The revised CONSORT statement lists the recommended key elements of statistical reporting to which investigators should adhere [150, 183, 184].

Recent evidence suggests that a detailed flowchart that clearly describes how patients progressed through a study improves the quality of data reporting, but has frequently not been provided by authors [185]. A complete flow diagram should consist of four sections. The *Enrollment Section* should contain an accounting of those assessed for eligibility with a description of patients who did not meet inclusion criteria or refused to participate. The *Allocation Section* should detail the total number of patients randomized as well as the number allocated to each in-

Table 4. Checklist of Items to Include When Reporting a Randomized Trial

Section and Topic	Descriptor
Title and Abstract	How participants were allocated to interventions, (e.g, "random allocation," "randomized," or "randomly assigned"
Introduction	
Background	Scientific background and explanation of rationale
Methods	
Participants	Eligibility criteria for participants and the settings and locations where the data were collected
Interventions	Precise details of the interventions intended for each group and how and when they were actually administered
Objectives	Specific objectives and hypotheses
Outcomes	Clearly defined primary and secondary outcome measures and, when applicable, any methods used to enhance the quality of measurements (e.g., multiple observations, training of assessors)
Sample size	How sample size was determined and, when applicable, explanation of any interim analyses and stopping rules
Randomization	
Sequence generation	Method used to generate the random allocation sequence, including details of any restriction (e.g., blocking, stratification)
Allocation concealment	Method used to implement the random allocation sequence (e.g., numbered containers or central telephone), clarifying whether the sequence was concealed until interventions were assigned
Implementation	Who generated the allocation sequence, who enrolled participants, and who assigned participants to their groups
Blinding (masking)	Whether or not participants, those administering the interventions, and those assessing the outcomes were blinded to group assignment. If done, how the success of blinding was evaluated.
Statistical methods	Statistical methods used to compare groups for primary outcome(s); methods for additional analyses, such as subgroup analyses and adjusted analyses

Results

Participant flow	Flow of participants through each stage (a diagram is strongly recommended). Specifically, for each group report the numbers of participants randomly assigned, receiving intended treatment, completing the study protocol, and analyzed for the primary outcome. Describe protocol deviations from study planned, together with reasons.
Recruitment	Dates defining the periods of recruitment and followup
Baseline data	Baseline demographic and clinical characteristics of each group
Numbers analyzed	Number of participants (denominator) in each group included in each analysis and whether the analysis was by "intention-to-treat." State the results in absolute numbers when feasible (e.g., 10/20, not 50%).
Outcomes and estimation	For each primary and secondary outcome, a summary of results for each group, and the estimated effect size and its precision (e.g., 95% confidence interval)
Ancillary analyses	Address multiplicity by reporting any other analyses performed, including subgroup analyses and adjusted analyses, indicating those prespecified and those exploratory.
Adverse events	All important adverse events or side effects in each intervention group

Comment

Interpretation	Interpretation of the results, taking into account study hypotheses, sources of potential bias or imprecision, and the dangers associated with multiplicity of analyses and outcomes
Generalizability	Generalizability (external validity) of the trial findings
Overall evidence	General interpretation of the results in the context of current evidence

---

tervention. A breakdown of those who received the intervention and those who did not receive the intervention should also be included. The *Follow-up Section* should describe the number of patients lost to followup or who discontinued the intervention. In the *Analysis Section*, the final number of patients analyzed as well as the number excluded from analysis should be listed. It is recommended that authors provide the reasons why patients did not complete the trial or were excluded from the analysis. The use of the CONSORT guidelines improves methodological quality and the quality of data reporting [150, 186]. Many journals now require that manuscripts describing clinical trials conform to the CONSORT guidelines. These can be found on the Web at www.consort-statement.org.

Investigators should adhere to the CONSORT statement on reporting of clinical trials.

Although this discussion focuses on the randomized controlled trial, recent recommendations similar to the CONSORT guidelines have been published for studies evaluating the accuracy of diagnostic testing (STARD initiative) [187, 188] and for the reporting of meta-analyses (QUOROM statement) [189]. The impact of implementing the recommendations of the Standards for Reporting of Diagnostic Accuracy (STARD) initiative and Quality of Reporting of Meta-analyses (QUOROM) statement remain to be validated. Nonetheless, it is anticipated that the acceptance and utilization of STARD and QUOROM will also improve the methodological quality and transparency of reporting of studies evaluating the operating characteristics of diagnostic tests and of meta-analyses, respectively. While the recommendations of the STARD initiative were intended for the design of studies to evaluate the ability of one or more tests to accurately diagnose a specific disease or condition, the same concepts can be applied to validation studies of the diagnostic criteria for the FGIDs.

It is recommended the STARD guidelines be used to report studies evaluating diagnostic tests and that the QUOROM guidelines be used to report meta-analyses.

— Primary Efficacy Analysis

A detailed discussion of data analysis for all trials cannot be provided here, as the type of statistical analysis will be determined by the particular study design and primary outcome measure(s). In general, a study should have one and no more than two primary outcome measures [183]. The EMEA has recommended two positive primary outcomes for IBS trials. However, the subcommittee feels that this recommendation may be overly conservative. The main analysis should focus on the chosen primary outcome measure(s) on which the overall conclusion of the study is based. This should determine whether the study has a positive or a negative result in support of a new treatment. Although the main outcome often is reported as a comparison between the end of treatment and baseline observations, it is also important that data are provided describing how patients changed throughout the course of the study. A result where patients are classified as responders some of the time and as failures at other times is far less convincing than results where patients have had a sustained response after the intervention. When two primary outcome variables are included in the trial, the investigators should specify in advance whether they will interpret the trial as positive if only one of the outcome measures is significant, or if they will require that both be significant. If significance of any primary outcome will provide evidence for efficacy of the treatment, the analysis should adjust for multiple comparisons. A commonly used technique is the Bonferroni correction [190].

The results of the primary outcome should be stated in absolute numbers to include both a numerator and denominator. It is not sufficient to list only percentages of (non)responders, (for example, not 20% but rather 10/50, 20%). For all outcome measures, the estimated effect of the intervention (difference between active and placebo treatment) and a 95% two-sided confidence interval should also be included [191–193].

The main result of the study must be based on the evaluation of the primary outcome measure as stated in the protocol before the study begins. The primary outcome should be stated in absolute numbers and should include a 95% confidence interval.

Statistically significant differences between study groups can also be expressed using a P value. If a P value is reported, actual values and not thresholds (e.g., $P=.04$ and not $P<0.05$) should be provided. The use of P values should be viewed as complementary to, and not a substitute for, confidence intervals. The reciprocal of the absolute risk reduction in a risk reduction trial or therapeutic gain in a treatment efficacy trial, 1/(% responding to active drug minus % responding to placebo), can also allow computation of the number of patients who need to be treated (NNT) to encounter a patient who will experience a clinical benefit. Although the NNT is reported infrequently in randomized controlled trials, its inclusion can frame the clinical importance of a study result [194].

When reporting P values, actual values and not thresholds should be provided. Investigators are encouraged to report the number needed to treat (NNT) in clinical trials. A number needed to harm (NNH) can be calculated based on the risk of adverse effects and be weighed against the NNT.

The statistical analysis should be based on an intention-to-treat (ITT) principle [191, 195]. Investigators should plan in advance how they will represent treatment dropouts in the ITT analysis. We recommend one of two strategies: either analyze the trial in terms of the proportion of responders and treat all dropouts as treatment nonresponders, or carry forward the last observation of the primary outcome variable that was available. In some cases, the last observation available will be the baseline score for the primary outcome variable. Further, a dual analysis in which dropouts are classed using the last value carried forward or, alternatively as a "treatment failure," should be examined to test for differences in results. Many studies also report a per-protocol (all patients who followed the protocol) or an all-patients-treated (all patients who received treatment following randomization) analysis. These analyses may provide insight as to whether a treatment works under optimal conditions but cannot replace the ITT analysis. What is critical in study reports, however, is a clear statement of the sample size/power calculations carried out prior to study initiation, the numbers of patients included in the ITT and per-protocol or all-patients-treated analyses, and how these were determined. The number of patients who were lost to followup should also be declared, as well as their reason for and time of attrition.

The effect of potential modifiers such as sex, age, duration or severity of disease, and presence of psychological stress can be assessed using a logistic regression analysis, where the binary dependent variable represents the a priori specified definition of a responder [196]. Such covariates also need to be prespecified.

The primary analysis should be the intention to treat (ITT) analysis and must include all patients randomized.

— Analysis of Secondary Outcome Measures and Subgroups

It is recommended that changes be reported for each of the symptoms that comprise the entry criteria. It is likely that several different symptoms of a particular FGID will be interdependent and hence may respond in a similar fashion. Reporting of such secondary outcome measures may support (or refute) the direction and magnitude of the interventional effect on the primary outcome measure. For example, if the primary outcome measure shows improvement, it is likely that some other cardinal disease symptoms will also show amelioration. Because these secondary outcome variables are used to support the effectiveness analysis of the primary outcome variable, they should also be analyzed by ITT and not per protocol.

When secondary variables are used for the purpose of supporting the primary outcome analysis, there are usually only a few, and it is unnecessary to adjust for multiple comparisons. However, investigators sometimes include a large number of secondary variables to (1) identify predictors of which patients respond to the intervention, or (2) explore other possible effects (benefits) of the intervention unrelated to the primary hypothesis of the study. In such cases, the type I error rate may be inflated by a large number of comparisons. One approach to overcome this problem is to adjust by using, for example, the Bonferroni correction [190]. This correction derives a new P value by dividing the original P value (usually set at 0.05) by the number of outcome comparisons. If there are large numbers of statistical tests, the Bonferroni correction may be too conservative [190] since it also increases the likelihood of a type II statistical error, rendering truly important differences nonsignificant. There are two suggested strategies for dealing with this problem: (1) the multiple secondary outcome measures can be analyzed using descriptive rather than inferential statistics (e.g., means and confidence intervals), and (2) investigators may choose a conservative alpha level such as .01 that protects against type I error without unduly inflating the type II error rate. Results should be reported for all prespecified outcomes, not only those demonstrating statistically significant differences between study groups.

Exploratory subgroup analyses are commonly performed in trials addressing the effectiveness of therapies for patients with FGIDs. This practice is controversial and some researchers question its validity [183, 197, 198], particularly when it is undertaken after an initial evaluation of the data set (post hoc subgroup analysis). The test of interaction is the most appropriate type of subgroup analysis [183, 199]. Such an analysis evaluates for a difference in treatment effect *between* complementary subgroups (for example older and younger subjects), rather than simply comparing P values generated by each individual subgroup. Details regarding the test of interaction can be found elsewhere [183, 199].

Specific plans to present and analyze harms data (coding, handling of recurrent events, specification of timing issues, handling of continuous measures, and statistical analyses) should be clearly described. Participant withdrawals from each arm of the trial should be detailed. Actual incidence rates and 95% confidence intervals should always be reported. When statistical comparisons are performed, ITT is the preferred analysis for harms data. Investigators should attempt to place benefits and harms of any intervention into perspective, together with study limitations, generalizability of the data, and other sources of information on harms. For further details on the recording and reporting of harms, the reader is referred to the reference [149].

The purpose for inclusion of all secondary variables and the plans for their analysis should be specified in advance. Adjustment for multiple comparisons is necessary only if there are large numbers of comparisons (e.g., greater than five) for any specific purpose.

— Sample Size and Power Calculations

The protocol should clearly specify the assumptions upon which the sample size calculation was based [200]. The elements of a sample size calculation include the minimum effect size (difference in the primary outcome between groups) that the trial is designed to detect, α (type I) error level, the statistical power or β (type II) error level, and, when evaluating changes (differences) in continuous outcomes (for example difference in severity scores), the standard deviation of the difference. Recent trials have been powered to detect differences as small as 10% [118], 12% [11, 13], or 15% [7, 83]. Often a power of 80% is used (beta error or type II error of 20%) and alpha (type I) error of 5%, using a two-sided test. An allowance for dropouts should also be made in determining the appropriate sample size, but efforts should be made to keep the dropout rate below 10% to 20%. When dealing with dropouts in studies of longer duration, it is reasonable to use the last observation of the patient while in the study in order not to lose all of the data gathered from this individual (i.e., last observation carried forward). The number and timing of the dropouts should be reported.

For responder analyses, the protocol should clearly state what constitutes a patient responder. Simply recording average changes in symptoms without stating what amount of change constitutes a treatment success is not sufficient. The sample size should be based on a priori consideration of what is the clinically important difference in the proportion of responders between active treatment and placebo. The study must have sufficient power to detect a clinically important difference in the proportion of responders [40, 201–203]. The smaller a difference is— that is felt to be meaningful—the larger the number of patients that must be enrolled in the study to avoid a type II error. It is inappropriate for an inadequately powered study that fails to find a statistically significant difference between interventions to conclude that the two interventions are equivalent [40, 49].

A sample size calculation should be routinely performed and should be based on the expected behavior of the primary outcome measure. The smallest effect that the study is powered to detect should be explicitly stated.

— Interim Analysis and Stopping Rules

There is no compelling reason to incorporate specific interim analyses for interventions in the FGIDs, since they are not life-threatening. Moreover, since the incidence of serious adverse events is expected to be low, any occurrence of a serious adverse event is likely to prompt the safety committee to re-evaluate the trial without carrying out an interim analysis. Thus, interim analyses in trials of FGIDs will normally only be done to assess the futility of continuing the trial. Plans for interim analyses should be clearly prespecified in the study protocol. Such analyses should be distinguished from monitoring to ensure therapeutic safety. If interim analyses are performed to evaluate futility or harms, appropriate statistical methods to adjust for multiple analyses are necessary [183, 204–206]. The most common method is to partition the alpha level initially selected for the trial so that the alpha level used for the interim analysis is subtracted from the alpha level intended for the final analysis. Consequently, most investigators use a very conservative alpha level, such as .001, for the interim analysis so that sufficient power is reserved for the final analysis. If an interim analysis has been preplanned, it is possible to take this alpha-sharing into account when calculating the sample size. Unplanned preliminary analyses should be avoided since premature presentation of results may affect the further conduct of the trial and can lead to the reporting of inaccurate observations [207].

There are few guidelines for conducting interim analyses to assess the futility of continuing a trial. However, to preserve the credibility of the investigators (a) such analyses should be overseen by a Data and Safety Monitoring Board (DSMB) that is independent from the investigators, (b) the analysis should test for equivalence rather than superiority of one treatment relative to the other, and (c) liberal equivalence margins for the effect size should be defined a priori and will likely be wider than those applied to serious harms.

Interim analyses are not recommended as they may jeopardize the trial integrity unless there is reason to believe participation in the trial (either in the active treatment or control group) places the patient at risk.

Ethical Issues

While there is an understandable desire to obtain positive results from well-designed and well-conducted studies, the main result of a trial must be presented according to the predetermined primary outcome measure(s). To select the primary outcome measure after the trial is concluded inflates the type I error rate to an unacceptable (and usually unknown) degree. It is misleading and unethical if the originally stated primary outcome measures are abandoned for others that favor the active treatment. A secondary analysis of data may also lead to the discovery of results that were not part of the original hypothesis [200]. Such data should be considered as purely exploratory (i.e., hypothesis-generating) for testing in future studies. Adherence to the study goals is strengthened if there is an independent advisory group for the trial, which is one function of a DSMB.

Changing the primary outcome measure(s) in the analysis phase of a study should not be done; it invalidates the statistical analysis and renders the conclusions of uncertain value by inflating the chances of a type I error.

Concern has been voiced in the popular press that negative treatment trials for FGIDs (or other disorders) have not always been published, which may have led to an overestimation of the efficacy of some treatments and an underestimation of safety concerns. Investigators have an ethical obligation to publish the results of all completed studies and to acknowledge the existence of all prematurely terminated studies, regardless of whether the results are positive or negative. Several journals are implementing a policy that will require investigators to register all clinical trials before they are initiated, using a publicly accessible trial registry; failure to register the trial before initiation will result in the manuscript being barred from publication by the subscribing journals [208]. Now that a concerted effort has been made to systematically review the medical literature through the Cochrane Collaboration, it is imperative that all relevant studies are published [209]. This underscores the obligation of journal editors to publish methodologically sound studies, whether results are negative or positive.

It is unethical to withhold publishing the results of a completed trial.

Recommendations for Future Research

In reviewing the relevant literature for this report, the committee identified a number of areas that require additional evaluation. These areas were identified as priorities for future research to improve study design for FGIDs and are listed in Table 5.

Conclusions

Significant gains have been made in study design since the first Rome process. However, there is considerable work still to be done to further improve the quality of the research methods for studies of the FGIDs. A list of recommendations for additional research is provided below. Trials should be registered before enrollment begins. Defining the study question is the most critical task. Adequate descriptions of population sampling, recruitment strategies, and inclusion criteria are required. A full description of concealed randomization is imperative, and blinding of the intervention (with use of a plausible control and blinded outcome assessment) are exceedingly important. The choice of the primary outcome measure(s) is critical and much work is still needed in this area. Use of the appropriate statistical methods must be undertaken, and a sample size should be calculated, a priori, based on the primary outcome measure. Results should be described and an unbiased interpretation of safety, efficacy, effect size, and number needed to treat or harm are important clinical considerations. Exploration of clinically important changes in outcome should also be performed within the trial and, where appropriate, extended validation of outcome measurement tools should be performed. Publication and communication of objectively interpreted results are the final and most important elements in completing a treatment trial.

Table 5. Recommendations for Future Research

1. Examine the periodicity and severity of symptoms in natural history studies.

2. Evaluate the multidimensional construct of symptom severity (e.g., frequency, number present, clustering, severity, contribution to "global severity," and changes in primary symptoms over time).

3. Examine the influence of disease modifiers (predictors) such as disease duration, baseline severity, psychological status, comorbidity, surgeries, and response to prior treatments.

4. Investigate what contributes to the placebo response in different FGIDs and how to minimize its impact on efficacy assessment.

5. Evaluate the impact of baseline observations and diagnostic testing on symptoms, data quality, and treatment response.

6. Further validate adequate and satisfactory relief during clinical trials.

7. Develop, validate fully, and determine minimal clinically important differences (MCID) for new outcome measures and disease-specific QOL instruments. Catalog and critically appraise them.

8. Further evaluate and validate definitions of treatment responder measure(s) including a 50% reduction in symptom severity, and ensure that the definitions are clinically relevant.

9. Develop and validate trial designs for testing on-demand treatments for intermittent symptoms.

10. Examine the impact of CONSORT and EMEA and FDA guidelines on study quality.

References

1. Irvine EJ, Whitehead WE, Chey WD, Matsueda K, Talley NJ, Shaw M, Veldhuyzen van Zanten SJO. Design of treatment trials for functional gastrointestinal disorders. In: Drossman DA, Corazziari E, Delvaux M, Talley NJ, Thompson WG, Spiller RC, and Whitehead WE, eds. The Functional Gastrointestinal Disorders: Diagnosis, Pathophysiology and Treatment. A multinational consensus. Third ed. McLean VA: Degnon Associates, 2006.
2. Veldhuyzen Van Zanten SJ, Talley NJ, Bytzer P, Klein KB, Whorwell PJ, Zinsmeister AR. Design of treatment trials for functional gastrointestinal disorders. Gut 1999;45 Suppl 2:II69–II77.
3. Talley NJ, Nyren O, Drossman DA, Heaton KW, Veldhuyzen van Zanten SJO, Koch MM, Ransohoff DF. The Irritable Bowel Syndrome: Toward optimal design of controlled treatment trials. Gastroenterology International 1993;189–211.
4. Kamm MA. Entry criteria for drug trials of irritable bowel syndrome. Am J Med 1999;107:51S-58S.
5. Spiller RC. Problems and challenges in the design of irritable bowel syndrome clinical trials: experience from published trials. Am J Med 1999;107:91S-97S.
6. Corazziari E, Bytzer P, Delvaux M, Holtmann G, Malagelada JR, Morris J, Muller-Lissner S, Spiller RC, Tack J, Whorwell PJ. Clinical trial guidelines for pharmacological treatment of irritable bowel syndrome. Aliment Pharmacol Ther 2003;18: 569–580.
7. Camilleri M, Northcutt AR, Kong S, Dukes GE, McSorley D, Mangel AW. Efficacy and safety of alosetron in women with irritable bowel syndrome: a randomised, placebo-controlled trial. Lancet 2000;355:1035–1040.
8. Northcutt AR, Camilleri M, Mayer EA, Drossman DA, Dukes GE, Ehsanullah RSB, Hamm LR, Harding JP, Heath AT, Jacques L, Wolfe S, Kong S, McSorley D, Mangel AW. Alosetron, a 5HT(3)-receptor antagonist, is effective in the treatment of female irritable bowel syndrome patients. Gastroenterol 1998;114:A812.
9. Lembo T, Wright RA, Bagby B, Decker C, Gordon S, Jhingran P, Carter E. Alosetron controls bowel urgency and provides global symptom improvement in women with diarrhea-predominant irritable bowel syndrome. Am J Gastroenterol 2001;96:2662–2670.
10. Muller-Lissner SA, Fumagalli I, Bardhan KD, Pace F, Pecher E, Nault B, Ruegg P. Tegaserod, a 5-HT(4) receptor partial agonist, relieves symptoms in irritable bowel syndrome patients with abdominal pain, bloating and constipation. Aliment Pharmacol Ther 2001;15:1655–1666.
11. Kellow J, Lee OY, Chang FY, Thongsawat S, Mazlam MZ, Yuen H, Gwee KA, Bak YT, Jones J, Wagner A. An Asia-Pacific, double blind, placebo controlled, randomised study to evaluate the efficacy, safety, and tolerability of tegaserod in patients with irritable bowel syndrome. Gut 2003;52:671–676.
12. Lefkowitz M, Ligizio G, Glebas K, Heggland JE. Tegaserod provides relief of symptoms in female patients with irritable bowel syndrome (IBS) suffering from abdominal pain and discomfort, bloating and constipation. Gastroenterology 2001;120: A22.
13. Nyhlin H, Bang C, Elsborg L, Silvennoinen J, Holme I, Ruegg P, Jones J, Wagner A. A double-blind, placebo-controlled, randomized study to evaluate the efficacy, safety

and tolerability of tegaserod in patients with irritable bowel syndrome. Scand J Gastroenterol 2004;39:119–126.

14. Fass R, Longstreth GF, Pimentel M, Fullerton S, Russak SM, Chiou CF, Reyes E, Crane P, Eisen G, McCarberg B, Ofman J. Evidence- and consensus-based practice guidelines for the diagnosis of irritable bowel syndrome. Arch Intern Med 2001;161: 2081–2088.

15. Cash BD, Schoenfeld P, Chey WD. The utility of diagnostic tests in irritable bowel syndrome patients: a systematic review. Am J Gastroenterol 2002;97:2812–2819.

16. Sonnenberg A, Vakil N. The benefit of negative tests in non-ulcer dyspepsia. Med Decis Making 2002;22:199–207.

17. Veldhuyzen Van Zanten SJ, Cleary C, Talley NJ, Peterson TC, Nyren O, Bradley LA, Verlinden M, Tytgat GN. Drug treatment of functional dyspepsia: a systematic analysis of trial methodology with recommendations for design of future trials. Am J Gastroenterol 1996;91:660–673.

18. Drossman DA, Thompson WG. The irritable bowel syndrome: review and a graduated multicomponent treatment approach. Ann Intern Med 1992;116:1009–1016.

19. Jones R. Likely impacts of recruitment site and methodology on characteristics of enrolled patient population: irritable bowel syndrome clinical trial design. Am J Med 1999;107:85S-90S.

20. Whitehead WE, Levy RL, Von Korff M, Feld AD, Palsson OS, Turner MJ, Drossman DA. Usual medical care for Irritable Bowel Syndrome. Aliment Pharmacol Ther 2004;30:1305–1315.

21. Talley NJ, Meineche-Schmidt V, Pare P, Duckworth M, Raisanen P, Pap A, Kordecki H, Schmid V. Efficacy of omeprazole in functional dyspepsia: double-blind, randomized, placebo-controlled trials (the Bond and Opera studies). Aliment Pharmacol Ther 1998;12:1055–1065.

22. Longstreth GF, Hawkey CJ, Mayer EA, Jones RH, Naesdal J, Wilson IK, Peacock RA, Wiklund IK. Characteristics of patients with irritable bowel syndrome recruited from three sources: implications for clinical trials. Aliment Pharmacol Ther 2001; 15:959–964.

23. Whitehead WE, Palsson O, Jones KR. Systematic review of the comorbidity of irritable bowel syndrome with other disorders: what are the causes and implications? Gastroenterology 2002;122:1140–1156.

24. Camilleri M, Atanasova E, Carlson PJ, Ahmad U, Kim HJ, Viramontes BE, McKinzie S, Urrutia R. Serotonin-transporter polymorphism pharmacogenetics in diarrhea-predominant irritable bowel syndrome. Gastroenterol 2002;123:425–432.

25. Berman SM, Chang L, Suyenobu B, Derbyshire SW, Stains J, Fitzgerald L, Mandelkern M, Hamm L, Vogt B, Naliboff BD, Mayer EA. Condition-specific deactivation of brain regions by 5-HT3 receptor antagonist Alosetron. Gastroenterol 2002;123:969–977.

26. Prather CM, Camilleri M, Zinsmeister AR, McKinzie S, Thomforde G. Tegaserod accelerates orocecal transit in patients with constipation-predominant irritable bowel syndrome. Gastroenterol 2000;118:463–468.

27. Guthrie E, Barlow J, Fernandes L, Ratcliffe J, Read N, Thompson DG, Tomenson B, Creed F. Changes in tolerance to rectal distension correlate with changes in psychological state in patients with severe irritable bowel syndrome. Psychosom Med 2004;66:578–582.

28. Drossman DA. Illness behavior in the Irritable Bowel Syndrome. Gastroenterology International 1991;77–81.

29. Drossman DA, Mckee DC, Sandler RS, Mitchell CM, Cramer EM, Lowman BC, Burger AL. Psychosocial factors in the irritable bowel syndrome. A multivariate study of patients and nonpatients with irritable bowel syndrome. Gastroenterol 1988;95:701–708.

30. Whitehead WE, Bosmajian L, Zonderman AB, Costa PT, Schuster MM. Symptoms of Psychologic Distress Associated with Irritable Bowel Syndrome—Comparison of Community and Medical Clinic Samples. Gastroenterol 1988;95:709–714.

31. Creed F, Levy R, Bradley L, Francisconi C, Drossman DA, Naliboff B, Olden K. Psychosocial Aspects of Functional Gastrointestinal Disorders. In: Drossman DA, Corrazziari E, Delvaux M, Spiller R, Talley N, Thompson WG, Whitehead W, eds. Rome III: The Functional Gastrointestinal Disorders. 3rd ed. McLean, VA: Degnon Associates, 2006:295–368.

32. Whitehead WE, Engel BT, Schuster MM. Irritable Bowel Syndrome—Physiological and Psychological Differences Between Diarrhea-Predominant and Constipation-Predominant Patients. Digestive Diseases and Sciences 1980;25:404–413.

33. Hahn BA, Kirchdoerfer LJ, Fullerton S, Mayer E. Patient-perceived severity of irritable bowel syndrome in relation to symptoms, health resource utilization and quality of life. Aliment Pharmacol Ther 1997;11:553–559.

34. Longstreth GF, Yao JF. Irritable bowel syndrome and surgery: a multivariable analysis. Gastroenterol 2004;126:1665–1673.

35. Hahn B, Watson M, Yan S, Gunput D, Heuijerjans J. Irritable bowel syndrome symptom patterns: frequency, duration, and severity. Dig Dis Sci 1998;43:2715–2718.

36. Whitehead WE. Control groups appropriate for behavioral interventions. Gastroenterol 2004;126:S159–S163.

37. Rockville MD. FDA updates warnings for cisapride. 2000.

38. Camilleri M. Safety concerns about alosetron. Arch Intern Med 2002;162:100–101.

39. Sackett DL. Bias in analytic research. J Chronic Dis 1979;32:51–63.

40. Detsky AS, Sackett DL. When was a "negative" clinical trial big enough? How many patients you needed depends on what you found. Arch Intern Med 1985;145:709–712.

41. Spilker B. Choosing and validating the clinical trial's blind. Guide to clinical trials. New York: Raven Press, 1991:15–20.

42. Spilker B. External influences on protocol design. Epilepsy Res Suppl 1993;10:115–124.

43. Spilker B.I. Randomization Procedures. Guide to Clinical Trials. New York: Raven Press, 1991:69–73.

44. Altman DG. Randomisation. Brit Med J 1991;302:1481–1482.

45. Chalmers TC CPSHeal. Bias in treatment assignment in controlled clinical trials. N Engl J Med 1983;309:1358–1361.

46. Altman DG. Comparability of randomised groups. The Statistician 1985;34:125–136.

47. Spilker B. [How to improve the quality of clinical trials and their publications]. Med Clin (Barc) 1992;98:303–304.

48. Tfelt-Hansen P, Block G, Dahlof C, Diener HC, Ferrari MD, Goadsby PJ, Guidetti V, Jones B, Lipton RB, Massiou H, Meinert C, Sandrini G, Steiner T, Winter PB. Guidelines for controlled trials of drugs in migraine: second edition. Cephalalgia 2000;20:765–786.

49. Tinmouth JM, Steele LS, Tomlinson G, Glazier RH. Are claims of equivalency in digestive diseases trials supported by the evidence? Gastroenterol 2004;126:1700–1710.

50. Temple RJ. When are clinical trials of a given agent vs. placebo no longer appropriate or feasible? Control Clin Trials 1997;18:613–620.

51. Calvert EL, Houghton LA, Cooper P, Morris J, Whorwell PJ. Long-term improvement in functional dyspepsia using hypnotherapy. Gastroenterol 2002;123:1778–1785.

52. Payne A, Blanchard EB. A controlled comparison of cognitive therapy and self-help support groups in the treatment of irritable bowel syndrome. J Consult Clin Psychol 1995;63:779–786.

53. Drossman DA, Toner BB, Whitehead WE, Diamant NE, Dalton CB, Duncan S, Emmott S, Proffitt V, Akman D, Frusciante K, Le T, Meyer K, Bradshaw B, Mikula K, Morris CB, Blackman CJ, Hu Y, Jia H, Li JZ, Koch GG, Bangdiwala SI. Cognitive-behavioral therapy versus education and desipramine versus placebo for moderate to severe functional bowel disorders. Gastroenterol 2003;125:19–31.

54. Guthrie E, Creed F, Dawson D, Tomenson B. A controlled trial of psychological treatment for the irritable bowel syndrome. Gastroenterol 1991;100:450–457.

55. Borkovec TD, Nau SD. Credibility of analogue therapy rationales. Journal of Behavior Therapy and Experimental Psychiatry 1972;3:257–260.

56. Weissman AN, Beck AT, Kovacs M. Drug abuse, hopelessness, and suicidal behavior. Int J Addict 1979;14:451–464.

57. Toner BB, Stuckless N, Ali A, Downie F, Emmott S, Akman D. The development of a cognitive scale for functional bowel disorders. Psychosom Med 1998;60:492–497.

58. Thompson WG. Placebos: a review of the placebo response. Am J Gastroenterol 2000;95:1637–1643.

59. Su C, Lichtenstein GR, Krok K, Brensinger CM, Lewis JD. A meta-analysis of the placebo rates of remission and response in clinical trials of active Crohn's disease. Gastroenterol 2004;126:1257–1269.

60. de Craen AJ, Moerman DE, Heisterkamp SH, Tytgat GN, Tijssen JG, Kleijnen J. Placebo effect in the treatment of duodenal ulcer. Br J Clin Pharmacol 1999;48:853–860.

61. Bland JM, Altman DG. Some examples of regression towards the mean. BMJ 1994;309:780.

62. Boyce PM, Talley NJ, Balaam B, Koloski NA, Truman G. A randomized controlled trial of cognitive behavior therapy, relaxation training, and routine clinical care for the irritable bowel syndrome. Am J Gastroenterol 2003;98:2209–2218.

63. Pitz M, Cheang M, Bernstein CN. Defining the predictors of the placebo response in irritable bowel syndrome. 3 ed. 2005:237–247.

64. Howarth PH, Stern MA, Roi L, Reynolds R, Bousquet J. Double-blind, placebo-controlled study comparing the efficacy and safety of fexofenadine hydrochloride (120 and 180 mg once daily) and cetirizine in seasonal allergic rhinitis. J Allergy Clin Immunol 1999;104:927–933.

65. Bachert C, Brostoff J, Scadding GK, Tasman J, Stalla-Bourdillon A, Murrieta M. Mizolastine therapy also has an effect on nasal blockade in perennial allergic rhinoconjunctivitis. RIPERAN Study Group. Allergy 1998;53:969–975.

66. Berger VW, Rezvani A, Makarewicz VA. Direct effect on validity of response run-in selection in clinical trials. Control Clin Trials 2003;24:156–166.

67. Woods JR, Williams JG, Tavel M. The two-period crossover design in medical research. Ann Intern Med 1989;110:560–566.
68. Louis TA, Lavori PW, Bailar JC, III, Polansky M. Crossover and self-controlled designs in clinical research. N Engl J Med 1984;310:24–31.
69. Hills M, Armitage P. The two-period cross-over clinical trial. Br J Clin Pharmacol 2004;58:S703–S716.
70. Committee for Proprietary Medicinal Products (CPMP). Notes for guidance on statistical principles for clinical trials. ICH/363/96 ed. London, UK.: European Agency for Evaluation of Medicinal Products, 1998.
71. Tack J, Muller-Lissner S, Bytzer P, Corinaldesi R, Chang L, Viegas A, Schnekenbuehl S, Dunger-Baldauf C, Rueegg P. A randomised controlled trial assessing the efficacy and safety of repeated tegaserod therapy in women with irritable bowel syndrome with constipation (IBS-C). Gut 2005;54:1707–1713.
72. Drossman DA, Camilleri M, Mayer EA, Whitehead WE. AGA technical review on irritable bowel syndrome. Gastroenterol 2002;123:2108–2131.
73. Holroyd KA, O'Donnell FJ, Stensland M, Lipchik GL, Cordingley GE, Carlson BW. Management of chronic tension-type headache with tricyclic antidepressant medication, stress management therapy, and their combination: a randomized controlled trial. JAMA 2001;285:2208–2215.
74. Keller MB, McCullough JP, Klein DN, Arnow B, Dunner DL, Gelenberg AJ, Markowitz JC, Nemeroff CB, Russell JM, Thase ME, Trivedi MH, Zajecka J. A comparison of nefazodone, the cognitive behavioral-analysis system of psychotherapy, and their combination for the treatment of chronic depression. N Engl J Med 2000;342:1462–1470.
75. Silvers D, Kipnes M, Broadstone V, Patterson D, Quigley EM, McCallum R, Leidy NK, Farup C, Liu Y, Joslyn A. Domperidone in the management of symptoms of diabetic gastroparesis: efficacy, tolerability, and quality-of-life outcomes in a multicenter controlled trial. DOM-USA-5 Study Group. Clin Ther 1998;20:438–453.
76. O'Donoghue DP DAP-TJBRL-JJE. Double-blind withdrawal trial of azathioprine as maintenance treatment for Crohn's disease. Lancet 1978;4:955–957.
77. Hanauer SB, Feagan BG, Lichtenstein GR, Mayer LF, Schreiber S, Colombel JF, Rachmilewitz D, Wolf DC, Olson A, Bao W, Rutgeerts P. Maintenance infliximab for Crohn's disease: the ACCENT I randomised trial. Lancet 2002;359:1541–1549.
78. Rutgeerts P, Feagan BG, Lichtenstein GR, Mayer LF, Schreiber S, Colombel JF, Rachmilewitz D, Wolf DC, Olson A, Bao W, Hanauer SB. Comparison of scheduled and episodic treatment strategies of infliximab in Crohn's disease. Gastroenterol 2004;126:402–413.
79. Committee for Proprietary Medicinal Products (CPMP), CPMP/EWP/785/97. Points to consider on the evaluation of medicinal products for the treatment of IBS. 785/97 ed. European Agency for the Evaluation of Medicinal Products, 2003.
80. Tack J et al. Tegaserod. Gut 2004.
81. Novicki J MPKReal. A randomized, double-blind, placebo-controlled trial of tegaserod in female patients suffering from irritable bowel syndrome with constipation. Aliment Pharmacol Ther 2002;16:1877–1888.
82. Bardhan KD, Forbes A, Marsden CL, Mason T, Short G. The effects of withdrawing tegaserod treatment in comparison with continuous treatment in irritable bowel syndrome patients with abdominal pain/discomfort, bloating and constipation: a clinical study. Aliment Pharmacol Ther 2004;20:213–222.

83. Camilleri M, Chey WY, Mayer EA, Northcutt AR, Heath A, Dukes GE, McSorley D, Mangel AM. A randomized controlled clinical trial of the serotonin type 3 receptor antagonist alosetron in women with diarrhea-predominant irritable bowel syndrome. Arch Intern Med 2001;161:1733–1740.

84. Rothmann MD, Tsou HH. On non-inferiority analysis based on delta-method confidence intervals. J Biopharm Stat 2003;13:565–583.

85. Thompson WG, Longstreth G, Drossman DA, Heaton K, Irvine EJ, Muller-Lissner S. Functional bowel disorders and functional abdominal pain. In: Drossman DA, Corazziari E, Talley NJ, Thompson WG, and Whitehead WE, eds. Rome II: The Functional Gastrointestinal Disorders. 2nd ed. McLean, VA: Degnon Associates, 2000: 351–432.

86. Bardhan KD. Intermittent and on-demand use of proton pump inhibitors in the management of symptomatic gastroesophageal reflux disease. Am J Gastroenterol 2003;98:S40–S48.

87. Zacny J, Zamakhshary M, Sketris I, Veldhuyzen van ZS. Systematic review: the efficacy of intermittent and on-demand therapy with histamine H2-receptor antagonists or proton pump inhibitors for gastro-oesophageal reflux disease patients. Aliment Pharmacol Ther 2005;21:1299–1312.

88. Kaplan MA, Prior MJ, McKonly KI, DuPont HL, Temple AR, Nelson EB. A multicenter randomized controlled trial of a liquid loperamide product versus placebo in the treatment of acute diarrhea in children. Clin Pediatr (Phila) 1999;38:579–591.

89. Dreverman JW, Van der Poel AJ. Loperamide oxide in acute diarrhoea: a double-blind, placebo-controlled trial. The Dutch Diarrhoea Trialists Group. Aliment Pharmacol Ther 1995;9:441–446.

90. Bytzer P. Assessment of reflux symptom severity: methodological options and their attributes. Gut 2004;53 Suppl 4:iv28–iv34.

91. Talley NJ, Venables TL, Green JR, Armstrong D, O'Kane KP, Giaffer M, Bardhan KD, Carlsson RG, Chen S, Hasselgren GS. Esomeprazole 40 mg and 20 mg is efficacious in the long-term management of patients with endoscopy-negative gastro-oesophageal reflux disease: a placebo-controlled trial of on-demand therapy for 6 months. Eur J Gastroenterol Hepatol 2002;14:857–863.

92. Talley NJ, Lauritsen K, Tunturi-Hihnala H, Lind T, Moum B, Bang C, Schulz T, Omland TM, Delle M, Junghard O. Esomeprazole 20 mg maintains symptom control in endoscopy-negative gastro-oesophageal reflux disease: a controlled trial of 'on-demand' therapy for 6 months. Aliment Pharmacol Ther 2001;15:347–354.

93. Simon TJ, Berlin RG, Gardner AH, Stauffer LA, Gould AL, Getson AJ. Self-Directed Treatment of Intermittent Heartburn: A Randomized, Multicenter, Double-Blind, Placebo-Controlled Evaluation of Antacid and Low Doses of an H(2)-Receptor Antagonist (Famotidine). Am J Ther 1995;2:304–313.

94. Fujii Y, Tanaka H, Kawasaki T. A comparison of granisetron, droperidol, and metoclopramide in the treatment of established nausea and vomiting after breast surgery: a double-blind, randomized, controlled trial. Clin Ther 2003;25:1142–1149.

95. Tillisch K, Labus JS, Naliboff BD, Bolus R, Shetzline M, Mayer EA, Chang L. Characterization of the alternating bowel habit subtype in patients with irritable bowel syndrome. Am J Gastroenterol. 100 ed. 2005:896–904.

96. Talley NJ, Weaver AL, Zinsmeister AR, Melton LJ, III. Onset and disappearance of gastrointestinal symptoms and functional gastrointestinal disorders. Am J Epidemiol 1992;136:165–177.

97. Talley NJ, McNeil D, Hayden A, Colreavy C, Piper DW. Prognosis of chronic unexplained dyspepsia. A prospective study of potential predictor variables in patients with endoscopically diagnosed nonulcer dyspepsia. Gastroenterol 1987;92:1060–1066.

98. Cremonini F, Delgado-Aros S, Camilleri M. Efficacy of alosetron in irritable bowel syndrome: a meta-analysis of randomized controlled trials. Neurogastroenterol Motil 2003;15:79–86.

99. Evans BW, Clark WK, Moore DJ, Whorwell PJ. Tegaserod for the treatment of irritable bowel syndrome. Cochrane Database Syst Rev 2004;CD003960.

100. Bytzer P, Blum A, De Herdt D, Dubois D. Six-month trial of on-demand rabeprazole 10 mg maintains symptom relief in patients with non-erosive reflux disease. Aliment Pharmacol Ther 2004;20:181–188.

101. Compliance in Health Care. Baltimore: Johns Hopkins University Press, 1979.

102. Eraker SA, Kirscht JP, Becker MH. Understanding and improving patient compliance. Ann Intern Med 1984;100:258–268.

103. Patient compliance in therapeutic trials. Lancet 1991;337:823–824.

104. Feinstein AR. Intent-to-treat policy for analyzing randomized trials. In: Cramer JA and Spilker B, eds. Patient Compliance in Medical Practice and Clinical Trials. NY: Raven Press, 1991:359–370.

105. Jensen MP, Turner LR, Turner JA, Romano JM. The use of multiple-item scales for pain intensity measurement in chronic pain patients. Pain 1996;67:35–40.

106. Von KM, Moore JC. Stepped care for back pain: activating approaches for primary care. Ann Intern Med 2001;134:911–917.

107. Max MB, Kishore-Kumar R, Schafer SC, Meister B, Gracely RH, Smoller B, Dubner R. Efficacy of desipramine in painful diabetic neuropathy: a placebo-controlled trial. Pain 1991;45:3–9.

108. Means B, Nigam A, Zarrow M, Loftus EF, Donaldson MS. Autobiographical memory for health-related events. DHHS Publication No. PHS 89–1077. ed. Washington, DC: U.S. Government Printing Office, 1989.

109. Sandha GS, Hunt RH, Veldhuyzen Van Zanten SJ. A systematic overview of the use of diary cards, quality-of-life questionnaires, and psychometric tests in treatment trials of Helicobacter pylori-positive and -negative non-ulcer dyspepsia. Scand J Gastroenterol 1999;34:244–249.

110. Stone AA, Shiffman S, Schwartz JE, Broderick JE, Hufford MR. Patient non-compliance with paper diaries. BMJ 2002;324:1193–1194.

111. Hufford MR, Stone AA, Shiffman S, Schwartz JE, Broderick JE. Paper vs. electronic diaries: Compliance and subject evaluations. Applied Clinical Trials (actmagazine com) 2002;38–43.

112. Spector SL, Kinsman R, Mawhinney H, Siegel SC, Rachelefsky GS, Katz RM, Rohr AS. Compliance of patients with asthma with an experimental aerosolized medication: implications for controlled clinical trials. J Allergy Clin Immunol 1986;77:65–70.

113. Mazze RS, Shamoon H, Pasmantier R, Lucido D, Murphy J, Hartmann K, Kuykendall V, Lopatin W. Reliability of blood glucose monitoring by patients with diabetes mellitus. Am J Med 1984;77:211–217.

114. Harding JP, Hamm LR, Ehsanullah RS, Heath AT, Sorrells SC, Haw J, Dukes GE, Wolfe SG, Mangel AW, Northcutt AR. Use of a novel electronic data collection sys-

tem in multicenter studies of irritable bowel syndrome. Aliment Pharmacol Ther 1997;11:1073–1076.

115. Bardhan KD, Bodemar G, Geldof H, Schutz E, Heath A, Mills JG, Jacques LA. A double-blind, randomized, placebo-controlled dose-ranging study to evaluate the efficacy of alosetron in the treatment of irritable bowel syndrome. Aliment Pharmacol Ther 2000;14:23–34.

116. Whitehead WE, Palsson OS, Levy RL, Feld AD, Von Korff M, Turner M. Reports of "satisfactory relief" by IBS patients receiving usual medical care are confounded by baseline symptom severity and do not accurately reflect symptom improvement. 2005.

117. Camilleri M, Mayer EA, Drossman DA, Heath A, Dukes GE, McSorley D, Kong S, Mangel AW, Northcutt AR. Improvement in pain and bowel function in female irritable bowel patients with alosetron, a 5-HT3 receptor antagonist. Alimentary Pharmacology & Therapeutics 1999;13:1149–1159.

118. Chey WD, Chey WY, Heath AT, Dukes GE, Carter EG, Northcutt A, Ameen VZ. Long-term safety and efficacy of alosetron in women with severe diarrhea-predominant irritable bowel syndrome. Am J Gastroenterol 2004;99:2195–2203.

119. Drossman DA, Corazziari E, Talley NJ, Thompson WG, Whitehead WE. Rome II. The Functional Gastrointestinal Disorders. Diagnosis, Pathophysiology and Treatment: A Multinational Consensus. McLean, VA: Degnon Associates, 2000.

120. Fallone CA, Guyatt GH, Armstrong D, Wiklund I, Degl'Innocenti A, Heels-Ansdell D, Barkun AN, Chiba N, Zanten SJ, El Dika S, Austin P, Tanser L, Schunemann HJ. Do physicians correctly assess patient symptom severity in gastro-oesophageal reflux disease? Aliment Pharmacol Ther 2004;20:1161–1169.

121. Guyatt GH, Veldhuyzen Van Zanten SJ, Feeny DH, Patrick DL. Measuring quality of life in clinical trials: a taxonomy and review. CMAJ 1989;140:1441–1448.

122. Guyatt GH, Feeny DH, Patrick DL. Measuring health-related quality of life. Ann Intern Med 1993;118:622–629.

123. Borgaonkar MR, Irvine EJ. Quality of life measurement in gastrointestinal and liver disorders. Gut 2000;47:444–454.

124. Bradette M, Moennikes H, Carter F, Krause G, Caras S, Steinborn C. Cilansetron in irritable bowel syndrome with diarrhea predominance (IBS-D): Efficacy and safety in a 6 month global study. 126 ed. 2004:A-42.

125. Creed F, Fernandes L, Guthrie E, Palmer S, Ratcliffe J, Read N, Rigby C, Thompson D, Tomenson B. The cost-effectiveness of psychotherapy and paroxetine for severe irritable bowel syndrome. Gastroenterol 2003;124:303–317.

126. Francis CY, Morris J, Whorwell PJ. The irritable bowel severity scoring system: a simple method of monitoring irritable bowel syndrome and its progress. Alimentary Pharmacology & Therapeutics 1997;11:395–402.

127. Blanchard EB, Schwarz SP, Suls JM, Gerardi MA, Scharff L, Greene B, Taylor AE, Berreman C, Malamood HS. Two controlled evaluations of multicomponent psychological treatment of irritable bowel syndrome. Behav Res Ther 1992;30:175–189.

128. Blanchard EB, Scharff L, Payne A, Schwarz SP, Suls JM, Malamood H. Prediction of outcome from cognitive-behavioral treatment of irritable bowel syndrome. Behav Res Ther 1992;30:647–650.

129. Mangel AW, Hahn BA, Heath AT, Northcutt AR, Kong S, Dukes GE, McSorley D.

Adequate relief as an endpoint in clinical trials in irritable bowel syndrome. J Int Med Res 1998;26:76–81.

130. Dunger-Baldauf C, Nyhlin H, Rueegg P, Wagner A. Subject's global assessment of satisfactory relief as a measure to assess treatment effect in clinical trials in irritable bowel syndrome (IBS). 98 (Suppl 1) ed. 2003:S269.

131. Muller-Lissner S, Koch G, Talley NJ, Drossman D, Rueegg P, Dunger-Baldauf C, Lefkowitz M. Subject's Global Assessment of Relief: an appropriate method to assess the impact of treatment on irritable bowel syndrome-related symptoms in clinical trials. J Clin Epidemiol 2003;56:310–316.

132. Bijkerk CJ, de Wit NJ, Muris JW, Jones RH, Knottnerus JA, Hoes AW. Outcome measures in irritable bowel syndrome: comparison of psychometric and methodological characteristics. Am J Gastroenterol 2003;98:122–127.

133. Talley NJ, Janssens J, Lauritsen K, Racz I, Bolling-Sternevald E. Eradication of Helicobacter pylori in functional dyspepsia: randomised double blind placebo controlled trial with 12 months' follow up. The Optimal Regimen Cures Helicobacter Induced Dyspepsia (ORCHID) Study Group. BMJ 1999;318:833–837.

134. Fraser A, Delaney B, Moayyedi P. Symptom-Based Outcome Measures for Dyspepsia and GERD Trials: A Systematic Review. Am J Gastroenterol 2005;100:442–452.

135. Gonsalkorale WM, Miller V, Afzal A, Whorwell PJ. Long term benefits of hypnotherapy for irritable bowel syndrome. Gut 2003;52:1623–1629.

136. Gonsalkorale WM, Toner BB, Whorwell PJ. Cognitive change in patients undergoing hypnotherapy for irritable bowel syndrome. J Psychosom Res 2004;56:271–278.

137. Patrick DL, Drossman DA, Frederick IO, Dicesare J, Puder KL. Quality of life in persons with irritable bowel syndrome: development and validation of a new measure. Dig Dis Sci 1998;43:400–411.

138. Drossman DA, Whitehead WE, Toner BB, Diamant N, Hu YJ, Bangdiwala SI, Jia H. What determines severity among patients with painful functional bowel disorders? Am J Gastroenterol 2000;95:974–980.

139. Wiklund IK, Junghard O, Grace E, Talley NJ, Kamm M, Veldhuyzen van ZS, Pare P, Chiba N, Leddin DS, Bigard MA, Colin R, Schoenfeld P. Quality of Life in Reflux and Dyspepsia patients. Psychometric documentation of a new disease-specific questionnaire (QOLRAD). Eur J Surg Suppl 1998;41–49.

140. Whitehead WE, Palsson OS, Levy RL, Feld AD, Von Korff M, Turner MJ. "Satisfactory relief" is an unsatisfactory method of defining an irritable bowel syndrome (IBS) treatment responder. 126 ed. 2004:A-88.

141. Nyren O, Adami HO, Bates S, Bergstrom R, Gustavsson S, Loof L, Sjoden PO. Self-rating of pain in nonulcer dyspepsia. A methodological study comparing a new fixed-point scale and the visual analogue scale. J Clin Gastroenterol 1987;9:408–414.

142. El-Omar EM, Banerjee S, Wirz A, McColl KE. The Glasgow Dyspepsia Severity Score—a tool for the global measurement of dyspepsia. Eur J Gastroenterol Hepatol 1996;8:967–971.

143. Moayyedi P, Duffett S, Braunholtz D, Mason S, Richards ID, Dowell AC, Axon AT. The Leeds Dyspepsia Questionnaire: a valid tool for measuring the presence and severity of dyspepsia. Aliment Pharmacol Ther 1998;12:1257–1262.

144. Veldhuyzen Van Zanten SJ, Tytgat KM, Pollak PT, Goldie J, Goodacre RL, Riddell RH, Hunt RH. Can severity of symptoms be used as an outcome measure in trials

of non-ulcer dyspepsia and Helicobacter pylori associated gastritis? J Clin Epidemiol 1993;46:273–279.

145. Rabeneck L, Wristers K, Goldstein JL, Eisen G, Dedhiya SD, Burke TA. Reliability, validity, and responsiveness of severity of dyspepsia assessment (SODA) in a randomized clinical trial of a COX-2-specific inhibitor and traditional NSAID therapy. Am J Gastroenterol 2002;97:32–39.

146. Talley NJ, Verlinden M, Jones M. Validity of a new quality of life scale for functional dyspepsia: a United States multicenter trial of the Nepean Dyspepsia Index. Am J Gastroenterol 1999;94:2390–2397.

147. Tack J, Talley NJ, Camilleri C, Holtmann G, Hu P, Malagelada J, Stanghellini V. Functional Gastroduodenal Disorders. In: Drossman DA, Corrazziari E, Delvaux M, Spiller R, Talley N, Thompson WG, Whitehead W, eds. Rome III: The Functional Gastrointestinal Disorders. 3rd ed. McLean, VA: Degnon Associates, 2006:419–486.

148. Guyatt G, Walter S, Norman G. Measuring change over time: assessing the usefulness of evaluative instruments. J Chronic Dis 1987;40:171–178.

149. Ioannidis JP, Evans SJ, Gotzsche PC, O'Neill RT, Altman DG, Schulz K, Moher D. Better reporting of harms in randomized trials: an extension of the CONSORT statement. Ann Intern Med 2004;141:781–788.

150. Moher D, Schulz KF, Altman D. The CONSORT statement: revised recommendations for improving the quality of reports of parallel-group randomized trials. JAMA 2001;285:1987–1991.

151. Heaton KW, O'Donnell LJ. An office guide to whole-gut transit time. Patients' recollection of their stool form. J Clin Gastroenterol 1994;19:28–30.

152. Lewis SJ, Heaton KW. Stool form scale as a useful guide to intestinal transit time. Scand J Gastroenterol 1997;32:920–924.

153. Reilly MC, Zbrozek AS, Dukes EM. The validity and reproducibility of a work productivity and activity impairment instrument. Pharmacoeconomics 1993;4:353–365.

154. Whitehead WE, Burnett CK, Cook EW, III, Taub E. Impact of irritable bowel syndrome on quality of life. Dig Dis Sci 1996;41:2248–2253.

155. Talley NJ, Weaver AL, Zinsmeister AR. Impact of functional dyspepsia on quality of life. Dig Dis Sci 1995;40:584–589.

156. Watson ME, Lacey L, Kong S, Northcutt AR, McSorley D, Hahn B, Mangel AW. Alosetron improves quality of life in women with diarrhea-predominant irritable bowel syndrome. Am J Gastroenterol 2001;96:455–459.

157. Bergner M, Bobbitt RA, Carter WB, Gilson BS. The Sickness Impact Profile: development and final revision of a health status measure. Med Care 1981;19:787–805.

158. Hunt SM, McKenna SP, McEwen J, Backett EM, Williams J, Papp E. A quantitative approach to perceived health status: a validation study. J Epidemiol Community Health 1980;34:281–286.

159. Ware JE, Brook RH, Davies-Avery A, et al. Model of Health and Methodology. Santa Monica: Rand Corporation, 1980.

160. Sackett DL, Chambers LW, MacPherson AS, Goldsmith CH, Mcauley RG. The development and application of indices of health: general methods and a summary of results. Am J Public Health 1977;67:423–428.

161. Stewart AL, Hays RD, Ware JE, Jr. The MOS short-form general health survey. Reliability and validity in a patient population. Med Care 1988;26:724–735.

162. Dimenas E, Glise H, Hallerback B, Hernqvist H, Svedlund J, Wiklund I. Quality of life in patients with upper gastrointestinal symptoms. An improved evaluation of treatment regimens? Scand J Gastroenterol 1993;28:681–687.

163. Hahn BA, Kirchdoerfer LJ, Fullerton S, Mayer E. Evaluation of a new quality of life questionnaire for patients with irritable bowel syndrome. Aliment Pharmacol Ther 1997;11:547–552.

164. Chassany O, Marquis P, Scherrer B, Read NW, Finger T, Bergmann JF, Fraitag B, Geneve J, Caulin C. Validation of a specific quality of life questionnaire for functional digestive disorders. Gut 1999;44:527–533.

165. Eypasch E, Williams JI, Wood-Dauphinee S, Ure BM, Schmulling C, Neugebauer E, Troidl H. Gastrointestinal Quality of Life Index: development, validation and application of a new instrument. Br J Surg 1995;82:216–222.

166. Wong E, Guyatt GH, Cook DJ, Griffith LE, Irvine EJ. Development of a questionnaire to measure quality of life in patients with irritable bowel syndrome. Eur J Surg Suppl 1998;50–56.

167. Miller GA. The magical number seven plus or minus two: some limits on our capacity for processing information. Psychol Rev 1956;63:81–97.

168. Jaeschke R, Singer J, Guyatt GH. Measurement of health status. Ascertaining the minimal clinically important difference. Control Clin Trials 1989;10:407–415.

169. Wyrwich KW, Tardino VM. A blueprint for symptom scales and responses: measurement and reporting. Gut 2004;53 Suppl 4:iv45–iv48.

170. MacKenzie CR, Charlson ME. Standards for the use of ordinal scales in clinical trials. Br Med J (Clin Res Ed) 1986;292:40–43.

171. Reading AE. A comparison of pain rating scales. J Psychosom Res 1980;24:119–124.

172. Kerns RD, Finn P, Haythornthwaite J. Self-monitored pain intensity: psychometric properties and clinical utility. J Behav Med 1988;11:71–82.

173. Huskisson EC. Measurement of pain. Lancet 1974;2:1127–1131.

174. Ohnhaus EE, Adler R. Methodological problems in the measurement of pain: a comparison between the verbal rating scale and the visual analogue scale. Pain 1975;1:379–384.

175. Guyatt GH, Townsend M, Keller JL, Singer J. Should study subjects see their previous responses: data from a randomized control trial. J Clin Epidemiol 1989;42:913–920.

176. Naliboff BD. Choosing outcome variables: global assessment and diaries. Gastroenterol 2004;126:S129–S134.

177. Guyatt GH, Townsend M, Berman LB, Keller JL. A comparison of Likert and visual analogue scales for measuring change in function. J Chronic Dis 1987;40:1129–1133.

178. Jensen M, Karoly P. Self-report scales and procedures for assessing pain in adults. In: Turk D and Melzack R, eds. Handbook of Pain Assessment. 2nd ed. New York: Guilford, 2001.

179. National Institute of Mental Health, CGI: Clinical Global Impressions. In: Guy W, ed. ECDEU Assessment for Psychopharmacology. Revised ed. Rockville: 1976:217–222.

180. Gordon S, Ameen V, Bagby B, Shahan B, Jhingran P, Carter E. Validation of irritable bowel syndrome Global Improvement Scale: an integrated symptom end point for assessing treatment efficacy. Dig Dis Sci 2003;48:1317–1323.

181. Begg C, Cho M, Eastwood S, Horton R, Moher D, Olkin I, Pitkin R, Rennie D,

Schulz KF, Simel D, Stroup DF. Improving the quality of reporting of randomized controlled trials. The CONSORT statement. JAMA 1996;276:637–639.

182. Altman DG. Better reporting of randomised controlled trials: the CONSORT statement. BMJ 1996;313:570–571.

183. Altman DG, Schulz KF, Moher D, Egger M, Davidoff F, Elbourne D, Gotzsche PC, Lang T. The revised CONSORT statement for reporting randomized trials: explanation and elaboration. Ann Intern Med 2001;134:663–694.

184. Moher D, Jones A, Lepage L. Use of the CONSORT statement and quality of reports of randomized trials: a comparative before-and-after evaluation. JAMA 2001; 285:1992–1995.

185. Egger M, Juni P, Bartlett C. Value of flow diagrams in reports of randomized controlled trials. JAMA 2001;285:1996–1999.

186. Huwiler-Muntener K, Juni P, Junker C, Egger M. Quality of reporting of randomized trials as a measure of methodologic quality. JAMA 2002;287:2801–2804.

187. Bossuyt PM, Reitsma JB, Bruns DE, Gatsonis CA, Glasziou PP, Irwig LM, Lijmer JG, Moher D, Rennie D, de Vet HC. Towards complete and accurate reporting of studies of diagnostic accuracy: the STARD initiative. BMJ 2003;326:41–44.

188. Bossuyt PM, Reitsma JB, Bruns DE, Gatsonis CA, Glasziou PP, Irwig LM, Moher D, Rennie D, de Vet HC, Lijmer JG. The STARD statement for reporting studies of diagnostic accuracy: explanation and elaboration. Clin Chem 2003;49:7–18.

189. Moher D, Cook DJ, Eastwood S, Olkin I, Rennie D, Stroup DF. Improving the quality of reports of meta-analyses of randomised controlled trials: the QUOROM statement. Quality of Reporting of Meta-analyses. Lancet 1999;354:1896–1900.

190. Perneger TV. What's wrong with Bonferroni adjustments. BMJ 1998;316:1236–1238.

191. DerSimonian R, Charette LJ, McPeek B, Mosteller F. Reporting on methods in clinical trials. N Engl J Med 1982;306:1332–1337.

192. Simon R. Confidence intervals for reporting results of clinical trials. Ann Intern Med 1986;105:429–435.

193. Guyatt G, Jaeschke R, Heddle N, Cook D, Shannon H, Walter S. Basic statistics for clinicians: 2. Interpreting study results: confidence intervals. CMAJ 1995;152:169–173.

194. Nuovo J, Melnikow J, Chang D. Reporting number needed to treat and absolute risk reduction in randomized controlled trials. JAMA 2002;287:2813–2814.

195. Gore SM, Jones G, Thompson SG. The Lancet's statistical review process: areas for improvement by authors. Lancet 1992;340:100–102.

196. Katz MH. Multivariable analysis: a primer for readers of medical research. Ann Intern Med 2003;138:644–650.

197. Smith DG, Clemens J, Crede W, Harvey M, Gracely EJ. Impact of multiple comparisons in randomized clinical trials. Am J Med 1987;83:545–550.

198. Oxman AD, Guyatt GH. A consumer's guide to subgroup analyses. Ann Intern Med 1992;116:78–84.

199. Assmann SF, Pocock SJ, Enos LE, Kasten LE. Subgroup analysis and other (mis)uses of baseline data in clinical trials. Lancet 2000;355:1064–1069.

200. Campbell MJ, Julious SA, Altman DG. Estimating sample sizes for binary, ordered categorical, and continuous outcomes in two group comparisons. BMJ 1995;311: 1145–1148.

201. Reed JF, III, Slaichert W. Statistical proof in inconclusive 'negative' trials. Arch Intern Med 1981;141:1307–1310.

202. Freiman JA, Chalmers TC, Smith H, Jr., Kuebler RR. The importance of beta, the type II error and sample size in the design and interpretation of the randomized control trial. Survey of 71 "negative" trials. N Engl J Med 1978;299:690–694.

203. Makuch RW, Johnson MF. Some issues in the design and interpretation of 'negative' clinical studies. Arch Intern Med 1986;146:986–989.

204. Berry DA. Interim analyses in clinical trials: classical vs. Bayesian approaches. Stat Med 1985;4:521–526.

205. DeMets DL, Pocock SJ, Julian DG. The agonising negative trend in monitoring of clinical trials. Lancet 1999;354:1983–1988.

206. Pocock SJ. When to stop a clinical trial. BMJ 1992;305:235–240.

207. Geller NL, Pocock SJ. Interim analyses in randomized clinical trials: ramifications and guidelines for practitioners. Biometrics 1987;43:213–223.

208. De Angelis C, Drazen JM, Frizelle FA, Haug C, Hoey J, Horton R, Kotzin S, Laine C, Marusic A, Overbeke AJ, Schroeder TV, Sox HC, Van Der Weyden MB. Clinical trial registration: a statement from the International Committee of Medical Journal Editors. N Engl J Med 2004;351:1250–1251.

209. Bero L, Rennie D. The Cochrane Collaboration. Preparing, maintaining, and disseminating systematic reviews of the effects of health care. JAMA 1995;274:1935–1938.

Chapter 16

Development and Validation of the Rome III Diagnostic Questionnaire

William E. Whitehead and the
Validation Working Team[1]
in association with the
Rome Questionnaire Committee[2]

[1] William E. Whitehead, Chair; Olafur S. Palsson, Syed Thiwan, Nicholas J. Talley, William D. Chey, E. Jan Irvine, Douglas A. Drossman
[2] W. Grant Thompson, Chair; Douglas A. Drossman, Nicholas J. Talley, Lynn S. Walker, William E. Whitehead

Background

As part of the effort to revise and update the Rome criteria, the Rome Foundation planned to develop a questionnaire that would embody the Rome III criteria for diagnosing functional GI disorders (FGIDs) and serve as an aid to researchers, clinicians, and epidemiologists. Such a questionnaire had been developed for the Rome II criteria. The Rome Foundation's board decided to change from the binary response scale used in the Rome II questionnaire ("no or rarely" vs. "often") to an ordinal frequency scale to improve upon some of the limitations of the previous questionnaire:

1. The Rome II questionnaire applied the same frequency threshold to all symptoms, usually to indicate whether the subject had a symptom at least 25% of the time or occasions. However, some symptoms such as belching and straining with defecation are thought not to be clinically meaningful unless they occur almost daily, whereas other symptoms such as digital facilitation of defecation are clinically significant if they occur at all. The use of an ordinal frequency scale would allow for the use of different frequency thresholds for different symptoms. This would also permit greater flexibility in developing diagnostic criteria, thus allowing investigators to set more restrictive criteria for study inclusion if desired.
2. Some of the symptom questions in the Rome II questionnaire were difficult to understand as they incorporated two or more frequency thresholds in the same criterion: for example, asking whether on at least one fourth of weeks in the last 3 months the patient had three or more bowel movements per day. Ordinal frequency scales would allow for grammatically simpler questions.
3. It is desirable for some research studies to be able to assess the relative severity (frequency and/or intensity) of symptoms in addition to making a diagnostic decision.

Based on these considerations, the Rome Foundation commissioned two survey studies. The first study compared four different response scales that have been used to elicit symptom reports with the goal of identifying the optimal scale for use in the Rome III questionnaire. The second study investigated the reliability, sensitivity, and specificity of the Rome III modular diagnostic questionnaire that was subsequently developed by the Rome Foundation. These two studies are described below.

Study 1: Comparison of Response Scales in the Rome II Questionnaire

— Aims

There were two aims:

1. to test the assumption that different frequency thresholds may be required to distinguish patients from controls for common symptoms such as straining to defecate as compared to rare symptoms such as a sensation of blocked defecation;
2. to compare the four different response scales: the binary scale used in the original Rome II Modular Questionnaire, a specific frequency scale (e.g., less than once a month, monthly, weekly, etc.), a subjective or relative frequency scale (e.g., rarely, occasionally, often, etc.), and a bothersome scale (e.g., not at all bothered, a little bit bothered, moderately bothered, etc.).

For each symptom question, we examined the distribution of responses in a sample of healthy controls and in a sample of patients with functional GI disorders and we computed the correlation between the four different response scales. We were particularly interested in how subjects who reported intermediate frequencies of symptom occurrence such as "less than once a month" or "occasionally" responded on the binary scale (e.g., "no or rarely" vs. "often"). The third aim of the study was to assess the sensitivity and specificity of different frequency thresholds for identifying patients diagnosed with IBS by physicians.

— Subjects

One hundred fifty-two healthy subjects who denied any current gastrointestinal diseases and any history of gastrointestinal surgery other than appendectomy or cholecystectomy were recruited by advertisement and invited to participate; 120 (78.9%) returned questionnaires and were included in the analysis. One hundred thirty-seven FGID patients identified from previously evaluated patients were sent questionnaires and 84 (61.3%) returned them. Fifty-two of the 84 FGID patients who returned the questionnaire had a clinical diagnosis of irritable bowel syndrome (IBS).

— Design

The Rome II questionnaire was transformed to four different questionnaires using response scales A–D below. These four questionnaires were completed in counterbalanced order. Subjects received the questionnaires in a numbered sequence and were asked to complete each questionnaire and put it in an envelope before going on to the next one (i.e., they were asked not to look back). When subjects had completed all four questionnaires, they returned them in a postage-prepaid envelope. They received $10 for completing all four questionnaires.

— Response Scales Used in the Four Different Questionnaire Versions

Scale A: Binary Scale Used in the Original Rome II Modular Questionnaire
"No or rarely"
"Often" [In a footnote to the questionnaire "often" is defined as "present during at least 3 weeks (at least 1 day in each week) in the last 3 months."]

Scale B: Specific Interval Frequency Scale
"Never"
"Less than once a month"
"Monthly"
"Weekly"
"Multiple times per week"
"Daily"

Scale C: Relative Frequency Scale
"Not at all or rarely"
"Occasionally"
"Often"
"Very often"
"Almost always"

Scale D: Bothersome Scale—How much were you bothered by <symptom>?
"Not at all"
"A little bit"
"Moderately"
"Quite a bit"
"Extremely"

Table 1. Response Frequencies for Frequent Symptoms of Constipation (Straining) and Infrequent Symptoms of Constipation (Digital Evacuation) as Reported on Four Different Response Scales

Scale	Threshold	Straining to Evacuate				Digital Facilitation of Defecation			
		Healthy n = 120	FGID n = 84	Specificity	PPV	Healthy n = 120	FGID n = 84	Specificity	PPV
A	Never or rarely	97	21			113	48		
	Often	23	60	81%	72%	7	33	94%	83%
B	Never	38	5			106	35		
	< once a month	41	12			7	9		
	Monthly	26	12			3	11	95%	86%
	Weekly	10	18			1	15		
	Multiple times per week	3	22	96%	87%	1	9		
	Daily	2	11			1	2		
C	Not at all or rarely	62	7			108	37		
	Occasionally	50	24			9	20	90%	78%
	Often	4	17	93%	86%	2	12		
	Very often	1	19			1	5		
	Almost always	3	13			0	6		
D	Not at all	63	6			108	33		
	A little bit	48	25			9	24	90%	80%
	Moderately	5	17	93%	85%	1	13		
	Quite a bit	2	21			2	6		
	Extremely	2	12			0	4		

PPV = positive predictive value
Scales: A = binary scale used in Rome II questionnaire; B = specific interval frequency scale;
    C = relative frequency scale; D = bothersome scale

— Results

Demographics

The average age of the healthy control sample was 31.8±1.3 years (mean ± standard error), 70.2% were female, and 77.7% were Caucasian. The average age of the FGID patients was 41.5±1.7 years, 82.3% were females, and 82.1% were Caucasian. The healthy controls were significantly younger than the patients.

Thresholds for Common Symptoms vs. Rare Symptoms to Distinguish FGID Patients from Controls

In Table 1 we compare a commonly occurring symptom of constipation (i.e., straining) to a less common symptom (i.e., digital facilitation of defecation). For each scale we identified a threshold that would misclassify 10% or less of the healthy controls as having the disorder (i.e., specificity ≥90%), and we calculated positive predictive value (PPV) of this threshold to discriminate patients from controls. The principal findings are (1) As expected, when symptoms are common in the population, the frequency threshold must be set higher to avoid misclassifying an unacceptably high proportion of healthy controls as patients (i.e., to preserve adequate specificity in the diagnostic criterion). (2) The number of ordinal scale step differences between thresholds on the subjective frequency scale (Scale C) is less than for the specific frequency scale (Scale B). However, common symptoms still require a different threshold than rare symptoms to achieve the same specificity. This provides support for the a priori hypothesis that, when patients are asked to rate symptom frequency on a subjective scale (i.e., rarely, occasionally, often) rather than a specific frequency scale (i.e., monthly, weekly, daily), they may be able to compensate for differences in the frequency of occurrence of the symptom when deciding what "rarely," "occasionally," or "often" mean. (3) The specific symptom frequency scale (Scale B) appeared to provide the highest PPV, although the PPV for the subjective symptom scale (Scale C) was also good. (4) The bothersome scale (Scale D) performed similarly to the subjective frequency scale (Scale C). However, the bothersome scale cannot be used for some symptom criteria such as whether abdominal pain is relieved by defecation.

Table 1 presents data for only two symptoms, but these are representative of what would be found for scale comparisons on other symptoms. The data for other symptoms can be obtained by contacting the authors.

Response Distributions and Correlations among Scales

For the purpose of comparing the response scales to each other, only data for the question on the frequency of abdominal pain will be presented because it is representative of all questions. Tables showing the relationship between response scales for other questions can be obtained by contacting the authors.

Table 2. Binary Scale Compared to Specific Frequency Scale for the Question on Frequency of Abdominal Pain. All Subjects Were Combined (Rho=0.77, p<.001; Wilcoxon Z=10.15, p<0.001.)

	Never	< Once a Month	Monthly	Weekly	Multiple Times per Week	Daily	TOTAL
Never or Rarely	60	35	16	7	0	0	118
Often	0	6	16	18	24	18	82
TOTAL	60	41	32	25	24	18	200

Table 3. Binary Scale Compared to Subjective Frequency Scale for the Question on Frequency of Abdominal Pain (Rho=0.79, p<0.001; Wilcoxon Z=8.46, p<0.001.)

	Not at All or Rarely	Occasionally	Often	Very Often	Almost Always	TOTAL
Never or Rarely	82	34	1	0	0	117
Often	2	23	22	21	14	82
TOTAL	84	57	23	21	14	199

Table 4. Binary Scale Compared to Bothersome Scale for the Question on Frequency of Abdominal Pain (Rho=0.79, p<0.001; Wilcoxon Z=9.20, p<0.001.)

	Not at All	A Little Bit	Moderately	Quite a Bit	Extremely	TOTAL
Never or Rarely	74	39	5	0	0	118
Often	1	17	20	28	16	82
TOTAL	75	56	25	28	16	200

Tables 2 through 6 show that all four response scales are correlated with each other (Spearman rhos of 0.77 to 0.84, all p<0.001). However, the response distributions were significantly different between scales (Z-scores for Wilcox tests of 3.80 to 10.15, all p<0.001). Note especially that subjects who had an intermediate frequency of abdominal pain were inconsistent with respect to whether they said "never or rarely" vs. "often" on the binary scale. This is shown in Table 2 where half of subjects who had abdominal pain once a month responded "never or

Table 5. Specific Frequency Scale Compared to Subjective Frequency Scale for the Question on Frequency of Abdominal Pain. (Rho=0.82, p<0.001; Wilcoxon Z=8.61, p<0.001.)

	Not at All or Rarely	Occasionally	Often	Very Often	Almost Always	TOTAL
Never	54	4	1	0	0	59
< Once a Month	22	19	0	0	0	41
Monthly	5	19	5	3	0	32
Weekly	3	10	9	3	1	26
Multiple Times per Week	0	5	6	11	2	24
Daily	0	1	2	4	11	18
TOTAL	84	58	23	21	14	200

Table 6. Specific Frequency Scale Compared to Bothersome Scale for the Question on Frequency of Abdominal Pain (Rho=0.84, p<0.001; Wilcox Z=7.30, p<0.001.)

	Not at All	A Little Bit	Moderately	Quite a Bit	Extremely	TOTAL
Never	53	7	0	0	0	60
< Once a Month	18	20	3	0	0	41
Monthly	3	17	6	4	2	32
Weekly	1	9	11	4	1	26
Multiple Times per Week	0	3	3	14	4	24
Daily	0	0	3	6	9	18
TOTAL	75	56	26	28	16	201

rarely" on the binary scale while the other half responded "often." Table 3 shows that 65% of subjects who reported having abdominal pain "occasionally" on the subjective frequency scale responded "never or rarely" on the binary scale while the other 35% responded "often." As shown in Table 4, subjects who reported being "a little bit" or "moderately" bothered by abdominal pain were also inconsistent in their responses to the binary scale.

— Conclusions

Study 1 demonstrates that ordinal frequency scales can more accurately portray the distribution of intermediate frequency responses in contrast to binary scales where the responses are inconsistent: half of the patients who had abdominal pain once a month on average responded "never or rarely" on the binary scale, and the other half responded "often." Ordinal scales also permit different frequency thresholds when symptoms are common vs. rare in the population (e.g., straining vs. digital facilitation of defecation). In comparing different ordinal scale response formats to each other, the data suggest that specific frequency scales perform best, but subjective frequency scales are also acceptable. Asking subjects to indicate how bothersome the symptom was in the last 3 months discriminates between patients and controls in a manner similar to the subjective frequency scale, but the bothersome scale is not appropriate to some of the symptom criteria for FGIDs.

Study 2: Development and Validation of the Rome III Diagnostic Questionnaire

— Choice of Response Scales for Rome III Diagnostic Questionnaire

Based on Study 1, the Rome Foundation Board decided to use two ordinal frequency scales to evaluate most of the symptom criteria in the Rome III diagnostic questionnaire under development. The first was a specific frequency scale similar to Scale B, and the second was a subjective frequency scale similar to Scale C in Study 1, which was modified slightly. The questionnaire committee felt that the subjective frequency rather than a specific frequency scale would be more easily understood by subjects when assessing some symptom criteria (e.g., "How often is your abdominal pain relieved by defecation?"). In addition to these two ordinal scales, the committee elected to retain some questions with the binary response format used in the Rome II questionnaire. One of the aims of Study 2 was to compare these binary response questions to alternative questions with an ordinal scale response format.

Specific Frequency Scale	*Subjective Frequency Scale*
Never	Never or rarely
Less than one day a month	Sometimes
One day a month	Often
One day a week	Most of the time
More than one day a week	Always
Every day	

— Development of Draft Symptom Questions for Rome III Diagnostic Questionnaire

The first draft of the questionnaire resulted from a series of meetings of the Rome Foundation Board extending over a 2-year period. The members of this group are Douglas Drossman (chair), Michel Delvaux, Enrico Corrazziari, Robin Spiller, Nicholas Talley, W. Grant Thompson, and William Whitehead, all of whom have experience in questionnaire development. The board also sought input from the Rome III committees assigned to revise the diagnostic criteria for their respective disorders. The committee chairs were asked to propose draft questions, to review questions that were proposed by the board, and to insure that the questions accurately reflected the diagnostic criteria that their working teams developed.

The Rome Foundation Board also established a Questionnaire Committee consisting of W. Grant Thompson (chair), Nick Talley, Lynn Walker, and William Whitehead, and Douglas Drossman participated as an ex officio member of this committee. The Questionnaire Committee held a two-day face-to-face meeting to review the questions again for clarity and consistency, to compare the questions to the diagnostic criteria produced by the working teams, and to develop a diagnostic algorithm for inferring diagnoses from the questionnaire. During and following this meeting, the Questionnaire Committee sent additional queries to the chairs of the working teams to clarify whether the questions accurately reflected the diagnostic criteria.

The final step in questionnaire development was a study to validate the Rome III Diagnostic Questionnaire. The Rome Foundation Board commissioned William Whitehead to organize a multicenter validation study whose aims are outlined below. Collaborators included Douglas Drossman, Olafur Palsson, and Syed Thiwan at the University of North Carolina, William Chey at the University of Michigan, E. Jan Irvine at the University of Toronto, and Nicholas Talley at the Mayo Clinic in Rochester.

— Aims of the Validation Study

1. Assess the understandability of the questionnaire items.
2. Determine the frequency of endorsement of the symptom questions (response distributions) in a large, age- and gender-stratified sample of healthy controls to insure that the thresholds selected were reasonable, and determine the frequency of false positive diagnoses of FGIDs in the healthy control sample. (The specificity of the diagnostic criteria is calculated as one minus the false-positive rate in the healthy controls.)

3. Assess the test-retest reliability of the questionnaire for all diagnoses and for individual questions.
4. Test the sensitivity and specificity of the questionnaire for identifying medically diagnosed patients with functional gastrointestinal disorders.
5. Compare two versions of the questionnaire, one of which retained some questions in binary format (Version 1) and the other of which included ordinal scaled questions for these items (Version 2).

— Methods

Healthy Control Sample

Healthy controls were recruited through a mass email to faculty, staff, and students at the University of North Carolina at Chapel Hill (UNC). This sample was stratified and screened for inclusion criteria by a webform link requesting demographic and gastrointestinal (GI) health information. Eligible subjects were automatically assigned a random ID number and sent a letter of implied consent with a questionnaire package containing both Version 1 and Version 2. Returning the questionnaires in a postage-paid pre-addressed envelope connoted their consent to participate. Out of 734 people invited to participate, 554 returned questionnaires (75.5%). A randomly selected subset of 53 healthy controls completed the questionnaires again 2 weeks after the first completion to assess test-retest reliability.

FGID Patient Sample

Patients with clinical diagnoses of FGIDs were recruited at UNC by (1) contacting patients who had participated in previous research studies and had indicated an interest in participating in future studies and (2) contacting patients attending the UNC Functional GI and Motility Disorders Clinic. Patients were required to have a physician diagnosis of a FGID. Eligible subjects were mailed an implied consent letter with questionnaires. Out of 412 patients invited to participate at UNC, 274 completed questionnaires (66.5%). An additional 138 FGID patients were recruited by three other participating institutions: the Mayo Clinic in Rochester, Minnesota; St. Michael's Hospital in Toronto, Ontario; and the University of Michigan in Ann Arbor. Participation rate was not ascertainable from these external sites. A randomly selected 51 FGID patients from the UNC site completed the questionnaire twice (2 weeks apart) to assess test-retest reliability in this sample. Complete data were available for 399 FGID patients including 328 with IBS, ten with functional dyspepsia, 27 with functional constipation, five with functional defecation disorder, 14 with functional diarrhea, eight with functional abdominal pain, and seven with fecal incontinence. Table 7 compares the demographic characteristics of the FGID sample to the control sample.

Data Analysis

To assess the understandability of the questions, all subjects were asked after completing Version 1 of the questionnaire to identify all questions that were difficult to understand and to indicate what about these questions was difficult. For each question, we manually tallied the cumulative number of people who found the question difficult. Subjects' responses regarding what was difficult to understand were used as a guide to revise the question if more than 1% indicated difficulty understanding it. Healthy controls and FGID patients were pooled in this analysis.

The frequency distributions of responses to each question by all healthy controls and FGID patients were examined using the Statistical Package for the Social Sciences (SPSS) "cross-tabulation" function. These distributions were used to validate that the diagnostic criteria incorporated frequency criteria that did not misclassify more than approximately 5% of healthy controls as abnormal and that the selected threshold discriminated healthy controls from FGID patients. This was an iterative process: for some diagnostic criteria the frequency thresholds were adjusted based on this analysis. Finally, diagnoses for the 23 FGIDs were made based on all diagnostic criteria, and the frequency of false-positive diagnoses was tabulated.

The test-retest reliability of the FGID diagnoses was tested by calculating the percent agreement between the occurrence or nonoccurrence of each diagnosis in each subject in the reliability sample. The FGID sample and the healthy control sample were pooled for this analysis.

The specificity of each set of diagnostic criteria was assessed by calculating the proportion of healthy controls who met the criteria for this diagnosis (i.e., the false-positive rate) and subtracting this proportion from 1.0. Specificity was defined as the proportion of the medically diagnosed group with each FGID who met Rome III diagnostic criteria based on the questionnaire. This analysis was limited to those FGIDs that were detected in the FGID patient sample.

Two versions of the questionnaire were completed by all subjects: Version 1, which included 31 questions with binary response scales identical to the old Rome II questionnaire and Version 2, which converted these 31 binary questions to ordinal scaled questions. We compared these two versions of the questionnaire with respect to specificity of diagnosis, test-retest reliability, and understandability of the questions.

— Results

Demographics of Patient and Control Samples

Table 7 shows that there were demographic differences between the patient and control groups: FGID patients were older, more likely to be females and

Table 7. Demographics of Samples for Study 2

	Controls n = 554	FGID n = 399
Age (years)	35.0±0.5	44.1±0.7*
Sex (% female)	72.7	84.9*
Race:		
Caucasian	79.8	90.5*
African American	10.1	7.0
Asian	9.3	2.2
Ethnicity (% Hispanic)	3.0	2.0
Education (% graduated college)	74.2	48.9*

* FGID group significantly (p<.05) different from controls

Caucasians, and also less well educated. To assess whether these demographic differences were likely to bias the results of the study, nonparametric Spearman correlations between each of these demographic variables and all symptom questions were calculated. Although there were significant correlations (21% of questions correlated with age, 18% with race, and 15% with sex and education), none of the correlations exceeded rho=0.27. This indicates that no more than 7% of the variability in an individual question could be explained by demographic factors.

Understandability of Questions

Eighteen questions were identified as difficult to understand by at least 1% of subjects (at least 10 individuals). Only four questions were listed by more than 2% of subjects. The poorest question was judged difficult to understand by 7% of subjects.

Eleven of 18 difficult questions were judged to be conceptually complex and were revised. The old and new questions are provided in Table 8.

Six questions were conceptually complex because they asked for more than one judgment about frequency: for example, "In the last 3 months, were there 21 days when you had more than 3 (4 or more) bowel movements a day?" These were binary questions that could be simplified by using an ordinal response scale, and this change was made. One other question, which was difficult for 1.2% of subjects, was not revised: "In the last 3 months, how often did you feel uncomfortably full after a regular-sized meal?"

Table 8. Original and Revised Versions of Questions that Subjects Identified as Difficult to Understand

Old Question	Revised Question
When food from your stomach came into your mouth, did you generally hold it in your mouth for a while and then swallow it again or spit it out?	When food came back up into your mouth, did it usually stay in your mouth for a while before you swallowed it or spit it out?
Did you stop bringing up food when it turned sour or acidic?	Did food stop coming back up into your mouth when it turned sour or acidic?
Did you only have pain (not discomfort)?	Did you only have pain (not discomfort or a mixture of discomfort and pain)?
In the last 3 months, how often did you bring up food from your stomach into your mouth?	In the last 3 months, how often did food come back up into your mouth?
Did any of the symptoms in questions 50–56 begin more than 6 months ago?	Did any of the symptoms of constipation listed in questions 52–58 above begin more than 6 months ago?
Did loose or watery stools begin more than 6 months ago?	Did you begin to have frequent loose, mushy, or watery stools more than 6 months ago?
In the last 3 months, how often did you have bloating or visible distention?	In the last 3 months, how often did you have bloating or distention?
For women: did this discomfort or pain occur only during your menstrual period?	For women: did this discomfort or pain occur only during your menstrual bleeding and not at other times?
When this discomfort or pain started, how often did you have more bowel movements?	When this discomfort or pain started, did you have more frequent bowel movements?
When this discomfort or pain started, how often did you have fewer bowel movements?	When this discomfort or pain started, did you have less frequent bowel movements?
When this discomfort or pain started, how often did you have looser stools?	When this discomfort or pain started, were your stools (bowel movements) looser?

Frequency of Reporting Symptoms and Frequency of Meeting Criteria for a Rome III FGID Diagnosis

The second aim was to investigate the frequency distribution of responses to the individual symptom questions by healthy controls and to assess the frequency with which healthy controls fulfilled these criteria. The frequency distributions of individual symptoms were examined and symptom frequency

Table 9. Proportion of Healthy Controls Meeting Rome III Diagnostic Criteria for FGIDs and Test-Retest Reliability of the Diagnoses

	Ordinal Scale	Binary Scale	Test-Retest % Agreement
Functional Chest Pain	2.8		92.3
Functional Heartburn	4.4		87.5
Functional Dysphagia	5.2		92.3
Functional Globus	3.0		97.1
Functional Dyspepsia	5.9		86.5
Postprandial Distress Syndrome	1.1		84.6
Epigastric Pain Syndrome	0	0	98.1
Chronic Idiopathic Nausea	0.9		96.2
Rumination	0.2	0.2	97.1
Functional Vomiting	0		98.1
Cyclic Vomiting	0.4	0.4	96.2
Aerophagia	6.8		82.7
Irritable Bowel Syndrome	12.2		81.7
Functional Constipation	3.5	4.6	93.3
Functional Diarrhea	1.1		96.2
Functional Bloating	12.7	12.6	84.6
Unspecified Functional Bowel Disorder	52.7		69.2
Functional Abdominal Pain	0	0	99.0
Functional Biliary Pain	0	0	98.1
Functional Fecal Incontinence	5.0		87.5
Functional Anorectal Pain	1.5		89.4
Proctalgia Fugax	5.7		81.7
Functional Defecation Disorder	1.5	41.6	95.2

n = 554

thresholds were selected that would yield a false-positive rate of approximately 5%. However, an exception was made for the diagnosis of IBS, where the working team selected a threshold for the frequency of abdominal pain (2 to 3 times per month or more often) that occurred in 12.2% of the healthy controls. This criterion led to a specificity of 87.8% and a sensitivity of 70.7% for IBS, whereas the selection of a more stringent threshold eroded the sensitivity of the diagnostic criteria to an unacceptably high rate. The frequency distribution of responses to individual symptoms is not included in this report.

Table 9 shows the proportion of healthy controls that met diagnostic criteria for each of the Rome III-defined FGIDs. The goal of limiting the false-positive rate to approximately 5% was achieved for all diagnoses except IBS, functional bloating, and nonspecific functional bowel disorder. The false-positive rate for unspecified functional bowel disorder is so high (and the corresponding specificity is so low) that this diagnosis is of questionable utility.

Test-Retest Reliability of Diagnostic Criteria

Table 9 also shows the test-retest reliability for each of the Rome III diagnoses, expressed as the proportion of subjects who received the same diagnosis on two occasions spaced approximately 2 weeks apart. For this analysis, 51 patients with FGIDs were pooled with 53 healthy controls. With only one exception (unspecified functional bowel disorder), the percent agreement was greater than 80%, and the median percent agreement across 23 diagnoses was 92.3%.

Sensitivity and Specificity of the Questionnaire for Identifying Medically Diagnosed Patients with FGIDs

The goal of the validation study was to recruit relatively large samples of patients who had been medically evaluated and had received clinical diagnoses of FGIDs; the sensitivity of the criteria was to be tested by calculating the proportion of these medically diagnosed patients who were identified by the Rome III Diagnostic Questionnaire. This was possible for IBS, which had a sensitivity of 0.707 and a specificity of 0.878, because the validation sample included 328 patients with a medical diagnosis of IBS. However, there were insufficient numbers of patients in other categories to estimate sensitivity: 27 with functional constipation, 14 with functional diarrhea, 10 with functional dyspepsia, 8 with functional abdominal pain, 7 with fecal incontinence, and 5 with functional defecation disorder.

Comparison of Questionnaire Version 1 Containing 31 Binary Scaled Items to Version 2 Substituting Ordinal Scales

Study 1 has already shown that subjects who have an intermediate frequency of a symptom are inconsistent with respect to whether they respond "never or rarely" vs. "often" when asked to respond to a binary-scaled question. Study 1 also showed that a different frequency threshold is required for commonly occurring symptoms such as straining, as compared to rare symptoms such as digital facilitation of defecation, to separate FGID patients from healthy controls. Therefore, the analyses for Study 2 were limited to (1) comparing the test-retest reliability of diagnoses based on the binary-scaled items to the reliability of diagnoses based on substituted ordinal-scaled items, and (2) comparing the sensitivity and specificity of diagnoses based on these alternative response scales against the gold standard of medical diagnosis.

When diagnoses based on ordinal scaled items were compared to diagnoses based on binary items, the test-retest reliability was equal or better. For one diagnosis, (functional defecation disorder), the reliability of the diagnosis incorporating ordinal scaled items was substantially better (95.2% vs. 77.9% agreement). For sensitivity and specificity, there were no differences between the questionnaire with ordinal-scaled questions vs. the questionnaire containing 31 binary-scaled symptom questions.

Discussion

The Rome III Diagnostic Questionnaire was developed through a rational process: The Rome Foundation drew on a large pool of academic investigators with expertise in questionnaire development and with knowledge of these disease entities. In order to select the most appropriate response format for questions, a large-scale study was carried out to compare the responses of subjects (both FGID patients and healthy controls) to the same symptom questions using four different response scales. Subsequently, the draft questionnaire was extensively evaluated for item understandability, test-retest reliability, and sensitivity and specificity in a new study involving 556 healthy controls and 412 patients with FGIDs. This development process and psychometric testing contrasts with the development of the Rome II Modular Questionnaire: this questionnaire did not undergo psychometric testing.

The principal innovation in the Rome III Diagnostic Questionnaire is the use of ordinal response scales for most questions. The decision to change from binary to ordinal response scales was made by the Rome Foundation Board because symptoms that define the FGIDs sometimes occur in healthy individuals, making it necessary to define a threshold frequency of occurrence that is clinically significant and that warrants diagnosis and medical management. The board also realized that the frequency of occurrence that is clinically meaningful (i.e., abnormal) varies across symptoms: for frequently occurring symptoms such as belching and straining with defecation, a high threshold is required, whereas for rare symptoms such as digital facilitation of defecation, a low frequency of occurrence may be clinically significant. To test these assumptions, the Rome Foundation commissioned Study 1 to collect data on the normal frequency of occurrence of these symptoms in healthy individuals and patients with FGIDs, and to compare different response scales.

Study 1 confirmed that the frequency of occurrence of FGID symptoms varied across symptoms in healthy individuals, and that different frequency thresholds were required to separate FGID patients from healthy controls. Study 1 also showed that an ordinal scale had distinct advantages over the binary scale used in the Rome II Modular Questionnaire: subjects who had symptoms "sometimes" or "2 to 3 times per month" differed with respect to whether they answered "never or rarely" vs. "often" on the binary scale.

Study 2 showed that with few exceptions, the questions drafted by the committee were understood with little difficulty by both healthy controls and patients with FGIDs. Only 18 questions were judged to be difficult by at least 1% of the sample, and only 6 questions were judged difficult by at least 2%. This analysis also showed that the binary response questions that were retained in the questionnaire were often among the more difficult to understand because they involved multiple judgments about frequency or circumstances of occurrence of symptoms, e.g., "In the last 3 months, were there 21 days when you had more than 3 (4 or more) bowel movements a day?" Seventeen of the 18 questions that were identified as difficult to understand by at least 1% of subjects were reworded to improve clarity.

A large sample of healthy controls was included in Study 2 to confirm that the frequency thresholds selected by the Rome working teams were appropriate. We tested these thresholds by computing the frequency distribution of responses in these healthy controls with the goal of limiting false-positive diagnoses to 5% or less. In a few cases, the working teams were asked to reconsider the thresholds they had set based on these data. By this iterative process, the goal of arriving at diagnostic criteria with reasonable specificity was achieved for 20 of 23 diagnoses (Table 9). The exceptions were IBS, functional bloating, and nonspecific functional bowel disorder, which had false positive rates of 12.2%, 12.7%, and 52.7% respectively.

The test-retest reliability of the diagnostic criteria as incorporated into the questionnaire was found to be excellent (Table 9). With the exception of unspecified functional bowel disorder, all diagnoses showed agreement of 80% or greater (median 92%) between questionnaires administered 2 weeks apart.

The sensitivity of the diagnostic criteria for IBS was acceptable at 0.707, and the specificity was also very good at 0.878. However, there were insufficient numbers of patients with other FGID clinical diagnoses to estimate the sensitivity of the diagnostic criteria and the questionnaire for these disorders.

It is also important to recognize the limitations of a study design that treats clinical diagnosis as the gold standard against which the accuracy of questionnaire-based diagnoses is judged: clinicians may disagree with each other in their evaluations of individual patients and even on the definitions they use for some of the FGIDs. In some studies this inter-rater variability is dealt with by having the raters discuss cases on which they disagree until they reach consensus, but this was not done in this study.

Study Limitations

In Study 1, the healthy control sample was significantly younger than the FGID patient sample, and in Study 2, where more complete demographic information was collected, the healthy controls were found to be not only younger and more likely to be male, but also better educated and with a higher proportion of them from racial minority groups. These demographic differences emerged because both groups had to be recruited and tested simultaneously due to project time constraints, which prevented close matching. However, question-by-question analysis of nonparametric correlations (Spearman's rho) between demographic variables and responses of the healthy subjects showed only 15% to 21% of questions to be significantly correlated ($p<.05$) with demographic variables. Specifically, age showed significant correlations with responses on 21% of questions, race with 18.7%, and gender and education each with 15.3% of questions. Furthermore, the significant correlations were universally weak; rho was less than 0.25 in all but one instance, where it was 0.27. Bias due to demographic differences in the group comparisons made in Study 2 is therefore likely to be sufficiently small for the conclusions to be valid.

A second limitation of the study is that many of the FGIDs are underrepresented in the validation sample of FGID patients in both studies. With small numbers of subjects it was not possible to estimate the sensitivity of the diagnostic criteria. To address this limitation, investigators will need to selectively recruit for these categories of patients, and they should consider standardizing the diagnostic evaluation.

A third limitation is that many of the FGIDs now require clinical evaluation and laboratory-based tests to confirm the diagnosis. Examples are functional biliary disorders and functional anorectal disorders. For these disorders, alternative study designs are needed that conceptualize the questionnaire responses as screening instruments for identifying possible cases and that evaluate whether the questionnaire reduces the cost of diagnostic evaluation or increases diagnostic accuracy.

Conclusions

The Rome III Diagnostic Questionnaire is a valid and reliable instrument for making provisional diagnoses of all FGIDs except unspecified functional bowel disorder. It can be used for clinical, epidemiological, or research (inclusion criteria) purposes, but users must recognize that laboratory diagnostic tests and clinical judgment are required to confirm some diagnoses.

Acknowledgements: This validation study was supported by a generous grant from the Rome Foundation and by grant R24 DK67674.

Chapter 17

The Road to Rome

W. Grant Thompson

The traditional medical diagnosis of disease requires observed anatomical or physiological abnormalities. Description of the disease's symptoms and signs follows naturally. Clinicians can then predict the anatomic diagnosis by recognizing these symptoms and signs in their patients. In the case of the functional disorders, such a process is impossible. Since there are no observed pathophysiological defects, we only know of the existence of the disorders through the words of our patients. The movement to define these disorders of unknown pathology represents a substantial change in thinking for doctors whose training concentrates on basic science and palpable "evidence." Since more than half of gut disorders encountered by gastroenterologists and primary care doctors are functional, we must face the reality that no current scientific evidence explains these disorders, and develop alternate methods to identify them.

For too long, functional diseases were described by what they are not, rather than as real entities. Yet they are real enough to patients. Not only does such an exclusive approach fail to provide the patient with the dignity of a diagnosis, but it also generates needless tests and consultations. The fruitless pursuit of an anatomical cause renders functional disorders "diagnoses of exclusion." Their very numbers and cost demand a more positive approach.

More seriously, there was a disconnect between the subjects chosen for randomized clinical trials (RCTs) and the labels used in clinical practice. Because clinical scientists failed to describe their subjects accurately, the results of their RCTs are of uncertain applicability to the patients encountered by practicing doctors. In a 1988 critique of 43 clinical trials of irritable bowel syndrome (IBS) treatments, Klein [1] observed that 58% of them reported "absolutely nothing about the criteria by which IBS patients were selected." There were important differences among the remainder, some not requiring abdominal pain, and others not even requiring a bowel habit abnormality. Klein concludes, "Not a single IBS treatment trial reported to date [1988], used an adequate operational definition of IBS."

Table 1 further illustrates this point. Many of these reports were published in prestigious journals and in some cases form the basis of regulatory approval of drugs that remain on national formularies. Most of these reports implied that the diagnosis of their subjects rested solely on the exclusion of structural disease. The trials shown in Table 1 include IBS or irritable colon syndrome (ICS) in their titles, yet they describe very different trial subjects. The listed trimebutine trials were the basis of regulatory approval in France, Canada, and elsewhere, yet the entered patients in these "IBS trials" were dissimilar. The trial reports in Table 1 fail to state entry criteria that would permit doctors to judge which patients should receive the tested treatments. This lack of definition was similar for dys-

Table 1. Irritable Bowel Syndrome Entry Criteria for Randomized, Controlled Trials Prior to 1988

Author	Year	Journal	Drug	Entry Criteria
Kasich [24]	1959	AJ Gastro	tricyclanol	irritable colon syndrome (ICS)
Connell [25]	1965	BMJ	mebeverine	ICS
Tasmen-Jones [26]	1973	N Zealand J Med	mebeverine	abdominal pain & altered bowel habit
Greenbaum [27]	1973	NEJM	diphenylhydrate	compatible history of irritable bowel syndrome (IBS)
Piai [28]	1979	Gastroenterology	profinium	compatible history of IBS
Moshal [29]	1979	J Int Med Res	trimebutine	constipation—10% had pain
Fielding [30]	1980	Irish Med J	trimebutine	diagnosed as suffering from the IBS
Luttecke [31]	1980	Curr Med Res Opin	trimebutine	IBS on the basis of their symptoms
Fielding [32]	1981	Digestion	timolol	IBS
Cann [33]	1983	Gut	domperidone	abdominal pain and bowel disturbance suggestive of IBS
Dew [34]	1984	Brit J Clin Pract	peppermint oil	typical symptoms of IBS
Flexinos [35]	1985	Eur J Clin Pharm	trimebutine	constipation or diarrhea or both
Pidgeon [36]	1985	Ir J Med Sci	cimetidine	IBS patients with excessive muscle spasm on sigmoidoscopy
Narducci [37]	1985	Am J Gastro	nifedipine	abdominal pain relieved by defecation and either constipation or diarrhea
Perez-Mateo [38]	1986	Int J Clin Pharm Res	Diltiazam	compatible clinical history, physical exploration
Prior [39]	1988	Aliment Pharm Ther	lidamadine	abdominal pain and distress with abnormal bowel habit
Dobrilla [40]	1990	Gut	cimetropium	abdominal pain "after all other organic causes . . . excluded"

pepsia and constipation. It was time to define and establish criteria for the functional gastrointestinal disorders.

There are many references to gut dysfunction in the ancient and early European literature. However, the first credible English-language descriptions of irritable bowel syndrome (IBS) appeared in the early nineteenth century. One such description of the IBS in 1818 [2] drew attention to three cardinal symptoms of IBS; abdominal pain, "derangement of . . . digestion," and "flatulence." A few years later, Howship [3] described a "spasmodic stricture" of the colon reflecting the enduring, but unsubstantiated belief that functional gut disorders are somehow the product of gut spasm. Midcentury brought more sophisticated treatises (and very unsophisticated cures such as purging and "electrogalvanism"). In 1849, Cumming [4] exclaims incredulously, "the bowels are at one time constipated and at another lax in the same person . . . how the disease has two such different symptoms I do not propose to explain." Were he to return to a modern IBS consensus meeting, he would discover that this enigma remains! Cumming's treatise contained one other comment in line with modern thinking about IBS. "One can tell, without more minute examination, what the nature of the complaint is." The authors of this book agree with Cumming's notion of a positive diagnosis, even though many doctors persist in recognizing IBS and the other functional gut disorders only after the patient has undergone exhaustive investigation.

Medicine's understanding of IBS progressed little during the next 120 years. Indeed, it may have lost ground! Edwardian physicians considered functional disorders to be diseases of the wealthy. In fact, only the affluent could afford to be the patients of those Harley Street doctors who published their observations in the medical literature [5]. Constipation became associated with uncleanness [6]. The notion of "autointoxication" due to retained colon contents prompted an urge to purge that persists to this day. In the 1920s and 1930s pejorative descriptors such as "psychogenic," "neurogenic," and "The Abdominal Woman" [7] did little to help patients with functional gut disorders. Proctalgia fugax was long thought to be a disease of young professional males, because only doctors had the temerity to describe their symptoms in letters to the editor of *The Lancet* [8]. Use of terms such as "spastic colitis" and "hyperacidity," inferred now-discredited etiologies for these disorders [6].

The first systematic attempt to bring discipline to this area was a 1962 retrospective review of IBS patients at Oxford by Chaudhary and Truelove [9]. The authors reported symptoms that we recognize to be those of the IBS (or ICS as they termed it). They even separated IBS from what we now call functional diarrhea, and noted that one quarter of their patients' complaints began with an enteric infection. Their report ushered a new era, and scientific publications on functional disorders increased rapidly thereafter. (Figure 1)

The table of contents of my book *The Irritable Gut* (1979) contained the first classification of the functional gastrointestinal disorders [10]. In 1978, Ken Heaton

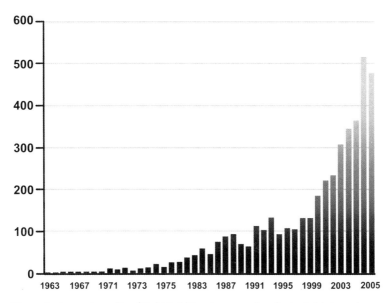

Figure 1. Annual results of PubMed literature searches for irritable bowel syndrome (IBS) and irritable colon syndrome (ICS) between the 1962 Chaudhary and Truelove report and 2005 (In the Figure, the data for 2005 was determined February 1, 2006—the publication deadline). Note the rapid rise in publications during that period. While half the publications in the 1960s had "irritable colon syndrome" in their titles, only one or two occur annually now—exclusively in the non-English literature.

and colleagues reported results obtained by questionnaire administered to Bristol outpatients with abdominal pain and disordered bowel habit [11]. The 6 out of 15 symptoms we found more common in IBS than organic gut disease (diagnosis determined by a chart review a year later) became the *Manning Criteria*. In 1984, Kruis and his colleagues from Germany reported a similar study [12]. Their report recalls the three cardinal IBS symptoms of pain, bowel dysfunction, and flatulence mentioned by Powell in 1818. If all three were present, IBS was highly likely. Kruis et al. stressed chronicity and other symptoms as well, but their major contribution was to record "alarm" symptoms that should alert the physician to organic disease. These two discriminate function studies, in addition to epidemiologic data provided by Drossman [13] and Whitehead [14], are the basis of the Rome criteria for IBS.

The inspiration for the Rome process was an IBS symposium at the 12th International Congress of Gastroenterology held in Lisbon in 1984. Despite being perhaps the earliest international symposium on IBS, the symposium attracted an audience that far outstripped the capacity of the assigned room. One panel member, Professor Aldo Torsoli, was an organizer of the next international con-

Table 2. History of the Rome Diagnostic Criteria

The Manning Criteria for IBS (1978) [11]

The Kruis Criteria for IBS (1984) [12]

The Rome Guidelines for IBS (1989) [15] *(Rome -2 IBS Criteria)*

The Rome Classification System for FGIDs (1990) [16] *(Rome -1)*

The Rome I Criteria for IBS (1992) [20] and the FGIDs (1994) [22]

The Rome II Criteria for IBS (1999) [41] and the FGIDs (1999) [23]

The Rome III Criteria (2006)

gress planned for Rome in 1988. Over coffee in Portugal, we discussed the need for guidelines for the management and study of IBS. A working team was set up to produce such guidelines for the next congress.

As chair, I collaborated with Doug Drossman (USA), Ken Heaton (UK), Gerhard Dotteval (Sweden), and Wolfgang Kruis (Germany) for two years. In 1987, we met in Rome to debate a draft proposal and reach consensus. We sent the penultimate draft to 16 expert colleagues in seven countries. The working team considered their comments and suggestions and presented the first Rome criteria at the 13th Congress in Rome in 1988. The guidelines were published the following year [15]. Guidelines were this report's objectives, and diagnostic criteria were subordinate. They might be known as the *Rome -2 IBS Criteria*, and attracted much interest among researchers and pharmaceutical companies. (See Table 2.)

Following that Rome meeting, Professor Torsoli and Dr. Enrico Corrazziari invited Dr. Doug Drossman to set up another committee to consider subgroups of IBS. After discussion, the project expanded to include all the functional gastrointestinal disorders. This working team, which included most of the this book's editors, met in Rome to classify the functional gastrointestinal disorders into 21 entities in five anatomical regions of the gut [16]. This was the first time that diagnostic criteria were proposed for all the functional gut disorders and included the first revision of the 1988 IBS criteria. This was *Rome -1*.

With sponsorship organized by Professor Torsoli, Doug Drossman gathered a succession of working teams over four years that further developed these criteria in the five anatomical regions (esophageal [17], gastroduodenal [18], biliary [19], bowel [20], and anorectal [21]) and discussed topics related to functional gut disorders. In 1994, their collective work was updated and published in *The Functional Gastrointestinal Disorders: Diagnosis, Pathophysiology and Treatment; A Multinational Consensus* [22].

While this work is now known as *Rome I*, it includes the *third* rendition of the

Rome IBS criteria [20]. From 1988 to 1992, three IBS working teams added duration parameters, and pain went from being unnecessary for the diagnosis of IBS (15), to being a suggested symptom (16), to eventually a requisite [20].

The Rome II process included 4 years of deliberations by over 50 investigators from 13 Western countries organized into 10 committees. The result was the second edition of *The Functional Gastrointestinal Disorders: Diagnosis, Pathophysiology and Treatment: A Multinational Consensus*. This iteration encompassed several important innovations. George Degnon became the Rome organization's executive director in 1994 and provided logistic and management support for a greatly expanded process generously funded by several pharmaceutical companies. Carlar Blackman became the administrative coordinator for the Coordinating Committee and the working teams. The organization became separated into an operational component (fundraising, meeting planning, book publishing) managed by Degnon Associates, and an academic component coordinated by Ms. Blackman and the Coordinating Committee. To ensure that the Rome process remained at arm's length from the sponsors, the Industry Research Council (IRC) was created with Dr. Bill Whitehead as chair. The IRC meets annually to allow Rome committee members, representatives of the sponsoring companies, and regulatory authorities to discuss progress and mutual concerns. Working team members do not communicate directly with the sponsors, and participating individuals must report their industry relationships. Rather than meeting independently, the working teams met together in Rome in 1998. This permitted interaction and harmonization among the committees. The Rome II criteria and essential supporting information were published in a *Gut* supplement in 1999 [23]. In addition to the anatomically determined criteria and clinical trials working teams, new teams addressed basic science, neurogastroenterology, psychosocial issues, and pediatric functional gut disorders. The second edition of the book, also published in 1999, included a glossary, proposed questionnaires, and the results of a Vienna symposium on the *Definition of a Responder* involving academics, regulators, and the pharmaceutical industry.

By 2000, there was great interest in the Rome process as more researchers and interest groups entered the field, and the pharmaceutical companies and regulators became concerned with how to define and test treatments for the functional gastrointestinal disorders. Thus, plans for Rome III began promptly. Dr. Robin Spiller and Dr. Michel Delvaux joined the now seven-member Coordinating Committee. The organization registered as a nonprofit educational foundation, and the Coordinating Committee became known as the *Rome Board*. The board held a retreat in London in February 2002 to plan its future. The board agreed upon a Rome III format and addressed a wide range of operational topics including relationships with industry; projects such as validation that went beyond publication of diagnostic criteria; the promotion of evidence as the basis of criteria change; and the encouragement of "developing world" participation. The board also initiated an ongoing project to develop an educational slide program for the functional gastrointestinal disorders.

For Rome III, the Board selected 87 participants from 18 countries in 14 committees and briefed the chairpersons in 2003, 2004, and 2005. Members were added from developing countries including China, Brazil, Chile, Venezuela, Hungary, and Romania. New working teams were created for gender, society, patient and social issues; and pharmacology and pharmacokinetics. Functional abdominal pain was split from functional bowel disease and two committees (neonate/toddler and child/adolescent), rather than one, served pediatrics. A subcommittee of the board consisting of myself (chair), Doug Drossman, Nick Talley, Lynn Walker and William Whitehead designed the adult and pediatric questionnaires as the criteria were developed. Rome III culminated in a meeting in Rome in November/December 2004. As the final drafts of the chapters were being prepared, Dr. Whitehead conducted a validation study of the criteria and the questionnaire designed by the questionnaire subcommittee, the results of which are included in this publication. Following peer review, the results of the process have been published as articles in *Gastroenterology* in May 2006 and in full as the third edition of *Rome III: The Functional Gastrointestinal Disorders* in September 2006. In addition, board members reported the Rome III process to the 2005 World Congress of Gastroenterology in Montreal, and the criteria themselves to the 2006 American Gastrointestinal Association meeting in Los Angeles.

The Rome criteria generate much energy and controversy. They are imperfect. Validation studies are difficult and rare. There is much debate among the Rome participants about terminology, notably the use of the term *functional*. How much physiological or structural evidence is necessary for an entity to cease being functional? How long, how often, and how severe must symptoms be before they constitute a functional gastrointestinal disorder? Tradition and the lack of viable alternatives make change difficult. Those interested in the functional disorders express disparate views on these and other issues—epidemiologists, primary care physicians, consultants, researchers, psychologists, physiologists, pharmaceuticals, regulators, third-party payers and, of course, the patients themselves. In Rome III, these voices were prominent in the background and in the reviews of the chapter manuscripts.

Despite the controversies, the criteria have gained such currency that they are the basis for entry into most research studies of functional gut disorders and have compelled an accurate description of entered patients in the remainder. They are the industry standard for entry into clinical drug trials, although they are sometimes modified to suit the characteristics of the product to be tested. They have given these disorders, particularly IBS, a profile. Patients can now be reassured they suffer from a legitimate disorder, not symptoms rendered imaginary by a negative test. The criteria have created a language with which the above-mentioned groups can communicate. The coming together of such disparate constituencies in a common effort is a major achievement, due in no small way to Rome's systematic recognition of the functional gut disorders.

This Rome III publication culminates a new 6-year effort to update the Rome criteria and, like Rome I and II, owes much to the energy and drive of Doug Drossman who describes the mechanics of this process in Chapter 1. The Rome II and Rome III processes were generously supported by industry, and attracted the interest and participation of many people in several disciplines from around the world. There can be no better testimony to the stature that the Rome criteria have achieved. However, Rome III is neither the end, nor even the beginning of the end. It is perhaps the end of the beginning of an ongoing process that will last as long as understanding the pathophysiology of functional gut disorders eludes us. Meanwhile, there is a great need to generate data that will sharpen the criteria and validate their use. Preliminary discussions have begun for Rome IV, but we must allow sufficient time for the accumulation of evidence to justify meaningful changes. The Delphi approach may be less useful now, but the need remains for consensus as to the meaning of the slowly accumulating, fragmented, and controversial evidence.

W. Grant Thompson M.D.
Ottawa, Canada
January 11, 2006

References

1. Klein KB. Controlled treatment trials in the irritable bowel syndrome: a critique. Gastroent 1988;95:232–241.
2. Powell R. On certain painful afflictions of the intestinal canal. Med Trans Royal Coll Phys 1818;6:106–117.
3. Howship J. Practical remarks on the discrimination and successful treatment of spasmodic stricture of the colon. London: Burgess and Hill, 1830.
4. Cumming W. Electro-galvanism in a peculiar affliction of the mucous membrane of the bowels. Lond Med Gazette 1849;NS9:969–973.
5. Hale-White W. Colitis. Lancet 1895;1:537.
6. Thompson WG. Gut Reactions. New York: Plenum, 1989.
7. Hutchison R. Lectures on Dyspepsia. London: Edward Arnold, 1927.
8. Thompson WG. Proctalgia fugax. Dig Dis Sci 1981;26:1121–1124.
9. Chaudhary NA, Truelove SC. The irritable colon syndrome. Q J Med 1962;31:307–322.

10. Thompson WG. The Irritable Gut. Baltimore: University Park Press, 1979.

11. Manning AP, Thompson WG, Heaton KW, Morris AF. Towards positive diagnosis of the irritable bowel. Br Med J 1978;2:653–654.

12. Kruis W, Thieme CH, Weinzierl M, Schussler P, Hall J, Paulus W. A diagnostic score for the irritable bowel syndrome. Its value in the exclusion of organic disease. Gastroent 1984;87:1–7.

13. Drossman DA, Sandler RS, McKee DC, Lovitz AJ. Bowel patterns among subjects not seeking health care. Use of a questionnaire to identify a population with bowel dysfunction. Gastroent 1982;83:529–534.

14. Whitehead WE, Winget C, Fedoravicius AS, Wooley S, Blackwell B. Learned illness behavior in patients with irritable bowel syndrome and peptic ulcer. Dig Dis Sci 1982;27:202–208.

15. Thompson WG, Dotevall G, Drossman DA, Heaton KW, Kruis W. Irritable bowel syndrome: Guidelines for the diagnosis. Gastroent Int 1989;2:92–95.

16. Drossman DA, Funch-Jensen P, Janssens J, Talley NJ, Thompson WG, Whitehead WE. Identification of subgroups of functional bowel disorders. Gastroent Int 1990; 3:159–172.

17. Richter JE, Baldi F, Clouse RE, Diamant NE, Janssens J, Stiano A. Functional oesophageal disorders. Gastroent Int 1992;5:3–17.

18. Talley NJ, Colin-Jones D, Koch KL, Koch M, Nyren O, Stanghellini V. Functional Dyspepsia: A classification with guidelines for diagnosis and management. Gastroent Int 1991;4:145–160.

19. Corazziari E, Funch-Jensen P, Hogan W, Tanaka J, Toouli J. Working team report on functional biliary disorders. Gastroent Int 1993;6:129–144.

20. Thompson WG, Creed FH, Drossman DA, Heaton KW, Mazzacca G. Functional bowel disorders and functional abdominal pain. Gastroent International 1992;5:75–91.

21. Whitehead WE, Devroede G, Habib FI, Meunier P, Wald A. Report of an international workshop on functional disorders of the anorectum. Gastroent International 1992;5:92–108.

22. Drossman DA, Richter JE, Talley NJ, Corazziari E, Thompson WG, Whitehead WE. Functional Gastrointestinal Disorders. Boston: Little, Brown, 1994.

23. Drossman DA, Corazziari E, Talley NJ, Thompson WG, Whitehead WE. Rome II: a multinational consensus document on functional gastrointestinal disorders. 45 ed. 1999.

24. Kasich A, Rafsky JC. Clinical evaluation of an anticholinergic in the irritable colon syndrome. Am J Gastroenterol 1959;4:229–234.

25. Connell AM. Physiological and clinical assessment of the effect of the musculotropic agent mebeverine on the human colon. BMJ 1965;2:848–851.

26. Tasman-Jones C. Mebeverine in patients with the irritable colon syndrome: double blind study. New Zealand Med J 1973;1:232–235.

27. Greenbaum DS, Ferguson RK, Kater LA, et al. A controlled therapeutic study of the irritable bowel syndrome. New Engl J Med 1973;288:612–616.

28. Piai G, Mazzacca G. Profinium Bromide in the treatment of the irritable bowel syndrome. Gastroent 1979;77:500–502.

29. Moshal MG, Herron M. A clinical trial of trimebutine in spastic colon. J Int Med Res 1979;7:231–234.

30. Fielding JF. Double blind trial of trimebutine in the irritable bowel syndrome. Ir Med J 1980;73:377–379.
31. Luttecke K. A trial of trimebutine in spastic colon. J Int Med Res 1978;6:86–88.
32. Fielding JF. Timolol treatment in the irritable bowel syndrome. Digestion 1982;22:155–158.
33. Cann PA, Read NW, Holdsworth CC. Oral domperidone: double blind comparison with placebo in irritable bowel syndrome. Gut 1983;24:1135–1140.
34. Dew MJ, Evans BK, Rhodes J. Peppermint oil for the irritable bowel syndrome. Br J Clin Pract 1984;38:394–398.
35. Flexinos J, Fioramonti J, Bueno L. Effect of trimebutine on colonic myoelectric activity in IBS patients. Eur J Clin Pharm 1985;28:181–185.
36. Pidgeon F, Craig F, Fielding JF. Lack of effect of cimetidine in the irritable bowel syndrome. Ir J Med Sci 1985;154:33–34.
37. Narducci F, Bassotti G, Gaburri M. Nifedipine reduces the colonic motor response to eating in patients with the irritable colon syndrome. Am J Gastroenterol 1985;80:317–319.
38. Perez-Mateo M, Sillero C, Cuesta A, Vazquez N, Berbegel J. Diltiazem in the treatment of irritable bowel syndrome. International Journal of Clinical Pharmacology Research 1986;5:425–427.
39. Prior A, Wilson KM, Whorwell PJ. Double-blind study of an α_2 agonist in the treatment of irritable bowel syndrome. Aliment Pharmacol Therap 1988;2:535–539.
40. Dobrilla G, Imbimbo BP, Piazzi L, Bensi G. Longterm treatment of IBS with cimetropium bromide: a double blind placebo controlled clinical trail. Gut 1990;31:355–358.
41. Thompson WG, Longstreth GF, Drossman DA, Heaton KW, Irvine EJ, Muller-Lissner SA. Functional Bowel Disease and Functional Abdominal Pain. Gut 1999;45:43–47.

Glossary

Prepared by
W. Grant Thompson, MD
and the Rome III Committees

abdominal distension: objective evidence that the abdomen is swollen, bloated, or full. This may be visible to the patient or to an observer.

abuse: threats or actions of an emotional, sexual, or physical nature in which a power differential exists between the perpetrator and the victim.

achalasia: the best recognized motor disorder of the esophagus, characterized by aperistalsis of the esophageal body and a failure of the lower esophageal sphincter to relax.

action potential: sometimes called "spike potential." A short-lasting, all-or-none change in membrane potential of a nerve or muscle cell that arises when a graded membrane depolarization passes a threshold; usually becomes a propagated nerve or muscle cell impulse.

adrenocorticotropic hormone (ACTH): the peptide hormone secreted by the pituitary that stimulates the adrenal grand to secrete cortisol, which in turn has many functions, including suppression of the immune system. ACTH is activated by corticotropin-releasing factor (CRF), which is produced by the hypothalamus in response to stress. CRF and ACTH are part of the hypothalamic-pituitary-adrenal (HPA) immune axis. This axis is involved with brain-body regulation and adaptation to stress. HPA reactivity to stress and release of ACTH may be dysfunctional in functional GI disorders.

adverse event: refers to an undesirable result of a treatment.

aerophagia: ingestion of air. See Mueller maneuver.

afferent nerve (afferents): nerve fibers (usually sensory) carrying impulses from an organ or tissue toward the central nervous system or the information processing centers of the enteric nervous system.

aganglionosis: congenital absence of ganglionic cells in the enteric nervous system in a segment of bowel. This may affect the anal canal and is the pathophysiological basis for Hirschprung's disease.

alarm symptoms: symptoms such as fever, bleeding, anemia, weight loss, or physical findings such as an abdominal mass that cannot be explained by functional gastrointestinal disorders. They help in the decision to undertake diagnostic studies to identify other disease.

allodynia: a form of visceral hypersensitivity where there is an abnormal pain response to an innocuous or nonnoxious visceral afferent signal.

anal fissure: crack in the skin or mucosa in or adjacent to the anal canal, causing symptoms of stinging or itching during defecation.

anal wink reflex/perianal wink reflex: a reflex contraction of the external anal sphincter that can be elicited by gentle stroking of the perianal skin.

anemia: reduced blood hemoglobin or red cell concentration.

anorectal angle: the (approximately) 90 degree angle between the rectum and the anal canal. This angle becomes more obtuse during defecation and more acute when holding back stool. The angle is formed by the contraction of the puborectalis muscle.

anoscopy: examination of the anus and lower rectum with a rigid cone or tube.

antidepressants: a class of drugs whose primary effect is to correct neurotransmitter imbalance in the central nervous system as occurs with major depression. They can also be useful in treating the functional GI disorders because of their effects on pain modulation and motility as well as in treating psychological comorbidities.

antipsychotics: agents that act mainly via dopaminergic pathways in the central nervous system to decrease symptoms of psychosis, such as delusions (including somatic delusions), hallucinations, and severe agitation.

antral dysrhythmia: abnormality of electrical rhythm in the gastric antrum (bradygastria/tachygastria); analogous to cardiac arrhythmia.

anxiety: a subjective sense of feeling fearful or worried, often accompanied by bodily symptoms such as palpitations, breathlessness, or abdominal churning. It occasionally can lead to panic.

anxiety disorder: excessive anxiety and worry that can not be controlled and is persistent with a range of symptoms. Mild forms include phobias; more severe forms amount to panic disorder.

anxiolytic: a drug that can decrease, via action on the central nervous system, the symptoms of acute or chronic anxiety, including panic disorder, obsessive-compulsive disorder, phobia, or generalized anxiety.

Apley's criteria: research criteria proposed by John Apley in 1958 and widely used for many years in studies of recurrent abdominal pain in children. They have now been updated with the pediatric Rome criteria.

area postrema: brain stem region outside the blood-brain barrier believed to be an emetic trigger zone.

Auerbach's plexus: ganglionated plexus of the enteric nervous system situated between the longitudinal and circular muscle coats of the muscularis externa of the digestive tract. May be referred to as the myenteric plexus.

axons: fibers that carry impulses away from the perikaryon of a nerve cell.

barostat: computerized electronic device for maintaining a constant pressure, enabling (1) assessment of gut intraluminal tone, by measuring volume changes that reflect variations in gut tone; (2) assessment of gut sensitivity by determining perception in response to isobaric distension of a specific gut region.

behavior: acts, activities, responses to reactions, movements, processes, operations, etc.—in short, any measurable response of an organism.

behavioral: any variable that can assess a person's total activity, especially that which can be externally observed.

belch: retrograde expulsion of gas or air (usually ingested) from the upper gut.

benzodiazepine: a class of drugs that act on the cerebral cortex and ascending reticular activating system (ARAS) to facilitate the effect of the inhibitor peptide gamma amino butyric acid (GABA), which in turn decreases central nervous system irritability and promotes smooth muscle relaxation, sleep, lessened arousal (decreased anxiety).

biliary sphincter of Oddi dysfunction: motility abnormalities of the sphincter of Oddi of the choledochus, which include sphincter of Oddi stenosis and sphincter of Oddi dyskinesia.

biliary-type pain (I, II, III): classification of patients with continued biliary-type pain, despite cholecystectomy, according to clinical presentation, laboratory results, and endoscopic retrograde cholangiopancreatography (ERCP) findings.

biofeedback: the use of electronic or mechanical devices to provide visual and/or auditory information (feedback) on a biological process for the purpose of teaching an individual to control the biological process.

biogenic amines: group of chemical substances that include the neurotransmitters, 5-hydroxytryptamine and norepinephrine.

biomedical model: the model of illness and disease commonly taught in Western medical education and research. It has two assumptions: (1) reductionism—that all conditions can be linearly reduced to a single etiology and (2) dualism—where illness and disease are dichotomized either to an "organic" disorder having an objectively defined etiology, or a "functional" disorder, with no specific etiology or pathophysiology.

biopsychosocial model: a model that proposes that illness and disease result from simultaneously interacting systems at the cellular, tissue, organismal, interpersonal, and environmental level. It incorporates the biologic aspects of the disorder with the unique psychosocial features of the individual, and helps explain the variability in symptom expression among individuals having the same biologic condition.

bipolar depression: an affective disorder in which the patient experiences both depressive and manic episodes.

blinding: (also called "masking") where participants in a clinical trial are not aware which treatment they are receiving. When only the subjects are blinded in a randomized controlled trial, it is said to be single-blind. When both subjects and investigators are blinded, the trial is said to be double-blind.

bloating: the sensation of abdominal distension, with or without objective evidence. (See abdominal distension).

bloating in the upper abdomen: tightness located in the upper abdomen. It should be distinguished from visible abdominal distension.

borborygmi: audible bowel sounds.

brain-gut axis: the bidirectional nervous connections between the brain (central nervous system, CNS) and gut (enteric and autonomic nervous systems) that serve various physiological functions. Visceral afferent fibers project to somatotypic, emotional, and cognitive centers of the CNS, producing a variety of interpretations to the stimuli based on prior learning and one's cognitive and emotional state. In turn, the CNS can inhibit or facilitate afferent nociceptive signals, motility, secretory function, or inflammation.

Bristol Stool Form Scale: a 7-point descriptor scale of stool form, ranging from watery to hard and lumpy. The scale correlates with whole gut transit time. (See Figure 1, Functional Bowel Disorders chapter.)

bulking agents: macromolecular substances that increase stool bulk and soften feces by water binding. They may be of plant origin (e.g. bran, plantago) or synthetic (e.g. polyethylene glycol). They cannot be split by the enzymes of the human gut, but may be partially digested by the colon flora.

burp: retrograde expulsion of gas or air (usually ingested) from the upper gut. Also to burp a baby.

Carnett's test: a test of abdominal pain. The test is positive if abdominal pain increases with abdominal muscle flexion, indicating a muscle wall etiology (e.g. cutaneous nerve entrapment, a hernia or a radicular source), or with central hypervigilance. If the pain is reduced with abdominal muscle flexion (negative test), the pain is usually visceral.

catastrophizing: an individual's tendency to focus on and exaggerate the threat value of painful stimuli and negatively evaluate one's ability to deal with pain. Catastrophic thoughts tend to dwell on pessimistic interpretations of a situation in which there is a possibility of an unpleasant outcome.

CCK–cholescintigraphy: see cholescintigraphy

Chagas disease: neuropathic degeneration of autonomic neurons resulting from autoimmune attack in patients infected with the blood-borne parasite *Trypanosoma cruzi*.

cholecystokinin (CCK): a messenger peptide in the digestive tract that may be released as a hormone from enteroendocrine cells or as a neurotransmitter from enteric neurons.

choledochoscintigraphy: quantitative scintigraphic measurement of the time for bile transit from the hepatic hilum to the duodenum in patients who have undergone cholecystectomy.

cholescintigraphy: quantitative scintigraphic measurement of gallbladder emptying after i.v. infusion of CCK-8.

closed-eye sign: physical finding often seen in chronic abdominal pain syndrome. The patient will close their eyes when their abdomen is palpated, thereby communicating chronic pain behavior. In contrast, patients with acute visceral pain are hypervigilant and will usually keep their eyes open.

coding: the translation or representation of a message by one of a set of signals.

cognitions: beliefs, attitudes, expectations, and other mental events.

cognitive behavioral therapy: several approaches or sets of techniques drawn from a large pool of cognitive and behavioral strategies. The theme that unifies these approaches in functional GI disorders centers on an exploration of how certain cognitions and behaviors affect gut symptoms and associated psychosocial distress.

colic: spasmodic pain from a hollow viscous. In contrast, biliary pain does not briefly remit and recur; hence, "biliary colic" is a misnomer.

compliance: the capability of a region of the gut to adapt to an increased intraluminal volume.

contractile activity: muscular activity of the gut wall, either of short duration (phasic contractions) or more sustained activity (tonic contractions).

coping: behaviors or mental activities that manage (i.e., master, tolerate, minimize) environmental and internal stressors that tax or exceed a person's resources. It may be adaptive (e.g., problem-focused) or maladaptive (emotion-focused, "catastrophizing") in terms of health status. Therefore, coping is a mediating psychosocial factor in illness that may positively or negatively affect health outcome.

cortical evoked potentials: electrical manifestation of cerebral responses to sensory stimuli recorded by electrodes placed on the scalp.

corticotropin-releasing factor (CRF): chemical substance released from neurons in the hypothalamus to stimulate ACTH; can also be released from enteric neurons. CRF is one of the mediators of effects of physical or emotional stress on the behavior of the gastrointestinal tract.

cyclic vomiting: recurrent stereotypical episodes of intense nausea and vomiting lasting hours to days separated by symptom-free intervals.

defecography: radiographic assessment of the shape of the rectum during attempted defecation. A mixture of barium sulfate and a thickening agent is inserted into the rectum prior to attempted defecation. This test can also be done with pelvic functional magnetic resonance imaging (fMRI).

dendrites: fibers that receive synaptic inputs and transmit electrical signals toward the perikaryon of a nerve cell.

depolarization: a change in electrical potential in the direction of a more positive potential across the membrane of cells. In excitable cells, depolarization to a threshold potential triggers an action potential.

depression: a feeling of pessimism, sadness, tearfulness and/or irritability. **depressive disorders**: depression accompanied by reduced activities, appetite, sleep pattern, feelings of fatigue or loss of energy, guilt, worthlessness. Suicidal ideas occur in severe forms.

descending corticofugal pathways: often associated with down-regulation of incoming afferent signals. It is part of a homeostatic system whereby higher brain centers can inhibit signals going cephalad from the dorsal horn. It is the efferent limb of the "gate control system."

diabetic peripheral neuropathy: peripheral nerve injury resulting from diabetes.

dietary fiber: naturally-occurring bulking agents, mostly of plant origin (cell wall constituents or energy stores).

discomfort: (upper abdomen) a subjective, unpleasant sensation or feeling that is not interpreted as pain according to the patient and which, if fully assessed, can include any of nausea, fullness, bloating, and early satiety.

disinhibitory motor disease: disordered gastrointestinal motility resulting from neuropathic degeneration of enteric inhibitory motor neurons.

dissociation: disruption of the usual integration of consciousness, memory, and perception of the environment. This may lead to a number of symptoms including loss of memory, blunted emotion, apparent loss of identity and unexplained bizarre bodily symptoms.

distension: see abdominal distension.

dorsal column nuclei: also called posterior column neuclei in reference to the nucleus gracilis and cuneatus in the medulla oblongata. Ascending sensory fibers in the dorsal spinal column synapse in these nuclei.

dorsal columns: two large ascending tracts in the spinal cord that terminate in the nucleus gracilis and nucleus cuneatus in the medulla oblongata. Historically believed to transmit sensory information from large diameter sensory afferents from the skin. Now believed to also transmit sensory information from the intestinal tract.

dorsal root ganglion: location of cell bodies of spinal afferent neurons.

dorsal vagal complex: combined structures of dorsal vagal motor nucleus, nucleus tractus solitarius, and area postrema in the medulla oblongata (brain stem).

dorsal vagal motor nucleus: location in the medulla oblongata (brain stem) of cell bodies of vagal efferent (motor) fibers to the digestive tract, excluding parts of the esophagus.

dualism: a concept, first proposed by Descartes, that separates mind and body. Cartesian dualism (the biomedical model) has been the dominant model of illness and disease, and is challenged by the biopsychosocial model.

dyschezia: difficult defecation, defined by straining, a feeling of incomplete evacuation, and/or digital facilitation of defecation (pressing around the anus or inside the vagina).

dyspepsia: pain or discomfort centered in the upper abdomen (Rome I and II).

dysphagia: a sensation of abnormal bolus transit through the esophageal body.

dyssynergic defecation: (also pelvic floor dyssynergia, anismus, spastic pelvic floor syndrome): chronic disorder of defecation, due to functional outlet obstruction by paradoxic puborectalis muscle and/or the external anal sphincter contraction.

early satiety: a feeling that the stomach is overfilled soon after starting to eat. The sensation is out of proportion to the size of the meal being eaten, so that the meal cannot be finished.

effector systems: the musculature, secretory epithelium, and blood/lymphatic vasculature in the digestive tract.

efferent nerve (efferents): nerve fibers carrying impulses away from the central nervous system which cause muscles to contract and glands to secrete (inhibitory efferent nerves).

electrical syncytium: a tissue (e.g., gastrointestinal and cardiac muscle) in which the cells are electrically coupled one to another at cell-to-cell appositions that do not include cytoplasmic continuity. It accounts for the three-dimensional spread of excitation in excitable tissues.

electrical slow waves: omnipresent form of electrical activity (rhythmic depolarization and repolarization) in gastrointestinal muscle cells.

electrogalvanic stimulation: transrectal low-frequency electrical stimulation, used to treat rectal pain by relaxing skeletal muscles in the pelvic floor.

electrogastrography: the recording of gastric electrical activity from surface electrodes positioned on the abdominal wall.

electromyographic (EMG): refers to recordings of the electrical potentials generated by muscle cells when they contract.

emotion: a state usually caused by an event of importance to the person. It typically includes (a) a conscious mental state with recognizable quality of feeling and directed toward some object; (b) a bodily perturbation of some kind; (c) recognizable expressions of the face, tone of voice, and gesture; (d) a readiness toward certain kinds of action.

emotion-focused coping: a method in which the individual seeks to manage distressing emotions evoked by a situation or condition (e.g., praying or denial).

endosonography: use of reflected sound waves to image tissues. Anal endosonography is done by placing the transducer/probe into the anal canal and imaging the internal and external anal sphincters.

enmeshment: a dysfunctional interaction style associated occurring usually in families where individuals have difficulty in establishing boundaries (i.e. separation) in behavior.

enteric minibrain: used in reference to the brain-like functions of the enteric nervous system.

enteric nervous system: division of the autonomic nervous system situated within the walls of the digestive tract and involved with independent integrative neural control of digestive functions.

enterocele: descent of loops of small intestine into the pelvis that bulge into the vagina during straining. An enterocele may cause pain and/or obstructed defecation.

episodicity: recurrences of pain at varying and unpredictable intervals, a feature typical of peptic ulcer disease.

epithelial barrier: formed by tight junctions between epithelial cells of the gastrointestinal mucosa that prevent the translocation of infectious agents and large molecules from the gut lumen into the body.

etiology: cause.

excitable cells: cells such as neurons and muscle with membranes capable of giving rise to action potentials and propagated impulses.

external anal sphincter: a ring of skeletal muscle surrounding the anal canal which can be voluntarily contracted to postpone defecation.

factor analysis: a statistical method to reduce a large number of highly intercorrelated symptoms or variables that have been measured in a group of subjects to a smaller number of symptoms that are relatively independent.

fart: to pass gas per rectum or, the act, sound, odor of gas passing per rectum.

farting: passing gas from the bowel via the anus.

fecal impaction: larger than normal, firm mass of stool in the rectum or colon that is difficult for the patient to evacuate. This may contribute to fecal incontinence (overflow).

fecaloma: mass of hard stool in the rectum, fecal impaction.

fever: body temperature in excess of 37 degrees C.

flatulence: usually a euphemism for farting, but may embrace gasiness, bloating, even belching. Therefore, it is of little value as a symptom.

flatus: gas (wind) passed per anum.

fullness: an unpleasant sensation like the persistence of food in the stomach. This may or may not occur post-prandially.

functional abdominal bloating: a group of functional bowel disorders that are dominated by a feeling of abdominal fullness or bloating and without sufficient criteria for another functional gastrointestinal disorder.

functional abdominal pain (FAP): continuous, nearly continuous, or frequently recurrent pain localized in the abdomen that is poorly related to gut function.

functional abdominal pain syndrome (FAPS): abdominal pain present for the last 3 months with onset at least 6 months previous, that is poorly related to gut function and is associated with some loss of daily activities. Also called "chronic idiopathic abdominal pain" or "chronic functional abdominal pain."

functional bowel disorder (FBD): a functional gastrointestinal disorder with symptoms attributable to the mid or lower gastrointestinal tract.

functional chest pain: is of presumed esophageal origin and is characterized by episodes of unexplained chest pain that is usually midline and of visceral quality.

functional constipation: a group of functional disorders that present as persistent, difficult, infrequent or seemingly incomplete defecation.

functional diarrhea: daily or frequently recurrent passage of loose (mushy) or watery stools without abdominal pain or intervening constipation.

functional dysphagia: dysphagia where there is no structural abnormality, pathological reflux, or pathology-based motility disturbance to explain the symptom.

functional fecal incontinence: recurrent uncontrolled passage of fecal material for at least one month in an individual with a developmental age of at least 4 years who has no evidence of neurological or structural etiologies for incontinence.

functional heartburn: episodic retrosternal burning in the absence of gastroesophageal reflux, pathology-based motility disorders, or structural explanations.

functional outlet obstruction: inability or difficulty to void the rectum due to pelvic floor dyssynergia, internal prolapse, or enterocele that become apparent only upon straining.

gallbladder dysfunction: a disorder of gallbladder motility not explained by an identifiable cause.

ganglia: a grouping of nerve cell bodies situated outside the central nervous system.

ganglionated plexus: an array of ganglia and interganglionic fiber tracts forming parts of the enteric nervous system.

gas: known as *wind* in the U.K. In the context of this book, gas refers to the gases in or escaping from the gut.

gastroesophageal reflux (GER): the retrograde flow of gastric contents into the esophagus.

gastrointestinal motility: the organized application of forces of muscle contraction that results in physiologically significant movement or nonmovement of intraluminal contents.

genetic polymorphism: multiple forms of the same gene.

globus: (globus pharyngis, globus pharyngeus) a sensation of something stuck or of a lump or tightness in the throat.

gut hypersensitivity: ambiguous term referring to both conscious perception of gut stimuli, and to afferent input within gastrointestinal sensory pathways, whether related to perception or reflex responses.

health beliefs (health concerns): cognitive theories of patients' beliefs about the causes of illness, and worries that they may have a disease.

health-related quality of life (HRQOL): the impact that illness has on quality of life, including the individual's perception of his/her illness.

heartburn: episodic retrosternal burning. Also, pyrosis.

hemoglobin: the oxygen-carrying protein in red cells.

holism: from the Greek holos, or whole, was proposed by Plato, Aristotle, and Hippocrates in ancient Greece. It postulates that mind and body are inseparable, so the study of medical disease must take into account the whole person rather than merely the diseased part. This concept fell into disfavor after Descartes proposed the separation between mind ("res cogitans") and body ("res extensa"). (See dualism.)

5-hydroxytryptamine: an important neurotransmitter in both central and peripheral digestive neurophysiology.

hyperalgesia: a form of visceral hypersensitivity where there is an increased pain response to a noxious stimulus.

hyperpolarization: a change in electrical potential in the direction of a more negative potential across the membrane of cells.

hypervigilance: an intensified version of being vigilant or paying attention to/or focusing on specific things.

hypnosis: a state of focused attention and heightened suggestibility that can be induced in a variety of ways. During this state, patients are responsive to suggestions for symptom improvement.

hypnotherapy: the use of hypnosis to improve psychological and/or physical symptoms. Hypnosis renders patients more responsive to suggestions for symptom improvement.

hypochondriasis: fear of disease (disease phobia) combined with the conviction that one has a disease, in the absence of objective evidence that one is present.

IGLEs: intraganglionic laminar endings. Sensory nerve endings associated with ganglia of the enteric nervous system.

illness behavior: a conduct or behavior in response to an individual's perceptions of being ill or not well. Examples of "illness behavior" may include visits to the doctor, taking time off work, staying in bed, and taking medications. This behavior is not necessarily an abnormal reaction to illness but a behavioral response based on a person's formulation and attribution of his/her illness.

imperforate anus: congenital malformation in which the colon does not open at the anus but ends in a blind sack.

incident cases: those who have sought health care for their FGID for the first time in the past year. (Incidence and prevalence are only meaningful when referring to population-based studies.)

indigestion: term used by patients for an unpleasant abdominal or substernal sensation from such a variety of illnesses that it is no useful diagnostically. Further symptom description is needed.

inhibitory junction potential: membrane hyperpolarization leading to decreased excitability in gastrointestinal muscles. Evoked by the release and action of inhibitory neurotransmitters from enteric motor neurons.

innervated: the structure referred to is supplied with intact nerves.

integration: process of assembling parts together to make a whole. Neural network processing resulting in output being a function of input other than one. Organization of behavior of individual digestive effector systems into harmonious function of the whole organ.

interganglionic fiber tracts: bundles of nerve fibers connecting adjacent ganglia of the enteric nervous system.

internal anal sphincter: smooth muscle sphincter surrounding the anal canal that provides a passive barrier to leakage of liquid and gas from the rectum.

interneuron: an internuncial neuron that is neither sensory nor motor. Connects neurons with neurons.

interpersonal therapy: a form of psychotherapy in which the therapist identifies aspects of the relationship between the patient and therapist that mirror difficulties in relationships outside of the therapy.

interstitial cells of Cajal: specialized cells of mesodermal origin believed to be the pacemaker cells for intestinal electrical slow waves.

intussusception: telescoping of any part of the intestine or rectum. This is more commonly seen in childhood in an idiopathic form and in adulthood often occurs in association with a bowel disease.

irritable bowel syndrome (IBS): a group of functional bowel disorders in which abdominal discomfort or pain is associated with defecation or a change in bowel habit, and with features of disordered defecation.

Kruis criteria: early symptom criteria for irritable bowel syndrome developed in the 1980s.

laxative: a compound that increases fecal water content. The primary mechanism is the inhibition of colonic water absorption or stimulation of active or passive colonic water secretion. Some laxatives are also prokinetics.

laxative abuse: laxative ingestion without proper indication or at higher than necessary doses.

learned illness behavior: patterning of pain behavior during childhood by parental modeling.

levator ani syndrome: chronic or recurring dull aching pain in the rectum or anal canal, with episodes lasting 30 minutes or longer, in the absence of organic etiologies.

life stress: stressful events that are part of life but occur rarely—e.g., bereavement, divorce, severe financial loss, severe illness in a family member, serious accident, etc.

Manning criteria: early symptom criteria for the irritable bowel syndrome developed in the late 1970s.

manometric: refers to pressure measurements (in this context, within the gut lumen).

marker test: test of whole-gut transit time. Ingested small radiopaque markers are followed through the gastrointestinal tract.

mask: See blinding.

mechanical obstruction: any physical obstacle to the caudal movement of intestinal contents, including tumors, scar tissue, or volvulus (twisting). Mechanical obstruction is distinguished from a functional obstruction, which is due to absent or abnormal contractions of the intestine.

meteorism: archaic. Flatulent dyspepsia with gas in the alimentary canal.

migrating motor complex (MMC): an organized, distinct, cyclically recurring and distally propagating sequence of contractile activity occurring in the small intestine during the fasting state; it may be associated with similar activities in the stomach and proximal colon.

morning rush syndrome: urgent diarrhea upon arising.

motility: movements within the intestinal tract, encompassing the phenomena of contractile activity, myoelectrical activity, tone, compliance, wall tension, and transit within the gastrointestinal tract.

motor neuron: a nerve cell that sends an axon to a muscle or, by extension, any effector.

Mueller maneuver: deep inspiration against a closed glottis.

myenteric plexus: ganglionated plexus of the enteric nervous system situated between the longitudinal and circular muscle coats of the muscularis externa of the digestive tract. Also called Auerbach's plexus.

myogenic: originating in muscle tissue.

myopathic pseudoobstruction: pathologic failure of propulsion in the gastrointestinal tract related to muscular degeneration and weakened contractility.

nausea: queasiness or sick sensation; a feeling of the need to vomit.

neural networks: aggregates of interconnected neurons that produce a range of behaviors associated with the central and enteric nervous systems.

neurogastroenterology: a subdiscipline of gastroenterology that encompasses all basic and clinical aspects of nervous system involvement in normal and disordered digestive functions and sensations.

neurogenic inflammation: inflammation initiated by activity in sensory nerves and the release of substance P.

neuropathic pseudoobstruction: pathologic failure of propulsion in the gastrointestinal tract related to enteric neuropathy and loss of nervous control mechanisms.

neuropil: a tangle of fine nerve fibers (dendrites and arborizations of axons) and their endings.

neurotransmitter: substance released from nerve cells at synapses that amounts to a chemical signal from one neuron to another or from motor neurons to effectors.

neuroticism: a personality trait characterized by a predisposition to experience anxiety, depression, anger, and a sense of hopelessness and helplessness about the future (negative affect).

nitric oxide: a putative inhibitory neurotransmitter released by enteric motor neurons to gastrointestinal muscles.

nociception: experience of a stimulus as harmful, in contrast to a pleasant sensation.

nodose ganglion: location of cell bodies of vagal afferent neurons.

nonpatients: for the purpose of this publication, those who have never sought health care for their functional gastrointestinal disorder.

nonspecific thalamocortical projection: a sensory pathway from the periphery to the cerebral cortex that involves multiple synaptic connections in the brain stem and thalamus.

nucleus ambiguous: located in the medulla oblongata (brain stem) of cell bodies of vagal efferent (motor) fibers to the esophagus.

nucleus rapine obscurus: a group of neurons in the brain stem that send projections to form synapses with neurons in the dorsal vagal complex.

nucleus tractus solitarius: located in medulla oblongata, contains cell bodies of second-order neurons in vagal afferent sensory pathway.

obsessive-compulsive disorder: an anxiety disorder characterized by recurrent, intrusive thoughts and compulsive, stereotyped repetitive behaviors or cognitions.

'on-demand' treatment: period of treatment in which the patient initiated therapy during a period when symptoms are present.

pain: a subjective, unpleasant sensation; some patients may feel that tissue damage is occurring. Other symptoms may be extremely bothersome without being interpreted by the patient as pain. By questioning the patient, pain should be distinguished from discomfort.

pain-prone personality: constellation of personality features, including personality disorders, exhibited by patients whose lives are dominated by pain. Common characteristics include childhood abuse or deprivation, a history of pain-related surgeries, care-seeking from multiple physicians, and disappointment with therapeutic results.

pancreatic sphincter of Oddi dysfunction: motility abnormalities of the sphincter of Oddi of the pancreatic duct.

paradoxic sphincter contraction: contraction of the external anal sphincter and/or the puborectalis muscle upon straining, impeding stool passage. Causes are painful anal disorders (fissures, perianal thrombosis, abscess) or pelvic floor dyssynergia.

paraneoplastic syndrome: neuropathic degeneration of autonomic neurons resulting from autoimmune attack in patients with small cell carcinoma of the lung.

parasympathetic system: division of the autonomic nervous system with its outflow from the central nervous system in certain cranial nerves and sacral nerves respectively and having its ganglia in or near the innervated viscera.

patients: (in this publication) people with symptoms of functional gastrointestinal disorders (FGIDs) who have ever sought health care for them.

pattern generator: interneuronal neural networks that generate rhythmic or repetitive behavior patterns of effector system behavior.

pelvic pain: a term used by gynecologists to describe pain in the lower abdomen. It is not clear where the pelvis begins and the abdomen begins. For clarity, and to avoid suggesting etiology, "lower abdominal pain" is preferred.

pelvic tension myalgia: synonym for levator ani syndrome.

perikaryon: the cell body of a neuron containing the nucleus.

personality disorder: an enduring pattern of inner experience and behavior that deviates markedly from the expectations of the individual's culture. It is persistent, starts in adolescence, is stable over time, and is not amenable to psychiatric treatment.

phasic contraction: a contraction that is not long maintained (transitory), in contrast to a tonic contraction.

phobia: An anxiety disorder characterized by (a) persistent fear of a specific situation out of proportion to the reality of the danger, (b) compelling desire to avoid and escape the situation, (c) recognition that fear is unreasonably excessive. It is not due to any other disorder.

physician-patient relationship (physician-patient interaction): ideally understood in terms of interpersonal behaviors that enhance or diminish mutual communication, satisfaction, and trust. In particular, physician behaviors may enhance or diminish mutual communication, satisfaction, and trust. Positive physician behaviors are characterized by empathy, respect, and positive regard.

placebo: pill, injection, sham incision or other harmless and ineffective treatment. Used in the past as a treatment to "harmlessly" please the patient, now the designation of a control treatment in a randomized clinical trial.

placebo effect: in randomized clinical trials, the difference in outcome between a placebo-treated group and an untreated group in an unbiased experiment. In clinical practice, change in a patient's illness attributable to the symbolic import of the treatment rather than a specific pharmacologic or physiologic property.

placebo response: response to a treatment that is the sum of the placebo effect, natural history of the disease being tested, parallel treatments, and time-dependent factors such as regression to the mean.

postprandial: after meals.

power propulsion: an intestinal motility pattern associated with defense and pathologic conditions. Rapid propulsion of luminal contents over extended lengths of intestine.

presynaptic inhibitory receptors: receptors on axons that suppress the release of neurotransmitters at neural synapses and neuro-effector junctions.

prevalent cases: Those who have ever sought health care for their FGID. (Incidence and prevalence are only meaningful when referring to population-based studies.)

problem-based coping: a method in which the individual tries to deal directly with situational stressors by changing the stressor or oneself. (e.g., by seeking social support, reappraising the stressor, etc.). In general, problem-focused coping is used in situations appraised by patients to be changeable or adaptable, and is an appropriate coping method for chronic illness.

proctalgia fugax: fleeting (only a few minutes in duration) pains in the rectum or anal canal, in the absence of known organic etiology.

progressive muscle relaxation: voluntary relaxation through systematically tensing and relaxing different muscle groups while attending to the sensations associated with tension and relaxation.

prokinetic: drug that acts on enteric nerve endings to enhance propulsion of contents through the gut. May act by direct muscle stimulation, release of motor neurotransmitters or blockade of inhibitory neurotransmitters.

pseudodiarrhea: frequent and/or urgent defecations with stools of normal form and even with firm/lumpy stools.

pseudoobstruction: pathologic failure of propulsion in the gastrointestinal tract in the absence of mechanical obstruction.

psychiatric diagnosis: a diagnosis of one of the psychiatric disorders. Now standardized in the Diagnostic and Standardized Manual of Mental Disorders, 4th edition (DSM IV) and World Health Organization (WHO) International Classification of Diseases.

psychodynamic therapy: the application of psychological theories derived from the works of Freud and others. The theories base current problems on past difficulties in relationships, especially with parents.

psychological distress: symptoms of anxiety or depression not amounting to anxiety or depressive disorders.

psychological state: a temporary or changeable phenomenon, for example, anxiety.

psychological traits: personality characteristics or an internal predisposition to respond in a particular way.

psychologist: specialist with a degree in one or more branches of psychology, who is licensed to practice and/or certified to teach in one of these specialties.

psychological: pertaining to psychology and any/all of its manifestations. Psychology is that branch of science which deals with the mind and mental processes, especially in relationship to human and animal behavior.

psychoneuroendocrinology: the study of the interrelationship between environmental stress and neuroendocrine functions.

psychoneuroimmunology: the study of the influence of environmental stress on immune cellular function and susceptibility to disease.

psychopharmacology: the study of drugs to treat symptoms of psychiatric disease.

psychophysiology: the study of the interactions between psychological factors (e.g., anxiety, stress) and physiological factors (e.g., muscle tension, cardiovascular arousal).

psychosocial: psychological and social difficulties (which often occur together).

psychosomatic: medical diseases believed to be caused by a pre-existent biologic susceptibility and disease-specific psychological characteristics.

psychotherapist: an individual who engages in behavioral treatment of emotional distress, using various modalities, including hypnosis and relaxation training as well as traditional talk therapy.

puborectalis muscle: a sling muscle that anchors to the symphysis pubis anteriorly and loops around the rectum to form the anorectal angle. This muscle is important to continence for stool.

pudendal nerve terminal motor latency: time between electrical stimulation of pudendal nerve with electrodes on the tip of a gloved finger, and the contraction of the external anal sphincter. This is used as a measure of the integrity of the pudendal nerve.

pyrexia: fever.

pyriformis syndrome: synonym for levator ani syndrome.

pyrosis: heartburn.

quality of life: a person's perception that they are able to meet their needs in self-care, physical activities, work and social interactions, and psychological well-being.

radiograph: x-ray image.

receptor (membrane): membrane surface proteins with unique conformations for specific binding of chemical signal substances and triggering of changes in the cell's behavior.

rectal prolapse: protrusion of the mucosal lining of the rectum through the anus.

rectocele: weakness in the tissues surrounding the rectum which permits it to bulge abnormally. The most common rectocele is one affecting the rectovaginal septum in women.

reflex: a neuronal event occurring beyond volition. In neurophysiology, a relatively simple behavioral response of an effector produced by influx of sensory afferent impulses to a neural center and its reflection as efferent impulses back to the periphery to the effector (e.g., muscle). The neural center may consist of interneurons. The simplest reflex circuit consists only of sensory and motor neurons.

Rome criteria: lists of symptoms among which a specified minimum number allows a diagnosis of a functional gastrointestinal disorder.

rumination: a regurgitation of recently ingested food into the mouth with subsequent remastication and reswallowing or spitting out. The regurgitation is effortless, unassociated with abdominal discomfort, heartburn, or nausea, and sometimes seems to be a pleasurable experience.

scintigraphic techniques: the use of radioisotopes, either ingested with food or released from swallowed capsules, (in this case) to measure transit times through different regions of the gastrointestinal tract.

scybala: hard, round, lumpy stools.

scybalous: fecal material formed into small balls resembling the stools of a rabbit, sheep or deer.

secretomotor neuron: motor neurons in the submucous plexus, which innervate and evoke secretion from the intestinal glands.

self-esteem: a personality trait where an individual is able to evaluate his/her abilities, achievements, and value in society in a way that promotes confidence and personal satisfaction.

sensory neuron: a neuron that conducts impulses arising in a sense organ or at sensory nerve endings.

sensory receptor: a cell or part of a cell specialized and normally functioning to convert environmental stimuli into nerve impulses or some response, which in turn evokes nerve impulses. Most sensory receptor cells are nerve cells, but some nonnervous cells can be receptors (e.g., intestinal enteroendocrine cells). One method of classifying receptors is by the form of adequate stimulus. Chemoreceptors, osmoreceptors, mechanoreceptors are normally stimulated by chemicals, osmotic pressure differences, and mechanical events respectively.

silent nociceptor: an unresponsive afferent that becomes responsive to mechanical stimulation during inflammatory states.

slow wave: membrane electrical potential that waxes and wanes in a rhythmic fashion. The slow wave determines the timing of a contraction but is not enough to produce a contraction in the absence of a burst of spike potentials triggered by the release of a neurotransmitter.

somatization: the behavior of reporting physical symptoms that are not associated with any known pathophysiological process, or that are excessive when compared to known pathophysiology.

specific thalamocortical projection: a sensory pathway from the periphery to the cerebral cortex that involves only two synaptic connections.

sphincter of Oddi dysfunction: unexplained motility abnormalities of the sphincter of Oddi not explained by an identifiable cause.

sphincter of Oddi dyskinesia: functional abnormalities of the sphincter of Oddi presenting at manometry as reversible elevated basal pressure or abnormal phasic contractions.

sphincter of Oddi stenosis: structural abnormality (scarring) of the sphincter of Oddi presenting as elevated basal pressure that does not decrease after administrating a smooth muscle relaxant.

stethoscope sign: abdominal tenderness on palpation that is not evident when similar pressure is applied during auscultation with a stethoscope, suggesting a functional source.

stool withholding: most common cause of functional constipation in children, a condition in which a child attempts to delay the act of defecation by contracting the pelvic floor and the gluteal muscle after having experienced a painful or frightening defecation.

stress: may be environmental stress or the feeling of being stressed. Also, any external or internal stimulus or sequence of stimuli that tend to disrupt homeostasis. Stress becomes an injury resulting in disease when mechanisms of homeostatic adjustment fail.

submucous plexus: a ganglionated plexus of the enteric nervous system situated between the mucosa and circular muscle coat of the small and large intestine. Consists of an inner ganglionated plexus called Meissner's plexus and an outer ganglionated plexus called Schabadasch's plexus.

sympathetic: division of the autonomic nervous system with its outflow from the central nervous system in the thoracolumbar segments of the spinal cord and having its ganglia in a pair of chains on either side of the spinal cord and in a grouping of three (celiac, superior and inferior mesenteric) in the abdomen.

synapse: a functional (noncytoplasmic) connection between neurons consisting of a presynaptic site of chemical transmitter release and a postsynaptic site of action of the released transmitter.

synthase: an enzyme that catalyzes synthesis of neurotransmitters in the enteric nervous system.

thyrotropin-releasing hormone: a hormone in the hypothalamic-pituitary axis that also functions as a neurotransmitter at synapses in the dorsal vagal complex in the brain stem.

toddler's diarrhea: common pediatric condition in which an otherwise healthy toddler or school-age child passes several poorly formed stools daily. It is also referred to as "functional diarrhea" or "chronic nonspecific diarrhea" of childhood.

tonic contraction: a degree of tension, firmness, or maintained contraction in a muscle, in contrast to a phasic contraction.

transit time: the time taken for food or other material to traverse a specified region of the gut.

unspecified functional bowel disorder: functional bowel symptoms that do not meet criteria for the previously defined categories.

vago-vagal reflex: a reflex for which both afferent and efferent fibers are contained in the vagus nerves.

vasoactive intestinal peptide: a putative inhibitory neurotransmitter released by enteric musculomotor neurons to gastrointestinal muscles. A putative excitatory neurotransmitter released by enteric secretomotor neurons; it stimulates mucosal secretion of H_2O, electrolytes, and mucus.

visceral hyperalgesia: gut hypersensitivity. The appreciation or exaggeration of gut symptoms with stimuli (such as balloon distension of the gut) that would ordinarily not be noticed or considered noxious.

viscoelastic: compliance of a hollow visceral organ (when used in gastroenterology).

visceral hypersensitivity: gut hypersensitivity. A condition in which the individual response to visceral afferent signals are amplified or increased. The appreciation as unpleasant of gut symptoms elicited by stimuli (such as balloon distension of the gut) that would ordinarily not be noticed or considered noxious.

wall tension: the force acting on the gut wall resulting from the interaction between intraluminal content and the reaction of the muscular and elastic properties of the wall.

whole-gut transit time: time required for transit from mouth to anus.

wind: a colloquial term in the UK, like gas in North America, for flatus.

Rome III Diagnostic Criteria for Functional Gastrointestinal Disorders

A. Functional Esophageal Disorders

A1. Functional Heartburn

Diagnostic criteria   Must include **all** of the following:*

1. Burning retrosternal discomfort or pain
2. Absence of evidence that gastroesophageal acid reflux is the cause of the symptom
3. Absence of histopathology-based esophageal motility disorders

* Criteria fulfilled for the last 3 months with symptom onset
   at least 6 months prior to diagnosis

A2. Functional Chest Pain of Presumed Esophageal Origin

Diagnostic criteria   Must include **all** of the following:*

1. Midline chest pain or discomfort that is not of burning quality
2. Absence of evidence that gastroesophageal reflux is the cause of the symptom
3. Absence of histopathology-based esophageal motility disorders

* Criteria fulfilled for the last 3 months with symptom onset
   at least 6 months prior to diagnosis

A3. Functional Dysphagia

Diagnostic criteria   Must include **all** of the following:*

1. Sense of solid and/or liquid foods sticking, lodging, or passing abnormally through the esophagus
2. Absence of evidence that gastroesophageal reflux is the cause of the symptom
3. Absence of histopathology-based esophageal motility disorders

* Criteria fulfilled for the last 3 months with symptom onset
   at least 6 months prior to diagnosis

A4. Globus

Diagnostic criteria   Must include **all** of the following:*

1. Persistent or intermittent, nonpainful sensation of a lump or foreign body in the throat
2. Occurrence of the sensation between meals
3. Absence of dysphagia or odynophagia
4. Absence of evidence that gastroesophageal reflux is the cause of the symptom
5. Absence of histopathology-based esophageal motility disorders

* Criteria fulfilled for the last 3 months with symptom onset
   at least 6 months prior to diagnosis

B. Functional Gastroduodenal Disorders

B1. FUNCTIONAL DYSPEPSIA

Diagnostic criteria*   *Must include:*

1. *One or more* of the following:
    a. Bothersome postprandial fullness
    b. Early satiation
    c. Epigastric pain
    d. Epigastric burning

AND

2. No evidence of structural disease (including at upper endoscopy) that is likely to explain the symptoms

* Criteria fulfilled for the last 3 months with symptom onset
  at least 6 months prior to diagnosis

B1a. Postprandial Distress Syndrome

Diagnostic criteria*   *Must include **one or both** of the following:*

1. Bothersome postprandial fullness, occurring after ordinary-sized meals, at least several times per week
2. Early satiation that prevents finishing a regular meal, at least several times per week

* Criteria fulfilled for the last 3 months with symptom onset
  at least 6 months prior to diagnosis

Supportive criteria

1. Upper abdominal bloating or postprandial nausea or excessive belching can be present
2. Epigastric pain syndrome may coexist

B1b. Epigastric Pain Syndrome

Diagnostic criteria*   *Must include **all** of the following:*

1. Pain or burning localized to the epigastrium of at least moderate severity, at least once per week
2. The pain is intermittent
3. Not generalized or localized to other abdominal or chest regions
4. Not relieved by defecation or passage of flatus
5. Not fulfilling criteria for gallbladder and sphincter of Oddi disorders

* Criteria fulfilled for the last 3 months with symptom onset
  at least 6 months prior to diagnosis

Supportive criteria

1. The pain may be of a burning quality, but without a retrosternal component
2. The pain is commonly induced or relieved by ingestion of a meal, but may occur while fasting
3. Postprandial distress syndrome may coexist

B2. BELCHING DISORDERS

B2a. Aerophagia

Diagnostic criteria   Must include **all** of the following:*

1. Troublesome repetitive belching at least several times a week
2. Air swallowing that is objectively observed or measured

* Criteria fulfilled for the last 3 months with symptom
onset at least 6 months prior to diagnosis

B2b. Unspecified Excessive Belching

Diagnostic criteria   Must include **all** of the following:*

1. Troublesome repetitive belching at least several times a week
2. No evidence that excessive air swallowing underlies the symptom

* Criteria fulfilled for the last 3 months with symptom onset
at least 6 months prior to diagnosis

B3. NAUSEA AND VOMITING DISORDERS

B3a. Chronic Idiopathic Nausea

Diagnostic criteria   Must include **all** of the following:*

1. Bothersome nausea occurring at least several times per week
2. Not usually associated with vomiting
3. Absence of abnormalities at upper endoscopy or metabolic disease
   that explains the nausea

* Criteria fulfilled for the last 3 months with symptom onset
at least 6 months prior to diagnosis

B3b. Functional Vomiting

Diagnostic criteria   Must include **all** of the following:*

1. On average one or more episodes of vomiting per week
2. Absence of criteria for an eating disorder, rumination, or major
   psychiatric disease according to DSM-IV
3. Absence of self-induced vomiting and chronic cannabinoid use and
   absence of abnormalities in the central nervous system or metabolic
   diseases to explain the recurrent vomiting

* Criteria fulfilled for the last 3 months with symptom onset
at least 6 months prior to diagnosis

B3c. Cyclic Vomiting Syndrome

*Diagnostic criteria   Must include **all** of the following:*

1. Stereotypical episodes of vomiting regarding onset (acute) and duration (less than one week)
2. Three or more discrete episodes in the prior year
3. Absence of nausea and vomiting between episodes

Supportive criterion

History or family history of migraine headaches

B4. Rumination Syndrome in Adults

*Diagnostic criteria   Must include **both** of the following:*

1. Persistent or recurrent regurgitation of recently ingested food into the mouth with subsequent spitting or remastication and swallowing
2. Regurgitation is not preceded by retching

Supportive criteria

1. Regurgitation events are usually not preceded by nausea
2. Cessation of the process when the regurgitated material becomes acidic
3. Regurgitant contains recognizable food with a pleasant taste

C. Functional Bowel Disorders

C1. Irritable Bowel Syndrome

Diagnostic criterion*

Recurrent abdominal pain or discomfort** at least 3 days/month in the last 3 months associated with *two or more* of the following:

1. Improvement with defecation
2. Onset associated with a change in frequency of stool
3. Onset associated with a change in form (appearance) of stool

* Criterion fulfilled for the last 3 months with symptom onset
  at least 6 months prior to diagnosis

** "Discomfort" means an uncomfortable sensation not described as pain.

In pathophysiology research and clinical trials, a pain/discomfort frequency of at least 2 days a week during screening evaluation is recommended for subject eligibility.

C2. Functional Bloating

Diagnostic criteria*   Must include **both** of the following:*

1. Recurrent feeling of bloating or visible distension at least 3 days/month in the last 3 months
2. Insufficient criteria for a diagnosis of functional dyspepsia, irritable bowel syndrome, or other functional GI disorder

* Criteria fulfilled for the last 3 months with symptom onset
  at least 6 months prior to diagnosis

C3. Functional Constipation

Diagnostic criteria*

1. Must include *two or more* of the following:
   a. Straining during at least 25% of defecations
   b. Lumpy or hard stools in at least 25% of defecations
   c. Sensation of incomplete evacuation for at least 25% of defecations
   d. Sensation of anorectal obstruction/blockage for at least 25% of defecations
   e. Manual maneuvers to facilitate at least 25% of defecations (e.g., digital evacuation, support of the pelvic floor)
   f. Fewer than three defecations per week
2. Loose stools are rarely present without the use of laxatives
3. Insufficient criteria for irritable bowel syndrome

* Criteria fulfilled for the last 3 months with symptom onset
   at least 6 months prior to diagnosis

C4. Functional Diarrhea

Diagnostic criterion*

Loose (mushy) or watery stools without pain occurring in at least 75% of stools

* Criterion fulfilled for the last 3 months with symptom onset
   at least 6 months prior to diagnosis

C5. Unspecified Functional Bowel Disorder

Diagnostic criterion*

Bowel symptoms not attributable to an organic etiology that do not meet criteria for the previously defined categories

* Criterion fulfilled for the last 3 months with symptom onset
   at least 6 months prior to diagnosis

D. Functional Abdominal Pain Syndrome

D. Functional Abdominal Pain Syndrome

Diagnostic criteria*   *Must include **all** of the following:*

1. Continuous or nearly continuous abdominal pain
2. No or only occasional relationship of pain with physiological events (e.g., eating, defecation, or menses)
3. Some loss of daily functioning
4. The pain is not feigned (e.g., malingering)
5. Insufficient symptoms to meet criteria for another functional gastrointestinal disorder that would explain the pain

* Criteria fulfilled for the last 3 months with symptom onset
   at least 6 months prior to diagnosis

E. Functional Gallbladder and Sphincter of Oddi Disorders

E. Functional Gallbladder and Sphincter of Oddi Disorders

*Diagnostic criteria   Must include episodes of pain located in the epigastrium and/or right upper quadrant and **all** of the following:*

1. Episodes lasting 30 minutes or longer
2. Recurrent symptoms occurring at different intervals (not daily)
3. The pain builds up to a steady level
4. The pain is moderate to severe enough to interrupt the patient's daily activities or lead to an emergency department visit
5. The pain is not relieved by bowel movements
6. The pain is not relieved by postural change
7. The pain is not relieved by antacids
8. Exclusion of other structural disease that would explain the symptoms

Supportive criteria

The pain may present with one or more of the following:

1. Associated with nausea and vomiting
2. Radiates to the back and/or right infra subscapular region
3. Awakens from sleep in the middle of the night

E1. Functional Gallbladder Disorder

*Diagnostic criteria   Must include **all** of the following:*

1. Criteria for functional gallbladder and sphincter of Oddi disorder
2. Gallbladder is present
3. Normal liver enzymes, conjugated bilirubin, and amylase/lipase

E2. Functional Biliary Sphincter of Oddi Disorder

*Diagnostic criteria   Must include **both** of the following:*

1. Criteria for functional gallbladder and sphincter of Oddi disorder
2. Normal amylase/lipase

Supportive criterion

Elevated serum transaminases, alkaline phosphatase, or conjugated bilirubin temporarily related to at least two pain episodes

E3. Functional Pancreatic Sphincter of Oddi Disorder

*Diagnostic criteria   Must include **both** of the following:*

1. Criteria for functional gallbladder and sphincter of Oddi disorder and
2. Elevated amylase/lipase

F. Functional Anorectal Disorders

F1. Functional Fecal Incontinence

Diagnostic criteria*

1. Recurrent uncontrolled passage of fecal material in an individual with a developmental age of at least 4 years and *one or more* of the following:
   a. Abnormal functioning of normally innervated and structurally intact muscles
   b. Minor abnormalities of sphincter structure and/or innervation
   c. Normal or disordered bowel habits, (i.e., fecal retention or diarrhea)
   d. Psychological causes

AND

2. Exclusion of *all* the following:
   a. Abnormal innervation caused by lesion(s) within the brain (e.g., dementia), spinal cord, or sacral nerve roots, or mixed lesions (e.g., multiple sclerosis), or as part of a generalized peripheral or autonomic neuropathy (e.g., due to diabetes)
   b. Anal sphincter abnormalities associated with a multisystem disease (e.g., scleroderma)
   c. Structural or neurogenic abnormalities believed to be the major or primary cause of fecal incontinence

* Criteria fulfilled for the last 3 months

F2. FUNCTIONAL ANORECTAL PAIN

F2a. Chronic Proctalgia

Diagnostic criteria Must include **all** of the following:*

1. Chronic or recurrent rectal pain or aching
2. Episodes last 20 minutes or longer
3. Exclusion of other causes of rectal pain such as ischemia, inflammatory bowel disease, cryptitis, intramuscular abscess, anal fissure, hemorrhoids, prostatitis, and coccygodynia

* Criteria fulfilled for the last 3 months with symptom onset
at least 6 months prior to diagnosis

*Chronic proctalgia may be further characterized into levator ani syndrome
or unspecified anorectal pain based on digital rectal examination.*

F2a.1. Levator Ani Syndrome

Diagnostic criterion
Symptom criteria for chronic proctalgia and tenderness during posterior traction on the puborectalis

F2a.2. Unspecified Functional Anorectal Pain

Diagnostic criterion

Symptom criteria for chronic proctalgia but no tenderness during posterior traction on the puborectalis

F2b. Proctalgia Fugax

*Diagnostic criteria   Must include **all** of the following:*
1. Recurrent episodes of pain localized to the anus or lower rectum
2. Episodes last from seconds to minutes
3. There is no anorectal pain between episodes

For research purposes criteria must be fulfilled for 3 months;
however, clinical diagnosis and evaluation may be made prior to 3 months.

F3. Functional Defecation Disorders

Diagnostic criteria*
1. The patient must satisfy diagnostic criteria for functional constipation**
2. During repeated attempts to defecate must have *at least two* of the following:
   a. Evidence of impaired evacuation, based on balloon expulsion test or imaging
   b. Inappropriate contraction of the pelvic floor muscles (i.e., anal sphincter or puborectalis) or less than 20% relaxation of basal resting sphincter pressure by manometry, imaging, or EMG
   c. Inadequate propulsive forces assessed by manometry or imaging

* Criteria fulfilled for the last 3 months with symptom onset
  at least 6 months prior to diagnosis

** **Diagnostic criteria for functional constipation:**
(1) **Must include *two or more* of the following:** (a) Straining during at least 25% of defecations, (b) Lumpy or hard stools in at least 25% of defecations, (c) Sensation of incomplete evacuation for at least 25% of defecations, (d) Sensation of anorectal obstruction/blockage for at least 25% of defecations, (e) Manual maneuvers to facilitate at least 25% of defecations (e.g., digital evacuation, support of the pelvic floor), (f) Fewer than three defecations per week.
(2) **Loose stools are rarely present without the use of laxatives.**
(3) **Insufficient criteria for irritable bowel syndrome.**

F3a. Dyssynergic Defecation

Diagnostic criterion

Inappropriate contraction of the pelvic floor or less than 20% relaxation of basal resting sphincter pressure with adequate propulsive forces during attempted defecation

F3b. Inadequate Defecatory Propulsion

Diagnostic criterion

Inadequate propulsive forces with or without inappropriate contraction or less than 20% relaxation of the anal sphincter during attempted defecation

G. Childhood Functional GI Disorders: Infant/Toddler

G1. Infant Regurgitation

*Diagnostic criteria   Must include **both** of the following in otherwise healthy infants 3 weeks to 12 months of age:*

1. Regurgitation two or more times per day for 3 or more weeks
2. No retching, hematemesis, aspiration, apnea, failure to thrive, feeding or swallowing difficulties, or abnormal posturing

G2. Infant Rumination Syndrome

*Diagnostic criteria   Must include **all** of the following for at least 3 months:*

1. Repetitive contractions of the abdominal muscles, diaphragm, and tongue
2. Regurgitation of gastric content into the mouth, which is either expectorated or rechewed and reswallowed
3. Three or more of the following:
   a. Onset between 3 and 8 months
   b. Does not respond to management for gastroesophageal reflux disease, or to anticholinergic drugs, hand restraints, formula changes, and gavage or gastrostomy feedings
   c. Unaccompanied by signs of nausea or distress
   d. Does not occur during sleep and when the infant is interacting with individuals in the environment

G3. Cyclic Vomiting Syndrome

*Diagnostic criteria   Must include **both** of the following:*

1. Two or more periods of intense nausea and unremitting vomiting or retching lasting hours to days
2. Return to usual state of health lasting weeks to months

G4. Infant Colic

*Diagnostic criteria   Must include **all** of the following in infants from birth to 4 months of age:*

1. Paroxysms of irritability, fussing or crying that starts and stops without obvious cause
2. Episodes lasting 3 or more hours/day and occurring at least 3 days/wk for at least 1 week
3. No failure to thrive

G5. Functional Diarrhea

*Diagnostic criteria   Must include **all** of the following:*

1. Daily painless, recurrent passage of three or more large, unformed stools
2. Symptoms that last more than 4 weeks
3. Onset of symptoms that begins between 6 and 36 months of age
4. Passage of stools that occurs during waking hours
5. There is no failure-to-thrive if caloric intake is adequate

G6. Infant Dyschezia

*Diagnostic criteria   Must include **both** of the following in an infant less than 6 months of age*

1. At least 10 minutes of straining and crying before successful passage of soft stools
2. No other health problems

G7. Functional Constipation

*Diagnostic criteria   Must include one month of **at least two** of the following in infants up to 4 years of age:*

1. Two or fewer defecations per week
2. At least one episode/week of incontinence after the acquisition of toileting skills
3. History of excessive stool retention
4. History of painful or hard bowel movements
5. Presence of a large fecal mass in the rectum
6. History of large diameter stools which may obstruct the toilet

Accompanying symptoms may include irritability, decreased appetite, and/or early satiety. The accompanying symptoms disappear immediately following passage of a large stool.

H. Childhood Functional GI Disorders: Child/Adolescent

H1. VOMITING AND AEROPHAGIA

H1a. Adolescent Rumination Syndrome

Diagnostic criteria   Must include **all** of the following:*

1. Repeated painless regurgitation and rechewing or expulsion of food that
    a. begin soon after ingestion of a meal
    b. do not occur during sleep
    c. do not respond to standard treatment for gastroesophageal reflux
2. No retching
3. No evidence of an inflammatory, anatomic, metabolic, or neoplastic process that explains the subject's symptoms

* Criteria fulfilled for the last 3 months with symptom onset at least 6 months prior to diagnosis

H1b. Cyclic Vomiting Syndrome

*Diagnostic criteria   Must include **both** of the following:*

1. Two or more periods of intense nausea and unremitting vomiting or retching lasting hours to days
2. Return to usual state of health lasting weeks to months

H1c. Aerophagia

Diagnostic criteria   Must include **at least two** of the following:*

1. Air swallowing
2. Abdominal distention due to intraluminal air
3. Repetitive belching and/or increased flatus

* Criteria fulfilled at least once per week for at least 2 months prior to diagnosis

H2. ABDOMINAL PAIN-RELATED FUNCTIONAL GI DISORDERS

H2a. Functional Dyspepsia

Diagnostic criteria   Must include **all** of the following:*

1. Persistent or recurrent pain or discomfort centered in the upper abdomen (above the umbilicus)
2. Not relieved by defecation or associated with the onset of a change in stool frequency or stool form (i.e., not irritable bowel syndrome)
3. No evidence of an inflammatory, anatomic, metabolic or neoplastic process that explains the subject's symptoms

* Criteria fulfilled at least once per week for at least 2 months prior to diagnosis

H2b. Irritable Bowel Syndrome

Diagnostic criteria   Must include **both** of the following:*

1. Abdominal discomfort** or pain associated with *two or more* of the following at least 25% of the time:
    a. Improvement with defecation
    b. Onset associated with a change in frequency of stool
    c. Onset associated with a change in form (appearance) of stool
2. No evidence of an inflammatory, anatomic, metabolic, or neoplastic process that explains the subject's symptoms

* Criteria fulfilled at least once per week for at least 2 months prior to diagnosis

** "Discomfort" means an uncomfortable sensation not described as pain.

H2c. Abdominal Migraine

Diagnostic criteria   Must include **all** of the following:*

1. Paroxysmal episodes of intense, acute periumbilical pain that lasts for 1 hour or more
2. Intervening periods of usual health lasting weeks to months
3. The pain interferes with normal activities
4. The pain is associated with 2 of the following:
    a. Anorexia
    b. Nausea
    c. Vomiting
    d. Headache
    e. Photophobia
    f. Pallor
5. No evidence of an inflammatory, anatomic, metabolic, or neoplastic process considered that explains the subject's symptoms

* Criteria fulfilled two or more times in the preceding 12 months

H2d. Childhood Functional Abdominal Pain

Diagnostic criteria   Must include **all** of the following:*

1. Episodic or continuous abdominal pain
2. Insufficient criteria for other FGIDs
3. No evidence of an inflammatory, anatomic, metabolic, or neoplastic process that explains the subject's symptoms

* Criteria fulfilled at least once per week for at least 2 months prior to diagnosis

H2d1. Childhood Functional Abdominal Pain Syndrome

Diagnostic criteria   Must satisfy criteria for childhood functional abdominal pain and have at least 25% of the time **one or more** of the following:*

1. Some loss of daily functioning
2. Additional somatic symptoms such as headache, limb pain, or difficulty sleeping

* Criteria fulfilled at least once per week for at least 2 months prior to diagnosis

H3. CONSTIPATION AND INCONTINENCE

H3a. Functional Constipation

Diagnostic criteria   Must include **two or more** of the following in a child with a developmental age of at least 4 years with insufficient criteria for diagnosis of IBS:*

1. Two or fewer defecations in the toilet per week
2. At least one episode of fecal incontinence per week
3. History of retentive posturing or excessive volitional stool retention
4. History of painful or hard bowel movements
5. Presence of a large fecal mass in the rectum
6. History of large diameter stools which may obstruct the toilet

* Criteria fulfilled at least once per week for at least 2 months prior to diagnosis

H3b. Nonretentive Fecal Incontinence

Diagnostic criteria   Must include **all** of the following in a child with a developmental age at least 4 years:*

1. Defecation into places inappropriate to the social context at least once per month
2. No evidence of an inflammatory, anatomic, metabolic, or neoplastic process that explains the subject's symptoms
3. No evidence of fecal retention

* Criteria fulfilled for at least 2 months prior to diagnosis

Comparison Table of Rome II & Rome III Adult Diagnostic Criteria

ROME III DIAGNOSTIC CRITERIA	ROME II DIAGNOSTIC CRITERIA
A. Functional Esophageal Disorders	*A. Functional Esophageal Disorders*
A1. Functional Heartburn *Diagnostic criteria** *Must include **all** of the following:* 1. Burning retrosternal discomfort or pain 2. Absence of evidence that gastroesophageal acid reflux is the cause of the symptom 3. Absence of histopathology-based esophageal motility disorders * Criteria fulfilled for the last 3 months with symptom onset at least 6 months prior to diagnosis	**A4. Functional Heartburn** *At least 12 weeks, which need not be consecutive, in the preceding 12 months of:* 1. Burning retrosternal discomfort or pain; and 2. Absence of pathologic gastroesophageal reflux, achalasia, or other motility disorder with a recognized pathologic basis.
A2. Functional Chest Pain of Presumed Esophageal Origin *Diagnostic criteria** *Must include **all** of the following:* 1. Midline chest pain or discomfort that is not of burning quality 2. Absence of evidence that gastroesophageal reflux is the cause of the symptom 3. Absence of histopathology-based esophageal motility disorders * Criteria fulfilled for the last 3 months with symptom onset at least 6 months prior to diagnosis	**A3. Functional Chest Pain of Presumed Esophageal Origin** *At least 12 weeks, which need not be consecutive, within the preceding 12 months of:* 1. Midline chest pain or discomfort that is not of burning quality; and 2. Absence of pathologic gastroesophageal reflux, achalasia, or other motility disorder with a recognized pathologic basis.

ROME III DIAGNOSTIC CRITERIA	ROME II DIAGNOSTIC CRITERIA
A3. Functional Dysphagia *Diagnostic criteria** *Must include **all** of the following:* 1. Sense of solid and/or liquid foods sticking, lodging, or passing abnormally through the esophagus 2. Absence of evidence that gastroesophageal reflux is the cause of the symptom 3. Absence of histopathology-based esophageal motility disorders * Criteria fulfilled for the last 3 months with symptom onset at least 6 months prior to diagnosis	**A5. Functional Dysphagia** *At least 12 weeks, which need not be consecutive, in the preceding 12 months of:* 1. Sense of solid and/or liquid foods sticking, lodging, or passing abnormally through the esophagus; and 2. Absence of pathologic gastroesophageal reflux, achalasia, or other motility disorder with a recognized pathologic basis.
A4. Globus *Diagnostic criteria** *Must include **all** of the following:* 1. Persistent or intermittent, nonpainful sensation of a lump or foreign body in the throat 2. Occurrence of the sensation between meals 3. Absence of dysphagia or odynophagia 4. Absence of evidence that gastroesophageal reflux is the cause of the symptom 5. Absence of histopathology-based esophageal motility disorders * Criteria fulfilled for the last 3 months with symptom onset at least 6 months prior to diagnosis	**A1. Globus** *At least 12 weeks, which need not be consecutive, in the preceding 12 months of:* 1. The persistent or intermittent sensation of a lump or foreign body in the throat; 2. Occurrence of the sensation between meals; 3. Absence of dysphagia and odynophagia; and 4. Absence of pathologic gastroesophageal reflux, achalasia, or other motility disorder with a recognized pathologic basis (e.g., scleroderma of the esophagus).
Rome III criteria do not include unspecified functional esophageal disorder as in Rome II.	**A6. Unspecified Functional Esophageal Disorder** *At least 12 weeks, which need not be consecutive, in the preceding 12 months of:* 1. Unexplained symptoms attributed to the esophagus that do not fit into the previously described categories; *and* 2. Absence of pathologic gastroesophageal reflux, achalasia, or other motility disorder with a recognized pathologic basis.

ROME III DIAGNOSTIC CRITERIA	ROME II DIAGNOSTIC CRITERIA
B. Functional Gastroduodenal Disorders	*B. Functional Gastroduodenal Disorders*

Note major changes in classification for dyspepsia and nausea and vomiting disorders

B1. Functional Dyspepsia

Diagnostic criteria*
Must include:

1. *One or more* of the following:
   a. Bothersome postprandial fullness
   b. Early satiation
   c. Epigastric pain
   d. Epigastric burning
AND
2. No evidence of structural disease (including at upper endoscopy) that is likely to explain the symptoms

* Criteria fulfilled for the last 3 months with symptom onset at least 6 months prior to diagnosis

B1a. Postprandial Distress Syndrome

Diagnostic criteria*
Must include **one or both** *of the following:*

1. Bothersome postprandial fullness, occurring after ordinary-sized meals, at least several times per week
2. Early satiation that prevents finishing a regular meal, at least several times per week

* Criteria fulfilled for the last 3 months with symptom onset at least 6 months prior to diagnosis

Supportive criteria

1. Upper abdominal bloating or postprandial nausea or excessive belching can be present
2. Epigastric pain syndrome may coexist

B1. Functional Dyspepsia

At least 12 weeks, which need not be consecutive, in the preceding 12 months of:

1. Persistent or recurrent symptoms (pain or discomfort centered in the upper abdomen);
2. No evidence of organic disease (including at upper endoscopy) that is likely to explain the symptoms; *and*
3. No evidence that dyspepsia is exclusively relieved by defecation or associated with the onset of a change in stool frequency or stool form.

B1a. Ulcer-like dyspepsia
Pain centered in the upper abdomen is the predominant (most bothersome) symptom.

B1b. Dysmotility-like dyspepsia
An unpleasant or troublesome nonpainful sensation (discomfort) centered in the upper abdomen is the predominant symptom; this sensation may be characterized by or associated with upper abdominal fullness, early satiety, bloating, or nausea.

B1c. Unspecified (nonspecific) dyspepsia
Symptomatic patients whose symptoms do not fulfill the criteria for ulcer-like or dysmotility-like dyspepsia.

ROME III DIAGNOSTIC CRITERIA	ROME II DIAGNOSTIC CRITERIA
B1b. Epigastric Pain Syndrome *Diagnostic criteria** *Must include **all** of the following:* 1. Pain or burning localized to the epigastrium of at least moderate severity, at least once per week 2. The pain is intermittent 3. Not generalized or localized to other abdominal or chest regions 4. Not relieved by defecation or passage of flatus 5. Not fulfilling criteria for gallbladder and sphincter of Oddi disorders * Criteria fulfilled for the last 3 months with symptom onset at least 6 months prior to diagnosis *Supportive criteria* 1. The pain may be of a burning quality, but without a retrosternal component 2. The pain is commonly induced or relieved by ingestion of a meal, but may occur while fasting 3. Postprandial distress syndrome may coexist	

ROME III DIAGNOSTIC CRITERIA	ROME II DIAGNOSTIC CRITERIA
B2. Belching Disorders *B2a. Aerophagia* *Diagnostic criteria** *Must include **all** of the following:* 1. Troublesome repetitive belching at least several times a week 2. Air swallowing that is objectively observed or measured * Criteria fulfilled for the last 3 months with symptom onset at least 6 months prior to diagnosis *B2b. Unspecified Excessive Belching* *Diagnostic criteria** *Must include **all** of the following:* 1. Troublesome repetitive belching at least several times a week 2. No evidence that excessive air swallowing underlies the symptom * Criteria fulfilled for the last 3 months with symptom onset at least 6 months prior to diagnosis	**B2. Aerophagia** *At least 12 weeks, which need not be consecutive, or more in the preceding 12 months of:* 1. Air swallowing that is objectively observed; *and* 2. Troublesome repetitive belching.

ROME III DIAGNOSTIC CRITERIA	ROME II DIAGNOSTIC CRITERIA
B3. Nausea and Vomiting Disorders	
B3a. Chronic Idiopathic Nausea	
Diagnostic criteria* *Must include* **all** *of the following:*	
1. Bothersome nausea occurring at least several times per week 2. Not usually associated with vomiting 3. Absence of abnormalities at upper endoscopy or metabolic disease that explains the nausea	
* Criteria fulfilled for the last 3 months with symptom onset at least 6 months prior to diagnosis	
B3b. Functional Vomiting	**B3. Functional Vomiting**
Diagnostic criteria* *Must include* **all** *of the following:*	*At least 12 weeks, which need not be consecutive, in the preceding 12 months of:*
1. On average one or more episodes of vomiting per week 2. Absence of criteria for an eating disorder, rumination, or major psychiatric disease according to DSM-IV 3. Absence of self-induced vomiting and chronic cannabinoid use and absence of abnormalities in the central nervous system or metabolic diseases to explain the recurrent vomiting	1. Frequent episodes of vomiting, occurring on at least three separate days in a week over three months; 2. Absence of criteria for an eating disorder, rumination, or major psychiatric disease according to DSM-IV; 3. Absence of self-induced and medication-induced vomiting; *and* 4. Absence of abnormalities in the gut or central nervous system, and metabolic diseases to explain the recurrent vomiting.
* Criteria fulfilled for the last 3 months with symptom onset at least 6 months prior to diagnosis	

ROME III DIAGNOSTIC CRITERIA	ROME II DIAGNOSTIC CRITERIA
B3c. Cyclic Vomiting Syndrome *Diagnostic criteria* *Must include **all** of the following:* 1. Stereotypical episodes of vomiting regarding onset (acute) and duration (less than one week) 2. Three or more discrete episodes in the prior year 3. Absence of nausea and vomiting between episodes *Supportive criteria* History or family history of migraine headaches	
B4. Rumination Syndrome in Adults *Diagnostic criteria** *Must include **both** of the following:* 1. Persistent or recurrent regurgitation of recently ingested food into the mouth with subsequent spitting or remastication and swallowing 2. Regurgitation is not preceded by retching *Supportive criteria* 1. Regurgitation events are usually not preceded by nausea 2. Cessation of the process when the regurgitated material becomes acidic 3. Regurgitant contains recognizable food with a pleasant taste *The Rome III criteria classify rumination as a functional gastroduodenal disorder. In the Rome II classification, rumination was considered a functional esophageal disorder.*	**A2. Rumination Syndrome** *At least 12 weeks, which need not be consecutive, in the preceding 12 months of:* 1. Persistent or recurrent regurgitation of recently ingested food into the mouth with subsequent remastication and swallowing; 2. Absence of nausea and vomiting; 3. Cessation of the process when the regurgitated material becomes acidic; *and* 4. Absence of pathologic gastroesophageal reflux, achalasia, or other motility disorder with a recognized pathologic basis as the primary disorder.

ROME III DIAGNOSTIC CRITERIA	ROME II DIAGNOSTIC CRITERIA
C. Functional Bowel Disorders	*C. Functional Bowel Disorders*
C1. Irritable Bowel Syndrome *Diagnostic criterion** Recurrent abdominal pain or discomfort** at least 3 days/month in last 3 months associated with *two or more* of the following: 1. Improvement with defecation 2. Onset associated with a change in frequency of stool 3. Onset associated with a change in form (appearance) of stool * Criterion fulfilled for the last 3 months with symptom onset at least 6 months prior to diagnosis **"Discomfort" means an uncomfortable sensation not described as pain. In pathophysiology research and clinical trials, a pain/discomfort frequency of at least 2 days a week during the screening evaluation is recommended for subject eligibility.	**C1. Irritable Bowel Syndrome** *At least 12 weeks, which need not be consecutive, in the preceding 12 months of abdominal discomfort or pain that has two out of three features:* 1. Relieved with defecation; *and/or* 2. Onset associated with a change in frequency of stool; *and/or* 3. Onset associated with a change in form (appearance) of stool. *Symptoms that Cumulatively Support the Diagnosis of Irritable Bowel Syndrome* – Abnormal stool frequency (for research purposes "abnormal" may be defined as greater than 3 bowel movements per day and less than 3 bowel movements per week); – Abnormal stool form (lumpy/hard or loose/watery stool); – Abnormal stool passage (straining, urgency, or feeling of incomplete evacuation); – Passage of mucus; – Bloating or feeling of abdominal distension.
C2. Functional Bloating *Diagnostic criteria** *Must include **both** of the following:* 1. Recurrent feeling of bloating or visible distension at least 3 days/month in the last 3 months 2. Insufficient criteria for a diagnosis of functional dyspepsia, irritable bowel syndrome, or other functional GI disorder * Criteria fulfilled for the last 3 months with symptom onset at least 6 months prior to diagnosis	**C2. Functional Abdominal Bloating** *At least 12 weeks, which need not be consecutive, in the preceding 12 months of:* 1. Feeling of abdominal fullness, bloating, or visible distension; *and* 2. Insufficient criteria for a diagnosis of functional dyspepsia, irritable bowel syndrome, or other functional disorder.

ROME III DIAGNOSTIC CRITERIA	ROME II DIAGNOSTIC CRITERIA

C3. Functional Constipation
 	
*Diagnostic criteria**
 	
1. Must include *two or more* of the following:
  a. Straining during at least 25% of defecations
  b. Lumpy or hard stools in at least 25% of defecations
  c. Sensation of incomplete evacuation for at least 25% of defecations
  d. Sensation of anorectal obstruction/blockage for at least 25% of defecations
  e. Manual maneuvers to facilitate at least 25% of defecations (e.g., digital evacuation, support of the pelvic floor)
  f. Fewer than three defecations per week
2. Loose stools are rarely present without the use of laxatives
3. Insufficient criteria for irritable bowel syndrome
 	
 * Criteria fulfilled for the last 3 months with symptom onset at least 6 months prior to diagnosis
	C3. Functional Constipation
	
	At least 12 weeks, which need not be consecutive, in the preceding 12 months of two or more of:
	
	1. Straining > 1/4 of defecations;
	2. Lumpy or hard stools > 1/4 of defecations;
	3. Sensation of incomplete evacuation > 1/4 of defecations;
	4. Sensation of anorectal obstruction/blockage > 1/4 of defecations;
	5. Manual maneuvers to facilitate > 1/4 of defecations (e.g., digital evacuation, support of the pelvic floor); *and/or*
	6. < 3 defecations per week.
	
	 Loose stools are not present, and there are insufficient criteria for IBS.

C4. Functional Diarrhea *Diagnostic criterion** Loose (mushy) or watery stools without pain occurring in at least 75% of stools * Criterion fulfilled for the last 3 months with symptom onset at least 6 months prior to diagnosis	**C4. Functional Diarrhea** *At least 12 weeks, which need not be consecutive, in the preceding 12 months of:* 1. Loose (mushy) or watery stools 2. Present > 3/4 of the time; *and* 3. No abdominal pain.
C.5. Unspecified Functional Bowel Disorder *Diagnostic criterion** Bowel symptoms not attributable to an organic etiology that do not meet criteria for the previously defined categories * Criterion fulfilled for the last 3 months with symptom onset at least 6 months prior to diagnosis	**C5. Unspecified Functional Bowel Disorder** Bowel symptoms in the absence of organic disease that do not fit into the previously defined categories of functional bowel disorders.

ROME III DIAGNOSTIC CRITERIA	ROME II DIAGNOSTIC CRITERIA
D. Functional Abdominal Pain Syndrome	*D. Functional Abdominal Pain*
D. Functional Abdominal Pain Syndrome *Diagnostic criteria** *Must include **all** of the following:* 1. Continuous or nearly continuous abdominal pain 2. No or only occasional relationship of pain with physiological events (e.g., eating, defecation, or menses) 3. Some loss of daily functioning 4. The pain is not feigned (e.g., malingering) 5. Insufficient symptoms to meet criteria for another functional gastrointestinal disorder that would explain the pain * Criteria fulfilled for the last 3 months with symptom onset at least 6 months prior to diagnosis	**D1. Functional Abdominal Pain Syndrome** *At least 6 months of:* 1. Continuous or nearly continuous abdominal pain; *and* 2. No or only occasional relationship of pain with physiological events (e.g., eating, defecation, or menses); *and* 3. Some loss of daily functioning; *and* 4. The pain is not feigned (e.g., malingering), *and* 5. Insufficient criteria for other functional gastrointestinal disorders that would explain the abdominal pain.
The Rome III Criteria do not include Unspecified Functional Abdominal Pain	**D2. Unspecified Functional Abdominal Pain** This is functional abdominal pain that fails to reach criteria for functional abdominal pain syndrome.

ROME III DIAGNOSTIC CRITERIA	ROME II DIAGNOSTIC CRITERIA
E. Functional Gallbladder and Sphincter of Oddi Disorders	*E. Functional Disorders of the Biliary Tract and the Pancreas*

E. Functional Gallbladder and Sphincter of Oddi Disorders *Diagnostic criteria* *Must include episodes of pain located in the epigastrium and/or right upper quadrant and all of the following:* 1. Episodes lasting 30 minutes or longer 2. Recurrent symptoms occurring at different intervals (not daily) 3. The pain builds up to a steady level 4. The pain is moderate to severe enough to interrupt the patient's daily activities or lead to an emergency department visit 5. The pain is not relieved by bowel movements 6. The pain is not relieved by postural change 7. The pain is not relieved by antacids 8. Exclusion of other structural disease that would explain the symptoms *Supportive criteria* The pain may present with one or more of the following: 1. Associated with nausea and vomiting 2. Radiates to the back and/or right infra subscapular region 3. Awakens from sleep in the middle of the night ***E1. Functional Gallbladder Disorder*** *Diagnostic criteria* *Must include all of the following:* 1. Criteria for functional gallbladder and sphincter of Oddi disorder and 2. Gallbladder is present 3. Normal liver enzymes, conjugated bilirubin, and amylase/lipase	**E1. Gallbladder Dysfunction** *Episodes of severe steady pain located in the epigastrium and right upper quadrant, and all of the following:* 1. Symptom episodes last 30 minutes or more, with pain-free intervals; 2. Symptoms have occurred on one or more occasions in the previous 12 months; 3. The pain is steady and interrupts daily activities or requires consultation with a physician; 4. There is no evidence of structural abnormalities to explain the symptoms; 5. There is abnormal gallbladder functioning with regard to emptying. **E2. Sphincter of Oddi Dysfunction** *Episodes of severe steady pain located in the epigastrium and right upper quadrant, and all of the following:* 1. Symptom episodes last 30 minutes or more, with pain-free intervals; *and* 2. Symptoms have occurred on one or more occasions in the previous 12 months; *and* 3. The pain is steady and interrupts daily activities or requires consultation with a physician; *and* 6. There is no evidence of structural abnormalities to explain the symptoms.

ROME III DIAGNOSTIC CRITERIA	ROME II DIAGNOSTIC CRITERIA
E2. Functional Biliary Sphincter of Oddi Disorder	
Diagnostic criteria *Must include* **both** *of the following:*	
1. Criteria for functional sphincter of Oddi disorder 2. Normal amylase/lipase	
Supportive criterion	
Elevated serum transaminases, alkaline phosphatase, or conjugated bilirubin temporarily related to at least two pain episodes	
E3. Functional Pancreatic Sphincter of Oddi Disorder	
Diagnostic criteria *Must include* **both** *of the following:*	
1. Criteria for functional gallbladder and sphincter of Oddi Disorder and 2. Elevated amylase/lipase	

ROME III DIAGNOSTIC CRITERIA	ROME II DIAGNOSTIC CRITERIA
F. Functional Anorectal Disorders	*F. Functional Disorders of the Anus and Rectum*

FI. Functional Fecal Incontinence

Diagnostic criteria*

1. Recurrent uncontrolled passage of fecal material in an individual with a developmental age of at least 4 years and *one or more* of the following:
   a. Abnormal functioning of normally innervated and structurally intact muscles
   b. Minor abnormalities of sphincter structure and/or innervation
   c. Normal or disordered bowel habits, (i.e., fecal retention or diarrhea)
   d. Psychological causes

AND

2. Exclusion of *all* of the following:
   a. Abnormal innervation caused by lesion(s) within the brain (e.g., dementia), spinal cord, or sacral nerve roots, or mixed lesions (e.g., multiple sclerosis), or as part of a generalized peripheral or autonomic neuropathy (e.g., due to diabetes)
   b. Anal sphincter abnormalities associated with a multisystem disease (e.g. scleroderma)
   c. Structural or neurogenic abnormalities believed to be the major or primary cause of fecal incontinence.

* Criteria fulfilled for the last 3 months

FI. Functional Fecal Incontinence

Recurrent uncontrolled passage of fecal material for at least one month, in an individual with a developmental age of at least 4 years, associated with:

1. Fecal impaction; *or*
2. Diarrhea; *or*
3. Nonstructural anal sphincter dysfunction.

ROME III DIAGNOSTIC CRITERIA	ROME II DIAGNOSTIC CRITERIA
F2. Functional Anorectal Pain	**F2. Functional Anorectal Pain**

F2. Functional Anorectal Pain

F2a. Chronic Proctalgia

Diagnostic criteria*
*Must include **all** of the following:*

1. Chronic or recurrent rectal pain or aching
2. Episodes last 20 minutes or longer
3. Exclusion of other causes of rectal pain such as ischemia, inflammatory bowel disease, cryptitis, intramuscular abscess, anal fissure, hemorrhoids, prostatitis, and coccygodynia

* Criteria fulfilled for the last 3 months with symptom onset at least 6 months prior to diagnosis

Chronic proctalgia may be further characterized into levator ani syndrome or unspecified anorectal pain based on digital rectal examination.

F2a.1. Levator Ani Syndrome

Diagnostic criterion
Symptom criteria for chronic proctalgia and tenderness during posterior traction on the puborectalis

F2a.2. Unspecified Functional Anorectal Pain

Diagnostic criterion
Symptom criteria for chronic proctalgia but no tenderness during posterior traction on the puborectalis

---

F2. Functional Anorectal Pain

F2a. Levator Ani Syndrome

At least 12 weeks, which need not be consecutive, in the preceding 12 months of:

1. Chronic or recurrent rectal pain or aching;
2. Episodes last 20 minutes or longer; *and*
3. Other causes of rectal pain such as ischemia, inflammatory bowel disease, cryptitis, intramuscular abscess, fissure, hemorrhoids, prostatitis, and solitary rectal ulcer have been excluded.

ROME III DIAGNOSTIC CRITERIA	ROME II DIAGNOSTIC CRITERIA
F2b. Proctalgia Fugax *Diagnostic criteria* *Must include **all** of the following:* 1. Recurrent episodes of pain localized to the anus or lower rectum 2. Episodes last from seconds to minutes 3. There is no anorectal pain between episodes For research purposes criteria must be fulfilled for 3 months; however, clinical diagnosis and evaluation may be made prior to 3 months.	**F2b. Proctalgia Fugax** 1. Recurrent episodes of pain localized to the anus or lower rectum; 2. Episodes last from seconds to minutes; *and* 3. There is no anorectal pain between episode

F3. Functional Defecation Disorders
 	
Diagnostic criteria*
 	
1. The patient must satisfy diagnostic criteria for functional constipation**
2. During repeated attempts to defecate must have *at least two* of the following:
  a. Evidence of impaired evacuation, based on balloon expulsion test or imaging
  b. Inappropriate contraction of the pelvic floor muscles (i.e., anal sphincter or puborectalis) or less than 20% relaxation of basal resting sphincter pressure by manometry, imaging, or EMG
  c. Inadequate propulsive forces assessed by manometry or imaging
 	
* Criteria fulfilled for the last 3 months with symptom onset at least 6 months prior to diagnosis
 	
** **Diagnostic criteria for functional constipation:**
(1) Must include *two or more* of the following: (a) Straining during at least 25% of defecations, (b) Lumpy or hard stools in at least 25% of defecations, (c) Sensation of incomplete evacuation for at least 25% of defecations, (d) Sensation of anorectal obstruction/blockage for at least 25% of defecations, (e) Manual maneuvers to facilitate at least 25% of defecations (e.g., digital evacuation, support of the pelvic floor), (f) Fewer than three defecations per week.
(2) **Loose stools are rarely present without the use of laxatives.**
(3) **There are insufficient criteria for irritable bowel syndrome.**
	F3. Pelvic Floor Dyssynergia
	
	1. The patient must satisfy diagnostic criteria for functional constipation in Diagnostic criteria C3;
	2. There must be manometric, EMG, or radiologic evidence for inappropriate contraction or failure to relax the pelvic floor muscles during repeated attempts to defecate;
	3. There must be evidence of adequate propulsive forces during attempts to defecate, *and*
	4. There must be evidence of incomplete evacuation.

ROME III DIAGNOSTIC CRITERIA	ROME II DIAGNOSTIC CRITERIA
F3a. Dyssynergic Defecation *Diagnostic criterion* Inappropriate contraction of the pelvic floor or less than 20% relaxation of basal resting sphincter pressure with adequate propulsive forces during attempted defecation **F3b. Inadequate Defecatory Propulsion** *Diagnostic criterion* Inadequate propulsive forces with or without inappropriate contraction or less than 20% relaxation of the anal sphincter during attempted defecation	

Rome III Diagnostic
Questionnaire for
the Adult Functional
GI Disorders
(including Alarm
Questions) and
Scoring Algorithm

This questionnaire was developed by the Rome Foundation Board based on the Rome III criteria for the functional gastrointestinal disorders (FGIDs) and in cooperation with the Rome III criteria committees. It builds on the Rome I and II questionnaires and captures the Rome III diagnostic criteria for all of the functional gut disorders. The Rome III innovations include alarm symptoms to help alert physicians to possible structural disorders that might require further investigation, a psychosocial module to help identify psychosocial difficulties that might require mental health referral (see Appendix D), and 5- to 7-point alphanumeric scales to measure frequency and/or severity. Note also that there are separate questionnaires for adolescents and the parents of children and toddlers.

This questionnaire is designed for clinical practice and research. It should help identify individuals who have one or more of the FGIDs. The instrument is a guide only, and cannot substitute for the clinical judgments necessary to arrive at a correct diagnosis and select evidence-based investigations and treatments.

The questionnaire is followed by a coding system that identifies provisional (or possible) diagnoses from the responses to the questions. The presence of an "alarm" symptom does not negate a diagnosis of an FGID, but it may indicate further inquiry or testing to rule out structural disease. Similarly, an indication of psychosocial difficulties will not alter the diagnosis, but should prompt more information and appropriate treatment. Thus, a clinical diagnosis will depend on the clinician's application of these criteria and the judicious exclusion of other diseases (e.g., with other studies as needed).

This is not an all-purpose questionnaire. It does not address structural disorders or FGIDs requiring physical findings or laboratory abnormalities in addition to symptoms (e.g., biliary disorders and functional defecation disorder); the questionnaire alone is insufficient for diagnosis.

The use of exclusion items (e.g., to exclude a diagnosis of functional constipation when irritable bowel syndrome criteria are fulfilled) will depend upon the purpose of the investigation. For clinical purposes, the questions should detect all possible diagnoses, while for a clinical trial a "pure" sample of individuals with a certain diagnosis may be preferred.

Many clinical scientists may prefer to study only one or a few of the disorders. To serve such a purpose, the questionnaire may be subdivided into question and coding modules for each of the esophageal, gastroduodenal, gallbladder/sphincter of Oddi, bowel, chronic abdominal pain, and anorectal disorders. The questionnaire and the coding for individual diagnoses are available at our website, www. RomeCriteria.org and may be downloaded as required.

> W. Grant Thompson, MD, Chair
> Douglas A. Drossman, MD, Nicholas J. Talley, MD, PhD
> Lynn Walker, PhD, William E. Whitehead, PhD
> *Questionnaire Subcommittee*

Information for Clinician/Investigator

This self-report questionnaire is designed to identify FGIDs using the Rome III criteria. It can be self-administered and takes about 15 to 20 minutes to complete. Response formats for questions include yes/no responses, a 5-point ordinal response scale for conditional questions (never or rarely to always), a 7-point ordinal response scale for frequency questions (never to every day), and a few other response scales specific to an item not fitting these (e.g., questions #76, 77, & 79). A series of "red flag" or alarm symptom questions are included at the end of the questionnaire (questions #82–93). While not part of the diagnostic algorithm, they are helpful in determining whether other diagnostic studies are needed to exclude other disease. Please see the scoring algorithm for information on specific diagnoses.

This questionnaire (with its algorithms) is intended for research and may be employed as an aid to diagnosis. However, it is not meant as an instrument for self-diagnosis nor does it obviate the need for medical evaluation including history and physical examination of individual patients.

Instructions for Respondent

The purpose of this survey is to learn more about the health problems that people sometimes have with their stomach and intestines. The questionnaire will take about 15 minutes to complete. To answer each question, fill in the circle directly to the left of the correct answer. You may find that you have not had any of the symptoms that we will ask you about. When this happens, you will be instructed to skip over the questions that do not apply to you. If you are not sure about an answer, or you cannot remember the answer to a question, just answer as best you can. It is easy to miss questions, so please check that you haven't left any out as you go.

ROME III ADULT QUESTIONNAIRE

Question	Answer

Symptoms in the Esophagus

1. In the last 3 months, how often did you have a feeling of a lump, fullness, or something stuck in your throat?

   ⓪ Never → *Skip to question 4*
   ① Less than one day a month
   ② One day a month
   ③ Two to three days a month
   ④ One day a week
   ⑤ More than one day a week
   ⑥ Every day

2. Have you had this feeling 6 months or longer?

   ⓪ No
   ① Yes

3. Does this feeling occur between meals (when you are not eating)?

   ⓪ No
   ① Yes

4. When you are eating or drinking, does it hurt to swallow?

   ⓪ Never or rarely
   ① Sometimes
   ② Often
   ③ Most of the time
   ④ Always

5. In the last 3 months, how often did you have pain or discomfort in the middle of your chest (not related to heart problems)?

   ⓪ Never → *Skip to question 8*
   ① Less than one day a month
   ② One day a month
   ③ Two to three days a month
   ④ One day a week
   ⑤ More than one day a week
   ⑥ Every day

6. Have you had this chest pain 6 months or longer?

   ⓪ No
   ① Yes

7. When you had your chest pain, how often did it feel like burning?

   ⓪ Never or rarely
   ① Sometimes
   ② Often
   ③ Most of the time
   ④ Always

ROME III ADULT QUESTIONNAIRE

Question	Answer	
8. In the last 3 months, how often did you have heartburn (a burning discomfort or burning pain in your chest)?	⓪ Never → ① Less than one day a month ② One day a month ③ Two to three days a month ④ One day a week ⑤ More than one day a week ⑥ Every day	*Skip to question* *10*
9. Have you had this heartburn (burning pain or discomfort in the chest) 6 months or longer?	⓪ No ① Yes	
10. In the last 3 months, how often did food or drinks get stuck after swallowing or go down slowly through your chest?	⓪ Never → ① Less than one day a month ② One day a month ③ Two to three days a month ④ One day a week ⑤ More than one day a week ⑥ Every day	*Skip to question* *13*
11. Was the symptom of food sticking associated with heartburn?	⓪ Never or rarely ① Sometimes ② Often ③ Most of the time ④ Always	
12. Have you had this problem 6 months or longer?	⓪ No ① Yes	
13. In the last 3 months, how often did you feel uncomfortably full after a regular-sized meal?	⓪ Never → ① Less than one day a month ② One day a month ③ Two to three days a month ④ One day a week ⑤ More than one day a week ⑥ Every day	*Skip to question* *15*

ROME III ADULT QUESTIONNAIRE

Question	Answer

Symptoms in the Esophagus (continued)

14. Have you had this uncomfortable fullness after meals 6 months or longer?

⓪ No
① Yes

15. In the last 3 months, how often were you unable to finish a regular-sized meal?

⓪ Never   →   *Skip to question*
① Less than one day a month   *17*
② One day a month
③ Two to three days a month
④ One day a week
⑤ More than one day a week
⑥ Every day

16. Have you had this inability to finish regular-sized meals 6 months or longer?

⓪ No
① Yes

Symptoms in the Stomach and Intestines

17. In the last 3 months, how often did you have pain or burning in the middle of your abdomen, above your belly button but not in your chest?

⓪ Never   →   *Skip to question*
① Less than one day a month   *26*
② One day a month
③ Two to three days a month
④ One day a week
⑤ More than one day a week
⑥ Every day

18. Have you had this pain or burning 6 months or longer?

⓪ No
① Yes

19. Did this pain or burning occur and then completely disappear during the same day?

⓪ Never or rarely
① Sometimes
② Often
③ Most of the time
④ Always

ROME III ADULT QUESTIONNAIRE

Question	Answer
20. Usually, how severe was the pain or burning in the middle of your abdomen, above your belly button?	① Very mild ② Mild ③ Moderate ④ Severe ⑤ Very severe
21. Was this pain or burning affected by eating?	⓪ Not affected by eating ① Worse pain after eating ② Less pain after eating
22. Was this pain or burning relieved by taking antacids?	⓪ Never or rarely ① Sometimes ② Often ③ Most of the time ④ Always
23. Did this pain or burning usually get better or stop after a bowel movement or passing gas?	⓪ Never or rarely ① Sometimes ② Often ③ Most of the time ④ Always
24. When this pain or burning started, did you usually have a change in the number of bowel movements (either more or fewer)?	⓪ Never or rarely ① Sometimes ② Often ③ Most of the time ④ Always
25. When this pain or burning started, did you usually have softer or harder stools?	⓪ Never or rarely ① Sometimes ② Often ③ Most of the time ④ Always

Symptoms in the Stomach and Intestines (continued)

26. In the last 3 months, how often did you have bothersome nausea?

⓪ Never → *Skip to question 28*
① Less than one day a month
② One day a month
③ Two to three days a month
④ One day a week
⑤ More than one day a week
⑥ Every day

27. Did this nausea start more than 6 months ago?

⓪ No
① Yes

28. In the last 3 months, how often did you vomit?

⓪ Never → *Skip to question 33*
① Less than one day a month
② One day a month
③ Two to three days a month
④ One day a week
⑤ More than one day a week
⑥ Every day

29. Have you had this vomiting 6 months or longer?

⓪ No
① Yes

30. Did you make yourself vomit?

⓪ Never or rarely
① Sometimes
② Often
③ Most of the time
④ Always

31. Did you have vomiting in the last year that occurred in separate episodes of a few days and then stopped?

⓪ Never or rarely → *Skip to question 33*
① Sometimes
② Often
③ Most of the time
④ Always

Question	Answer	
32. Did you have at least three episodes during the past year?	⓪ No ① Yes	
33. In the last 3 months, how often did food come back up into your mouth?	⓪ Never → ① Less than one day a month ② One day a month ③ Two to three days a month ④ One day a week ⑤ More than one day a week ⑥ Every day	*Skip to question 39*
34. Have you had this problem (food coming back up into your mouth) 6 months or longer?	⓪ No ① Yes	
35. When food came back up into your mouth, did it usually stay in your mouth for a while before you swallowed it or spit it out?	⓪ Never or rarely ① Sometimes ② Often ③ Most of the time ④ Always	
36. Did you have retching (heaving) before food came into your mouth?	⓪ Never or rarely ① Sometimes ② Often ③ Most of the time ④ Always	
37. When food came into your mouth, how often did you vomit or feel sick to your stomach?	⓪ Never or rarely ① Sometimes ② Often ③ Most of the time ④ Always	

Question	Answer

Symptoms in the Stomach and Intestines (continued)

38. Did food stop coming back up into your mouth when it turned sour or acidic?

ⓞ Never or rarely
① Sometimes
② Often
③ Most of the time
④ Always

39. In the last 3 months, how often did you experience bothersome belching?

ⓞ Never → *Skip to question 41*
① Less than one day a month
② One day a month
③ Two to three days a month
④ One day a week
⑤ More than one day a week
⑥ Every day

40. Did this bothersome belching start more than 6 months ago?

ⓞ No
① Yes

41. In the last 3 months, how often did you have discomfort or pain anywhere in your abdomen?

ⓞ Never → *Skip to question 52*
① Less than one day a month
② One day a month
③ Two to three days a month
④ One day a week
⑤ More than one day a week
⑥ Every day

42. Did you have pain only (not discomfort or a mixture of discomfort and pain)?

ⓞ Never or rarely
① Sometimes
② Often
③ Most of the time
④ Always

ROME III ADULT QUESTIONNAIRE

Question	Answer
43. For women: Did this discomfort or pain occur only during your menstrual bleeding and not at other times?	⓪ No ① Yes ② Does not apply because I have had the change in life (menopause) or I am a male
44. When you had this pain, how often did it limit or restrict your daily activities (for example, work, household activities, and social events)?	⓪ Never or rarely ① Sometimes ② Often ③ Most of the time ④ Always
45. Have you had this discomfort or pain 6 months or longer?	⓪ No ① Yes
46. How often did this discomfort or pain get better or stop after you had a bowel movement?	⓪ Never or rarely ① Sometimes ② Often ③ Most of the time ④ Always
47. When this discomfort or pain started, did you have more frequent bowel movements?	⓪ Never or rarely ① Sometimes ② Often ③ Most of the time ④ Always
48. When this discomfort or pain started, did you have less frequent bowel movements?	⓪ Never or rarely ① Sometimes ② Often ③ Most of the time ④ Always

Question	Answer

Symptoms in the Stomach and Intestines (continued)

49. When this discomfort or pain started, were your stools (bowel movements) looser?	⓪ Never or rarely ① Sometimes ② Often ③ Most of the time ④ Always
50. When this discomfort or pain started, how often did you have harder stools?	⓪ Never or rarely ① Sometimes ② Often ③ Most of the time ④ Always
51. How often was this pain or discomfort relieved by moving or changing positions?	⓪ Never or rarely ① Sometimes ② Often ③ Most of the time ④ Always
52. In the last 3 months, how often did you have fewer than three bowel movements (0–2) a week?	⓪ Never or rarely ① Sometimes ② Often ③ Most of the time ④ Always
53. In the last 3 months, how often did you have hard or lumpy stools?*	⓪ Never or rarely ① Sometimes ② Often ③ Most of the time ④ Always

Those who wish to use the new criteria for subclassifying IBS patients into subtypes based on stool consistency may substitute the following response scale in Questions 53 and 61:

⓪ Never or rarely
① About 25% of the time
② About 50% of the time
③ About 75% of the time
④ Always, 100% of the time

ROME III ADULT QUESTIONNAIRE

Question	Answer
54. In the last 3 months, how often did you strain during bowel movements?	⓪ Never or rarely ① Sometimes ② Often ③ Most of the time ④ Always
55. In the last 3 months, how often did you have a feeling of incomplete emptying after bowel movements?	⓪ Never or rarely ① Sometimes ② Often ③ Most of the time ④ Always
56. In the last 3 months, how often did you have a sensation that the stool could not be passed, (i.e., was blocked), when having a bowel movement?	⓪ Never or rarely ① Sometimes ② Often ③ Most of the time ④ Always
57. In the last 3 months, how often did you press on or around your bottom or remove stool in order to complete a bowel movement?	⓪ Never or rarely ① Sometimes ② Often ③ Most of the time ④ Always
58. In the last 3 months, how often did you have difficulty relaxing or letting go to allow the stool to come out during a bowel movement?	⓪ Never or rarely ① Sometimes ② Often ③ Most of the time ④ Always
59. Did any of the symptoms of constipation listed in questions 52–58 above begin more than 6 months ago?	⓪ No ① Yes

ROME III ADULT QUESTIONNAIRE

Question	Answer

Symptoms in the Stomach and Intestines (continued)

60. In the last 3 months, how often did you have 4 or more bowel movements a day?

⓪ Never or rarely
① Sometimes
② Often
③ Most of the time
④ Always

---

61. In the last 3 months, how often did you have loose, mushy, or watery stools?*

⓪ Never or rarely → *Skip to question 64*
① Sometimes
② Often
③ Most of the time
④ Always

---

62. In the last 3 months, were at least three-fourths (3/4) of your stools loose, mushy, or watery?

⓪ No
① Yes

---

63. Did you begin having frequent loose, mushy, or watery stools more than 6 months ago?

⓪ No
① Yes

---

64. In the last 3 months, how often did you have to rush to the toilet to have a bowel movement?

⓪ Never or rarely
① Sometimes
② Often
③ Most of the time
④ Always

Those who wish to use the new criteria for subclassifying IBS patients into subtypes based on stool consistency may substitute the following response scale in Questions 53 and 61:

⓪ Never or rarely
① About 25% of the time
② About 50% of the time
③ About 75% of the time
④ Always, 100% of the time

ROME III ADULT QUESTIONNAIRE

Question	Answer
65. In the last 3 months, how often was there mucus or slime in your bowel movement?	⓪ Never or rarely ① Sometimes ② Often ③ Most of the time ④ Always
66. In the last 3 months, how often did you have bloating or distension?	⓪ Never → *Skip to question 68* ① Less than one day a month ② One day a month ③ Two to three days a month ④ One day a week ⑤ More than one day a week ⑥ Every day
67. Did your symptoms of bloating or distention begin more than 6 months ago?	⓪ No ① Yes

Symptoms in the Gall Bladder or Pancreas

Question	Answer
68. In the last 6 months, how often did you have steady pain in the middle or right side of your upper abdomen?	⓪ Never → *Skip to question 75* ① Less than one day a month ② One day a month ③ Two to three days a month ④ One day a week ⑤ More than one day a week ⑥ Every day
69. Did this pain last 30 minutes or longer?	⓪ Never or rarely ① Sometimes ② Often ③ Most of the time ④ Always

Question	Answer

Symptoms in the Gall Bladder or Pancreas (continued)

70. Did this pain build up to a steady, severe level?

    ⓪ Never or rarely
    ① Sometimes
    ② Often
    ③ Most of the time
    ④ Always

71. Did this pain go away completely between episodes?

    ⓪ Never or rarely
    ① Sometimes
    ② Often
    ③ Most of the time
    ④ Always

72. Did this pain stop you from your usual activities, or cause you to see a doctor urgently or go to the emergency department?

    ⓪ Never or rarely
    ① Sometimes
    ② Often
    ③ Most of the time
    ④ Always

73. Have you had your gallbladder removed?

    ⓪ No   →   *Skip to question 75*
    ① Yes

74. How often have you had this pain since your gallbladder was removed?

    ⓪ Never or rarely
    ① Sometimes
    ② Often
    ③ Most of the time
    ④ Always

ROME III ADULT QUESTIONNAIRE

Question	Answer

Symptoms in the Rectum or Anal Canal

75. In the last 3 months, how often have you accidentally leaked liquid or solid stool?
   - ⓪ Never → *Skip to question 78*
   - ① Less than one day a month
   - ② One day a month
   - ③ Two to three days a month
   - ④ One day a week
   - ⑤ More than one day a week
   - ⑥ Every day

76. In the last 3 months, when this leakage occurred, about what amount was leaked?
   - ① A small amount (staining only)
   - ② Moderate amount (more than staining, but less than a full bowel movement)
   - ③ Large amount (a full bowel movement)

77. In the *last year,* when this leakage occurred, what was the composition of leakage?
   - ① Liquid/mucus only
   - ② Stool only
   - ③ Both liquid/mucus and stool

78. In the last 3 months, how often have you had aching, pain, or pressure in the anus or rectum when you were not having a bowel movement?
   - ⓪ Never → *Skip to question 82*
   - ① Less than one day a month
   - ② One day a month
   - ③ Two to three days a month
   - ④ One day a week
   - ⑤ More than one day a week
   - ⑥ Every day

79. How long did the aching, pain or pressure last?
   - ① From seconds to up to 20 minutes and disappeared completely
   - ② More than 20 minutes and up to several days or longer

Question	Answer

Symptoms in the Rectum or Anal Canal (continued)

80. Did the pain in your anus and rectum occur and then completely disappear during the same day?

   ⓪ No
   ① Yes

81. Did the aching, pain, or pressure in the anal canal or rectum begin more than 6 months ago?

   ⓪ No
   ① Yes

Other Questions

82. In the last 3 months, how often have you noticed blood in your stools?

   ⓪ Never or rarely
   ① Sometimes
   ② Often
   ③ Most of the time
   ④ Always

83. In the last 3 months, how often have you noticed black stools?

   ⓪ Never or rarely
   ① Sometimes
   ② Often
   ③ Most of the time
   ④ Always

84. In the last 3 months, how often have you vomited blood?

   ⓪ Never or rarely
   ① Sometimes
   ② Often
   ③ Most of the time
   ④ Always

ROME III ADULT QUESTIONNAIRE

Question	Answer
85. Have you been told by your doctor that you are anemic (a low blood count or low iron)? (If female, *not* due to your menstrual period.)	⓪ No ① Yes
86. In the last 3 months, how often have you taken your temperature and found it to be over 99 degrees Fahrenheit (38 degrees Centigrade) on different days?	⓪ Never or rarely ① Sometimes ② Often ③ Most of the time ④ Always
87. In the last 3 months, have you unintentionally lost over 10 pounds (4.5 kilograms)?	⓪ No ① Yes
88. If you are over age 50, have you had a recent major change in bowel movements (change in frequency or consistency)?	⓪ No ① Yes ② Does not apply
89. Do you have a parent, brother, or sister who has (or had) one or more of the following:	
89.1 Cancer of the esophagus, stomach, or colon	⓪ No ① Yes
89.2 Ulcerative colitis or Crohn's disease	⓪ No ① Yes
89.3 Celiac disease	⓪ No ① Yes

Other Questions (continued)

90. In the past 3 months, how often did you have persistent or worsening hoarseness of the voice?

⓪ Never or rarely
① Sometimes
② Often
③ Most of the time
④ Always

91. In the past 3 months, how often did you have persistent or worsening neck or throat pain?

⓪ Never or rarely
① Sometimes
② Often
③ Most of the time
④ Always

92. In the past 3 months, how often did you have chest pain on exertion, or chest pain related to heart problems?

⓪ Never or rarely
① Sometimes
② Often
③ Most of the time
④ Always

93. In the last 3 months, how often have you had difficulty swallowing?

⓪ Never or rarely
① Sometimes
② Often
③ Most of the time
④ Always

Introduction

The diagnostic criteria for each of the FGIDs are listed below. Following each criterion there is **bold and italicized text** to indicate (a) the questions in the Rome III Diagnostic Questionnaire that capture this information and (b) the frequency threshold that defines a clinically significant frequency of occurrence for this symptom. For example, for heartburn, "question 8>3" means that the frequency should be more than that for response #3 or at least one day a week.

For some of the FGID diagnoses, the working teams concluded that clinical evaluation or laboratory tests are required to make the diagnosis. These criteria are identified in red. There are no questions in the questionnaire for these criteria. Note that since there are no questions in the modular questionnaire for supporting criteria, they are not included in this document.

For functional fecal incontinence and functional defecation disorder, the working team concluded that the diagnosis could only be made based on laboratory tests. However, a set of questions have been included in the questionnaire that can be used for screening purposes in order to identify cases that may require laboratory testing.

Functional Esophageal Disorders

A1. Functional Heartburn

Diagnostic criteria*
*Must include **all** of the following:*

1. Burning retrosternal discomfort or pain
   Heartburn = at least one day per week (question 8>3)

2. Absence of evidence that gastroesophageal acid reflux is the cause of the symptom
   No question. Requires ambulatory pH study.

3. Absence of histopathology-based esophageal motility disorders
   No question. Requires objective testing.

   * Criteria fulfilled for the last 3 months with symptom onset at least 6 months prior to diagnosis
   Yes. (question 9=1)

A2. Functional Chest Pain of Presumed Esophageal Origin

Diagnostic criteria*
*Must include **all** of the following:*

1. Midline chest pain or discomfort that is not of burning quality
   Chest pain occurs at least 2 to 3 days a month (question 5 > 2)

2. Absence of evidence that gastroesophageal reflux is the cause of the symptom
   When you had chest pain, how often did it feel like burning? Never. (question 7=0)

3. Absence of histopathology-based esophageal motility disorders
   No question.

   * Criteria fulfilled for the last 3 months with symptom onset at least 6 months prior to diagnosis
   Yes. (question 6=1)

A3. Functional Dysphagia

Diagnostic criteria*
*Must include **all** of the following:*

1. Sense of solid and/or liquid foods sticking, lodging, or passing abnormally through the esophagus
   Food or drink sticks or goes down slowly at least once a month (question 10 > 1)

2. Absence of evidence that gastroesophageal reflux is the cause of the symptom
   Was the sensation of food sticking associated with heartburn? Never or rarely. (question 11=0)

   Heartburn occurred less often than once a week. (question 8 < 4)

3. Absence of histopathology-based esophageal motility disorders
   No question.

   * Criteria fulfilled for the last 3 months with symptom onset at least 6 months prior to diagnosis
   Yes. (question 12=1)

A4. Globus

Diagnostic criteria*
*Must include **all** of the following:*

1. Persistent or intermittent, nonpainful sensation of a lump or foreign body in the throat
   Sensation of lump in throat occurs more than once a month. (question 1 > 2)

2. Occurrence of the sensation between meals
   Sensation of lump occurs between meals. Yes. (question 3=1)

3. Absence of dysphagia or odynophagia
   Food gets stuck one day a month or less often. (question 10 < 3)

   It hurts to swallow. Never or rarely. (question 4=0)

4. Absence of evidence that gastroesophageal reflux is the cause of the symptom
   Heartburn occurs 1 day a month or less often (question 8 < 3)

5. Absence of histopathology-based esophageal motility disorders
   No question.

   * Criteria fulfilled for the last 3 months with symptom onset at least 6 months prior to diagnosis
   Yes. (question 2=1)

B. Functional Gastroduodenal Disorders

B1. Functional Dyspepsia

Diagnostic criteria*
Must include:

1. *One or more* of the following:
   a. Bothersome postprandial fullness
      Uncomfortably full after regular-sized meal, more than 1 day/week (question 13 > 4)

      Onset more than 6 months ago (question 14=1)

   b. Early satiation
      Unable to finish regular-sized meal, more than 1 day/week (question 15 > 4)

      Onset more than 6 months ago. Yes. (question 16=1)

   c. Epigastric pain
      Pain or burning in middle of abdomen, at least 1 day/week (question 17 > 3)

      Onset more than 6 months ago. Yes. (question 18=1)

   d. Epigastric burning
      (This criterion is incorporated in the same question as epigastric pain)

AND

1. No evidence of structural disease (including at upper endoscopy) that is likely to explain the symptoms
   No question.

   * Criteria fulfilled for the last 3 months with symptom onset at least 6 months prior to diagnosis
   Yes. (question 18=1)

B1a. Postprandial Distress Syndrome

Diagnostic criteria*
Must include **one or both** *of the following:*

1. Bothersome postprandial fullness, occurring after ordinary-sized meals, at least several times per week
   Uncomfortably full after regular-sized meal, more than 1 day/week (question 13 > 4)

2. Early satiation that prevents finishing a regular meal, at least several times per week
   Unable to finish regular sized meal more than 1 day/week (question 15 > 4)

   * Criteria fulfilled for the last 3 months with symptom onset at least 6 months prior to diagnosis
   Requires a "Yes" to both. (question 14=1) & (question 16=1)

B1b. Epigastric Pain Syndrome

Diagnostic criteria
Must include **all** *of the following:*

1. Pain or burning localized to the epigastrium of at least moderate severity, at least once per week
   Pain or burning in middle of abdomen, at least 1 day/week (question 17 > 3)

   Pain is at least moderate severity (question 20 > 2)

2. The pain is intermittent
   Pain or burning often disappears completely in the same day (question 19 > 1)

3. Not generalized or localized to other abdominal or chest regions
   Chest pain occurs once a month or less often (question 5 < 3)

   Heartburn occurs once a month or less often (question 8 < 3)

4. Not relieved by defecation or passage of flatus
   Never or rarely gets better after defecation (question 23=0)

5. Not fulfilling criteria for gallbladder and sphincter of Oddi disorders

6. Criteria fulfilled for the last 3 months with symptom onset at least 6 months prior to diagnosis
   Yes. (question 18=1)

B2. Belching Disorders

B2a. Aerophagia

Diagnostic criteria*
*Must include **all** of the following:*

1. Troublesome repetitive belching at least several times a week
   Bothersome belching more than 1 day a week (question 39 > 4)

2. Air swallowing that is objectively observed or measured
   No question.

   * Criteria fulfilled for the last 3 months with symptom onset at least 6 months prior to diagnosis
   Yes. (question 40 = 1)

B2b. Unspecified Excessive Belching

Diagnostic criteria*
*Must include **all** of the following:*

1. Troublesome repetitive belching at least several times a week
   Bothersome belching more than 1 day a week (question 39 > 4)

2. No objective evidence that excessive air swallowing underlies the symptom

   * Criteria fulfilled for the last 3 months with symptom onset at least 6 months prior to diagnosis
   Yes. (question 40 = 1)

B3. Nausea and Vomiting Disorders

B3a. Chronic Idiopathic Nausea

Diagnostic criteria*
*Must include **all** of the following:*

1. Bothersome nausea occurring at least several times per week
   Nausea more than once a week (question 26 > 4)

2. Not usually associated with vomiting
   Vomiting less than 1 day a week (question 28 < 4)

3. Absence of abnormalities at upper endoscopy or metabolic disease that explains the nausea
   No question.

   * Criteria fulfilled for the last 3 months with symptom onset at least 6 months prior to diagnosis
   Yes. (question 27 = 1)

B3b. Functional Vomiting

Diagnostic criteria*
*Must include **all** of the following:*

1. On average one or more episodes of vomiting per week
   Vomiting occurs at least once a week (question 28 > 3)

2. Absence of criteria for an eating disorder, rumination, or major psychiatric disease according by DSM-IV
   Patient does not meet criteria for Rumination Disorder.
   No questions for eating disorder or major psychiatric disease.

3. Absence of self-induced induced vomiting and chronic cannabinoid use and absence of abnormalities in the central nervous system or metabolic diseases to explain the recurrent vomiting
   Never or rarely makes himself or herself vomit (question 30 = 0)

   * Criteria fulfilled for the last 3 months with symptom onset at least 6 months prior to diagnosis
   Yes. (question 29 = 1)

B3c. Cyclic Vomiting Syndrome

Diagnostic criteria
*Must include **all** of the following:*

1. Stereotypical episodes of vomiting regarding onset (acute) and duration (less than one week)
   Vomiting occurs more often than 'never or rarely' (question 28 > 0)

2. Three or more discrete episodes in the prior year
   At least 3 episodes during the year. Yes. (question 32 = 1)

3. Absence of nausea and vomiting between episodes
   Occurred in separate episodes and then stopped at least sometimes (question 31 > 0)

B4. Rumination Syndrome in Adults

Diagnostic criteria*
*Must include **both** of the following:*

1. Persistent or recurrent regurgitation of recently ingested food into the mouth with subsequent spitting or remastication and swallowing
   Bring up food at least 1 day/week (question 33 > 3)
   Hold food in mouth before spitting or swallowing often (question 35 > 1)

2. Regurgitation is not preceded by retching
   Was bringing up food preceded by retching? No. (question 36=0)

   * Criteria fulfilled for the last 3 months with symptom onset at least 6 months prior to diagnosis
   Yes. (question 34=1)

C. Functional Bowel Disorders

C1. Irritable Bowel Syndrome

Diagnostic Criterion*
Recurrent abdominal pain or discomfort** at least 3 days/month in last 3 months associated with *two or more* of criteria #1–#3 below

Pain or discomfort at least 2 to 3 days/month (question 41>2)

*For women, does pain occur only during menstrual bleeding?
(question 43=0 or 2)*

1. Improvement with defecation
   Pain or discomfort gets better after defecation at least sometimes (question 46>0)

2. Onset associated with a change in frequency of stool
   Onset of pain or discomfort associated with more stools at least sometimes (question 47>0), OR

   Onset of pain or discomfort associated with fewer stools at least sometimes (question 48>0)

3. Onset associated with a change in form (appearance) of stool
   Onset of pain or discomfort associated with looser stools at least sometimes (question 49>0), OR

   Onset of pain or discomfort associated with harder stools at least sometimes (question 50>0)

   * Criterion fulfilled for the last 3 months with symptom onset at least 6 months prior to diagnosis
   Yes. (question 45=1)

   ***"Discomfort" means an uncomfortable sensation not described as pain.*
   In pathophysiology research and clinical trials, a pain/discomfort frequency of at least 2 days a week during screening evaluation is recommended for subject eligibility.

C2. Functional Bloating

*Diagnostic criteria**

*Must include **all** of the following:*

1. Recurrent feeling of bloating or visible distension at least 3 days/month in 3 months

   Bloating or distention at least 2 to 3 days/month (question 66 > 2)

2. There are insufficient criteria for a diagnosis of functional dyspepsia, irritable bowel syndrome, or functional constipation.

   Insufficient criteria for functional dyspepsia, &

   Insufficient criteria for IBS, &

   Insufficient criteria for other functional GI disorder

   * Criteria fulfilled for the last 3 months with symptom onset at least 6 months prior to diagnosis
   Yes. (question 67=1)

C3. Functional Constipation

*Diagnostic criteria**

1. Must include *two or more* of the following:

   a. Straining during at least 25% of defecations

      At least often. (question 54 > 1)

   b. Lumpy or hard stools in at least 25% of defecations

      At least often. (question 53 > 1)

   c. Sensation of incomplete evacuation for at least 25% of defecations

      At least sometimes. (question 55 > 0)

   d. Sensation of anorectal obstruction/blockage for at least 25% of defecations

      At least sometimes. (question 56 > 0)

   e. Manual maneuvers to facilitate at least 25% of defecations (e.g., digital evacuation, support of the pelvic floor)

      At least sometimes. (question 57 > 0)

   f. Fewer than three defecations per week

      At least often. (question 52 > 1)

2. Loose stools are rarely present without the use of laxatives.

   Loose stools occur never or rarely (question 49=0)

3. There are insufficient criteria for IBS

   Diagnostic criteria for IBS not met

   * Criteria fulfilled for the last 3 months with symptom onset at least 6 months prior to diagnosis
   Yes. (question 59=1)

C4. Functional Diarrhea

*Diagnostic criterion**

Loose (mushy) or watery stools without pain occurring in at least 75% of stools
  AND

  Watery stools at least ¾ of time (question 62=1)

  Pain or discomfort never occurs (question 41=0)

  * Criterion fulfilled for the last 3 months with symptom onset at least 6 months prior to
  diagnosis
  Yes. (question 63=1)

C5. Unspecified Functional Bowel Disorder

*Diagnostic criterion**

Bowel symptoms not attributable to an organic etiology that do not meet criteria
  for the previously defined categories.

  * Criterion fulfilled for the last 3 months with symptom onset at least 6 months prior to
  diagnosis

  [(question 41>0) & (question 41<3) & (question 45=1)] OR

  [(question 66>0) & (question 66<3) & (question 67=1)] OR

  [(question 54>0) & (question 54<2) & (question 59=1)] OR

  [(question 53>0) & (question 53<2) & (question 59=1)] OR

  [((question 55>0) & (question 55<2) & (question 59=1)]) OR

  [(question 57>0) & (question 57<2) & (question 59=1)] OR

  [((question 52>0) & (question 52<2) & (question 59=1)]) OR

  [(question 60>0) & (question 60<2) & (question 63=1)] OR

  [((question 58>0) & (question 58<2) & (question 59=1)] OR

  [(question 64>0) & (question 64<2)]

D. Functional Abdominal Pain Syndrome

Diagnostic criteria*
*Must include **all** of the following:*

1. Continuous or nearly continuous abdominal pain
   Pain or discomfort occurs every day (question 41=6)

   Subject experiences only pain, not discomfort (question 42>0)

2. No or only occasional relationship of pain with physiological events (e.g., eating, defecation, or menses)
   Pain is affected by eating sometimes or less often (question 21<2)

   Pain stops or lessens with defecation sometimes or less often (question 46<2)

   Pain onset is associated with more frequent stools sometimes or less often (question 47<2)

   Pain onset is associated with fewer stools sometimes or less often (question 48<2)

   Pain onset is associated with looser stools (question 49<2)

   Pain onset is associated with harder stools (question 50<2)

   Pain or burning is associated with a change in stool consistency never, rarely, or sometimes (question 25<2)

   Pain or burning is associated with a change in stool frequency never, rarely, or sometimes (question 24<2)

   For women, pain is not limited to menstrual bleeding, or question is not applicable (question 43=0 or 2)

3. Some loss of daily functioning
   Pain limits activity at least some of the time (question 44>0)

4. The pain is not feigned (e.g., malingering)
   No question

5. Insufficient symptoms to meet criteria for another functional gastrointestinal disorder that would explain the pain
   Epigastric pain syndrome criteria not met, &

   IBS criteria not met, &

   Anorectal pain criteria not met

* Criteria fulfilled for the last 3 months with symptom onset at least 6 months prior to diagnosis
Yes. (question 45=1)

E. Functional Gallbladder and Sphincter of Oddi Disorders

Diagnostic criteria

Must include episodes of pain located in the epigastrium and/or right upper quadrant
Steady pain which may occur less than once per month or more often (question 68>0)

AND *all* of the following:

1. Episodes lasting 30 minutes or longer
   At least often (question 69>1)

2. Recurrent symptoms occurring at different intervals (not daily)
   At least often (question 71>1)

3. The pain builds up to a steady level
   At least often (question 70>1)

4. The pain is moderate to severe enough to interrupt the patient's daily activities or lead to an emergency department visit
   At least often (question 72>1)

5. The pain is not relieved by bowel movements
   Never or rarely. (question 46=0)

6. The pain is not relieved by postural change
   Never or rarely. (question 51=0)

7. The pain is not relieved by antacids
   Never or rarely. (question 22=0)

8. Exclusion of other structural disease that would explain the symptoms.
   No question.

E1. Functional Gallbladder Disorder

Diagnostic criteria
*Must include **all** of the following:*

1. Criteria for functional gallbladder and sphincter of Oddi disorders
   Yes.

2. Gallbladder is present
   Gallbladder has not been removed

   No. (question 73=0)

3. Normal liver enzymes, conjugated bilirubin and amylase/lipase
   No question. Laboratory studies needed.

E2. Functional Biliary Sphincter of Oddi Disorder

Diagnostic criteria
Must include **both** *of the following:*

1. Criteria for functional gallbladder and sphincter of Oddi disorders
   Yes.

   Gallbladder has been removed (question 73=1)

   Pain has recurred at least sometimes since gallbladder was removed (question 74>0)

2. Normal amylase/lipase
   No question. Laboratory studies needed.

E3. Functional Pancreatic Sphincter of Oddi Disorder

Diagnostic criteria
Must include **both** *of the following:*

1. Criteria for functional gallbladder and sphincter of Oddi disorder
   Yes.

2. Elevated amylase/lipase
   No question.

F. Functional Anorectal Disorders

F1. Functional Fecal Incontinence

Diagnostic criteria*

1. Recurrent uncontrolled passage of fecal material in an individual with a developmental age of at least 4 years
   Leakage of liquid or solid stool occurred at least once a month (question 75>1)

   No other criteria listed below are incorporated into the questionnaire. Clinical and laboratory assessment are required to confirm that the fecal incontinence is functional.

   AND *one or more* of the following:
   a. Abnormal functioning of normally innervated and structurally intact muscles
   b. Minor abnormalities of sphincter structure and/or innervation
   c. Normal or disordered bowel habits, (i.e., fecal retention or diarrhea)
   d. Psychological causes
   AND
2. Exclusion of *all* of the following:
   a. Abnormal innervation caused by lesion(s) within the brain (e.g., dementia), spinal cord, or sacral nerve roots, or mixed lesions (e.g. multiple sclerosis),

or as part of a generalized peripheral or autonomic neuropathy, e.g. due to diabetes

b. Anal sphincter abnormalities associated with a multisystem disease, (e.g., scleroderma)

c. Structural or neurogenic abnormalities believed to be the major or primary cause of FI.

* Criteria fulfilled for the last 3 months

F2. Functional Anorectal Pain

F2a. Chronic Proctalgia

Diagnostic criteria*
*Must include **all** of the following:*

1. Chronic or recurrent rectal pain or aching
   Pain or aching occurs more than once a month (question 78 > 2)

2. Episodes last 20 minutes or longer
   Pain or aching lasts more than 20 minutes (question 79 = 2)

3. Exclusion of other causes of rectal pain such as ischemia, inflammatory bowel disease, cryptitis, intramuscular abscess, anal fissure, hemorrhoids, prostatitis, and coccygodynia.
   No question.

   * Criteria fulfilled for the last 3 months with symptom onset at least 6 months prior to diagnosis
   Yes. (question 81 = 1)

Chronic proctalgia may be further characterized into levator ani syndrome or unspecified anorectal pain based on digital rectal examination.

F2a1. Levator Ani Syndrome

Diagnostic criterion

Symptom criteria for chronic proctalgia and tenderness during posterior traction on the puborectalis
   No Question. Physical examination needed

F2a2. Unspecified Functional Anorectal Pain

Diagnostic criterion

Symptom criteria for chronic proctalgia but no tenderness during posterior traction on the puborectalis
   No question. Physical examination needed

F2b. Proctalgia Fugax

Diagnostic criteria
*Must include **all** of the following:*

1. Recurrent episodes of pain localized to the anus or lower rectum
   Pain or aching in anorectal area occurs at least 1 day/month (question 78 > 1)

2. Episodes last from seconds to minutes
   Pain or aching lasts seconds to minutes, up to 20 minutes (question 79 = 1)

3. There is no anorectal pain between episodes
   Pain in anus or rectum occurs and then completely disappears during the same day (question 80 = 1)

   For research purposes criteria must be fulfilled for 3 months; however, clinical diagnosis and evaluation may be made prior to 3 months.

F3. Functional Defecation Disorders

The diagnostic criteria define functional defecation disorders solely in terms of laboratory tests. However, the following questions may identify possible cases that would require further investigation to confirm or refute a diagnosis. A response of at least 'often' to any of these questions identifies a possible case of functional defecation disorders:

Straining during bowel movements (question 54 > 1)

Feeling of incomplete evacuation (question 55 > 1)

Sensation of blocked stools (question 56 > 1)

Manual maneuvers to facilitate defecation (question 57 > 1)

Difficulty relaxing to allow defecation (question 58 > 1)

AND criteria for functional constipation are fulfilled
AND onset of constipation symptoms began more than 6 months previously.
Yes. (question 59 = 1)

Diagnostic Criteria* for Functional Defecation Disorders

1. The patient must satisfy diagnostic criteria for functional constipation**
2. During repeated attempts to defecate must have *at least two* of the following:
   a. Evidence of impaired evacuation, based on balloon expulsion test or imaging
   b. Inappropriate contraction of the pelvic floor muscles (i.e., anal sphincter or puborectalis) or less than 20% relaxation of basal resting sphincter pressure by manometry, imaging, or EMG
   c. Inadequate propulsive forces assessed by manometry or imaging
      No question.

* Criteria fulfilled for the last 3 months with symptom onset at least 6 months prior to diagnosis

** Functional constipation criteria:
1. *Two or more* of the following: *(a) Straining during at least 25% of defecations, (b) Lumpy or hard stools in at least 25% of defecations, (c) Sensation of incomplete evacuation for at least 25% of defecations, (d) Sensation of anorectal obstruction/blockage for at least 25% of defecations, (e) Manual maneuvers to facilitate at least 25% of defecations (e.g., digital evacuation, support of the pelvic floor) and/or, (f) Fewer than three defecations per week.*
2. Loose stools are rarely present without the use of laxatives.
3. Insufficient criteria for IBS.

F3a. Dyssynergic Defecation

Diagnostic criterion

Inappropriate contraction of the pelvic floor, or less than 20% relaxation of basal resting sphincter pressure, with adequate propulsive forces during attempted defecation.

No question.

F3b. Inadequate Defecatory Propulsion

Diagnostic criterion

Inadequate propulsive forces with or without inappropriate contraction or less than 20% relaxation of the anal sphincter during attempted defecation.

No question.

Rome III Psychosocial Alarm Questionnaire for the Functional GI Disorders

The following questions are screening questions within a clinical context and are not designed for survey purposes. They help identify psychosocial problems commonly faced by patients with FGIDs. For each question there are two possible recommendations:

a. There is a problem (**boldfaced items**) that the physician should acknowledge, discuss with the patient, and agree to an appropriate action, which might include referral to a mental health specialist and/or initiation of pharmacotherapy.

b. A "more serious" situation, (marked with ▐) that the physician is advised to either address personally, or consider referring to a mental health professional (psychiatrist, psychologist or other) simultaneous with or prior to treatment of the FGID. These are referred to as "*red flag*" situations to stress their importance.

Note: Further research is needed to determine accurately the most appropriate action according to the nature and severity of psychosocial problems.

This questionnaire was produced by the Psychosocial Aspects of Functional GI Disorders subcommittee for Rome III: Francis Creed, MD (Chair), Rona Levy, PhD (Co-Chair), Lawrence Bradley, PhD, Douglas A. Drossman, MD, Carlos Francisconi MD, Bruce D. Naliboff, PhD, and Kevin W. Olden, MD.

ROME III PSYCHOSOCIAL ALARM QUESTIONNAIRE

Question	Answer	Scoring
1. Question for anxiety: In the last week have you felt tense or "wound up?"	○ *Most of the time* 🏴 ○ ***A lot of the time*** ○ *Occasionally* ○ *Not at all*	***Most of the time*** or ***a lot of the time*** indicates a problem (probable anxiety disorder). **Rationale for Scoring** This question is taken from the Hospital Anxiety and Depression Scale (HADS). The answers ***"Most of the time"*** or ***"A lot of the time"*** identify the majority of depressive or anxiety disorders in this population. These patients had a mean HADS anxiety score of 13.3 (sd=3.6) compared with 6.0 (sd=2.5) for those who scored ***"Occasionally"*** or ***"Not at all"*** [1, 2]. 🏴 *Red flag.* Patients answering ***"Most of the time"*** represent 24% of patients with functional gastrointestinal disorders and their HADS anxiety score was 15.7 (sd=3.2) (range: 10–21) [1, 2]. (Note: A HADS anxiety score of 10 or more indicates a probable case of anxiety, so this level of anxiety merits referral to behavioral management for these patients prior to treatment of the FGID.)

ROME III PSYCHOSOCIAL ALARM QUESTIONNAIRE

Question	Answer	Scoring
2. Question for depression: In the last week have you felt downhearted and low?	○ *Most of the time* 🚩 ○ *A good bit of the time* ○ *Some of the time* ○ *Not at all*	***Most of the time*** and ***A good bit of the time*** indicate a problem (probable depressive disorder). **Rationale for Scoring** This question is taken from the Short Form-36 (SF-36, question 9f). The answers *"Most of the time"* and *"A good bit of the time"* identify FGID patients, whose mean HADS depression score was 9.0 (sd=3.0) compared to 5.0 (sd=3.6) for the remainder [1, 2]. 🚩 *Red flag.* Patients answering to this question *"Most of the time"*: represent 12.8% of patients with FGID and their mean HADS depression score was 9.4 (sd=2.6) [1, 2]. In addition, nearly all the patients who scored *"Most of the time"* to this question also scored *"Most of the time"* to the anxiety question. So, by using both the anxiety and depression questions, our red flag criterion includes the top 15% of the most anxious/depressed patients with FGID.

956

ROME III PSYCHOSOCIAL ALARM QUESTIONNAIRE

Question	Answer	Scoring
3. Question for suicidal ideas: Have you recently felt so low that you felt like hurting or killing yourself?	○ *Often* 🏳 ○ *Occasionally* ○ *Not at all*	***Often*** or ***Occasionally*** indicates a problem and the physician should ask the patient to describe more fully their current feelings and any specific plans. **Rationale for Scoring** This question has not been tested empirically but has clinical face validity. The physician should not be frightened of asking more questions of patients who answer **"Often"** or **"Occasionally."** All the evidence suggests that better prevention of suicide starts with doctor's preparedness to ask such questions.
4. Question for pain severity: During the last *four* weeks how much bodily pain have you had?	○ *Very severe* ○ *Severe* ○ *Moderate* ○ *Mild* ○ *None*	***Very severe*** or ***Severe*** indicate a problem. **Rationale for Scoring** Patients answering *"Severe"* or *"Very severe"* to this question (question 7 of SF-36) represent 24% of patients with functional gastrointestinal disorders and their mean SF summary physical component score was 30.1 (sd=8.5) [1, 2], which is 2 standard deviations below the population norm.

ROME III PSYCHOSOCIAL ALARM QUESTIONNAIRE

Question	Answer	Scoring
5. Question for impairment: During the last four weeks how much did pain (or other symptoms) interfere with your normal activities (including work both outside the home and housework)?	○ *Extremely* ○ *Quite a bit* ○ *Moderately* ○ *A little bit* ○ *Not at all*	***Extremely*** or ***Quite a bit*** indicate a problem. **Rationale for Scoring** Patients answering *"Quite a bit"* or *"Extremely"* to this question (question 8 of SF-36) represent 26% of patients with functional gastrointestinal disorders and their mean SF summary physical component score is 28.9 (sd=8.2) [1, 2], which is 2 standard deviations below the population norm.
6. Question for impaired coping: When I have pain (or other symptoms) I say to myself "it is terrible and I feel it will never get better."	○ *Always* 🏳 ○ *Sometimes* ○ *Never*	***Always*** or ***Sometimes*** indicate a problem. **Rationale for Scoring** This question is the one-item form of the Coping Strategies Questionnaire. It has been used in a study of chronic pain [3] but has yet to be validated in patients with FGID.

ROME III PSYCHOSOCIAL ALARM QUESTIONNAIRE

Question	Answer	Scoring
7. Question for abuse: It is quite common for people to have been emotionally, physically, or sexually victimized at some time in their life and this can affect how people manage with their medical condition. Has this ever happened to you?	O *Yes* O *Never*	*If the response is **Yes**, then the physician should ask:* "Is this causing you distress in your life", ***and*** "Would you like to see someone discuss this in more detail?" *If the patient agrees that he/she is very distressed and would like to see someone, then this should be a* ⚑ *"red flag" situation (i.e., the physician should consider early referral to a mental health professional, provided the patient agrees).* This comes from a published literature review and recommendations [4].

References

1. Biggs AM, Aziz Q, Tomenson B, Creed F. Effect of childhood adversity on health related quality of life in patients with upper abdominal or chest pain. Gut 2004; 53: 180–186.
2. Fiddler M, Jackson J, Kapur N, Wells A, Creed F. Childhood adversity and frequent medical consultations. General Hospital Psychiatry 2004; 26:367–377.
3. Jensen MP, Keefe FJ, Lefebvre JC, Romano JM, Turner JA. One- and two-item measures of pain beliefs and coping strategies. Pain 2003; 104: 453–469.
4. Drossman DA, Talley NJ, Olden KW, Leserman J, Barreiro MA. Sexual and physical abuse and gastrointestinal illness: Review and recommendations. Ann Intern Med. 1995; 123:782–94.

Rome III Diagnostic Questionnaire for the Pediatric Functional GI Disorders

The Questionnaire on Pediatric Gastrointestinal Symptoms—Rome III Version (QPGS-RIII)* is an adaptation and abbreviation of the Questionnaire on Pediatric Gastrointestinal Symptoms (QPGS) (Walker, Caplan-Dover, & Rasquin-Weber, 2000; Walker et al., 2005) that was developed with the support of a grant from the Rome Foundation and that has undergone preliminary validation (Caplan, Walker, & Rasquin, 2005a, b). The original QPGS assesses the Rome II symptom criteria for pediatric functional gastrointestinal disorders and additional gastrointestinal symptoms. The QPGS-RIII is an adaptation and abbreviation of the original QPGS. It was developed with input from the Rome III Child and Adolescent Committee and the Rome III Questionnaire Committee. Although the format and many items from the original QPGS have been retained, several new items have been included and the scoring has been revised to reflect changes in symptom criteria based on Rome III. Some items included in the original QPGS for research purposes have been deleted from the QPGS-RIII for brevity.

The parent-report version of the QPGS-RIII is suitable for use by parents of children four years of age and older. The self-report version is suitable for administration to children ten years of age and older and is preferable to the parent-report version when parents have limited knowledge of their children's symptoms. The questionnaire uses 5-point scales to measure frequency, severity, and duration of symptoms. In addition, it may be scored to assess whether a patient meets the criteria for each of the individual functional gastrointestinal disorders.

The questionnaire is followed by a coding system that identifies provisional diagnoses from the responses to the questions. The QPGS-RIII cannot substitute for the medical evaluation and clinical judgment required for an accurate diagnosis.

* Developed by Lynn S. Walker, Arlene Caplan, and Andrée Rasquin

References

Caplan, A., Walker, L. S., & Rasquin, A. (2005). Development and preliminary validation of the Questionnaire on Pediatric Gastrointestinal Symptoms to assess functional gastrointestinal disorders in children and adolescents. J Pediatric Gastroenterol Nutrition, 4, 296–304.

Caplan, A., Walker, L. S., & Rasquin, A. (2005). Validation of the Pediatric Rome II Criteria for functional gastrointestinal symptoms using the Questionnaire on Pediatric Gastrointestinal Symptoms. J Pediatric Gastroenterol Nutrition, 41, 305–316.

Walker, L. S., Lipani, T. A., Greene, J. W., Caines, K., Stutts, J., Polk, D. B., Caplan, A., & Rasquin-Weber, A. (2004). Recurrent abdominal pain: Subtypes based on the Rome II criteria for pediatric functional gastrointestinal disorders. J Pediatric Gastroenterol Nutrition, 38, 187–191.

Walker, L. S., Caplan, A., & Rasquin, A. (2000). Manual for the Questionnaire on Pediatric Gastrointestinal Symptoms. Nashville, TN: Department of Pediatrics, Vanderbilt University Medical Center.

Questionnaire on Pediatric Gastrointestinal Symptoms, Rome III Version (QPGS-RIII)

(Adapted from the Questionnaire on Pediatric Gastrointestinal Symptoms, Walker, Caplan-Dover, & Rasquin-Weber, 2000)

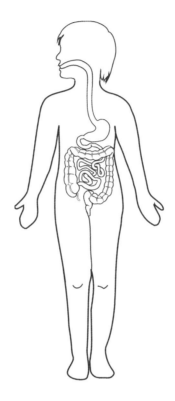

Instructions

This questionnaire is about your child's digestive system (esophagus, stomach, small intestine, and colon) and problems you can have with it. Certain problems may apply to your child and others will not.

Please try to answer *all* of the questions as best as you can. If it is *impossible* for you to answer a particular question, please answer "I don't know" where indicated.

If you have any questions, the research assistant will be glad to help!

Section A. Pain and Uncomfortable Feelings In the Upper Abdomen Above the Belly Button

The shaded area in the pictures below shows an area ABOVE your child's belly button where children sometimes hurt, feel pain, or have an uncomfortable feeling. Some words for these feelings are stomachaches, nausea, bloating, a feeling of fullness, or not being hungry after eating very little.

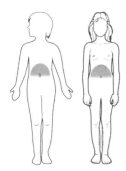

Above the Belly Button

The questions in this section are about pain and uncomfortable feelings ABOVE the belly button that your child may have had in the last 2 months. Children can have pain and uncomfortable feelings in more than one area of the belly. In a different section of the questionnaire, you will be asked about the areas around and below your child's belly button.

1. In the last 2 months, how often did your child have pain or an uncomfortable feeling in the upper abdomen *above the belly button*?
   0. __ Never
   1. __ 1 to 3 times a month
   2. __ Once a week
   3. __ Several times a week
   4. __ Every day

If your child has not had ANY pain or uncomfortable feelings above the belly button in the past 2 months, please go to Section B.

2. Which of the following feelings did your child have *above the belly button*? (You may check one or more than one.)
   a. Pain   0. __ No   1. __ Yes
   b. Nausea   0. __ No   1. __ Yes
   c. Bloating   0. __ No   1. __ Yes
   d. Feeling of fullness   0. __ No   1. __ Yes
   e. Not being hungry after eating very little   0. __ No   1. __ Yes

3. In the last 2 months, how much did your child hurt or feel uncomfortable *above the belly button*?

    1. ___ A little
    2. ___ Some (between a little and a lot)
    3. ___ A lot
    4. ___ A very lot
       ___ I don't know

4. When your child hurt or felt uncomfortable *above the belly button*, for how long did it last?

    1. ___ Less than an hour
    2. ___ 1 to 2 hours
    3. ___ 3 to 4 hours
    4. ___ Most of the day
    5. ___ All the time

5. For how long has your child had pain or an uncomfortable feeling *above the belly button*?

    1. ___ 1 month or less
    2. ___ 2 months
    3. ___ 3 months
    4. ___ 4 to 11 months
    5. ___ 1 year or longer

PARENT-REPORT FORM
CHILDREN 4 YEARS OF AGE AND OLDER

Circle a number for your answer to each question below. **In the last 2 months, when your child hurt or felt uncomfortable above the belly button, how often**	0% of the time Never	25% of the time Once in a while	50% of the time Sometimes	75% of the time Most of the time	100% of the time Always	I don't know (check box)
6. Did the hurt or uncomfortable feeling get better after your child had a poop?	0	1	2	3	4	☐
7. Were your child's poops softer and more mushy or watery than usual?	0	1	2	3	4	☐
8. Were your child's poops harder or lumpier than usual?	0	1	2	3	4	☐
9. Did your child have more poops than usual?	0	1	2	3	4	☐
10. Did your child have fewer poops than usual?	0	1	2	3	4	☐
11. Did your child feel bloated in the belly?	0	1	2	3	4	☐
12. Did your child have a headache?	0	1	2	3	4	☐
13. Did your child have difficulty sleeping?	0	1	2	3	4	☐
14. Did your child have pain in the arms, legs, or back?	0	1	2	3	4	☐
15. Did your child feel faint or dizzy?	0	1	2	3	4	☐
16. Did your child miss school or stop activities?	0	1	2	3	4	☐

Section B. Belly Aches and Abdominal Pain
Around and Below the Belly Button

The questions in this section are about the areas AROUND and BELOW your child's belly button. These areas are shown shaded in the pictures below. Children sometimes have a belly ache or pain in these areas. Belly aches are sometimes milder than pain. Some children call their belly aches or pains "stomach aches" or "tummy aches."

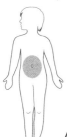
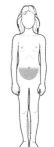

Around the Belly Button   *Below the Belly Button*

1. In the last 2 months, how often did your child have a belly ache or pain *in the area around or below the belly button*?
   0. ___ Never
   1. ___ 1 to 3 times a month
   2. ___ Once a week
   3. ___ Several times a week
   4. ___ Every day

If your child has not had ANY belly aches or pain in the areas around or below the belly button in the past 2 months, please go to Section C.

2. In the last 2 months, how much did your child usually hurt *in the area around or below the belly button*?
   1. ___ A little
   2. ___ Some (between a little and a lot)
   3. ___ A lot
   4. ___ A very lot
      ___ I don't know

3. When your child hurt or felt uncomfortable *around or below the belly button*, for how long did it last?
   1. ___ Less than an hour
   2. ___ 1 to 2 hours
   3. ___ 3 to 4 hours
   4. ___ Most of the day
   5. ___ All the time

4. For how long has your chi ld had belly aches or pain *around or below the belly button*?
   1. ___ 1 month or less
   2. ___ 2 months
   3. ___ 3 months
   4. ___ 4 to 11 months
   5. ___ 1 year or longer

Circle a number for your answer to each question below. **In the last 2 months, when your child had a belly ache or pain around or below the bellow button, how often**	0% of the time Never	25% of the time Once in a while	50% of the time Sometimes	75% of the time Most of the time	100% of the time Always	I don't know (check box)
5. Did it get better after having a poop?	0	1	2	3	4	☐
6. Were your child's poops softer and more mushy or watery than usual?	0	1	2	3	4	☐
7. Were your child's poops harder or lumpier than usual?	0	1	2	3	4	☐
8. Did your child have more poops than usual?	0	1	2	3	4	☐
9. Did your child have fewer poops than usual?	0	1	2	3	4	☐
10. Did your child feel bloated in the belly?	0	1	2	3	4	☐
11. Did your child have a headache?	0	1	2	3	4	☐

Circle a number for your answer to each question below. **In the last 2 months, when your child had a belly ache or pain around or below the bellow button, how often**	0% of the time Never	25% of the time Once in a while	50% of the time Sometimes	75% of the time Most of the time	100% of the time Always	I don't know (check box)
12. Did your child have difficulty sleeping?	0	1	2	3	4	☐
13. Did your child have pain in the arms, legs, or back?	0	1	2	3	4	☐
14. Did your child feel faint or dizzy?	0	1	2	3	4	☐
15. Did your child miss school or stop activities?	0	1	2	3	4	☐

16. In the last **year**, how many times did your child have an episode of **severe intense pain** around the belly button that lasted **2 hours or longer** and made your child **stop everything** that he or she was doing?

0. ___ Never (*if never, please go to the next section*)
1. ___ 1 time
2. ___ 2 times
3. ___ 3 to 5 times
4. ___ 6 or more times

16a. During the episode of severe intense pain, did your child have any of the following?

a. No appetite   0. ___ No   1. ___ Yes
b. Feeling sick to his/her stomach   0. ___ No   1. ___ Yes
c. Vomiting (throwing up)   0. ___ No   1. ___ Yes
d. Pale skin   0. ___ No   1. ___ Yes
e. Headache   0. ___ No   1. ___ Yes
d. Eyes sensitive to light   0. ___ No   1. ___ Yes

16b. Between episodes of severe intense pain, does your child return to his or her usual health for several weeks or longer?

0. ___ No
1. ___ Yes

Section C. Bowel Movements ("Poop," "Stool," "Number 2")

This section asks about your child's bowel movements. There are many words for bowel movements, such as "poop," "stool," "BMs," and "going to the bathroom for number 2." Your family may use another special word when they talk about poops.

1. In the last 2 months, how often did your child usually have poops?
   1. ___ 2 times a week or less often
   2. ___ 3 to 6 times a week
   3. ___ Once a day
   4. ___ 2 to 3 times a day
   5. ___ More than 3 times a day
   ___ I don't know

2. In the last 2 months, what was your child's poop usually like?
   1. ___ Very hard
   2. ___ Hard
   3. ___ Not too hard and not too soft
   4. ___ Very soft or mushy
   5. ___ Watery
   6. ___ It depends (his/her poops are not always the same)
   ___ I don't know

   2a. If your child's poops were usually hard, for how long have they been hard?
   0. ___ Less than 1 month
   1. ___ 1 month
   2. ___ 2 months
   3. ___ 3 or more months

3. In the last 2 months, did it hurt when your child had a poop?
   0. ___ No
   1. ___ Yes
   ___ I don't know

Circle a number for your answer to each question below. **In the last 2 months, how often**	0% of the time Never	25% of the time Once in a while	50% of the time Sometimes	75% of the time Most of the time	100% of the time Always	I don't know (check box)
4. Did your child have to rush to the bathroom to poop?	0	1	2	3	4	☐
5. Did your child have to strain (push hard) to make a poop come out?	0	1	2	3	4	☐
6. Did your child pass mucus or phlegm (white, yellowish, stringy, or slimy material) during a poop?	0	1	2	3	4	☐
7. Did your child have a feeling of not being finished after a poop (like there was more that wouldn't come out)?	0	1	2	3	4	☐

8. In the last 2 months, did your child have a poop that was so big that it clogged the toilet?

0. ___ No

1. ___ Yes

9. Some children hold in their poop even when there is a toilet available. They may do this by stiffening their bodies or crossing their legs. In the last 2 months, while at home, how often did your child try to hold in a poop?

0. ___ Never

1. ___ 1 to 3 times a month

2. ___ Once a week

3. ___ Several times a week

4. ___ Every day

10. Did a doctor or nurse ever examine your child and say that your child had a huge poop inside?

0. ___ No

1. ___ Yes

11. In the last 2 months, how often was your child's underwear stained or soiled with poop?

    0. ___ Never. *If never, please go to Section D.*

    1. ___ Less than once a month

    2. ___ 1 to 3 times a month

    3. ___ Once a week

    4. ___ Several times a week

    5. ___ Every day

    11a. When your child stained or soiled underwear, how much was it stained or soiled?

    1. ___ Underwear was stained (no poop)

    2. ___ Small amount of poop in underwear (less than a whole poop)

    3. ___ Large amount of poop in underwear (a whole poop)

    11b. For how long has your child stained or soiled underwear?

    1. ___ 1 month or less

    2. ___ 2 months

    3. ___ 3 months

    4. ___ 4 to 11 months

    5. ___ 1 year or longer

Section D. Other Symptoms

Circle a number for your answer to each question below. **In the last 2 months, how often did your child**	0% of the time Never	25% of the time Once in a while	50% of the time Sometimes	75% of the time Most of the time	100% of the time Always	I don't know (check box)
1. Burp (belch) *again and again* without wanting to?	0	1	2	3	4	☐
2. Pass a lot of gas *very frequently*?	0	1	2	3	4	☐
3. Develop a clearly swollen belly during the day (you could see it was swollen)?	0	1	2	3	4	☐
4. Swallow or gulp extra air? (You might hear a clicking noise when your child swallows.)	0	1	2	3	4	☐

5. IN THE PAST YEAR, how many times did your child vomit (throw up) *again and again without stopping for 2 hours or longer?*

0. ___ Never. *If never, please go to Section E.*

1. ___ Once

2. ___ 2 times

3. ___ 3 times

4. ___ 4 or more times

5a. For how long has your child had episodes of vomiting again and again without stopping?

1. ___ 1 month or less

2. ___ 2 months

3. ___ 3 months

4. ___ 4 to 11 months

5. ___ 1 year or longer

5b. Did your child usually feel nausea when he or she vomited again and again without stopping?

0. ___ No

1. ___ Yes

5c. Was your child in good health for several weeks or longer between the episodes of vomiting again and again?

0. ___ No

1. ___ Yes

6. In the past 2 months, how often did food come back up into your child's mouth after eating?

0. ___ Never. *If never, please go to Section E.*

1. ___ 1 to 3 times a month

2. ___ Once a week

3. ___ Several times a week

4. ___ Every day

6a. Does this usually happen less than an hour after your child eats?

0. ___ No

1. ___ Yes

6b. Does food come back up into your child's mouth while your child is sleeping?

0. ___ No

1. ___ Yes

6c. Does your child usually feel nausea and vomit when food comes back up into his or her mouth?

0. ___ No

1. ___ Yes

6d. Does it usually hurt your child when the food comes back up into his or her mouth?

0. ___ No

1. ___ Yes

6e. What does your child usually do with the food that comes back up into his or her mouth?

0. ___ Swallow it.

1. ___ Spit it out.

Questionnaire on Pediatric Gastrointestinal Symptoms, Rome III Version (QPGS-RIII)

(Adapted from the Questionnaire on Pediatric Gastrointestinal Symptoms, Walker, Caplan-Dover, & Rasquin-Weber, 2000)

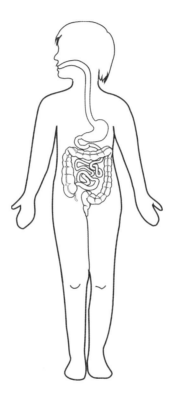

Instructions

This questionnaire is about your digestive system (esophagus, stomach, small intestine, and colon) and problems you can have with it. Certain problems may apply to you and others will not.

Please try to answer *all* of the questions as best as you can.

If you have any questions, the research assistant will be glad to help!

Section A. Pain and Uncomfortable Feelings In the Upper Abdomen Above the Belly Button

The shaded area in the pictures below shows an area ABOVE your belly button where children sometimes hurt, feel pain, or have an uncomfortable feeling. Some words for these feelings are stomachaches, nausea, bloating, a feeling of fullness, or not being hungry after eating very little.

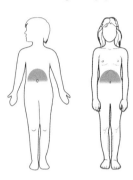

Above the Belly Button

The questions in this section are about pain and uncomfortable feelings ABOVE the belly button that you may have had in the last 2 months. Children can have pain and uncomfortable feelings in more than one area of the belly. In a different section of the questionnaire, you will be asked about the areas around and below your belly button.

1. In the last 2 months, how often did you have pain or an uncomfortable feeling in the upper abdomen *above the belly button*?
   0. __ Never
   1. __ 1 to 3 times a month
   2. __ Once a week
   3. __ Several times a week
   4. __ Every day

If you have not had ANY pain or uncomfortable feelings above the belly button in the past 2 months, please go to Section B.

2. Which of the following feelings did you have *above the belly button*? (You may check one or more than one.)

   a. Pain   0. __ No   1. __ Yes
   b. Nausea   0. __ No   1. __ Yes
   c. Bloating   0. __ No   1. __ Yes
   d. Feeling of fullness   0. __ No   1. __ Yes
   e. Not being hungry after eating very little   0. __ No   1. __ Yes

3. In the last 2 months, how much did you hurt or feel uncomfortable *above the belly button*?
   1. ___ A little
   2. ___ Some (between a little and a lot)
   3. ___ A lot
   4. ___ A very lot

4. When you hurt or felt uncomfortable *above the belly button*, for how long did it last?
   1. ___ Less than an hour
   2. ___ 1 to 2 hours
   3. ___ 3 to 4 hours
   4. ___ Most of the day
   5. ___ All the time

5. For how long have you had pain or an uncomfortable feeling *above the belly button*?
   1. ___ 1 month or less
   2. ___ 2 months
   3. ___ 3 months
   4. ___ 4 to 11 months
   5. ___ 1 year or longer

SELF-REPORT FORM FOR CHILDREN AND ADOLESCENTS (10 YEARS OF AGE AND OLDER)

Circle a number for your answer to each question below. **In the last 2 months, when you hurt or felt uncomfortable above the belly button, how often**	0% of the time Never	25% of the time Once in a while	50% of the time Sometimes	75% of the time Most of the time	100% of the time Always
6. Did the hurt or uncomfortable feeling get better after you had a poop?	0	1	2	3	4
7. Were your poops softer and more mushy or watery than usual?	0	1	2	3	4
8. Were your poops harder or lumpier than usual?	0	1	2	3	4
9. Did you have more poops than usual?	0	1	2	3	4
10. Did you have fewer poops than usual?	0	1	2	3	4
11. Did you feel bloated in your belly?	0	1	2	3	4
12. Did you have a headache?	0	1	2	3	4
13. Did you have difficulty sleeping?	0	1	2	3	4
14. Did you have pain in the arms, legs, or back?	0	1	2	3	4
15. Did you feel faint or dizzy?	0	1	2	3	4
16. Did you miss school or stop activities?	0	1	2	3	4

SELF-REPORT FORM FOR CHILDREN AND ADOLESCENTS (10 YEARS OF AGE AND OLDER)

Section B. Belly Aches and Abdominal Pain Around and Below the Belly Button

The questions in this section are about the areas AROUND and BELOW your belly button. These areas are shown shaded in the pictures below. Children sometimes have a belly ache or pain in these areas. Belly aches are sometimes milder than pain. Some children call their belly aches or pains "stomach aches" or "tummy aches."

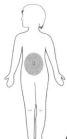

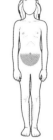

Around the Belly Button   *Below the Belly Button*

1. In the last 2 months, how often did you have a belly ache or pain *in the area around or below the belly button?*
   0. __ Never
   1. __ 1 to 3 times a month
   2. __ Once a week
   3. __ Several times a week
   4. __ Every day

If you have not had ANY belly aches or pain in the areas around or below the belly button in the past 2 months, please go to Section C.

2. In the last 2 months, how much did you usually hurt *in the area around or below the belly button?*
   1. __ A little
   2. __ Some (between a little and a lot)
   3. __ A lot
   4. __ A very lot

3. When you hurt or felt uncomfortable *around or below the belly button*, for how long did it last?
   1. __ Less than an hour
   2. __ 1 to 2 hours
   3. __ 3 to 4 hours
   4. __ Most of the day
   5. __ All the time

4. For how long have you had belly aches or pain *around or below the belly button*?
   1. __ 1 month or less
   2. __ 2 months
   3. __ 3 months
   4. __ 4 to 11 months
   5. __ 1 year or longer

Circle a number for your answer to each question below. **In the last 2 months, when you had a belly ache or pain around or below the bellow button, how often**	0% of the time Never	25% of the time Once in a while	50% of the time Sometimes	75% of the time Most of the time	100% of the time Always
5. Did it get better after having a poop?	0	1	2	3	4
6. Were your poops softer and more mushy or watery than usual?	0	1	2	3	4
7. Were your poops harder or lumpier than usual?	0	1	2	3	4
8. Did you have more poops than usual?	0	1	2	3	4
9. Did you have fewer poops than usual?	0	1	2	3	4
10. Did you feel bloated in the belly?	0	1	2	3	4
11. Did you have a headache?	0	1	2	3	4

SELF-REPORT FORM FOR CHILDREN AND ADOLESCENTS (10 YEARS OF AGE AND OLDER)

Circle a number for your answer to each question below. **In the last 2 months, when you had a belly ache or pain around or below the bellow button, how often**	0% of the time Never	25% of the time Once in a while	50% of the time Sometimes	75% of the time Most of the time	100% of the time Always
12. Did you have difficulty sleeping?	0	1	2	3	4
13. Did you have pain in the arms, legs, or back?	0	1	2	3	4
14. Did you feel faint or dizzy?	0	1	2	3	4
15. Did you miss school or stop activities?	0	1	2	3	4

16. In the last **year**, how many times did you have an episode of **severe intense pain** around the belly button that lasted **2 hours or longer** and made you **stop everything** that you were doing?
    0. __ Never (*if never, please go to the next section*)
    1. __ 1 time
    2. __ 2 times
    3. __ 3 to 5 times
    4. __ 6 or more times

    16a. During the episode of severe intense pain, did you have any of the following?
    a. No appetite   0. __ No   1. __ Yes
    b. Feeling sick to his/her stomach   0. __ No   1. __ Yes
    c. Vomiting (throwing up)   0. __ No   1. __ Yes
    d. Pale skin   0. __ No   1. __ Yes
    e. Headache   0. __ No   1. __ Yes
    d. Eyes sensitive to light   0. __ No   1. __ Yes

    16b. Between episodes of severe intense pain, do you return to your usual health for several weeks or longer?
    0. __ No
    1. __ Yes

Section C. Bowel Movements ("Poop," "Stool," "Number 2")

This section asks about your bowel movements. There are many words for bowel movements, such as "poop," "stool," "BMs," and "going to the bathroom for number 2." Your family may use another special word when they talk about poops.

1. In the last 2 months, how often did you usually have poops?
   1. __ 2 times a week or less often
   2. __ 3 to 6 times a week
   3. __ Once a day
   4. __ 2 to 3 times a day
   5. __ More than 3 times a day

2. In the last 2 months, what was your poop usually like?
   1. __ Very hard
   2. __ Hard
   3. __ Not too hard and not too soft
   4. __ Very soft or mushy
   5. __ Watery
   6. __ It depends (my poops are not always the same)

   2a. If your poops were usually hard, for how long have they been hard?
      0. __ Less than 1 month
      1. __ 1 month
      2. __ 2 months
      3. __ 3 or more months

3. In the last 2 months, did it hurt when you had a poop?
   0. __ No
   1. __ Yes

Circle a number for your answer to each question below. **In the last 2 months, how often**	0% of the time Never	25% of the time Once in a while	50% of the time Sometimes	75% of the time Most of the time	100% of the time Always
4. Did you have to rush to the bathroom to poop?	0	1	2	3	4
5. Did you have to strain (push hard) to make a poop come out?	0	1	2	3	4
6. Did you pass mucus or phlegm (white, yellowish, stringy, or slimy material) during a poop?	0	1	2	3	4
7. Did you have a feeling of not being finished after a poop (like there was more that wouldn't come out)?	0	1	2	3	4

8. In the last 2 months, did you have a poop that was so big that it clogged the toilet?
   0. __ No
   1. __ Yes

9. Some children hold in their poop even when there is a toilet they could use. They may do this by stiffening their bodies or crossing their legs. In the last 2 months, while at home, how often did you try to hold in a poop?
   0. __ Never
   1. __ 1 to 3 times a month
   2. __ Once a week
   3. __ Several times a week
   4. __ Every day

10. Did a doctor or nurse ever examine you and say that you had a huge poop inside?
    0. __ No
    1. __ Yes

11. In the last 2 months, how often was your underwear stained or soiled with poop?

　0.＿＿ Never. *If never, please go to Section D.*

　1.＿＿ Less than once a month

　2.＿＿ 1 to 3 times a month

　3.＿＿ Once a week

　4.＿＿ Several times a week

　5.＿＿ Every day

　11a. When you stained or soiled underwear, how much was it stained or soiled?

　　1. ＿ Underwear was stained (no poop)

　　2. ＿ Small amount of poop in underwear (less than a whole poop)

　　3. ＿ Large amount of poop in underwear (a whole poop)

　11b. For how long have you stained or soiled your underwear?

　　1. ＿ 1 month or less

　　2. ＿ 2 months

　　3. ＿ 3 months

　　4. ＿ 4 to 11 months

　　5. ＿ 1 year or longer

Section D. Other Symptoms

Circle a number for your answer to each question below.	0% of the time	25% of the time	50% of the time	75% of the time	100% of the time
In the last 2 months, how often did you	Never	Once in a while	Sometimes	Most of the time	Always
1. Burp (belch) *again and again* without wanting to?	0	1	2	3	4
2. Pass a lot of gas *very frequently*?	0	1	2	3	4
3. Develop a clearly swollen belly during the day (you could see it was swollen)?	0	1	2	3	4
4. Swallow or gulp extra air? (You might hear a clicking noise when you swallow.)	0	1	2	3	4

5. IN THE PAST YEAR, how many times did you vomit (throw up) *again and again without stopping for 2 hours or longer?*
   0. __ Never
   1. __ Once
   2. __ 2 times
   3. __ 3 times
   4. __ 4 or more times

   5a. For how long have you had episodes of vomiting again and again without stopping?
   1. __ 1 month or less
   2. __ 2 months
   3. __ 3 months
   4. __ 4 to 11 months
   5. __ 1 year or longer

   5b. Did you usually feel nausea when you vomited again and again without stopping?
   0. __ No
   1. __ Yes

   5c. Were you in good health for several weeks or longer between the episodes of vomiting again and again?
   0. __ No
   1. __ Yes

6. In the past 2 months, how often did food come back up into your mouth after eating?
   0. __ Never
   1. __ 1 to 3 times a month
   2. __ Once a week
   3. __ Several times a week
   4. __ Every day

   6a. Does this usually happen less than an hour after you eat?
   0. __ No
   1. __ Yes

6b. Does food come back up into your mouth while you are sleeping?

0. __ No

1. __ Yes

6c. Do you usually feel nausea and vomit when food comes back up into your mouth?

0. __ No

1. __ Yes

6d. Does it usually hurt when the food comes back up into your mouth?

0. __ No

1. __ Yes

6e. What do you usually do with the food that comes back up into your mouth?

0. __ Swallow it.

1. __ Spit it out.

```
┌─────────────────────────────────────────────────────┐
│  SCORING INSTRUCTIONS FOR PARENT-REPORT FORM          │
│  AND CHILD/ADOLESCENT SELF-REPORT FORM                │
└─────────────────────────────────────────────────────┘
```

Questionnaire on Pediatric Gastrointestinal Symptoms, Rome III Version (QPGS-RIII)

(Adapted from the Questionnaire on Pediatric Gastrointestinal Symptoms, Walker, Caplan-Dover, & Rasquin-Weber, 2000)

Scoring Instructions for Parent-report Form and Child/Adolescent Self-report Form

Note. Items are labeled by section (e.g., A1 is item #1 in Section A of the QPGS-RIII). For each disorder, the patient must meet the criteria for all items indicated. Cut-points for symptom frequencies to meet diagnostic criteria are based on provisional recommendations by the Rome III Child and Adolescent Committee).

I. Functional Dyspepsia
__ (A 1) Upper abdominal pain or discomfort "several times a week" or more often
__ (A 5) Duration of upper abdominal pain or discomfort is "2 months" or longer
__ (A 6) Not exclusively relieved with defecation; A6 is "sometimes" or less often
__ Not associated with change in stool form: "never" or "once in a while" indicated for
    __ (A 7) softer stools **and** __ (A 8) harder stools
__ Not associated with change in stool frequency: "never" or "once in a while" indicated for
    __ (A 9) more stools **and** __ (A 10) fewer stools

SCORING INSTRUCTIONS FOR PARENT-REPORT FORM AND CHILD/ADOLESCENT SELF-REPORT FORM

II. Irritable Bowel Syndrome

Lower abdominal pain associated with bowel symptoms

__ (B 1) Periumbilical/lower abdominal pain/discomfort "once a week" or more often

__ (B 4) Duration of periumbilical/lower abdominal pain/discomfort is "2 months" or longer

__ At least two of the following "sometimes" or more often:

    __ (B 5) Relief with defecation

    __ Change in bowel movement form: __ (B 6) softer **or** __ (B 7) harder

    __ Change in bowel movement frequency: __ (B 8) more **or** __ (B 9) fewer

AND/OR

Upper abdominal pain associated with bowel symptoms

__ (A 1) Upper abdominal pain or discomfort "once a week" or more often

__ (A 5) Duration of upper abdominal pain/discomfort is "2 months" or longer

__ At least two of the following "sometimes" or *more* often:

    __ (A 6) Relief with defecation

    __ Change in bowel movement form: __ (A 7) softer **or** __ (A 8) harder

    __ Change in bowel movement frequency: __ (A 9) more **or** __ (A 10) fewer

Note. Additional symptoms suggestive of IBS but not required: C4, C5, C6, C7.

III. Abdominal Migraine

__ (B16) In the past year, 2 or more episodes of severe pain lasting 1 hour or longer and causing restriction in daily activities

__ (B16a) Two or more of the following during episodes:

    __ a. No appetite   __ d. Pale skin

    __ b. Nausea   __ e. Headache

    __ c. Vomiting   __ f. Eyes sensitive to light

__ (B 16b) Symptom-free periods between pain episodes ("yes")

IV. Functional Abdominal Pain

Lower abdominal location

__ (B1) Periumbilical/lower abdominal pain "once a week" or more often

__ (B4) Duration of abdominal pain is "2 months" or longer

__ Does not meet criteria for other functional gastrointestinal disorders associated with abdominal pain (functional dyspepsia, IBS, abdominal migraine, functional abdominal pain syndrome).

Upper abdominal location

__ (A1) Upper abdominal pain "once a week" or more often

__ (A5) Duration of abdominal pain is "2 months" or longer

__ Does not meet criteria for other functional gastrointestinal disorders associated with abdominal pain (functional dyspepsia, IBS, abdominal migraine, functional abdominal pain syndrome).

V. Functional Abdominal Pain Syndrome

Lower abdominal location

__ (B1) Periumbilical/lower abdominal pain "several times a week" or more often

__ (B4) Duration of abdominal pain is "2 months" or longer

__ **EITHER** __ Two or more other somatic symptoms "once a week" or more often

      __ (B11) Headache

      __ (B12) Difficulty sleeping

      __ (B13) Pain in arms, legs, or back

      __ (B14) Faint or dizzy

  OR   __ (B15) Misses activities "once in a while" or more often

__ Does not meet criteria for other functional gastrointestinal disorders associated with abdominal pain (functional dyspepsia, irritable bowel syndrome, abdominal migraine)

Upper abdominal location

__ (A1) Upper abdominal pain "several times a week" or more often

__ (A5) Duration of abdominal pain is "2 months" or longer

__ **EITHER** __ Two or more other somatic symptoms "once a week" or more often

      __ (A12) Headache

      __ (A13) Difficulty sleeping

      __ (A14) Pain in arms, legs, or back

      __ (A15) Faint or dizzy

  OR   __ (A16) Misses activities "once in a while" or more often

__ Does not meet criteria for other functional gastrointestinal disorders associated with abdominal pain (functional dyspepsia, irritable bowel syndrome, abdominal migraine)

VI. Functional Constipation
___ Two or more of the following:
> ___ (C 1) Two or fewer stools per week
> ___ **Either** ___ (C2) hard or very hard stools **or** ___ (C3) painful stool
> ___ (C8) Passage of very large stool
> ___ (C9) Stool retention "once a week" or more often
> ___ (C10) History of large fecal mass in rectum
> ___ (C11) Soiling "once a week" or more often

___ Does not meet criteria for irritable bowel syndrome

VII. Nonretentive Fecal Incontinence
___ Child is 4 years of age or older
___ (C11) Soiling "once a week" or more often
___ (C11a) Amount of stool is small or large (not just a stain)
___ (C11b) Soiling for 2 months or longer
___ No evidence of fecal retention (does not meet criteria for functional constipation)

VIII. Aerophagia
___ Two or more of the following are "several times a week" or "every day":
> ___ **Either**: ___ (D1) belching **or** ___ (D2) flatus
> ___ (D3) Abdominal distention
> ___ (D4) Swallowing air

X. Cyclic Vomiting Syndrome
___ (D 5) Three or more episodes of repeated vomiting in the past year
___ (D 5a) Duration is 2 months or longer
___ (D 5b) Presence of nausea is "yes"
___ (D 5c) Occurrence of wellness intervals is "yes"

IX. Adolescent Rumination Syndrome
___ (D6) Food comes back up "several times a week" or "every day."
___ (D6a) Episodes occur shortly after eating ("Yes")
___ (D6b) Episodes do not occur during sleep ("No")
___ (D6c) Episodes are not accompanied by nausea or vomiting ("No")
___ (D6d) Episodes are not painful ("No")

Photographs
of the Rome III
Members

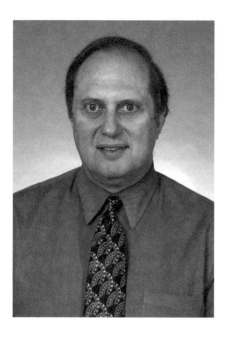

Douglas A. Drossman, MD
President, Rome Foundation Board
of Directors
Member, Psychosocial Aspects in
the FGIDs
Member, Functional Abdominal
Pain Syndrome

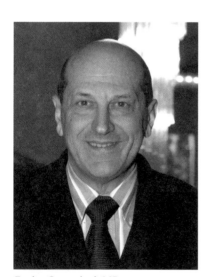

Enrico Corazziari, MD
Member, Rome Foundation Board of
Directors
Co-Chair, Functional Gallbladder and
Sphincter of Oddi Disorders

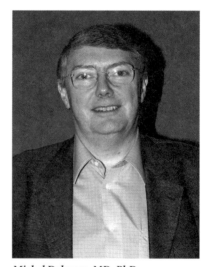

Michel Delvaux, MD, PhD
Member, Rome Foundation Board of
Directors
Member, Principles of Applied
Neurogastroenterology: Physiology/
Motility-Sensation

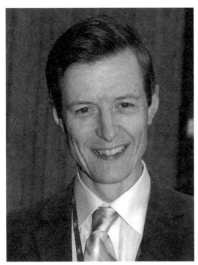

Robin C. Spiller, MD
Member, Rome Foundation Board of
    Directors
Member, Functional Bowel Disorders

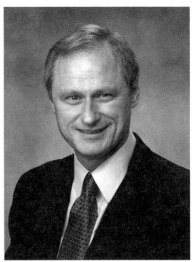

**Nicholas J. Talley, MD, PhD, FRACP,
    FRCP**
Member, Rome Foundation Board of
    Directors
Co-Chair, Functional Gastroduodenal
    Disorders
Member, Design of Treatment Trials in
    the FGIDs

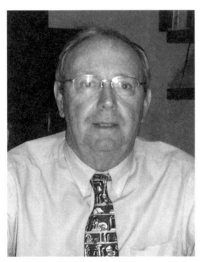

W. Grant Thompson, MD, FRCPC
Member, Rome Foundation Board of
    Directors
Co-Chair, Functional Bowel Disorders

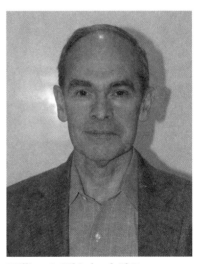

William E. Whitehead, PhD
Member, Rome Foundation Board of
    Directors
Co-Chair, Design of Treatment Trials in
    the FGIDs

993

Rome III Administration

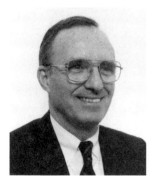

George K. Degnon, CAE
Publisher, Degnon Associates
Executive Director, Rome
  Foundation

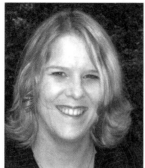

Carlar J. Blackman
Managing Editor, Rome III
  Book
Administrative Director, Rome
  Foundation

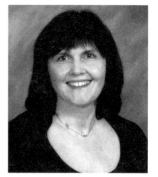

Kathy Haynes
Administrator
Rome Foundation

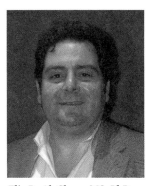

Elie D. Al-Chaer, MS, PhD, JD
Member, Fundamentals of Neurogastroenterology: Basic Science

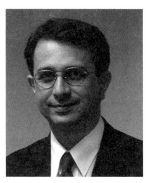

Qasim Aziz, PhD, FRCP
Member, Fundamentals of Neurogastroenterology: Basic Science
Member, Functional Abdominal Pain Syndrome

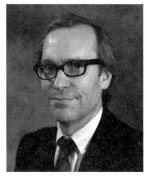

Fernando Azpiroz, MD, PhD
Co-Chair, Principles of Applied Neurogastroenterology: Physiology/ Motility-Sensation

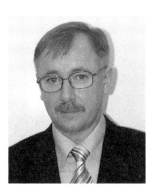

András Bálint, MD, PhD
Member, Functional Esophageal Disorders

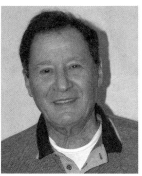

Jose Behar, MD
Chair, Functional Gallbladder and Sphincter of Oddi Disorders

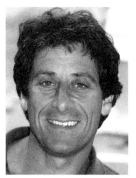

Marc A. Benninga, MD, PhD
Member, Childhood Functional Gastrointestinal Disorders: Neonatal/ Toddler

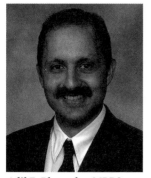

Adil E. Bharucha, MBBS, MD
Co-Chair, Functional Anorectal Disorders

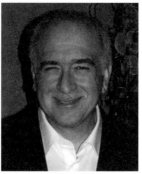

Laurence A. Bradley, PhD
Member, Psychosocial Aspects of FGIDs

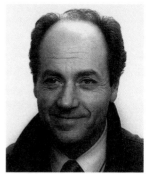

Lionel Bueno, PhD
Co-Chair, Pharmacological and Pharmacokinetic Aspects of FGIDs

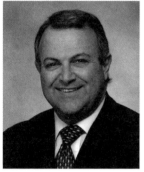

Michael Camilleri, MD
Chair, Pharmacological and Pharmacokinetic Aspects of FGIDs
Member, Functional Gastroduodenal Disorders

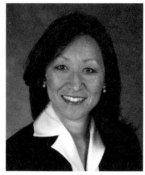

Lin Chang, MD
Co-Chair, Gender, Age, Society, Culture and the Patient's Perspective

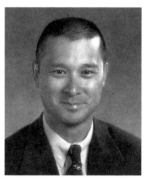

William D. Chey, MD, FACG, FACP
Member, Functional Bowel Disorders
Member, Design of Treatment Trials in the FGIDs

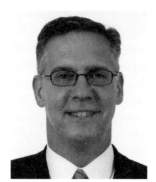

Ray E. Clouse, MD
Co-Chair, Functional Esophageal Disorders
Chair, Functional Abdominal Pain Syndrome

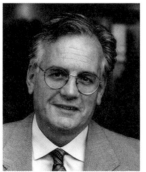

Stephen M. Collins, MD
Member, Fundamentals of Neurogastroenterology: Basic Science

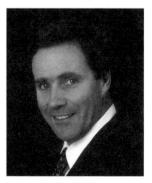

Ian J. Cook, MD, FRACP
Member, Functional Esophageal Disorders

996

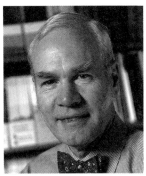

Francis Creed, MD
Chair, Psychosocial Aspects
of FGIDs

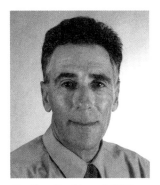

**Geoffrey Davidson, MBBS,
MD, FRACP**
Member, Childhood Func-
tional Gastrointestinal
Disorders: Neonatal/
Toddler

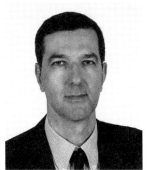

Fabrizio De Ponti, MD, PhD
Member, Pharmacological and
Pharmacokinetic Aspects
of FGIDs

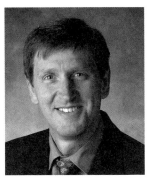

Carlo Di Lorenzo, MD
Chair, Childhood Functional
Gastrointestinal Disorders:
Child/Adolescent

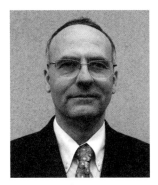

Dan L. Dumitrascu, MD
Member, Functional
Abdominal Pain Syndrome

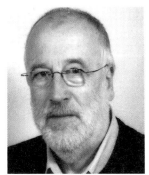

Paul Enck, PhD
Member, Functional Anorectal
Disorders

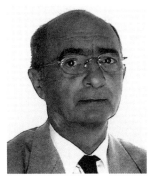

Jean Fioramonti, PhD
Member, Pharmacological and
Pharmacokinetic Aspects
of FGIDs

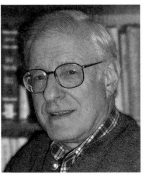

David Fleisher, MD
Member, Childhood
Functional Gastrointestinal
Disorders: Neonatal/
Toddler

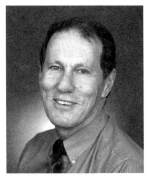

David Forbes, MBBS
Member, Childhood
Functional Gastrointestinal
Disorders: Child/
Adolescent

997

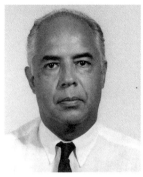

Carlos Francisconi, MD
Member, Psychosocial Aspects
of FGIDs

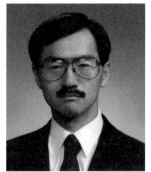

Shin Fukudo, MD, PhD
Member, Gender, Age, Society,
Culture and the Patient's
Perspective

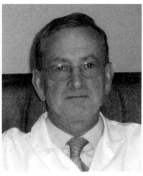

Jean Paul Galmiche, MD
Chair, Functional Esophageal
Disorders

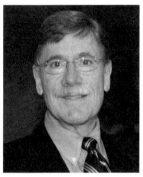

Gerald F. Gebhart, PhD
Member, Principles of Applied
Neurogastroenterology:
Physiology/Motility-
Sensation

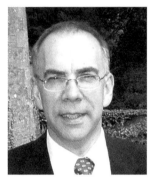

David Grundy, PhD
Co-Chair, Fundamentals of
Neurogastroenterology:
Basic Science

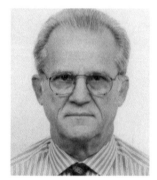

Moises Guelrud, MD
Member, Functional
Gallbladder and Sphincter
of Oddi Disorders

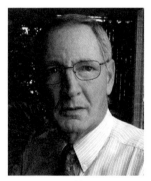

Ernesto Guiraldes, MD
Member, Childhood
Functional Gastrointestinal
Disorders: Child/
Adolescent

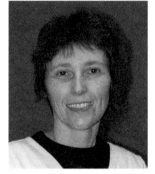

Elspeth Guthrie, MD
Member, Gender, Age, Society,
Culture and the Patient's
Perspective

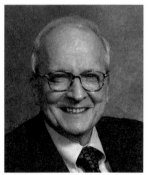

Walter J. Hogan, MD
Member, Functional
Gallbladder and Sphincter
of Oddi Disorders

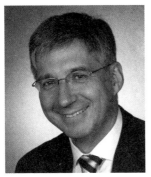

Gerald Holtmann, MD
Member, Functional
    Gastroduodenal Disorders

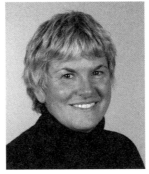

Lesley A. Houghton, PhD
Member, Functional Bowel
    Disorders

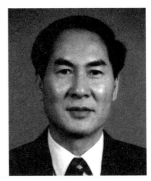

Pinjin Hu, MD
Member, Functional
    Gastroduodenal Disorders

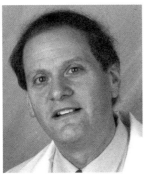

Jeffrey S. Hyams, MD
Member, Childhood
    Functional Gastrointestinal
    Disorders: Child/
    Adolescent

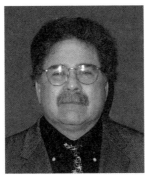

Paul E. Hyman, MD
Co-Chair, Childhood
    Functional Gastrointestinal
    Disorders: Neonatal/
    Toddler

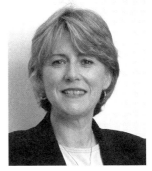

**E. Jan Irvine, MD, FRCP(C),
MSc**
Chair, Design of Treatment
    Trials in the FGIDs

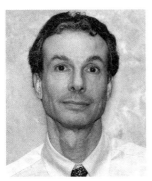

Peter J. Kahrilas, MD
Member, Functional
    Esophageal Disorders

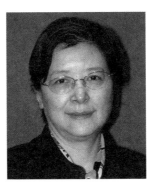

Meiyun Ke, MD
Member, Fundamentals of
    Neurogastroenterology:
    Basic Science

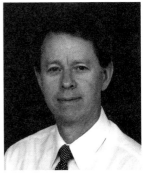

John E. Kellow, MD, FRACP
Chair, Principles of Applied
    Neurogastroenterology:
    Physiology/Motility-
    Sensation

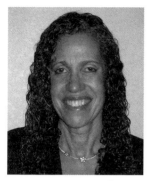

Rona L. Levy, MSW, PhD, MPH
Co-Chair, Psychosocial
Aspects of FGIDs

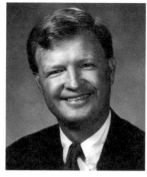

G. Richard Locke, III, MD
Member, Gender, Age, Society,
Culture and the Patient's
Perspective

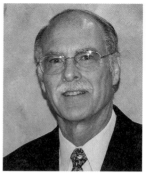

George F. Longstreth, MD
Chair, Functional Bowel
Disorders

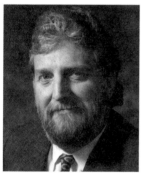

R. Bruce Lydiard, PhD, MD
Member, Pharmacological and
Pharmacokinetic Aspects
of FGIDs

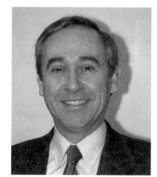

Juan-R Malagelada, MD, PhD
Member, Functional Gastroduodenal Disorders

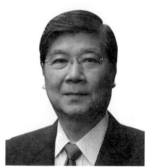

Kei Matsueda, MD, PhD
Member, Design of Treatment
Trials in the FGIDs

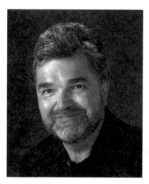

Emeran A. Mayer, MD
Co-Chair, Functional
Abdominal Pain Syndrome

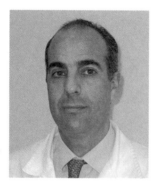

Fermín Mearin, MD, PhD
Member, Functional Bowel
Disorders

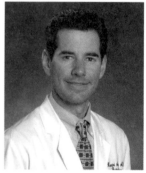

Howard M. Mertz, MD
Member, Principles of Applied
Neurogastroenterology:
Physiology/Motility-
Sensation

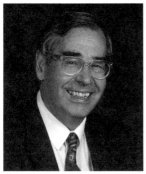

Peter J. Milla, MD
Chair, Childhood Functional
Gastrointestinal Disorders:
Neonatal/Toddler

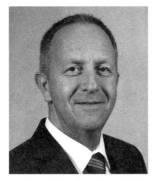

Hubert Mönnikes, MD, PhD
Member, Functional Abdominal Pain Syndrome

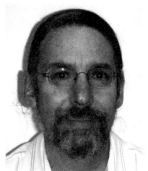

Bruce D. Naliboff, PhD
Member, Psychosocial Aspects
of FGIDs
Member, Functional Abdominal Pain Syndrome

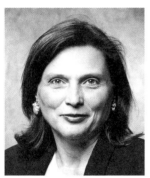

Nancy Norton, BS
Member, Gender, Age, Society,
Culture and the Patient's
Perspective

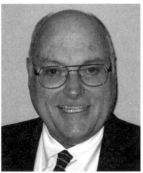

Kevin W. Olden, MD
Member, Psychosocial Aspects
of FGIDs

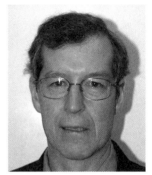

William G. Paterson, MD
Member, Functional
Esophageal Disorders

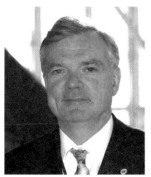

**Eamonn M. M. Quigley, MD,
FRCP, FACP, FACG, FRCPI**
Member, Principles of Applied
Neurogastroenterology:
Physiology/Motility-
Sensation

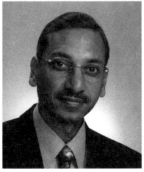

**Satish S.C. Rao, MD, PhD,
PRCP (LON)**
Member, Functional Anorectal
Disorders

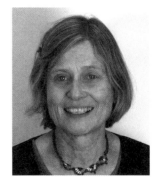

Andrée Rasquin, MD
Co-Chair, Childhood
Functional Gastrointestinal
Disorders: Child/
Adolescent

1001

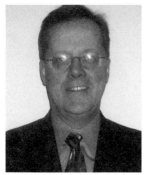

Michael Shaw, MD
Member, Design of Treatment
Trials in the FGIDs

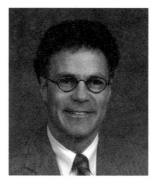

Stuart Sherman, MD
Member, Functional
Gallbladder and Sphincter
of Oddi Disorders

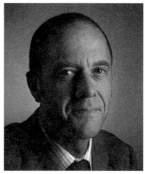

André J.P.M. Smout, MD, PhD
Member, Principles of Applied
Neurogastroenterology:
Physiology/Motility-
Sensation
Member, Functional
Esophageal Disorders

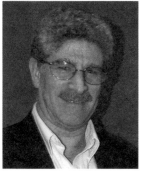

Ami D. Sperber, MD, MSPH
Member, Gender, Age, Society,
Culture and the Patient's
Perspective

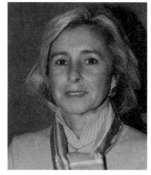

Annamaria Staiano, MD
Member, Childhood
Functional Gastrointestinal
Disorders: Child/
Adolescent

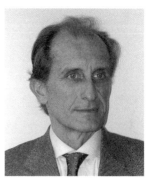

Vincenzo Stanghellini, MD
Member, Functional
Gastroduodenal Disorders

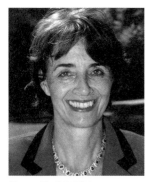

Yvette Taché, PhD
Member, Fundamentals of
Neurogastroenterology:
Basic Science

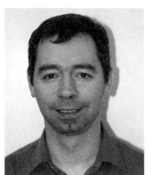

Jan Tack, MD, PhD
Member, Pharmacological and
Pharmacokinetic Aspects
of FGIDs
Chair, Functional
Gastroduodenal Disorders

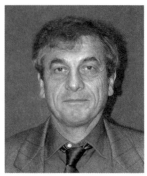

Jan Taminiau
Member, Childhood
Functional Gastrointestinal
Disorders: Neonatal/
Toddler

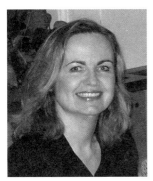

Brenda B. Toner, PhD
Chair, Gender, Age, Society,
   Culture and the Patient's
   Perspective

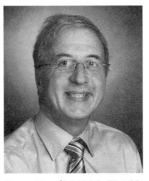

**James Toouli, MBBS, FRACS,
   PhD**
Member, Functional
   Gallbladder and Sphincter
   of Oddi Disorders

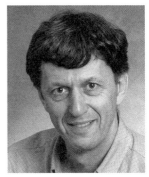

**Sander J. O. Veldhuyzen van
   Zanten, MD, PhD**
Member, Design of
   Treatment Trials in the
   FGIDs

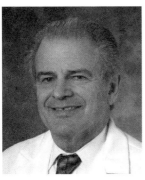

Arnold Wald, MD
Chair, Functional Anorectal
   Disorders

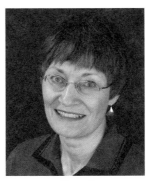

Lynn S. Walker, PhD
Member, Childhood
   Functional Gastrointestinal
   Disorders: Child/
   Adolescent

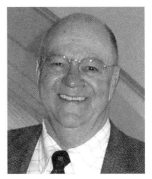

**Jackie (Jack) D. Wood, MSc,
   PhD**
Chair, Fundamentals of
   Neurogastroenterology:
   Basic Science

Reviewers

---

*We are grateful to the following reviewers and consultants
for their careful review of the Rome III committee manuscripts*

Lars Agreus, MD, PhD, Karolinska Institutet, Huddinge, SWEDEN

Fernando Azpiroz, MD, University Hospital Vall d'Hebron, Barcelona, SPAIN

John Baillie, MD, Wake Forest University Medical Center, Winston-Salem, NC, USA

Shrikant Bangdiwala, PhD, University of North Carolina at Chapel Hill, Chapel Hill, NC, USA

Ronald G. Barr, MA, MDCM, FRCPC, Montreal Children's Hospital, Montreal, Quebec, CANADA

Gabrio Bassotti, MD, PhD, Clinica di Gastroenterologia ed Epatologia, Perugia, ITALY

John T. Boyle, MD, Rainbow Babies and Children's Hospital, Cleveland, OH, USA

John V. Campo, MD, Ohio State University, Columbus, OH, USA

Bernard J. Coulie, MD, PhD, J&J Pharm. Res. & Dev, Beerse, BELGIUM

Francis Creed, MD, University of Manchester, Manchester, UK

Roberto DeGiorgio, MD, PhD, University of Bologna, Bologna, ITALY

Nicholas E. Diamant, MD, University of Toronto, Toronto, Ontario, CANADA

James A. DiSario, MD, University of Utah Medical Center, Salt Lake City, UT, USA

Douglas A. Drossman, MD, University of North Carolina at Chapel Hill, Chapel Hill, NC, USA

Paul Enck, PhD, Universtatsklinikum Tubingen, Tubingen, GERMANY

Robert S. Fisher, MD, Temple University School of Medicine, Philadelphia, PA, USA

Thomas Frieling, MD, Heinrich-Heine Universitat Dusseldorf, Dusseldorf, GERMANY

Luca Frulloni, MD, PhD, Cattedra di Gastroenterologia, Verona, ITALY

David Grundy, PhD, University of Sheffield, Sheffield, UK

Ernesto Guiraldes, MD, Pontificia Universidad Catolica de Chile, Santiago, CHILE

William L. Hasler, MD, University of Michigan, Ann Arbor, MI, USA

Margaret Heitkemper, PhD, RN, FAAN, University of Washington, Seattle, Washington, USA

Pali S. Hungin, MD, Durham University, Durham, UK

John M. Inadomi, MD, University of California, San Francisco, San Francisco, CA, USA

Michael Jones, MD, Northwestern University Medical School, Chicago, IL, USA

Roger Jones, MD, Kings College, London, UK

Brian E. Lacy, MD, PhD, Dartmouth-Hitchcock Medical Center, Lebanon, NH, USA

Shiu-Kum Lam, MD, The University of Hong Kong, Hong Kong, HONG KONG

Jane Leserman, PhD, University of North Carolina at Chapel Hill, Chapel Hill, NC, USA

Rona Levy, MSW, PhD, MPH, University of Washington, Seattle, WA, USA

Vera Loening-Baucke, MD, University of Iowa, Iowa City, IO, USA

George F. Longstreth, MD, Kaiser Permanente, San Diego, CA, USA

R. Bruce Lydiard, MD, Medical University of South Carolina, Charleston, SC, USA

Robert Madoff, MD, University of Minnesota, Saint Paul, MN, USA

Gary Mawe, MD, University of Vermont College of Medicine, Burlington, VT, USA

Emeran A. Mayer MD, Center for Neurovisceral Sciences & Women's Health, University of California, Los Angeles, Los Angeles, CA, USA

Bruce Naliboff, PhD, Center for Neurovisceral Sciences & Women's Health, University of California, Los Angeles, Los Angeles, CA, USA

Susan Orenstein, MD, University of Pittsburgh Medical Center, Pittsburgh, PA, USA

Fabio Pace, MD, University Hospital L. Sacco, Milano, ITALY

P. Jay Pasricha, MD, University of Texas Medical Branch, Galveston, TX, USA

Roberto Penagini, MD, Cattedra di Gastroenterologia, Milano, ITALY

Satish SC Rao MD, PhD, University of Iowa, Iowa City, IO, USA

Nicholas W. Read, MD, Northern General Hospital, Sheffield, UK

Colin Rudolph, MD, PhD, Children's Hospital, Milwaukee, WI, USA

Keith A. Sharkey, MD, University of Calgary, Calgary, Alberta, CANADA

Daniel A. Sifrim, MD, PhD, Katholieke Universiteit, Leuven, BELGIUM

Vincenzo Stanghellini, MD, University of Bologna, Bologna, ITALY

Peter Sullivan, MD, University of Oxford, Oxford, UK

Jan F. Tack, MD, PhD, University Hospitals Gasthuisberg, Leuven, Vlaanderen, BELGIUM

David G. Thompson, MD, Hope Hospital, Manchester, UK

Brenda Toner, PhD, University of Toronto, Toronto, Ontario, CANADA

Marcello Tonini, PhD, University of Pavia, Pavia, ITALY

Gigi Veereman-Wauters, MD, PhD, Katholieke Universiteit, Leuven, BELGIUM

William E. Whitehead, PhD, University of North Carolina at Chapel Hill, Chapel Hill, NC, USA

Peter J. Whorwell, MD, Wythenshawe Hospital, Manchester, UK

Ashraf F. Youssef, MD, PhD, TAP Pharmaceutical Products, Inc, Lake Forest, IL, USA

Index

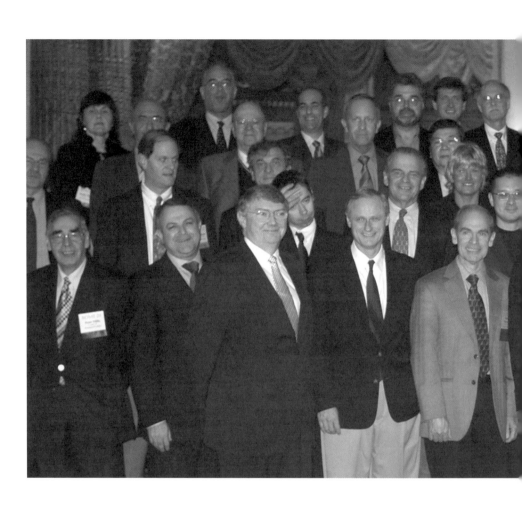

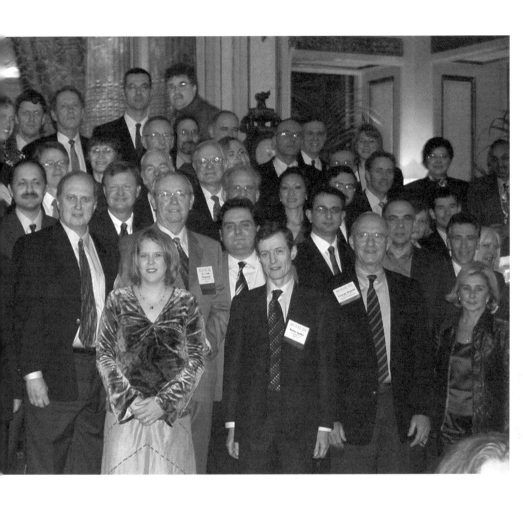